EMOTIONAL DISORDERS IN CHILDREN AND ADOLESCENTS

Medical and Psychological Approaches to Treatment

CHILD BEHAVIOR AND DEVELOPMENT
Dennis P. Cantwell, Series Editor

EMOTIONAL DISORDERS IN CHILDREN AND ADOLESCENTS
Medical and Psychological Approaches to Treatment

G. Pirooz Sholevar, Ronald M. Benson and Barton J. Blinder, Editors

CLINICAL TREATMENT AND RESEARCH IN CHILD PSYCHOPATHOLOGY

A.J. Finch, Jr. and Philip C. Kendall, Editors

AUTISM
Diagnosis, Current Research and Management

Edward R. Ritvo, Betty Jo Freeman, Edward M. Ornitz and Peter Tanguay, Editors

THE HYPERACTIVE CHILD
Diagnosis, Management, Current Research

Dennis P. Cantwell, Editor

EMOTIONAL DISORDERS IN CHILDREN AND ADOLESCENTS

Medical and Psychological Approaches to Treatment

Edited by

G. Pirooz Sholevar, M.D.
Clinical Professor and Director
Division of Child, Adolescent and
Family Psychiatry
Thomas Jefferson University
Philadelphia, Pennsylvania

with

Ronald M. Benson, M.D.
Clinical Associate Professor and Director
Youth and Outpatient Services
Children's Psychiatric Hospital
University Medical Center
Ann Arbor, Michigan

and

Barton J. Blinder, M.D.
Clinical Associate Professor
Department of Psychiatry and Human Behavior
School of Medicine
University of California at Irvine
Irvine, California

MTP PRESS LIMITED
International Medical Publishers

Published in the UK and Europe by
MTP Press Limited
Falcon House
Lancaster, England

Published in the US by
SPECTRUM PUBLICATIONS, INC.
175-20 Wexford Terrace
Jamaica, N.Y. 11432

Softcover reprint of the hardcover 1st edition 1980

ISBN-13: 978-94-011-6686-7 e-ISBN-13: 978-94-011-6684-3
DOI: 10.1007/978-94-011-6684-3

Contributors

JULES C. ABRAMS, M.D.
Professor and Director of Graduate Education in Psychology
Hahnemann Medical College and Hospital
Philadelphia, Pennsylvania

PAUL L. ADAMS, M.D.
Professor and Vice Chairperson
Department of Psychiatry
University of Louisville
Louisville, Kentucky

PAULA BRAM AMAR, Ph.D.
Clinical Assistant Professor
Department of Psychiatry and Human Behavior
Thomas Jefferson University
Philadelphia, Pennsylvania

ASHLEY J. ANGERT, D.O.
Clinical Assistant Professor
Department of Psychiatry and Human Behavior
Thomas Jefferson University
Philadelphia, Pennsylvania
and
Assistant Director
Developmental Center for Autistic Children
Philadelphia, Pennsylvania

RUSSELL S. ASNES, M.D.
Associate Professor of Clinical Pediatrics
College of Physicians and Surgeons
Columbia University
New York, New York

JULES R. BEMPORAD, M.D.
Director of Children's Services
Associate Professor of Psychiatry
Massachusetts Mental Health Center
Harvard Medical School
Cambridge, Massachusetts

RONALD M. BENSON, M.D.
Clinical Associate Professor and Director
Youth and Outpatient Services
Children's Psychiatric Hospital
University Medical Center
Ann Arbor, Michigan

JOHN M. BERECZ, Ph.D.
Associate Professor of Psychology
Andrews University
Berrien Springs, Michigan

IRVING H. BERKOVITZ, M.D.
Senior Psychiatric Consultant for Schools
Los Angeles County Department of Mental Health
and
Associate Clinical Professor
Child Psychiatry
University of California at Los Angeles
and
Member and Faculty Southern California Psychoanalytic Society-Institute
Los Angeles, California

BARTON J. BLINDER, M.D.
Clinical Assistant Professor
Department of Psychiatry and Human Behavior
University of California at Irvine
Irvine, California

HILDE BRUCH, M.D.
Professor Emeritus of Psychiatry
Baylor College of Medicine
Houston, Texas

J. ALEXIS BURLAND, M.D.
Clinical Professor
Department of Psychiatry and Human Behavior
Thomas Jefferson University
and
Philadelphia Psychoanalytic Institute
Philadelphia, Pennsylvania

DENNIS P. CANTWELL, M.D.
Professor
Department of Psychiatry
University of California, Los Angeles
School of Medicine
Los Angeles, California

THEODORE B. COHEN, M.D.
Clinical Professor of Psychiatry and Human Behavior
Thomas Jefferson University
Philadelphia, Pennsylvania

CHARLES W. DAVENPORT, M.D.
Associate Professor and Director
Division of Child Psychiatry
Medical College of Ohio
Toledo, Ohio

JOHN Y. DONALDSON, M.D.
Associate Professor of Psychiatry
University of Nebraska Medical Center
and
Clinical Director
Children's/Adolescent Services
Nebraska Psychiatric Institute
Omaha, Nebraska

MERRITT H. EGAN, M.D.
Clinical Associate Professor of Psychiatry
College of Medicine
University of Utah
Salt Lake City, Utah.

RUDOLF EKSTEIN, Ph.D.
Clinical Professor of Medical Psychology
University of California, Los Angeles
and
Training Analyst
Los Angeles Psychoanalytic Society and Institute
and
Training Analyst
Southern California Psychoanalytic Society and Institute
Los Angeles, California

MILTIADES GEORGE EVANGELAKIS, M.D.
Clinical Professor
Department of Psychiatry
School of Medicine
University of Miami
Miami, Florida
and
Director
Department Education, Training and Research
South Florida State Hospital
Hollywood, Florida

LINDA FEINFELD, M.D.
Clinical Assistant Professor
Department of Psychiatry and Human Behavior
Thomas Jefferson University
Philadelphia, Pennsylvania

STUART M. FINCH, M.D.
Department of Psychiatry
University of Arizona College of Medicine
Tucson, Arizona

RONALD C. HANSEN, M.D.
Assistant Professor
Department of Pediatrics
University of Arizona College of Medicine
Tucson, Arizona

CHARLES JAFFE, M.D.
Assistant Director
Adolescent Services
Institute for Psychosomatic and Psychiatric Research and Training
Michael Reese Hospital and Medical Center
Chicago, Illinois

RICHARD L. JENKINS, M.D.
Emeritus Professor of Psychiatry
University of Iowa
Iowa City, Iowa

IRVIN A. KRAFT, M.D.
Clinical Professor of Psychiatry
Baylor College of Medicine
Houston, Texas
and
Clinical Professor
School of Public Health
University of Texas Health Science Center
Houston, Texas

RICHARD A. KRESCH, M.D.
Instructor in Clinical Psychiatry
Columbia University
College of Physicians and Surgeons
New York, New York
and
Director of Psychiatry
St. Mary's Hospital for Children
Bayside, New York

CECILY LEGG, M.S.W., R.N.
Children's Psychiatric Hospital
University of Michigan
Ann Arbor, Michigan

RONALD A. MANN, Ph.D.
Assistant Clinical Professor in Psychiatry
University of California at Los Angeles
Los Angeles, California

FRANK J. MENALASCINO, M.D.
Professor of Psychiatry
University of Nebraska Medical Center
and
Associate Director
Nebraska Psychiatric Institute
Omaha, Nebraska

GILBERT G. MORRISON, M.D., Ph.D.
Clinical Professor of Psychiatry and Child Psychiatry
College of Medicine
University of California, Irvine
and
Supervisor and Training Psychoanalyst
Southern California Psychoanalytic Institute

and
Instructor in Psychoanalysis
Southern California Psychoanalytic Institute
Los Angeles, California

GENE RICHARD MOSS, M.D.
Associate Clinical Professor in Psychiatry
University of Southern California
Los Angeles, California

HUMBERTO NAGERA
Director of the Child Analytic Study Program
Chief of the Youth Service
Department of Psychiatry
University of Michigan Medical School
Ann Arbor, Michigan

DANIEL OFFER, M.D.
Chairman
Department of Psychiatry
Director
Institute for Psychosomatic and Psychiatric Research and Training
Michael Reese Hospital and Medical Center
and
Professor of Psychiatry
Pritzker School of Medicine
University of Chicago
Chicago, Illinois

THEODORE A. PETTI, M.D.
Assistant Professor of Child Psychiatry
Program Director
Children's Psychiatric Intensive Care Service
Western Psychiatric Institute and Clinic
University of Pittsburgh
Pittsburgh, Pennsylvania

DONALD B. RINSLEY, M.D.
Clinical Professor of Psychiatry
University of Kansas School of Medicine
and
Associate Chief for Education, Psychiatry Service
Topeka Veterans Administration Medical Center
and
Senior Faculty Member, Adult and Child Psychiatry
Menninger School of Psychiatry
Topeka, Kansas

ALAN J. ROSENTHAL, M.D.
Director
Children's Health Council
Palo Alto, California
and
Clinical Associate Professor of Psychiatry
Department of Psychiatry and Behavioral Science
Stanford University School of Medicine
Stanford, California

BERTRUM A. RUTTENBERG, M.D.
Professor
Department of Psychiatry and Human Behavior
Thomas Jefferson University
and
Director
Developmental Center for Autistic Children
Philadelphia, Pennsylvania

CHARLES A. SARNOFF, M.D.
Lecturer
Columbia University
College of Physicians and Surgeons
Psychoanalytic Center for Training and Research
New York, New York

CHARLES E. SCHAEFER, Ph.D.
Supervising Psychologist
The Children's Village
Dobbs Ferry, New York

RODNEY J. SHAPIRO, M.D.
Director
Family and Marriage Clinic
Associate Professor of Psychiatry and Psychology
Department of Psychiatry
University of Rochester Medical School
Rochester, New York

G. PIROOZ SHOLEVAR, M.D.
Clinical Professor and Director
Division of Child, Adolescent and Family Psychiatry
Jefferson Medical College
Thomas Jefferson University
and
Hahnemann Medical College and Hospital
Philadelphia, Pennsylvania

MOISY SHOPPER, M.D.
Clinical Associate Professor of Child Psychiatry
St. Louis University
School of Medicine
and
Faculty
St. Louis Psychoanalytic Institute
St. Louis, Missouri

M. DUNCAN STANTON, Ph.D.
Associate Professor of Psychology
Department of Psychiatry
University of Pennsylvania School of Medicine
and
Director
Addicts and Families Program
Philadelphia Child Guidance Clinic
and
Director of Family Therapy
Drug Dependence Treatment Center
Philadelphia VA Hospital
Philadelphia, Pennsylvania

JOHN A. SOURS, M.D.
Clinical Assistant Professor of Psychiatry
College of Physicians and Surgeons
Columbia University
and
Supervisor and Training Psychoanalyst
Columbia Psychoanalytic for Training and Research
and
Supervising Child Psychoanalyst
New York Psychoanalytic Institute
New York, New York

JOSEPH L. TAYLOR, ACSW
Executive Director
Association for Jewish Children of Philadelphia
Philadelphia, Pennsylvania

JAMES M. TOOLAN, M.D.
Assistant Professor of Clinical Psychiatry
University of Vermont
Burlington, Vermont
and
Consulting Psychiatrist, Marlboro College
Marlboro, Vermont

ROBERT G. WAHLER, Ph.D.
Professor and Director
Child Behavior Institute
University of Tennessee
Knoxville, Tennessee

DAVID ZINN, M.D.
Director of Adolescent Services
Clinical Assistant Professor
University of Chicago
Chicago, Illinois

JOEL P. ZRULL, M.D.
Professor and Chairman
Department of Psychiatry
Medical College of Ohio
Toledo, Ohio

Contents

EMOTIONAL DISORDERS IN CHILDREN AND ADOLESCENTS

Medical and Psychological Approaches to Treatment

Part I
Individual Psychotherapies

Treatment of Emotional Disorders in Children and Adolescents

CHAPTER 1

Individual Psychotherapy

Paul L. Adams

Individual Psychotherapy

Unique Skill

There is nothing more specific, more intrinsic, to treatment of emotional disorders in children than individual psychotherapy. It is *the* novelty that must be contended with by anyone who attempts to function well in the field of child treatment. It is the acid test for someone who can "make it" in being helpful and therapeutic with children. We can take family histories, perform physical examinations, order laboratory studies, dispense drugs appropriate to a child's weight and needs—all on the basis of earlier acquired skills *and knowledge*. Almost everything else we do in child psychiatry is derivative or modified from psychiatric work with adults. Only in individual psychotherapy do we glimpse what is radically new and different: that sharp demarcation between the state of the child and the state of the adult. A truly skillful therapist can work with a whole range of ages, perhaps, all across the life cycle, but the singular epoch to test the mettle of the attending therapist is childhood. And therapy with the individual child is a unique art and craft. There is even some promise of semi-scientific work and study looming in the future.

Terminology

"Individual psychotherapy" is a nonspecific label. The terms tells us only that one child is being seen by a therapist. The term does not say what they do together, nor does it set any limits on what they may do. It is like the Zen sign in the post office: the postmaster is neither required to give change for bills, nor authorized to refuse. Take your chances and hope for the best.

Critics of individual psychotherapy are legion. Some denounce it as a fruitless expenditure of time, energy and money. Some contend that since it is not of universally proven efficacy in unselected cases, it is no better than the passage of time and the evolution of the natural history of emotional crises in the human cycle of experienced stresses and problems. Some see it as dangerous from a political standpoint because it questions both individual and societal status quo. Some have philosophic objections, claiming that it is not a suitable endeavor for mass society, where normlessness, alienation and loneliness are the major facts of life, problems that are not readily soluble by individual verbal therapy. Some point out that all therapies do some good, have some ameliorative consequences on suffering, but that one type is about as good as another, and that proves, they say, that no claims can be made for any particular type of therapy (Eysenck, 1966).

Ford and Urban (1964) concluded that individual verbal psychotherapy is done when two people get together, interacting (mainly by talking) in a prolonged series of emotionally charged encounters, with the whole intent being one of changing the behavior of one of the dyad. That is a good enough summation of what it is that happens in individual child therapy, too, it would seem. It is largely a talking cure—dialogue about dreams and wakeful experiences—although selected times may be given over to play, to role-taking, to walks, to eating together, to caressing and holding, and perhaps even to massage. In Norway, under the influence of Nik Waal, a Reichian analyst, it is quite acceptable for a child guidance clinic therapist to undertake massage and muscle palpation in the interest of "vegetotherapy," and yet to make the main burden of the therapy one that is carried forward verbally.

Individual therapy as it is discussed in this chapter is the kind of therapy that is verbal, dynamically oriented but adaptable to short and medium terms of time and effort. That is, it is practicable in child psychiatry clinics, child guidance clinics, child-and-family agencies, and community mental health programs, as well as in private consulting rooms. It may be that this kind of individual therapy can be employed along with, or in series with, child analysis, behavior therapy, crisis intervention, group therapies, and other modalities. It is not altogether certain that the form of individual therapy described in this chapter is fully compatible with all these other forms, but it does seem likely.

Dynamisms and Motives in Individual Psychotherapy

Insight-oriented psychotherapy takes very seriously the question *why* and the question *how*. Causation of behavior, the precipitants and triggers of behavior, the remote genesis of behavior, the driving force, reinforcers and punishers, the motive power—all are important in individual verbal psychotherapy between adult and child. Yet these are diverse schools. Some therapists may rely fully on the general orthodox Freudian dynamisms of Eros and Thanatos, while others may not be able to swallow the death instinct and will substitute *aggression* for it (Brenner, 1955). Horneyans will be content with basic anxiety about love loss (and anxiety-influenced patterns of moving toward, moving away from and moving against others) as the wrap-up of motivation. Adlerians will stress the desire to move into a "relative plus" position in one's self-esteem as well as becoming relatively more competent and sociable in one's interpersonal dealings. Sullivanians point out the primacy of dynamics referable to the child's wish for gratification of animal needs, as well as its needs for security and comfort interpersonally. Maslow (1943) developed a more complicated and a more personal, humanistic, and comprehensive pyramid of dynamics. Maslow's scheme encompassed Marxian, Freudian, Sullivanian, Adlerian, and other systems of psychodynamics, adding some of the optimism of Rousseau as to human fulfillment and perfectibility. Maslow added at the peak of his epigenetic pyramid, *self-actualization*, a term derived from Kurt Goldstein and now widely adopted by humanistic psychologists of many and varied stripes.

Caveat Concerning Context

In this discussion of the individual child in direct psychotherapy some risky assumptions may seem to be made. For example, it may erroneously be concluded that the only sensible and effective way is to work with one child alone. In reality, that assumption is not made. The present task, sacrificing but not forgetting completeness, is to try to make as many rational statements as can be made in a brief chapter about what transpires when one works directly with a child. But that is not to say nor to imply that no other work needs to be done. At times, work with children in groups is important, and most of the time work with family groups is essential. Collaborative work, alongside a colleague who sees the parents, is a tried and true procedure in child guidance and child therapy. In what is said on the topic of direct work with the single child, it may appear that a message is being sent that *context* can be ignored when we dwell on one child and his inner world. Far from that: a full awareness of the larger context is a virtue, an aid, and an adjunct to individual psychotherapy with the child. Only when we can see the child and the therapy in a fuller biocultural milieu—and make the outer world explicit, too—do we commence being truly of aid and comfort to distressed young children.

History

The history of individual child psychotherapy is enwrapped with a diversity of social developments and intellectual movements which are child-focused. The history of child psychotherapy is the subject of a forthcoming publication by Professor John F. Kenward (1977) of the University of Chicago, which will give a more judicious assessment of the fuller story. Articles by Crutcher (1943), Harms (1960), Selesnick (1965), Anthony (1973),

Kanner (1973), and de Mause (1975) will be helpful to the interested student in the meantime.

It will suffice to point out now that individual child therapy is eclectic or pluralistic and has a diversified heritage—in the work of educators, nonparticipant child watchers, participant observers of children, psychometrists, reformers, pediatricians, norm-finding surveyors of customs and opinions, revolutionaries, psychoanalysts, social scientists, social workers, legal scholars, and behavioristic psychologists. Probably others have played a vital role in the development of dynamically oriented, ego-centered, verbal psychotherapy with one child. But it is a proud heritage that started with John Amos Comenius, a Moravian bishop uprooted by the Thirty Years' War who was an apostle of kindness and permissiveness in educating and enculturating children. Comenius was a refugee, too, from religious persecution in Bohemia; so from this beginning on, humaneness with children seems repetitively bound up with liberation movements. Lacking, however, from later longings for justice are the colorful phrasings of Comenius, the beauty of Moravian music, the joyous simplicity of the Eastertime love feast, and the whole pietistic spirit of German Protestantism.

Sustenance for positive valuations on children during the last two centuries flowed over from the liberal, anti-monarchical or anti-totalitarian philosophers; from the movement against slavery; from the movement to protect domestic animals against cruel treatment (here the spin-off was direct, for children were first protected in the United States against cruel beatings on the grounds that they were animals after all [Kahn, 1963]); from the movement to end child labor, to provide free education for all (and to test IQ); from the women's movement to obtain equality and justice regardless of gender; from the workers' movement for socialism or economic equality, whereby no person was given special advantage based on inherited great wealth; from the *Heilpaedogogik* movement (special or remedial education); from the psychoanalytic movement, even if psychoanalysis came to scorn direct social action and to set itself up as a substitute for social action (seeing itself as an ethical culture substitute for the neurotic excesses of socialism, democracy, Judaism, and Christianity [Fromm, 1959]), and most particularly from child analysis, Hermione von Hug-Hellmuth, Anna Freud, Melanie Klein, and the followers of the latter two. In the United States during the twentieth century additional sustenance for child therapy has come from the child guidance and mental hygiene movements, from Otto Rank's influence on therapy and functional casework, from the support given to child psychiatry within medical schools, from the new humanistic field of psychohistory, from the so-called kiddie lib movement (for civil liberation of children), but alas, hardly anything at all from the NIMH-fostered community mental health movement. Recently the field of child therapy has begun to derive as much as it has given to such off beat developments as humanistic therapy, growth or human potential gatherings, transactional analysis, Gestalt therapy, and other trends included under Maslow's "Third Force" rubric. Many of these are dealt with in sections devoted to therapy in the *Basic Handbook of Child Psychiatry* (Noshpitz et al., 1979).

Multiple historical roots can be traced for a flexible, eclectic, or pluralistic type of dynamoverbal psychotherapy that values highly the life and destiny of one small child. Some of this converging multiplicity and diversity is discernible in the assumptions that underlie the therapy I shall describe.

Axioms and Assumptions

In science, facts are tested statements about observed events and relationships. Theories are systems of facts, more general, but still *statements*, however, that correspond to replicable, consensually validated experience. When theories become so well accepted because they are highly useful or simply earn the status of being statements to which most sensible people do not take exception, theories drop out of the spotlight and come to be taken for granted. Hence, theory merges into the realm of axioms, undisputed facts, implicitly held assumptions. Thereafter, only new hypotheses can call facts and theories out of the shadows.

Now, psychotherapy is not scientific yet, but it is so much an art that its footing as a secure craft is not always earned. Still, there are certain assumptions not commonly spelled out—axioms—that underlie individual verbal psychotherapy with one child and one adult. Undoubtedly, there would be disagreement and controversy about the most careful and judicious statement of these axioms. If for no other reason, we object to any critique, articulation, and formulation of our axioms because it is "nicer" to leave axioms unsaid, unstated, sacred.

1. The first axiom underlying individual psychotherapy is that *a child is a person of value*. Some groups of people in our era and masses of people

in milieus and epochs different from our own have not valued children positively. That puts it mildly. When people do not want to serve and supply children with resources they need, people will not do psychotherapy. Instead, they will work for and with adults exclusively, even to a child's detriment, for they find children to be gross, immature, weak, and too crudely incipient, too inexperienced.

2. A second axiom underpinning this kind of therapy is that *a child depends on adults to provide security to the child.* Children are consumers of security, both economic and mental, and if a child is lucky, the fundamental unit for giving and receiving security is the family unit.

3. *Adults can communicate with children; they can have empathy for children.* Adults have been children and can reach back across the chasm of forgetting and repression to the times when they lived in a sensorimotor, prelogical cognitive stage. It is a sign of maturity and mental health, and above all of therapeutic skill, if an adult is able to be childlike in imagination and thereby establish warm rapport with a young child.

4. *Talking is an important vehicle for interpersonal relatedness.* Distinctively human, speech allows us to project ideas and feelings from one cerebral cortex to another. In talking with one another, we can hurt and insult, or we can bring healing help. Hence the talking cure becomes a possibility for child-adult relations.

5. *Early intervention is preferable*; preventive work is superior to remedial and rehabilitative work. Childhood presents us with an opportunity to do early intervention and to turn the course of the blighted life cycle around toward health.

6. *Problematic behavior can be changed.* The biologic foundations given by heredity may be durable and nearly immutable, but the *behavior* of an individual is subject to reinforcers and extinguishers, and is relatively malleable.

7. *All behavior loses some of its weirdness when it is understood in its existential context.* The context must be specified if the behavior is to be rendered understandable and alterable.

8. It is easier to augment competent acts than to diminish defective behavior. Behaviorists and Rankians join the majority in stressing the positive aspects of a child's behavior (Saslow, 1975; Allen, 1963).

9. *When a child's behavior is healthier, the child will also feel better and think better.* Therapy has affective, cognitive, and behavioral effects. Therapy is both rational and humanistic.

10. Medical ethics and practice provide a system of guides for psychotherapy, even if the therapist is nonmedical. Values on confidentiality, respect, moral rectitude, professional constraints, and endeavors (with eclecticism and empiricism) to do anything that is honorable to be of use to the patient—all are values that undergird both medicine and the kind of child psychotherapy I am considering. The reader will note that this is in strong contradistinction to Sigmund Freud's contentions that lay analysis is superior to medical analysis, or that a therapist should not touch the body of his analysand, and so on.

Limits on Applicability

A therapy mode that is marked by diversity, is pluralistic and flexible, and relies basically on the help that comes through dialogue, through sharing of one's humanity with an imaginative other person, does not have too many areas where it is not of some helpfulness to unhappy children. Nonetheless, there are some therapy prospects that are considerably more auspicious, relatively speaking. These must be stated, along with the relatively unfavorable traits. Limits (some of which may be needlessly so) include age of child, developmental stage, IQ, gender, class, ethnicity, family type, diagnostic grouping, ego strengths, physique, temperament and id strengths.

The child under five years of age is not an ideal candidate for this general therapy approach, and responds better to more play, less talk, and more concentrated work through the parents. An alternative way of putting this and some subsequent ideas would be not to emphasize the child's lacks, and to put more of the onus for limitations on the adults, the therapists. In sum, our frailties are not to be projected as the child's faults and deficiencies.

Developmental stage is limiting whenever the child is far behind his expected stage of development—that is, in comparison to his chronologic age. Low IQ—below 70, for example—generallly makes the work more difficult. Also, *ego strengths* that are impaired set up obstacles to the usefulness of this general type of therapy. Specifically, handicaps in perception, in intellection, and in conation impede therapeutic success (Murray and Kluckhohn, 1954). Obversely, intactness of reality testing, judgment, sense of reality, regulation and control of drives, object relations, thought processes, adaptive regression in the service of the ego, defensive functioning, stimulus barrier, autonomous functioning, synthetic and integrative functioning, and mastery-competence will enhance the therapeutic prospects (Bellak, 1973).

In a society that features economic inequality, racism, and sexism, and sees to it that each intertwines with childism to victimize the child, the child who is female, who is black or from some other ethnic minority, or who is poor is a relatively disadvantaged patient. Class, sex, and ethnicity are treated not as mere differences, but as impairments. Disadvantage lowers the child's chances for ever getting in contact with the mental health system (or non system), for proceeding beyond initial contact or brief evaluation, for being accepted without bias and prejudice if a trial of psychotherapy is offered, and for staying during a lengthy period without being cooled out (Adams and McDonald, 1966).

Id strengths, too, can be so lacking in depressed, inhibited, physically ill, leukemic, hungry, poisoned, sexually abused, and worm-infested children that they are not prime candidates for psychotherapy. A modicum of energy, of zesty appetites and cravings, of strong feelings and vivid imaginations helps therapy to move along. If a child is too listless, he is hardly amenable to the adventure that is individual psychotherapy (Adams, 1974). *Temperament* and *physique* set limits, too, but perhaps chiefly through their contribution to the child's endowment with id strengths.

Methods

Six levels in therapeutic transactions between one child and one therapist may be conceptualized as follows:

1. Symmetry or asymmetry of adult-child relation.
2. Models of adult-child interaction.
3. Personal styles of therapist and consonance or dissonance with child's style.
4. Therapy processes or methods.
5. Therapy operations or procedures.
6. Therapy techniques or modalities.

1. *Symmetry in the relationship.* Individual psychoterapy is an interaction, a series of systematized transactions. Individual psychotherapy can be highly asymmetrical, as in brainwashing or hypnosis, for one person dictates the correct thoughts to the other, extinguishing all resistance and sinful deviance. Individual psychotherapy can be nondirective, so that only by the therapist's changes of posture and muscle tonus, or only by his focusing selectively on one item of the passing welter of topics, can the child catch onto what the therapist might possibly want of him. Or individual psychotherapy may be in a large zone between these extremes, with something being done by the therapist and some things being said explicitly by adult to child but without badgering and intruding.

Difficult to explain to someone who is not initiated, the power imbalance referred to herein is set up by our society, by the way we customarily deal with children. The child is to be seen, not heard. Children are expected to approach adult strangers with a spirit of reserve and deference. Childism is the fundamental form of exploitation and victimization which all human beings suffer in some degree, and childism as a weak-strong dyadic interplay becomes the prototype for our co-optation into being exploiter and victim, by turns, in different interpersonal transactions or in different times during the interactions we have with a given individual. Tutored in childism, we easily go over to sexism and racism (Pierce and Allen, 1975). Many of us, by being bought out or selling out, come to justify our persecution in childhood as "good for us," a needed discipline to break our imperious wills, and so on (Schatzman, 1974). The name often given to this adaptive or defensive device is *identification with the aggressor.*

The power imbalance producing asymmetry in early psychotherapy sessions with a child not only is set up through societal pervasion by childism but is also fostered by the doctor-patient relationship as it is known to most adults and children. For in our folklore and cultural axioms the doctor is *agent*, the client is *patient*. "Patient" connotes long-suffering and passivity; "doctor" connotes activity and enterprise. The doctor teaches actively; the patient learns in quiet submission. Or more often, the doctor refrains from much teaching and the patient knows to wait until he is told what to do or is otherwise acted upon—however little he may obey the doctor's "orders." Children come to psychotherapy with prefigured passivity. The adult therapist's obligation is to help them see the therapist as realistically as possible. This entails a brief time of role induction: talking about other doctors and other therapists, and showing how by contrast the therapist will expect the child to have more say-so than the child ordinarily has (Hoehn-Saric et al., 1964). In short, asymmetry in the therapeutic relationship between adults and child is a beginning fact to be dealt with but is not a virtue to be enshrined.

2. *Models of adult-child interaction.* We concep-

tualize children, childhood, and child phychotherapy through stylized filters. We are so much subjugated by our conventional thought forms that we do not get the whole picture at all. We see things only partially and indistinctly, and we selectively discern certain things while selectively overlooking other matters. We are the prisoners of our own thought forms, stereotypes, metapsychologies, and personal cognitive idiosyncrasies. We think as if our thoughts corresponded intimately and veridically with reality. Since our thought models are so weighty in our therapeutic problem-solving with children, I will comment more than is customary on four of these countertransference models that regularly enter into our professional relations with children. They enter. They intrude. Oftentimes, they interfere. They haunt us, at times, and embarrass us when we are caught red-handed using a favorite model inappropriately. Our cognitive models cast shadows, as would clouds or (more optimistically!) guardian angels, as they hover around us and our work as adults in relatedness with children.

Parent

When a therapist relates "parentally" to a child in treatment, the therapist moves into the professional work as though the work were not professional, but personal, having to do with one or another variant of fathering or mothering to the child patient. Often this seems to set up a facilitating and holding environment for a child that can provide a footing for a later, sounder relationship that will be analyzed and become more business like. Not all parental approaches are "holding," benign, and enhancing of therapy, however. As a case in point, the parent who relates to the child through *projective identification* is not a useful model to follow. The child catches on sooner or later, and says, in compliant word and nonverbal deed, to the would-be therapist, "Help me, a sinner, to get right." The therapist who goes at the child with projective identification is a moral reformer, and may be the therapist who prefers to do Reality Therapy or other therapies with delinquent children who need, if anyone does, some moral habilitation or rehabilitation.

Therapists who relate, in the way shown by parents, through *identification and role-modeling* are on safer ground and more therapeutic. They stand ready to be exemplars for the child when called on, to teach whatever they know that the child may find useful, and to serve as handy reminders that childhood, however painful, is not lethal. A specimen of human survival, especially if the adult has survived and lived a full life, can be a good thing for a child to encounter. These adults, especially when they are child therapists, identify with the children with whom they are in close relations. At least they do not reject and hate the child, but they sometimes turn children off by the misty-eyed boosting of the child. Also, these therapists, again mimicking certain parents, tend to be highly future-oriented, hardly a cognitive mode that appeals to a child. They are forever inflicting their private images of the life cycle on the child patient, and most child patients see such a leap into the future as a questionable vote of confidence for the child here and now, or there and then. At least the "identifying" therapist is like a relatively harmless parent. He will never beat, kill, or sexually exploit a child—which is progress of magnitude—but he may never get going on meaningful therapy, either. Loving identification is not always enough for therapy.

Much more negative again is the therapist who apes a parent in *role reversal,* as he encounters a child in treatment. Such a therapist elicits from the child a message that the child will take care of the therapist, thus "I will take better care of you, I promise." Sometimes the child may emit this message strictly out of transference from his own parent onto the therapist, but at times the therapist also makes strong unconscious bids for the child to be less "self-seeking, narcissistic, aggressive, disobedient, inattentive and so on." Adults cannot easily deceive children when the adults pour their hearts and souls into their therapeutic work, expecting rewards of love and caring from their child patients. Role reversal as a part of as-if playing (role-playing) during treatment may be a useful device, but it is clearly categorized and labeled as play, and discussed somewhat soberly during or after the play sequence has ended. That kind of role-playing may find a child assuming adult roles in imagery and fancy, giving child roles to the therapist for the duration of the play. But that is very different from, as an example, the unmarried child therapists whose only religion, family, and love life consist in the gratifications received from their grateful patients.

Ideally, the best model for parentlike relation by the therapist is the model of the *empathic, helping* parent. To such a therapist the child responds, again with an implicit message: "You meet my needs and we love and trust each other." In real life, the child may see the therapist as a transference extension not of a parent but of a grandparent. The child senses that this kind of therapist is out to serve him well, willing to stand in his shoes, eager to see how the world looks from the child's-eye view, and will never willfully manipulate, con, exploit, or do violence to the child. Chances are, a helping, empathic (or empathetic) therapist is one "protector" from whom the child will not need protection, and he may not even need to get a lawyer to look after his interests as opposed to the therapist's. Empathy is the adult stance that is therapeutic, not cramping and warping of the child, but permitting the child to grow and unfold in dependence and security. Empathy entails some liberties freely allocated and waxing with each added day or year, and empathy affirms the child's conviction that as a child one can be dependent, ever consuming security from dependable grown-ups. To work in therapy with a child who knows from the onset, or learns through the course of therapy, that children are dependent and adults are dependable is joyous for most child therapists.

Teacher or Tutor

It is not uncommon for persons who have been schoolteachers to get into the child-therapy field. They carry very naturally and gracefully some of the habitual patterns and approaches that they used as teachers and do some helpful work as therapists without giving up all of their earlier trappings. It has often been said that Anna Freud and the other child analysts functioned according to the model of the piano teacher in Vienna. They saw children within their own homes, but apart from the family, and they came regularly and punctually, all adding up to traits that children had come to expect of their piano teachers. Tutors at heart who engage in child therapy can be empathetic and healing, attentive and serving in a non-intrusive way, *or* they can be taskmasters who overemphasize the cognitive and push children to perform. Anna Freud and her followers epitomize in some ways the serving, and healing, tutor-therapists, whereas behavior therapists are good examples of the tutorial therapists who rush to adequacy and competence, worrying not at all about the unconscious and intrapsychic meanings to the child.

Martin Buber, the Jewish existentialist philosopher, thought a great deal about teaching, and about psychotherapy, both of which Buber regarded as instances of human growth through a life of dialogue and consensual validation. Buber (1955) said sagely that education of two varieties occurs—one is funneling, pouring facts and generalizations into the relatively passive recipient; the other is pumping, encouraging the expression (literally, squeezing out) of what the learner finds shareable within him. The Kleinians may do both of these operations, pumping and funneling, with vigor.

When a therapist "thinks like a teacher," the therapist is frequently alert to reference-group norms in a way that is hard to ken by people who never taught groups of children. These therapists often have a good eye for clinical research. They steadily go about comparing one child to others and to a class as a whole, and hence they are keenly adept in using a developmental perspective.

Casual Caretaker

Some therapists bring another kind of ideational freight to the child-therapy enterprise, for they are so unobtrusive, so nondirective, that a child may crave that the therapist did have something to teach to the child. These therapists do not hold a parental model or an educational model uppermost. Instead, they seem unduly impressed by roles such as babysitter, recreation leader, Scout leader and camp counselor. A psychoanalytically oriented Boy Scout leader might do no harm (a first principle, to be sure), but he may not get into the real essence of psychotherapy with an individual child.

However, there are worse models than the casual caretaker. Or, again, each and every therapist who acknowledges the limits of time, of will, of human understanding, and of the capabilities for change has some of the air of a casual caretaker about him. Children in professional therapy are with us for a purpose and for a brief time, all things considered. We do well to adopt a certain amount of watchful waiting as we live and work together with them in a healing relationship.

Policeman or Judge

Some therapists have the model of advancing law and order uppermost in their minds as they engage in therapy. They concentrate on power interactions and on one-upmanship, and worry a great deal about assertive casework and rational Reality Therapy. They fret about the use of authority as they work with their young clients, and in general, they feel comfortable about carrying a big stick and about making children toe the line.

A disturbed child might benefit from association with a therapist who has some values, who believes in something and is not namby-pamby about asserting his own values. Assuredly, the model of the judge or cop is not all negative. There is always a measure of asymmetry present whenever a therapist meets a child and offers professional help to the child. The adult has more power, more know-how, and sometimes more accessible brute strength.

As an attempt to ferret out an ideal authoritative, but not authoritarian, relationship, Erich Fromm distinguished between *rational and irrational authority*. Rational authority is realistically, reasonably based, and longs to level the imbalance between child and adult. Irrational authority, by contrast, is unreasonably and unlovingly based. Irrational authority does not aim to end the asymmetry between adult and child, but to perpetuate it. The ultimate warrant of irrational authority is "Do as I say for I can make you do it."

All of these models—parent, teacher, casual caretaker and authority—enter into most therapeutic relationships. Even when our intentions are to be professional and somewhat neutral, and to build an artificial, as-if relationship with the child, we get sidetracked into countertransference that is dadlike, momlike, teacherish, babysitterlike or coplike. All too often our countertransferences are not analyzed. They elicit from children a welter of transference, pseudo-transference and counter-countertransference. Full inspection, analysis, or scrutiny of these shadowy images would help all therapy to be more appropriate to what the child so insistently requires from a therapeutic adult.

3. *Stylistic or temperamental similarities and differences*. From birth onward, in complicated ways that are not fully understood and spelled out, each human being has certain ways in which he expresses emotions and feelings. Some display, from infancy until old age, a penchant for deep, strong emotions, whereas others run more superficially. Also, as the ancient Greeks attested, certain people who have deep emotions may be rather coarcted in the range of feelings they manifest (melancholic) *or* another person may be ready to go with a rather broad range of emotions (choleric). Likewise, the person whose feelings are shallow may have a narrow range of expression (phlegmatic) or a broad scope for manifesting feelings (sanguine). Children are described conveniently today by these categories, although we no longer postulate that humors such as phlegm, blood, and bile are responsible for these largely heredo-constitutional differences. Therapists, too, have their own biological endowments and preprogrammed temperaments. Differences and similarities of temperament impede, enrich, enhance, distract, and otherwise influence the course of therapy as an interaction between the therapist and the child.

Carl G. Jung disliked work with extroverts. Child therapists generally prefer not to work with acting-out delinquents. Aichhorn was an exception to the latter. William Healy appears to have been another exception to the latter. Otto Rank preferred work with artistic, creative patients. Some therapists resonate with hysterics, others with obsessives, and so on. Therapists have their likes and dislikes that run deeper than mere "unanalyzed predilections" when it comes to patients they seem able to help with both enthusiasm and gracefulness. This is probably not a matter of "auras" and "karma" and may not even be a question of how Intuition-Thinking-Sensation-Feeling are distributed—as the Jungians depict these basic, in-our-bones orientations. Hysterics find obsessives *cold*; obsessives find hysterics *primitive*. Schizophrenics see manics as too wild; manics see schizoid people as too woolly and flaky. Therefore, the two myths, of child and therapist, cannot clash to a degree that precludes an alliance.

Children sometimes sense that a therapist is benign and benevolent enough but that for fundamental temperamental reasons they two might never hit it off. The therapist can be very useful to the child by considering his viewpoint seriously, attempting whatever accommodations he can to meet the child's needs, and helping the child to respect and admire the differences between them. A rule of thumb in psychotherapy is that differences discussed can have a liberating effect but differences concealed from candid discussion can give insuperable barriers to the course of therapy.

4. *Processes for change to occur*. There are certain processes whereby behavioral, cognitive, and affective change occur in a child in therapy. Most conceptualization of these processes is derived from psychoanalysis. The major examples are: *transference analysis* (open consideration of how present behavior is an extension of earliest experiences, how distortions are carried forth from the individual child's babyhood in his particular family, how the ways the child faces life inclusive of therapy is a reflection and rehash of these early attitudes of self-regard and patterns of interpersonal relations);

reality testing (the child probes his cognitive and

behavioral "errors," he checks on his fantasies and projections, he curbs his antisocial leanings, he sees his denials of observable facts undergo an atrophy of disuse—how he comes to feel that people and events take on a new vibrancy and sense of aliveness);

ego strengthening (nothing succeeds like success, and as the child makes changes, his optimism grows for being able to master added difficulties, or as the child learns to bring some of his longings and cravings into shared awareness with the therapist, he takes heart that self-understanding and self-acceptance are more fully possible for him);

insight and outsight (the child learns about his own motives and interior wishes and makes connections that were not possible previously; too, the child learns how his behavior includes others in imagination and reality and that the contexts in which he lives are determinative of many of his successes and failures—in Adlerian terminology, he learns how sociability enhances a happy existence);

catharsis (by injunction and by example, by rehearsal and replaying of emotion-laden scripts, the therapist aids the child in derepression and an outpouring of feelings because that release is a cleansing force—the child encompasses a picture of himself as an expressive animal, pleased to emote, to abreact, and to gain release from inner tension and conflict);

sublimation (not all lusts and longings can be unleashed directly, the child learns, but by being incorporated and made intrinsic to himself they are controllable, as he must control them for his peaceable life with others or even with his own self-esteem—besides, he can obtain satisfactions through mostly acceptable behavior).

5. *Operations or procedures.* If the foregoing processes are the instruments, the vehicles for bringing about changes, then the modus operandi for individual psychotherapy consists of a number of operations for advancing therapy. In the actual operations of child therapy, semi-abstract as they may be, we try (1) to teach, (2) to comfort or to heal, and whenever the occasion demands, (3) to advocate for the child patient. Our didactic efforts, of course, can be comforting and healing; advocacy can be comforting and healing also. By convention we do not ordinarily include advocacy as a therapeutic operation. Advocacy can be instructive or didactic; it can also be comforting to an exploited child. The operations overlap but are distinctive to a degree. This tripartite swarm of therapeutic operations will be subdivided into five that may be seen as principally teaching or tutorial operations, four that are mainly healing-comforting, and four that are mainly advocating-protecting.

Teaching Operations

A professionally trained, empathetic adult may have something worth teaching a child. Teaching is done in the forms of: *imparting information, giving advice, identifying actuality, clarifying,* and *confronting.*

Imparting information is a basic operation of individual dynamoverbal psychotherapy with a child. It is often relegated to the dung heap, as if it were not worthy of an elegant psychotherapy, but it is as important and salient as to offer professional psychotherapeutic help, to aid a child to grow with fewer arrests and hangups. All psychotherapy gives information, the least in the more headless versions of Gestalt therapy or in the more mindless versions of relationship therapy.

It is not possible to work psychotherapeutically and hold back information from a child who wants to know about where babies come from, why a plant in the sun is green but one under a rock is white, why dreams are important, whether parents become children as a child grows to womanhood or manhood (so the child can beat up his parents and get revenge).

Giving advice is another operation that has received a bad, but unmerited, reputation with some of the schools of dynamic psychotherapy. Naturally, direct unvarnished advice, as that which a parent gives a clumsy child, is not helpful. But advice that has preambles, precautions, and safeguards is a part of the therapeutic way of working. Orthodoxy comes easily in psychotherapy, and it is especially easy to withold advice from a child. The therapist can be stingy and justify it as good technique, or as proper deference to the child's parent(s), or as a way of promoting the child's rugged individualism and independence.

What are the kinds of advice children may ask? An obsessive child, for instance, may ask if you have seen anyone with his "kind of troubles" before; to that, one responds not by a direct answer. An obsessive may ask you how to diminish his ritualistic symptoms, and here I think some more direct advice is warranted. A therapist may ask the child if anyone's advice has helped any in the past, and thereby confront the child with his desire to lead the therapist into voicing foolish remarks and counsels. The therapist may ask what the child feels would be helpful to relieve the tension he feels, and when the child has already prescribed something sensible, say, "That sounds like a decent thing." The therapist does better if, instead of the preceding examples, he seems to want to help the child but rephrases the child's request to one such as "I believe you want me to help you get more natural and easygoing, and I will try to help you to feel more natural, more at ease, less uptight." That is advice giving, too. The advice does not fit the question, but it attempts to fit the message.

Identification. When the child gets confused, seems to be mystified, fearful, or alienated, the therapist helps to dispel this state of murkiness by speaking candidly so that the child is led to candor, too, and knows surely and vividly what it is that he is really experiencing over and above the games, the phony scripts, and the conventional roles laid on him by parents and adults other than the therapist. Identification is a detective-like operation, trying to read between the lines, to speak outright truth, to follow small clues until they turn up some genuine experience. This attitude of inquiry or investigation sometimes delights a child, but also at times mobilizes a ferocious resistance. Identification is a device for letting the child realize what he knows in his heart but has been afraid to let into full awareness during his everyday existence.

Clarification is an extension of identification, but with some additions. If in using identification the child says, "If I say what I really felt, it was a wish co run away and never see my father again," in using clarification the child will not only identify the affect clearly but will move on to a bit of unraveling of mysteries hardly visualized theretofore. The child clarifies by explaining the context in which his school failure on one particular examination occurred, by speaking more truth than poetry about his mother's alcoholism during a family session and thereby demonstrating to the parents he will not keep the pact to remain quiet that the family made before enrolling in family group therapy. Clarification is an operation taking the child away from fog, from feeling behavior is inexplicable, and from being perplexed by ambivalence and inner conflict. Clarification takes the child toward better understanding, problem-solving that is reliable, and some acceptance of the malaise and ambivalence which is all too human here in the briar patch.

Confrontation is a brisk educational operation, often making for speedy learning and change in the child. It is the kind of device that August Aichhorn employed when he suddenly faced the neurotically delinquent child with some information (derived from collateral sources) that the child previously either had disclaimed, or, lying, had denied outright. Confronting consists of a sudden juxtaposition of another truth or another perspective that the child refrained from seeing or adopting. Once the therapist assertively puts in his few words, the child, too, must face the situation from a new vantage point. Soilers, bed-wetters, assaultive children, thieves, truants, school refusers, liars, and obsessives glean most from confrontation, in usual clinical experience. They seem to be simmering in denial, so confrontation seizes their attention; it entails the therapist taking initiative for getting down to serious business, and more or less demanding that the child see the therapist's point quickly and change quickly from half-truthful pussyfooting to more open honesty. Confrontation arouses counter-anger in the child, who senses some anger in the therapist, but after a time the child patient understands that the therapist may state things flatly in order to get dialogue started, not to subordinate and overpower the child. "Now, wait a minute, I thought you told me"—that is confrontation. If there is a good alliance, there is no real problem; and sometimes confrontation is needed to get an alliance established.

Comforting Operations

Psychotherapy also involves coming to the rescue, instilling security and comfort where danger and unpleasure had previously reigned. The doctor is not only a teacher but also a healer, and in his repertoire of therapy operations are four comforting procedures that will be considered briefly: *alliance, promoting regression, reassurance,* and *interpretation.*

Alliance forming begins with rapport externally and with an inward split between sick and well, good and bad, competent and defective. Then the final step comes when the child affiliates his more positive behavior and striving with the personal aid and comfort that he imputes to the therapist. That is a therapeutic alliance that will enhance the work of both teaching and healing, and will make the therapist more accessible to the child if needed to be a child advocate.

The alliance is in evidence when the child asks the therapist to help him solve a specific problem, particularly a newly enunciated one, or when the recalcitrant child begins to show enthusiasm for coming to therapy, or when a child who proclaims dreamlessness begins to report dreams to the therapist. Without a therapeutic alliance, little can be accomplished, but with an alliance, much may be done that serves the child well.

Reassurance is another operation that is universally adopted by child therapists but seldom admitted as worthy by many therapists. The operation of reassurance spans from a purr of reinforcing approval (if that suffices to give the child a needed vote of confidence) to a dare made to the child that if he works on it harder, you can help him understand some inner turmoil that besets him. Sometimes a challenge can reassure more than a compliment. I have even made bets with children that if they cooperate in specific ways they will get better. Reassurance is not necessarily a pat on the back, but it could be. The main thing in reassuring is to convey to the child that his therapist has faith that he is a good egg and will surmount his difficulties, and that indeed his therapist cannot accept any other premises and assumptions.

Promoting regression is a comforting procedure for many hurt children. Until they have had some compensatory babying, thay cannot benefit from other therapeutic operations such as confrontation or reassurance or interpretation. Departures from talking for doll play, for puppet play, for play in a sandbox or with water (the regresser par excellence, in the opinion of many clinicians), taking feeding breaks, setting aside times for rocking and holding, or times for massage and cuddling of younger children—all these will facilitate the child's acting younger than his real age or his previous level of action.

Damaged and neglected children (as seen in some groups of poor, mentally retarded, hyperactive, physically and sexually abused children) may require some compensatory acts of loving kindness before "regular" therapy can take hold, and indeed may need to regress more than once interspersed with a more businesslike talking cure.

Interpretation has been defined by Edith Buxbaum (1954) as "explaining irrational behavior in terms of fantasies and past experiences." Very little of the interpretation is therapist-initiated, according to this concept, for most of the work is intrapsychic—the child sees his symptoms in relation to his fantasies and earlier childhood experiences. In this work, the therapist plays a helpful role, perhaps, but the best interpretations are those elicited spontaneously in the child. Still, in all, the therapist is not passively mute but may converse, help to clarify, and add some things of value to the interpretative act.

Dream interpretation is likewise something produced within the child; not a bright idea planted by the therapist first and foremost. The child is asked what his dream means, and if he sees meaning that ties current symptoms with infantile experience or present fantasies, he has given a valuable interpretation of his dream without invoking any of his oneirocritical virtuosity. Once the interpretation has jelled and been worked through, the child feels both liberated and comforted.

Advocacy

Children, being dependent on parents and other adults, may be preyed upon, exploited, or demeaned consciously and unwittingly by adult figures in their real lives. The therapist is a good counterpoint to some of childhood's tragic aspects, and the empathetic therapist is ready to go to bat to advocate for the child's protection and liberties in four customary areas: *home, school, court,* and the *political arena.* The therapist is an ally and teacher who knows far better what serves the child best than many of the people who staff those areas. Parents, schools, and courts are generally more powerful than the child and therapist combined in protecting the child. Powerlessness sometimes feeds the militancy of a therapist's advocacy, however, and by working assiduously in the political arena, the therapist may work toward an ultimate restructuring of institutions so that children are truly served and not victimized. Many of the professional organizations of psychiatrists, psychologists, social workers, and other therapists are more politically astute and energetic than they were in former times. Therapeutic alliances blend easily into coalitions for social action on behalf of children.

6. *Therapy techniques or modalities.* Finally, on a concrete level there are techniques (such as play, talk, operant conditioning, dream study, home visits, family sessions, and concurrent peer group therapy) that make up the substance of individual verbal child therapy. Also, there are certain requirements of space and setting, of supplies and equipment that give the practical underpinning and framework by which the healing and teaching operations are carried forward. These have been considered sufficiently in the literature (Adams, 1974, for example), so they will not be dealt with further at this point.

Comparisons with Other Therapies

Pharmacotherapy—behavior therapy—analysis—play therapy—this therapy. That spectrum displays, on the left, three therapies that rely on a mechanistic mystique. In the sense of their sharing underlying mechanistic assumptions, psychoanalysis, behavior therapy, and psychopharmacotherapy are blood brothers. But at the same time, psychoanalysis, play therapy, and dynamically oriented verbal child therapy fall close to each other because they all share in humanistic and biosocial traditions. Finally, if we see the spectrum as forming a circle and not as on a ramrod-straight line, we can see that dynamically oriented individual therapy is situated next to pharmacotherapy, with which there are no basic contradictions or inconsistencies.

Individual psychotherapy can draw freely upon the more relevant offerings of pharmacotherapy, behavior therapy, psychoanalysis with children, and play therapy. Indeed, borrowing, adoption, adapting, and incorporation of other schools are some of the central features of a flexible, open-minded approach to child therapy.

Systematic studies of any of these different forms of psychotherapy, of their outcomes with varied groups of children, and of their relative costs in time and money would be highly instructive. Today, they are largely lacking.

Summary and Conclusions

There are many kinds of relatively unadulterated therapy, but the one I have elected to practice is one that is flexible and nondoctrinaire. I prefer to work without the rituals and controls of orthodoxy, and to be free to use any devices that I feel apt and helpful to the child I seek to serve. One can, however, respect orthodoxy and "simon-purity" because there *are* some values worthy of our espousal as we undertake to help children to solve their problems and overcome their blocks, regressions, and fixations. Doing a little bit of everything, but doing it all badly in the long run, is far from a blessing. It would be better, some say, to master a single method and apply it well with true craftsmanship and grace. These are sensible arguments, I believe.

I do not believe that flexible, dynamically oriented, individual and verbal psychotherapy is a second-rate or easy form of therapy, designed for the lazy or the inept. It probably takes more skill to be flexible, and help, than to be rigid, and take it slowly. It probably takes more wisdom to deal with the here and now than to dig slowly for antique buried treasures. Simply dispensing drugs or doing strictest behavior therapy might be less taxing on one's limited energies; adhering strictly to psychoanalytic technique might give greater security to the therapist than being so available and vulnerable in a freewheeling therapeutic approach. Play therapy may be more fun, more gratifying to child and adult alike. But flexible talking therapy, drawing in other methods as they are called for, precludes a therapeutic staleness and allows for a wider versatility in the therapeutic offering of an adult therapist in helping an unhappy child.

References

Adams, P. (1974) *A Primer of Child Psychotherapy*, Boston: Little, Brown.

Adams, P., and N. McDonald. (1966) Clinical cooling out of poor people. *Am. J. Orthopsychiat.* 38:457-464.

Allen, F. (1963) *Positive Aspects of Child Psychiatry.* New York: Norton.

Anthony, E. (1973) The state of the art and science of child psychiatry. *Arch. Gen. Psychiat.* 29: 299-305.

Bellak, L. (1973) *Ego Functions in Schizophrenia, Neurotics, and Normals.* New York: Wiley.

Brenner, C. (1957) *An Elementary Textbook of Psychoanalysis.* Garden City, N.Y.: Doubleday-Anchor Books.

Buber, M. (1955) *Between Man and Man.* Boston: Beacon Press.

Buxbaum, E. (1954) Technique of child therapy: A critical evaluation. *Psychoanal. Study Child.* 9:297-333.

Crutcher, R. (1943) Child psychiatry: A history of its development. *Psychiatry.* 6:191-201.

de Mause, L., ed. (1975) *The History of Childhood.* New York: Harper Torchbooks.

Eysenck, H. (1966) *The Effects of Psychotherapy.* New York: International Science Press.

Ford, D., and H. Urban. (1964) *Systems of Psychotherapy.* New York: Wiley.

Fromm, E. (1959) *Sigmund Freud's Mission: An Analysis of His Personality and Influence.* New York: Harper & Row.

Harms, E. (1960) At the cradle of child psychiatry. *Am. J. Orthopsychiat.* 30:186-190.

Kahn, A. (1963) *Planning Community Services for Children in Trouble.* New York: Columbia University Press.

Kanner, L. (1973) Historical perspective on developmental deviations. *J. Autism Childhood Schizo.* 3:197-198.

Kenward, J. (1977) History of child therapy. Unpublished paper written for Group for Advancement of Psychiatry, Committee on Child Psychiatry.

Maslow, A. (1943) A theory of human motivation. *Psycholog. Rev.* 50:370-396.

Murray, H., and C. Kluckhohn. (1954) Outline of a conception of personality. In C. Kluckhohn et al., *Personality in Nature, Society and Culture.* New York: Knopf, pp. 3-49.

Noshpitz, J., et al., eds. (1979) *Basic Handbook of Child Psychiatry.* New York: Basic Books.

Pierce, C., and G. Allen. (1975) Childism. *Psychiat. Ann.* 5:266-270.

Saslow, G. (1975) Application of Behavior Therapy. In G. Usdin, ed. *Overview of the Psychotherapies.* New York: Brunner/Mazel, pp. 68-91.

Schatzman, M. (1974) *Soul Murder: Persecution in the Family.* New York: New American Library.

Selesnick, S. (1965) Historical perspectives in the development of child psychiatry. In J. H. Masserman, ed., *Current Psychiatric Therapies.* New York: Grune & Stratton.

Treatment of Emotional Disorders in Children and Adolescents

CHAPTER 2

Child Psychoanalysis

Humberto Nagera

Brief Historical Account

Child psychoanalysis as a treatment method for the emotional disturbances of children of various ages can be said to have started in 1909. The now famous case of Little Hans was published by Freud on that date. Yet it will be more appropriate to state that Hans was the first known child in whom the psychoanalytic method as it was known and developed in those days was applied to a child. As one would expect, the technique that was employed was significantly different in various respects from the technique that has since evolved and that nowadays characterizes the practice of child psychoanalysis. Furthermore, the therapist of the case was the father of the child, whom Freud supervised closely for the duration of the treatment. This in itself was naturally a somewhat unconventional approach by today's present standards. Nevertheless, I should hasten to add that the parental role in the conduct of a child psychoanalysis is quite distinct and relevant in contradistinction to the role played by relatives in the case of adult analysis, a point that will be discussed later on in this paper.

Not much is known about the vicissitudes of the development of child analysis as a technique of treatment up to the twenties. At that time Melanie Klein was active in this field, first in Germany, and later on in England, where she was instrumental in the development of the Kleinian school of psychoanalysis. Simultaneously, Anna Freud and some collaborators were actively engaged in the psychoanalytic treatment of children in Vienna.* Through these various efforts, the technique of child analysis was developed and reached the form with which we are acquainted today. It should be noticed that there were from the beginning significant differences in the theoretical tenets of Melanie Klein and Anna Freud, differences that could not but influence significantly various aspects of technique. We can say that two well-differentiated schools of child analysis were developed and established. It should be noticed too that though the differences in the Kleinian and Freudian approach to child psychoanalysis still exist, there has been through the years a convergent move, at least in regard to certain aspects of the field.

Except for the early efforts (perhaps somewhat informal) at training in Vienna and elsewhere, child psychoanalysis took many years to become of age. It is only relatively recently that it became a formalized, well-organized training program attached to the adult training programs at various institutes in the world and more particularly so in this country.

As such, it has developed its own curriculum, with its specialized faculty, continuous case seminars, seminars on technique, supervision of cases of various ages for specified periods of time, and

* For a historical review of such developments, see the Preface of Anna Freud's *The Psychoanalytical Treatment of Children* (1946).

so forth—in short, a status quite similar to the training in adult psychoanalysis. In many ways and to this day, child psychoanalysis has remained subservient to adult psychoanalysis. Thus, for example, it is still the rule that training as a child psychoanalyst requires previous training in adult analysis. True, in many training centers the child aspects of the training can be initiated after the candidate has reached a certain degree of progression in his adult training, at which point they can run concomitantly.

Exceptions to the above rule have existed for some years, at the Hampstead Child Therapy Clinic and Course in London (Anna Freud's clinic), at Leyden (Holland), and in Cleveland in this country. In those centers it was possible to undertake training directly in child analysis, but except for those from Leyden, their graduates are not officially recognized by the established psychoanalytic associations as child psychoanalysts.

Similarities and Differences between Child and Adult Psychoanalysis

The basic theoretical principles as understood for adult psychoanalysis and the theory of technique are all applicable to child psychoanalysis. Yet the special characteristics of the functioning of the mind of children of different ages and stages of development have determined the use of special technical procedures and devices in child analysis. Because of this, the noninitiated may conclude that such massive apparent differences must imply that child and adult analysis are two totally different procedures with little, if anything, in common.

Take, for example, the issue of so-called free associations, one of the fundamental rules in adult analysis. Children, as we all know, are quite incapable of free associations. In its place, the child analyst has substituted the child's natural tendency to play. Though quite dissimilar in appearance, the child's play is as effective as the free associations of the adult in leading the analysts to identification of the unconscious mental contents and determinants, thus elucidating the nature of unconscious fantasies and conflicts. Because of the above, the term "play therapy" is frequently and perhaps unfortunately utilized. It leads many to assume that just playing with children would bring about the necessary therapeutic changes. Clearly, play is to be understood as an unconscious derivative, more or less distanced, that must be interpreted as necessary and appropriate with due regard for timing, wording, and the like, as is the case with free associations. Among factors contributing to the apparent differences between child and adult analysis is the question of motivation and understanding. The adult patient has substantial reasons to seek help actively. He may suffer from painful symptoms, from severe anxiety, or from inhibitions that interfere in a distressing form with the capacity to work, to relate to others, to love, to enjoy an active sexual life, and so forth. In contrast, though some children may present with obvious neurotic suffering, this is not always the case. Given that the child is still in a protected situation and environment, many of the above symptoms do not have the impact on him that they would have on an adult. Further, the symptoms of the child may constitute a nuisance for the parents, teachers, and other adults, while for the child they may even be somewhat enjoyable, as indeed is true for example in some cases of bedwetting. His limited understanding of cause and effect, of consequences for the future, and so forth, in combination with his protected situation conspire against his being strongly motivated for treatment and change. Given, too, that he has a limited capacity to handle psychological pain, it is easy to understand that he does not always welcome being placed in a "treatment situation," and is not willing to cooperate, or actively fights it.

Such lack of personal motivation on the side of the child patient would be an enormous hindrance to the treatment. The child analyst thus endeavors to establish a meaningful relationship with his or her patient. This relationship becomes an important motivating factor in sustaining the child's interest in the person of the analyst and in continuing to come to his treatment, especially at those times when he is confronted and faced with painful interpretations, verbalizations, and confrontations during the analysis. This special relationship is in every way similar to the so-called treatment alliance described in the analytic treaatment of adults. On its success largely depends the outcome of the treatment. The child analyst must manage to become an important and significant person, not only in the child's perception but in his life. This is not an easy task, since he must do so without the use of seductive behaviors of various kinds toward the child, without reinforcing the secondary gains of the child, and without losing in the child's eyes the necessary authority and distance to carry out the treatment through its various stages and occasional painful steps.

In years now long past, the necessity of building such a relationship led Anna Freud to the description of an introductory phase, a preparatory period, preceding the actual analytic work per se. It was assumed that such a period could last from a few days to a few months. An extensive description of such a preparatory phase can be found in Anna Freud's *Psychoanalytical Treatment of Children* (1946). Though the idea of the necessity of such a prepratory phase has been abandoned, the concepts that it embodied are still relevant, and particularly so, the development of a meaningful analytic relationship with the child. Instead, that mandatory preparatory phase has now blended into the initial stages of a child analysis.

In part the conceptualization of a necessary preanalytic period was based on the argument of how able were children, particularly young ones, to develop transferences, transference neurosis, and the like, since they do have by right, reasons of age and stage of development the closest of relationships to their primary objects. How and why, then, will they develop transferences? This argument, rampant in the early stages of the development of child analysis, seems now to have settled down considerably. Here again, some found a most significant difference between child and adult psychoanalysis. In my view, children of all ages are very capable of the transferential phenomena on which we rely so heavily in adult analysis. Obviously, some corrections and reformulations may be necessary in this regard to describe accurately and understand the problems of the transference manifestations in children. They may take into account the age of the child, stage of development, the quality of the parent-child relationship, and the fact that indeed the child is right in the middle of his interactional developmental transactions with his primary objects. In short, it is widely accepted that the transference shows special characteristics, nuances, and so forth; also accepted is the fact that it forms an essential element of the analysis of children. But there remains the still somewhat controversial question of childrens' ability to develop a "transference neurosis." (See, for example, Anna Freud, 1946.)

The Question of Age:

How early can a child be in analysis is a frequently heard question. Here we must clearly differentiate child psychoanalysis proper in a dyadic situation from other forms of intervention utilizing analytic principles and knowledge, on behalf of children, with or without the participation of parents.

In my judgment child psychoanalysis can start quite early in the life of the child if this is indicated.* Rather than refer to a given age, what is important are those preconditions in terms of the development of the child without which the application of such technique becomes an impossibility. Two necessary preconditions are that the child must have both a minimum capacity for verbalization and a minimuum capacity for comprehension of language and basic propositions. This would be rare save for exceptional children much before two or two and a half years of age. The child analyst may face some additional problems related to the idiosyncracies of child development. For example, it is not uncommon that a very verbal and bright two- or two-and-a-half-year-old child may not feel

---

* See Bolland and Sandler et al. (1965).

It should be noted that the age of the child has enormous relevance to the way the analysis evolves and the technical characteristics of it. Children can be roughly divided into three main groups: those under five, the latency child, and the adolescent child. Each group for reasons of its various developments will pose specific technical problems characteristic for that age group. Thus, for example, though generalizations might prove misleading in the long run and certainly in specific cases, it can be said that the child under five tends to be more spontaneous and less well defended, frequently surprising us with statements that seem to come out of the pages of a textbook. In a manner of speaking, there is less distance between the unconscious system and consciousness. Similarly, because superego structuralization may be just proceeding in relation to certain impulses, these and the fantasies accompanying them may be quite accessible and undefended. In contrast, the latency child is generally well defended, at times excessively so, and in that sense lacks the occasional spontaneity and freshness of those children under five. The latency child uses massive amounts of denial, displacement, externalization, and projection. Analysis in this age group tends to run contrary to what the developmental forces are trying to accomplish. Development is trying to repress certain drives, socializing others, and so forth, while the analysis by its very nature keeps some such issues alive temporarily, in the search for a more favorable resolution.

With its manifold developmental tasks to be mastered, and their consequent turmoil and stresses, the adolescent stage constitutes a technical problem all of its own, quite distinct from those of the latency child and the adult. Its discussion is outside the scope of this presentation.

comfortable in separating from the mother in order to go with a stranger (the therapist). This is aggravated, of course, if beyond the natural developmental reluctance the situation is complicated by specific problems related to separation anxiety. Yet the lack of ability to separate in a very young infant need not be a counterindication to his treatment, since it is possible to deal with it by various parameters such as accepting the mother temporarily in the consulting room or have her sit outside the office door. In this way, the child can touch home as required. Soon most children will be comfortable and would have developed some kind of therapeutic alliance, as the trust of the parent is transferred to the therapist.

Frequency

The frequency of sessions for child analysis is no different from the frquency of sessions for adult analysis. Four or five sessions a week are the usual norm, and any diminution from this is generally considered a dilution in the direction of psychoanalytic psychotherapy.

The child analyst is frequently burdened in most cases by the fact that the child patient needs to be brought to him. This undoubtedly constitutes an enormous stress in the resources of a family, and more particularly the mother. Coupled with this, there is a reluctance to accept the realization that a small child might need such frequency of sessions, a fact not uncommonly related in the parent's mind (wrongly so) to the severity of the disturbance, that in many cases they naturally fail to identify. Hence the child's analyst needs to clarify all these issues, as well as to be most cooperative with the family in terms of time of appointments and so forth.

Technique

I have already discussed the role that play has as a substitute for free associations and also the fact that the development, management, utilization, and analysis of the transference is quite similar to that of adult analysis, with only a few qualifications. The countertransference phenomena, though no different from the range observable in adult work, does pose some special problems. There is no question that many reasons contribute to making countertransference the special problem that it is. The age of the child, his tenderness, his helplessness in the face of many life situations, unreasonable and at times cruel, unconcerned parents, the special sensitivities and motivations of child analysts—all contribute to it. But no less important is the child's seductiveness, and above all his incredible tendency toward action and motility. In contrast with adults, the child frequently does not interpose thoughts between wishes and actions. The wish is not verbalized but becomes action, and his loving feelings quickly become kisses, embraces, or at times quite inappropriate attempts at bodily contacts. By the same token, his negative feelings can become immediately actualized. Thus if he feels like destroying some of your valuable property, he will not say so, but will actually destroy it; if he means to hurt you, the first you may know about it is his attempts in this direction. In other words, and especially more so with children with specific types of pathology, the analyst is always kept on the alert. The sessions can trigger off all sorts of countertransferential responses and prove quite exhausting. The child analyst cannot rely on sitting comfortably in a chair while the patient talks. He must move with him, sit on the floor, be ready to protect the child or himself, and so forth.

It will follow from the above that the consulting quarters of a child analyst should be well adapted to these potential hazards, a situation that will tend to minimize unnecessarily unpleasant situations and loss of valuables, while allowing the child a "reasonable" freedom of action and behavior.

The question of parameters is a much-argued problem among different "schools" of child analysis. The purist does not tolerate any, while other analysts adopt a more flexible posture in this regard, if the parameters are not capricious but justifiable by special situations, peculiarities of the development of the child, and so forth. There is much debate as well about such things as Christmas cards, birthday cards, birthday gifts and the like, or providing certain goodies on occasion or gratifying some specific wishes of the child.

I agree with the view that parameters should not be included lightly into the treatment situation and that it is desirable to avoid them. Nevertheless, each case should be considered on its own merits and carefully scrutinized in terms of advantages and disadvantages, gains expected from its introduction and losses to result from it. This type of assessment is particularly important, since it is relatively easy to introduce them for countertransferential reasons and then proceed to rationalize them on any given theoretical grounds.

The role of the parents cannot be sufficiently emphasized. Here again, in this regard, there tend to be significant differences among child analysts. Some child analysts try to avoid contact with the parents if at all possible. In my view, this is rather difficult to do for a number of reasons. Perhaps the most important is that given some children's frequent difficulty in chronicling current events to the therapist, it becomes essential, especially with very young children, to keep some form of more or less formal contact with the parents, at the very least on an ad hoc basis. Further, as part of the treatment of the child it might be necessary to engage the parents in a dialogue that may have various purposes such as counseling, guidance, etc. There are also to be considered the many arrangements necessary in terms of times, vacations, missed sessions, absences of the therapist, and so forth, as well as the occasional situation of jealousy, or rivalry that gets established with the therapist. All the above are significantly different from the treatment of adults, since children are not free agents but quite dependent in this regard.

Some therapists prefer to handle all the above by means of a third party in the form of a colleague or social worker who can handle the parents' end of the treatment of the child. There can be little question that in specific situations the above arrangement may be the only viable solution. Yet in many cases it is possible for the child therapist to handle the parents as well. In this case, he ought to discuss with the child such meetings in sufficient detail, as well as the reasons for it. The child's confidence must be respected at all times, a situation that must be carefully discussed with him. Betrayal of such trust usually will handicap the further treatment of the child to the point of making it unworkable. In many situations there is no ideal solution to this technical problem, so general rules should not be applied and each and every case should be carefully weighed on its own merits.

Further, parental support is needed at times when the child becomes highly resistant. He may not wish to come to his sessions any longer because they have turned painful, or he may prefer to avoid discussing and looking at certain issues as a revenge for disappointment with the therapist, who may have refused to gratify certain wishes of the child. It is my personal experience that many children in analysis, especially those of the latency period, will hit one or more such rough spots. At such point, the treatment alliance breaks down and the special relationship to the therapist is not enough to sustain it. Such rough spots tend to be temporary and things get on the right track again rather quickly through the analysis and handling of whatever may have motivated the crisis. But the child needs to be there. I think it is a useful technical device to forewarn parents, at the initial stage of this eventuality, and have found mostly cooperative parents who send a clear message to the child that they consider the treatment important and expect him or her to continue to attend the sessions.

Another important point to consider is that a successful treatment of a child, particularly a young child, is difficult if not impossible in the absence of a reasonably sustaining environment and family structure. Chaos in the family, lack of a minimum of stability, or severe forms of parental acting out are quite detrimental. With a slightly older child, who has already acquired the capacity to keep some distance from the family, the situation might be more hopeful. But this presupposes an intelligent, well-motivated child who has a good relationship to the therapist. Thus, for example, a young child who is exposed to her mother's overt sexual behavior with various men at their home may make for an impossible analysis.

There are some special technical problems that occasionally confront a child analyst. They are generally due to somewhat unusual situations coupled with the immaturity of the child as well as his or her developmental needs at the time. Thus the young child of a single parent (through absence, death, or otherwise) may strongly wish to invest the therapist with the role of the dead mother or father. Though these situations require special care and handling, they are on the whole manageable, especially if the child analyst can keep well under control his or her own countertransference responses. They are mentioned here mostly to highlight the importance of the developmental point of view in child analysis. The child's present developmental stage and the way his or her developmental needs and, indeed, rights are addressed and met are essential considerations for the child analyst. He must plan and proceed in treatment having them constantly in the foreground of his mind. Since the child is not a finished product, whatever psychopathology he may have acquired must of necessity be seen in terms of the fact that his development must continue very actively in a variety of directions against that background.

Such issues as timing, wording, interpreting, verbalizing, confronting, educating, dream analyses, analysis of resistances or of the transference, and so forth are as much an integral part of child analysis as they are of adult analysis. Some qualifications are nevertheless necessary. Appropriate wording is clearly of enormous importance for both adults and children, but particularly so for the latter, since it is easy to talk over a child's head. In my opinion this happens only too frequently with the novice. The child analyst must come down to the level of development of the child, to his level of discourse. Once he understands that, his interpretations and verbalizations will be very much to the point and reflect the world of the child and its conflicts as the child sees them.

As in all analysis there are certain educational aspects to it. This is true of child analysis, but contrary to prevailing opinion among the not too well informed, the educational role of the child analyst is limited and well circumscribed. Child analysts are not educators, and educational interventions are not the basis of child psychoanalysis.

The role played by dreams in child analysis is not without interest. I have known some children who consistently bring their dreams and work with them much as an adult would. Nevertheless, this is not the general rule, and many children won't pursue their dreams and work with them as some adults do. In this they are not very different from many other adult patients, in whose analysis dreams, important as they are, play a limited role.

Indications

This is another area of disagreement and discussion. I have heard the opinion that in the most ideal of all worlds, child analysis as a procedure should be available to all children for its preventive value as well as to ensure the most ideal unfolding of development possible. Quite apart from the merits of the idea (or its lack of merit), the reality is that child psychoanalysts are an exotic breed. They are certainly not abundant; indeed, there are not enough of them to go around to attend to those children under the most peremptory of needs.

Child analysis ideal indication (as with adults) is in the resolution of the multiplicity of forms of psychopathology related to neurotic conflicts and the various infantile neuroses. Frequently it is reserved for "bad" cases where nothing else would be credited with the possibility of working, such as borderline or psychotic conditions, including cases of infantile autism. In my judgment these are poor positive indications for child analysis.

Child analysis may also be well justified in all those cases where the severity of presenting developmental disturbances, developmental conflicts, partial neurotic conflicts (before the first infantile neuroses gets organized)* make it clear that the further normal development of the child is or would be compromised, or would be forced into a variety of psychopathological outcomes. The intervention here should be restricted to the removal and resolution of such conflicts as may cause the child to deviate from the path of normalcy. Once this is accomplished the child should be turned over to the progressive developmental forces that are contained in him. They may carry the day for him, and if future obstacles are encountered, a further intervention may be granted.

Much the same reasoning applies to the aims of child psychoanalysis. As Anna Freud (1945) has repeatedly pointed out, the essential task is to remove the obstacles that impede his developmental path and to allow his progressive developmental forces and ego resources to complete the task of development.

A final word about the length of a child analysis. A frequent misconception is that because children are short in years their analysis is not necessarily very time-consuming. Of course, there is some truth in the above statement, but the length of a child's analysis depends on many other variables, such as the severity of the conflicts, the intensity of the developmental interferences either present or that led to the observable conflicts, fixations and so on, the favorable and unfavorable circumstances in which the analysis is carried out (to include such things as family structure, supporting environment, familial or parental psychopathology, need to utilize the patient), the ego resources of the child, as well as other genetic givens in terms of strength of impulse, adhesiveness of the libido, and so forth.

References

Bolland, J., and J. Sandler et al. (1965) *The Hampstead Psychoanalytic Index: A Study of the Psychoanalytic Case Material of a Two-Year-Old Child.* Psychoanalytic

* See H. Nagera, (1966), *Early Childhood Disturbances, the Infantile Neuroses and the Adulthood Disturbances, Monograph No. 2 of the Psychoanalytic Study of the Child.* New York: International Universities Press.

Study of the Child Monographs: No. 1. New York: International Universities Press.

Freud, A. (1945) Indications for child analysis. In *The Psychoanalytic Study of the Child*, Vol. 1. New York: International Universities Press, pp.127–149.

Freud, A. (1946) *The Psychoanalytical Treatment of Children*. London: Imago.

Freud, S. (1909) Analysis of a phobia in a five-year-old boy. *Standard Edition of Freud*, Vol. 10. London: Hogarth Press, pp.3–129.

Klein, M. (1932) *The Psychoanalysis of Children*. London: Hogarth Press; New York: Grove Press, 1960.

Nagera, H. (1966) *Early Childhood Disturbances, the Infantile Neuroses and the Adulthood Disturbances*. Psychoanalytic Study of the Child Monographs: No. 2. New York: International Universities Press, 1966.

Treatment of Emotional Disorders in Children and Adolescents

CHAPTER 3

Behavior Modification: Applications to Childhood Problems

Robert G. Wahler

Behavior modification as a therapeutic strategy for troubled children has undergone a rapid metamorphosis in its brief existence. As a formal strategy, the approach began little more than twenty years ago with the appearance of a few simple laboratory derived procedures. Since that time, one can discern a growth pattern in which behavior modification became synonymous with operant conditioning; then, following a period of in-house procedural evaluation, a gradual separation of learning theory as a necessary part of the overall strategy became evident. Currently, the term "empirical" provides the best description for a set of guidelines summarized by the label. The theoretical simplicity that marked behavior modification as a uniform approach to childhood problems no longer portrays this strategy. The present chapter outlines this metamorphosis and attempts to provide a reasonably concise description of what has evolved.

Historical Origins

Child behavior modification is a specialty area within the larger field of behavior therapy. As such, this smaller area shares some of the historical roots of the overall behavioristic approach—namely, the guidance of experimental psychology and the ensuing respect for empirical data. Like the larger behavior therapy movement, emergence of the child-oriented strategy entailed some shifts from laboratory empiricism to a somewhat "softer" empiricism based in more natural settings. The laboratory–real world transition had two initially separate, but eventually related, research thrusts. One of these, seldom recognized as a determining force of the present-day behavior modification, is commonly described as *behavior ecology*. The second, more obviously related research avenue bears the label *applied behavior analysis*. An appreciation for both movements provides the clearest understanding of that child-clinical strategy addressed in this chapter.

Behavior ecology developed from the empirical work of two investigators who were disciples of the field theorist Kurt Lewin (1951). Roger Barker and Herbert Wright strongly believed that Lewinian hypotheses, or any set of hypotheses for that matter, required scientific explorations in natural environments rather than those of the laboratory. So pronounced and convincing were their anti-laboratory arguments that this emphasis is often cited as a major contribution to psychology—along with their discoveries of what children actually do in the real world (see Barker, 1968).

Many of the Barker-Wright findings and arguments were based on naturalistic observations of normal children in a variety of community environments, such as school playgrounds, homes, and the local drugstore (e.g., Barker and Wright, 1954). The sum and substance of their findings center on two notions that became crucial underpinnings of child behavior modification: (1) Child behavior seems largely governed by the environment setting in which the child is observed (home, school classroom, playground). (2) The principles accounting for these environment-behavior relationships are yet unknown.

Finding number 1 was surprising in view of the popularity of personality theories of that day. Contrary to the trait notions of human behavior, the Barker-Wright data showed little consistency in child behavior from setting to setting. A child's behavior in the local drugstore of Midwest was quite different from that same child's behavior at home. Environmental settings were thus shown to possess powerful behavior-eliciting functions—evidently far more powerful than any supposed child internalized determinants of behavior.

Finding number 2 was actually an underscoring of the complexity inherent in behavior-environment relationships. The Barker-Wright data indicated no direct, simple relationships between what children did in an environmental setting and how the stimuli in that setting were structured. In other words, contrary to the also-popular learning theory views of the day (e.g., Skinner, 1953), a one-to-one correspondence between child responses and environmental stimuli did not materialize. The total matrix of physical and social events composing a setting was somehow geared to the functioning of each child's behavior. But just how these environment-behavior relationships operated was by no means clear.

Shortly after the Barker-Wright behavior ecology movement was underway, another group of researchers, with quite different intentions, began a similar undertaking. This group, spearheaded by Sidney Bijou and Donald Baer, examined the fit between child behavior in the laboratory and that behavior in the free field. Unlike the Barker-Wright group, these latter investigators were strongly tied to learning theory (i.e., Skinner, 1953) as a set of guidelines to account for what children did. A Bijou-Baer elaboration of Skinnerian arguments outlined how principles of operant and respondent learning could provide a reasonable account of child development (Bijou and Baer, 1961). In fact, the early observational and experimental work by this research group lent good support to these contentions. The free field behaviors of normal children as well as disturbed children could be tied to reinforcement contingencies provided by social and physical properties of the children's natural environments. Out of these findings, a combined clinical and research strategy known as applied behavior analysis emerged.

Obviously, the Bijou-Baer production of direct, simple relationships between child behaviors and environmental events contradicted the more ambiguous relationships described by the Barker-Wright group. In part, this difference may have been due to research strategies separating the two groups. The Barker-Wright group was opposed to any sort of tampering with child-environment systems; they pointed out that *experimental* manipulations in essence turned the natural environment into a scientist-contrived laboratory—a direct violation of their naturalistic bent. However, the experimental analysis orientation of Bijou and Baer urged such scientist probes as necessary to sort out functional connections between child behaviors and environmental stimuli. Of course, because such probes were guided by reinforcement theory, only brief segments of the behavior-environment stream of events were likely to be observed. Since reinforcement concepts dealt with a one-to-one relationship between stimuli and the responses they control, measurement was geared to a narrow scope of events.

Thus applied behavior analysis emerged from the laboratory in much the same fashion as did the behavior ecology movement. Both rejected a reliance on the laboratory as a proving ground for the understanding of child behavior. However, applied behavior analysts did keep two facets of the Skinnerian laboratory as guidelines: (1) a reliance on reinforcement theory as an explanation of what children did; (2) a continued reliance on the single-event measurement systems so characteristic of the laboratory. These facets, along with the experimental intervention orientation, kept applied behavior analysis and behavior ecology on very separate paths. It is not surprising that early work leading to child behavior modification was almost exclusively the contribution of applied behavior analysis.

Early Success: Ramifications for Clinical Psychology

Forays into the behavior problems of children were bound to occur when development psychology accepted Bijou-Baer interpretations of how children progress through the life span. If the development of a behavior, or the absence of another, follow reinforcement principles, might not the same process account for childhood behavior problems? As alluded to in *Child Development* (Vol. 2, Bijou and Baer, 1965), the absence of a significant behavior (such as talking) might well be due to an unfortunate lack of reinforcement contingencies or to an equally unfortunate presence of punishment contingencies. Similarly, the excessive occurrences of disturbing behaviors (such as hitting people) are probably a result of misplaced reinforcers dispersed by the child's parents, teachers, and peers. The reasons for and solutions to these childhood problems are bound to be in a careful examination and control of stimuli in the child's immediate environment.

Laboratory studies had already shown that desirable, cooperative behaviors between people (in this case children—Azrin and Lindsley, 1956) could be established by programming reinforcers following designated behaviors by both parties. Thus if the interpersonal behavior of children could be predictably shaped and modified in the laboratory, could not a similar process be produced in real life? A few years after the Azrin and Lindsley demonstration, Williams (1959) did just that in a systematic effort to remedy a tantrum problem in a two-year-old boy. In essence, Williams employed an extinction procedure based on his assumption that the boy's excessive and inappropriate crying was being reinforced by his parents. When the parents were instructed to ignore crying at bedtime, the boy's duration of crying subsided gradually over a series of ten bedtimes.

The Williams study provided a needed empirical documentation of clinical success—with a minor problem of childhood. The study showed the value of conceptualizing child behavior problems as a function of the child's dyadic interchanges with others. Most importantly, the dyad appeared to operate according to those principles of reinforcement previously outlined in the laboratory (Azrin and Lindsley, 1956; Skinner, 1953). With the theoretical credence offered shortly thereafter by Bijou and Baer (1961), many members of the child-clinical field took notice. Over the next decade, child development journals as well as clinical journals were frequent sources of other empirical documentations.

The range of clinical problems subjected to reinforcement procedures was initially rather limited. First in order were a number of nursery school studies in which teachers were taught to alter their social reinforcement contingencies for the benefit of their children. Not only were such child problems as regressed crawling (Harris et al., 1964), isolate behavior (Allen et al., 1964), and crying (Hart et al., 1964) shown to change undesirable directions following the contingency shifts, but such studies also showed that the problem behaviors could be re-created by having the teachers return to their former schedules of dispensing social reinforcers. These studies, while again dealing with rather simple childhood problems, offered further proof that sound clinical procedures were available.

Later applications were aimed at more serious child problems, and they occurred in more numerous environments. For example, when the above nursery school studies were getting underway, Wolf, Risley, and Mees (1964) had begun their extensive study of a severely disturbed (autistic) child. Not only did these investigators demonstrate reinforcement-produced modifications in the boy's tantrums, bedtime problems, and speech, but these therapeutic changes were mediated through training a number of adults in hospital and home environments. This most impressive therapeutic endeavor marked the onset of other, more elaborate hospital and home treatment programs for psychotic children (Lovaas, 1966).

While the procedural armamentarium of these behavior modifiers expanded to include punishment contingencies (time-out, electric shock) and the use of imitative procedures, the basic operant approach offered all necessary guidelines.

Another important development in reinforcement or operant treatment procedures entailed the use of this strategy in community settings more complex than those previously entered by the child behavior modifier. The complexity factor was due to several considerations: (1) The mediators, or direct dispensers of child-directed reinforcers, were not always so sympathetic to the behavior modifier's philosophy of change (e.g., public school teachers; Madsen, Becker, and Thomas, 1968). (2) More than one setting required intervention for a single child (e.g., home *and* school; Tharp and Wetzel, 1969).

The complexity involved in these broader applications of operant principles actually seemed to foster continued pursuit of this approach to child treatment. Philosophical conflicts were welcomed by behavior modifiers, and led to a good many discussions and decisions on ethical issues (Martin, 1969).

The necessity of extending formerly narrow scoped environmental coverage to larger portions of the troubled child's environment opened doors to some mental health centers (Gardner, 1972). The concept of community behavior consultant (à la Tharp and Wetzel, 1969) became a reality in some cities (Briscoe, Hoffman, and Bailey, 1975). In terms of a continued documentation of the hows and whys of producing changes in troubled children, the volume of research generated grew too big for the single appropriate journal of the 1960's (*Behavior Research and Therapy*). The late 1960's was a time frame for a number of new journals on behavior modification (*Journal of Applied Behavior Analysis, Behavior Therapy, Behavior Therapy and Experimental Psychiatry*). In addition, a plethora of books and books of readings continued to outline the success of these applications to children, as well as outlining the necessary assessment and treatment guidelines. In family or home settings, books such as *Families* (Patterson, 1969) presented such guidelines based on the training of parents as change agents for their own children's problems (e.g., Patterson and Reid, 1970; Wahler et al., 1965). In school classroom settings, popular texts by O'Leary and O'Leary (1972) appeared at about the same time. In these latter settings, the focus of childhood change was often preventive in the sense that teachers were taught to extend these new helping procedures to *all* children in their classrooms. Once again, the guidelines in these texts were based on ample classroom research (e.g., O'Leary and Drabman, 1971). Research documentation on the utility of operant procedures spread to every imaginable community setting frequented by children. Other settings included recreation centers (Pierce and Risley, 1974), day care facilities for infants and toddlers (Twardosz, Cataldo, and Risley, 1974), and for those more seriously disturbed children, hospitals (Lovaas and Koegel, 1973) and halfway houses (Phillips, Wolf, and Fixen, 1968).

The flurry of research activity described above produced a new theoretical niche in the field of child-clinical psychology and psychiatry. Clinical training programs across the country were considered incomplete unless at least partial coverage of child behavior modification was included; some programs in the late 1960's adopted this strategy as the principal thrust of training (e.g., University of Hawaii). Even undergraduate texts in abnormal psychology provided discussions of operant conceptions regarding the development and treatment of childhood problems.

The Child-Clinical Strategy: Assessment and Treatment

By the early 1970's, child behavior modification could be considered a clinical specialty in the sense that one could describe the procedural steps and rationale encompassing this strategy. We turn now to an outline of the practical features of assessment and treatment growing directly from the burgeoning research of the 1960's.

Assessing or measuring the troubled child's problems became a process predictable on the basis of reinforcement theory. Factors to look for in assessment are logically those relating to the reinforcement of more desirable behaviors. As an outcome in preparation for treatment, an assessment must specify those environmental conditions necessary to change the troubled child's behavior. And one must always keep in mind that these conditions will be *specific to the environmental setting* in question. Unlike other assessment strategies (e.g., psychodynamic), this one is geared to specific settings. For example, assessment in a home setting will not be of much benefit in creating treatment procedures in that child's school classroom.

The Interview

Consider first the kind of interview goals deemed important in beginning an assessment for troubled children. Regardless of the environment in question, or the child problem in question, a verbal dialogue between the behavior modifier and the people who live with the child is a preliminary step. The interview exchange not only sets the stage for empirical assessment, but also marks the starting point for a necessary rapport between behavior modifier (consultant) and the child's caregivers (mediators such as parents and teachers). As in any clinical endeavor, the troubled people (mediator and child) must alter a pattern of behavior of some years' standing in most cases. Even though one or both of these parties are seeking help because the pattern has become aversive, neither is apt to change unless the clinician (consultant) has instructional value for at least one of the mediators in a setting. That instructional value is partly due to the consultant's professional status and partly due to "rapport." In addition to the humanistic concerns that are part of any help intending relationship, rapport building in the interview is advanced by an educational process specific to the operant framework. Not only should this process of teaching the mediator(s) to reconceptualize the child's problems facilitate the gathering of appropriate information, but the mediator should also come to anticipate the whys and hows of later assessment and intervention. Such anticipatory "sets" are bound to enhance the instructional value of the consultant.

In examining mediator conceptions of child problems, Goldiamond (1968) has discussed the importance of altering these beliefs. As he notes, a good many parents and other caregivers come to the initial interview with some common, not very useful views about the cause of childhood behavior problems. They may either view the causes as developmental (events in the past) or as a function of events internal to the child (in his or her mind). Following the interview guidelines of Wahler and Cormier (1970), the mediator must be "educated" on the importance of looking at *current* events in the child's *environment*. By shifting mediator focus to the here-and-now reinforcement contingencies operating at home, in the school, and so forth, an important first step has occurred. When the mediator comes to share the consultant's belief system (reinforcement theory), some insightful new looks at the child are possible. The motivational properties of this sort of teamwork cannot be overemphasized. Just as the experienced psychodynamic client becomes a "believer" in that conceptual system, so must the operant-guided mediator come to believe in the importance of reinforcement theory.

Obviously the above kind of rapport may only be initiated through the interview. At least it should become clear just what constitutes the conceptual ground rules for further discussions. In addition, that first interview should yield information about those behavior and stimulus events that constitute the targets of measurement and intervention. From the standpoint of child behaviors, three sets require definition and discussion between consultant and mediator: (1) Those problem behaviors *likely* to occur in the presence of the mediator. For example, whining, nagging, clinging, and noncompliance with mediator instructions are commonly cited problems. This set of child behaviors will probably represent the starting points of intervention, since they are most readily accessible to the mediator. (2) Those problem behaviors *unlikely* to occur in mediator presence. Here, we have reference to stealing, fighting, truancy, and other episodes that are typically detected in the aftermath of occurrence. Typically, this means that other members of the community will alert the caregiver concerning the presence of problems (e.g., neighbors, police). Later, the caregiver may be able to detect occurrences by questioning of the child or the initially complaining community members—or by simply noting likely outcome factors such as the child's torn clothing, possession of objects not belonging to the child, an so forth. (3) Finally, the interview should permit a specification of the child's foremost behavior deficiencies; those that should occur in caretaker presence, but do not. Typical examples here are sustained work, cooperative social interchanges, play and in more serious disorders, receptive and/or expressive language. In the later intervention phase, these deficient behaviors would hopefully take the place of problem behaviors comprising set number 1.

In reference to the above child behavior sets, the consultant interviewer will also find it useful to initiate caretaker recollection on how these adults deal with the child. What do they typically do when stealing is suspected, or how is frequent whining or self-stimulation dealt with? How does the caregiver attempt to remedy behavior deficiencies? In terms of rapport building, this line of inquiry ought to allow caregiver venting of those failure-induced frustrations that fostered the help-seeking process in the first place. In addition, another set of information is provided for the soon-to-be-initiated measurement process: presumably the caregiver is currently responding to the child in ways that are maintaining the child's problems (e.g., complying with the child's nagging or clinging; screaming at the child's noncompliances with caretaker instructions). Once again, measurement leading to planned change first requires a specification of critical behaviors—in this case, caregiver behaviors.

As a prelude to measurement, the consultant interviewer and caregiver must finally agree on some target settings for the measurement phase. That is, during what times of day are child-caregiver problem interchanges most likely to occur? Setting specification is based on the obvious fact that global setting such as "home" and "school" are actually composed of numerous subsettings, each of which can be roughly scaled in terms of the likelihood of child-caregiver problem interchanges. Target subsettings (e.g., fixing dinner, story time) should be selected with problem interchanges in mind *and* by considering the caregiver's measurement chores. Since the bulk of measurement must be borne by the caregiver, that adult must have reasonable opportunity to monitor the action during the setting time period.

The Child's Contribution to the Interview

Given that the targeted problem child's difficulties do not include serious language deficiencies, that person's contributions to all phases of the helping process should be considered virtually equivalent to the caregiver's role. With the prevailing operant model designating child and caregiver as *mutual* parties in any problem, it simply makes good sense to view child reinforcement support of caregiver behavior as well as vice versa. However, despite the obvious bi-directional properties of the operant, the child's contribution as a useful member of assessment and intervention procedures did not see much practical emphasis until the late 1960's and early 1970's. In large part, the earlier differential emphasis on adult roles in treatment was due to the technological demands of both the measurement and intervention phases. Since fairly young children were the usual choices for behavior modification, there was a logical tendency for the consultant to emphasize the training of adult members of the problem dyad. Then, along with later technological refinements (see the discussion of "self-control" procedures below) and the extension of these helping procedures to include older children, the child's neglected role was brought into better perspective.

When a reasonable level of rapport is possible between child and consultant, the interview has been commonly employed in several child-oriented directions. Of major importance is the child's report on his or her reward goals in the environmental setting under consideration. Since one of the aims of treatment will be to produce gains in the child's behavior deficiencies, these reinforcers available to support these gains must be specified. In essence, the child is asked to list those sorts of things worth working for (e.g., television watching, outings with friends). This topic area, incidently, can be related to a discussion of how the child currently strives to gain these reinforcers as well as reinforcers not specified but suspected to support the child's problem behavior (e.g., parent attention). Thus a fairly verbal child might prove capable of drawing conclusions about *why* he or she does the kinds of things that led to the caregiver's decision to seek psychological help. However, this sort of "contingency insight" is difficult to produce in an initial interview, and like any interview outcome, depends largely on the consultant's skill with children.

In addition to the above listing of child-judged reinforcers, the overall purpose of talking with children is geared to the teamwork effort to come. As noted in this section, the troubled child is a party equal to the caregiver in the reinforcement trap, maintaining those interpersonal problems under consideration. Thus, if the child can be given this perspective early in the assessment phase, later tasks centering on intervention ought to proceed more smoothly.

The Measurement Process

The measurement phase might best be viewed as a means of concretizing information obtained via interview. Such data reflecting important child behaviors and caregiver reactions might serve as a basis for initiating treatment. However, the success of any reinforcement-based treatment depends on the accuracy with which the participants arrange contingencies. While the usual mediators (parent or teacher) would know via interview data which child behaviors to consequate in certain ways, and which child behaviors to avoid, their success in doing so presumes that the interview data can provide necessary moment-to-moment guidelines. Unfortunately, the capability of people to translate summary reports (interview data) into more fine-grained actions in real-life settings is questionable. In fact, the degree of distortion in such translations has been found to be so great as to preclude successful applications (see Wahler and Leske, 1973). Thus a measurement phase in which the parties involved gain experience in concrete, moment-to-moment detection of relevant behaviors will probably be prerequisite to treatment.

In an ideal measurement process, caregiver, child, and consultant would all take part. With all parties sharing and comparing their independently acquired findings, correction of inaccuracies as well as a continued sense of teamwork are likely. Undoubtedly, however, the caregiver or mediator will be required to handle the bulk of measurement. Since the child may be unable or unwilling to do so, and the consultant will simply not have the time, the mediator will have to produce the lion's share of data. Of course, mediator training will require at least periodic evaluations through consultant measurement checks.

Measurement procedures used in applied behavior analysis have varied from elaborate coding systems appropriate only for consultant use (e.g., Patterson et al., 1969), to some simple techniques appropriate for use by extremely busy public school teachers (e.g., Kubany and Sloggett, 1973). For a complete compilation of measurement approaches, the reader should consult a recent chapter by Evans and Nelson (1977). For purposes here, we intend to present only some commonly used procedures for mediators, children, and consultant.

Mediators should gain competence in two sorts

of measurement: one aimed at their interactions with the troubled child, and another aimed at a daily log of significant child problem behaviors. The interaction measures are geared to those times of the day specified by the mediator as likely setting events for problem interactions. During these time periods (probably once per day) the mediator must be prepared to note child problem behaviors, as well as those mediator responses occurring as antecedents and/or consequences for these behaviors. Now, as outlined in Wahler's (1976) summary of caregiver-child problem interactions, the bulk of these interactions can be described as mand-compliance/punishment interchanges. These interchanges, recently documented for aggressive children by Patterson (1974), may be initiated by either child or caregiver. The initiator's approach to the other party can usually be specified as *manding* in the sense that it seems aimed at producing compliance in the other person. For example, child clinging to a parent or child whining often function as means of getting the adult to start or stop some specific action (e.g., start attending to child; stop attending to someone else). From the other side of the coin, parent instructions to the child have a similar function aimed at starting or stopping some child behavior. Following the mand by child or adult, the other person may either comply with the mand or react by punishing or ignoring the mand giver. In problem interchanges, the latter two responses will lead to an escalation in rate and intensity of the mands—as shown by Patterson (1974).

Using the mand sequence as a measurement framework, it is feasible for the caregiver to keep track of these episodes during the measurement period. Since mands are instructional in function, they are also good attending cues for one to monitor the sequence from start to finish. Thus the mediator may be told: "If you find it necessary to issue a mand to your child, or if your child issues a mand to you, that is your cue to remember the sequence that follows. When the entire episode is concluded (by mand cessation), write down the responses of both parties." In this fashion, most caregivers ought to find themselves capable of sampling problem interchanges during specific time periods of each day.

Those child problem behaviors often occurring outside the usual social interactions by child and caregiver can be charted in summary fashion on a day-to-day basis. Such problems (e.g., night fears, fighting, enuresis, property destruction), while important aspects for therapeutic change, pose a different intervention strategy than the above interaction problems. A problem behavior such as stealing is difficult to change through caregiver contingencies because its detection will usually follow some time after the actual occurrence. It is also true that sampling these behaviors may be a good deal more intermittent—again because of occurrences outside the caregiver's scope of direct observation. One is therefore forced to settle for a rough approximation of occurrences for these behaviors. While the caregiver should be prepared to chart each detection on a one-by-one basis, a yes-no statement for each detection should also be noted at the end of every day. In this way, should the caregiver neglect to chart detections during the day, at least one is assured of a weekly incidence report.

If the child is capable and willing to take part in the measurement process, procedures similar to those described for caregivers should be employed. However, since the tack of therapy will be somewhat different for the cooperating child, the focus of measurement must be different. Goal setting is perhaps the most important aspect of measurement for the child to grasp. The concept is typically discussed in reference to child behavior deficiencies, both those evident within caregiver-child interactions (e.g., child cooperative behavior) and those outside the interactions (e.g., independent work). In either case, consultant and child work toward an agreement on improving these deficiencies as daily goals. Once the child sets some particular goals as frequencies of expected occurrences, the stage is prepared for his or her recording. When the intervention phase is initiated later, the arrangement of child-selected reinforcers for these goal attainments would follow as a logical step.

The consultant's own recording of mediator-child problem interactions rounds out the measurement phase. Considerations on strategy are somewhat more complex in that both type of measurement *and* the environmental setting in which to base that measurement must be decided. It is clear, however, that the consultant's personal measurement is an essential means of validating mediator recording throughout the helping process.

Economic factors may prevent the consultant's visits to the natural setting in which child-mediator problems are focused. Ideally, of course, the natural setting should be the setting of choice—and in cases where the mediator cannot readily leave that setting (e.g., teacher in school classroom), the consultant may have no other choice. In home settings, however, it is likely that parent and child could come to the consultant's clinic setting for observation. Fortunately, comparative data are available to justify the use of such continued settings. Both Hanf (1968) and Forehand and co-workers (1975) have offered findings to show that parent-child interactions in a clinic playroom can be taken as similar to these interactions at home. Thus if parent (and child) records of manding episodes at home are at all representative of ongoing problems, consultant sampling of the interactions should reveal a similar picture.

Consultant measures might be as simple as those used by the mediator to objectify problem interactions. For a more complete picture of the interaction pattern, the consultant may choose to employ one of several coding systems now available commercially (Wahler, House, and Stambaugh, 1976; Patterson et al., 1968). It is of interest to note that these comprehensive measures consider problem behavior as potentially affecting five classes of everyday child activities: *opposition-compliance*, or the degree to which a child violates adult-imposed rules and instructions; *social interaction*, or the proportion of child activity involving other people; *work*, or those responsibilities set by adults for the child; *play*, or self-entertainment entailing complex interactions with objects; *autistic behavior*, or self-directed actions of a repetitive, simple nature. The comprehensive coding systems essentially specify problem behaviors as made up of excessive or infrequent occurrences of one or more of these five response classes. Peer and adult reactions to the five classes are commonly specified through two broad stimulus classes detailed as *instructions* and *social attention*. In essence, then, problem interchanges would be measured through five broad categories of target child activity and stimulus contingencies made up of two even broader categories.

The Treatment Process

By the time an adequate measurement phase has produced concrete samples of child problem behavior and its suspected support contingencies, the focal points of treatment will be obvious. Those stimulus contingencies provided by caregivers, siblings and other people who live in the child's environment must become nonfunctional for the problem behavior. These people and the child must work toward some new arrangement of their living conditions; arrangements conducive to the development of more adaptive behaviors by all parties concerned. The setting of such arrangements is considered within the same sort of framework governing assessment. That is, if at least one party in the trouble-inducing dyad can be taught to alter his or her interaction style, therapeutic outcomes should follow. Typically, that one party is the caregiver because that person is usually most willing to end the problem-supporting interchange. Of course, if the child, siblings, peers, and relatives are also willing to learn some new interaction styles, they, too, would become students in the following reeducation lessons.

Social Learning Concepts

Most consultants believe that changes in social interactions are fostered by understanding the conceptual system guiding proposed changes. By using the measurement data as examples, the concepts of reinforcement, extinction, and/or punishment are made understandable as guidelines to promote alterations in behaviors reflected by that data. The actual teaching of these concepts can be facilitated by one of several texts written for parents and teachers (*Living with Children* by Patterson and Gullion, 1968; *Parents Are Teachers* by Becker, 1971). In the outlining of learning concepts, these texts provide working illustrations of how reinforcement, punishment, and extinction operate in daily life. Then these concepts are discussed as most effectively (and ethically) applied in the solution of children's day-to-day problems. *Positive reinforcement* is presented in terms of the central means of solving such problems. This concept is viewed in conjunction with *extinction* through the following logic: ideally, a parent or teacher should arrange the availability of social and material reinforcers so that only the child's desirable behaviors are effective in obtaining them. This positive reinforcement process will then ensure that the child's problem or undesirable behaviors will occur under extinction conditions—that is, these behaviors result in neutral, nonreinforcing stimuli. If the caregiver can conduct arrangements of this sort, desirable child behaviors should increase in frequency, and undesirable behaviors should drop in frequency. All three of the above texts recommend this process as a formal contractual arrangement between caregiver and child. In essence, both parties would agree to, or at least understand, the contractual procedures.

Punishment is also discussed at length in the

concept texts. It is important to note in this discussion that ethical considerations are again at the forefront, this time in terms of its use only under certain conditions, and the use of only certain forms of punishment. In the latter use category, *time-out* and *response cost* are presented as possible means of suppressing problem behaviors. In both cases, the format entails a temporary loss of reinforcers for the child, contingent upon the child's emitting problem behaviors. In time-out the loss occurs because the child is isolated for a brief time interval (usually five to ten minutes). In response cost, material or token reinforcers already acquired by the child through contract arrangements are taken away—with the understanding that they may be re-earned through desirable behaviors. Both forms of punishment should of course be covered in contract arrangements prior to their actual use.

Conditions calling for the use of any form of punishment are also spelled out in the concept texts. Sometimes extinction is simply not feasible to arrange in the treatment setting (e.g., home). For example, the child's problem behavior may be self-injurious (head banging) or injurious to others (hitting). When such conditions are clearly to be encountered in the treatment setting, time-out or response cost will have to be considered in the treatment contract. Once again, it is emphasized that the punishment procedures are viewed as temporary measures; positive reinforcement always represents the stable, long-term ingredient of a successful treatment program.

Setting the Treatment Contingencies

Once the intent of treatment and its conceptual underpinnings are clear, the actual practice of contractual arrangements should be pursued. In the spirit of any contract, this phase usually begins with group discussion led by the behavior modification consultant. The group, made up of the child and those people to be active participants in the behavior change program, are first told about the consultant's recommended treatment contingencies. In essence, these would entail positive reinforcement for some aspects of the child's behavior and extinction or time-out for other aspects. Next, these proposed arrangements are presented for discussion in terms of their "fit with reality" as viewed by each member of the group: Is the use of time-out fair? Can its conditions be met (i.e., social isolation)? Is the listing of positive reinforcers complete? While all group members are encouraged to contribute their individual opinions, the consultant's directorship implies that he or she must offer the final opinion. Obviously, the treatment contingencies must be appropriate to change the problems outlined in the consultant's assessment. But at the same time, the consultant will not actually implement the contingencies. Thus the final treatment package must meet with the approval of those people who will implement the package. Unless the child's parents and teachers and the child (in cases of self-management procedures) believe in the treatment approach, there is little utility in the consultant's "final word." This process of compromise and belief generation remains a clinical art, not yet subjected to the empirical scrutiny of applied behavior analysis.

Given a consensus on the proposed treatment contingencies, the practice of such new interactions must proceed under the consultant's supervision. Ideally, these practice rounds should occur in the natural environment of child and mediator (home or school), although there is evidence to suggest that clinic settings may suffice (Forehand and King, 1977). In this latter, economically cheaper strategy, clinic-to-home generalization of practiced parent-child interactions has been shown to occur. In any case, all parties who have agreed to set reinforcement, extinction, or time-out contingencies must prove their capabilities to do so. Of course, the consultant's teaching role now becomes critical—as model and shaper of mediator behavior. Once the practice rounds show the mediators to approximate accurately the new contingencies, consultant supervision now shifts to a monitoring and feedback function for the mediators. Research indicates that this more natural practice would best be conducted in the natural environment to maximize generalization possibilities (Forehand and Atkeson, In press). A continuation of this intervention training of course assumes that the mediators continue to display their newly taught contingencies. If not, a resumption of consultant modeling of correct mediator behavior and shaping of mediator practice is called for. If the practiced interactions do continue correctly under consultant monitoring, a fading of consultant supervision would follow. Gradually, the consultant's role would diminish until the mediators themselves provide their sole feedback through baseline initiated measurement procedures. It is important to stress at this point that all measurement procedures must continue throughout the treatment phase. Ideally, then, the mediators should become capable of sustaining these consultant-taught contingencies. The task-setting contingencies will then be largely complete, although periodic monitoring checks by the consultant should be followed as a rule of thumb (Patterson, 1974).

When the troubled child is expected to take part in contingency setting, some changes in the above procedures are necessary. The cooperative child as self-manager will be required to complete several steps as outlined by Mahoney (1974). Step number 1 typically involves goal setting in which child, consultant, and caregivers reach a consensus on some aspect of child behavior to be increased or decreased in frequency. The goal-setting operation essentially specifies the extent of change to be produced over specific points in time. This part of goal setting must be left largely to the child's discretion, for it is he or she who will be responsible for meeting these goals. While others can and should contribute advice, the responsibility message should be loud and clear: if self-management is to become a part of treatment, the child has *full* control over this intervention.

When the goal-setting operation is concluded, the consultant must temper any previously discussed caregiver roles in treatment. In other words, the caregiver as mediator is largely incompatible with the self-management procedures to follow. Rather than having these adults function as the controllers of reinforcement, they should merely make these events available to the child. Prior to the child's goal setting of behavioral objectives, the usual child-controlled selection of positive reinforcers will have been completed. The behavior change practice of self-management would then be initiated by the child's specification of what kind and how many of these reinforcers are to be made freely available when a goal is reached. Obviously, an interaction obtains between caregiver surveillance of goal-reinforcer outcomes and child implementation of the same. As Bandura has argued, self-management does not mean that external sources of behavior control are absent (Bandura, Mahoney, and Dirks, 1976). Caregiver monitoring is bound to influence the child's success in obtaining goals. Ideally, this influence will be therapeutic and limited to caregiver observation. But in the absence of research on interactions between self and caregiver roles in behavior modification, the therapeutic-detrimental poles of such influence are unknown. At this point, research shows that cooperative children can use self-management techniques to produce desirable changes in their own behaviors; and the extent of these changes is about as noteworthy as those produced by caregiver control of contingencies. Obviously, the clinical practitioner needs to know more about how these two strategies interact.

Before moving on to the final section of this chapter, note should be taken of treatment considerations for special childhood disorders. In those disorders characterized by severe and chronic behavior deficits such as autism, far more intensive teaching procedures must be added to the above strategies. For example, the teaching of language and self-help skills would entail contingency arrangements more akin to a text on educational practice than one dealing with clinical work. The interested reader should consult recent surveys of behavioristic educational strategies such as that of Rincover and Koegel (1977).

Generalization Issues

The preceding few pages describe clinical practice as derived from two decades of learning theory guided research. Like any approach to behavior change, this current product is by no means considered final in the sense that a foolproof means of helping troubled children is now available. Hopefully, behavior modification procedures will continue to evolve as new research adds and detracts from existing clinical practice. The very fact that this book deals with a *number* of clinical strategies is a position view on the state of the art: no one strategy has yet solved the task of assessing and treating human problems. The clinical field has no therapeutic panacea; while behavior modification offers some useful means of therapeutic intervention, it too faces some obstacles in the way of clinical success. These obstacles are best summed under the heading of generalization issues.

When a contingency treatment operation is completed, the consultant will need to consider generalization phenomena in evaluating an overall picture of therapeutic success. Behavior change per se is of little value unless one can be assured that such changes will have impact over time, settings, and the behavior repertoire of the troubled child. Let us consider these success criteria separately.

Time or Maintenance Generalization

Once a contingency plan produces the desired changes in child behavior, it is important to anticipate the durability of these outcomes. Since the contingency plan does involve people other than the child, there is reason to believe that a mutually supportive system will have been created. That is, the mediator's newly developed positive behaviors directed to the child should maintain the child's newly acquired behaviors. In turn, that new behavior pattern produced by the child should positively reinforce the mediator's new style of interacting with the child. If both parties do in fact offer each other reinforcement for these therapeutically learned styles, generalization over time should be assured.

Setting Generalization

It is obvious that the troubled child moves through a number of stimulus settings during a day's time. The child will enter and leave school, the playground, other children's homes, the home yard, and the child's own home. Even within each of these settings, one could describe subsettings. For example, home as a setting is actually composed of smaller settings such as dinner time, television watching, sleeping, and so forth. It is also true that a troubled child's problem behaviors may occur in a number of these settings, yet mediator therapeutic training or the child's therapeutic self-management training is geared to only a few of these settings. In some fashion, then, therapeutic success in the training focused settings must have impact in other settings in which the child displays problems. Hopefully, the therpeutic coverage of more than one setting plus the teaching of social learning concepts will produce a generalized approach by all parties to the new settings. In much the same fashion that one would teach language concepts, it is assumed that setting concepts will be mastered by child and mediators—a mastery that might ensure setting generalization.

Response Generalization

Just as the child's environment is broken into numerous stimulus components, a similar component description of the child's behavior is possible. Children can do a variety of things, and as such, it is possible to derive a listing of their most likely to unlikely actions—a repertoire description, if you will. In terms of the troubled child's problem responses, a consultant will soon realize that not all problems can become the planned targets of therapeutic training. Those responses occurring outside the scope of mediator coverage (perhaps stealing) or those occurring so infrequently that trained intervention is unlikely (fire setting) are just not feasible to deal with directly. Presumably, the conceptually trained mediator and/or child can exert the same contingency-oriented "rules of thumb" in dealing with responses not included in the therapeutic program. Hopefully, then, the full range of problems describing the troubled child's repertoire will be affected. That is, therapeutic generalization will be evident across the child's response repertoire.

Of course, the above three generalization criteria are as open to empirical scrutiny as are other aspects of behavior modification programs. Unfortunately, it has only been in recent years that this sort of assessment has allowed a look at how well the various operant strategies have attained these criteria. We turn now to an examination of those findings that have emerged.

When the behavior modification consultant expands assessment procedures to cover a broad view of time, settings, and behaviors, some perplexing as well as disappointing data turn up. On the perplexing side, some forms of treatment-produced generalization have been shown to occur, but the phenomena make little sense within an operant framework. Here we have reference to response generalization, in which planned changes in one or more of a troubled child's responses are followed by unplanned changes in other aspects of that child's repertoire. For a detailed review of these findings, the reader should consult Wahler, et al. (1977). At this point let us cite one example of such behavior covariations. Sajwaj, Twardosz, and Burke (1972) implemented a teacher-controlled contingency management program in a preschool setting. The program was aimed at a child whose nagging directed to adults was seen as a rather serious problem for all concerned. The contingency plan called for teacher use of extinction for the nagging. Results indicated a reduction in the frequency of nagging along with some unexpected effects on other behaviors: the boy's play with girls' toys dropped in frequency, and his disruptive behavior in group activities increased in frequency. Now it was shown that these "side effects" were clear products of the nagging intervention. That is, when extinction conditions were removed, the side effects were reversed; when the treatment conditions were once again implemented, the two side effects once again materialized. The perplexing part of this generalization phenomenon was twofold:

(1) the phenomenon could not be predicted from the baseline assessment; (2) there was no evidence that teacher or peers did anything to influence directly the occurrences of the side effect behaviors. While more recent work by Wahler (1975) and Kara and Wahler (In press) indicate that prediction of side effects may be possible, an operant explanation for the findings has yet to be shown. At the very least, such findings should orient the behavior modification consultant to broader assessments of specific interventions.

Generalization of the setting or stimulus type seems to be the exception rather than the rule. Thus far, the settings under consideration have been major ones for most children such as the home, school classroom, school playground, and hospital or institutional locations. Smaller, more idiosyncratic settings within these boundaries have yet to be studied in terms of stimulus generalization from one setting to another. A review of the literature by Forehand and Atkeson (1978) suggests that contingency operations in one major setting will not produce effects in any second major setting. Child behavior change appears specific to the setting in which the change was produced. For example, in one of the earliest studies of this sort, Wahler (1969) studied two children whose problems were evident in two settings: their homes and school classrooms. In baseline assessment phases, professional observers monitored the children's 19problem behaviors in both settings (work deficit and noncompliance with adult instructions). Then both children became the targets of contingency intervention in their homes—with their mothers serving as mediators. Over a period of four weeks, results showed a rapid and stable improvement in these problems at home. Unfortunately, these same problem behaviors in the school classrooms showed no change from baseline levels. In essence, these children's home-based therapeutic experiences were not transmitted across their home-school stimulus boundaries. Only when the children's teachers were trained to mediate a similar contingency plan did therapeutic changes occur in the school settings. It seems evident that a behavior modification consultant cannot count on a "natural" spread of desirable treatment effects across environmental settings.

Of all three types of therapeutic generalization, it would seem that time or maintenance generalization is the most likely to follow a contingency treatment plan. Given that a successfully implemented plan will produce mutual positive reinforcement for child and mediator, one ought to expect durable treatment effects. And to be sure, the largest share of predicted generalization effects is of this variety. Patterson (1974) and Wahler and Moore (1975) have all consistently reported stable improvements in up to two years of follow-up. However, both Patterson (1974) and Wahler and Moore (1975) presented data to show that not all child-mediator dyads can be expected to show such durable effects. In fact, Wahler and Moore (1975) and Wahler, Leske, and Rogers (in press) were able to specify a grouping of families whose parents may find it difficult to start and maintain contingency operations with their troubled children. These parents were poorly educated, financially impoverished people who usually lived in crowded, problem-infested inner-city areas. Even though these parents were willing to function as mediators, it was also obvious that problem contingencies in their lives extended well beyond their children. As the findings of Wahler, Leske, and Rogers (in press) suggest, *any* sort of within family change based on instructive or manding interventions is likely to fail over time. Given a historical pattern of harassment by social welfare agencies, kinfolk, and neighbors, a contingency management approach to such parents is apt to be reacted to as part of that same pattern. Somehow, the competing influences of these extra-family manding agents must be considered in conjunction with the interfamily contingencies that directly lead to childhood problems.

Behavior Ecology:
The Missing Link in Behavior Modification? .

In the above discussion of generalization problems, we have come full circle to the initial part of this chapter—namely, the potentially beneficial impact of behavior ecology on the field of applied behavior analysis. Recall that behavior ecology developed as a means of understanding the full scope of *natural* influences on child behavior (see Barker, 1964). In the author's opinion, those critical generalization problems just reviewed are caused by precisely such influences. The unpredictable nature of side effects, the stubborn stimulus boundaries of environmental settings, and the difficulties of promoting treatment durability are mysterious and frustrating because their causal contingencies are unknown. More than likely, these contingencies are observable *if* the consultant would choose to observe them. But this choice will require a laborious, much expanded look at the social and physical environments of children. This kind of "looking" orientation is precisely the definition of behavior ecology.

Recently, there have been signs of an impending cooperative interchange between behavior ecology and applied behavior analysis. In 1977, two groups of scientists representing these strategies met to discuss such a liaison. A review of that discussion can be found in *Ecological Perspectives in Behavior Analysis* (Warren and Warren, 1977). In line with this discussion, it becomes apparent that liaison primarily means changes in assessment strategy for the behavior modifier. Prior to liaison, assessment had been heavily influenced by the operant-laboratory beginnings of applied behavior analysis. That is, measurement was restricted to the operants making up a child-caregiver problem interchange. This being the case, one need only keep track of a child problem behavior and its deficient counterpart, plus a single set of caregiver behaviors considered to function as reinforcers for the child. Thus the consultant's measures entailed records on a very small portion of the child's environment. The spirit of behavior ecology, however, calls for the widest possible coverage of the environments common to children. Obviously, operant conceptions of environment-behavior interactions cannot limit the breadth of this assessment. Since the ultimate goal of this search is to understand generalization phenomena, one might view behavior ecology as a means of constructing some new conception of how environment-behavior interchanges operate. While the operant might fit that new conception, it has not yet permitted an understanding of some generalization phenomena (side effects). At present, the behavior ecology liaison must proceed in the absence of any guiding theoretical model.

Specific approaches to liaison are already evident. For example, coding systems permitting the measurement of multiple child and adult behaviors are now on the clinical market (see Wahler, House, and Stambaugh, 1976). Such systems allow a "shotgun" approach to measurement: not only are targeted problem operants recorded, but other, potentially generalized behaviors can be monitored as well. Along with the multiple behavior emphasis, it has also become clear that applied behavior analysts are conducting these measures in more than one environment, and for longer time periods (e.g., see the review by Forehand and Atkeson, In press). Given that the current liaison continues this spirit of expanded assessment, childhood generalization problems are bound to be better understood. Coincident with this understanding, better means of helping troubled children should result.

References

Azrin, N.H., and O.R. Lindsley. (1956) The reinforcement of cooperation between children. *J. Abnor. Soc. Psychol.* 52:100–102.

Bandura, A. (1971) Vicarious and self-reinforcement processes. In R. Glaser, ed., *The Nature of Reinforcement.* New York: Academic Press, pp. 228–278.

Bandura, A., M.J. Mahoney, and S.J. Dirks. (1976) Discriminative activation and maintenance of contingent self-reinforcement. *Behav. Res. Ther.* 14:1–6.

Barker, R.G. (1968) *Ecological Psychology.* Stanford: Stanford University Press.

Barker, R.G., and H.F. Wright. (1954) *Midwest and Its Children: The Psychological Study of an American Town.* Evanston, Ill.: Row, Peterson.

Becker, W.C. (1971) *Parents Are Teachers: A Child Management Program.* Champaign, Ill.: Research Press.

Bijou, S.W., and D.M. Baer. (1961) *Child development,* Vol. 1. New York: Appleton-Century-Crofts.

Bijou, S.W., and D.M. Baer. (1965) *Child development,* Vol. 2. New York: Appleton-Century-Crofts.

Briscoe, R.V., D.B. Hoffman, and J.S. Bailey. (1975) Behavioral community psychology: Training a community board to problem solve. *J. Appl. Behav. Anal.* 8:157–168.

Evans, I.M., and R.O. Nelson. (1977) Assessment of child behavior problems. In A.R. Ciminero, K.S. Calhoun, and H.E. Adams, eds., *Handbook of Behavioral Assessment.* New York: Wiley-Interscience.

Forehand, R., and B.M. Atkeson. Generalization of treatment effects with parents as therapists: A review of assessment and implementation procedures. *Behav. Ther.* in press.

Forehand, R., and H.E. King. (1977) Non-compliant children: Effects of parent training on behavior and attitude change. *Behav. Mod.* 1:93–108.

Forehand, R., H.E. King, S. Peed, and P. Yoder. (1975) Mother-child interactions: Comparisons of a non-compliant clinic group and a non-clinic group. *Behav. Res. Ther.* 13:79–84.

Gardner, J.M. (1972) Teaching behavior modification to nonprofessionals. *J. Appl. Behav. Anal.* 5:517–521.

Goldiamond, I. (1976) Self-reinforcement. *J. Appl. Behav. Anal.* 9:509–514.

Hanf, C. (1968) Modifying problem behaviors in mother-child interactions: Standardized laboratory situations. Paper presented at the meeting of the Association of Behavior Therapies, Olympia, Washington.

Harris, F.R., M.K. Johnston, C.W. Kelley, and M.M. Wolf. (1964) Effects of positive social reinforcement on regressed crawling of a nursery school child. *J. Educat. Psychol.* 55:35–41.

Harris, F.R., M.M. Wolf, and D.M. Baer. (1964) Effects of

adult social reinforcement on child behavior. *Young Children* 20:8–17.

Hart, B.M., K.E. Allen, J.S. Buell, F.R. Harris, and M.M. Wolf. (1964) Effects of social reinforcement on operant crying. *J. Exper. Child Psychol.* 1:145–153.

Kara, A., and R.G. Wahler. Some organizational properties of a young child's behavior. *J. Exper. Child Psychol.* in press.

Lewin, K. (1951) *Field Theory in Social Science: Selected Theoretical Papers,* D. Cartwright, ed. New York: Harper.

Lovaas, O.I. (1966) Program for establishment of speech in schizophrenic and autistic children. In J.K. Wing, ed., *Early Childhood Autism: Clinical, Educational and Social Aspects.* London: Pergamon Press.

Lovaas, O.I., and R.L. Koegel. (1973) Behavior therapy with autistic children. *Seventy-second Yearbook of the National Society for the Study of Education.* Chicago: University of Chicago Press, pp. 230–258.

Madsen, C., W. Becker, and D. Thomas. (1968) Rules, praise and ignoring: Elements of elementary classroom control. *J. Appl. Behav. Anal.* 1:139–150.

Mahoney, M.J. (1974) *Cognition and Behavior Modification.* Cambridge, Mass.: Ballinger.

O'Leary, K.D., and R.S. Drabman. (1971) Token reinforcement programs in the classroom: A review. *Psycholog. Bull.* 75:379–398.

O'Leary, K.D., and S.G. O'Leary. (1972) *Classroom Management: The Successful Use of Behavior Modification.* New York: Pergamon Press.

Patterson, G.R. (1977) A three-stage functional analysis for children's coercive behaviors: A tactic for developing a performance theory. In B. Etzel, J. LeBlanc, and D. Baer, eds., *New Developments in Behavioral Research: Theory, Method and Application.* Hillsdale, N.J.: Lawrence Erlbaum Associates.

Patterson, G.R. (1974) Intervention for boys with conduct problems: Multiple settings, treatments and criteria. *J. Consult. Clin. Psychol.* 42:471–481.

Patterson, G.R., and M.E. Gullion. (1968) *Living with Children: New Methods for Parents and Children.* Champaign, Ill.: Research Press.

Patterson, G.R., R.S. Ray, D.A. Shaw, and J.A. Cobb. *A Manual for Coding Family Interactions,* 6th rev. (1969) Available from ASIS National Auxiliary Publications Service, in care of CCM Information Service, 90 Third Avenue, New York, N.Y. 10022. Document #01234.

Patterson, G.R., and J.B. Reid. (1970) Reciprocity and coercion: Two facets of social systems. In C. Neuringer and J.L. Michael, eds. *Behavior Modification in Clinical Psychology.* New York: Appleton-Century-Crofts, pp. 133-177.

Pierce, C., and T.R. Risley. (1974) Recreation as a reinforcer: Increasing membership and decreasing disruptions in an urban recreation center. *J. Appl. Behav. Anal.* 7:403-411.

Rincover, A., and R.L. Koegel. (1977) Research on the education of autistic children: Recent advances and future directions. In B. Lahey and A. Kazdin, eds., *Advances in Clinical Child Psychology,* Vol. I. New York: Plenum Press.

Rubany, E.S., and B.B. Sloggett. (1973) A coding procedure for teachers. *J. Appl. Behav. Anal.* 6:339–344.

Sajwaj, T., S. Twardosz, and M. Burke. (1972) Side effects of extinction procedures in a remedial preschool. *J. Appl. Behav. Anal.* 5:163–175.

Skinner, B.F. (1953) *Science and Human Behavior.* New York: Macmillan.

Tharp, R.G., and R.J. Wetzel. (1969) Behavior Modification in the Natural Environment. New York: Academic Press.

Twardosz, S., M.F. Cataldo, and T.R. Risley. (1974) Open environment design for infant and toddler day care. *J. Appl. Behav. Anal.* 7:529–546.

Wahler, R.G. (1976) Deviant child behavior within the family: Developmental speculations and behavior change strategies. In H. Leitenberg, ed., *Handbook of Behavior Modification.* New York: Appleton-Century-Crofts.

Wahler, R.G. (1969) Setting generality: Some specific and general effects of child behavior therapy. *J. Appl. Behav. Anal.* 2:239–246.

Wahler, R.G. (1975) Some structural aspects of deviant child behavior. *J. Appl. Behav. Anal.* 8:27–42.

Wahler, R.G., and W.H. Cormier. (1970) The ecological interview: A first step in outpatient child behavior therapy. *J. Behav. Ther. Exper. Psychiat.* 1:279–289.

Wahler, R.G., A.E. House, and E.E. Stambaugh. (1976) *Ecological Assessment of Child Problem Behavior.* New York: Pergamon Press.

Wahler, R.G., G. Leske, and E.S. Rogers. (1977) The insular family: A deviance support system for oppositional children. Banff International Conference on Behavior Modification.

Wahler, R.G., and D.M. Moore. (1975) School-home behavior change procedures for oppositional children. Paper presented at the Association for the Advancement of Behavior Therapy, San Francisco.

Wahler, R.G., G.H. Winkel, R.F. Peterson, and D.C. Morrison. (1965) Mothers as behavior therapists for their own children. *Behav. Res. Ther.* 3:113–124.

Walker, H.M. (1970) *The Walker Problem Behavior Checklist.* Los Angeles, Calif.: Psychological Services.

Warren, A.R., S.F. Warren, eds. (1977) *Ecological Perspectives in Behavior Analysis.* Baltimore: University Park Press.

Williams, C. (1959) The elimination of tantrum behavior by extinction procedures. *J. Abnorm. Soc. Psychol.* 59:269.

Wolf, M.M., T. Risley, M. Johnston, F.R. Harris, and K.E. Allen. (1967) Application of operant conditioning procedures to the behavior problems of an autistic child: A follow-up and extension. *Behav. Res. Ther.* 5:103–111.

Wolf, M.M., T. Risley, and H.L. Mees. (1964) Application of operant conditioning procedures to the behavior problems of an autistic child. *Behav. Res. Ther.* 1:305–312.

Treatment of Emotional Disorders in Children and Adolescents

CHAPTER 4

Behavioral Approaches in Adolescent Psychiatry*

Gene Richard Moss
Ronald A. Mann

Introduction

Behavior Technology and Psychiatry

The psychiatric literature reveals that until recently learning theory and its clinical application, behavior therapy, have exerted minimal influence on the practice of psychiatry. This lack of impact seems especially remarkable because psychiatrists generally have agreed upon the significance of learning as a factor both in the development of nonorganic psychiatric disorders and in their treatment through psychotherapy.

Several alternative explanations may account for the failure of learning theory to gain recognition among psychiatrists. Amidst social, political, economic, and intellectual factors, it may be simply that psychiatrists have felt more satisfied with traditional psychodynamic theories and therapies when compared to learning theory alternatives. Traditional psychodynamic theories have offered consistent, comprehensive and satisfying description of human behavior; furthermore, traditional psychodynamic therapies have offered comprehensive treatment methods consistent with theory, methods perhaps more satisfying to the psychiatrist in the treatment of human behavioral disorders.

In contrast to the wealth of clinical data accumulated by psychodynamic methodology, learning theory must seem pale indeed. Whereas traditional inquiry has emphasized the integrity of the human personality with all its intricate complexities, learning theory often has concentrated on seemingly trivial and superficial aspects of human behavior. Its theoretical constructs have been derived from animal experimentation and understandably have appeared mechanistic and inapplicable to human level of organization. Until recently, clinical application of learning theory had been limited to such an extent that it had not been developed into a body of specific treatment procedures that could be designated behavior therapy.

In spite of the seeming deficiencies of learning theory, there has been increasing pressure for psychiatrists to acquaint themselves with it. This pressure in large measure can be attributed to the challenge from behavior therapists for traditional psychotherapists to demonstrate empirically that their theories are the most valid and parsimonious and that their therapies the most effective and swift. The pressure to investigate learning theory has also come from within the psychodynamic movement. For example, towards the end of his career, Franz Alexander (1963) turned his attention

*The authors wish to express their appreciation to Gary R. Rick, Ph.D. for his assistance in the preparation of this chapter.

to learning theory, which he believed to hold great promise for psychotherapy. Alexander challenged his psychoanalytic colleagues by speculating that they may have retained their singular approach as an unconscious defense against their own anxiety and urged them to investigate learning theory as an additional means to further knowledge and therapeutic efficacy.

Adolescence and Society

Historically, adolescence has been considered a time of turmoil, both physiological and behavioral. It is during adolescence that great changes occur both in the biology of the individual and in his way of responding to the world. Adolescence is heralded by puberty, typically occurring at approximately the ago of 12 or 13. Adolescence, however, extends well beyond puberty, and its termination has come to be defined on a legal basis occurring somewhere between the ages of 18 to 21, depending upon the locality.

Recently, the problems associated with adolescence have become of increasing social concern; for example, the continually increasing crime rate reflects, in part, a large increase in the frequency of crimes committed by adolescents. Socially, adolescent problems generally fall into one or more of the following three categories: (1) problems within the family; (2) problems within the school; or (3) problems within the community.

Many of these behavioral problems reflect patterns of either *behavioral excesses* or *behavioral deficits* in the repertoire of the adolescent. *Behavioral excesses* may be defined as any behavior for which the rate of occurrences and/or duration of occurrences exceeds socially defined standards of acceptability, desirability, or appropriateness within a given context (Mann, 1976). Many behaviors that meet the above criteria are considered inappropriate by various members of society for a variety of reasons. Behaviors may be considered undesirable and excessive because they are dangerous to the individual himself or to others; because they interfere with the desired behaviors of others; because they provoke undesirable responses from others; or because they violate religious tenets or cultural norms.

Legal systems define through laws a large number of behaviors as undesirable and excessive. Ideally, excessive behaviors are judged illegal only when they cause harm to the self, to others, or to the property of others. When such behaviors occur, they are likely to prompt police, juvenile authorities, or other social agencies to arrest, incarcerate, detain, or institutionalize those individuals engaging in such undesirable and excessive behaviors.

Behavioral deficits represent the converse of behavioral excesses. Behavioral deficits may be defined as any behavior for which the rate of occurrences and/or duration of occurrences falls below socially defined standards of acceptability, desirability, or appropriateness within a given context. A behavioral deficit may be maladaptive in that either individually defined or socially defined goals cannot be met due to a lack of necessary, prerequisite skills in the behavioral repertoire.

In summary, behaviors are defined as undesirable due to excess or deficit by various members of society such as parents, teachers, peers, subcultures, law enforcement agencies, and so forth. Frequently occurring or excessive behaviors are labeled as inappropriate when they exceed the standards of acceptability within a given context or community. Infrequently occurring or deficient behaviors are labeled as inappropriate when they fail to meet the standards or expectations within a given context or community. Whether excess or deficit, the behavioral problems of the adolescent may be of such major proportions that they require immediate and dramatic change.

Historical and Theoretical Considerations

The roots of behavioral technology can be traced back to the late nineteenth and early twentieth centuries. The theoretical and experimental foundation of respondent (or classical) conditioning procedures can be attributed to Pavlov (1927), and the early clinical applications of respondent procedure can be attributed to Watson and his coworkers (1924). The theoretical and experimental foundations of operant procedure can be attributed earliest to Thorndike (1911), with later elaboration attributed to Skinner (1938).

Respondent Procedure

Ivan Pavlov, a contemporary of Sigmund Freud, began his scientific career with investigation of circulation and the heart. Pavlov, a physiologist, won the Nobel Prize in 1904 for his work on the physiology of digestion, and it was not until he was past his fiftieth year that Pavlov began his work on conditioned reflexes. Perhaps his major contribution can be viewed as the care with which he explored numerous empirical relationships and determined certain essential parameters, providing background and terminology for countless succeeding experiments by others.

Pavlov developed the first systematic procedure to contitioned animal behavior in his legendary experiments with the dog, the meat, and the bell. When presented to the dog, the meat elicited an innate, reflex-like salivation response. The meat is referred to as the unconditioned stimulus (UCS), and the innate, reflex-like salivation is referred to as the unconditioned response (UCR). Pavlov demonstrated that by pairing the UCS with a second stimulus (a bell) previously neutral with respect to the UCR, the previously neutral stimulus by itself acquired the property of eliciting a response similar but not identical to the UCR. In this case, by pairing the presentation of the meat with the bell, eventually the bell alone elicited salivation. The previously neutral stimulus is referred to as the conditioned stimulus (CS), and the response elicited by the CS is referred to as the conditioned response (CR). Both the CR and UCR thus fall roughly into the same class but are distinguished by the stimulus that elicits them. Although usually similar, the CR and UCR are seldom, if ever, precisely identical. The CS is said to acquire its conditioned properties through *reinforcement*, a term that refers to the procedure of following the CS by the UCS. As the CS is presented alone—that is, without the UCS—the CR will tend to weaken and eventually disappear. This procedure of nonreinforcement of previously reinforced responses is referred to as respondent *extinction*.

The procedural format described above is referred to as *respondent conditioning* (i.e., classical or Pavlovian conditioning). It is characterized by the pairing of two stimuli, the UCS with the CS. The applications of respondent conditioning have been largely in the area of psycho-physiology, especially autonomic responses.

Recognized as one of the founders of behaviorism in the United States, John Watson attempted to apply the principles of respondent procedure clinically in an attempt to explain behavioral pathology in humans. Watson and Rayners's classic study with Little Albert (1920) represents one of the earliest attempts experimentally to induce behavioral pathology. Watson and Rayner paired the visual presentation of a rabbit with the presentation of a loud noise associated with a startle response in an 11-month-old infant. The rabbit initially was neutral with respect to the startle response; however, by pairing the rabbit (CS) with the loud noise (UCS), the experimenters were able to produce a reaction (CR) similar to the startled response from the loud noise (UCR). This early pioneering study represented the application of a respondent procedure to the learning of conditioned emotional responses in humans. Watson believed that most human behavioral learning could be explained by the classical or respondent paradigm. It was left for Skinner to draw the distinction between the respondent and operant paradigms, operant paradigms representing the basis for most clinical applications.

Operation Procedure

In 1938 B.F. Skinner published his now-famous treatise *Behavior of Organisms*. This work went far to resolve both theoretically and experimentally many behavioral phenomena not adequately described by prior S-R analyses. In particular, it halted the fruitless attempt to describe all behaviors on the basis of Pavlovian or respondent conditioning principles. Skinner forced the recognition of two major types of behavior, specifically operants and respondents, only the latter of which had been described previously by respondent principles. Skinner outlined the distinctions between these behaviors solely by delineating their different relationship to the controlling environment. This analysis generated two major paradigms for producing behavioral change or learning, operant procedure and respondent procedure.

Skinner's functional analysis of behavior outlined empirical definitions and relationships quantified objectively. Perhaps his most influential contributions were his persuasive arguments for the importance of quantifying behavior in terms of rate. Frequency of occurence became the basic datum for the functional analysis of behavior.

Operant procedure is based upon the *Law of Effect* initially described by Thorndike (1911). The Law of Effect refers to the change in strength of a response as a result of its consequences. If the occurence of a response is followed by a stimulus that increases the frequency or magnitude of that response, such a stimulus is referred to as a positive reinforcer. A negative reinforcer is defined as a stimulus the removal or postponement of which strengthens a response. An example of negative reinforcement is found in the experimental paradigm of the conditioned avoidance response (CAR), in which the presentation of an aversive or unpleasant stimulus is contingent upon the failure of a response to occur. Removal of the aversive stimulus, the negative reinforcer, contingent upon the occurence of a response serves to strengthen that response. Punishment, on the other hand, is defined as the presentation of an aversive stimulus contingent upon the occurrence of a response, the effect of which is to decrease the frequency or magnitude of the response at least in the presence of the punishing stimulus. Reinforcement, whether positive or negative, always serves to increase the frequency or strength of a response; whereas the effects of punishment are to decrease the frequency or strength of a response.

In contrast to the eliciting in a reflex-like fashion of a response by an antecedent stimulus as described by respondent procedure, operant procedure describes responses by the organism as emitted without necessarily being elicited by a prior stimulus. Such responses are referred to as *free operants*. If a prior stimulus should become the occasion for an operant—that is, if the occurrence of a specific stimulus increases the probability of occurrence of a specific response—the antecedent stimulus is referred to as a *discriminative stimulus* (S^D), and the operant is referred to as a *discriminated operant*. The S^D is said to acquire its behavioral control because it has become the occasion on which the operant previously has been reinforced. Operants are said to be emitted then either reinforced, positively or negatively, or punished by the contingent environmental stimuli. Although a reinforcer need not follow every response for response strength to be maintained, repetitive reinforcement is necessary. An operant thus is said to be any behavior that is affected by its stimulus consequences.

The particular pattern formed by the emitted responses, referred to as behavioral topography, has been documented in the animal laboratory to be a function of the schedule according to which reinforcement is presented (Ferster and Skinner, 1957). Schedules of reinforcement fall under two categories: (1) continuous, variable or fixed; and (2) ratio or interval.

Nonreinforcement of previously reinforced operants is referred to as *operant extinction. Resistance to extinction*—that is, the tendency to emit responses after reinforcement has been withdrawn—is a reflection of the previous schedule of reinforcement. In general, intermittent or a periodic reinforcement generates greater resistance to extinction than does continuous reinforcement. Although extinction procedures result in an eventual decreased frequency leading to a virtual elimination of the occurrence of an operant, the decrease usually is not immediate. In fact, the typical sequence is an actual increase in frequency of response immediately following the institution of an extinction procedure followed subsequently by a decrease. Although originally described from work in the animal laboratory, these concepts associated with schedules of reinforcement play an enormous role in the management of human affairs.

Perhaps one of the greatest contributions of operant technology to the understanding of human behavior has been the distinction made between topographical and functional analyses. Standard psychiatric classification has been based largely upon description of process through behavioral topography. Topographical analysis classifies according to effects upon an observational device, such as the camera or the human eye (Goldiamond and Dyrud, 1968). This approach concerns itself with the form of the behavior rather than with the controlling variable—i.e., the antecedents and consequences associated with the behavior. Topographically, for example, one might classify a patient as hysterical or compulsive or depressed by observing the form of the behavior without reference to events occurring before or after.

An alternate approach based upon description of procedure through behavioral function is to be found in a *functional analysis*, which specifies the controlling variables in the form of antecedents and consequences that can be identified objectively and that are potentially manipulable (Ferster, 1965). Antecedents include both the past history and current stimuli that provide the occasion for the behavior to occur. Consequences are the objective events that the behavior produces, such as reinforcers or punishers that increase or decrease its future probability. Although originally developed in the experimental laboratory, functional analysis applied clinically emphasizes an operational therapeutic technology by referring to manipulable and observable events.

Worthy of repeated emphasis is the principle that behavior similar in topography may fall into different functional classes, and conversely, behaviors differing in topography may fall into the same functional class. Clinically, different complex behavioral topographies referred to by such labels as depression, phobia, compulsion, etc., may belong to the same functional class—i.e., under control of similar antecedents and consequences. Conversely, any given topography—e.g., depressive behavior—

may belong to different functional classes—i.e., under the control of different antecedents and consequences.

From an operant point of view, the most powerful demonstrations of behavioral change are likely to require the discovery and control of relevant consequences of the behavior to be changed. Such a demonstration requires that a number of criteria be satisfied. Among these, the most important are: (1) a reliable measurement of the behavior; (2) discovery or supplying of relevant consequences; (3) precise and systematic control of relevant consequences; and thereby, (4) an orderly and socially significant change in the behavior under study.

Due to the relative ease of controlling consequences and measuring behaviors in controlled or confined settings as opposed to outpatient settings, numerous applied clinical demonstrations of behavioral change have been performed with institutionalized psychiatric patients or residential clients. Experimental research on behavioral treatments with adolescents in institutional settings has provided substantial evidence for the effectiveness of token economies or point systems. The same cannot be boasted for studies conducted in the outpatient context, however.

Applications

Inpatient and Residential

Applications of behavioral technology to the psychiatric hospitalization of adolescents have been based upon implementation of a token economy or point system where tokens or points function as conditioned or secondary reinforcers that can be exchanged for goods, services, or privileges—similar to the use of money. Token reinforcement procedures have been demonstrated to be effective with a variety of populations and a variety of behavioral problems. Such procedures were developed by Allyon and Azrin (1968) to establish and maintain work and self-care behaviors of chronically institutionalized psychotic patients. Other investigators have used these procedures to remediate problem behaviors among so-called character-disordered patients hospitalized on a psychiatric ward for delinquent soldiers (Coleman and Baker, 1969) and to weaken institutionalized behaviors of chronic psychiatric patients (Winkler, 1970). Token programs have been used with patients in a maximum security correctional hospital (Lawson et al., 1971) and with chronic veteran psychiatric patients (Atthowe and Krasner, 1968), as well as with young veteran psychiatric patients on a rapid-turnover ward (Mann and Moss, 1973). Similar techniques have been utilized in settings other than psychiatric, such as in classrooms to deal with "emotionally disturbed" and "mentally retarded" children (Birnbrauer et al., 1965; O'Leary and Becker, 1967); to improve social, academic, and self-help behaviors of predelinquent children (Phillips, 1968; Phillips et al., 1971); and to weaken problem behaviors and strengthen academic behaviors of children in special classrooms (Wolf, Giles, and Hall, 1968). Evaluation of token reinforcement procedures has demonstrated that therapists, nurses, and teachers can generate therapeutic changes in a wide variety of behaviors by controlling the consequences of those behaviors (Allyon and Michael, 1959).

Behavioral treatments have been applied to adolescent behavior problems since the early 1960's (Stumphauzer, 1976). Reviews of this literature have concluded that there is an overall positive pattern of results (Davidson and Seidman, 1974), and that behavioral treatments tend to be more effective, efficient, and specific than traditional treatments (Foreyt et al., 1975).

Applications of behavioral technology have evolved through the following phases over time: (i) demonstration studies—whereby the token economy was demonstrated to be a flexible and effective treatment; (ii) component analysis—whereby the relevant variables were teased out from the total package in terms of (a) generalization, (b) treatment effects, and (c) behavioral economics; (iii) the constructional orientation—whereby methods were developed to generate successful living in the natural environment; and (iv) evaluation research—whereby behavioral approaches were compared to more traditional approaches in terms of (a) effects and (b) cost analysis.

Demonstration Studies

Early research with delinquents in community settings demonstrated that operant conditioning principles could be used effectively to recruit adolescent delinquents and maintain their attendance at traditional counseling and therapy sessions (Schwitzgebel, 1964). In 1968, Ayllon and Azrin reported the effectiveness of a token economy system in the management of chronic adult mental hospital patients (Allyon and Azrin, 1968). Tokens were used as generalized conditioned reinforcers to reinforce specific behaviors. Subsequent studies demonstrated the application of behavioral technology and the token system to a wide variety of populations in a wide variety of settings. Point systems or token economies were demonstrated to be effective with juveniles in detention facilities, with the retarded in institutions, with the retarded in the classroom, with delinquents in the classroom, with delinquents in residential settings, with delinquents in a summer camp setting, and with preadolescents on a psychiatric ward.

These early studies are marked both by their lack of experimental elegance and by problems of implementing a new type of program; nevertheless, despite these problems, this literature clearly demonstrated that token economies and other behavioral techniques could bring about administrative control of an institutional setting. Token systems freed the institution from such common problems as tardiness, sloppiness and aggression. On the other hand, while administrative control could be established, it was not clear to what extent therapeutic effectiveness necessarily followed. The extent to which therapeutic behavioral change obtained in an institution generalizes to the natural environment was not part of this early literature.

Component Analysis

In the early 1970's, behavioral research began to analyze various component aspects of treatment programs that might increase the likelihood of successful living in the natural environment. Among these component aspects were the following: (a) methods to improve generalization; (b) methods to maximize the effects of treatment; and (c) parameters of the token economy.

Generalization. In order for token economies to have socially relevant, therapeutic effects rather than merely administrative effects, there must be generalization of effects to the community after discharge from the institution. Accordingly, behaviors established in token environments must transfer to other situations and conditions. It is also desirable that positive changes spread to new behaviors other than those originally rewarded (response generalization). In their review of token economies, Kazdin and Bootzin indicated that in the absence of evidence of generalization some researchers had concluded that token economies were prosthetic rather than therapeutic (1972). They pointed out, however, that generalization may not be expected to occur unless specific provisions be included in a program. While they listed several ways to increase generalization, they concluded that the most fruitful approach would come from systematic programming of the natural environment. To date, few studies have been concerned primarily with generalization.

Effects of Treatment. A great deal of empirical research on the treatment effects of token economies as a function of their components has come from Achievement Place, a residential home for pre-delinquents in Lawrence, Kansas (Phillips, 1968). Numerous studies utilizing component analysis were conducted at Achievement Place, investigating such areas as social, academic, and self-care behaviors; self-government parameters; and student management skills. One important aspect of the studies was the demonstration that a series of empirical investigaions can produce a system that is maximally efficient, rated favorable by its consumers, and judged valid by society (Phillips et al., 1973).

A report of the replication of the Achievement Place type of program with Mexican-American youths in California was made by Liberman and his colleagues (1975). The results of these studies indicate that the specific procedures of token economies must be empirically individualized for different settings and populations. The data also suggest that a token system may function as a reward and discriminative stimulus for the staff members as well as the treatment population. The token economy system may cue the staff to prompt and socially reward behavior in a way that treatment effects may continue after the use of tokens is withdrawn.

Behavioral Economics. The term "behavioral economics" was first used by Kagel and Winkler (1972) to describe the study of the effects of economics on behavior. Winkler suggested that one method of promoting extra-institutional generalization would be to pattern a token system after the economic pattern used in the natural environment. More recently, Gagnon and Davidson (1976) questioned the relevance of institutionalized economics to those of the outside marketplace. They contended that token economies achieve institutional orderliness at the price of establishing a set that does not correspond to human relationships outside the hospital. The institutional economy is equitable and of high predictability, based upon an administrative monopoly entirely controlled by the staff. The marketplace, on the other hand, often is inequitable and of low predictability, established upon the principle of supply and demand. They further pointed out that institutionalized patients are not economically irrational but may be treated as such by token economies. To date, few empirical investigations have been conducted in this area.

Behavioral economics remains in its infancy. The contention that token economies would yield greater generalization if they were similar to the marketplace awaits empirical demonstration. Another question that remains unanswered concerns the type of economic experience for which a token economy should prepare its consumer. For those who may be faced with chronic unemployment, transitory low-paying jobs, or welfare roles, it seems doubtful that a token economy can do much, in Gagnon and Davidson's words, to "survive the fact that life is unjust" (1976). If, as appears likely, former consumers in token economies are able to adapt to reasonable economic conditions, it then becomes less a question of an institutional economy preparing its consumers for dealing with a poorly predictable economy of the natural environment than a question of society dealing with its own problems. A token economy might be more effective, in this regard, in developing job-related skills necessary to obtain and to maintain employment.

Constructional Orientation

One method offered for the development of successful living in the natural environment is the development of specific adaptive skills suited to the specific environment. Goldiamond (1974) defined the *constructional* orientation as one whose solution to problems is the construction of repertoires that can transfer to new situations.

Studies in this area have demonstrated that a variety of socially adaptive behaviors can be acquired and strengthened. Applications have included learning delay of gratification, increasing verbalization about current events, learning to ask questions in educational situations, learning effective negotiation behavior, improving employment interview skills, learning to communicate more effectively with authority figures. A variety of behavioral procedures were utilized in these studies, including token and verbal reinforcement, peer modeling, prompts, and discrimination training.

Evaluation Studies

Although there is a paucity of comparative research in the literature, a few studies have compared the application of behavioral technology and the token economy to more traditional treatment approaches. The few studies conducted indicate that both staff and patients may have a more positive attitude toward token economy wards than milieu-oriented wards, that specific behavioral goals may be achieved more effectively with behavioral techniques, and that relapse or recidivism rates may be lower with behavioral approaches.

Comparative outcome studies often are subjective and methodologically difficult. Experimenter biases, the Hawthorne effect, and numerous other factors suggest a cautious interpretive analysis of comparative treatment research; nevertheless, the above studies do provide at least some evidence that behavioral programs and token systems are relatively effective and provide for maintained improvement outside the institution.

A more objective and relevant evaluation criterion for institutional research, cost analysis, has been suggested by Krapfl (1974). *Cost effectiveness* is a measure of the amount of behavioral change in proportion to institutional costs. *Cost-benefit analysis* is concerned with the amount of cost that is saved by the institution through the implementation of a program. Foreyt and co-workers (1975) reported a cost-benefit analysis of a token economy program. In order to do this, an estimate of the probable number of years patients would be hospitalized was compared to the costs of the hospitalization corrected by an interest rate that discounted future costs to their present value. While these calculations are subject to strong assumptions about life-expectancy, treatment effects, and economic fluctuations, a reasonably objective range of cost benefits was believed to have been obtained. For 74 patients in the program, Foreyt et al calculated a new savings of 2½ to over 10½ million dollars! A cost-benefit ratio represents the benefits of a program in relation to its extra costs. In this study, cost-benefit ratio estimates ranged from 90:1 to 360:1. These results are startling even if one were to accept only a fraction of the low estimates reported.

An extension of this study conducted by Rockwood and Foreyt (1976) indicated how economic criteria could be used to select patients for treatment. Results indicated that securing the early release through intensive token economy treatment of younger patients and patients who have been hospitalized for longer periods of time produced the greatest economic benefit. The authors pointed out that this should not be the sole criterion for patient selection; however, it can be one criterion of an overall social benefit analysis.

Outpatient

Research conducted in institutional settings has had a number of inherent advantages over research conducted in extra-institutional settings. (1) Subjects of the research were in a restricted environment that facilitated direct observation of behavioral change with far greater ease than could be accomplished in the natural environment. (2) The institutional environment lent itself to systematic management of rewards and penalites under direct staff supervision. (3) Such systematic management allowed investigators to analyze the functional relationship between treatment variables and therapeutic behavioral change.

In contrast, research conducted in more natural environments has proven very difficult. (1) Subjects of the research are not available for direct behavioral observation. Consequently, reports by the patient, parents, or significant others must be relied upon. (2) The natural environment resists the high level of systematic management of the institution. (3) Due to the lower level of control and prediction, investigators have found themselves hard-pressed to document variables associated with behavioral change. Presumably because of these inherent difficulties, there has been a paucity of research in this area. The research that has been conducted generally has failed to document direct therapeutic efficacy.

Early research in the natural environment initially concerned itself with the development of service delivery systems for adolescents with behavioral problems. Some of the earlier work ironically utilized shaping and other operant procedures successfully to enlist the involvement of juvenile delinquents in traditional therapy (Schwitzgebel, 1964).

Subsequent studies applied behavioral techniques directly in an attempt to achieve behavioral change. Undesirable behaviors such as truancy, arson, theft, and assault were demonstrated amenable to change through implementation of home-based point systems and contingency contracting (Tharp and Wetzel, 1969). More recent studies implementing point systems and contingency contracts through parents or other agents of behavioral change have indicated effective application not only to delinquent behaviors but to behaviors such as communication skills, problem solving, schoolwork, and completion of household chores. Other studies, however, have cast doubt upon the universal application of behavioral procedures on an outpatient basis and have suggested that other nonspecific factors may exert significant effects (Weathers and Liberman, 1975; Stuart and Lott, 1973).

While these studies suggest that contingency contracts may be effective, they shed little light on some important aspects of contracting; for example, there has been no systematic evaluation of reward and response cost parameters. Furthermore, contracting has been presented as a procedure without alterable parameters. Weathers and Liberman, 1975; for instance, state, "Contingency contracting . . . cannot be considered an effective intervention strategy." It is not known, however, to what extent the contracts were correctly and consistently implemented, and if applied, the nature of their consequent parameters.

Behavioral interventions traditionally have been applied to individuals or small groups. A recent approach, referred to as *behavioral ecology*, is attempting to deal with entire urban communities. To date, only a few programs have been described (Burchard et al., 1976). Implementation of these programs may require that the records of police, schools, mental health, and other agencies be used to analyze reinforcement systems throughout the community. That these investigators have been developing means to monitor community-wide behaviors as a prerequisite to applying community-wide contingencies raises interesting philosophical and ethical issues.

Program Methodology

Inpatient

As the behavioral problem of an adolescent often is of such major proportions that he can no longer remain within the community, control and therapy of adolescent problems often require a degree of behavioral control that can be attained only in a closed setting—i.e., in a hospital or other institution. In attempting to deal with adolescent problems, the therapist often finds himself without sufficient leverage to control the behavior of the adolescent in his natural environment. Accordingly it becomes necessary to place the adolescent into a setting where sufficient leverage can obviate further destructive effects from the problems with which the adolescent is struggling and permit initiation of appropriate evaluative and therapeutic modalities.

Psychiatric treatment programs in a hospital setting can be subdivided into four categories: (1) a basic hospital program designed to provide a consistent therapeutic milieu in which the adolescent can operate without conflicting or destructive demands placed upon him by his immediate environment; (2) an individualized treatment program involving a variety of modalities, such as individual therapy, group therapy, somatic therapies (where indicated), vocational guidance, development of social skills, etc.; (3) a program of family therapy through which the dynamics of the family are analyzed in order to pinpoint problem areas and in order to target specific remedial alternatives, if practicable; and (4) the implementation of community liaison with the patient's school, probation officer, vocational rehabilitation counselor, etc., in order to develop constructive environmental support outside the home. The integration of these four treatment modalities is paramount; however, it should be stressed that a consistent therapeutic environment staffed by trained personnel is a necessary foundation for successful treatment. Without a highly structured, consistent hospital environment, the hospital staff itself can fall into the same trap as other adults in the adolescent's natural environment; for example, staff arguing amongst themselves as to what to do, staff attempting to become "good guys versus bad guys," etc. Optimally, the adolescent's control of his own personal destiny should be a consequence of his meeting the clear and consistent expectation of a specific therapeutic program rather than his manipulating others to meet his idiosyncratic maladaptive demands. Such a structured program that sets a consistent standard by which to evaluate the behavior of the adolescent patient offers the therapist, whatever his theoretical orientation, objective criteria by which to judge clinical change.

Because adolescent patients are often a population difficult to manage and treat effectively, many psychiatric units are reluctant to accept them as patients. The more disturbing behaviors associated with many adolescent patients include abuse and destruction of hospital property as well as threatening and assaultive behaviors to one another and to staff. Consequently, operant reinforcement procedures similar to those cited previously have been designed in an attempt to establish effective adolescent inpatient programs. The following provides a methodological model for a behaviorally-oriented adolescent inpatient program that illustrates necessary program requirements and design (Moss and Brown, 1978; Moss and Mann, 1978):

Patients

Program methodology can be designed to provide a hospital treatment program for adolescents presenting problems ranging from psychotic behavior to multiple runaway to child molesting to school truancy—often with extreme behavioral problems in the home. Patients may exhibit drug abuse problems involving alcohol, barbiturates, marijuana, amphetamines, or even heroin. They may face legal proceedings or already be on probation. Whatever the nature of the presenting complaints, clearly adolescents requiring psychiatric hospitalization will have been engaging in maladaptive, undesirable behaviors not under the stimulus control of parents, teachers, community norms, or legal statutes.

Upon admission, each patient should receive a complete evaluation, including psychiatric interview; family assessment; medical history and physical examination; psychological testing with emphasis upon intellectual potential, achievements, and learning disabilities; laboratory tests (CBC, urinalysis, SMA-12, and serology); and chest x-ray. EEG may be considered optional. Additional diagnostic procedures should be implemented as indicated. With these data and with baseline observations by staff of the patient's behavior in the hospital, specific treatment goals can be specified for the patient (Moss and Boren, 1971).

General Program Methodology and Goals

Program methodology is based upon the premise that adolescents with various behavioral problems can be assisted in their development through the use of a controlled environment, implementing principles of reinforcement in a consistent and systematic fashion. This of course includes selected therapies and activities as well as constructive, therapeutic patient-staff relationships. In general, the methodology is designed to foster independence, on the one hand, and to improve relations with family, peers, and the community, on the other.

In order to accomplish these objectives, program

methodology utilizes operant principles of reinforcement to provide an atmosphere of consistent expectation in which the adolescent patient can learn to function more effectively as an individual and as a member of the community. Thus the program should enhance the strength of adaptive, desirable behaviors through the use of positive reinforcement while weakening the strength of maladaptive, undesirable behaviors through the use of both extinction and punishment procedures; nevertheless, the conceptual framework of the program should not be to mold the adolescent into a "good patient" but rather to help him to develop his own individual creative skills in a positive and constructive manner consistent with the broad limits of social tolerance.

The major and most important aspect of a behaviorally oriented, adolescent program is the point or token system (i.e., the token reinforcement procedures), which provides the foundation for all other treatment modalities. As desirable behaviors typically are rewarded in the community, and undesirable behaviors are punished, similarly in the adolescent program adaptive desirable target behaviors are reinforced by the presentation of points and social praise. Maladaptive or undesirable behaviors, on the other hand, are punished by imposing penalties, which include penalty fines.

In addition to the point or token system, a variety of other therapeutic modalities should be provided for each adolescent patient. Chief among these therapeutic modalities is the individual and family therapy offered by the attending psychiatrist. It is during these sessions that a functional analysis of the patient's problems is conducted with an assessment of family behavioral dynamics. Individualized home programs can be designed based upon principles of contingency contracting (Mann, 1975). As the time for discharge approaches, specific plans for discharge are formulated, usually involving outpatient follow-up. Furthermore, special adolescent group therapies and family group therapy sessions should be conducted regularly. Adjunctive therapies, including occupational, recreational, and industrial therapies, should be offered under the direct supervision of a registered occupational therapist. Finally, a tutorial program involving accredited schoolwork should be available to all adolescent patients and conducted by a fully licensed schoolteacher with expertise in special education. When practicable, the adolescent may be able to attend his own regular school from the hospital. Chemotherapy should be kept to a minimum, with patients receiving medication for specific diagnostic entities—e.g., schizophrenia—as appropriate.

Point or Token System

The point system can be based on a five-day work week that begins Monday and ends Friday, similar to that found in the community. Accordingly, patients can earn points during the five working days and can spend their points seven days a week. Defined target behaviors for which points can be earned include grooming, beds made, clean room, attendance at school and completion of homework, attendance and participation in adolescent group therapies, and attendance and participation in occupational and recreational therapies.

Patients can exchange their earned points for various goods and services. In other words, the points derive their reinforcing power because the adolescents can convert them into desired goods or privileges. The points are similar to currency that has no intrinsic value but derives its value by virtue of the fact that it can be used to purchase goods and services. Thus the earned points are the currency of a behaviorally oriented adolescent program. It should be pointed out that privileges can be purchased by the adolescents only if they have an adequate number of points to buy them. No credit should be extended in the program. The various privileges that can be purchased with points may include a room on the open unit; electronic equipment in the room (i.e., TV, stereo, radio); off-ground passes with staff; smoking privileges; day passes, overnight passes, and weekend passes with parents; as well as staying up late at night.

The point economy should be designed in such a manner that if a patient performs most of the specified behaviors and does not emit, too often, behaviors penalized by point fines, he can purchase most of the goods and services provided. The economy should be geared so that a patient's behavior rather than just staff decision determine whether the patient is "well enough" or "ready" to be allowed, for example, to leave a locked ward or to go on overnight or weekend passes. Accordingly, overnight, day, and weekend passes appear relatively expensive compared to the price of other privileges. A patient is required to emit a high frequency of target behaviors systematically during the week and to follow the rules of the unit with few penalties in order to acquire the number of points necessary to purchase off-ward passes. Thus decisions that typically consume valuable staff meeting time due to differences of clinical opinion as to which patient was "well enough," etc., can be avoided. If a patient possesses the required amount of points—i.e., he has demonstrated a certain degree of "organized behavior"—he may be able to purchase off-ward passes with the aproval of his physician.

Rules

Program methodology should be designed to reinforce adaptive, constructive behaviors and to extinguish or punish maladaptive, destructive behaviors. Accordingly, a penalty system is an integral part of the adolescent program through which the adolescent learns the negative consequences of maladaptive behavior. Its implementation should include the use of posted rules.

Breaking hospital rules or engaging in undesirable behaviors results in penalties that include ward restrictions, the loss of points (i.e., penalty fines), and/or specified periods of time in a "time-out room" (i.e., time out from positive reinforcement). Penalties must be enforced consistently for behaviors considered to be maladaptive. Such behaviors include assaultive behaviors, destruction of patient or hospital property, and stealing. Penalties are imposed if patients appear intoxicated, are found to have a positive drug screen (using urinalysis techniques), or are found using illicit drugs, including alcohol. Other penalties may be levied for eating, drinking, or smoking in patient rooms; possession of contraband items such as weapons, sharp objects, or drugs; or using offensive language at inappropriate times.

A behaviorally oriented adolescent program tends to minimize differential treatment of patients by staff which typically can occur due to personal favoritism or prejudice. If a patient engages in specified target behaviors, he is paid the required number of points regardless of whether he is liked or disliked by any particular staff member. The minimizing of differential treatment of patients by staff can also be facilitated by providing the opportunity for patients to complain formally or to present grievances at a regularly scheduled "gripe meeting." At these meetings, patients' complaints can be investigated. Patients previously penalized due to staff error can have their point penalties refunded. Thus one source of patient-staff conflict in everyday social interactions is minimized. More importantly, the adolescent is provided the opportunity to learn to express grievances against authority in a constructive manner.

Although in a behaviorally-oriented program there are a number of undesirable behaviors leading to penalties, the number of behaviors leading to penalties should be fewer than the number of behaviors leading to reward. This ratio of reward to penalty tends to lend a more positive tone to the program in contrast to the oft-seen punitive atmosphere of some adolescent units.

Group Therapies

In addition to the normal routines and target behaviors of the point system, a behaviorally oriented adolescent program should provide each adolescent with an opportunity to attend group therapy sessions on a regular basis. The emphasis of these sessions is based upon behavioral principles, with the adolescents being taught to solve problems in terms of objective behavioral criteria. Adolescents can be paid points for on-time attendance and for participation.

In addition to adolescent group therapies, the program can provide the opportunity for parents to attend regularly scheduled family group therapy sessions. At these sessions, both parents and patients should be encouraged to discuss objectively the specific behavioral changes each believes the other should make to facilitate more harmony in the home or community. Patients should be paid points only if both the patient and at least one family member arrive on time. Additional points may be paid to the patient for participation. Patients neither should earn points nor attend family group therapy if a parent does not attend. Thus parents are encouraged to attend family therapy not only by program personnel but by their offspring as well.

Individual and Family Therapies

Complementary to the behavioral treatment program offered by the institution is the individual and family therapy offered by the attending psychiatrist. It is the attending psychiatrist who assumes overall responsibility for the patient's evaluation and treatment during his hospital stay.

In addition to the overall supervision of the patient's diagnostic evaluation and treatment plan, the attending psychiatrist is charged with the responsibility for providing individual and family therapy. For the behaviorally oriented psychiatrist, the initial task is to arrive at a psychiatric diagnosis based upon a functional analysis of the problem behaviors. It is upon this foundation that an individually tailored treatment plan is specified, and discharge planning begun. Frequent regularly scheduled therapy sessions with the patient, the parents, and all together usually are mandatory. In those instances where out-of-home placement is indicated, communication and planning with appropriate social agencies must be undertaken. Usually the behaviorally oriented psychiatrist will develop an individually tailored contingency contract prior to the patient's discharge. Design of such a contingency contract may require many family therapy sessions, during which a host of family conflicts may have to be resolved. Following discharge, both the patient and the parents usually will be followed in outpatient psychiatric treatment.

Outpatient Follow-up

Outpatient treatment following discharge from a behaviorally oriented adolescent hospital program essentially becomes an extension of the methodology implemented by the psychiatrist in the individual and family therapy sessions conducted during the patient's hospital stay. Preparation for discharge and outpatient follow-up should begin early in the course of hospitalization and be an integral part of the hospital treatment plan. Such preparation may have included a contingency contract to be implemented in the home, appropriate school placement and programs, as well as appropriate social and recreational activities. Thus the adolescent transitions from a hospital program implemented by staff to a home program implemented by parents with both being under the supervision of the psychiatrist.

Therapeutic tasks include the following: instruction of parents in basic principles of operant technology and contingency management; revision, as appropriate, of the contingency contract with both the adolescent and the parents; prescription of alternatives to solve conflicts between the adolescent and the rest of the family; provision of informational feedback to the adolescent and parents regarding the antecedents and consequences of their behaviors (i.e., discrimination training); instruction to all parties in methods to evaluate the consequences of behavior prior to its occurrence; mediation of family disputes; and education of the adolescent, especially in the use of positive behavioral control versus aversive control. Consequently, although the psychiatrist remains the agent of the patient, his role may expand to represent the best interests of the family as a whole in that context.

As the therapeutic gains made in the hospital and subsequent outpatient treatment stabilize, the frequency and duration of therapy sessions can be reduced gradually through a fading procedure. Successful termination can be accomplished only if the adaptive behaviors of the adolescent come under the control of reinforcers current in his natural environment.

Summary

In this chapter applications of behavior technology to adolescent psychiatric hospitalization and subsequent outpatient follow-up have been reviewed. Basic theoretical considerations pertaining to respondent and operant technologies have been discussed with emphasis upon clinical applications of operant methodology. A review of applications pertaining to inpatient and residential treatment has been presented as well as a review of the relatively few reports pertaining to outpatient care. Finally, specific program methodology derived from ongoing adolescent hospital programs has been offered.

References

Alexander, F. (1963) The dynamics of psychotherapy in the light of learning theory. *Am. J. Psychiat.* 120:440–449.

Allyon, T., and N.H. Azrin. (1968) *The Token Economy: A Motivational System for Therapy and Rehabilitation.* New York: Appleton-Century-Crofts.

Allyon, T., and J. Michael. (1959) The psychiatric nurse as a behavioral engineer. *J. Exper. Anal. Behav.* 2:323–334.

Atthowe, J.M., Jr., and L. Krasner. (1968) A preliminary report on the application of contingent reinforcement procedures on a "chronic" psychiatric ward. *J. Abnor. Psychol.* 73:37–43.

Birnbrauer, J., M.M. Wolf, J. Kidder, and C.E. Tague. (1965) Classroom behavior of retarded pupils with token reinforcement. *J. Exper. Child Psychol.* 2:219–235.

Burchard, J.D., P.T. Harig, R.B. Miller, and J. Amour. (1976) New strategies in community-based intervention. In E. Ribes-Inesta and A. Bandura, eds., *Analysis of Delinquency and Aggression.* Hillsdale, N.J.: Lawrence Erlbaum.

Coleman, A.D., and S.L. Baker. (1969) Utilization of an

operant conditioning model for the treatment of character and behavior disorders in a military setting. *Am. J. Psychiat.* 125:1395–1403.

Davidson, W.S., and E. Seidman. (1974) Studies of behavior modification in juvenile delinquents: A review, methodological critique, and social perspective. *Psycholog. Bull.* 81:998–1011.

Ferster, C.B. (1965) Classification of behavioral pathology. In L. Krasner and L.P. Ullman, eds., *Research in Behavior Modification.* New York: Holt, Rinehart and Winston.

Ferster, C.B., and B.F. Skinner. (1957) *Schedules of Reinforcement.* New York: Appleton-Century-Crofts.

Foreyt, J.P., C.E. Rockwood, J.C. Davis, W.H. Desvousges, and R. Hollingsworth. (1975) Benefit-cost analysis of a token economy. *Prof. Psychol.* 6:26–33.

Gagnon, J.H., and G.C. Davidson. (1976) Asylums, the token economies, and the metrics of mental life. *Behav. Ther.* 7:528–534.

Goldiamond, I. (1974) Toward a constructional approach to social problems. *Behaviorism* 2:1–84.

Goldiamond, I., and J.E. Dyrud. (1968) Some applications and implications of the behavioral analysis for psychotherapy. *Res. Psychother.* 3:54–89.

Kagel, J.H., and R.C. Winkler. (1972) Behavior economics: Area of cooperative research between economics and applied behavior analysis. *J. Appl. Behav. Anal.* 5:335–342.

Kazdin, A.E., and R.R. Bootzin. (1972) The token economy: An evaluative review. *J. Appl. Behav. Anal.* 5:343–372.

Krapfl, J.E. (1974) Accountability through cost-benefit analysis. In D. Harshbarger and R.F. Maley, eds. *Behavior Analysis and Systems Analysis: An Integrative Approach.* Kalamazoo, Mich.: Behaviordelia.

Lawson, R.B., R.T. Green, J.S. Richardson, G. McClure, and R.J. Padina. (1971) Token economy program in a maximum security correctional hospital. *J. Nerv. Ment. Dis.* 152:199–205.

Liberman, R.P., C. Ferris, P. Salgado, and J. Salgado. (1975) Replication of Achievement Place model in California. *J. Appl. Behav. Anal.* 8:287–300.

Mann, R.A. (1976) Behavioral excesses in children. In H. Hersen and A.S. Bellack, eds., *Behavioral Assessment: A Practical Handbook.* New York: Pergamon Press.

Mann, R.A. (1975) Contingency contracting and operant behavior change: An exercise in applied behavior analysis. *Resources in Education*, October.

Mann, R.A., and G.R. Moss. (1973) The therapeutic use of a token economy to manage a young and assaultive inpatient population. *J. Nerv. Ment. Dis.* 157:1–9.

Moss, G.R., and J.J. Boren. (1971) Specifying criteria for completion of psychiatric treatment: A behavioristic approach. *Arch. Gen. Psychiat.* 24:441–447.

Moss, G.R., and R.A. Brown. (1978) *Adolescent Psychiatric Hospitalization: A Procedure Manual.* Newport Beach, Calif.: Behavioral Medicine Associates.

Moss, G.R., and R.A. Mann. (1978) A behavioral approach to the hospital treatment of adolescents. *Psychiat. Clin. North America* 1(2):263–275.

O'Leary, K.D., and W.C. Becker. (1967) Behavior modification of an adjustment class: A token reinforcement program. *Except. Children* 9:637–642.

Pavlov, I.T. (1927) *Conditioned Reflexes.* London: Oxford University Press.

Phillips, E.L. (1968) Achievement Place: Token reinforcement procedures in a home-style rehabilitation setting for "pre-delinquent" boys. *J. Appl. Behav. Anal.* 1:213–223.

Phillips, E.L., E.A. Phillips, D.L. Fixsen, and M.M. Wolf. (1971) Achievement Place: Modification of the behaviors of pre-delinquent boys within a token economy. *J. Appl. Behav. Anal.* 4:45–59.

Phillips, E.L., E.A. Phillips, M.M. Wolf, and D. Fixsen. (1973) Achievement Place: Development of the elected manager system. *J. Appl. Behav. Anal.* 6:541–561.

Rockwood, C.E., and J.P. Foreyt. (1976) Selecting patients for token economy treatment. *J. Behav. Ther. Exper. Psychiat.* 7:129–132.

Schwitzgebel, R.K. (1964) *Streetcorner Research: An Experimental Approach to Juvenile Delinquency.* Cambridge, Mass.: Harvard University Press.

Skinner, B.F. (1938) *Behavior of Organisms.* New York: Appleton-Century-Crofts.

Stuart, R.B., and L.B. Lott. (1973) Behavioral contracting with delinquents: A cautionary note. *J/ Behav. Ther. Exper. Psychiat.* 3:161–169.

Stumphauzer, J. (1976) Modification of delinquent behavior: Beginnings and current practices. *Adolescence* 11:13–28.

Tharp, R.G., and R.J. Wetzel. (1969) *Behavior Modification in the Natural Environment.* New York: Academic Press.

Thorndike, E.L. (1911) *Animal Intelligence: Experimental Studies.* New York: Macmillan.

Watson, J.B. (1924) *Behaviorism.* New York: Norton and Co.

Watson, J.B., and R. Rayner. (1920) Conditioned emotional reactions. *J. Exper. Psychol.* 3:1–14.

Weathers, L., and R.D. Liberman. (1975) Contingency contracting with families of delinquent adolescents. *Behav. Ther.* 6:356–366.

Winkler, R.C. (1970) Management of chronic psychiatric patients by a token reinforcement system. *J. Appl. Behav. Anal.* 3:47–55.

Wolf, M.M., D.K. Giles, and R.V. Hall. (1968) Experiments with token reinforcements in a remedial classroom. *Behav. Res. Ther.* 6:51–64.

Treatment of Emotional Disorders in Children and Adolescents

CHAPTER 5

Application of Biofeedback Training with Children

Paula Bram Amar

Introduction

Like many newly coined shorthand terms, the word "biofeedback" conveys an impression of the ultra-modern or mysterious. The concept of biofeedback training, moreover, carries with it an aura of control, which although not mysterious may sound imposing. The reality is more ordinary, perhaps even mundane.

The term "biofeedback" refers to monitoring an ongoing biologic process and feeding back information about the specific process to the individual in whose body it occurs. We have all used biofeedback devices regularly throughout our lives. For example, when I step on a bathroom scale, the dial face gives me back precise information about my body weight. The scale gives me in pounds information that I would otherwise have only as an approximation. I can then use the information given to modify my behavior—that is, either to reach for another helping of pie, or renounce pie altogether. That is biofeedback. A stethoscope will amplify an ordinarily faint signal; a thermometer will make changes in body temperature visible in a precise and uniform way. All of these could be considered rudimentary biofeedback devices.

What is new and significant about biofeedback training as a clinical tool is that more subtle, less consciously available physiologic processes are being monitored, displayed, and brought under conscious control. Biofeedback training means *monitoring* a physiologic signal *electronically* and *displaying* the amplified signal back to the person in an understandable and appealing way. Without electronics and engineering there would be no biofeedback.

In working with children's psychophysiologic disorders, we see a fascination on the part of the child with playing the "electronic biofeedback game." If the feedback display is made appealing through interfacing with slide projectors, electric trains, phonographs, and so on, then the child's cooperation can be maintained and motivation can be high.

In addition, since most psychophysiologic disorders have unpleasant symptoms, children are usually highly motivated to reduce the severity of the discomfort. Similarly, since children seem to learn physiologic control rapidly (perhaps because they have fewer inhibiting habits to unlearn), they are, with specific exceptions, excellent candidates for biofeedback training.

At a time when considerable sensationalism has been attached to all techniques of self-control including biofeedback, and where in the popular mind there is a confusion between biofeedback and "mind control," it becomes necessary to separate biofeedback from the myths about it. This is true in describing appropriate therapeutic use of biofeedback in treatment of psychophysiologic disorders, whether in adults or children.

Biofeedback training is one of many approaches

to the treatment of psychophysiologic disorders. It implies a model of psychosomatic disorder that Schwartz (1977) has called psychophysiological disregulation. It is an approach resting on the principles of operant conditioning, on information theory, and on cognitive self-control, dependent upon electronic engineering, and rooted in preventive medicine, which suggests that stress reduction or production of a low arousal state in a particular organ system will allow that system to regulate itself in a more optimal fashion. The theoretical model of treatment is a disregulation/regulation model (Schwartz, 1977). The therapist acts as a teacher or coach, thus placing the child in a familiar learning role.

In this chapter we will explore the history of biofeedback training, its experimental base, and its clinical application. The material presented includes a review of the current state of the art in biofeedback training, a description of the modification of self-control techniques to children's applications, and the case history of the treatment of an eleven-year-old child with multiple psychophysiologic disorders, including tension and migraine headaches. Attention will be given to the therapist's role in biofeedback training, as well as to suggestion, placebo effects, and the maintenance of therapeutic gain.

History

Until quite recently it was believed that while we could bring the striated muscles of our body under voluntary control, we could not consciously control the autonomic nervous system. Respiration, cardiac rate, systolic and diastolic blood pressure, sweating, blushing, intestinal contraction, blood flow, and vasodilation were considered to be beyond or outside the control of the higher cortical centers. They were also considered nonconditionable despite Pavlov's classic experimental production of salivation to a neutral stimulus.

In part, this belief derives from an accident in the history of science. Physiologists looked at, studied, and made inferences about the working of the interior of the body; they were the basic scientists upon whom medicine relied. Psychologists, on the other hand, were concerned with external behavior mediated by skeletal muscle. Consequently the work of Skinner and others in operant conditioning was never applied to the attempt to condition smooth muscle or gland. Indeed, Skinner even wrote that the conditioning of smooth muscle was not possible. And so a myth developed and was given the status of a fact: that the laws of learning, the processes of operant conditioning, apply only to external behaviors mediated by skeletal muscle and not to internal events—the working of smooth muscle and gland.

In the mid-1960's research being conducted by Neal Miller and students in experimental psychology at Rockefeller University began to break down that myth. By 1969 Miller and his research group had published a series of articles demonstrating conditioning of cardiac rates in curarized laboratory animals, using as a reward electrical stimulation of the brain as the contingent reinforcer.

Miller's animal studies provided the experimental evidence necessary to proceed with this work in humans. In addition to demonstrating increase and decrease in heart rate, Miller and his associate Leo DiCara presented studies in which blood pressure was conditioned. Both increases and decreases in systolic blood pressure were produced in curarized rats, independent of changes in heart rate or respiration. The same investigators then demonstrated conditioned changes in vasodilation, increasing blood flow into one ear while decreasing blood flow into the other. Glandular responses have been conditioned in a series of experiments on the intestinal contractions of curarized rats performed by Banuiozizi in 1972, and Miller has shown conditioning of urine formation by the kidneys in curarized rats who were rewarded by electrical brain stimulation.

With these animal studies, the foundation was laid to experimentally condition autonomic nervous system responses in humans. While experimental psychologists worked in their laboratories, physiologist Elmer Green of the Menninger Foundation was studying the physiologic self-control exhibited by yogis and adepts of the esoteric disciplines. In 1970, Green and his staff published their account of Swami Rama, who was able to increase and decrease his heart rate and direct blood flow to such an extent that an 11-point temperature shift was recorded between the right and left side of his right hand. Rama could also alter the electrical rhythms of his brain activity. When his brain was producing patterns that we have come to recognize on the electroencephalograph as stage 4 sleep; he was awake and conscious and was able later to report everything that had gone on in his presence.

This degree of control led Elmer and Alyce Green to speculate that if Rama could achieve such control, then perhaps others could also be able to learn to control physiologic states. They began to run a series of experiments in which individuals were asked to increase vasodilation in their finger to demonstrate conscious control over blood flow. These first experimental subjects were given training by sitting in a comfortable room and chair with a thermistor taped to a finger. They were asked to watch a light display. When a red light went on, the temperature in the finger was going up. They were instructed to keep the red light on as much of the time as possible. All of the original group were able to learn this much control. There was a serendipitous finding: a subject in this hand-warming experiment who had suffered from years of migraine headaches began to experience fewer headaches of less severity as she learned to warm her hands.

By 1972, Elmer and Alyce Green, Joseph Sargent, and Dale Walters at Menninger had trained 62 migraine patients in this technique of increased blood flow to the hands while decreasing blood flow in the mid-forehead region. Of these 62 patients, 74 percent were much improved 150 days after treatment was completed. However, 26 percent showed no reduction of headache activity or of drug use to control their headaches. We do not yet understand in what way the nonimproved patients differ from those who show improvement.

At about the same time Johann Stoyva and Thomas Budzynski at the University of Colorado Medical Center began to publish reports of successful treatment of tension headache through operant conditioning of tension levels of the frontalis muscle of the forehead. Bernard Engles at the research center at Baltimore City Hospital published reports of operant control of cardiac rates in cardiac arrhythmia patients; David Shapiro, Gary Schwartz, and Bernard Tursky published reports of control of blood pressure in human hypertension patients; and Barbara Brown and Joe Kamiya in independent laboratories in California reported operant control of brain wave rhythms in humans.

Stoyva and Budzynski have shown that giving headache patients feedback from the electromyographic activity of their frontalis muscle can help them to learn to relax. For this purpose feedback from the frontalis muscle is sufficient training. In a clinical application, 23 of 30 patients with tension headaches were improved by being trained to relax their frontalis muscles. These findings have now been replicated by Haynes and others at the University of South Carolina. With patients suffering from migraine headache, Sargent, Green, and Walters report that 46 of 62 patients benefited significantly from being trained to warm their hands, aided by feedback of information about the temperature of their hands. However, headaches are notoriously subject to placebo effects, and further studies are needed with additional controls and with longer-term follow-ups. Also, since the experimenters combined biofeedback training with autogenic training techniques based on autosuggestion, we are unable to specify the exact process through which headache control was achieved.

At the present time clinical investigators are continuing to apply biofeedback training to a number of specific medical problems. There is general agreement that a highly convincing therapeutic application of biofeedback has been in the treatment of premature ventricular contractions (PVCs). This work done by Weiss and Engel and by Engel and Bleecker utilizes computer-programmed equipment to operate a light display that allows the patient to identify a premature heart-beat and learn to hold his heart rate within a steady narrow range.

Sterman reports studies demonstrating that rewarding epileptic patients (child and adult) for a sensorimotor rhythm produced a marked decrease in their seizures, which after several months reached the lowest levels in their clinical histories. This work has been replicated with epileptic children by Lubar at the University of Tennessee, who has also begun application of brain-wave training to control hyperactivity in children.

Brudny, Grynbaum, and Korein used electromyographic feedback to train nine patients to control their spasmodic torticollis. Feedback from muscle contraction was first used to train the patients to decrease progressively the spasm of the contracted muscle and then to increase the contraction in the contralateral muscle. All patients showed some improvement. Three of them were able to control the abnormal positions of their heads for several hours without feedback, and three others have remained symptom-free for from several months to over one year. Because these latter three patients had had the symptoms for 3, 10, and 15 years, respectively, and had not responded to previous treatment, it seems unlikely that their marked improvement was attributable to any placebo effect. Ken Russ at Jewish Hospital in St. Louis has demonstrated similar results.

There have been clinical reports of biofeedback training in cases of fecal incontinence, of asthma control through feedback training, and of reduced insulin requirements in a juvenile diabetic through biofeedback-enhanced relaxation training. Case reports have been published on treatment of tic, muscle spasm, Raynaud's phenomenon, dysmenorrhea, and hyperactivity. Many of these applications are on the level of single case reports. Few studies have been completed with adequate control groups and follow-up.

Among the few adequately controlled clinical studies are those of Sargent, Green, and Walters in treatment of migraine; Budzynski and Stoyva in treatment of tension headache; Sterman et al. in seizure control in epilepsy, and Engel et al. in control of cardiac arrhythmia. This is a fertile area of research with many current clinical studies in progress and new advances appearing yearly.

Theory

An adequate review of the principles of operant conditioning, information theory, cognition and self-control, and physiologic disregulation lie beyond the scope of this chapter, and the interested reader is referred to basic works in these areas.

The key operant conditioning concept in biofeedback training can be stated as follows: *Any behavior that is immediately positively reinforced will increase in frequency.* Human beings, unlike laboratory animals, derive considerable satisfaction from their awareness of having done a task they set out to do. Even a small amount of progress in a desired direction is rewarding. Consequently, a person who sees a small light go on to indicate that he has produced brain waves of a given frequency or vasodilation of a given vessel or muscle potential decrease or increase of a given muscle rewards himself with an awareness of control that is pleasurable. This "inner smile" may be as potent a reward as praise or money, lollipops, or the smile of approval of another person. This inner smile or sense of accomplishment is intrinsically rewarding. It is, to switch conceptual frameworks, ego-syntonic, and therefore increases the likelihood of further change in the desired direction. These changes are reinforced on a 1:1 ratio schedule of reinforcement, which enhances rapid acquisition of skills, which are then shaped from small changes to changes of the magnitude necessary to produce symptom remission.

The two information-theory concepts upon which biofeedback training rests are the concept of feedback itself, of which biofeedback is simply one case; and the idea, as summarized by Gaardner (1976) that *"a variable cannot be controlled unless information about the variable is available to the controller."* Thus the biofeedback instrument, by electronically amplifying and displaying information about a subtle internal process, permits that process to change via a loop from person to monitoring instrument to person.

The disregulation model of psychosomatic illness, as developed by Schwartz (1975, 1976, 1977), states simply that *the body maintains itself in health through homeostasis.* When the normal homeostatic system breaks down either through assault from outside the body or from hypo- or hyperactivity in a particular system, illness results. The proponents of this model suggest that it is this diregulation that is being treated by giving the person information about the moment-to-moment operation of that disregulated system and giving him the responsibility to regulate that system with the aid of an information displaying electronic amplifier. Biofeedback rests primarily on both information display and on operant conditioning.

Applicability

At the present time, the range of application of biofeedback training is quite wide. Most of these applications, while based in theory, are empirical and are reported as single case studies or at best as weakly controlled experiments. As noted earlier, it will be some years before the controlled studies with sufficient follow-up are available.

Even less has been adequately documented in the treatment of children. The most compelling controlled experimental work has been done by B. Sterman at Sepulveda Veterans Hospital, by Barbara Brown in the same setting, and by Joel Lubar at the University of Tennessee, all working on the control of seizure activity in epileptic children. To motivate the children and hold their interest, Brown uses an electric train set which is set in operation by brain waves of the appropriate frequency. Lubar has developed a system with an interface to a portable TV showing cartoons, which is then activated by brain-wave activity in the desired range. The Lubars have also reported some success in training hyperactive children for attention span.

Individual reports have been made of treatment of children as young as four years. While our own experience has been largely with children of school age, in theory age is not a specific limiting factor; it has been suggested that the younger the patient is, the more readily he learns a new set of physiologic habits and can replace the older habit. Obviously, the younger the child, the more skilled the therapist must be in developing strategies for holding the child's interest and in obtaining home practice without arousing power or control issues between parent and child. Similarly, the younger child with a developmental predisposition toward magical thinking may attribute power or control to the biofeedback device, and this could be considered a limiting factor in biofeedback training in prelatency age children. Whether this does occur, and if so, under what circumstances, remains to be answered by carefully planned research. It is our feeling that training with prelatency age children should be undertaken only if symptom severity is such as to limit the child's normal development.

Biofeedback training can also be conceptualized as ego training—that is, training in self-control and self-regulation. This aspect of biofeedback training has been considered by Rickles, writing on the psychodynamics of biofeedback training (1976).

At this point it seems useful to comment on the family system of the child with a psychophysiologic disorder. It has been our observation, along with others working in treatment of children's psychophysiologic disorders, that one must not only treat the child but also treat a family system that may tend to maintain the illness through reinforcement of illness behavior (secondary gain). A well-meaning parent may have to learn how to provide attention to a child at times other than when the child has a headache or an asthmatic attack. Parents must also be helped to face any need they may have for a dependent child so that as the child's symptom subsides, the parent can build a comfortable relationship with the more independent child. Family dynamics could thus be a crucial factor in accepting a child in biofeedback training and one which must be evaluated accordingly.

Limitations

We have seen that biofeedback training is not a treatment per se but an application of information theory and operant conditioning to the development of control over a disregulated Physiological system. The more specific the symptom, the greater the likelihood of monitoring and displaying information about the specific event; therefore the possibility of conditioning the alternative response. Conversely, then, the more general the symptom, the less likely it is that biofeedback training will be helpful. For example, although relaxation training is useful in a general way toward reducing the autonomic arousal that produces increased acid secretion in ulcer, the more specific treatment would be to monitor acid secretion with a tiny, swallowed PH meter that would provide moment-by-moment information on acid secretion, a treatment not generally available.

One limitation on biofeedback training is thus a technical limitation. Without appropriate monitoring equipment or a way to monitor a specific system, one cannot effect change as readily or with any degree of certainty. Thus we do better with migraine headache than with generalized aches and pains or with a tummy ache, unless the tummy ache is the result of intestimal motility that *can* be monitored and specifically displayed.

Another limitation rests in the ability of the child to attend to the task at hand and to make the necessary effort to learn the control task. This general limitation may be modified both by the ingenuity of the therapist and by the development of attractive motivating reinforcement equipment.

Some more specific cautions and limitations also must be kept in mind before attempting biofeedback training. There have been reported cases of insulin requirements dropping markedly in diabetics acquiring feedback-assisted relaxation. In one such case where blood levels were not monitored regularly, an insulin overdose occurred.

Although there have been no reports of individuals disregulating a normally regulated system, controlled studies ruling out that possibility have not been done. Indeed, because biofeedback training as a therapeutic form is in its infancy, it should be approached cautiously, with due regard for all of the possible limitations and only after other less experimental forms of treatment have been considered and either attempted or ruled out.

Methods

Most biofeedback training takes place either in a laboratory experimental setting or in clinical practice. Although some psychiatrists, social workers, and technicians are now being trained in biofeedback techniques, most of the experimental and clinical work is being done by psychologists with backgrounds in psychophysiology and by clinical psychologists.

The material presented here is the result of the author's experience in direct clinical work in a university-based mental health setting in which biofeedback training was perceived as one approach to be used either alone or in combination with other forms of therapy. The mandate of our clinic was to treat everyone referred with a psychosomatic or psychophysiologic disorder; to find or devise a treatment plan; and to use that treatment plan in the attempt to facilitate change, growth, or simply symptom relief. Our understanding was that while no one should be turned away, a patient who did not present a specific psychophysiologic disorder could be treated in other sections within our mental health center and need not be seen in a clinic primarily devoted to psychophysiologic disorders. The patients treated in the clinic included children as well as adults, although adults represented the larger proportion. Consequently, we did not develop specific electronic devices for holding the interest of children.

Each treatment room was developed to look rather like a living room, with a recliner chair, a table to hold biofeedback consoles, several additional chairs, a desk, and so forth. The room is usually softly lit and kept free of distraction at the outset of treatment, although additional light and distraction may be added in the final stages of training in order to facilitate eventual transfer of the newly learned skill to the larger environment outside the office. The therapist sits with the child, first demonstrating the equipment and explaining its function, then modeling for the child the skill to be learned, and finally, serving as a coach or teacher. In that respect the role of the therapist could be likened to that of a coach, and biofeedback training to skill training in any set of complex learned behaviors. Biofeedback requires practice and gradual shaping.

Since latency age children are often entranced by and certainly familiar with games and skill learning in general, biofeedback becomes a rather natural part of their routine. The role the therapist will play is a familiar one, as is their own, and with some initial attention to explanation and to exploration of the setting, the child seems to swim naturally in the biofeedback training setting.

In order to minimize the secondary gain associated with sickness for the child, parents are asked to develop ways and times of paying attention to the child other than when they are practicing or when they are sick. The children are asked to keep records both of their practice sessions and of the frequency and intensity of their symptom. They are asked to bring their symptom records and homework practice sheets with them to each session, but not to review them with their parents. Similarly, parents are told what it is that the child is being asked to do, but are asked not to tell the child to practice or to request to see the child's symptom check sheets. We do this in order to place control in the hands of the child and to minimize the possibility of the kinds of power struggles parents may get into around piano or other lessons. Particularly since biofeedback is a process of developing self-regulation, or self-control, we want to enlist the child's cooperation in the process of working in his own behalf. Where we encounter resistance from parents toward the child assuming control or see early signs of power struggle over practice, biofeedback training is delayed and these issues are dealt with in more traditional therapy, family therapy, counseling, and so on.

Once the child and his family have been introduced to the concepts of biofeedback training and have become familiar with the setting, the equipment, and the information-gathering procedures, then biofeedback can begin. The child is asked to sit in a quiet, softly lit room either watching a light display for feedback or listening to a sound display which indicates desired change. In the beginning, change in the desired direction can be backed up with a material reinforcer—a small toy or a candy—or just with praise. We have not run controlled studies to demonstrate superiority of one form of back-up reinforcer over another or of one form of feedback information, but it is our impression that children respond quite well to smiles and praise of their performance, and that where material reinforcers are needed to sustain attention, they can be quickly phased out.

Acquisition and Transfer of Biofeedback Training Skill

There are four clearly distinct stages or phases of learning: acquisition, transfer, generalization, and retention. Fischer (1973) offers a framework for learning that appears to be a useful tool in looking at the way in which humans learn a new behavior or set of behaviors, with implications for evaluating transfer of biofeedback learning.

Essentially what has been stated here is that Phase 4 or mastery or overlearning leads to positive transfer of learning in which the learned behavior quickly generalizes to a new and like situation. *But* where the new behavior has been only partially learned, negative transfer may occur in which the new, imperfectly learned behavior may actively interfere with competing behaviors. Studies demonstration these findings lie beyond the scope of this chapter.

Below we see a chart adapted from Fischer's

work, based on the verbal statements of patients in biofeedback training. We have come to use these spontaneous verbal statements as feedback to the therapist for determining phase of treatment.

Assuming that the new behavior (relaxation or vasodilation or some other newly learned skill) has reached Phase 4, another aspect of the transfer situation must be considered. That is, how closely does the new situation in which the learned behavior is to occur resemble the one in which it developed. The more closely the training situation approximates the new situation, or the environment approximates the training setting, the greater will be the transfer. To state it in the reverse, the greater the *difference* between the training setting and the environment in which the new behavior is to occur, *the weaker* the transfer will be.

In behavior therapy, it has been clearly demonstrated that systematic desensitization results in decrease and eventual extinction of a *maladaptive* emotional response (fear or unusual anxiety). But the transfer of a newly learned behavior (assertiveness or cooperative play or even calm in exposure to the fearful stimulus) relies on practice and exposure in vivo. No water/drowning phobic has ever been cured without entering a swimming pool.

So we have three major elements involved in the transfer of biofeedback training:

1. Overlearning of the new behavior.
2. Degree of approximation of the learning setting to the setting in which it will be practiced.
3. Degree of practice or exposure to life situations.

Therapist

It has been noted that the role of the therapist is that of teacher or coach. In addition, the therapist has the added responsibility of serving to reassure, reinforce the newly emerging skill, trouble-shoot and avert problems either in skill aquisition or in family interactions, and maximize transfer out to the child's environment.

Considerable attention has been devoted in recent years to the question of adequate training for the therapist using biofeedback techniques. While some believe that there should be specific certification proceedures for a "biofeedbacker," most professionals in the Biofeedback Society of America believe that biofeedback is a tool to be utilized by an already qualified and certified professional who should, in addition to his professional training, have become familiar with psychophysiology, the electronics of biofeedback instrumentation, operant conditioning, and information theory, as well as related areas in psychodynamics, family dynamics, and behavioral approaches to medical prob-

Table 1. Four Phases in Development of a Well-Learned Action

Phase	*Organization*	*Transition Rule*
0	Behavior shows no particular organization with regard to task to be learned.	
Recognition of Problem 1	Behavior is relatively disconnected and irregular in performance, although parts of task may be performed well. Excitement is present. Behavior is goal-directed.	S. recognizes there is a task to be done or a goal to obtain.
Definition of Behavior 2	Response is slow to begin, but once underway is performed rapidly without pause.	General outline of task is defined.
New Behavior Components Practiced 3	Task is performed smoothly, ease of starting, but with spontaneous pauses during performance.	Components are differentiated.
Mastery 4	Performance is smooth and regular. Responding becomes habit, effortless—overlearned.	Components are integrated.

Source: K. Fischer, *The Organization of Simple Learning*, 1973.

lems. These areas of additional training are not, however, a substitute for warmth, empathy, and the intuitive factors playing so important a role in all therapies. It is quite likely that biofeedback research, like all other outcome research in psychotherapy, will be open to the question of the role of undefined therapist variables affecting outcome. This is but one more reason for placing biofeedback training in the hands of otherwise qualified and well-trained psychotherapists rather than create an altogether new discipline.

When biofeedback techniques begin to be taught more regularly in psychiatry residencies, in clinical psychology internships, and in social work practicums, there will be a gradual delineation of which areas of knowledge are vital to biofeedback therapeutic applications and which are not.

A Case Study

The following brief case report is typical of our experience in treatment of children with specific psychophysiologic disorders. It illustrates a frequently encountered set of problems in a receptive but not unusually motivated child in a fairly typical family structure. Although abbreviated for the sake of clarity, and altered slightly for confidentiality, the case is one that might be seen in any general practice using biofeedback training, and follows an expected course.

Susie was 11 years old when she was first seen in our clinic on referral from her parents and her family physician with a history of migraine focusing over the left eye, accompanied by vomiting and visual scotoma. She had also had a history of childhood allergy syndrome, including allergies to trees, grass, dust, mold, eggs, milk, and chocolate. Her allergies had produced asthma, and at age 2 she had been hospitalized with an acute asthmatic attack. There had been no further acute asthmatic attacks.

Susie was a tense, nail-biting child with a history of severe stomachache—sometimes accompanying her headache, but sometimes separate. The oldest child, with a much more easygoing younger brother, she was advanced in school, an all-A student, a girl scout who enjoyed camping trips and related activities. As a matter of fact, she was a thoroughly likable, intelligent, but hard-driving young lady. Like most of the children we saw in the clinic, Susie was intrigued at the prospect of doing biofeedback training and was particularly pleased at being asked to monitor and chart her own headaches, as well as maintain her own practice chart. Her mother was supportive and encouraging of Susie's efforts.

Biofeedback electromyographic training was begun on a twice-weekly basis. She learned Jacobson's technique of progressive relaxation rapidly and by the second session was displaying EMG readings at 1.4 microvolts per 32 seconds as monitored on

Table 2. Biofeedback Training

Phase	*Organization of Behavior*	*Verbal Statement*
0	No particular organization.	
1	Patient recognizes there is a problem. Begins biofeedback training. Observes fluctuation in feedback signal but has no control. Excitement and enthusiasm are present.	"What should I do?" "I don't know why it happens."
2	Change in desired direction is slow, but accelerates during training sessions.	"I think I know what to do, but I don't know how I'm doing it."
3	Change in desired direction is smooth, but frequent pauses occur.	"I do better when you don't watch me." "Sometimes I get it at home."
4	Performance is smooth, regular, consistent, and effortless—occurs automatically.	"I know what I'm doing." "I have control."

the BIFS electromyograph feedback instrument. She also spontaneously reported some hand warming and tingling sensations in her finger tips when she practiced her relaxation at home. Her mother confirmed that during the first weeks of treatment she did her relaxation homework twenty minutes daily as requested with no encouragement from her parents. In fact, her mother said that when practicing she looked "relaxed enough to be a plate of wet spaghetti." By the third week of EMG training, she was reporting spontaneous hand warming, and when monitored on the temperature training unit, was indeed producing a 5-degree finger temperature shift in 15 minutes (without training). When feedback in the form of a sound signal as well as a visual temperature reading was given, she rapidly learned to accomplish a 5- to 10- degree shift. We added distraction by bringing observers into the room, and Susie asked to demonstrate before her mother and younger brother as well. She practiced hard and seemed to enjoy what she was doing. Four weeks from the beginning of active treatment, Susie came in and reported having aborted a headache the previous Saturday. She said that when she felt the headache coming on, she went to her room, lay down, and warmed her hands as she has learned to do, and the headache went away. Her mother verified that this had happened in exactly the way she had described it. Susie had also begun to teach her mother how to do hand warming, and her mother, who also had headaches, had aborted a headache. Her mother also reported that Susie's hands were noticeably warmer to the touch after practicing, and both she and her mother were convinced that she had learned to do the task.

After 8 weeks of training, Susie had continued to produce very low EMG levels and to warm her hands 3 to 5 degrees within a 5-minute period. Her mother also reported: "It's good to see Susie so relaxed and happy. She hasn't had a headache in a month, and I have never seen her look so content." It is interesting that they also reported that her nail-biting had diminished, although no treatment for this symptom had been initiated. She seemed also to be happier and less tense. Susie, however, continued to have stomachaches. It was considered that she had accomplished the task of control over her migraine, and that perhaps at sometime in the future an attempt might be made to find a solution for her stomachache. In the meantime, Susie's physician had begun to work on the stomachache as specific allergy response. A follow-up conference had continued to be able to abort her headaches and had very few of them to abort. A semi-restricted allergy diet has been of help in controlling her stomachaches. She has continued to do her relaxation, and it would appear that her ability both to control muscle relaxation and to maintain hand temperature control has continued. Although Susie's treatment follows the fairly standard pattern for migraine treatment, it is of interest generally to notice the rapidity with which this young lady learned both the task of relaxation and hand temperature control. On the basis of this and other experiences in treating children, we may speculate that children are able to learn these tasks rapidly and well, and perhaps by catching and re-regulating a poorly controlled system in childhood, at an age where learning is more rapid and new habits become more easily conditioned, we may be able to relieve a great deal of subsequent misery.

As in this case, a typical course of biofeedback training will run about 24 sessions—that is, twelve weeks of twice-weekly one-hour sessions. Follow-up with booster biofeedback sessions on a monthly basis may be necessary for about six months. It should also be explained to both parents and child that there is no set time period for learning a biofeedback skill. Some individuals learn more quickly, some more slowly; all who try learn to some extent, but not always in the same time. Since many children try to compete against others or against the biofeedback device itself, and since the effort of competing is counterproductive in learning a skill that can only be mastered through passive attention, the therapist must minimize an expectation of fast response and thereby prevent the sense of failure that can occur in the beginning phase. In most behavioral self-control programs, the attempt is made to arrange the teaching process in small enough steps to guarantee success—both day by day and in the long run.

As one particular intervention in behavioral self-control, biofeedback training develops in a step progression from the simple to the complex. Just as we do not expect a child to start reading by paragraphs in an encyclopedia, we do not expect a patient to make 5-degree hand temperature shifts in the first five minutes.

We begin by teaching the patient to recognize changes of tenths of a degree and to accomplish a change either up or down of two- or three-tenths of a degree. As in sports training, once the basic idea is mastered, then one can work for greater minutes before learning to make the same shift in five minutes. She learned to take time to practice relaxing when she had no headache before trying to use her newly developed skill when she felt the headache coming, and always before it was fully developed.

Summary and Conclusion

Biofeedback training with children is, as we have suggested, an extension of previously developed behavioral self-control systems. It represents a direct intervention in the functioning of a disregulated physiologic system with the specific goal of enhancing system regulation, establishing a new internal equilibrium, and reducing or eliminating a specific system. Change, however, generalizes and produces change in other systems as the person establishes a new internal balance and a new relation to the family and to others in the larger environment.

Thus biofeedback training, while a specific intervention in the physiologic sense, may nevertheless initiate a more general change in the psychological sense. The practitioner using biofeedback thus functions as more than a rehabilitation technician. Biofeedback training, as we see it, is a tool to be incorporated into a treatment program including family intervention and assistance to the child in incorporating prohealth behavior into his everyday life.

We do not yet fully understand the role which placebo effect and suggestion play in biofeedback training, and considerable research effort will probably go into clarifying this issue. From a clinical standpoint, however, the issue is less vital. If these techniques work to remediate symptoms that interfere with normal development and healthy function, then we as clinicians are justified in using them while we wait to learn whether the "active" ingredient is biofeedback or suggestion. Here the issue is one of weighing the value to be gained from treatment against the uncertainties of a newly developing modality of treatment. Certainly if another more well established treatment is available, that is the first treatment choice.

Biofeedback training as a treatment form is new; it has not yet fully emerged from the experimental stage, and even less so in application to children. As Neal Miller, the experimental psychologist and grandfather of biofeedback training, urged the members of the Biofeedback Research Society at their seventh annual meeting: "Be bold in what you attempt in biofeedback and modest in what you claim." The clinical practitioner using biofeedback in treatment of children is similarly enjoined to be knowledgeable, daring in concept, imaginative in practical application, and conservative in general approach. We are at the forefront of a new approach to treatment, an approach that brings together physiology, psychodynamics, family systems theory, and information and learning theory. Such a convergence will bring with it as many questions as answers. Inevitably, the coming years will have to justify the answers offered, as well as answer the questions raised.

References

Amar, P.B. (1976) Biofeedback; Myth or method? *Medical Comm.* 4:3.

Amar, P.B. (1974) Biofeedback in multimodality treatment. Unpublished Presentation, Biofeedback Research Society Annual Meeting, Colorado Springs, Colorado.

Amar, P.B. Transfer of training: From clinic to everyday world. Abs. *Proceedings Biofeedback Research Society,* 1977.

Benson, H. (1975) *The Relaxation Response.* New York: Morrow.

Borkovec, T.D. (1976) Physiological and cognitive processes in the regulation of anxiety. In G. Schwartz and D. Shapiro, eds., *Consciousness and Self-Regulation: Advances in Research.* New York: Plenum Press, pp. 261 -312.

Budzynski, T.H., J.M. Stoyva, and C.S. Adler. (1970) Feedback-induced muscle relaxation: Application to tension headache. *Behav. Ther. Exper. Psychiat.* 1: 205–211.

Budzynski, T.H., J.M. Stoyva, C.S. Adler, and D.J. Mullaney. (1973) EMG biofeedback and tension headache: A controlled outcome study. *Psychosom. Med.* 35: 484–496.

Brudny, J., B.B. Grynbaum, and J. Korein, (1974) Spasmodic torticollis; Treatment by feedback display of EMG—A report of nine cases. *Arch. Phys. Med. Rehab.* 55:403.

Diamond, S., and J. Franklin. (1976) Biofeedback: Choice of treatment in childhood migraine. *Biofeedback and Self-Regulation* 1:3.

Engel, B.T., and E.R. Bleecker. (1974) Application of operant conditioning techniques in the control of the cardiac arrhythmias. In P.A. Obrist et al., eds., *Cardiovascular Psychophysiology.* Chicago: Aldine, pp. 456–476.

Finley, W.W., and C.A. Niman. (1977) Electrophysiologic behavior modification of frontal EMG in cerebral palsied children. *Biofeedback and Self-Regulation* 2:1.

Fischer, K. (1973) *The organization of Simple Learning.* Chicago: Markham Press.

Fowler, J.E., and T.H. Budzynski, (1976.) Effects of an EMG biofeedback relaxation program on the control of diabetes: A case study. *Biofeedback and Self-Regulation* 1:1.

Friar, L.R., and J. Beatty. (1976) Migraine: Management by trained control of vasoconstriction. *J. Clin. Consult. Psychol.* 44:46–53.

Gaardner, K., and P. Montgomery. (1977) *Clinical Biofeedback: A Procedural Manual.* Baltimore: Williams & Wilkins.

Greenfield, N.S., and R.A. Sternbach, eds. (1972) *Handbook of psychophysiology.* New York: Holt, Rinehard and Winston, 1972.

Jacobson, E. (1938) *Progressive Relaxation,* 2nd ed. Chicago: University of Chicago Press.

Johnson, W.G., and A. Turin. (1975) Biofeedback treatment of migraine headache: A systematic case study. *Behav. Ther.* 6:394–397.

Kotses, H., and K.D. Glaus. (1976) The effect of operant conditioning of the frontalis muscle on the peak respiratory flow in asthmatic children. *Biofeedback and Self-Regulation* 1:3.

Lubar, J., and W.W. Bahler. (1976) Behavioral management of epileptic seizures following EEG biofeedback training. *Biofeedback and Self-Regulation* 1:1.

Lubar, J., and M. Shouse. (1976) EEG and behavioral changes in hyperkenetic child concurrent with training of the sensorimotor rhythm. *Biofeedback and Self-Regulation* 1:3.

Mackintosh, J.J., (1974) *The Psychology of Animal Learning.* New York: Academic Press.

Marks, I., and M. Gelder. (1965) Controlled retrospective study of behavior therapy. *Brit. J. Psychiat.* 1:201–216.

Meichenbaum, D. (1976) Cognitive factors in biofeedback therapy. *Biofeedback and Self-Regulation* 3:551–573.

Miller, N.E., L.V. DiCara, H. Solomon, J.M. Weiss and B. Dworkin. (1970) Learned modifications of autonomic functions: A review and some new data. *Circ. Res.* 26/27 (suppl. 1):3.

Miller, N.E. (1969) Learning of visceral and glandular responses. *Science* 163:434.

Miller, N.E. (1972) Interactions between learned and physical factors in mental illness. *Semin. Psychiat.* 4:239.

Miller, N.E. (1975) Clinical applications of biofeedback; Voluntary control of heart rate, rhythm, and blood pressure. In H. Russek, ed., *New Horizons in Cardiovascular Practice.* Baltimore: University Park Press.

Sargent, J.D., E.E. Green, and E.D. Walters. (1972) The use of autogenic feedback training in a pilot study of migraine and tension headaches. *Headache* 12: 120–124.

Sargent, J.D., E.E. Green, and E.D. Walters. (1973) Preliminary report on the use of autogenic feedback techniques in the treatment of migraine and tension headaches. *Psychosom. Med.* 35:129–135.

Sargent, J.D., E.D. Walters, and E.E. Green. (1973) Psychosomatic self-regulation of migraine headaches. In L. Birk, ed., *Biofeedback: Behavioral Medicine.* New York: Grune & Stratton, pp. 55–68.

Schwartz, G.E. (1977) Psychosomatic disorders and biofeedback: A psychobiological model of disregulation. in J. Maser, and M. Seligman, eds., *Psychopathology: Experimental Models.* San Francisco: W.H. Freeman.

Sterman, B.D. (1973) Neurophysiological and clinical studies of sensorimotor EEG biofeedback training: Some effects on epilepsy. *Semin. Psychiat.* 5:507.

Stoyva, J.M., and T.H. Budzynski. Cultivated low arousal—an anti-stress response? In L. V. DiCara, ed., *Recent Advances in Limbic and Autonomic Nervous Systems Research.* New York: Plenum Press, pp. 369–394.

Weiss, T., and B.T.Engel, (1973) Operant conditioning of heart rate in patients with premature ventricular contractions. In L. Birk, ed., *Biofeedback: Behavioral medicine.* New York: Grune & Stratton, pp. 79–100.

Wickramasekera, I. (1973) Temperature feedback for the control of migraine.*J. Behav. Ther. Exper. Psychiat.* 4:343–345.

Wolpe, J. (1958) *Psychotherapy by Reciprocal Inhibition.* Stanford: Stanford University Press.

Yates, A. (1970) *Behavior Therapy.* New York: Wiley.

CHAPTER 6

Pharmacotherapy

Joel P. Zrull

Introduction

In 1906 the author of a textbook on pediatrics recommended the following treatment for habit chorea or habit spasm: adequate diet, Fowler's solution (containing arsenic) quinine and strychnine (Carr, 1906). He suggested that if this was not effective, bromides could be added. Another author suggested that hysteria should be treated with aromatic spirits of ammonia and apomorphine in emetic doses (Chapin and Pisek, 1911). Bromides might be helpful and valerian, asafetida, and paraldehyde were substitutes for apomorophine. Their diagnostic categories were somewhat obscure and the medications available were multiple. The state of the art from these perspectives is quite the same today. There also remains difficulty viewing treatment of the child as unique, not always acknowledging that whatever is done to alter his state may likewise alter his development.

This chapter then will approach the clinical use of psychoactive medications, concentrating on it as a form of therapy with children and drawn from what has been learned these seventy years since Dr. Carr's book. It will include understanding the emotional effects of being on a drug, relating the applicability of the use of medications to developmental considerations, producing a clinical methodology for treating children with psychoactive medications, and finally, placing psychopharmacotherapy in relationship to other therapies. The latter part of the chapter will list some of the medications currently being used to treat children's behavior. It should, however, be apparent that this portion of the chapter will be as effusive as the quotes from Drs. Carr, Chapin, and Pisek, since in a few more years many of these medications will in likelihood be obsolete.

Historical Perspectives

The use of behavior-altering medications with children has been described for many years, attested to by the earlier quotations. However, the development of a systematic pharmacotherapy specifically for children began only in the 1930's. Tracing the use of central nervous system stimulants in child therapy could be seen as a history of childhood psychopharmacotherapy. In 1937, Bradley gave a description of the use of amphetamine for a disorder unique to children and with a response equally as unique to them.Through the 1940's, Bradley and other workers continued the exploration of the use of amphetamine with hyperactive children, broadening the numbers of children treated with the medication (Bakwin, 1948; Bender and Cottington, 1942; Cutts and Jasper, 1939; Lindsley and Henry, 1942; Molitch and Eccles, 1937; Moskowitz, 1971). In the 1950's, d-amphetamine was introduced and the fewer side effects with this medication made it even more usable. (Bradley, 1950; Ginn and Hohman, 1953). Late in the 1950's and early 1960's, methylphenidate was recognized as a competitor to d-amphetamine, one which had somewhat lessened side effects (Conners and Eisenberg, 1963; Knobel, 1962; Zimmerman and Burgermeister, 1958). The interest of investigators turned to the methodology being used (Fisher, 1959; Forster, 1961), including how the children were classified (Fish, 1960; Fish and Shapiro, 1965; Laufer and Denhoff, 1957), the use of blind studies (Chessick and McFarland, 1963; Conners, Eisenberg, and Barcai, 1962; Cytryn, Gilbert, and Eisenberg, 1960; Zrull et al., 1966). and careful dose-response evaluations.

During this era, the use of these medications also came under public scrutiny, and another type of investigation ensued (Report, 1971). In 1971, a blue-ribbon panel appointed by the Department of Health, Education and Welfare looked into the overuse of psychoactive medications when the classrooms in a large Midwestern city were thought to be populated by significant numbers of children given medications for disturbed behavior. This investigation gave support to the premises that medications when used for specific reasons, after thorough diagnostic study, and in the context of a total treatment plan were significant aids in the treatment of children's behavior problems.

In the 1970's, the use of other stimulant drugs was introduced with l-amphetamine (Arnold et al., 1972), imipramine (Huessy and Wright, 1970), caffeine (Schnackenberg, 1973), and pemoline (Conners et al., 1962). During this present decade increasing clarity of the classification of those behaviors responding to the CNS stimulants has occurred (Cantwell, 1975; Wender, 1975). Because the medications now have been used for prolonged periods, follow-up studies are beginning to appear (Mendelson, Johnson, and Stewart, 1971; Minde, Weiss, and Mendelson, 1972; Weiss et al., 1975). These have been helpful in further delineating side effects (Safer, Allen, and Barr, 1972). Advances in the understanding of the central nervous system have allowed further speculation about the etiology of the disorder (Satterfield, Cantwell, and Satterfield, 1974; Wender, 1975). With continuing refinements, the mode of action of the drugs will also come under further scrutiny, the future, no doubt, holding more understanding of brain behavior processes.

CNS stimulants, of course, were not the only medication being used with children during these forty years. Other classes of medications have been used effectively with children and added to the understanding of children's behavior problems. During the 1940's and 50's investigators were looking into the use of anticonvulsants in childhood behavior problems, especially those with aggressive outbursts (Fisher, 1959; Pasamanick, 1951).

The 1950's also saw the introduction of tranquilizers such as diphenhydramine (Fish, 1960, 1968), meprobamate (Kraft et al., 1959), hydroxyzine (Piuk, 1963), and in the 1960's, the benzodiazepines (D'Amato, 1962; Greenblatt and Shader, 1974; Pilkington, 1916; Piuk, 1963), leading to their use in children. However, the results of the use of these medications were not as dramatic or easily defined as those with CNS stimulants.

Major tranquilizing agents were introduced in the 1950's, and during that period until now the use of drugs such as the phenothiazines (Alderton and Hoddinott, 1964; Campbell, 1975; Fish, 1960; Fish, Shapiro, and Campbell, 1966; Garfield et al., 1962; Gatski, 1955; Millichap, 1968; Shaw et al., 1963; Tarjan, Lowery, and Wright, 1957; Werry et al., 1966), thioxanthenes (Campbell et al., 1970; Fish, Shapiro, and Campbell, 1966; Oettinger, 1962; Pilkington, 1916; Simeon et al., 1974), butyrophenones (Claghorn, 1972; Cunningham, Pillai, and Rogers, 1968; Engelhardt et al., 1973; Faetra, Dooher, and Dowling, 1970), and others have been investigated. These medications have been used for a variety of symptoms determined by their use in adults such as hallucinations and other psychotic manifestations, extreme agitation, and aggressive behavior. More specific to children, the drugs have also been investigated for hyperactivity (Alderton and Hoddinott, 1964; Millichap, 1968; Werry et al., 1966) and tics (Lucas, 1967; Lucas, Kauffman, and Morris, 1967; Shapiro et al., 1973). The length of the use of this medication is adding to the investigation of longer-term effects of medication on children (McAndrew, Case, and Treffert, 1972).

The use of antidepressants with children has been more difficult to investigate, since the existence of clinical depression in children has been less well defined. Earlier use of antidepressant drugs in children was in enuresis (MacLean, 1960; Pouissant and Ditman, 1965) and hyperactivity (Huessy and Wright, 1970; Winsberg et al., 1972, 1975), studies showing their efficacy in these two areas. More recent clinical studies exploring depression in the child (Cytryn and McKnew, 1972, 1974; Poznanski, Krahenbuhl, and Zrull, 1976; Poznanski and Zrull, 1970) may produce greater interest in determining the use of antidepressants with children (Frommer, 1967; Gittelman-Klein and Klein, 1970; Lucas, Lockett, and Grimm, 1965). The emergence of data describing manic-depressive disturbances in children has prompted the investigation of the use of lithium carbonate (Annell, 1969; Dyson and Barcai, 1970), which has also been studied in the agitated psychotic child (Campbell et al., 1972).

Theoretical Considerations: Emotional Aspects

It is generally understood that the effect of a medication taken by an individual has both a physiologic and emotional aspect. The emotional aspect is the most perplexing, since measuring it must take into account a series of events and states of mind. These begin with the attitude of the physician prescribing the medication and extend at least to the outcome of the response within the individual and his interactions.

The attitude of the physician cannot be overemphasized. If he views the child as bad and the medication is given in a disciplinary fashion, it will be felt by the child, who will no doubt view treatment as punishment. The physician who uses the medication to ensure that the patient does not return can be sure a certain number of his patients and their parents will feel rejected. Little faith in the use of a drug or lack of knowledge about it will also be communicated. Seeing the medication as an accepted therapeutic device to help a child and his family solve problems under his care should be the least a physician should offer.

The process of measuring response of a child to medication he receives is complicated by the manner in which he arrives at the office of the physician. Children seldom determine on their own that treatment for their behavior is needed and thus must come at the direction of someone in their environment. It could be one of many caretakers, but most often, the child is brought to the doctor at the direction of his parent or teacher. It then becomes problematic as to whom is the responder to the medication. Depending on the level of development of the child, his willingness to cooperate, his state of emotional intactness, and only if he is asked about his response, the child may become the observer of his own responses. It is still, however, a dramatic event for the physician when the child himself says he feels better on a medication, or acknowledges its need when he sees a change in his behavior. Communication about the medication and inquiries about responses are prequesities to the child's involvement in the process.

The physician, of course, can rely on his own observation of the child as a method of determining response. However, the child is not usually being given the medication for behavior seen in the doctor's office, and outside observations are necessary. Understanding this and requesting the information is all part of the process of giving psychoactive medication to children.

The parents or teacher being those who often request help for a child also become potential responders to the medication. If the parents request help, they often do it to relieve their own problems in handling the child's behavior, or what they perceive as the child's anguish. Obviously the observations depend on the parents' subjective responses as well as any objective changes they see in the child. If the teacher requests help for the child, a further measure of complexity is introduced. If the parents disagree with the teacher (or the physician disagrees), the parental response can be expected to reflect these feelings to some degree and thus affect the outcome.

The teacher, too, has her own attitude that must be understood to be able to review critically and utilize her observations. She may be looking for a way to manage her classroom better and medicating the child may be seen as the way to do it. Her attitude about what her classroom should be like and the way the children should act within it will reflect in her responses to the child's medication. Her expectations for the specific child and his potential will color her responses. At the same time, her observations are critical and can be the most objective.

Needless to say, the child who is being treated as an inpatient or in a residential center has the milieu to replace the parents. The milieu, too, has expectations of its own, and these must be understood in determining responses as observed by its members. Discussions about the use of medication and in-service training can add to the objectivity of their observation. In any event, the behavior being dealt with is subjectively felt by all of the responders, and in some measure, subjective responses are as important as those that are entirely objective.

To understand those emotional factors better in the response to medication, it is important to be aware of the conscious, or unconscious, meaning of taking medication. The child often perceives himself as going to the doctor because of something "bad" that he did. Thus the continuing use of medication may be a reminder that he has done something bad, or continues to be bad. It may also be presented to him as a controlling force over his behavior. If rebellious, he may need to react to that control. If dependent, he may assume that all the control is in the capsule and he no longer needs to exercise his own.

The child may also harbor concerns about whether he is or is not "crazy" and the medication be seen as that which prevents his craziness. As long as he takes the medication, it is an indication that others see him as potentially "crazy." Medication may be seen as the only source of survival, and dependency thus develops. This is less frequently seen in children than in adults, primarily because they are not usually involved with treatment by their own will.

Side effects are the basis for many erroneous and most often unconscious fantasies about medication. A sense of well-being can be interpreted as strength derived from the medication and suggest that the child may be more powerful while on the drug. Feelings of dizziness, drowsiness, nausea, or other such malaise may suggest the medication is harmful and produce fantasies about poisoning. In any event, the child who is better informed about why he is taking medication, and what it is to do, is better able to make effective use of it.

Parents also view medication in light of their own expectations, fears and knowledge. The parents may be suspicious of the use of medication and fear that their child will be "drugged." During the time he is being treated these parents no doubt will be concerned as to whether he will be addicted or at least see the use of medication as a crutch. This often reflects the parents' own responses to similar medications. Side effects, of course, enhance the parents' suspiciousness relative to medications. To be sure, it is appropriate for the parent to be concerned about harmful effects of the medication, but not to the extent that it inhibits positive results.

Control over the child's behavior is often a central issue in treating him. If the parents perceive the drug as producing control, they will respond according to their interpretation of that control. With guilt over their own inability to control, or with the fear of losing their control, they may find the medication's effectiveness unacceptable and attempt to stop or undermine treatment. On the other hand, they may be dependent or exhausted to the extent that they abrogate all control to the medication, and in essence feel little direct responsibility for the child. As with the child, thorough understanding of the medication and its use will help to divert from untoward results.

Many of the factors discussed above lead to and produce the elusive effect known as placebo. This obviously can enhance or detract from the physiologic effects of medication. Authors have demonstrated placebo effects of from 30% to 50% in studies of drugs using placebo as one of a series of treatments. It is clear that placebo effect is influenced by the attitudes and emotional state of the child receiving the medication, his parents, other caretakers, and the prescribing physician. All of these must be taken into account as the physician approaches the prescription of medication for the treatment of children's emotional and behavioral problems.

Applicability: Developmental Considerations

Probably the most unique aspect of giving medications to children is that the child is in the process of physical and psychological growth. It is conceivable that besides any immediate alteration in behavior produced by the drug, the child's development may be altered in a fashion that is progressive, inhibiting, or retrogressive. Other than the studies relating growth retardation to the use of CNS stimulants, little definitive material has been written. Thus, the discussion of this area must be largely speculative.

In the past, few clinicians or investigators used medications with the preschool child. However, as familiarity has been developed in using medication, the use of them with younger children has increased. It is hard to determine what the long-term effect of drugs on the ever-developing neural processes and endocrinologic system will be. However, as modes of action of the medications are further understood, these outcomes will no doubt be clearer.

The effect on the psychologic interactions of the infant or toddler, however, can in some measure be predicted. The infant who suddenly changes from a squirming, hypertonic, irritable bit of animal life to a calm, responsive, cooing baby will no doubt be positively disposed to his mother's care. The mother, in turn, will be more positively oriented toward her baby. On the other hand, if the child regresses to a sleepy, hypotonic, motionless state, his ability to respond to the development-producing aspects of mothering will be limited. The understanding of the use of medications must include finding the zone of effectiveness most productive to development.

More is known about the effect of these medications on the development of the school-age child. It is known that some drugs will enhance the cognitive performance of children, although it is not clear whether the child will in fact learn better, or whether he will retain better what he has learned. The child whose behavior has altered from intrusive, aggresive, antagonizing, or disturbing to receptive, happy, and acceptable, with channeled aggression, will better be able to react to family and peers alike. This of course ensures the development of those relationships necessary to the development of the individual. However, if the child is sleepy or affectively blunted while on the medication, he may not be available for, or more enthusiastic about, the learning situation or the interactive experiences at home or at play.

The adolescent presents a problem with his developmentally unstable endocrine system and rapidity of physical growth. Determining dosages that will be productive represents a challenge to the clinician. The concerns of the adolescent over his emotional intactness may cause paralyzing anxiety, and the use of a medication that quells this anxiety may make him able to continue in his development, both in relationships and learning. A medication that produces a sense of depersonalization, on the other hand, may add to the already inhibiting anxiety. Growth of the adolescent's self-concept and ego ideal depend on a sense of well-being and adequacy. The medication can produce thisif wisely used, or it may increase dependency and floings of inadequacy detrimental to his growth.

It appears that, as with many of the treatment methods in psychiatry, a proper balance must be reached. In regard to development, this is especially true and should determine some of the principles in the use of medication with children.

Clinical Methods

The use of psychoactive medication is directed at the alteration of behavior, unpleasant feelings, and incapacitating states of mind. As such, it cannot be used to treat a diagnosis, but rather certain aspects of an individual's mental and emotional functioning. In an attempt to objectify the use of psychoactive drugs, discrete symptoms should become the target for the medication. For instance, if anxiety is manifested by whininess in a child, his whining could be expected to be altered by the medication, If the anxiety was manifested by difficulty in sleeping, the expected symptom change would be the return to normal sleep patterns. In depression, a change from unhappiness to a sense of well-being would be the looked-for change. If, however, the depression were manifested by irritability, aggressive behavior, or poor concentration, these would become target symptoms. In the hyperkinetic syndrome, any one or more of the symptoms of hyperactivity, short attention span, and emotional lability would be noted for change. Delusions, hallucination, silliness or isolation could be targeted in the child with psychosis. These are not exhaustive lists, but represent some of the symptoms that could be the specific target of the medication. The target symptom, however, must always be viewed within the context of a thorough understanding of the child, his development, his current functioning, his problems, his family, and his daily life.

To enable the physician to evaluate further the effectiveness of his treatment, he must be knowledgeable about and familiar with the use of the medication prescribed. A reasonable repertoire would be one containing basic medications that are consistently used. This list of drugs should obviously be kept at the least possible number to alleviate effectively the symptoms encountered in the children seen by the doctor. It can be understood from the foregoing that if combinations of drugs are to be used in children, the following evaluation is made more complex. However, if this is employed, the necessity for keeping track of target symptoms becomes even more essential. The target symptoms for each medication must be delineated and then followed consistently. The effects of each medication should be thoroughly understood by the physician and his familiarity with the drugs used becomes essential.

As in most treatment, pharmacotherapy can be divided into initial, ongoing, and termination phases. Initiating drug therapy requires no less rigor than beginning psychotherapy. A thorough understanding of the history of the presenting problem and an evaluation of the child's development, including a past medical history, family history, and school history, should be obtained from the parents and child where possible. The child's current functioning should be assessed and an evaluation of his mental status should be done. Physical examination is equally important and helpful in determining dosage levels, and should include a thorough neurological examination. The use of an electroencephalogram would depend on the indications found within the physical and neurological examinations. Depending on the medications anticipated to be used, appropriate laboratory studies should be obtained as a baseline.

Psychological or educational testing may be helpful diagnostically, but can also serve as a baseline, especially when cognitive functioning is to be a target symptom. Following the diagnostic evaluation and when the treatment plan is being formulated, target symptoms should be delineated. In this way, if medications are to be used, a reasonable choice can be made.

The interpretative interview with the parents and child, where appropriate, should include a discussion of the medication including why it is being used, what one can expect as a result of its use, and any side effects that might be expected. The interview should also include the parents' and child's discussion of their concerns and expectations. Since the placebo effects can be enhancing to the effectiveness of the drug, suggestions should be used appropriately. The dosage schedule should be discussed with the parents and child and indications obtained that they understand the schedule.

Pharmacotherapy should be viewed as supportive therapy and coupled with an interrelationship with the therapist. The therapist may be the treating physician or an adjunctive therapist. The therapy may consist of brief follow-up visits or longer psychotherapeutic interviews. They may be spaced at weekly intervals or longer, but never less frequently than once a month. Initially, visits are best at weekly intervals to determine if an adequate response is being obtained and if there are any serious side effects. Side effects must be asked about throughout treatment.

A definite plan for follow-up with school personnel is essential in the initial phase of treatment and should be continued into the ongoing phase. This is a sensitive period when the patient and his family require the close attention of the therapist. An ongoing phase of treatment is attained when a response is obtained and maintenance at that level is continued.

As more precise laboratory measures for monitoring actual changes in the CNS become available, they should be included in the weekly to monthly visits. For instance, if EEG is changed by a medication, it should be used as a follow-up at appropriate intervals to insure proper dose-response levels. Where biochemical determinations of blood or urine samples can be clinically meaningful, such as in lithium or tricyclic drug administration respectively, they, too, should be part of the follow-up. Psychologic and educational testing may also be precise enough to be part of the follow-up during the ongoing phase of treatment. The above measures move the monitoring of the medication from observation of symptom removal to a clearer awareness of the functionality of the child while on medications.

Termination is an important part of pharmacotherapy and must be contemplated at the initiation of treatment. Criteria should be outlined at that time, and may include definite time periods, a certain level of functioning, or behavioral and emotional changes agreed upon between child, parent, and therapist. Termination may be preceded by a series of planned vacations from appropriate types of medication. For instance, if a short-acting CNS stimulant is being given to control hyperactivity at school which is recessed for the summer, the medication may also be recessed. The recesses may be as frequent as each weekend when the child is not attending school. In any event, pharmacotherapy should have a planned beginning and termination.

Comparison

Pharmacotherapy with children should be viewed as a form of supportive therapy. As previously stated, it of necessity involves an interrelationship with a therapist, whether it be the physician or another therapist. However, the use of medication with the child can also be seen as behavioral modification, for a change in behavior (R) can be related to the administration of a pill (S). Medications may produce relaxation and thus function as a form of relaxation therapy. Drugs have been used to reveal preconscious thought, in much the same way as hypnosis.

It must be understood, however, that the use of medications should in no way substitute for more definitive therapy. Thus if a phobic reaction is to be treated effectively, intensive psychotherapy or sophisticated behavioral modification should more likely be the treatment of choice. The use of a medication does not eliminate the need for the development of a relationship between the therapist and the child with serious ego impairment. The school phobic and his family still require crisis intervention directed to the entire family. Medication should in no way make it less important for parents to acknowledge their involvement in their child's disturbance.

A note of caution about the use of medication must be sounded. Its use can be that of an expedient economic alternative to what are more costly forms of therapy. It may also be used as an expedient restraint, instead of expending the effort and time thought to be more extensive than the potential outcome warrants.

Because of these and other factors, there has been criticism leveled suggesting that chemotherapy as a restraint has become the primary mode of treatment for families from lower socioeconomic strata, excluding them from more appropriate or definitive therapies. Every effort should be made to provide a child with the treatment indicated by a thorough diagnostic study of him and his family. The type of expediency mentioned above has little place in the delivery of psychiatric services.

On the other hand, many psychiatrists and therapists given to single and often narrow therapeutic approaches still deny children appropriate pharmacologic relief from disturbance as they ply their art. Even though other forms of therapy are being conducted, the use of medication can be a useful adjunct. Frequently medication allows the child to be settled enough to make use of his therapist, or alert enough to be aided through educational approaches. The child with aggressive outbursts may not be acceptable in a group therapy situation until his behavior can be controlled by medication. The milieu in many hospitals or residential settings can function only if certain symptoms within the patients are alleviated with medication.

Summary

All too often, medication is given after a very cursory understanding of the problem. The follow-up is then conducted in a perfunctory fashion, and termination is left to the whim of the patient or his parent. In this fashion, pharmacotherapy is merely an expedient way of dealing with what usually is a complex problem involving the child, his family and his environment. The results are often poor, or at best erratic. However, done within the context outlined above of understanding the child, his development, background, problems, family interactions, and mental and physical status, the use of medication can be a useful and predictable addition to treatment.

As greater understanding of the neurophysiology and neurochemistry of mental and emotional disorders emerges, a more predictable objective view of pharmacotherapy will follow. It is this function and careful individual diagnosis and treatment planning which will maintain child psychiatry and the treatment of children's behavior disorders in its status as a medical specialty.

Psychoactive Drugs Commonly Used With Children

The following list consists of drugs commonly used with children. It is not meant to be exhaustive, but illustrative. As noted earlier, the medications discussed here will not necessarily be lasting, but characterize the current clinical use. Some drugs are being used more on an experimental basis at the present and will not be included. The description of the medications included in this chapter is meant to highlight their clinical use and not discuss their pharmacology.

CNS Stimulants

D-amphetamine. This medication has been used primarily for treating children with the hyperkinetic syndrome, especially the symptoms of hyperactivity and short attention span. Some changes in school performance have also been demonstrated, although learning improvement does not seem to show lasting changes. It has also been used in enuresis, although not as effectively as imipramine.

Children from three years of age have been treated with d-amphetamine at dosages beginning at 2½ mg. b.i.d. The response to the medication is usually rapid and dramatic. A trial of two weeks is characteristic, and adjustment upward to dosages of 40 mg. per day in the older children is not unusual to obtain an optimum result.

D-amphetamine produces side effects in most children, but often children develop tolerance to the side effects rather rapidly. The most problematic and least tolerated side effect is an adverse reaction that produces extreme agitation, and with this, the medication should be stopped. More commonly there is sleeplessness (although drowsiness has been described), loss of appetite, whininess, nervousness, and occasionally diarrhea. Growth suppression has been described with the use of d-amphetamine at dosages of 20 mg. per day or more over prolonged periods of time. Paranoid psychosis has been described with high doses of d-amphetamine or with sudden withdrawal of the medication. There are no major contraindications for its use, except for psychosis, which is usually worsened by CNS stimulants.

Methylphenidate. This medication has been used with hyperkinetic children, much as d-amphetamine. Side effects from methylphenidate are said to be milder and thus make its use more attractive. Interestingly, some children who will not respond to d-amphetamine may respond to methylphenidate, and vice versa. Needless to say, one should try both medications prior to moving to another class of medications. This drug has been used as an appetite suppressant and antidepressant with adults, but has no place as this in the treatment of children.

Dosages of methylphenidate commonly begin at 10 mg. b.i.d., but again, can be adjusted upward. Levels of 80 mg. to 100 mg. per day have been used, but going above that limit should be done with extreme caution, trying not to exceed 4½ mg. per kilogram per day. Again, children at a preschool level have been placed on this drug.

Side effects are similar to d-amphetamine, but thought to be fewer. Occasionally, methylphenidate causes nasuea, but it does not usually cause diarrhea. Growth suppression has been noted with the use of this medication at dosages of 40 to 50 mg. per day and higher over prolonged periods of use. No major contraindications are noted other than previously mentioned.

Magnesium Pemoline. This medication is somewhat of a newcomer to the marketed CNS stimulants and is used primarily for children with hyperkinesis. At first it was thought to have fewer side effects, and being a long-acting drug, could be given once a day. So far, studies have shown it to be in the same range of effectiveness as the other two CNS stimulants.

The dosages are often given once a day at levels of 25 to 50 mg. per day. Dosages of as high as 125 mg. per day have been used. This medication has not been used with the very young child.

The side effects of magnesium pemoline are similar to those of the other CNS stimulants, although no one has noted growth suppression with it. There are no major contraindications other than previously noted.

Antipsychotics

Phenothiazines

Chlorpromazine. This, the oldest of the major tranquilizers, has had a long use with children for a variety of symptomatology. At the present, however, its main use is that of an antipsychotic agent and directed at such symptoms as bizarreness, silliness, agitation, delusional thinking, hallucinations, uncontrolled aggression, and other psychotic symptoms, but also has a use in children who are exceptionally aggressive, along with being hyperactive. This medication is often used adjunctively in the treatment of anorexia nervosa, especially in the hospitalized patient.

The medication has been used with children of all ages, including preschool children. Dosages usually range from 20 to 100 mg. per day, although as much as 200 mg. per day has been given, usually on a b.i.d. or a q.i.d. schedule. In the adolescent, dosage schedules follow those of adults. Below twelve, 0.25 mg. per pound b.i.d. or q.i.d. should not be exceeded. Chlorpromazine has been used intramuscularly in children. The dosage here normally does not exceed 40 mg.

The side effects of chlorpromazine are well known. Most inhibiting to its use in children is a sedative effect, making continuing cognitive development precarious. Children also experience dizziness, dry mouth, evidence of orthostatic hypotension, photosensitivity, and extrapyramidal signs. Anti-Parkinson drugs have been utilized in children to eliminate or control the latter. Leukopenia has been noted, but laboratory studies do show an initial depression that after a week or two remits and normal white counts are seen again. Unremitting leukopenia is an indication to stop the medication. Liver difficulties have also been noted. Convulsions have occurred only rarely.

However, the use of any of the phenothiazines is questionable in the treatment of a child with a convulsive disorder.

Thioridazine. The use of this medication is primarily for children with psychotic symptomatology. However, it has been used as an anxiolytic agent, and in children with hyperactivity because of a described energizing effect. The dosages range from 20 to 100 mg. per day given in four doses. This medication has also been used with the very young child. Side effects with thioridazine are much the same as all phenothiazines, but there seems to be less in the way of extrapyramidal signs. Leukopenia and liver problems are much less frequent.

Fluphenazine. This medication has been used to treat psychotic manifestations in children also. It is often considered after a trial of the two previously mentioned phenothiazines.

Dosage levels are considerably less with this medication and are in the range of 0.25 mg. to 2 mg. b.i.d. It has been used at somewhat higher levels also. This medication has not had wide use with the very young child.

The side effects are typical of phenothiazines, although the extrapyramidal signs may be more pronounced than with thioridazine. Tardive dyskinesia has been noted to occur in children treated with this medication.

Trifluoperazine. This medication is used with the psychotic child and has also been used with the hyperactive or agitated child.

Dosage levels range at the 1 mg. to 2 mg. b.i.d. level, although somewhat higher dosages are used in older children or adolescents. It, too, has not had wide use with very young children.

The extrapyramidal signs are greater with trifluoperazine, although drowsiness is less. The other side effects are much like the others.

Thioxanthenes

Thiothixene. This medication, along with chlorprothixene has also been used with children presenting psychotic symptoms and uncontrollable or aggressive behavior. They are, however, a derivative of the phenothiazines.

Dosages of thiothixene range on the average from 6 to 30 mg. per day, and it has not been used on the very young child.

Side effects are much like those of the phenothiazines. The advantage to this medication is the slight sedative effect and lessened extrapyramidal signs in children.

Butyrophenones

Haloperidol. This medication is used alternatively to phenothiazines in the treatment of psychotic manifestations in children and adolescents. It seems especially effective with the aggressive and assaultive behavior encountered in these children. It also has a good effect on withdrawal or isolated behavior. Haloperidol has been shown to have a surprisingly good result with children demonstrating Gilles de la Tourette syndrome.

Dosages range from 0.5 mg. b.i.d. to a total dose of 16 mg. per day. The medication should be started at a low dose such as 0.25 mg. b.i.d. and worked up by 0.5 mg. increments until the desired effect is attained. It has not had wide usage with the very young child.

The side effects are much like those of the phenothiazenes. However, drowsiness is generally less. Extrapyramidal signs and photosensitivity can be more pronounced with Haloperidol.

Anxiolytics

Benzodiazepines

Chlordiazepoxide. This medication has had fairly long use as a minor tranquilizer in the treatment of anxiety symptoms in children. Typically, the nervous child, the fearful child, or those with sleep problems, are treated with this medication. It should be understood that these symptoms are most often best treated by psychotherapy or behavioral techniques. Results with medication in these types of disorders have been less dramatic than those mentioned earlier. Chlordiazepoxide has been tried with hyperactive children, but the results are not dramatic.

Dosages of chlordiazepoxide are usually 5 to 10 mg. b.i.d. on the average, but do range to use at the same dosage on a q.i.d. schedule.

Side effects often include drowsiness, which is probably the most inhibiting factor in the use of chlordiazepoxide. Children have also been known to have nausea, ataxia, agitation, and in rare instances, syncope.

Diazapam. This medication has a shorter history than its close relative above. It is, however, about twice as potent and is used for the same symptoms.

Dosages run about half of that of chlordiazepoxide at 2 to 5 mg. b.i.d. Because of its slow-acting effect, it is usually given on a b.i.d. schedule.

Side effects are those of chlordiazepoxide. Some greater ataxia has been noted, and on rare occasions, syncope has been noted.

Antihistamine Sedatives

Hydroxyzine. The anxiety symptoms of sleeplessness, fearfulness, and nervousness are often the target of this medication. It has had a long history of use and has even been tried reasonably ineffectively with hyperactive children.

Dosages of 10 to 20 mg. b.i.d. in children under six years have been used, and in children over six the dosages range from 25 to 50 mg. b.i.d.

Side effects consist primarily of sedation and dry mouth.

Diphenhydramine. This antihistamine has also had a long history of use in child psychopharmacologic treatment. However, results with its use have not been well delineated. It has been frequently used for its sedative quality in sleeplessness in the very young. It has been used with the fearful, nervous, and hyperactive child.

It is given in dosages of 10 to 20 mg. t.i.d. and as much as 100 mg. per day in older children. As a sedative, it is frequently given in doses of 25 mg. h.s., or in older children 50 mg. h.s.

Antidepressants

Tricyclics

Imipramine. The present limited use of antidepressant medications for depression in children parallels the reawakened interest in this disorder in children. The depressive affect or its equivalents, including irritability, aggressiveness, self-destructive behavior, or others may all be indications for treatment with imipramine. Imipramine has also been utilized for children with hyperkinetic syndrome. School phobia has been another indicated use for this medication. Finally, imipramine has had long use in the treatment of enuresis.

Dosages are usually in the range of 1 to 2 mg. per kilogram per day. This translates into a range of 10 to 60 mg. for younger children and 25 to 100 mg. for older children. This is often initiated on a q.i.d. schedule. For enuresis the dosage is given at bedtime, starting at 25 mg. for children under twelve and 50 mg. for children over twelve. These dosages may be increased to 50 mg. in the younger child and 100 mg. in the older child. Since these drugs are slow-acting, two weeks may be required for an adequate trial.

Side effects include dry mouth, insomnia, dizziness, urticaria, excess perspiration, and hypertension. Recently reports of EKG changes at higher levels have limited the dosages of imipramine with children and require monitoring if used especially for longer terms. Leukopenia and liver problems have been reported with imipramine.

Amitryptiline. This medication has primarily been used in children with school phobia and older children or adolescents with depressive symptomatology. It is somewhat shorter acting than imipramine and earlier results can be expected.

The dosages of this medication do range from 25 to 100 mg. per day given in a variety of patterns including single doses at bedtime.

The side effects are similar to imipramine. The compound likewise has an affinity for the myocardium, and caution in the use of it should be exercised.

Nortryptiline. This compound is similar in all ways to amitryptiline.

MAO Inhibitors

These compounds have found little use in the United States because of the seriousness of their side effects.

Lithium Salts

*Lithium Carbonate.*This medication has found some use, especially in adolescents and older children in controlling agitation, mania, and other similar behavior. It has also been used in the agitated psychotic child. Investigators, especially in Europe, feel content in diagnosing cyclical affective disorders in children and find fairly broad use of lithium carbonate.

Dosage is primarily determined on the basis of maintaining blood levels from 0.5 mEq/L to 1.5 mEq/L, but usually around 1.0 mEq/L. Dosages from 50 mg. to 1,800 mg. per day in divided doses have been reported.

Side effects of lithium can be serious, and its use must be carefully monitored on an inpatient basis to begin with. Gastrointestinal symptoms, including diarrhea, occur, while tremors, excess thirst, and polyuria are also problems. Thyroid problems have arisen with its use. Depression can occur with the use of lithium carbonate. Toxicity produces convulsions, coma, and death. Leukocytosis is described with lithium, and if persistent, should contraindicate the medication's use.

Anticonvulsants

Diphenylhydantoin. This medication has been used with children who have uncontrolled behavior or aggressive outbursts, specifically where the EEG findings indicate some convulsant activity.

The dosage is in the range used for the anticonvulsant effect of the medication, 50 mg. to 200 mg. per day in divided doses.

The side effects include anorexia, nausea, gum hyperplasia, epigastric pain, hirsutism, skin rash, lymphadenopathy, and ataxia, when one reaches toxic levels.

*Phenobarbital.*This medication has little use in childhood emotional disorders, except as an anticonvulsant. The incidence of serious agitated reactions is quite high.

References

Alderton, H.R., and B.A. Hoddinott. (1964). A controlled study of the use of thioridazine in the treatment of hyperactive and aggressive children in a children's psychiatric hospital. *Can. Psychiat. Assn. J.* 9:239–242.

Annell, A-L. (1969) Manic-depressive illness in children and effect of treatment with lithium carbonate. *Acta Paedopsychiat.* 36:292–301.

Arnold, E., P. Wender, K. McCloskey, and S. Snyder. (1972) Levoamphetamine and dextroamphetamine: Comparative efficacy in the hyperkinetic syndrome. *Arch. Gen. Psychiat.* 27:816–822.

Bakwin, H. (1948) Benzedrine in behavior disorders for children. *J. Pediat.* 32:215–216.

Bender, L., and F. Cottington. (1942) The use of amphetamine sulfate in child psychiatry. *Am. J. Psychiat.* 99:116–121.

Bradley, C. (1937) The behavior of children receiving benzedrine. *Am. J. Psychiat.* 94:577–585.

Bradley, C. (1950) Benzedrine and dexedrine in the treatment of children's behavior disorders. *Pediatrics* 5:24–37.

Campbell, M. (1975) Psychopharmacology in childhood psychosis. In R. Gittleman-Klein, ed., *Recent Advances in Child Psychopharmacology.* New York: Human Sciences Press

Campbell, M., B. Fish, J. Korein, T. Shapiro, P. Collins, and C. Koh. (1972) Lithium and chlorpromazine: A controlled crossover study of hyperactive severely disturbed young children. *J. Aut. Child. Schizo.* 2:234–263.

Campbell, M., B. Fish, T. Shapiro, and A. Floyd. (1970) Thiothixene in young disturbed children: A pilot study. *Arch. Gen. Psychiat.* 23:7–72.

Cantwell, D.P., ed. (1975) *The Hyperactive Child: Diagnosis, Management and Current Research.* New York: Spectrum Publications.

Carr, W.L. (1906) *Practice of Pediatrics.* New York: Lea Brothers and Co.

Chapin, H.D., and G.R. Pisek. (1911) *Diseases of Children.* New York: William Wood & Co.

Chessick, R., and R. McFarland. (1963) Problems in psychopharmacologic research. *J.A.M.A.* 185:237–241.

Claghorn, J.L. (1972) A double-blind comparison of haloperidol (Haldol) and thioridazine (Mellaril) in outpatient children. *Curr. Ther. Res.* 14:785–789.

Conners, C.K., and L. Eisenberg. (1963) The effects of methylphenidate on symptomatology and learning in disturbed children. *Am. J. Psychiat.* 12:458–464.

Conners, C.K., L. Eisenberg, and A. Barcai. (1962) Effect of dextroamphetamine on children. *Arch. Gen. Psychiat.* 17:478–485.

Conners, C.K., E. Taylor, G. Meo, M. Kurtz, and M. Fournier. (1972) Magnesium pemoline and dextroamphetamine: A controlled study in children with minimal brain dysfunction. *Psychopharmacologica* 26:321–336.

Cunningham, M.A., V. Pillai, and W.J. Rogers. (1968) Haloperidol in the treatment of children with severe behavior disorders. *Brit. J. Psychiat.* 114:845–854.

Cutts, K.K., and H.H. Jasper. (1939) Effect of benzedrine sulfate and phenobarbital on behavior problem children with abnormal EEG. *Arch. Neur. Psychiat.* 41:1138–1145.

Cytryn, L., A. Gilbert, and L. Eisenberg. (1960) The effectiveness of tranquilizing drugs in supportive psychotherapy in treating behavior disorders of children: A double-blind study of eighty outpatients. *Am. J. Orthopyschiat.* 30:113–129.

Cytryn, L., and D.H. McKnew, Jr. (1972) Proposed classification of childhood depression. *Am. J. Psychiat.* 129: 149–155.

Cytryn, L., and D.H. McKnew, Jr. (1974) Factors influencing the changing clinical expression of the depressive process in children. *Am. J. Psychiat.* 131:879–881.

D'Amato, G. (1962) Chlordiazeproxide in management of school phobia. *Dis. Nerv. Syst.* 23:292–295.

Dyson, W.L., and A. Barcai. (1970) Treatment of children of lithium-responding parents. *Curr. Ther. Res.* 12:286–290.

Engelhardt, D.M., P. Palizos, J. Waizer, and S.P. Hoffman. (1973) A double-blind comparison of fluphenazine and haloperidol in outpatient schizophrenic children. *J. Aut. Child. Schizo.* 3:128–137.

Faetra, G., L. Dooher, and J. Dowling. (1970) Comparison of haloperidol on fluphenazine in disturbed children. *Am. J. Psychiat.* 126:1670.

Fish, B. (1960) Drug therapy in child psychiatry: Pharmacologic aspects. *Comp. Psychiat.* 1:212–227.

Fish, B. (1968) Drug use in psychiatric disorders of children. *Am. J. Psychiat.* Suppl. 124:31–36.

Fish, B., and T. Shapiro. (1965) A typology of children's psychiatric disorders: I. Its application to a controlled evaluation of treatment. *J. Am. Acad. Child Psych.* 4:32–52.

Fish, B., T. Shapiro, and M. Campbell. (1966) Long-term prognosis with the response of schizophrenic children to drug therapy: A controlled study of trifluoperazine. *Am. J. Psychiat.* 123:32–39.

Fisher, S. (1959) *Child Research in Psychopharmacology.* Springfield, Ill.: Charles C. Thomas.

Forster, F. (1961) *Evaluation of Drug Therapy.* Madison: University of Wisconsin Press.

Frommer, E.A. (1967) Treatment of childhood depression with antidepressant drugs. *Brit. Med. J.* 1:729–732.

Garfield, S.L., M.M. Helper, C.S. Willcott, and R. Muffly. (1962) Effects of chlorpromazine on behavior in emotionally disturbed children. *J. Nerv. Ment. Dis.* 135:147–154.

Gatski, R.L. (1955) Chlorpromazine in the treatment of emotionally maladjusted children. *J.A.M.A.* 157:1290–1300.

Ginn, S.A., and L.B. Hohman (1953) The use of d-amphetamine in severe behavior problems of children. *South. Med. J.* 46:1124–1127.

Gittelman-Klein, R., and D. Klein. (1970) Controlled

imipramine treatment of school phobia. *Arch. Gen. Psychiat.* 25:204–207.

Greenblatt, D.J., and R.I. Shader. (1974) Benzodiazepines. *New Eng. Med. J.* 291:1011–1015.

Huessy, H., and A.L. Wright. (1970) The use of imipramine in children's behavior disorders. *Acta Paedopsychiat.* 208:1613–1614.

Knobel, M. (1962) Psychopharmacology for the hyperkinetic child. *Arch. Gen. Psychiat.* 6:198–202.

Kraft, I.A., I.M. Marcus, W. Wilson, D.V. Swander, N.W. Rumage, and E. Schulhoffer. (1959) Methodological problems in studying the effect of tranquilizers in children, with specific reference to meprobamate. *South. Med. J.* 52:179–185.

Laufer, M.W., and E. Denhoff. (1957) Hyperkinetic behavior syndrome in children. *J. Pediat.* 50:463–474.

Lindsley, D.B., and C.E. Henry. (1942) The effect of drugs on behavior and the EEGs of children with behavior disorders. *Psychosom. Med.* 4:140–149.

Lucas, A. (1967) Gilles de la Tourette's disease in children, treatment with haloperidol. *Am. J. Psychiat.* 124:147–149.

Lucas, A.R., P.E. Kauffman, and E.M. Morris. (1967) Gilles de la Tourette's disease: A clinical study of 15 cases. *J. Am. Acad. Child Psychiat.* 6:700–722.

Lucas, A.R., H.S. Lockett, and E. Grimm. (1965) Amitryptiline in childhood depressions. *Dis. Nerv. Syst.* 26:105–110.

MacLean, R.E.G. (1960) Imipramine hydrochloride (Tofranil) and enuresis. *Am. J. Psychiat.* 117:551.

McAndrew, J.B., Q. Case, and D. Treffert. (1972) Effects of prolonged phenothiazine intake on psychotic and other hospitalized children. *J. Aut. Child. Schizo.* 2:75.

Mendelson, W., N. Johnson, and M.A. Stewart. (1971) Hyperactive children as teenagers: A follow-up study. *J. Nerv. Ment. Dis.* 153:273–279.

Millichap, J.G. (1968) Drugs in management of hyperkinetic and perceptually handicapped children. *J.A.M.A.* 206:1527–1530.

Millichap, J.G. (1974)Drugs in management of minimal brain dysfunction. *Ann. N.Y. Acad. Sci.* 205:321–334.

Millichap, J.G., and E.E. Boldrey. (1967) Studies in hyperkinetic behaviors: II. Laboratory and clinical evaluations of drug treatments. *Neurology* 17:467–471.

Minde, K., G. Weiss, and M. Mendelson. (1972) A five-year follow-up of 91 hyperactive school children. *J. Am. Acad. Child Psychiat.* 11:595–610.

Molitch, M., and A.K. Eccles. (1937) The effect of benzedrine on the intelligence scores of children. *Am. J. Psychiat.* 94:587–590.

Moskowitz, H. (1971) Benzedrine therapy for the mentally handicapped. *Am. J. Ment. Def.* 45:540–543.

Oettinger, L. (1962) Chlorprothixine in the management of problem children. *Dis. Nerv. Syst.* 23:568–571.

Pasamanick, B. (1951) Anticonvulsant drug therapy of behavior problem children with abnormal electroencephalograms. *Arch. Neur. Psychiat.* 65:752–766.

Pilkington, L. (1916) Comprehensive effects of lithium and taractan on behavior disorders of mentally retarded children. *Dis. Nerv. Syst.* 22:573–575.

Piuk, C.L. (1963) Clinical impressions of hydroxyzine and other tranquilizers in a child guidance clinic. *Dis. Nerv. Syst.* 24:483–488.

Pouissant, A.F., and K.G. Ditman. (1965) A controlled study of imipramine (Tofranil) in the treatment of childhood enuresis. *J. Pediat.* 67:283–290.

Poznanski, E., V. Krahenbuhl, and J. Zrull. (1976) Childhood depression: A longitudinal perspective. *J. Am. Acad. Child. Psychiat.* 15:491–501.

Poznanski, E., and J.P. Zrull. (1970) Childhood depression: Clinical characteristics of overtly depressed children. *Arch. Gen. Psychiat.* 23:8–15.

Report of the Conference on the Use of Stimulant Drugs in the Treatment of Behaviorally Disturbed Young School Children. *Psychopharmacol. Bull.* 7:23–29.

Safer, D., R. Allen, and E. Barr. (1972) Depression of growth in hyperactive children on stimulant drugs. *New Eng. J. Med.* 287:217–220.

Satterfield, J., D. Cantwell, and B. Satterfield. (1974) Pathophysiology of the hyperactive child syndrome. *Arch. Gen. Psychiat.* 31:839–844.

Schnackenberg, R. (1973) Caffeine as a substitute for schedule II stimulants in hyperkinetic children. *Am. J. Psychiat.* 130:796–798.

Shapiro, A.K., E. Shapiro, H. Wayne, J. Clarkin, and R.D. Brunn. (1973) Tourette's syndrome: Summary of data on 34 patients. *Psychosom. Med.* 34:419–435.

Shaw, C.R., H.J. Lockett, A.R. Lucas, C.H. Lamontagne, and E. Grimm. (1963) Tranquilizer drugs in the treatment of emotionally disturbed children: I. Inpatients in a residential treatment center. *J. Am. Acad. Child Psychiat.* 2:725–742.

Simeon, J., B. Saletu, M. Saletu, T.M. Itil, and J. Da Silva. (1974) Thiothixene in childhood psychosis. In I.S. Forrest, S.J. Carr, and E. Usdin, eds., *Phenothiazines and Structurally Related Drugs: Advances in Biochemical Psychopharmacology.* New York: Raven Press.

Tarjan, G., V.E. Lowery, and S.W. Wright. (1957) Use of chlorpromazine in two hundred seventy-eight mentally deficient patients. *J. Dis. Child.* 94:294–300.

Weiss, G., E. Kruger, U. Danielson, and M. Elman. (1975) Effect of long-term treatment of hyperactive children with methylphenidate. *Can. Med. Assn. J.* 112:159–165.

Wender, P.H. (1971) *Minimal Brain Dysfunction in Children.* New York: Wiley-Interscience.

Wender, P.H. (1975) Speculations concerning a possible biochemical basis of minimal brain dysfunction. *Int. J. Ment. Health* 4:11–28.

Werry, J.S. G. Weiss, V. Douglas, and J. Martin. (1966) Studies in the hyperactive child III: The effect of chlorpromazine upon behavior and learning ability. *J. Amer. Acad. Child Psychiat.* 5:292–312.

Winsberg, B., I. Bialer, S. Kupietz, and J. Tobias. (1972) Effects of imipramine and dextroamphetamine on behavior of neuro-psychiatrically impaired children. *Am. J. Psychiat.* 128:1425–1431.

Winsberg, B., S. Goldstein, L. Yepes, and J. Perel. (1975) Imipramine and electrocardiographic abnormalities in hyperactive children. *Am. J. Psychiat.* 132:542–545.

Zimmerman, F., and B. Burgermeister. (1958) Action of methylphenidate and reserpine in behavior disorders in children and adults. *Am. J. Psychiat.* 115:323–328.

Zrull, J.P., J.C. Westman, B. Arthur, and W.A. Bell. (1963) A comparison of chlordiozepoxide, d-amphetamine and placebo in the treatment of the hyperkinetic syndrome in children. *Am. J. Psychiat.* 120:590–591.

Zrull, J.P., J. C. Westman, B. Arthur, and D.L. Rice. (1964) A comparison of diazepam, d-amphetamine, and placebo in the treatment of the hyperkinetic syndrome in children. *Am. J. Psychiat.* 121:588–589.

Zrull, J.P., J.C. Westman, B. Arthur, and D.L. Rice. (1966) An evaluation of methodology used in the study of psychoactive drugs for children. *J. Am. Acad. Child Psychiat.* 5:284–291.

Treatment of Emotional Disorders in Children and Adolescents

CHAPTER 7

Brief Psychotherapy

Alan J. Rosenthal

Introduction

The practice of brief psychotherapy with children varies with the relatively few practitioners who employ it in both form and content. It is a pragmatic treatment approach based on several theoretical orientations and utilizing multiple methods and techniques. Nevertheless, a number of elements generally are recognized as fundamental to this psychotherapeutic approach:

Duration: Brief psychotherapy is time-limited. It is brief relative to more traditional, open-ended dynamically oriented psychotherapies. Its duration may vary from 3 hours (Shulman, 1960) to as long as 6 months (Proskower, 1969) depending on theoretical formulation and technique, or external time constraints, such as the departure of therapist or patient, limitations of insurance coverage, or clinic policies.

Focus: In time-limited psychotherapy, therapist and patient must focus on specific issues and develop particular goals consistent with the realities of time and psychopathology. While all psychotherapists should define goals and assess progress toward them, this is an essential element of brief psychotherapy (Rosenthal and Levine, 1971; Parad and Parad, 1968).

Reality, "Here and Now" Orientation: Time-limited therapy does not allow lengthy excursions into the patient's past for detailed analysis of early conflicts. The patient's past is explored, but primarily to understand and relate it to present life situations. Brief therapy concentrates on present, "here and now" issues, both interpersonal and intrapsychic. This is not to say that brief therapy is limited to crisis intervention or symptom removal. It may focus on more chronic conflicts as well, but does so with a present, reality oriented approach.

Family-Oriented Approach: Brief therapy with children, because of the child's obvious dependence on significant others for growth and development and for meeting physical and emotional needs, requires a family-oriented approach. In this sense, it moves beyond "individual psychotherapy." Parents and other family members must be involved in the brief therapy process, as much or even more than the child himself. Flexibility in involving other family members as indicated by the treatment focus and goals is a significant feature of this therapeutic approach and will be discussed later.

History

The development of brief therapy, with adults as well as with children and families, has probably been hindered by a widespread bias among mental health professionals that the most valuable and preferred mode of treatment is long-term psychoanalytic psychotherapy. Other treatment modalities, including brief therapy, often have been relegated to positions of second-class or inferior status. Actually brief psychotherapy was practiced by Freud and his followers, and has been encouraged by many psychoanalytic and psychiatric practitioners and writers—Breuer and Freud (1957), Fenichel (1954), and Alexander (1951), to name only a few. In 1941, the Chicago Institute for Psychoanalysis examined the topic in a national scientific meeting on brief psychotherapy. This approach received further emphasis as emergency and brief therapy achieved importance to the military during World War II (Kardiner, 1941), and as a result of Lindemann's development of crisis intervention techniques in the 1940's (1944). Since that time, the use of brief psychotherapy has continued to increase, particularly with adults. Numerous articles and volumes have been written about the topic (Wolberg, 1965; Small, 1971; Barton, 1971; Lewin, 1970; Phillips and Weiner, 1966), and brief therapy has become a more accepted treatment modality in general psychiatric practice.

Although practiced in community child guidance clinics for many years, therapy of relatively short duration with children was not originally identified as "brief therapy." From the reports of a number of early practitioners, it appears that at least some of the child psychotherapy they employed was relatively brief—that is, up to 6 months in duration. Witmer (1946) compiled reports of several session-by-session case studies by different child therapists handled within a 6-month period. Blanchard (1946), Rank (1946), and Allen (1946) in particular report cases treated within 20 sessions. Allen (1942) also describes a number of cases that he treated with relatively short-term therapy in *Psychotherapy with Children*, published in 1942. Early reports by Solomon (1948) and by Levy (1939) describe techniques in play therapy particularly applicable to brief therapy.

In addition to these reports, many community clinics and social service agencies, confronted with large caseloads and long waiting lists, have employed this technique for years, and some have reported successful results with brief therapy (Phillips and Johnston, 1954; Alpern, 1956). Labeled as such, brief psychotherapy with children and families has been used at least since 1949 (Bruch) but while sporadic reports in the literature advocated its use in the following decade, it was not until the 1960's that reports of its success appeared with more frequency (Shulman, 1960; Cytryn, Gilbert, and Eisenberg, 1960; Coddington, 1962; Kaffman, 1963; Kennedy, 1965; Hare, 1966; Mackay, 1967; Springe, 1968; Lester, 1968). These and other studies have begun to focus on treatment techniques in brief therapy with children (Rosenthal and Levine, 1971; Parad and Parad, 1968), types of problems treated with this modality (Lester, 1968; Rosenthal and Levine, 1970), and evaluation of treatment outcome and therapeutic results (Phillips and Johnston, 1954; Kaffman, 1963; Kennedy, 1965; Hare, 1966; Rosenthal and Levine, 1970; Shaw, Blumenfeld, and Senf, 1968; Phillips, 1960).

As pressures in community mental health increase for expanded treatment services to broader populations and larger numbers of emotionally disturbed children and families, reports of the use of brief therapy also increase. More recently, a volume devoted entirely to brief therapy with children and their parents has been published (Barton and Barton, 1973). This modality now appears to be developing a more recognized position in child and family psychotherapeutic practice.

Theoretical Contributions

As a pragmatic approach, brief therapy draws upon a variety of psychological schools of thought, and utilizes interventions from widely diverse theoretical orientations. While brief therapy is not synonymous with crisis intervention, its effects are based partially on elements of crisis theory. The child's and family's greater motivation for change, and the greater fluidity of intrapsychic and interpersonal dynamics during times of crisis allow the opportunity to effect change more rapidly (Berlin, 1970; Waldfogel, Tessman, and Hahn, 1959). Effective brief therapy provides aid at times of stress when pressure to alter behavior, relationships, and maladaptive patterns is at a peak.

Brief therapy emphasizes the self-healing capacities of children and families (Phillips and Johnston, 1954; Barton and Barton, 1973). While areas of conflict and pathological behaviors are explored and interpreted with a view toward change, the family's psychological strengths receive significant attention and support (Rosenthal and Levine, 1971; Berlin, 1970; Barton and Barton, 1973). Adaptive coping mechanisms are encouraged and developed, and family members learn to use these in response to present and future stress. Brief therapy places explicit responsibility for dealing with problems upon the child and parents. As family members learn to cope with and overcome current conflicts, they are also guided in anticipating and successfully preventing or managing future conflicts. Recognition of the family's basic capabilities to manage its situation, and with the therapist's interventions, allowing their psychological strengths to maintain the self-healing process, are basic to the practice of brief psychotherapy.

Other theoretical bases of brief therapy also

relate to its reality, here-and-now orientation. Brief therapy is a directive process in which the therapist actively intervenes in family members' relationships and behavior. Directive guidance can precipitate behavioral change, and it is well documented that persisting changes in affect, psychodynamics, and intrapsychic and interpersonal patterns can follow such brief therapeutic contacts (Wolberg, 1965; Phillips and Johnston, 1954; Kaffman, 1963; Berlin, 1970; Thomas, Chess, and Birch, 1968; Kelleher, 1968; Malan, 1963; Heinicke and Goldman, 1960; *Psychiatric News*, 1975). Affective insights may occur after the brief therapy process, and help to maintain the behavioral changes that began during the process itself. This does not imply that brief therapy will "cure" all present and future psychological distress. On the contrary, many families will experience additional stress as their development progresses, as children enter new developmental stages, as parents age, as economic, vocational, and sociocultural shifts occur, as unforeseen tragedy strikes. These later periods of stress may require additional brief therapy, usually not as lengthy as the initial course, to resolve the issues involved and to guide the family back to independent functioning. Further, the need for additional brief therapy does not imply its failure initially. Families vary in their abilities to cope with stress, and many will require periodic "booster" sessions of therapy following the initial course of brief therapy to manage later crises. This approach allows for therapeutic contact over a longer period of time, and avoids the implication of failure for those requesting additional therapeutic assistance.

Brief therapy employs techniques from varied theoretical positions. Intrapsychic conflicts of child and parents are explored and interpreted directly. Interpersonal relations, parent-child, marital, and others are analyzed in detail. Directions for improving communication, relationships, feelings, reduction of symptoms, and developing methods of reinforcing and maintaining improvement are provided. Brief therapy utilizes theory and interventions of analytically oriented psychotherapy, behavior modification (Werry and Wollershein, 1967; Wagner, 1968), communication theory, Gestalt therapy, marital and family therapy, educational approaches (Barton and Barton, 1973), and others.

Applicability

Controversy exists over the indications and contraindications for brief therapy. Many emotionally disturbed children and families are not responsive to traditional long-term psychotherapy. Brief therapy may be indicated for these families. Long-term psychotherapy may be inappropriate for some because of particular educational, sociocultural, or attitudinal and personality characteristics, or because of particular types of psychopathology—for example, certain characterologic or conduct disorders. In such situations, a brief, directive therapeutic approach, with regular follow-up, may be useful.

These indications for brief therapy, however, are indications by default. Conversely, it has been argued that all children and families requesting treatment should receive brief therapy initially, and only after determining this is insufficient should we commit ourselves to lengthier approaches (Barton and Barton, 1973). Nevertheless, particular situations do appear more conducive to brief therapy approaches than others. These situations may relate to the child and family, to the therapist, or to the external environment itself.

The Child and Family

Prevention

The so-called normal problems of child and family development that may reveal themselves in primary prevention services can usually be managed in a brief therapy setting (Barton and Barton, 1973; Augenbraun, Reid, and Friedman, 1967). Parent or child discussion groups or individual family consultations can provide the support, direction, and insight necessary for most families to cope with the situation successfully (Barton and Barton, 1973). Programs in secondary prevention, which emphasize the early identification of problems, may also uncover situations appropriate for brief therapy. The milder the presenting problems and the shorter their duration, the greater is the indication for brief therapy. In addition, prevention programs for target populations, such as mothers and infants at risk because of complications of pregnancy, prematurity (Caplan, Mason, and Kaplan, 1965), birth trauma, deprivation, and others can identify potential or beginning conflicts which might be managed in a brief therapy setting.

Acute Crisis

As mentioned previously, family crises provide an opportunity for change; individuals are in distress, relationships and psychodynamic mechanisms are more fluid, and motivation for change is usually high. Brief therapy is an appropriate approach during and following these crises (Berlin, 1970). Brief therapy programs may provide outreach services to target populations in crisis, such as families experiencing severe illness or death, divorcing families, and those experiencing other types of social or personal distress. Separation from or loss of a family member are particular indications for brief therapy (Kliman, 1971). As will be discussed later, termination, with its related aspects of separation and loss, is a major issue in the process of brief therapy. Because of this emphasis, brief therapy is a useful approach to help the child and family cope with a separation or loss experience.

Childhood Adjustment and Neurotic Problems

A wide variety of behavioral problems in childhood can be treated with brief therapy. This approach has been effective in cases of phobic, particularly school phobic (Kennedy, 1965; Waldfogel, Tessman, and Hahn, 1959), depressive, withdrawn, or aggressive or regressive behavior; with delinquent, "hard-to-teach" children (Minuchin, Chamberlain, and Graubard, 1967; Gordon, 1970), and with problems of drug abuse (Gottschalk et al., 1970); in families with parent-child conflicts (Phillips and Johnston, 1954) or with marital discord, but with a reasonable degree of family and environmental stability (Rosenthal and Levine, 1970). More severe symptomatology and more chronicity of child or parental problems are associated with a less favorable prognosis in brief therapy and constitute a lesser indication for its use (Rosenthal and Levine, 1970; Barton and Barton, 1973)

More Severe Disturbances

While more severe and chronic disturbances have a poorer prognosis in brief therapy, it may be quite appropriately used when the focus and goals of therapy are carefully and realistically selected and pursued. Families with a psychotic child, a significantly mentally retarded child, severe marital discord or parental psychopathology, or multi-problem families can benefit from brief therapeutic interventions focused on a specific area of difficulty or recent crisis situation (Argles and Mackenzie, 1970). In such cases of course, continued care and therapeutic contact usually are required. These families may receive ongoing care from a social service or child treatment center, while more intensive but brief therapy is reserved for them during times of particular stress or for particular focal issues.

Other Family Indications

In addition to the above clinical situations, several individual and family characteristics have been identified which are associated with a favorable prognosis in brief therapy.

Motivation. As mentioned previously, motivation for change is a significant factor in successful brief therapy (Rosenthal and Levine, 1971; Berlin, 1970; Waldfogel, Tessman, and Hahn, 1959). Motivation is often strong during an acute crisis, but whether the difficulties are acute or chronic, the child's and parent's desire for therapeutic change is an indication for brief therapy

Parental Flexibility and Capacity for Change. Regardless of their expression of motivation, parental personality structure and capability for shifts in behavior and attitude are critical factors in brief therapy. Their presence is an indication for its use (Lester, 1968).

Developmental Progression of Child. The child who has the capacity to move through developmental stages without *severe* blocks or fixations in development, with relatively stable early attachments, with the ability to relate reasonably well, and without incapacitating handicaps or illness, has a more favorable prognosis in brief therapy (Lester, 1968).

Parental and Family Stability. While parental pathology and marital discord are not in themselves contraindications to the use of brief therapy, some degree of stability in parents and family structure is important in its use. A background of impending divorce or family dissolution, chronic ambiguity about the child's placement or living situation, or other factors indicating an uncertain or unstable family structure may not allow a sufficiently firm foundation on which to develop psychotherapeutic change (Rosenthal and Levine, 1970). Of course, an acute situation of instability, as may occur in divorce, illness, or death, may be a clear indication for the use of brief therapy to help the child and family cope with the crisis and regain some stability.

The Therapist

Motivation of the therapist for brief therapy is associated with a favorable outcome in this approach (Rosenthal and Levine, 1970, 1971). A number of reports indicate that therapists who believe that only a brief period of time is necessary for treatment are successful in brief therapy (Frank, 1961). Therapists who remain skeptical of the approach because of past training, experience, peer pressures, clinic policies, and so forth are less successful in spite of attempts to employ brief therapy. Lower therapist motivation is associated with brief therapy failures, and referrals for further treatment following the brief therapy period (Rosenthal and Levine, 1971).

Therapist style in conducting therapy is a further factor in successful brief therapy. Therapists with inactive, non-directive, or relatively inflexible styles have less success with brief therapy. Therapeutic flexibility and an active, often directive approach are associated with a more favorable treatment outcome (Rosenthal and Levine, 1970; Barton and Barton, 1973).

The Environment

Stability of the family's external environment is a further factor associated with successful brief therapy. As well as a predictable family structure, predictability in the family's living situation, housing and neighborhood, economic situation, and social structure form a firm base upon which therapeutic change can occur.

Complications and Contraindications

The potential complications of a brief therapy approach result from inexperience with the method or absence of adequate supervision, or from errors in evaluation and development of therapeutic goals. Brief therapy is not an arbitrarily abbreviated form of traditional long-term psychotherapy. It has a particular set of methods and techniques, and inexperience or failure to become familiar with them may lead to therapeutic disappointments. Supervision or peer consultation will help to avoid a variety of pitfalls in the brief therapy process: assessment of family and therapist motivation; selection of treatment goals; issues of termination; transference and future planning. In addition, regular peer consultation provides stimulation and reinforcement for the therapist to continue the practice of brief therapy. Without such reinforcement, therapists frequently revert to more comfortable, less intense, open-ended therapy based on past training and experience.

Rapid evaluation and setting realistic treatment goals are crucial to the brief therapy process. Errors in evaluation of the child and family may result in inappropriate treatment goals, beyond the capability of the child or family to achieve. Even more, urging the family toward goals beyond their capacity may push them into deeper difficulties or despair. These potential complications are avoidable however, given sufficient therapist preparation and adequate consultation as the brief therapy process progresses.

Brief therapy is contraindicated when the potential for achieving therapeutic goals during the treatment period is low. Such situations may include severe and chronic psychosis; significant mental retardation; the need for institutionalization; absence of early, stable attachments; lifelong severe characterologic problems; absence of any family or environmental stability; absence of family motivation; absence of therapist motivation (Rosenthal and Levine, 1971; Kaffman, 1963). Lester (1968) identifies developmental retardation, an internalized and complicated neurotic structure, multiple phobias, and characterologic disorders as situations having an unfavorable prognosis in brief therapy with children and families; these disorders constitute a relative contraindication to its use.

Brief therapy may be useful even with children and families with these difficulties (with the exception of absence of motivation), provided limited and realistic therapeutic goals are set (Kaffman, 1963).

Methods

Time Limit

A specified period of time in which formal therapy will occur is basic to the practice of brief therapy. The time period may be similar for virtually all children and families selected for this approach (Rosenthal and Levine, 1970), or it may be individually determined depending on each family's problems and needs (Proskower, 1969). The existence of limited time places a certain therapeutic pressure (Rosenthal and Levine, 1971) or expectation for improvement on both the therapist and family. If guided appropriately by the therapist—

that is, not allowed to become excessive or demanding—this pressure appears to enhance the therapeutic process itself. Preset time limits in therapy have been associated with favorable treatment outcome, fewer dropouts from therapy, and greater patient motivation. (Parad and Parad, 1968).

The therapist must specify explicitly the nature of the time limit to the family as treatment begins. Their agreement and cooperation to work on therapeutic issues within this time frame form the basis of the treatment contract.

Treatment Focus and Goals

As mentioned previously, brief therapy must be goal-oriented (Proskower, 1969; Rosenthal and Levine, 1971; Parad and Parad, 1968; Mackay, 1967). Given a limited time period for therapy, a rapid child and family evaluation and delineation of problem areas are essential. Based on this evaluation, which should include both psychodynamic and behavioral formulations, therapeutic goals which become the focus of the brief therapy are selected.

The selection of treatment goals in brief therapy may involve selecting out inappropriate therapeutic goals as well. Particular aspects of family psychopathology may be unrelated to the presenting problems and may be unsuitable for treatment in a brief therapy setting. Such psychopathology is sometimes evident during the initial family evaluation or is uncovered later in the brief therapy process. The therapist may have to avoid dealing with this psychopathology in order to focus sufficiently on the brief therapy treatment goals. Of course, treatment goals can and should be altered if other psychopathology becomes more prominent and pressing. In any event, additional treatment following or outside of the brief therapy should be recommended if indicated.

At this point the family is informed, in frank language they can both accept and understand, of the therapist's evaluation and treatment focus or goals. Often, and particularly when family motivation is high, the evaluation is consistent with the family's view of their difficulties, and delineating treatment goals becomes a shared process, beginning a collaborative relationship between therapist and family. When the evaluation is inconsistent with the family's perceptions or attitudes, the therapist may delineate acceptable formulations and treatment goals; at the same time, he may also propose, tactfully but directly and with sufficient explanation, additional formulations or treatment goals which he and the family may wish to pursue as therapy progresses. When such formulations are reasonably accurate, families, in our clinical experience, either perceive them as sound or are willing to consider them further in therapy. Reluctance to consider particular formulations, while perhaps indicating resistance, should also raise suspicions of erroneous formulations or questionable motivation for therapeutic change.

Formulations presented to the family by the therapist may be intrapsychic, interpersonal, communicational, or behavioral and symptomatic. Similarly, treatment goals may focus on any or several of these levels. While a focus on presenting symptoms and "here-and-now" problems is essential, approaching underlying psychopathology, either intrapsychic or interpersonal, is frequently indicated and useful. Therapeutic intervention with both symptoms and underlying psychopathology in a brief therapy setting can effect significant behavioral and attitudinal changes and often has lasting therapeutic benefit (Wolberg, 1965; Phillips and Johnston, 1954; Kaffman, 1963; Berlin, 1970).

Rapport

The development of rapport or positive transference is an important feature of most psychotherapy, but is essential in brief therapy (Proskower, 1969; Rosenthal and Levine, 1971; Shaw, Blumenfeld, and Senf, 1968). With limited time, the early establishment of rapport and a therapeutic alliance are necessary if the collaborative work of therapist and family is to occur. The sharing of a treatment focus and goals is the beginning of the therapeutic alliance, and maintaining this positive relationship is crucial in the brief therapy process.

Therapist Activity

Brief therapy is characterized by active, often directive interventions (Rosenthal and Levine, 1971; Wagner, 1968). Conveying formulations and setting treatment goals with the family is an active process, and the therapist maintains this stance throughout the brief therapy period (Rosenthal and Levine, 1971; Barton and Barton, 1973). The therapist's activities may include interpretations and confrontations, based on formulations and goals, as well as support, advice and direction.

The therapist must utilize his rapport with the

family, the limited therapy time period, the family's motivation, and their collaborative definition of treatment goals, to urge them into active participation in the therapy process both within and between therapy sessions. Family members are requested to undertake homework assignments related to their particular difficulties and treatment goals. Homework may involve family members consciously attempting to change a piece of behavior; structuring discussion of a conflictual issue; reading materials in child development (Fraiberg, 1959), temperament and parent-child "fit" (Thomas, Chess, and Birch, 1968; Chess, Thomas, and Birch, 1965), family communication (Gordon, 1970), behavior modification (Patterson and Gullion, 1968; Patterson, 1971; Smith and Smith, 1966; Becker, 1971), and parent-child relationships (Ginott, 1965; Salk, 1973); restructuring tasks and activities at home to alter stereotypic patterns of behavior; or assigning activities to enhance parental and marital relationships.

Behavioral change may precede emotional and attitudinal change (Wolberg, 1965; Phillips and Johnston, 1954; Kaffman, 1963; Berlin, 1970; Mackay, 1967; Kelleher, 1968; Malan, 1963; Heinicke and Goldman, 1960; *Psychiatric News*, 1975). As motivated family members engage in new behaviors, albeit somewhat structured and mechanical at first, their hope and desire for further change is enhanced, and the process becomes self-reinforcing. During therapy sessions homework assignments are reviewed, particularly the interpersonal encounters of family members, always relating them to treatment formulations and goals. Reviewing failures of homework assignments often leads to productive exploration of other intrapsychic, characterologic, and interpersonal issues. Modifying difficult assignments to become more manageable, exploring affective levels in carrying out assignments, and reviewing successful assignments, emphasize the responsibility family members must take themselves in the therapy process.

In developing and assigning homework tasks, the therapist must assess the psychological strengths of the child and parents, and help them to utilize these strengths in coping with their difficulties. Emphasis on psychological strengths, coping mechanisms, and adaptive interactions further places therapeutic responsibility on the family members, enhances independence and self-esteem, and fosters a self-healing process that can continue beyond the brief therapy period.

In the process of brief therapy, the therapist should:

1. Provide insight and education into the origins and factors maintaining psychopathology—intrapsychic, interpersonal, communicational, symptomatic, or environmental reinforcement.
2. Begin a process of therapeutic change through structured, assigned behavioral tasks for family members.
3. Gradually shift responsibility for maintaining and expanding behavioral change to the family, helping them to utilize psychological strengths, and adaptive coping mechanisms, whether old or new.
4. Anticipate with the family potential pitfalls or future times of crisis, and plan adaptive responses if not the prevention of problems, based on the insights and new behaviors learned and practiced during the brief therapy period.

While differing views exist, our own preference for a single therapist, as opposed to co-therapists conducting brief child and family therapy is supported in the literature (Kaffman, 1963). The single therapist can more easily maintain a cohesive view and consistent approach in the brief therapy process, and can avoid the often time-consuming but necessary coordination of collaborative conferences. With this in mind, peer group consultation for the therapist becomes even more important.

Termination

Because of the time limitation, termination is a central issue throughout the brief therapy process (Rosenthal and Levine, 1971; Mackay, 1967). It is introduced during the initial session as the time limit is explained. For many families requesting psychotherapy, loss or anticipated loss is a significant dynamic feature of their concerns or difficulties. Termination in brief therapy is handled as a reality issue, but where appropriate, also as a representation of previous significant loss. The therapist reminds the family of the approaching termination throughout the brief therapy period, and actively explores related feelings and behavior. Final sessions should include some review of the therapy, insights or knowledge gained, new attitudes or patterns of behavior developed, and progress in approaching the goals of treatment. Future difficulties should be anticipated with the family, with preparation for coping with potential crises.

Finally, brief therapy should not be viewed, nor

perhaps should any psychotherapy, as marking the end of emotional upsets or crises in an individual's or family's life. Hopefully, the family will be better able to handle crises after therapy, but they may require "booster" sessions to reinforce insights and behavior. Returning for further sessions is not necessarily a failure of brief therapy, and the opportunity to return if additional family crises arise is an integral part of the brief therapy process (Rosenthal and Levine, 1971; Kerns, 1970).

Therapy Structure

Length and Frequency

While variations exist according to therapist preference and the nature of the family psychopathology, brief therapy generally has a time limit of between 2 and 6 months (Proskower, 1969), with 3 months being a commonly used period (Rosenthal and Levine, 1970; Parad and Parad, 1968).

Frequency of therapy sessions is one to two hours per week, including sessions with the child, parents, or the entire family. For adequate evaluation, individual interviews with the child and each parent, as well as with the parents conjointly are helpful. Following the evaluation, family members selected to be involved in further therapy sessions depend on the treatment focus and goals.

Family-Oriented Approach

As well as selecting particular goals during the brief therapy process, the particular family members to be involved in the therapeutic sessions also require selection. This, of course, depends on the case formulation and treatment goals. The focus of therapy may be on marital difficulties, in which case the parents would be involved in most sessions. If parent-child relationships and child management are central issues, the parent and child would be involved, both individually and conjointly. The therapist must maintain a good deal of flexibility in providing therapeutic sessions for individual or combinations of family members as the treatment goals indicate.

A family-oriented approach is usually maintained in brief therapy, and family members other than the child presented as the identified patient are seen as often or more often than the child himself (Rosenthal and Levine, 1970; Barton and Barton, 1973). The issues addressed during therapy reflect a family orientation, and usually consist of such topics as child-rearing practices, family communication, parent-child relationships, marital relationships, sibling rivalries, and child or parent intrapsychic conflicts that affect other family members (Rosenthal and Levine, 1971).

Other Activities of the Therapist

During the brief therapy process, other activities by the therapist are appropriate to stimulate therapeutic change during treatment, and to maintain it following termination. For example, the use of medication indicated for symptomatic treatment of hyperkinesis, anxiety, and other symptoms may enhance the brief therapy process (Cytryn, Gilbert, and Eisenberg, 1960).

Other simultaneous activities often involve some form of environmental manipulation. They may involve brief consultations, by telephone or office visit, with supportive individuals significant in the child's and family's life—pediatricians, clergy, close relatives, associates, welfare workers, etc. Schoolteachers or counselors may be valuable allies in providing therapeutic approaches for the child in his class and school activities (Heinicke and Goldman, 1960). Any individuals sufficiently involved in the family's life who can provide ongoing support for therapeutic change may be included, with the family's approval, through brief consultation in the therapeutic process.

Depending on the therapeutic goals delineated, other activities during and following brief therapy may be indicated. Structured peer group activities for the child, outside-of-home activities for the single parent or the marital couple, and total family activities may help to support and maintain therapeutic change begun during the brief therapy period.

Follow-up

Follow-up appointments after the termination of brief therapy may be scheduled for several purposes. Obviously, 2 to 3 months of therapy will not fully resolve the difficulties that many children and families face upon entering treatment. The opportunity for follow-up visits becomes important if further crises in the family arise, or if some aspects of changes made during therapy require further reinforcement. Often one to three further visits, several months following the brief therapy, is sufficient to accomplish this.

Follow-up visits may also be used as check-up appointments to assure that therapeutic changes are continuing. Family members often require structured guidance in maintaining behavior change, at least for a period of time before these changes become more internalized. One or two "checks" may provide this guidance, prevent therapeutic deterioration and stimulate further therapeutic movement. These follow-up appointments are useful as well in evaluating the longer term benefits of brief therapy. Occasional appointments or at least some contact (telephone or mail) with the family over a year or longer following brief therapy may satisfy any or all of these reasons for follow-up.

The following clinical vignettes illustrate these techniques of brief therapy:

Case #1:

Dennis, an 11 year old boy, and his parents presented themselves at the clinic because Dennis had run away from home and threatened to kill himself. This incident was precipitated by the parents' preparation for departing on a planned weekend vacation. Dennis and his sister were to remain at home. The initial interviews with Dennis individually, and with his parents as a couple, elicited the following historical and dynamic information.

Separation had been a difficult issue in the history of this family. Neither parent had completely resolved the conflicts around separating from his and her own parents. When they met and married they formed an almost inseparable bond themselves. Dennis' birth precipitated a severe crisis in the family as he literally came between his parents and interrupted their relationship. His father reacted with jealousy and resentment. His mother was torn between giving to her infant son and to her husband, with the result that she felt inadequate both as a mother and a wife. A period of stormy marital conflict ensued, but gradually diminished as Dennis developed. Nevertheless, father's resentment and mother's inadequate feelings remained. These reactions resulted in Dennis' parents being unable to separate from him during his first three years of life. Separation problems emerged as Dennis entered nursery school, and again as he entered public school, but were not long-lasting. The family always took vacations together, and the parents infrequently left their children.

On the rare occasions they did leave the children, Dennis' reaction was one of severe protest. His runaway and suicide threat was the most severe of these and alarmed his parents so that they sought professional help.

On the basis of this information, the issue of separation was identified by therapist and family as a central focus of therapy. During the ten-week brief therapy period, a number of treatment goals related to "separation" were delineated, and therapist and family attempted to approach these collaboratively. During individual and conjoint sessions with Dennis' parents, his father's jealousy and resentments and his mother's feelings of inadequacy and ambivalence about separation were identified. From these discoveries, the parents resolved to redevelop their own identities and relationship as a marital couple and through the pursuit of some individual interests. Mother began an adult education class she had been interested in for some time. The parents began to explore new activities as a couple, apart from their children. These included both recreation and discussion of conflictual areas between them. These activities were initially homework assignments, carefully structured with the therapist's help. As the parents continued and grew more comfortable with these "new" activities, their structure and careful planning became less important for their continuation.

Dennis himself expressed ambivalent feelings about the issue of separation. He had strong urges to achieve more independence with his peer group, but had misgivings about his ability to relate to them, in part a result of his mother's difficulty in allowing him to develop more independence and self-sufficiency. Dennis had a strong interest in animals, and after some discussion, his parents allowed him to join the school biology club. This involved after school meetings and a number of evening and weekend field trips. With this beginning, Dennis established a few new friendships, one of which led him into two other peer activities, soccer and bicycling. These experiences led to further peer interactions, and helped Dennis to establish some greater independence.

The process of termination with this family regenerated their feelings of separation and loss. The therapist related these feelings to the central issues of the therapy as another example of managing separation situations. During the course of the therapy, increasing responsibility was placed on the family to discover and implement methods of handling their concerns. As the progress of therapy was reviewed during the termination process, it became more evident to the family the degree of responsibility they had taken, and that their dependence and initial dismay at "losing" their therapist was an over-reaction. Therapy was terminated as the parents planned and took a week's vacation by themselves without protest or problems with them or the children.

The family members were free of symptoms at termination, had significant insights into the dynamic issues they faced, and had developed a number of successful coping mechanisms to manage present and future difficulties. A follow-up appointment was scheduled two months later, at which time further therapeutic progress was evident. Dennis' independence and peer relationships had improved, and the parents were pleased with the continued development of their own relationship. About 6 months later, the family called because of a minor crisis. Dennis had arranged to spend a month vacationing with a friend and his family, but became uncertain about leaving a few days before departure. After a 15 minute telephone consultation with the therapist, the family was able to discuss and resolve the situation themselves. They reviewed the separation issues, determined that they had some ambivalence about the trip themselves, and dealt with their concerns about it. They were able to resolve the issues and Dennis left on the trip comfortably. After one week, Dennis called his parents long distance and "wondered" if he should return home early. His parents assured him that all was well with them and he was able to finish the vacation successfully. The parents called 4 months later to indicate continued progress in these areas. Although they realized future circumstances involving separations might generate problems again, they felt they could recognize these as they arose and manage them satisfactorily.

Case #2:

Timmy is a 5-year-old boy whose parents visited the clinic because of their concern about his dressing up in his 3-year-old sister's clothing. Timmy had done this infrequently but intermittently over the past two years, usually in the privacy of his bedroom. His parents initially tried to ignore it, and then became disapproving, but not punitive of this behavior. Although he had no effeminate characteristics, they requested an evaluation because of this concern about his sexual development.

The parents were interviewed jointly in the initial evaluation, and Timmy was seen individually in a play diagnostic session. The therapist was impressed by a variety of evidence during the play session that Timmy's identifications and gender role were developing along masculine lines. At the same time, his play indicated a great deal of generalized aggressive and angry affect. During the next meeting with Timmy's parents, a number of formulations and treatment goals, based on information from these evaluation interviews were delineated.

The therapist informed his parents that while Timmy appeared to be developing along masculine-oriented lines, another issue that impressed him which they had not raised previously, and one that might be related to the dressing up, was Timmy's excessive angry and aggressive feelings and behavior. Both parents immediately confirmed this impression and stated that while they had some minor concerns about his dressing up, they were more often quite disturbed by his very aggressive behavior with other children, particularly his sister and other girls.

The parents and therapist together formulated hypotheses about Timmy's behavior. Timmy's father was raised by controlling, dominating parents who inhibited his expressions of anger and assertiveness. He was determined that Timmy should develop traits of assertiveness, and regularly reinforced his aggressive and defiant behavior, often failing to set appropriate limits. Timmy's mother identified with her own rather perfectionistic mother, and tended to overcontrol Timmy with excessive demands and expectations. These often inconsistent parental messages contributed to Timmy's aggressive behavior toward others. To further complicate the situation, Timmy's younger sister was the apple of his father's eye. His resentment, jealousy, and both rivalrous and envious feelings resulted in anger and aggressiveness on one hand, and dressing up to be like his sister on the other. Several areas of conflict in the parents' relationship also emerged as we discussed their personality characteristics and manner of relating to each other.

With these formulations, several treatment goals were identified: to help his father develop more appropriate reinforcement and limit setting for Timmy; to help his mother relinquish some of her over controlling approach, and allow Timmy more autonomous choices within appropriate and consistent limits; to help both parents relate to Timmy with more warmth and empathy, recognizing his feelings and frustration; to explore the parents' inconsistencies in child management as well as their relationship with each other, with a view toward beginning indicated therapeutic intervention.

The parents were assigned readings in parent-child communication and relationships, in child development, and in child management and behavior modification. They were helped to develop reinforcements for appropriate behavior at particularly difficult times for Timmy and the family—at dinner time, bedtime, and while playing with his sister. Consistent limits and reinforcement helped his mother to avoid overcontrol, and his father to avoid encouraging Timmy's defiance and aggressiveness. At the same time, the parents began to communicate and relate more positively with Timmy, recognizing and accepting his anger and frustration. Their time with him began to be more enjoyable rather than being taken up with continual parent-child conflicts. As the parents applied appropriate reinforcements and began to meet Timmy's emotional needs for acceptance and autonomy, his defiance and aggressiveness both decreased significantly. Increased activities with Timmy's peer group also promoted this improvement. Further, the difficult experience of altering their behavior in these ways forced both parents to examine their own personal relating styles with the children and with each other. In several ways, the mother's overcontrol and the father's inhibition and tendency toward passive-aggressiveness (including subtly encouraging his son's defiance) resulted in significant stress in their marriage. The parents began to examine these issues during the brief therapy period, and following it entered couples' therapy elsewhere to improve their marital relationship.

While most of the sessions during the nine-week brief therapy period involved the parents, both individually and as a couple, several hours were spent with Timmy in play therapy, exploring his feelings of anger, aggressiveness, and jealousy. With some directive guidance and suggestions, Timmy began to discover alternative behaviors for expressing his angry feelings, and had the opportunity to strengthen them as his parents altered their approach with him in relating and reinforcement. Timmy's parents were enthusiastic about the changes in the family, and were reinforced themselves to continue to work on and maintain them. Follow-up telephone calls indicated that Timmy's improvement persisted and the parents had made progress in a brief course of marital couple therapy. About two months after the brief therapy, Timmy once again experimented with "dressing up"; he soon lost interest in this as his other needs were being met however, and there have been no further reports of this activity.

Case #3:

Sara, seven years old, and her parents were referred to the clinic by her school teachers because of her disruptive behavior. Although quite petite, Sara virtually terrorized others in her class with rages of screaming, throwing books, and overturning desks. She was regularly sent to the principal's office and her mother called to take her home. Her rages appeared associated with having to follow teachers' directions and with academic frustration. While having high intellectual capabilities, she was performing well below her potential academically. Sara also had great difficulties in relating to other children and her controlling behavior alienated most of her peers.

Sara is an only child, and her parents had had difficulties with her for several years. Her school problems in fact had existed since nursery school. Her father, a lawyer, was a strict disciplinarian who expected and demanded high levels of adult-like behavior from his intelligent, somewhat precocious daughter. Her mother, a former school teacher, tended to ignore any misbehavior by Sara until it reached an intolerable level. She then over-reacted with screaming rages, often throwing and breaking plates and utensils. During a play diagnostic session Sara, while relating well to the therapist, was both manipulative and controlling, and had difficulty conforming even to limits of time and space. Each parent, during evaluation sessions with them, displayed evidence of significant individual psychopathology. Sara's father was often bothered by obsessive-compulsive symptoms and tended to have mildly paranoid thoughts. Her mother was significantly depressed and felt overwhelmed in her daily life.

In attempting to develop formulations and treatment goals with the parents, the therapist pointed out several obvious relationships between the parents' behavior, their expectations of Sara, and inconsistencies in handling her, and Sara's disruptive and manipulative school behavior. The parents were willing to acknowledge these relationships, but were quite resistant to any further examination of their own personality characteristics or interpersonal relations. They tended to see the situation largely as Sara's problems, and requested help to change her behavior. The therapist agreed that therapy with Sara was indicated and that he would be willing to begin with this, but also explicitly stated his belief that parent-child interactions and parental personality characteristics contributed to the situation. He urged regular sessions with the parents to "coordinate" the treatment approach and to explore their parent-child interactions further. The parents agreed to this and therapy began.

Sara was seen in play therapy once a week for the 12 week brief therapy period. Sara's father had three individual sessions; her mother had six sessions, and the couple was seen jointly for the final two sessions. Although father's resistance remained high, he was able to accept, in the individual sessions, that his high expectations of Sara contributed to her frustration and anger at being unable to accomplish goals immediately, her fear of failure, and her consequent resistance to take directions and her need to control others. With support, father was able to reduce some of his demands on Sara, and to tolerate less than perfect performance from her. While he did alter some of his behavior in this way, which clearly helped in Sara's gradual improvement, he remained resistant to further therapy and refused further individual appointments. Sara's mother on the other hand seemed to welcome the opportunity for individual therapy sessions. She accepted readily therapeutic intervention for her depression and was eager for guidance to improve her relationship with her daughter. Readings in parent-child communication and in child management helped her to develop more appropriate approaches in relating to Sara, both in general interactions and limit setting. Increased confidence in these areas encouraged her to begin to communicate more openly with her husband about their relationship as well as about their handling of Sara's difficulties. Her husband accepted her attempts to communicate, and their relationship began to develop more openness and warmth. The final two sessions of the brief therapy period included additional support and guidance for their therapeutic progress in this area.

Play therapy for Sara consisted of gradual attempts to challenge her need for total control and help her to accept appropriate limits more comfortably, using her positive relationship with the therapist to reinforce these difficult changes for her. Her anxiety at loss of control and accepting limits began to decrease in the therapy sessions, and with simultaneous support by her parents and teachers, this began to generalize to home and school situations as well. The therapist consulted with Sara's teachers once at school and twice by telephone to help them provide similar therapeutic approaches. As these changes developed, she began to improve academically, and to tolerate more sharing relationships with her peer group, which further reinforced the changes she, her parents, and her teachers were making. Follow-up visits were scheduled every six to eight weeks for six months, and several further telephone conversations with Sara's teachers were held. While her course was uneven, she continued to show improvement as her school and peer relationships improved. It is anticipated that Sara's parents will continue to require periodic consultations as further issues in her development and in their own relationship arise.

Comparison

Other Therapeutic Modalities

The use of brief therapy with children and families does not preclude their involvement in more traditional long term psychotherapy, nor in any other type of treatment. At times in fact a course of brief therapy will stimulate a family member's desire to enter additional therapy for further personal insight, change and growth.

The question of need for other therapy for the child and family following the brief therapy period is complicated. Many feelings are generated by termination, both within the therapist and family members. Feelings of loss, sadness, abandonment, guilt, dependence, return of symptoms, or others may influence therapist or family to press for further therapy. This decision of course must be made on the basis of therapeutic need, rather than because of transference or counter-transference issues. In these cases, peer group consultation for the therapist can be quite helpful to perceive the issues involved and reach a clinically indicated decision. If further therapy is indicated, it is possible of course to contract for a further brief therapy period, again with specific goals and treatment focus.

Comparative Evaluation

The evaluation of treatment outcome in psychotherapy presents numerous methodological difficulties. Volumes which review psychotherapy outcome studies repeatedly point out their limitations and inadequacies (Meltzoff and Kornreich, 1970; Stollak, Guerney, and Rothberg, 1966). Relatively few studies of therapeutic results of brief therapy with children and their families exist, and those that do have numerous methodological problems. While partially limited by lack of adequate controls, by global or general assessment criteria, or by inadequate follow-up, a number of studies do provide useful indications of the efficacy and results of brief therapy.

Maher and Katkovsky (1961) reported improvement in nervousness, fighting, and destructive behavior in children and their parents receiving three or less hours of semi-directive therapy. When compared with an untreated control group, other symptoms or behavioral difficulties were not improved. Coddington's experience in pediatric practice indicated that the majority of cases referred to him for psychotherapy could be successfully managed by a brief, direct type of psychotherapy (Coddington, 1962). Brief family therapy by Kaffman was reported successful in 75% of 29 cases treated (Kaffman, 1963). Success was based on the disappearance of the presenting symptoms or problems. Kaffman suggests that brief therapy is indicated when motivation is high, when emotional conflict has not been internalized, and when a positive relationship can be developed with the therapist.

School phobia has been successfully treated with brief treatment according to a number of reports (Kennedy, 1965; *Psychiatric News*, 1975; Minuchin, Chamberlain, and Graubard, 1967). Success is measured by the child's prompt return to school. Success rates of 80% to 90% in this condition are not unusual provided that treatment is initiated early, that is, while symptoms are acute and family motivation is high.

Other studies of treatment outcome in brief psychotherapy with children report success rates of 70% to 80%. Hare (1966) was able to achieve a 72% improvement rate with unselected cases in a child guidance clinic. Shaw, Blumenfeld and Senf (1968), Eisenberg, Conners and Sharpe (1965), Nebl (1971), and Lessing and Shilling (1966) report similar results, and indicate that improvement is maintained in most treated children during follow-up periods. In studies by Phillips (1960) and Phillips and Johnston (1954), children and their parents treated with brief therapy have even higher improvement rates than those treated with conventional long term therapy.

Our own studies (Rosenthal and Levine, 1970, 1971) as well as these others suggest that brief therapy with children and their parents is as effective as long term psychotherapy when measured by improvement of presenting symptoms and ongoing conflicts. Further, they indicate that beneficial results are sustained during follow-up periods of one to two years. These success rates however, are achieved under particular conditions. The authors emphasize the structure of brief therapy with children and the factors leading to its success (Phillips and Johnston, 1954). Among the factors cited repeatedly in these reports are family motivation, acuteness of problems, therapist motivation, some measure of family stability, clearly defined time limits, therapeutic goals and focus of treatment, working intensively with parents as well as children, and supporting healthy psychological mechanisms in the family to enable the development of successful coping for the future.

While more methodologically sophisticated approaches are needed in treatment outcome studies of brief therapy with children, numerous reports provide evidence of its efficacy and beneficial results. Given proper patient selection, appropriate therapist motivation and style, and structure of the brief therapy process, this approach holds great promise in reaching many more emotionally disturbed children and families.

Summary and Conclusion

Rationale

Estimates of emotional disturbance in childhood and adolescence range from 10% to 20% (Joint Commission on Mental Health of Children, 1969; Gorman, 1969; Tarjan, 1969). Only 10% of those requiring psychotherapeutic intervention actually receive it (Alderton, 1969). It has become increasingly clear that the ranks of professionals are insufficient to meet the mental health needs of children in our society. Traditional treatment approaches cannot provide the intervention necessary, and a variety of alternate methods of delivering mental health care have been explored. Brief psychotherapy is one such method.

The community mental health movement has helped to bring mental health care to many segments of our child population. With the need and demand for services far exceeding the capacity to provide them, however, waiting lists in community clinics remain lengthy. Many children and families must wait long periods of time for an opening for evaluation or treatment. Brief therapy is one approach to delivering services more rapidly, decreasing the waiting list, and providing intervention closer to the time of the family's request for service.

Community clinics often experience high dropout rates—that is, patients leaving therapy after a few visits (Frank et al., 1957; Freedman et al., 1958). Presumably many of these patients do not respond to traditional insight-oriented, open-ended therapy. Many others, although they remain in treatment, do not improve with this therapeutic approach. Brief therapy, as an alternative approach to patients for whom traditional psychotherapy is inappropriate or ineffective, has been shown to reduce dropout rates (Parad and Parad, 1968) and maintain ongoing though intermittent therapeutic relationships with resistant patients.

Brief therapy also has an important role in programs of primary and secondary prevention. Exploring issues of child development, parent-child relationships, and parenting skills with individual or groups of families often uncovers potential or relatively minor conflict areas (Barton and Barton, 1973; Thomas, Chess, and Birch, 1968; Augenbraun, Reid, and Friedman, 1967). Approaching these in the context of a discussion group or of brief individual consultations may help to prevent the development of more serious conflicts later.

B. Advantages

Clinical experience indicates that children and families readily accept brief therapy, and in fact that this approach results in fewer dropouts from therapy (Parad and Parad, 1968). Offering therapy immediately after the family applies for service, when motivation is high, is an important factor in this. Following the evaluation and the decision that brief therapy is indicated, the family should be informed of the time limit, the focus on particular treatment goals, and the collaboration during the therapy process of therapist and family. The family must understand the responsibility they will be asked to assume during the therapy—attempting behavior changes, completing homework assignments, and confronting issues in therapy that may be uncomfortable or even painful. At the same time, the fact that particular difficulties and treatment goals can be approached in a three month period with intensive work, casts an optimistic and hopeful tone over the therapy and may enhance motivation further. It must be explained, of course, that problems will not disappear or "be cured" in a three month period, but that the family may gain insights into them and develop the coping mechanisms to handle them themselves in the future.

Brief therapy also has the advantage of economy, both from the family's and from the therapist's standpoint. For the family in therapy, the point of termination is known; families can plan for the financial expense of therapy and predict the time involved. Families may return for follow-up visits as needed, but usually without the uncertainty of an open-ended financial or time commitment.

Viewed by the therapist, brief therapy is an efficient as well as effective approach. Treatment goals must be explicitly and clearly specified. The time limit exerts its "therapeutic pressure" toward achieving these goals. The family is given direct responsibility for change within the therapy and afterward. Family members in a sense become "therapists" with each other to maintain and expand gains made during the brief therapy process (Kliman, 1971).

In addition, a brief therapy approach allows for the extension of therapeutic services. More families may be seen in therapy; waiting lists may be reduced and waiting periods for therapy diminished. While the greater practice of brief therapy would not in itself resolve the problem of the many untreated emotionally disturbed children and families, it would provide an additional approach to reach more of them therapeutically.

C. Conclusions

As issues in community mental health and health care delivery have achieved prominence, brief focused therapy with children and families has emerged as a useful and beneficial approach in psychotherapeutic practice. For many therapists, brief therapy requires a new orientation (Heinicke and Goldman, 1960). As described here, it requires an intensive and pragmatic approach, utilizing theory and active techniques from numerous and often diverse areas of psychology and psychotherapy. Consequently, brief therapy offers difficulties or complications that may not be encountered in long-term open-ended psychotherapy. Rather than a second-class approach to be practiced by the inexperienced, brief therapy is the treatment of choice for many, and its intensity and complexities are best handled by the more experienced clinician who has the opportunity for regular peer consultation.

Brief therapy recognizes the family's health, psychological strengths, capabilities and responsibility for maintaining and continuing therapeutic progress during and following the brief therapy process. Its successful practice requires a brief therapy "set"

(Rosenthal and Levine, 1970, 1971) or orientation by both therapist and family. The elements of this set must include:

- therapist motivation
- family motivation
- "therapeutic pressure" of time-limited therapy
- collaborative effort in defining the therapeutic focus and working toward specific treatment goals
- encouraging family responsibility for therapeutic progress
- here-and-now, reality orientation
- rapidly developed therapeutic alliance
- termination as a central issue of therapy
- flexible, family-oriented approach
- therapist activity in directing and structuring the therapy, and developing adaptive family coping mechanisms
- follow-up contacts and the opportunity to return if further stress or family crises arise.

While brief therapy is not a panacea for the emotional ills of children and families, it clearly offers the promise of an effective as well as efficient psychotherapeutic approach for many of our emotionally disturbed. With continued recognition and acceptance by child and family psychotherapists, brief therapy will provide relief for many more of the large number of emotionally disturbed families in our society.

References

Alderton, H.R. (1969) The therapeutic paradox. *Can. Psychiat. Assn. J.* 14(3):287–293.

Alexander, F. (1951) Principles and techniques of briefer psychotherapeutic procedures. *Proc. Assn. Res. Nerv. Ment. Dis.* 31:16.

Allen, F.H. (1946) Case 8. Betty Ann Meyer. In H. L. Witmer, ed., *Psychiatric Interviews with Children.* Cambridge, Mass.: Harvard University Press, pp. 259–331.

Allen, F.H. (1942) *Psychotherapy with Children.* New York: Norton.

Alpern, E. (1956) Short clinical services for children in a child guidance clinic. *Am. J. Orthopsychiat.* 26(2):314–325.

Argles, P., and M. Mackenzie. (1970) Crisis intervention with a multi-problem family: A case study. *J. Child Psychol. Psychiat.* 11(3):187–195.

Augenbraun, B., H.L. Reid, and D.B. Friedman. (1967) Brief intervention as a preventive force in disorders of early childhood. *Am. J. Orthopsychiat.* 37(4):697–702.

Barton, H.H., ed. (1971) *Brief Therapies.* New York: Behavioral Publications.

Barton, H.H., and S.S. Barton, eds. (1973) *Children and Their Parents in Brief Therapy.* New York: Behavioral Publications.

Becker, W.C. (1971) *Parents Are Teachers—A Child Management Program.* Champaign, Ill.: Research Press.

Berlin, I.N. (1970) Crisis intervention and short-term therapy: An approach in a child psychiatric clinic. *J. Am. Acad. Child Psychiat.* 9(4):595–606.

Blanchard, P. (1946) Case 1. Tommy Nolan. In H.L. Witmer, ed., *Psychiatric Interviews with Children.* Cambridge, Mass.: Harvard University Press, pp. 59–92.

Breuer, J., and S. Freud. (1957) *Studies on Hysteria.* New York: Basic Books. (originally published in 1895)

Bruch, H. (1949) Brief psychotherapy in a pediatric clinic. *Quart. J. Child Behav.* 1(1):2–8.

Caplan, G., E.A. Mason, and D.M. Kaplan. (1965) Four studies of crisis in parents of prematures. *Com. Ment. Health J.* 1(2):149–161.

Chess, S., A. Thomas, and H.G. Birch. (1965) *Your Child Is a Person.* New York: Parallax.

Coddington, R.D. (1962) The use of brief psychotherapy in a pediatric practice. *J. Pediat.* 60(2):259–265.

Cytryn, L., A. Gilbert, and L. Eisenberg. (1960) The effectiveness of tranquilizing drugs plus supportive psychotherapy in treating behavior disorders of children: A double-blind study of 80 outpatients. *Am. J. Orthopsychiat.* 30(1):113–128.

Eisenberg, L., C.K. Conners, and L. Sharpe. (1965) A controlled study of the differential application of outpatient psychiatric treatment for children. *Jap. J. Child Psychiat.* 6(1):1–8.

Fenichel, O. (1954) Brief psychotherapy. In H. Fenichel and D. Rapaport, eds., *The Collected Papers of Otto Fenichel.* New York: Norton.

Fraiberg, S.H. (1959) *The Magic Years.* New York: Scribner's.

Frank, J.D. (1961) *Persuasion and Healing.* Baltimore: Johns Hopkins Press.

Frank, J. D., L.H. Gliedman, S.D. Imber, et al. (1957) Why patients leave psychotherapy. *A.M.A. Arch. Neurol. Psychiat.* 77(3):283–299.

Freedman, N., D.M. Engelhardt, L.D. Hankoff, et al. (1958) Drop-out from outpatient psychiatric treatment. *A.M.A. Arch. Neurol. Psychiat.* 80(11):657–666.

Ginott, H.G. (1965) *Between Parent and Child.* New York: Macmillan.

Gordon, T. (1970) *Parent Effectiveness Training.* New York: Peter H. Wyden.

Gorman, M. (1969) An action program for the mental health of our children. Paper read at the San Francisco Mental Health Association meeting, San Francisco, California.

Gottschalk, L.A., G.C. Morrison, R.B. Drury, and A.C. Barnes. (1970) The Laguna Beach experiment as a community approach to family counseling for drug abuse problems in youth. *Comp. Psychiat.* 11(3):226–234.

Hare, M.K. (1966) Shortened treatment in a child guidance clinic: Results in 119 cases. *Brit. J. Psychiat.* 112(6):613–616.

Heinicke, C.M., and A. Goldman. (1960) Research on psychotherapy with children. *Am. J. Orthopsychiat.* 30(3):483–494.

Joint Commission on Mental Health of Children. (1969) *Crisis in Child Mental Health: Challenge for the 1970's.* New York: Harper & Row.

Kaffman, M. (1963) Short-term family therapy. *Fam. Proc.* 2(2):216–234.

Kardiner, A. (1941) *The Traumatic Neuroses of War.* New York: Hoeber.

Kelleher, D. (1968) A model for integrating special education and community mental health services. *J. Special Ed.* 2:263–272.

Kennedy, W.A. (1965) School phobia: Rapid treatment of 50 cases. *J. Abnor. Psychol.* 70(4):285–289.

Kerns, E. (1970) Planned short-term treatment: A new service to adolescents. *Social Casework* 51(6):340–346.

Kliman, G. (1971) Discussion. *Am. J. Psychiat.* 128(2):145–146.

Lessing, E.E., and F.H. Shilling. (1966) Relationship between treatment selection variables and treatment outcome in a child guidance clinic: An application of data processing methods. *J. Am. Acad. Child Psychiat.* 5(2):313–348.

Lester, E.P. (1968) Brief psychotherapy in child psychiatry. *Can. Psychiat. Assn. J.* 13(4):301–309.

Levy, D.M. (1939) Release therapy. *Am. J. Orthopsychiat.* 9(4):713–736.

Lewin, K.K. (1970) *Brief Psychotherapy.* St. Louis: Warren H. Green.

Lindemann, E. (1944) Symptomatology and management of acute grief. *Am. J. Psychiat.* 101(2):141–148.

Mackay, J. (1967) The use of brief psychotherapy with children. *Can. Psychiat. Assn. J.* 12(3):269–279.

Maher, B.A., and W. Katkovsky. (1961) The efficacy of brief clinical procedures in alleviating children's problems. *J. Indiv. Psychol.* 17:205–211.

Malan, D.H. (1963) *A Study of Brief Psychotherapy.* Springfield, Ill.: Charles C. Thomas.

Meltzoff, J., and M. Kornreich. (1970) *Research in Psychotherapy.* New York: Atherton Press.

Minuchin, S., P. Chamberlain, and P. Graubard. (1967) A project to teach learning skills to disturbed, delinquent children. *Am. J. Orthopsychiat.* 37(3):558–567.

Nebl, N. (1971) Essential elements in short-term treatment. *Social Casework* 52(6):377–381.

Parad, H.J., and L.G. Parad. (1968) A study of crisis-oriented planned short-term treatment: Part I. *Social Casework* 49(6):346–355.

Parad, L.G., and H.J. Parad. (1968) A study of crisis-oriented planned short-term treatment: Part II. *Social Casework* 49(7):418–426.

Patterson, G.R. (1971) *Families.* Champaign, Ill.: Research Press.

Patterson, G.R., and M.E. Gullion. (1968) *Living with Children.* Champaign, Ill.: Research Press.

Phillips, E.L. (1960) Parent-child psychotherapy: A follow-up study comparing two techniques. *J. Psychol.* 49(1):195–202.

Phillips, E.L., and M.S.H. Johnston. (1954) Theoretical and clinical aspects of short-term parent-child psychotherapy. *Psychiatry* 17(3):267–275.

Phillips, E.L., and D.N. Weiner. (1966) *Short-Term Psychotherapy and Structured Behavior Change.* New York: McGraw-Hill.

Proskower, S. (1969) Some technical issues in time-limited psychotherapy with children. *J. Am. Acad. Child Psychiat.* 8(1):154–169.

Psychiatric News. (1975) Bio-feedback said to place responsibilities on patient. 10(14):28–29.

Rosenthal, A.J., and S.V. Levine. (1970) Brief psychotherapy with children: A preliminary report. *Am. J. Psychiat.* 127(5):646–651.

Rosenthal, A.J., and S.V. Levine. (1971) Brief psychotherapy with children: Process of therapy. *Am. J. Psychiat.* 128(2):141–146.

Rank, B. (1946) Case 3. Jerry Hoskins. In H.L. Witmer, ed., *Psychiatric Interviews with Children.* Cambridge, Mass.: Harvard University Press, pp. 136–156.

Salk, L. (1973) *What Every Child Would Like His Parents to Know.* New York: Warner.

Shaw, R., H. Blumenfeld, and R. Senf. (1968) A short-term treatment program in a child guidance clinic. *Social Work* 13(3):81–90.

Shulman, J.L. (1960) One-visit psychotherapy with children. *Prog. Psychother.* 5:86-93.

Small, L. (1971) *The Briefer Psychotherapies.* New York: Brunner/Mazel.

Smith, J.M., and D.E.P. Smith. (1966) *Child Management: A Program for Parents and Teachers.* Ann Arbor, Mich.: Ann Arbor Publishers.

Solomon, J.C. (1948) Trends in orthopsychiatric therapy: Play technique. *Am. J. Orthopsychiat.* 18(3):402–413.

Springe, M.P. (1968) Work with adolescents: Brief psychotherapy with a limited aim. *J. Child Psychother.* 2(1):31–37.

Stollak, G.E., B.G. Guerney, and M. Rothberg, eds. (1966) *Psychotherapy Research: Selected Readings.* Chicago: Rand McNally.

Tarjan, G. (1969) And what of the children. *Hosp. Com. Psychiat.* 20(4):223–227.

Thomas, A., S. Chess, and H.G. Birch. (1968) *Temperament and Behavior Disorders in Children.* New York: New York University Press.

Wagner, M.K. (1968) Parent therapists: An operant conditioning method. *Ment. Hyg.* 52(3):452–455.

Waldfogel, S., E. Tessman, and P.B. Hahn. (1959) A program of early intervention in school phobia. *Am. J. Orthopsychiat.* 29(2):324–332.

Werry, J.S., and J.P. Wollersheim. (1967) Behavior therapy with children: A broad overview. *J. Am. Acad. Child Psychiat.* 6(2):346–370.

Witmer, H.L., ed. (1946) *Psychiatric Interviews with Children.* Cambridge, Mass.: Harvard University Press.

Wolberg, L.R. (1965) *Short-Term Psychotherapy.* New York: Grune & Stratton.

Treatment of Emotional Disorders in Children and Adolescents

CHAPTER 8

Play Therapy

Charles E. Schaefer

Introduction

Play is a universal activity of childhood that has definite purposes. One of the most firmly established principles of psychology is that play is a process of development for a child. Through play, children develop their intellectual, emotional, perceptual-motor, and social skills. According to Piaget (1969), active experimentation and repetition in play enables children to "mentally digest" and assimilate novel situations and experiences. White (1966) stresses that problem-solving and competence skills develop through play activities. Children deal with daily experiences by creating similar situations in play and then mastering these events by experiment and planning. In play the child is in control of the happenings, and there is less anxiety because it is a low-risk situation. Erikson (1963) also views play as a kind of "emotional laboratory" in which the child learns to master his environment and come to terms with the world. Psychologists and educators now take play very seriously and are actively engaged in extensive research to uncover further its potential for normal child development. In recent years there have been a number of excellent volumes reviewing and synthesizing the literature on the psychology of play (Millar, 1968; Ellis, 1973) and presenting a sampling of the prime contributions (Bruner et al., 1976).

Apart from its obvious growth-producing role, play has an equally powerful therapeutic value for children with emotional or behavior problems. Erikson (1963) states that to "play it out" is the most natural and self-healing process in childhood. Among the curative powers of play are the following: it releases tensions and pent-up emotions; it allows for compensation in fantasy for loss, hurts, and failures; it facilitates self-discovery of more adaptive behaviors; it promotes awareness of conflicts revealed only sumbolically or through displacement; and it offers the opportunity to reeducate children to alternate behaviors through role-playing or storytelling. The therapeutic usefulness of play is also based on the fact that play is the child's natural mode of self-expression, just as talk is the natural form of communication for the adult. Ginott (1961) noted that "the child's play is his talk and toys are his words." Play also represents a way of establishing rapport and friendly contact with a child, since it is an activity that is interesting, enjoyable, and natural to children. Thus play can be used as a *medium* for achieving such external goals as building a relationship, setting limits, or applying reinforcement contingencies. On the other hand, it can be used for its intrinsic therapeutic processes such as catharsis, problem-solving, and assimilation of stressful experiences. Both as a medium and a process then, play has unique therapeutic functions. Both aspects of play therapy will be discussed in this chapter.

In a recent article, Nickerson (1973) listed the following reasons why play activities remain the main therapeutic approach for both individual and group work with children:

1. Play is a child's natural medium for self-expression, experimentation, and learning.

2. Feeling at home in a play setting, the child can readily relate to toys and play out concerns with them.
3. A play medium facilitates a child's communication and expression.
4. A play medium also allows for a cathartic release of feelings, frustrations, and so on.
5. Play experience can be renewing, wholesome, and constructive in a child's life.
6. The adult can more naturally understand the child's world by observing him at play, and can more readily relate to the child via play activities than through an entirely verbal discussion.

History

Sigmund Freud was the first therapist to recognize the value of play for uncovering a child's unconscious conflicts, wants, and desires. He first used play in treating the famous case of "Little Hans," a boy whose father was worried about his sudden fear of horses. The father observed the boy's play, dreams, and talk while Freud interpreted the meanings of these expressions to the father. It is not surprising, then, that child psychoanalysts were the early pioneers in the use of play for the diagnosis and treatment of childhood emotional problems. Hermine Hug-Hellmuth, a psychoanalytically-oriented educator, began using play as part of her treatment of children in 1920, but it was not until some ten years later that Melanie Klein and Anna Freud formulated the theory and practice of psychoanalytic play therapy. Although both women adhered to an analytic framework, their use of play differed substantially in actual practice. In particular, their use of interpretation varied greatly, as will be discussed later.

In the early thirties, two other approaches to play therapy appeared—namely, nondirective and structured therapy. About this time Slavson (1947) combined nondirective and group approaches with preadolescent children so as to allow them to work out their tensions and anxieties in games and activities within a group context. The nondirective approach is based on the philosophy of an early student of Freud—Otto Rank—who stated that constructive drives toward growth, development, and self-realization are inherent in human nature and can be counted on to produce change when given the opportunity for expression. The psychiatrist Frederick Allen espoused Rank's philosophy and applied it to the playroom, wherein he tried to develop an accepting, warm, and respectful relationship with a child (Allen, 1934). Carl Rogers later articulated the nondirective approach in greater detail, and Axline (1947a) wrote extensively of her use of this strategy with children. Axline stated that play is therapeutic because of the freedom of expression and growth it offers the child within the context of a safe, secure relationship with the therapist.

Structured play therapy involving the use of structured play materials and situations also appeared in the early thirties. David Levy (1939) began reporting success with his method of "release therapy," wherein he structured the play situation so as to encourage the child to reexperience traumatic events and release pent-up emotions and anxieties. Hambidge (1955) later termed this approach "structured play therapy."

Since the importance of setting limits was minimized by the previous approaches, Bixler (1949) and Ginott (1959) asserted that the early and consistent setting of limits in play therapy is just as important as establishing a warm relationship or interpreting underlying conflicts. By "saying what you mean and meaning what you say," they felt that the therapist can make authority a positive in the playroom. Finally, behavior therapy methods became popular in the playroom beginning in the early sixties. Behavior modification procedures, especially the contingent application of rewards for prosocial behaviors, are now used extensively in both individual and group play situations. Clearly, the trend of late is for therapists to become much more active and directive in the playroom.

Applicability

Since play is the universal language of childhood, the therapeutic use of child's play is common with children of all ages (two to adolescence) and differing types of problems (normal situational reactions to severe retardation and psychosis). Because boys and girls from all socioeconomic levels love to play, an inability to play has been found to be an index of severe emotional disturbance. The type of play encouraged in therapy should of course be suited to the child's current level of functioning. The infant and toddler love sensory-motor play, while the preschool and/or primary grade child is more prone to pretend or make-believe play. Games with rules and active physical activities are usually the choice of the grade school child, while team games are preferred by children age 10 and older.

With the possible exception of the highly verbal child who may prefer to talk and the child too inhibited to play, there are few contraindications to the use of play therapy with children.

Flexibility seems to be the key to effective use of play therapy—that is, one should match the play therapy approach with the particular needs of the child. With a wide assortment of approaches and techniques currently available, the clinician may find it rather difficult to decide which strategy is best for an individual child. At the present state of the art, one has to rely more on clinical judgment and experience more than research data to resolve this question. It has been this writer's experience that the psychoanalytic approach is best suited for middle- or upper-class children who exhibit long-standing neurotic disorders and little insight into their intrapsychic conflicts. The structured play therapy approach has been used effectively with children who show emotional reactions to specific environmental factors, such as sibling rivalry, death, divorce, or other loss. The nondirective or relationship method seems particularly appropriate for encouraging insecure, inhibited, or withdrawn children to gain self-confidence and trust in others. The play or activity group approach is designed to develop socialization skills in shy or aggressive children. The limit-setting approach is best employed with impulsive, undisciplined children with poor self-control, while the behavioral approach is applicable to a broad spectrum of behavior problems. The behavior modification technique has proven especially useful with habit and conduct problems.

Major Approaches to the Therapeutic Use of Play

Six major approaches to the therapeutic use of play have been reported in the literature—namely, psychoanalytic, structured, relationship, group, limit-setting, and behavioral. These six main theoretical approaches or schools of thought will be described in this section, beginning with the pioneering efforts of the child analysts and ending with the more recent applications of learning theory principles to the playroom. Quite diverse in nature, these approaches explain the therapeutic changes that occur during the play sessions in terms of different psychological processes and levels of psychic functioning. Also noteworthy is the fact that several approaches focus on the content and inherent therapeutic processes of play itself, while others use play primarily as a medium through which to apply other interventions. For this reason the term "therapeutic use of child's play" seems a more apt way of classifying the six major approaches than the more popular term "play therapy."

Psychoanalytic Approach

In general, the psychoanalytic approach to play emphasizes the use of the therapist's interpretation of a child's words and actions, as well as the analysis of the transference relationship, to help children achieve insight into their unconscious conflicts. Melanie Klein (1937) was the first analyst to use interpretation frequently in the psychoanalysis of children and to explore deeply their unconscious. Through play activities she encouraged the child to express fantasies, anxieties, and defenses which she then interpreted. Klein felt that an analysis of the child's transference relationship with the therapist was the main way to provide insight into the child's underlying conflict. By analyzing how the child transfers to the therapist earlier experiences and feelings toward his parents, psychoanalysts attempt to understand the child's psyche and reveal this insight to the child. Thus Klein might try to interpret a sign of negative transference by stating, "You're afraid of what I might do to you when we are alone like this?" In addition to transference, Klein would interpret the hidden meaning of a child's use of toys; for example, she might suggest that by putting a doll representing a sister out of the doll house, the child is expressing the desire to be alone with the parents and to be an only child again. If the father doll is then put out of the room Klein might interpret this as meaning that the child wants the father out of the way so he can have his mother all to himself at times. Cars colliding might be interpreted as some sexual activity between a child and a friend. The validity of an interpretation is inferred from the child's reaction; a telling look, a roguish smile, or a vehement denial may be taken as confirmation that the interpretation is on target.

Believing play to be the medium in which children express themselves most freely, Klein stocked the playroom with a wide variety of toys and materials designed to promote self-expression—particularly about the family situation. She advocated keeping toys simple, small, unstructured, and nonmechanical. Typically she would offer the child freedom to select toys representing the common interests of childhood: little wooden men and women, animals, cars, houses, balls, marbles, and other types of creative materials—paper, scissors, plasticine, paints, and pencils. She kept each child's playthings locked in a drawer that was part of the private and intimate relationship between child and therapist. Although Klein did not allow physical attacks on herself, she did encourage the child to express deep-seated hostilities in other ways including verbal attacks on the therapist. She did not show annoyance at verbal assaults but would interpret their deeper motives so as to keep the situation under control.

In contrast to Melanie Klein, Anna Freud (1946) used interpretations much more sparingly. She employed play to a considerable extent during the early stages of treatment to get to know the child and to influence the child to like her. She would supplement play observations with information from parents in order to gain a broad perspective on the child's problem. Only after she had gained extensive knowledge about a child would she offer direct interpretations to the child concerning the real meaning of the play behavior. Although Anna Freud now believes that a transference neurosis is possible in the treatment of children, she continues to believe that it cannot be equal to the adult variety (Freud, 1965). Moreover, Anna Freud is careful to note that psychoanalytic treatment is not suitable for all types of children. It may be contraindicated for the psychotic and for children who have a marked difficulty in establishing a relationship due to severe emotional deprivation in early life. The presence of severe infantile neurosis and verbal facility are regarded as two prerequisites for analytic treatment. Since children are typically seen in analysis three or four times a week for an extended period, parents must have high motivation for treatment and ample financial resources. Most analysts now treat most latency age children (age 7 to 11) and often supplement play with such constructive projects as playwriting and drawings.

Anna Freud disagreed with the use of interpretations by Klein, which she felt to be excessive and extreme. Klein would see symbolic meanings, especially sexual meanings, in a great many play activities. For example, Klein would state: "In his [Egon's] case, as in all analyses of boys, making a cart move along meant masturbation and coitus, making carts hit together meant coitus, and comparison of a larger cart with a smaller meant rivalry with his father or his father's penis." (Klein, 1937, p. 26). Anna Freud, on the contrary, believes that play may not necessarily be symbolic of anything. A child could enjoy making a tower just because he recently saw one.

Among the criticisms of the psychoanalytic play technique are that interpretations are difficult to make accurately and that they often impede the development of a therapeutic relationship. It has also been said that children's capacity for insight into hidden meanings is limited, and that insight alone rarely leads to constructive behavior change. On the other hand, child analysts report that they have found even very young children to possess an insight ability that is greater than that of adults. Analysts also find that interpretations often help a child gain insight into repressed feelings and motives, which frequently lead to the development and anticipation of new adaptive modes of behavior. In comparison with other methods, the psychoanalytic use of play is both active in the sense of offering interpretations and nondirective in the sense of not attempting to reeducate or pressure the child towards alternate courses of action.

Structured Approach

Levy (1939) stimulated considerable interest in this method by reporting success with children between the ages of two and ten with "release" therapy. Rather than allowing children to play freely with a wide variety of toys and materials, Levy controlled the play by selecting a few definite toys which he felt the child needed to work out a particular problem. The probable cause of a child's difficulty was determined from the case history. For instance, if Levy noted that a specific event such as watching a monster movie seemed to precipitate night terrors, he would help the child release his fears and anxieties by playing with toy monsters in the therapy sessions. The child is asked to say what the dolls are thinking and feeling during the play. This controlled situation may be repeated several times to allow release of pent-up feelings. The therapist notes or reflects the feelings that the child expresses both verbally and nonverbally in play. Moreover the therapist plays with and sometimes for the child in order to bring out and release the assumed emotions.

Three forms of release therapy have been developed: 1. simple release of instinctual drives by encouraging the child to throw objects around the playroom, burst balloons, or suck a nursing bottle; 2. release of feelings in a standardized situation such as stimulating feelings of sibling rivalry by presenting a baby doll at a mother's breast; 3. release of feelings by re-creating in play a particular stressful experience in a child's life. To illustrate the latter form of release therapy, Carl Rogers once advised his daughter to use release play therapy at home when his 1½-year-old granddaughter exhibited a strong fear of a specific situation (Fuch, 1957). The granddaughter became extremely frightened of bowel movements after experiencing painful eliminations in infancy due to rectal fissures. Since medical tests revealed no current organic difficulty, Rogers advised his daughter to encourage the child to express her fears in play. The mother set aside a special time and place each day to play with the child and provided the following play objects: family dolls, brown clay, toy toilet, diaper, baby oil and cotton, and a nursing bottle. The mother refrained from initiating or directing the play in any other manner; instead, she tried to reflect the child's feelings and understand the child's thoughts and motives. After a few days of play therapy the child stopped fussing about doing BMs and soon conquered her fear of elimination. Her mother reported that the child's anxieties about bowel movements never reappeared. This case demonstrates that the specific fears and anxieties of normal children can be treated effectively by release play therapy conducted by parents in the home.

According to the psychoanalytic theory of play (Waelder, 1933), children frequently use play to repeat specific experiences that are too large or difficult to assimilate immediately. The process of repetition is an important element in release therapy because by repeatedly playing out a difficulty or loss the natural slow healing process of nature can take place. By play repetition a child can relive and gradually assimilate a stressful event and integrate it rather than denying or being overwhelmed by it. In play a child has control of the situation, so events seem less overpowering and can be mastered. Play allows a child to vicariously try out new roles or possible solutions, anticipate the future, and generally become an active problem solver. Through play repetition a child passes from passivity to activity and thus psychically masters the impressions that were originally received in a merely passive manner. Moreover, play tends to relax a tense child and allow for substitute sources of gratification in fantasy.

Hambidge (1955) maintains that repetition is the single most important factor in structured or release therapy because only by repeated exposure to a stimulus will the child gradually show the following three signs of successful release therapy: 1. directly manipulate the dolls rather than tell them what to do; 2. become so absorbed in play that he or she is oblivious of surroundings; and 3. play out primary impulses such as aggression rather than stop out of defensiveness.

Apart from the cognitive processing that occurs through repetition, it is well known that simple repetition or reexperiencing of a stressful event allows for release of tension. Over fifty years ago Josef Breuer discovered the principle of catharsis. He observed that mental patients who were able to recall the origins of a symptom and to give uninhibited expression to the accompanying emotions were greatly improved in their overall adjustment. Expression of emotions tends to give a feeling of release from both physiological and psychological tension, and this good feeling gives one courage to attack problems so that creative energy is activated. Playing out or talking out intense emotions also lessens the likelihood one will act out hurt feelings. This emotional purging has come to be recognized as one aspect of a more general process in which the patient—with the accepting, encouraging, and supportive friendship of the therapist—is helped to give full expression to previously bottled-up conflicts, fears, and anxieties. This general process is called ventilation, and it seems to account for a significant portion of the total therapeutic impact of all psychotherapies (Schofield, 1964). It is well known that simple repetition or reexperiencing of a stressful event allows for release of tension.

In summary, structuring a child's play so he reexperiences a stressful situation not only allows for a release of pent-up emotions but also assists the child to cognitively assimilate the event and master it. In general it takes frequent repetition of the stimulus for this working-through process to occur. The encouragement of a supportive therapist or parent is needed to get the child to keep facing strong hurtful emotions and gradually overcome them.

A pitfall to avoid in release therapy is to come on too strong so that emotional "flooding" occurs—that is, a release of a massive amount of negative feelings so that the child is overwhelmed and regresses or disintegrates. Structured or release therapy should only be employed when a positive therapeutic relationship is firmly established and the child is judged to possess sufficient ego strength to tolerate an emotional upheaval. It should be recognized that the feelings of troubled children are quite deep and powerful. It has been found, for instance, that emotionally disturbed children differ from normal children not in the content of their play (normal children reveal just as many bloodthirsty killings and mutilations) but in the intensity of negative feelings. Moustakas (1955) observed that normal 4-year-olds expressed more open and direct hostility to their siblings than the disturbed group, but the intensity ratings for such expressions were significantly higher for the latter.

A major advantage of structured play therapy is that it increases the specificity of treatment. It can save hours of time by not indulging in periods of diffuse, haphazard, and uneventful therapy. As a result, the most recent trend in play therapy is toward the use of structured techniques to encourage a child to express emotions without undue delay. Among the more recent techniques for structuring play therapy are the mutual storytelling technique (Gardner, 1971), and dramatic or role-playing techniques such as costume play therapy (Marcus, 1966) and hand puppets (Woltmann, 1972). Most play therapists now incorporate a mixture of free and structured play in their work with children.

Relationship Approach

Rooted in the writings of Otto Rank, Frederick Allen, and Carl Rogers, nondirective therapy emphasizes the importance of the relationship between therapist and child. The therapist endeavors to create a playroom atmosphere in which the child feels fully accepted, respected, and understood. In this way it is felt that the child is free to experience and realize his own inner world and activate his self-curative powers and innate potential for growth. Self-awareness and self-direction by the child are the goals of this approach. The therapist operates by avoiding criticism, advice, interpretations, and directions; rather, the child is provided with a well-stocked playroom and given the freedom to play as he wishes or to remain silent. The therapist is not a passive onlooker but actively observes and reflects the child's thoughts and feelings and tries to understand empathically the world from the child's perspective. Thus, empathy, warmth, genuineness, encouragement, and listening skills are the key aspects of this new child-adult relationship.

A basic premise of nondirective therapy is that when a child's feelings are expressed, identified, and accepted, the child can accept them more and is better able to integrate and deal with them. The therapist helps by not only providing toys and materials that elicit self-expressions but by reflecting or being a mirror to the feelings of the child and accepting these negative feelings so the child can also accept them without thinking himself abnormal or "bad" because he has them.

The therapeutic process in play seems to pass through four distinct phases. At first the child exhibits diffuse, undifferentiated emotions that are very negative in nature. Thus disturbed children either want to destroy everything or to be left alone in silence. As the therapeutic relationship grows, the children are able to express anger more specifically, such as towards a parent or sibling. When these negative feelings are accepted, the child begins to accept himself more and feel worthwhile. This leads to the third stage, wherein the child is able to express positive feelings. He shows considerable ambivalence in this stage, so that his kindly feelings are interspersed with hostile ones. He will hug a doll one moment and yell at it or attempt to hurt it the next. The ambivalent feelings tend to be intense and irrational in the beginning, but as the positive emotions become stronger, the child enters the final stage, in which he is able to separate and express more realistically his positive and negative emotions.

According to Axline (1969), the eight basic principles which guide the nondirective therapist are simple:

1. The therapist must develop a warm, friendly relationship with the child as quickly as possible.
2. The therapist must accept the child exactly as he or she is.
3. The therapist must be permissive and allow the child freedom to express feelings completely.
4. The therapist reflects back the child's *feelings* to help the child gain insight into his own behavior.
5. The therapist shows a deep respect for the child's ability to solve his own problems when given the opportunity. Responsibility for decision-making and change is left with the child.
6. The therapist does not attempt to direct a child's behavior or conversation in any way. The child takes the initiative and the therapist follows. The child is in charge in the playroom.
7. The therapist does not attempt to hurry the therapy, which is seen as a gradual process.
8. The therapist sets only those limits necessary to make the child responsible for the relationship.

In recent years Moustakas (1966) has stressed the importance of genuineness or authenticity in the therapist-child relationship. In the existential tradition he highlights the need to tune in to concretely felt here-and-now experiences in the relationship. For example the therapist should try to own and express personal reactions; the therapist might say, "I'm happy about that. How do you feel about it?" In this way the child is helped to differentiate his own feelings, find meaning in his life, and to discover his unique selfhood. Loss of self, according to Moustakas, is the central problem of the disturbed child. Moustakas currently calls his form of relationship therapy "experiential or existential child therapy." Rather than playing a role, the therapist communicates his or her real self to the child.

Relationship therapy is based upon a particular theory of personality which assumes that an individual has within himself not only the ability to solve his own problems but also a growth force that makes mature behavior more satisfying than immature bahavior. Once a child experiences a relationship in which he feels accepted, respected, and understood, his creative forces are released which drive him towards a full, healthy, self-directed life. According to Axline (1969, p. 74): "The relationship that is created between the therapist and the child is the deciding factor in the success or failure of the therapy." Research has supported this position that the most important aspect of effective psychotherapy is the interpersonal skills of the therapist, the relationship itself rather than techniques. The critical interpersonal skills of the therapist seem to be empathy or the ability to "be with" the child, nonpossessive warmth, and genuineness or coming across as a real person (Truax and Carkhuff, 1967).

Because of the apparent simplicity of the concepts and the popularity of the writing of Axline and others, nondirective counseling has come to be regarded as *the* approach to play therapy. This is unfortunate because it tends to encourage the forcing of children into a rigid mold rather than flexibly selecting methods to fit the needs of the child. There are signs, however, that many therapists are now attempting to accelerate the nondirective therapy process by introducing structured techniques at selected intervals. Another trend in nondirective play therapy is to train paraprofessionals, such as parents (Stover and Guerney, 1967) and college students (Linden and Stollak, 1969), to be play therapists. Preliminary studies by Guerney and Stollak indicate that it is possible to train a wide variety of people to use nondirective methods with children.

Group Approach

Most group therapies for children, up to adolescence, include some aspect of play. Children respond well to some type of play period or feeding situation during the therapy session. Talking about problems just does not seem interesting enough and does not drain off enough physical energy, so at some point in therapy, active physical activity becomes necessary.

Applying a nondirective approach to the group situation, Slavson (1947) experimented with group psychotherapy with preadolescent children (ages 7 to 14). As opposed to talk or interview methods, these were activity groups for children to release emotional and physical tensions through games and arts and crafts projects wherein few limits were set. The therapist modeled prosocial acts by such behaviors as cleaning up the room at the end of the session. Activity group therapy seems particularly appropriate for children with poor social skills because peer group pressure is often a more powerful influence than adult interactions at this age.

In 1950, Schiffer (Rothenberg and Schiffer, 1966) adapted activity group principles to younger children in early latency (ages 6 to 9). In this "therapeutic play group" approach the leader had to be more involved and less permissive so as to prevent intense acting-out behaviors. Still, the leader tolerated considerable emotional release and intervened only when the frustration tolerance of any child or of the group was being overly taxed, or to protect the children from injury. A maximum of six children met with the therapist for an hour a week in a playroom. Typically a child remained in this surrogate family environment for two or more years so that the child could gradually work through deep-seated tensions and anxieties. Careful attention was paid to group composition so that a therapeutic mix of aggressive and shy, withdrawn children was achieved. Refreshments were served at each meeting and play, game, and craft activities were selected for their expressive qualities and ability to promote social interaction.

The unique aspect of this play group approach as opposed to individual therapy is that the child has to learn to share an adult with other children. The theory and practice of group psychotherapy with children will be discussed further in another chapter of this book.

Limit-setting Approach

The limit-setting approach to play sessions regards the setting of limits as the major rather than minor part of the therapeutic process. By restricting a child's behavior, it is felt that you give him a sense of security, preserve his sense of reality, and maintain the physical and psychological well-being of the child and therapist. Bixler (1949) and Haim Ginott (1959) have been the leading advocates of limit setting in play therapy.

In regard to the actual practice of setting limits, there is general agreement among therapists that limits should be *minimal* in therapy. Most child therapists will set some limits on blatant physical aggression, such as kicking the therapist, marring walls, and throwing or breaking objects. A survey of play therapists (Ginott and Lebo, 1963) revealed that the most widely used limits concern the protection of playroom property (breaking windows, furniture, and fixtures and painting walls or doors), child's safety (drinking dirty water and climbing on high sills), therapist's safety (attacking the therapist or painting his clothing), and socially unacceptable behaviors (urinating and defecating on the floor and cursing at passers-by).

Most play therapists will also insist that the child remain within the playroom during the session and leave when the time is up. On the other hand, child therapists tend to allow children to verbalize profanities, write four-letter words, draw obscene objects, and use racial slurs.

Limits or playroom rules should be well defined in the therapist's mind so that the line between acceptable and unacceptable behavior can be quickly and clearly spelled out. It seems best to establish limits on an *all-or-none* basis; for example, the rule should be "No hitting the therapist" as opposed to the vague "No hitting the therapist so as to hurt him." All-or-none limits are easier to distinguish and generate more security on the part of both therapist and child. There is general agreement among child therapists that limits should not be posted or set in advance; rather, they should be communicated immediately when the child begins or threatens to break them. In this manner the child learns what he is permitted to do as he explores and tests the limits of this new relationship. An honest explanation of the reason for a rule should be offered the child when the limit is first introduced (Straughan, 1964)

Therapists differ with respect to the actual method one should use to set limits. Some try to distract the child when he begins to act up by directing his attention to other play activities. Others will quickly terminate the play session after certain unacceptable behaviors. Bixler (1949) recommended a graduated, three-step sequence for enforcement, with the latter steps initiated only if the earlier ones are ineffective. First the therapist should reflect the desire or attitude of the child when his behavior exceeds the limit: "You are very angry and you would like to hit me because I will not let you take the crayons home." Next the therapist should verbally express the limit in a clear way: "You may not hit me, but you may hit the Bobo." Bixler has found that the majority of children cease their misbehavior at this point. Finally, the therapist should control the child's behavior by physical means, such as holding the child's hands while firmly sitting him in a chair. If the child continues to fight, the therapist should put the child out of the playroom and end the session. In enforcing limits it is important for the therapist to exhibit a nonjudgmental, nonpunitive attitude wherein disapproval is expressed toward the child's behavior but acceptance is shown toward's the child's attitude, motives, and feelings (Ginott, 1961).

In conclusion, it should be clearly recognized that not to enforce a limit is to invite more aggressive antisocial acts in the future. Clinical experience indicates that children want to have their antisocial behavior controlled and express relief when limits are firmly and consistently enforced. A number of nondirective therapists maintain that no predetermined set of limits can ever be applied in therapy because one must flexibly apply limits based upon the needs of the individual case. Each therapist must think this issue out, because the clearer and more confident one is in this regard, the easier and more successfully one will use limits. Certainly limits (discipline, authority) are part of therapy itself, especially for the aggressive child, and not some adjunct, peripheral issue that is of little import. Experience indicates that your relationship with a child will be strengthened in the long run if you can effectively limit certain behaviors while showing understanding and acceptance of the whole child.

Behavioral Approach

Basically, behavior therapy refers to the systematic application of learning theory principles to the modification of deviant behavior. It embraces a variety of techniques, including positive and negative reinforcement, modeling, and reciprocal inhibition. Behavior therapy works on changing present maladaptive behaviors and does not attempt to understand past causes. No emphasis is placed on energy release or expression of feelings. The basic assumption of learning theory is that behaviors represent responses learned in relation to specific stimulus situations. It is felt that symptoms can be unlearned and this process will not result in symptom substitution. In addition to unlearned maladaptive behaviors, behavior therapists make an active effort to teach or reinforce a child to engage in more constructive alternative courses of action.

The last two decades have witnessed a mushrooming of behavior therapy work with children. When treatment involves unlearning maladaptive behaviors and relearning more appropriate behavior, this treatment has come to be termed behavior therapy. In the playroom, operant conditioning methods are typically employed whereby the therapist will ignore deviant behavior and give concrete (candy, tokens, toys) and social (praise) rewards for prosocial behaviors. Working with a mother and daughter in a playroom, Russo trained the mother to give no attention to the children's temper outbursts and to reward cooperative acts by verbal praise and by such overt behaviors as enthusiastically joining in the activity (Russo, 1964). To ensure generalization of treatment effects, behavior therapists prefer to train parents and peers to use operant techniques with the target child in a play situation. Play is used in this approach as a means of eliciting desired behavior and applying other therapeutic processes, not as a therapeutic end in itself.

Behavior therapy has been found to be suited to a wide variety of behavior problems in children. It can be used effectively with children who exhibit intellectual, cultural, and language difficulties. Behavior therapy seems best for childhood disorders that result from faulty learning and manifest themselves in specific symptoms, such as phobias, stealing, bedwetting, or soiling.

Play Materials

It is advantageous to have an attractive, well-stocked play therapy room set aside, but this is not absolutely necessary. The room should be well-lighted and brightly colored, and have a sink, protected windows, a one-way mirror, and audio or videotape capabilities. It is possible, on the other hand, to conduct play therapy in a corner of an office (Durfee, 1942) or to pack essential toys in a portable suitcase (Cassell, 1972). Thus play therapy is an extremely flexible modality that can be adapted to very small budgets and facilities.

The selection of play materials is an important consideration if play is to be used therapeutically. Certain toys and materials have been found to elicit more self-expression of thoughts and feelings than others, and specific toys (checkers, cards) have been found to elicit cooperative social behaviors while others (crayons, jigsaw puzzles, clay) tend to result in isolate play (Quilitch and Risley, 1973). An inadequate selection of toys in terms of the child's age and level of maturity can drive the child from the playroom and seriously hamper the therapeutic process. In general, toys should be kept simple, durable (nonmechanical), and unstructured, capable of being adapted to many roles and purposes. The toys should be familiar to the child and within his cognitive and manipulative skills. Strange, unfamiliar toys tend to produce "novelty shock," while overdifficult materials generate anxiety and defensiveness.

A wide variety of toys and materials in good condition should be available on easily visible shelves so that the child can select in accord with his own interests. Play materials that have been used with some degree of success include: 1. dramatic toys (doll house; doll family; puppets, small animals; countryside objects such as trees and fences; cars; and costumes); 2. visual expressive materials (paints, easel, crayons); 3. manipulative materials (blocks, peg-pounding set, Bobo, plasticine or clay, sand and water); 4. games (table games, cards, checkers); and 5. special-purpose toys (nursing bottle).

Play Therapy Research

Although few in number, the available outcome studies of play therapy have yielded positive results. Seeman, Barry, and Ellinwood (1964) found that teachers and classmates perceived children who received individual, nondirective play therapy as significantly less maladjusted after therapy. Dorfman (1958) studied personality outcomes of nondirective play therapy, using both the own control and matched control techniques. Her findings indicated significant positive changes associated with play therapy. Axline (1947b) found that as a result of play therapy, significant improvement in reading performance occurred.

The most recent trend has been to study therapist

variables related to successful play therapy. Stover and co-workers (1967, 1971) found, for example, that mothers receiving training in nondirective play therapy exhibited more reflective statements, gave fewer commands, and increased empathy and involvement with their children in the play sessions. In addition, children of trained parents increased their verbalizations of negative feelings toward their parents, while control children did not. Landisberg and Snyder (1946) found that young children (ages 5, 6) increased their expressions of feelings during play therapy and conclude that for the younger child the value of play therapy may be cathartic. Other studies have shown that clients of behavior therapy and psychotherapy tend to agree that the personality of the therapist is the most important factor in treatment. Sloan and co-workers (1977), for instance, conclude that behavior therapy clients place more emphasis on the therapeutic relationship (trust, understanding, encouragement) than do the behavior therapists themselves.

Notwithstanding the outcome and process studies conducted to date, we still cannot state with any degree of certainty that a specific play therapy approach is superior to other approaches with children exhibiting certain problems. The crucial question remains: what kinds of childhood problems are best treated by what kinds of therapy, by what kind of therapists, and under what conditions. With respect to play therapy, we need a much broader base of process and outcome studies before we can begin to answer this question

Summary and Conclusions

Since play therapy capitalizes on a child's most natural medium of self-expression and way of solving problems, it remains one of the prime methods of individual child therapy. Quite multifaceted in nature, play therapy currently encompasses six different approaches: psychodynamic, structured, relationship, group, limit-setting, and behaviorial. Some of these major approaches tap the natural self-curative powers of play, while others use play primarily as a medium for the application of other therapeutic processes. There is growing realization that the content of play can be utilized to achieve a number of therapeutic goals including: release of pent-up emotions; insight into hidden meanings and motives; substitute source of gratification; a sense of control and mastery of one's life; re-creation of problem situations so one can accept, work through, and find alternate solutions; reeducation by means of role-playing and behavior rehearsal; a sense of adventure and excitement; and opportunity for a child to relax and enjoy life.

A common element in all forms of play therapy is the use of the therapist-child relationship. There is general consensus that the first task of the therapist is to establish a friendly, accepting, and trusting relationship with the child. Empathy, warmth, and genuineness seem to be the key therapist variables underlying a positive relationship. Coupled with this special relationship is the need to establish and consistently enforce limits on the child's behavior in the playroom. Some therapists consider limit-setting to be the key aspect of successful therapy with acting-out children.

Among the recent trends in the field of play therapy is the greater use of structured play therapy techniques. Costumes, puppets, family dolls, and storytelling are commonly used now to promote self-expression by the child and thereby expedite the therapeutic process. Another trend involves training and supervising members of a child's natural environment (parents, peers, and college students) to be play therapists for a child. In this way it is hoped that the therapeutic gains will generalize to the child's local community.

Play therapy is still a young field, and as a result suffers from a number of growing pains. Due to the popularity of the writings of Axline and Moustakas, many professionals equate play therapy with nondirective counseling. As a result they view play therapy as a rather passive, diffuse, even frivolous process that should not be taken too seriously. Also, few play therapists have been trained in more than one approach, so they lack the skills necessary to apply play therapy strategies differentially based upon the needs of the individual child. Moreover, much more extensive and well-controlled research needs to be conducted on both the process and outcome variables (including long-term follow-up studies) of play therapy.

On a more positive note, there is a considerable body of literature regarding both the theory and clinical practice of play therapy. A recent handbook on play therapy by this writer (Schaefer, 1976) presents a comprehensive overview of the clinical literature, as well as a description of the six major approaches to the therapeutic use of child's play. There has also been a dramatic increase of late in empirical studies on the relationship between play and normal child development. Clearly the potential of play for psychic growth and healing has barely been tapped to date. Although a number of the positive functions of play are now known, many others are yet to be discovered. In sum, play therapy is a multifaceted, ever-evolving field that remains as exciting to study and practice as ever.

References

Allen, F.H. (1934) Relationship therapy through play. *Am. J. Orthopsychiat.* 4: 193.

Axline, V.M. (1947a) *Play Therapy*. Boston: Houghton Mifflin.

Axline, V.M. (1947b) Nondirective therapy for poor readers. *J. Consult. Psychol.* 11: 61.

Axline, V. *Play Therapy*. (1969) New York: Ballantine.

Bixler, R.H. (1949). Limits are therapy. *J. Consult. Psychol.* 13: 1–11.

Bruner, J.S., A. Jolly, and K. Silva, eds. (1976) *Play—Its Role in Development and Evolution*. New York: Basic Books.

Cassell, S. (1972) The suitcase playroom. *Psychother. Theory Res. Prac.* 9, 346–348.

Clement, P.W., and D.C. Milne. (1967) Group play therapy and tangible reinforcers used to modify the behavior of eight year old boys. *Behav. Res. Ther.* 5: 301–312.

Dorfman, Elaine. (1964) 1958 study cited in Seeman et al., Interpersonal assessment of play therapy outcome. *Psychother.: Theory Res. Prac.* 1: 64–66.

Durfee, M.B. (1942) Use of ordinary office equipment in play therapy. *Am. J. Orthopsychiat.* 12: 495–503.

Ellis, M.J. (1973) *Why People Play*. Englewood Cliffs, N.J.: Prentice-Hall.

Erikson, E.H. (1963) Chapter 6. In *Childhood and Society*. New York: Norton.

Freud, A. (1946) *The Psycho-Analytical Treatment of Children*. London: Imago.

Freud, A. (1965) *Normality and Pathology in Childhood*. New York: International Universities Press.

Fuch, N.R. (1957) Play therapy at home. *Merrill-Palmer Quart.* 3: 89–95.

Gardner, R.A. (1971) *Therapeutic Communication with Children: The Mutual Storytelling Technique*. New York: Science House.

Ginott, H.G. (1959) The theory and practice of therapeutic intervention. *J. Consult. Psychol.* 23: 160–166.

Ginott, H.G. (1961) *Group Psychotherapy with Children*. New York: McGraw-Hill.

Ginott, H.G., and D. Lebo. (1963) Most and least used play therapy limits. *J. Gen. Psychol.* 103: 153–159.

Hambidge, G. (1955) Structured play therapy. *Am. J. Orthopsychiat.* 25: 601–617.

Klein, M. (1937) *The Psychoanalysis of Children*, 2nd ed. London: Hogarth Press.

Landisberg, S., and W.U. Snyder. (1946) Nondirective play therapy. *J. Clin. Psychol.* 2: 203–214.

Levy, D.M. (1939) Release therapy. *Am. J. Orthopsychiat.* 9: 713–736.

Linden, J.I., and G.E. Stollak. (1969) The training of undergraduates in play technique. *J. Clin. Psychol.* 25: 213–218.

Marcus, I.D. (1966) Costume play therapy. *Am. Acad. Child Psychiat. J.* 5: 441–451.

Millar, S. (1968) *The Psychology of Play*. London: Penguin.

Moustakas, C.E. (1953) *Children in Play Therapy*. New York: McGraw-Hill.

Moustakas, C.E. (1955) The frequency and intensity of negative attitude expressed in play therapy: a comparison of well-adjusted and disturbed children. *J. Genet. Psychol.* 86: 309–325.

Moustakas, C. (1966) *The Child's Discovery of Himself*. New York: Ballantine.

Nickerson, E.T. (1973) Psychology of play and play therapy in classroom activities. *Educating Children*, Spring: 1–6.

Piaget, J. (1969) *The Mechanisms of Perception*. New York: Basic Books.

Quilitch, H.R., and T.R. Risley. (1973) The effects of play materials on social play. *J. Applied Behav. Anal.* 6: 573–578.

Rothenberg, L., and M. Schiffer. (1966) The therapeutic play group—a case study. *Except. Children.* 32: 483–486.

Russo, S. (1964) Adaptations in behavioral therapy with children. *Behav. Res. Ther.* 2: 43-47.

Schaefer, C.E. (1976) *Therapeutic Use of Child's Play*. New York: Jason Aronson.

Schofield, W. (1964) *Psychotherapy: The Purchase of Friendship*. Englewood Cliffs, N.J.: Prentice-Hall.

Seeman, J., E. Barry, and C. Ellinwood. (1964) Interpersonal assessment of play therapy outcome. *Psychother. Theory Res. Prac.* 1: 64–68.

Slavson, S.R. ed. (1947) *The Practice of Group Therapy*. New York: International Universities Press.

Sloan, R.B., F.R. Staples, and A.A. Cristol. (1977) Patients' attitudes toward behavior therapy and psychotherapy. *Am. J. Psychiat.* 134: 134–137.

Stover, L., and B.G. Guerney. (1967) The efficacy of training procedures for mothers in filial therapy. *Psychother. Theory Res. Prac.* 4: 110–115.

Stover, L., B. Guerney, and M. O'Connell. (1971) Measurements of acceptance following self-direction, involvement and empathy in adult-child interaction. *J. Psychol.* 77: 261–269.

Straughan, J.H. (1964) Treatment with child and mother in the playroom. *Behav. Res. Ther.* 2: 37–41.

Sutton-Smith, B. (1971) Child's play—very serious business. *Psychol. Today.* 5: 67–69.

Truax, C.B., and R.R. Carkhuff. (1967) *Toward Effective Counseling and Psychotherapy*. Chicago: Aldine.

Waelder, R. (1933) The psychoanalytic theory of play. *Psychoanal. Quart.* 2: 208–224.

White, R.W. (1966) *Lives in Progress*, 2nd ed. New York: Holt, Rinehart and Winston.

Woltmann, A.G. (1972) Puppetry as a tool in child psychotherapy. *Int. J. Child Psychiat.* 1: 84–96.

Part II

Family, Group, and Milieu Therapies

Treatment of Emotional Disorders in Children and Adolescents

CHAPTER 9

Group Therapy with Children and Adolescents

Irvin A. Kraft

Introduction

"I'm scared. My dream scared me."

"Tell us about it and stay in the present tense—like 'I am . . .' "

"I am driving a huge truck that weighs 30,950 tons. The whole back end is an atomic bomb. I have to drive it into a mountain. The mountain is like a cone, like a fish-head. It can open up and swallow even the Empire State Building. So I drive my truck into it. Then I jump out just in time, and it is swallowed up in the mountain, and it blows the whole mountain all to pieces."

Vincent, age 10, looked around, as if to check out with his group-mates how they would deal with his dream. Mark, also 10, commented at once that he'd be real scared to blow up a mountain. Of the four other latency age boys in the group, several began hitting at each other and one dangled his hands in front of the video camera.

"Vincent, be the big truck and tell us how you, the truck, feel."

"Okay, I'm big. I'm real fast. I head right into the mountain."

"I'm real strong. I'm mad at the mountain."

And, so into the dream. Brantly became more agitated and stuttered out that lots of people would get hurt. "I don't like that." After about 7 to 10 minutes of these interactions, the leader commented that Vincent's mother, with whom he did not live and who was grossly psychotic intermittently, surely seemed like a swallowing monster a lot of the time. Also, he might well want to blow her up.

"What's wrong with this family is that *they* won't discipline us," 14-year-old Helen said.

Her father dropped his jaw, grew apoplectic, and stuttered, "Why, you twerp! I've told you a thousand times what to do."

"No, you haven't, you think you have. In any other family you couldn't get away with calling your parents 'stupid.' It's like they're afraid to discipline us or something." Her aggressively hostile, intensely manipulative behavior within her family signaled for someone to take charge.

Helen continued this vein in her peer group of seven 13- to 14-year-old girls who met once each week with two female leaders. Each entered this group after structured family sessions to obtain treatment contracts that clearly delineated the expectations, overt and covert, of all involved. Helen, who rarely missed a group session once she began, recognized and accepted the group's response to her behavior. "Helen, you just aren't going to run us the way you do your parents. We don't have to take your crap. So shut up about what Lou [the co-leader] just said." Helen flushed but really seemed relieved and quieter when she slumped back in her chair.

In subsequent family sessions, at about 6-week

intervals, her parents reported their own enhanced assertiveness and sense of greater responsibility for consistency of discipline. They mentioned that Helen seemed different nowadays.

"I smoke dope because I like it. Nothing wrong with me." Dave looked around his group of eight adolescent boys and girls belligerently, as if defying anybody to tell him anything else could be involved.

Marian responded with her shrill voice, "You know damn well you kid yourself that that's the way you do your own thing. You do it because it drives your parents up the wall, and you think the guys at school will take you in."

What happens in these groups that reflects similarities in therapeutic techniques and in group dynamics? Which ones (or do all?) offer the most challenge to the beginning group therapist? Or the advanced one? Do you see yourself as leader of any of these groups?

As you can perceive, group psychotherapy of children and adolescents fails to fall into the patterns we traditionally know for adults. There exists a different ambiance, outlook, and set of expectations in doing these kinds of group therapy. What are some of the qualities required of a therapist to do group therapy with children or adolescents? Do they differ from those needed to do adult group psychotherapy?

How do these and other types of children/adolescent group psychotherapy fit the criteria for Yalom's (1975) curative factors in group therapy? Do the standards for patient selection involve factors more multiple and complex, say, as compared with adult patient selection?

What roles do parents, teachers, and others intimately involved in the caretaking and stroke-giving of youngsters play in their recovery once the boy or girl is found to be disturbed? Does group therapy of parents, for example, afford boys and girls opportunities for retrieving appropriate developmental paths and patterns?

As always, what does group therapy offer in comparison with more traditional dyadic psychotherapy? Does group therapy of youngsters differ significantly from family therapy, in which the child or adolescent will be part of a special group, the family? Since the child or adolescent is usually still very much part of his nuclear family, in what ways do his group therapy experiences fit in with the open energy system in his family?

Along with these questions, there remain the controversial areas of diagnosis, psychodynamics, internalization of conflicts, structuralization, and transferences: how are these and correlated phenomena described and handled in group psychotherapy of children and adolescents?

Countertransference, both negative and positive, are more inherently likely in this type of group psychotherapy than with adults, since greater and more stressful pushes and pulls arise from the sucking bogs of the complications and involvements of adolescence and childhood. This group psychotherapy intertwines with the child, his family, his school and teachers, possibly the probation department, and other sectors which add to the administrative and therapeutic burdens of the therapist. Sometimes a leader feels mired more than admired, so that he finds himself negatively anticipating the next session. The therapist needs to be self-scrutinizing and vigilant for these negative countertransference signals.

This chapter looks at these and many other facets. We ask you to keep them and other questions in mind as you peruse this material. The practice of group psychotherapy of children and adolescents tends to assail stereotypical, therapeutic leader behavior and makes demands of time, patience, knowledge, and skills more vigorously and trenchantly than does adult group psychotherapy.

What do the above examples (and a number of others which could have also been illustrated) have in common? How do they differ? What changes occur with different patient ages, if that is a way of deciding on patient selection and on technique? Immediately, we see that these and other groups have an age factor built into patient selection.

Patient Selection

Most therapists in this field begin with the assumption that different ages have different developmental-behavioral configurations and thus even different emphases in problems common to all of youth: school performance, discipline difficulties at home, neurotic traits, and so forth. More perhaps than any other factor, the characteristics of the different developmental stages have influenced the growth of group psychotherapy techniques. Because the standard diagnostic nomenclature inadequately discriminated among the psychiatric disorders of childhood, therapists grouped children by age and then by the nature of presenting difficulties. Since they assumed children could not adequately utilize verbalization meaningfully much before puberty or adolescence, play and activities dominated their approaches. Aside from psychotic children and several types of sexual deviates, the categories that appeared were: (1) preschool and early school age, (2) late latency, ages 9 to 11, (3) pubertal, ages 12 and 13, (4) early adolescence, ages 13 and 14, and (5) middle adolescence through late adolescence, ages 14 to 17. (Kraft, 1968; Soble and Geller, 1964).

Once you decide which age group interests you, a first step would consist of asking yourself why. Is it because patients in that grouping are more available to you? Do you have some predilection or leaning in that direction, perhaps from your own memories and autobiography? In any case, self-scrutiny here, as in most of psychiatry, offers a basic and significant input.

Curative factors operate only under circumstances and sets favorable and not inimicable to their existence. If, for example, patient selection is faulty, and the leader puts several grossly psychotic or sexually deviant children into a latency age group of boys and girls, he lessens his effectiveness. Thus ordinarily one excludes from an outpatient group the grossly psychotic, very active sexual deviates, children who are murderers or extremely assaultive, the extreme sociopaths, and low-functioning retardates. Inevitably some exceptions arise, either ffrom expediency or from a therapist's experimental bent. We must always keep in mind, however, that ultimately the clinician must decide on the basis of his self-knowledge, the external circumstances, and his clinical hunches whether to include a child who would ordinarily be excluded.

Now, with those variables answered to your satisfaction, how do you go about selecting the patients? First, will you mix genders? Will you try for homogenous or heterogenous symptom presentations? Will you utilize IQ as a valuable selective factor? Will your site and setting influence the group population unduly? Clinics, the parents' ability to pay, third-party payments, private practice: these and other vectors figure into your secondary and tertiary considerations subsequent to your initial decision.

As part of your beginning thinking and feeling that concluded with your decision to do a group, you might well review the indications and contraindications for such a therapeutic measure.

Indications

Very few disturbed children would not benefit at some point from a group therapy experience. This seems evident if we accept the wide range of diagnostic categories for which, to date, groups have been used. As always, sound clinical judgment determines when to use group therapy. For example, one therapist may conclude that group therapy might not be indicated for a severely neurotic youngster of six, at least not before a period of intensive individual therapy. At the same time, the experience of some therapists demonstrates that concomitant group participation augmented individual therapy. In general, if basically adequate group therapy is available for a certain age child, then you should seriously consider it as part of that child's total treatment recommendation.

Criteria for group psychotherapy of children demonstrate less clarity than they possess for adults. Most types of group therapy for children and adolescents seem ego syntonic. At their meetings, the children usually avoid unconscious material, as they focus on here-and-now productions that often seem superficial and banal. This patient population, however, involves itself intensively in expected and usual life patterns, as well as in each patient's life with his own growth, development, and consolidation of ego functions well in the foreground. Multiple reasons rest behind referral to group psychotherapy. Comparatively few reasons exist for not referring a child to a group (as either a main or an adjunctive procedure). Thus exclusion criteria dominate the process of selection except when training and theoretical bias skew the therapist's viewpoint against group psychotherapy, so that he does not consider it at all in his treatment recommendations.

Contraindications

Contraindications to using a group method rest on your clinical judgment. The major factor is your impression as to the patient's ability to tolerate stress. Severely borderline adolescents sometimes find outpatient group treatment too stressful, although they might well be able to handle it as part of a total inpatient regimen. We utilized an office setting for schizophrenic boys in their early teens who did well; and they did even better when we added patients who were comparatively only mildly upset. The therapist's acumen and skill remain overriding factors in deciding what contraindications obtain beyond the exclusion criteria mentioned above.

Data exchange for living, especially in the to-and-from transmission with the child's parents and other caretaking persons, strongly affects the behavioral patterns of children and adolescents. No one set of techniques replies to the varied needs of the different age groups nor to the reported experiences of a number of investigators. You will then presumably decide what your own internal and external forces dictate for you. Perhaps a brief historical review will add perspective to your enterprise.

History

Group therapy in general and with adults began with Pratt's work in 1907 in Boston. In Europe, Adler initiated group methods in his child guidance clinics in 1918. A gap of 16 years intervened until Slavson, in 1934, originated activity group therapy with latency age children. Early on, Slavson and his students differentiated group psychotherapy from children participating in group activities such as camping and scouting. They believed group psychotherapy implied the presence of an objectively stated theory of personality and behavior, and that its implications afforded testing opportunities. Accordingly, the leader acted and spoke from his theoretical position, usually utilizing deliberately designed situations for the group. As a corollary, the investigators assumed the behavior of the children in group comprised responses to the treatment.

The clinicians doing activity group psychotherapy, as well as later forms of group therapy for children based their work on classical psychoanalytic theory as exemplified by Bender's (Bender and Waltman, 1936) use of group therapy with children on a hospital ward in 1936. Once additional, basic therapeutic group techniques became known, therapists utilized other factors: various age groupings of children required different methods of treatment. Adolescent work required other important considerations. Also, settings in which patients were treated influenced the choice of techniques; these included residential treatment centers, public schools, pediatric specialty clinics, units for delinquents, and hospitals.

By the 1950's, therapists experimented with elaborations and variations of technique, although still within the basic framework of psychoanalytic theory. Adolescent group psychotherapy expanded beyond its initial confinement to situations for delinquents and inpatient units, and clinicians used it in a wide range of outpatient settings, including private practice. The cultural and social phenomena of the mid and late 1960's flooded clinical facilities and their staffs with new and often different patients, unusual phenomena, and novel treatment challenges (Sadock, 1975). The adolescent and youth counterculture, new and old role expansions in femininity and masculinity, and the many byways of drug abuse pressed the psychiatric caretakers to reexamine their therapy procedures. Many of these issues remain, and the emerging methods still need to be refined for eventual utilization in routine situations.

Interview-activity techniques appeared (Duffy and Kraft, 1966-67; Kraft, 1961) with variations, such as interactional emphasis, employment of selected encounter group techniques (Kraft and Vick, 1973; Rachman, 1971), transactional analysis methods, psychodrama exercises, modified marathon regimes, Gestalt modalities, and behavioral therapy programs. Along with this stimulating experimentation, there was a state of concomitant confusion; this has not yet been replaced by any truly systematic synthesis.

Theoretical Considerations

In general, group psychotherapy accommodates itself to a number of theoretical positions and their subsequent variations of techniques. Now, newer formulations, such as reality therapy, Gestalt therapy, and transactional analysis, nudge the traditional dominance of Adlerian concepts, classical psychoanalytic principles, and client-centered psychotherapy. Yet if one examines closely the conceptual frameworks of therapists, certain assumptions tend to be found in common. These include Freudian constructs of the mind (such as the ego and the defenses), psychic determinism (which coexists more and more uneasily with a philosophical allegiance to the free will of other theoreticians), infantile sexuality, and the unconscious.

Along with these notions, we find an additional factor extremely important for work with children. Activity—such as artwork, play, dancing, gestures, and interactions—allows the inner fantasies of the child to seek expression and resolution in development, in family transactions, and in other aspects of growth-promoting adaptation (Schacter, 1973). The child exerts his will and engages in family power plays to further his constant search for need gratification within his time-space complex. To the perceptive therapist, the behaviors of the child reveal and communicate content, whose meaning is inferred within the therapist's theoretical orientation. To deal with the healthy as well as the sick (distorted) complexities of the child's behavior calls for special skills and empathic qualities. From his background and his training, the therapist evolves his individualized treatment style.

Development also plays a cogent role in all treatment considerations. All therapy, and especially group psychotherapy, attempts restoration of the child as closely as possible to his own path of individuation and normal development. At most stages of childhood and adolescence, positive peer interactional experiences promote such growth.

Additional Theoretical Contributions

A child processes the data of forces that he uses for development, and he often seems overwhelmed by rapidly oscillating, changing inputs, so that he lacks adequate dwelling, reflective, and associative time for purposive decision making. A therapist assumes responsibility in group psychotherapy of children and adolescents for helping the patient sift and sort out faddish messages. Gibson (1973) pointedly tells us that "we have arrived at the stage where the time required to make decisions (i.e., assemble and examine all necessary information), even simple ones by human beings, is considerably longer than the time required to transmit the information over a communication system." He further makes the point that either valid or misleading information gets transmitted with equal ease and fidelity. In life, and in group psychotherapy, more and more time becomes allotted to securing accurate information, be it cultural, interpersonal, and/or intrapsychic, in order to aid in reality-oriented decision-making.

As children develop, they learn to operate in varying systems, their changing behavioral patterns call for rearrangements of equilibria. In their group psychotherapy experience, they find settings and techniques with which to glimpse at varying levels of abstraction the roles of their family, which is primarily that of a message center and information processor. The systems of negotiation then become the focus rather than the individual psychopathology, as in negotiations with the small group, including the family, and larger interest groups, such as scouts. The group leader and the group itself confront this structured segment of their lives primarily in the here-and-now of the group session.

The leader's operational assumptions and his definitions of how people function determine how he handles these transactions. He may construe a child's behavior in the group as the resultant of intrapsychic and social forces. He could then point out to that child and to the group how the family system elsewhere required the patient to be disturbed in order to maintain family balance. In group interaction it is quickly evidenced that the patient demonstrates the schisms, secret alliances, and power plays of his family of origin (Melville, 1973). Combating this trend, especially with children and adolescents, is the built-in capacity for identification as part of growth. Bandura (1969) describes modeling behavior and its importance in personality formation. A study by Patterson and Anderson (1964) postulated that peers serve as effective agents to provide social reinforcers. As a therapy group anneals and grows, group values permeate the behavior of the patient. These serve to counter the nonadaptive family-sponsored behaviors. The latency child also takes in data from his social, educative, and group experiences. Under normal circumstances this will enhance his industriousness and transfer sufficient libidinal energy to out-of-home activities to lead him somewhat from the family canopy.

Early on, children and parents sense this; they feel buffeted. Diminished time together reduces their ability to monitor and filter the bombardment of overt and covert stimuli. These include both information for rational decision-making and subliminal messages designed not to inform but to influence. The family must fulfill the tasks of providing emotional support to its members and of training the children in competency (age and gender adequate control of the body and the symbolic environment). These functions falter amid the welter of megamachine living (Mumford, 1972). Increased tension and decreased control lead to faulty communication, especially in the interpersonal areas, and in time, to familial disorganization. The family offers the child initial training in adaptation at one level of a hierarchical organization into which he will gradually fit. Survival, however, may not be equivalent to health.

Setting and Its Practical Considerations

To return to the more technical aspects of your adventure into the group experience, the settings for therapy deserve discussion. Settings vary widely, yet must be consistent with the practicalities of the therapist's working arrangements. Often, this requires a room whose primary purpose is to service group functions, with durable furnishings and an unencumbered carpeted and undercushioned area of a minimal size of 8 feet by 10 feet. Some therapists use sturdy chairs and perhaps a strong, low central table, whereas others prefer a rather bare room. They may have tools, models, games, or other artifacts available to the group. As with the basic rule that the therapist does not permit injuries to self or to others in the group and doesn't allow destruction of furniture, lights, or windows, he also clearly delineates what will be permitted and what will not be allowed in the use of tools, furniture, food, audiovisual instruments, and the like.

The literature is not sufficiently explicit about those practical details that the beginner learns with difficulty. For example, the optimal size for a group tends to be 6 to 8 children. In deference to usual school circumstances, most groups for school-aged children meet in the mid to late afternoon, although some therapists report that Saturday mornings work out well (Brandes, 1971).

The sessions with younger children tend to be weekly, lasting one hour or even less, except in the use of classical activity group psychotherapy, where the time is 1½ hours or more. In those cities with urban sprawl and poor public transportation, this means a parent, usually the mother, brings the child and waits for the group to end. Clinics often utilize this opportunity for a mothers' group or some other work with the mother, which proves more complex for the privately practicing child clinician.

The group usually takes 5 to 10 minutes to settle into its work. The children, especially boys, exchange information, boasts, taunts, and challenges. The therapist has the option of several approaches for openings, which children quickly pick up on (with comments, usually derogatory) and then accept. This may reflect the interest of the therapist, who, for example, might inquire about dreams occurring since the last session or about those emotional events that might have stirred anyone in the past week.

In effect, this encourages the group to be an activity-interactional type with emphasis on verbalizations. In contrast, others may want the children to do things together (such as games) and deemphasize their more personal and possibly introspective verbal productions. The last 10 to 15 minutes of the session could entail some free or organized play activity involving all the members. Some therapists find this an extremely useful means of ascertaining other facets of the children. For example, 15 minutes of kickball on a nearby playground can elucidate productive interactions, revealing body-damage concerns, skills, and competitiveness. Having food to share (doughnuts, popcorn, cookies, cokes, or milk) enables observation of how food is used with each other and individually.

Whether to have more than one therapist is best answered with reference to the overall setting: private office, clinic, or inpatient. Most reports suggest two therapists, preferably of opposite gender. Within broad limits, each therapist can hew to his own therapeutic approach and the children handle the differences nicely.

The major emphasis emanating from the therapist is confidentiality and seeing the child as a person, not a culprit delegated to the therapist for correction and change. When indicated, he protects the weak child from the overly aggressive ones by taking the heat off verbally or by actually physically intervening. He intervenes at times in other circumstances, as with contagion of excitement, by pointing out the group process underlying the turmoil. At other points he may be authoritative in forcibly telling someone to sit down or to halt what he is doing until the emotional elements behind it are explored.

We usually tell the children that none of their verbalizations will undergo censure. Beginning about 1968 we added that drug usage (marijuana, alcohol, LSD, etc.) would not be allowed in the sessions. The therapists reserved the responsibility and the attendant freedom to notify the parents if a serious matter arose that significantly affected health, such as suicidal behavior. The children in turn will be notified of telephone calls or other contacts their parents make with the therapists about them. The therapists explain too that they are trying to get the parents better to understand them and to change situations; in the service of that goal, many therapists feel free to tell parents of the general concerns of the patient, while not quoting his words per se. Although some children test out these regulations, especially the latter, no one seriously bothers to oppose them.

Curative Factors

Let us examine for this field of group therapy what Yalom (1975) describes as the curative factors. These vectors listed below play significant roles in this type of psychotherapy. Please keep in mind that the reality and developmental features of children and adolescents (such as a real dependency on parents) may create alterations.

1. Instillation of hope. In adults the phenomenon of placebo effect remains basic to this. In children, however, assessment difficulties become apparent, for many children do not see themselves as troubled or as not coping adequately. We find that adolescents seem better able to view themselves as needing to change and being capable of change, and thereby given to hope. Once young children do get involved with group, hope (of sorts) begins to manifest itself in combination with other curative factors.

2. Universality. Since children and adolescents seek peer conformity, they find the group immensely reassuring as they discover others of like age with feelings and experiences similar to their own.

3. Imparting of information. As is observed below, clinical judgment always determines when, how much, and what should be said. Thus at times with an adolescent group the therapist might well utilize didactic information, such as concepts of dyadic relationships; and with younger age patients the leader might at times intrigue them with information from science, biology, or other fields (e.g., dinosaurs—their habitat and their behaviors).

4. Altruism. Even with the counterculture surge "to do one's own thing," for the child or adolescent, to do something for others still fosters good feelings in both doer and recipient. The patients might not see their interactions as altruistic, yet they do utilize this in the group process.

5. Corrective recapitulation of the primary family group. We find a most interesting facet of child and adolescent group psychotherapy exists in the more immediate applicability within the patient's primary family of what he learns now in the group. Again, as with most therapy with children and to a lesser extent with adolescents, the patients relive the distortions of their original family experiences in portions of their present group experience. These corrective experiences also occur in the lower levels of awareness.

6. Development of socializing techniques. Social learning plays a large role in a number of different kinds of child and adolescent group psychotherapy. Modeling of the therapist's behavior as well as that of other group members often occurs. Deliberate use is made of this tendency in varying formats, especially in groups for the retarded and for pubertal and early adolescent girls. Children consciously and deliberately watch each other as the group goes along, and then they will often pick out the current "hero" to emulate. Sometimes parents complain about new behavioral tactics and new language, especially more basic words, that their child enacts and quotes from his group.

7. Imitative behavior. This includes role modeling, as above, but in the sense that the patient will observe how one group member deals with emotional situations which he himself must also encounter. He then imitates the model, with "It worked for him, so why not for me?" With children and adolescents, role playing in brief psychodramatic exercises and other activities often leads to experiences in behaving a certain way, as demonstrated by others in the group. What works then tends to become incorporated into a behavioral repertory, especially when the patient practices first in the group with its vociferous comments and approval.

8. Interpersonal learning. Since the range of group structures is so much greater for the child population, this factor presents evaluation difficulties, especially if we compare them with adult groups. Evidence emerges, especially from adolescent groups, that patients do become aware of their own behaviors, appreciating some of their qualities, and sensing their effects upon others in the group. Generally, our youths develop more rewarding relationships with peers and often even with parents.

9. Group cohesiveness. Although not often verbalized, this factor soon appears. In outpatient settings where the parents support their attendance, the children tend not to miss sessions; the resulting continuity provides a good basis for cohesiveness. The "group" becomes quite important to the members, usually with a core who attend regularly and with a few who are more peripheral and less regular. An interesting finding, in interviewing patients years later, is how often they remember the group and members, but not the therapist.

10. Catharsis. Under appropriate conditions, it is helpful for children and youth to express strong emotions, especially when hostile to authority figures. However, it is probably the interpersonal process involved in the group more than the "release" of feelings that enables the patient to utilize the experience for growth.

11. Existential factors. So many children see their parents and other grown-ups as unfair and unjust that the fact of their inherent dependency becomes lost amid their distortions. Facing life alone, for example, has limited meaning to 8-year-olds. Probably a sense of being responsible for one's behavior

is the most meaningful of Yalom's five items of existential factors. In any case, these factors have less applicability in groups for younger patients, the retarded, and for the mild behavior disorders.

Techniques

In recent years, therapists have made increased use of group psychotherapy within such settings as hospitals, private offices, and community clinics. Experimentation in this field has expanded as well.

We now return to the different age levels and the group treatment methods appropriate to them. The paragraphs that follow will emphasize a pragmatic discussion of the major modalities employed for each developmental period.

Preschool and Early School Age Groups

Most of the work during the preschool years utilizes play therapy with or without accompanying supervised observational interaction by mothers. The therapist aims at individual emotional expression with the materials, as in one-to-one treatment, but with the process facilitated by peer interactions. When indicated, interpretations are used in keeping with the theoretical proclivities of the therapist (Ginott, 1961; Slavson, 1950; Slavson and Schiffer, 1975). The mothers may observe and/or meet as a parallel group with another therapist. This tends to emphasize their cognitive grasp of their child's problem, and to enhance their understanding and skills in parenting.

The therapist usually structures the situation by using a specific approach, such as artwork puppets (Bender and Waltman, 1936), or a permissive play ambiance. Children project their fantasies onto puppets, and they find a means to express their feelings, an experience of considerable value. The child utilizes the group setting perhaps more as a site for the observation and imitation of others than as an opportunity for direct interactions.

A useful tool for infants to 3-year-olds is Nielson's method (1970). This is conducted in a family living project in which the mothers sit in a group with a therapist while watching their own children interacting with school personnel and with one another. The focus of these informal, leisurely meetings is on the nature of play, and on its role and importance in the child's development. Hopefully, other workers will study this in different settings, such as Sunday school nurseries or day care centers.

Hansen, Niland and Zani (1969) used modeling theory to show that socially isolated, early elementary students of low socioeconomic background would respond well to peer "models." When compared to control groups, they retained their gains. Behavioral intervention of this sort interrupted their somewhat fixed interactional repertories.

Play group therapy emphasizes the propensities of the children to interact with one another and the therapist in a permissive playroom setting. Slavson suggests a woman therapist who would induce the children to produce verbal and played out fantasies; she would also use active restraint when the children translated excessive tension into hyperkinetic patterns. The room offers the traditional artifacts of toys, water, plasticine, toy guns, and a doll's house. Children usually respond by reproducing their home difficulties and acting out aggressive impulses. By catalyzing each other, the children obtain libido-activating stimulation from their play materials.

Group play therapy effects basic changes in the child's intrapsychic equilibrium in his capacity for relationship, and in his reality testing through catharsis, insight, and sublimation (Ginott, 1961). The child finds significant opportunities to change in a positive direction as he identifies himself with other group members and with the therapist. Ginott (1961) places little emphasis on the group as a unit, since each child assumes the focus of the therapy. Frequent shifts occur in the play relationships, attachments to toys and peers, and the subgroups that come and go.

Haizlip, McRee, and Corder (1975) found that only one of ten randomly selected clinics provided group therapy for the younger child. In those that they studied as well as in their own program, staff resistance was expressed in terms of theoretical issues and a lack of referrals; underlying these were more basic anxieties deriving from insufficient experience with this age group.

There are reports of programs (Lovell, 1973; Poole and Ruck, 1972) with children under five in general hospital physiotherapy units. These were retarded children with histories of insufficient environmental stimulation and/or minimal cerebral damage. The groups utilized maternal participation with staff to help the children control behavior, enhance mobility, and increase peer communication.

A basic requirement for selection as a group member is the presence of social hunger, a need to be liked and to be accepted by other children. If the child had never experienced a primary relationship with a mother figure, Ginott (1961) excluded him and referred him for individual psychotherapy. He also rejected children who felt murderous toward their siblings, sociopathic youngsters, those with perverse sexual experiences, extremely aggressive patients, and habitual thieves. The symptom picture of those who were selected included: phobic reactions, effeminacy in boys, excessive shyness and withdrawal, separation anxiety, and the milder primary behavior disorders.

Speers and Lansing (1965) went beyond these criteria and utilized group therapy along with art therapy and parent group therapy for autistic children. They began with four children under the age of five who showed withdrawal from reality and severe disturbances in self-identity. Among these children, language deficits, lack of bowel and bladder control, severe sleeping and eating disturbances, and stereotyped behavior were prominent. The investigators reported that within their group setting these psychotic children were able to change through obtaining the rudiments of self-identity. At the outset, the physical and psychological closeness of the group members panicked some of the children; over time, however, it helped them establish relationships. After the austistic defenses had been repeatedly penetrated, a group ego developed much in the form that E.J. Anthony had originally described for older children in group therapy. This provided part of a therapeutic symbiosis for each patient. Safety in the group fostered emancipation from the sick relationship with the mother.

Another variation of group therapy has been employed for preschool youngsters with special disability problems, such as retardation, brain damage, and cerebral palsy. The usual emphasis was to offer the child opportunity for age- and ability-appropriate activities, especially communication with peers. An essential ingredient of such groups was the active involvement of the mothers; the end result was to enhance both the physical care of the child and their communication with him (Flint and Deloach, 1975; Poole and Ruck, 1972).

We can move on to see how these considerations fit in with the next age level appropriate to group therapy.

Latency Age Groups

The basic techniques for this age group were discussed above in the section on settings. We wish to emphasize here that in addition to activities and play, verbalization techniques enhance group experience. In this fashion, activity-interview group therapy differs from the "pure" activity type in that the therapist actively intercedes and interprets to the children the meanings of both their verbal productions and their actions. These groups are able to accept more severely disturbed youngsters. The therapist encourages the telling of dreams, the expression of dynamically laden material, and peer-to-peer interpretations.

Composition of the Latency Group

Most of the time late latency children (ages 9–11) undergo activity-interview therapy rather well. When the flow of patients permits, you can place girls as well as boys in the group, for, as is generally the case, in work with latency children the sex ratio runs about three boys to one girl. As a result, finding enough girls becomes a problem for these groups. If possible, you should have about equal numbers of each sex, for the girls act as a modulating influence and diminish the extremes of the boys' behavior. Selecting the patients depends more on the overall structure of the group than on the characteristics of each patient. Six is the optimum number of group members, although some therapists (especially if they operate with co-therapists) undertake eight members.

The leader's gender doesn't seem to produce any significant differences. Sometimes the therapist talks to, or with, and sometimes for the children. As they relate their daily experiences, when they make comments about their parents or discuss their interactions with other group members, the therapist occasionally offers psychodynamic generalizations (Schamess, 1976). The therapist's discipline of origin may be any of the traditional fields, or he may come from the newer paraprofessional training programs in mental health. A co-therapist of the same or opposite sex can be useful in these groups, as Laybourne reports a creative use on a pediatric ward (Laybourne, Shupe, and Sikkema, personal communication).

It is helpful to differentiate types so as not to include more than a limited number of withdrawn and taciturn members. Also, such groups fail to function adequately if they include the incorrigible or psychopathic child, the homicidal child, and the child with overt sexual deviance. For example, a child prostitute or molestee can upset his co-patients and their parents—when the word spreads. Severely threatened, ritualistic, socially peculiar children who cannot establish effective communication with other group members at any useful level do poorly in these groups; they do better if placed in more homogeneous groups with their own kind. Too many retardates in the group impede interaction and tend to enhance motoric patterns for all the group members. On the other hand, children with physical deformities, protruding teeth, tics, or behavior based on maturational brain dysfunction generally find the group situation helpful. Groups respond supportively when its members perceive the victim's sensitivities and feelings as one or two patients vehemently taunt them about their disabilities.

As freedom of expression and activity evokes responses among the members, different roles emerge. We find the instigators, who enable the group to stay alive dynamically; the neutralizers, who, in response to their stronger superegos, keep impulsive acts down and help regulate behavior; the social neuters, who seem impotent to accelerate or impede the flow of group activity; and the isolates, who are so neurotically constricted that they initially find the group too frightening to join in its activities.

In general, within the group, the child reproduces his customary and usual adaptational patterns. For example, all his life he may have utilized helplessness to elicit dependency fostering and psychological feeding responses from adults and peers. In the group, however, he is likely to find peers and the therapist "failing" him.

The therapist's neutrality impedes these characteristic patterns; in time he creates enough frustration to initiate different behavior. Similarly, the provocative, extremely aggressive child finds no rejection or punishment for his behavioral distortions; instead, he meets with acceptance and controls. In time, he also reacts differently to the therapist and to his fellow group members.

Frequently therapists report that latency age children become caught up in irrepressible behavior with strong contagious elements. Impulsive, acting-out children usuallly cow their more inhibited, conforming group-mates, though sometimes even these more reserved children catch on and join the bedlam. A recent report (Strunk and Witkin, 1974) recounts such an experience. The therapists cope with it by eliminating the play period and its regressive magnetism; instead, they take a very active role in an hour-long discussion session and emphasize self-control as a value. Their work illustrates what often occurs—i.e., given clearly defined limits and expectations, the children in a therapeutic group will feel more comfortable and adopt more age-appropriate behavior.

A related technique, with the primary emphasis on the associative element rather than on the activities involved, is the club formed by the children themselves (Celia, 1970; Lieberman, Yolom, and Miles, 1973; Olsson and Myers, 1972). The members name the club, determine its goals, and elect its leadership. The very fact that the club is chosen, not imposed, generates enthusiasm and enables members to participate actively in the therapeutic process itself—as agents rather than "patients." The club forms a therapeutic milieu that allows members to face competitors and to dramatize conflicts which, without the support of an integrated group, might have destroyed them. Parental participation is sometimes encouraged. Therapeutic clubs have been successful with disadvantaged children of minority groups, with psychotic children, and with severely disturbed pubertal boys. The reported results include the strengthening of impulse control, reality testing, and self-esteem, and the improvement of object relations.

Most therapists agree that the function of group psychotherapy at this age is to aid the organization of drives into socially acceptable behavior modes (Sand et al., 1973). The child enhances his coping patterns as well as finding his place in the group. Thus, beyond certain fundamental rules established by the therapist, children develop their own group behavioral standards. These take forms that are both open and explicit, as well as covert and concealed, a pattern that holds true for all group process.

In some groups videotaping of the initial 20 minutes of the group interview has been utilized. Dreams, negative and positive reports about any aspect of the children's lives, and specific comments about what the therapist defines as each child's major problem area might be recorded. Then, if meaningful material emerges, the group reviews the tape and any further material which enters is also noted. The TV equipment usually presents no deterrent to group process (Melnick and Tims, 1974), even if it is in the same room.

Behavior modification approaches (Pratt et al., 1975) to the latency child vary in terms of the nature of the proffered rewards, the extent to which they are provided and how they are used. Rose (1972) developed an extensive program based on earning points that could be translated into material rewards. His patients reflected varying kinds of emotional problems. In such a program the therapists must find the details and exigencies of such an approach rewarding for themselves as well; otherwise they would be better advised to utilize the more traditional group procedures. A variation of this counter-condition is test anxiety through Wolpe's systematic desensitization procedures in a classroom setting (Barabasz, 1973; Stamps, 1973).

An increased interest in sexual disconformities in adults has led to efforts to change the life-styles of effeminate boys, aged 4–9. No work appears on similar projects with masculine girls, if in fact they can be identified as such. Green and Fuller (1973) describe a first effort in working with seven effeminate boys concomitant with a mothers' group, a fathers' group, individual psychotherapy each for mother, father, and boy, and a home-based token economy system for reinforcing masculine behavior. This total push produced reductions in effeminate patterns and an increase in closeness of the father-son relationships. The team believed the group experiences proved essential for the boys and for parents.

Group therapy for boys with absent fathers (Sugar, 1975) strives to meet their unresolved dependency and other oral conflicts, their oedipal distress at replacing the father, and the associated general authority conflicts. Obviously, the therapist must be male and able to bear up well and respond flexibly to both the overt and even more powerful covert demands such a group makes upon him. Sessions with mothers and sons helped highlight the core problems; optional ways of handling them could then be offered.

Activity-interview techniques can be modified especially for girls. In late latency with its overlap with early pubescence, girls readily discover common problems and concerns, which center about maturational problems and quests, such as clothing, makeup, boys, closeness with fathers, and physical changes. Change in such girls reflects both inherent and social maturational factors along with group cognitive and experiential learning. One study (Shere and Techman, 1971) utilized repeated Rorschach testing to assess progress and found positive changes in the girls' records.

In working with latency age children, primarily boys, and especially those who are hyperactive, the therapist often ends up letting the members have at it with movement (Cermak, Stein, and Abelson, 1973; Egan, 1975). Sometimes, if allowed to get very involved in activities, the group gets physically out of control. Schachter (1973) attempts to harness this by suggesting that games stimulate emotional responses as in real-life situations. When the therapist perceives such an expression of feelings, he can freeze the action and have the participants stop and get in touch with the feelings. Similar work has also made use of TV tapes and replay to enhance the recognition of the feelings being discussed (VanScoy, 1972).

Group therapy in school settings has been controversial. Some therapists contend that group permissiveness carries over to classroom behavior, creating separation and dissonance. Pasnau, Williams, and Tallman (1971), after twelve years of experience, suggest this does not necessarily occur. Teachers can be used as leaders under continuing supervision and friendly psychiatric liaison is encouraged by this. Moreover, small activity groups provide a service to children as a bridge between classroom and clinic (Harris and Trujillo, 1975). Schiffer (1969) describes over twenty years of work with therapeutic play groups in elementary schools. He sees the group following a psychodynamic evolutionary time table over several years; it develops from a preparatory to a therapeutic to a reeducative and finally to a termination phase.

Anderson and Marrone (1976) describe nine years of experience in a program that utilized teachers as well as others: "Many teachers can be brought to a level of competency in dealing with emotionally disturbed children in the group therapy process . . . . " They suggest the model works also for normal children in affectively-oriented educational programs.

In the form of group counseling, group therapy lends itself readily to school settings. DeLara (1969) uses gender and problems as criteria for the selection of homogenous groups of six to eight students which meet once a week during school hours. Six to eight students might gather over a time span of two to three years. The commonality of the presenting problems underlie the ultimate success of the groups. Groups of retardates fit this classification (Etters, 1975).

Yet, contrary to other school group therapy reports, Minde and Werry (1969) found that intensive group treatment of a verbal nature in a low socioeconomic neighborhood school demonstrated no overall treatment effect. Other inner-city work shows mixed results. Barcai's work demonstrated that children were capable of acquiring verbalizing skills when taught carefully in a remedial manner (Barcai et al., 1973).

In clinic and school settings, where large numbers of children need to be processed or screened, various group screening methods have been devised. In the procedure used by Gratton and Pope

(1972) the three investigators put five to six children into a diagnostic group for an hour a week for three weeks. They also conducted weekly group psychotherapy for twelve weeks with two groups of five children each. This was carried out in keeping with play therapy models with the goals of modifying the child's classroom behavior. Their work, and that of others, indicate that group techniques can be applied to school settings in flexible ways in order to achieve limited goals of social behavior alterations. Rhodes (1973) found that conventional verbal treatement along with clear behavioral limits worked well in a short-term (six to eight sessions) program when carried out by very active therapists in an elementary school setting. The therapy directed itself to exploring the child's classroom difficulties and to gathering information for further referrals.

In a day hospital setting, Kraft and Delaney (1968) utilized what can be called "discovery" therapy, employing a form of dance-movement therapy. If offers an opportunity for the child to function with others in a literally hamonious fashion so that through rhythmic and expressive movements positive relationships emerge between individuals and the group as a whole. Feelings of isolation and alienation diminish as the group members spontaneously share their feelings actively and aesthetically. The casual and enjoyable associations that come about through their rhythmic movements allow the children sufficient individual freedom to permit their dancing and moving by themselves without feeling that they disrupt group activity. The changing actions of the group bring on one-to-one relationships as well as group relationships. These result in a sense of acceptance and influence on others that bolsters feelings of independence and self-esteem. This enhanced sense of personal strength and identity often provides the first steps toward participation in other forms of individual or group therapy.

The rhythmic movements make it possible to express emotions in ways that hurt no one; at the same time they allow for the discharge of tension. This leads to relaxation and the freedom to go on to other things. Rhythmic action allows expressive behavior without great physical strain. It provides control over emotion rather than allowing the emotion itself to take control. Movement communication makes use of the natural kinesthetic responses to musical rhythm and leads to satisfying structured action. In responding to rhythm, the child becomes aware of his body; it moves in time and space and in a way that he wants it to. For children who have difficulties in relating directly to what is outside of the self, this technique allows them a combination of relationship and shared action which occurs in the here and now. The movements transcribe themselves into functions that are at once expressive and reality-oriented.

In group dance therapy, physical movement allows the children a means of "speaking" with each other, a method of tuning into and sharing what people are "saying" with their actions. Movement communication establishes direct relationships, makes initial contacts, and offers access to sharing the experience of feelings. This provides an opportunity for "working through," of obtaining emotional release with symbolic body action via the rhythmic, expressive, physical movements of the group. Being in a group feels safer and more conducive to individual risk-taking.

Art therapy is another relatively new technique employed in group therapy. Once again, providing the patient with the opportunity to speak freely and to express himself while occupied with an activity—in this case, an art or a craft—has proved to be of great value. Socialization is enhanced through the group, and patients are able to express emotional conflicts symbolically through artistic productions. Such material helps the therapist clarify the diagnosis. Family participation can be encouraged, or may occur spontaneously. Art therapy thus helps to reestablish lines of communication within the family. This is particularly likely to occur when the therapeutic group becomes the family itself rather than a children's group. Originally, art therapy relied heavily on psychoanalytic concepts; at present, other theoretical constructs serve as the bases for interpretation and diagnosis. This therapeutic form has become an increasingly common technique in psychiatric hospitals, clinics, and special schools. Art therapy is especiallly valuable with younger children; for them it is a more "natural" mode of expression, and they find it easier to say graphically what they lack the ability to communicate verbally.

Pediatric hospitals or pediatric wards of general hospitals have been utilized for group support and brief therapy. This has been demonstrated at cancer centers by Adams (1976). Almost any affliction lends itself to this process for its limited goals.

Pubertal Groups

Similar group therapy methods can be used with pubertal children, who are often grouped by gender.

Although their problems resemble those of late latency children, they are also beginning to feel the impact and pressures of early adolescence. This is especially true of girls. In a way, these groups offer help during a transitional period.

Group structure appears to satisfy the social appetites of preadolescents, who tend to compensate for feelings of inferiority and self-doubt by the formation of groups. This form of therapy takes advantage of the "natural" pressure toward socialization during these years. Since children of this age experience difficulties in conceptualizing, pubertal therapy groups tend to use play, drawing, psychodrama, and other nonverbal modes of expression. The therapist's role is active and directive, as opposed to the more passive role classically assigned him (Crowdes, 1975).

Activity group psychotherapy has been the recommended type of group therapy for preadolescent children (Soo, 1974). The children are usually of the same sex and with not more than eight to the group. They are encouraged to act freely in a setting especially designed and planned for its physical and milieu characteristics. Slavson (Slavson, 1950; Slavson and Schiffer, 1975) pictures the group as a substitute family in which the passive neutral therapist becomes the surrogate for the parents. He assumes different roles, mostly in a nonverbal manner as each child interacted with him and with other group members. More recently, however, therapists regard it as a form of a peer group, with all its attendant socialization processes, rather than as a reenactment of the family.

Activity therapy involves games, structure forms of play, and projects which must be planned and carried out. For children with neurotic-type difficulties, the work is designed to achieve maximal elicitation of fantasies and expression of feelings about others. In order to reduce the potential for frustration and failure, the equipment supplied the child is minimal. Anxiety, however, is allowed to develop, and the therapist works to help the group members cope with it. In the ego-impaired group the sessions are highly structured and anxiety is reduced to a minimum, although the structure is progressively loosened as their frustration tolerance rises. For these children, all destructive behavior is actively discouraged. In the neurotic-type groups, on the other hand, limit setting is maintained only to protect personal safety and to prevent property damage.

This therapeutic medium can help children with deficient and distorted self-images, inadequate role identifications, habit and conduct problems, and mild psychoneuroses. Neurotic traits that may be present in behavior disorders as exemplified by the passive, dependent, infantilized child, tend to alter as these personality traits persistently fail to achieve satisfaction, are worked with, and are gradually replaced by other behaviors.

The group procedure has been used as a diagnostic tool in child guidance work; small, short-term groups when brought together provide data on peer interactions. In effect, the clinic sets up a group milieu to furnish the staff with pertinent observations, observations of the patient's behavior, while concomitantly engaging the child in a therapeutic experience (Churchill, 1965).

In selecting patients, one can strive for homogeneity; for example, brain-damaged youngsters can be placed in one group and neurotic children in another, where both groups are modifications of activity group therapy. The neurotic group emphasizes the verbalization of fantasy and the expression of feelings. The ego-impaired group devoted itself to structured physical activity and to carefully designed group discussions about current events (Gerstein, 1969).

Another form of homogeneity is to give group treatment in an outpatient clinic to patients, usually boys, who have been recommended for residential or day treatment. The children gain impulse control, enhanced reality testing, and elevated self-esteem (Lilleskov et al., 1969).

Psychiatric inpatient facilities offer other opportunities for selecting fairly homogeneous populations; yet even here the therapist cannot use only one procedure as the basic treatment process. He must match his armamentarium of techniques flexibly to the behavior patterns of the group members (Josselyn, 1972; VanScoy, 1971). In most latency groups that are not designedly varieties of activity therapy, the therapist involves himself in determining goals and structures of the therapy, and actively pursues topics or activities.

Egan (1975) suggests a modification in the form of activity discussion group therapy. Certain dynamisms occur in the groups: first, identification with the therapist, with group members, and with the group as a "family." Second, reinforcement and other behavioral techniques modify behavioral patterns. Third, direct (verbal) or indirect or derivative insight develops. In contrast to routine activity group therapy, the physical characteristics of the room include gymnastic and other equipment, which discourage practitioners who occupy cramped quarters.

When boys (especially those in residential treatment) reach the preadolescent age range, their aggressive feelings often perplex them and drive them to impulsive actions; group therapy, especially when it is combined with other techniques, can help in many ways. It affords opportunities for positive interpersonal transactions that can serve to diminish their basic mistrust, it provides ways to enhance low self-esteem, and it can affect dependency-independency conflicts for the better. Bardill (1972) utilized behavioral contracting as a means of scheduling the exchange of positive reinforcements. Great pains were taken to clarify explicitly the expectations of each party to the contract. Points were awarded for certain specified behaviors during therapy.

In contrast to the residential setting, Barcai et al. (1973) worked in a school setting with fourth- and fifth-grade students from a low socioeconomic area. The goal of the undertaking was to increase the students' school achievements. The therapist set up groups, counseling, remediation, and art. They found that performance improved differentially in relationship to the specificity of interventions used and the climate of the classroom. They hypothesized that underachievement could be tied to lack of reward for language-oriented communication in their homes. Hence, specific interventions would effect more change than generalized interest and care. Their work agrees with findings reported elsewhere of the generalization effects of psycholinguistic remediation programs (Battin and Kraft, 1968).

To show that the specificity of intervention, when insistent and constant, plays a major role in change are experiences with a transactional analysis (TA) approach with a late latency group of boys and with groups of 13-year old girls and with the 14-year old girls in a clinic setting. In this technique the initial interviews occupy an important place. At this point, the therapists set up contractual guidelines with the parents. They are told how much involvement there will be for them with the leaders, and what types of data will be given to them about what their child does and says in the group. A commitment is usually obtained from the patients for at least a 3-month group stay before they make any decision about terminating therapy. One successful modality for this is a 4-session series of family meetings (Parker, Hogan, and Kraft, 1977). This has been used in both all-girls and all-boys groups. Strong emphasis is placed on the confidentiality that the therapists will enforce for themselves, and the patients for themselves. It is made clear, however, that there will be an active response to any hints about destructive behavior a patient plans to direct at himself or at others. If there are data whose seriousness requires telling the parents, as when a girl is not certain but that she might be pregnant, the patient is urged to tell them herself, usually in a family session. She can do this along with the therapists' help, with tutoring and protection.

It is stated as well that the therapists are available to patient and parents at all times: any hour and any day.

The child is asked: "Why are you here? What is it you want to change about yourself? What is it you'd like to see altered in your family?" The therapy contract is then constructed on the basis of his replies. When resistances emerge ("Talk to my parents; they send me and pay for it"), in this TA framework it is assumed that the rebellious adapted child ego state prevails; it is stroked, and the contractural negotiations proceed. The children catch on quickly to the ego-states paradigm and work astutely with game classification, both on each other and the therapists. This approach is used consistently with them, endeavoring to achieve symptom amelioration and behavioral change.

In sum, when the physical situation of the office permits in latency and puberty, activity groups provide an opportunity for an emotionally corrective experience. This is accomplished by utilizing a highly permissive setting to encourage freedom of expression of pent-up feelings along with regression (Singer, 1974). Interview activity and other variants along the spectrum of therapeutic techniques also provide opportunities for effective experiential insight. Consistency, warmth, flexibility, and empathic qualities of the therapist, coupled with adequate knowledge of personality theory and of therapeutic techniques, provide the ingredients for good group therapy in this and other age bands.

Parent Groups

As is true with most treatment procedures for children, parental difficulties present obstacles. Sometimes uncooperative parents refuse to bring a child or to participate in their own therapy; in certain cases, severely disturbed parents use the child as their channel of communication to work out their own needs. Then the child finds himself in the intolerable position of receiving positive group experiences at the clinic that create havoc at home.

Parent groups have, therefore, been a source of

valuable aid to the children's group therapy (Epstein, 1970). The parent of a child in therapy often has difficulty in understanding the nature of his child's ailment, in discerning the line of demarcation between normal and pathological behavior, in relating to the clinical establishment, and in coping with feelings of guilt. A parents' group assists them in these areas. More than that, it helps members formulate guidelines for action. Participation in discussion groups has been valuable for mothers of disadvantaged children; as mothers acquired changed attitudes and new understanding of their children, this in turn improved the behavior of the children. In fact, in one group the most lasting changes in the younger children occurred when the changes in parental attitudes were greatest. By the same token, the greatest failures occurred where the mothers were least influenced. In the community at large, parent groups were designed to further understanding of preschool development and emotional needs. Health personnel then tried to interest the mothers to join, but their efforts were largely in vain.

Pasnau et al. (1976) utilized a parallel, concomitant parents in a couples group to their group of neurotic latency boys. They emphasize the importance of the parents' meeting being at the same time and place. They suggest this format enhances a focus on family interaction, diminishing the identified patient syndrome, that it adds to a family model—e.g., pointing out that the parents have a separate relationship from the children.

Kernberg and Ware (1975) use a group workshop technique to teach parents and also child care personnel about child development. This brought basics for "empathic understanding for children, namely, to get in touch with the child within oneself."

An interesting variation has been described by Bellucci (1975) who initiated group treatment for newly placed adopted children, ages 10 to 13, who had been shifted through at least five foster homes. They used the techniques of short-term content-oriented sessions, emphasizing support, clarification, interpretation, and didactic material.

Fishman and Fishman (1975) explored a group approach to teaching behavior modification principles and techniques to mothers of physically handicapped children. Their results in this brief therapy proved encouraging for further usage of a group adaptation of the child management training approach. A similar concept underlay work by Flint and Deloach (1975) with parents of handicapped children in the form of small and large group sessions with a lecture-discussion format. A dissimilar approach to the same purposes by Kelley (1974) was used in an inner-city school with the parents in open-ended discussion-centered groups. Other reports (Rinn et al., 1975; Schaefer, Palkes, and Stewart, 1974) add to the general upsurge of interest in groups for parents education to help disordered children.

Adolescent Groups

In early and middle adolescence, boys and girls tend to differ in social awareness and responsivity. Therapists assume that the main streams of emotional striving are present in both genders and run throughout these two periods. However, as the youth acquires more social tools within his peer group and with adults, the strivings are expressed and handled somewhat differently. Adolescent deviancy proceeds by characteristic stages that seem to occur and be gone through as if of necessity. This has been studied extensively; unfortunately, each observer attaches significance to only one element or another that commands his attention. Goldberg (1972), for example, suggests in the search for identity that some adolescents lack the ability to love adequately, thereby feeling that they miss out on something. As a result of this lack, they use other people primarily in the service of their own narcissism rather than as objects loved for their own qualities.

As Josselyn points out (1972), peer identity processes are important keys to the successful transit of latency and adolescence. In the teens especially, the youngster's recognition of "himself as a child of his past and an adult of his future" becomes fundamental to maturity. For the normal youth, the turmoil of adolescence is the process of abandoning his childhood patterns for adult ones.

When cultures undergo rapid and massive changes, the trial and error necessary for learning and growth become hindered; there is simply not enough time and opportunity. The current almost total emphasis on twosomes "going steady," in contrast to multiple dating, adds to the difficulties of learning about one's self through brief and varying heterosexual encounters. Therapeutic efforts that employ mixed gender groups offer opportunities for some degree of honest experimentation with feelings and thoughts (Berkowitz, 1972; Brandes, 1971; Singer, 1974; Soble and Geller, 1964).

Drugs usually fail as a pathway to insightful growth. Theoretically, the deep drug user seeks oneness with the universe, or he spends hours searching for himself in an unshackled inner world to provide overall meaning to existence (Bratter, 1974; Rachman, 1971). By way of contrast, peer group affiliations offer an opportunity for identification, working on self-esteem, devices to enhance ego strength, personal consistency, and a feeling of environmental mastery. Again, when the adolescent fails to obtain these structural elements in his family, he sometimes can retrieve his lost opportunity through group psychotherapy. Working in this helpful psychosocial therapeutic context, he heads on more directedly to adulthood.

Today, over a decade later many an adolescent embraces the counterculture mores and strictures, summed up in "Do your own thing!" Ironically, as with drug use, he again places himself in situations where there is less opportunity for growth. To the extent that he adheres rigidly to the countergroup, gains in separateness and independence are less likely to occur. When girls' groups were formed (Kraft and Vick, 1973), they presently developed a degree of cohesiveness that came in direct conflict with the call of the countergroups. This was especially true when the latter were involved with extensive drug usage. Interestingly, the clamorous craving for excitement that is so characteristic of these patients (Rosenthal, 1971) was satisfied by the use of encounter and other modalities in the group.

Techniques of group therapy with adolescents vary rather widely; usually they correlated with the therapist's background and present outlook. In 1955, Ackerman readily placed both genders, ranging in age from 15 to 23, in the same group. Each of his patients had previously undergone individual psychotherapy, and the group therapy experience supplemented it. Ackerman suggested that the group functioned to "provide a social testing ground for the perceptions of self and relations to others." He emphasized the importance of nonverbal behavioral patterns as material for group discussion.

Subsequent reports tended to agree that group therapy dealt more with conscious and preconscious levels than did the individual intensive, more deeply introspective approach. Hulse (1960) listed clarification, mutual support, facilitation of catharsis, reality testing, superego relaxation, and group integration as ego-supportive techniques. Adolescent group therapy provides constructive experiences, support for youth's attempt to behave differently, opportunities to look at his problems in everyday life, and a chance to see how he impacts on others (Berkowitz and Sugar, 1975).

Composition of the Adolescent Group

Group therapy with adolescent patients can be conducted in an outpatient clinic (Hodgman and Stewart, 1972), private office, hospital (Herrick and Binger, 1974; Lewis, et al., 1970; Masterson, 1972; Rizzo, Ossario, and Saxon, 1975), or in special settings, such as a detention home, with modifications appropriate to the setting (Sugar, 1975). The setting itself strongly influences the total group process. One group format is that of an open-ended interview-interaction. The preferred number of adolescents for these groups is eight to ten; circumstances often require the screening of perhaps 30 or more youths in order to produce a group of 15. Of these, about six will form a core group with constant attendance and effort; another three or four will constitute an intermediate group who attend more than they miss; and the remainder will make up a peripheral group who attend occasionally. Attendance and therapeutic achievement become difficult to predict for the individual patient, since these factors do not seem to relate to age, presenting problem, and diagnosis. Some therapists suggest separation of patients in early (ages 13 and 14), from later adolescent patients, since boys of 13 and 14 and 17-year-old girls live in quite different worlds and find one another difficult to deal with in these groups. Robinson (1970) used role play with retarded adolescent girls in a vocational school setting to teach appropriate job behavior and to enhance their management of interpersonal relationships.

Here again, the diagnostic categories fail to distinguish among patients sufficiently to serve as guideposts to patient selection. Certain behavioral patterns—such as overt homosexuality, a flagrant sociopathic history, drug addiction, and psychosis—contraindicate inclusion in these groups. However, group techniques for these patients do exist, particularly with alcoholism, homosexuality, and drug addiction, but they require special conditions (Bratter, 1973).

Aims and Techniques

Mixed group psychotherapy offers the adolescent an opportunity to relearn peer-relating techniques in a protected and supported situation (Shapiro and Berkowitz, 1975). Under favorable circumstances, diminution of anxiety over sexual feelings and consolidation of sexual identity can be expected to occur. In time, as he begins to participate in the group interaction, the youth feels the pull of group cohesiveness. He reacts to the group's pace and its changes. The group shifts its content level frequently and rapidly, often within a single session. In the course of this he experiences relationship, catharsis, insight, reality testing, and sublimation. The boy or girl presently begins to identify himself with other group members and often with the therapist. In the course of these processes, the mechanism of identification affords him major opportunities for therapeutic gain. The individual adolescent constitutes the focus of treatment, but he/she and the therapist are continually involved with the group as a sounding board and testing ground.

Inevitably, the adolescents employ numerous diversionary tactics to avoid discussing threatening subjects. One favorite maneuver changes the focus by a question or a comment about some unrelated topic. Sometimes diversion masks itself behind physical activity, such as throwing a gum wrapper at the wastebasket or showing the others a picture in a textbook. As the group persists in time and shared experiences, these and other behaviors frequently evoke precise confrontations and/or interpretations from other group members; if not, the therapist calls attention to them.

Several investigators (Duffy and Kraft, 1966-67; Kraft, 1961; Marvitt, Lind, and McLaughlin, 1974; Schulman, 1956) comment that the therapist must be active, ego-supportive, and in control of the group situation at all times. Cautiously given interpretations avoid a patient misconstruing the interpretation as personal criticism. Such interpretations frequently focus on reality rather than on symbolism. They involve simple direct references to basic feelings; statements about the unconscious intent of behavior can be made when the meaning lies quite close to awareness.

The therapist can be of either gender. Co-therapists and observers do not deter group process and interaction. When the co-therapists are of different sexes, differential responses emerge to each. Leadership involves goal identification for the group, showing the group how to function, keeping it task oriented, furthering its cohesiveness, serving as a model, and representing a value system. In carrying out these tasks, the leader may offer clarification of reality, analysis of transactions, brief educational input, empathic statements acknowledging his own feelings as well as those of the members (Weiner and King, 1977), and at times, delineating the feeling states at hand in the group.

The content of the discussions varies enormously, ranging over school examination, sibling competition, parental attitudes, difficulties with self-concepts, and sexual concerns. Sexual acting out or impulse eruption rarely occur. For most paitents, brief group responses to significant experiences that the patient narrates fulfill his needs, for he can return to the subject later if necessary. The group usually prefers short discussions, since the anxiety level is too high to dwell on a significant topic at length.

One valuable type of therapy is the encounter group. Here the emphasis falls on intense activity, and the therapy utilizes psychodrama, role play, and other more active forms of interaction (Kraft and Vick, 1973; Miller, 1973; Olsson and Myers, 1972; Osario, 1970; Vick and Kraft, 1973). The raw material offers numerous opportunities from which insight can develop. The group becomes the vehicle for heightened emotional interaction between therapist and patient and between patient and patient. Encounter techniques insist that it is not enough merely to be present while a patient goes through some emotional turmoil; in order to increase group interactions, the leader expects the group to experience and share the feelings of each member. A key concept is "free role experimentation." This facilitates the resolution of the adolescent ego identity crisis by allowing the adolescent to experiment with a wide variety of feelings, thoughts, and behavior in the group setting. Group cohesion is fostered, however, by common emotional experiences, in which all share, by field trips undertaken together, and by other group activities. One of the most useful of these is the camping trip, which is popular with adolescents and serves to bind them together (Leatherman and Nehring, personal communication).

Recently minithons have been tried with a mixed group of adolescents. This consists of meeting for four to six hours of the usual group session, a 30-to-45-minute break is taken for food and stretch, and the group then resumes for several additional hours. Essentially, the longer time allows for more intensive exploration of a number of topics without everyone succumbing to malaise and fatigue. Greater depth and more intensity to themes seem to happen.

Transactional analysis is being used increasingly with adolescent therapy groups. It emphasizes treatment directed toward specific goals, which are defined in terms of observable change in behavior, as well as attitudinal changes. The concepts of transactional analysis provide a common vocabulary and frame of reference that are readily intelligible and acceptable to adolescents and preadolescents and that can be the focus of group discussions and analysis. Group members learn to detect "games" in their own behavior and those of others, to analyze transactions, and to put into practice various techniques which enable them to solve "crossed transactions" and to acquire "stroking."

For example, a very common transactional interplay or game is "kick me," which involves the adolescent offering some verbal or behavioral hook or ploy to a peer or adult. The other person then responds in a predictable fashion which consists of some sort of put-down or criticism of the adolescent, who then righteously feels badly and offended. The leader and/or group members point out how he has maneuvered himself into this to obtain a negative stroke, since he feels undeserving of straight or positive strokes, which are egosyntonic, and supportive actions or verbalizations.

Ulterior transactions are those in which the true message is covert and perhaps subtle. Adolescents love to detect these in their peers, parents, and authority figures. One such incident involved an adolescent girl who kept telling the group she did not behave enticingly to boys or to her father, but the group picked up her tone and manner, which conveyed the sexual seductiveness she really portrayed. Behavior is changed primarily by increasing the groups members' understanding of themselves and of each other. Transactional analysis uses role play, Gestalts, psychodrama, and other group therapy techniques involving verbalization and analysis, and relies as well on verbal contracting, in which the patient specifies the goals toward which he will work and the length of time he expects it will take him to achieve them.

Behavioral contracting is a technique which involves scheduling the exchange of positive reinforcements between two or more persons. Although in many ways similar, transactional analysis differs from behavior modification's original "black box" basis. A good contract fulfills five requirements: (1) the privileges each party expects for fulfilling his responsibilities; (2) the responsibilities essential to securing each privilege; (3) a system of sanctions for failure to meet responsibilities; (4) a bonus clause; and (5) a feedback system to keep track of reinforcement given and received (Rose, 1972). It is crucial that the expectations of each party to the transactions be clearly understood.

The theory of modeling shows that adolescents will respond to new stimulus situations in a manner consistent with that of the models even if they had never observed the models responding to these particular stimuli. Modeling influences thus produce not only specific mimicry, but also generative and innovative behavior. Group therapists working with disadvantaged children succeeded in introducing "star" students into the group and encouraging the members to model some aspects of their behavior on that of the "stars." Peers have also been used as agents who dispense social reinforcers. This has resulted in significant change in the behavior of group members, especially when reinforced by friends rather than by nonpreferred peers.

In brief, the tendency to regard the group as an object acted on by the therapist is now giving way to a trend to view the group itself as an active therapeutic factor. Transactional analysis, encounter therapy, modeling, and peer reinforcement all seem to be part of this trend.

Group Therapy for Delinquent Adolescents

In Western society, many special caretaking facilities have been devised for children and adolescents. In many instances group psychotherapy techniques have been adapted to these different settings. Among others, the delinquent has received a good deal of attention, including group work field workers who work directly with neighborhood gangs and group psychotherapy with probationers.

The customary procedures for group psychotherapy require modification when employed for delinquent adolescents, as these changes are in response to the contingencies arising from the character disorders of the delinquents. These adolescents differ in their dyssocial patterns from those who violate the legal, moral, and social values of the community during an adjustment reaction of adolescence or a transitional neurotic acting-out incident. The adolescent with a delinquent character structure persistently truants, steals, vandalizes, runs away, or engages in other activities which usually mean removal to an institution.

Institutional Group Therapy

Schulman (1956) pointed out that the complexities of group psychotherapy are increased by the characterological antagonisms and chronic uncooperativeness of delinquent patients. These factors combine with those inherent in institutional settings to make it difficult to study the role of group therapy for the antisocial adolescent. Psychotherapists have pressed for the humanization of institutions, and whenever possible, for the use of alternatives such as homes and halfway houses.

Several reports indicate favorable results with this group of patients (Brandt, 1973). In Gersten's 1951 study, group psychotherapy with male delinquents in an institution resulted in improved intellectual and school functions. Psychological tests indicated some enhancement of emotional maturity (Gersten, 1951). Another report by Thorpe and Smith in 1952 described sequential steps in the youngsters' responses. At first there were episodes of testing, and later a series of acceptance operations. In 1954, Peck and Bellsmith used group methods for delinquent adolescents with reading disabilities. Richardson and Meyer (1972) used the peer group as a catalyst for change by encouraging a high level of interaction within various autonomous groups. In some instances, they used the therapist roles to harass the patient in his "hot seat," and had the group itself verbally pummel the transgressor until he "gave out" to the group.

Schulman (1956) emphasized a threefold purpose in blending psychotherapy into the totality of care for these patients: (1) intellectual insight and reality testing occur in the group milieu; (2) alloplastic symptoms and superego development can be observed; and (3) the group situation readily tests the developmental stage of new attitudes, since the patient continues to perform in a homogenous group of delinquents.

These character distortions use aggression predominantly to reduce internalized anxiety. The delinquents show a weak ego structure and a defective superego. Schulman suggested that their inherent difficulty with society and its authority symbols serves as the nidus for a therapeutic relationship. Modifications of the traditional therapist-patient relationship can then allow the delinquent to develop a shallow emotional attachment. Schulman initially used variations in activity and unexpected refreshments; later he modified this to focus on the authority-dependency relationship built into the institutional situation. From the beginning, the adolescent knows that his getting out of the institution depends on the therapist, who then assumes a certain omnipotence and thereby becomes a person with whom the youngster can identify. As the therapist continues to evoke a sense of early life experience for the adolescent—but without the inconsistencies, exploitations, and dishonesties that were formerly present—he becomes somewhat of an ego-ideal for the embryonic superego.

Other therapists challenge this type of therapy precisely because it is based on the authority-dependency relationship. As they see it, the goal for the patient is real autonomy, not merely good adjustment to the institution; they stress that the delinquent's release must depend on him. They strive to present a leader role characterized by permissiveness and support, and at times their stance may be contrary to the overall patterns of the institution. However, they maintain that despite their stated aims, these institutional arrangements do not so much prepare the delinquent for life in society as incapacitate him. Thus the permissive approach in their view promotes therapeutic readiness.

Schulman and others described the sexual preoccupations of adolescent female delinquents; they assert that the therapist needs to control this in order to avoid group deterioration through continuous perseveration. This sort of deterioration occurs in the male group as well, often with the onus falling on some group scapegoat. Directed discussion by the therapist can change the tone of the session and/or block group disintegration.

Among the many variables that need to be examined, one of the most pertinent seems to be the duration of the group therapy process. Generally, the longer the group can function effectively, the better the chances for positive change among its members. Other techniques employing audiovisual methods such as videotapes are beginning to be employed and show considerable promise.

Resistances in both adolescent and children group therapy have been studied by Marshall (1972). He views as resistance lengthy silences, stereotyped and repetitive talk and play, and objections and refusal to attend sessions. Marshall advocates "joining" techniques, such as hypervaluation, which means going along, for example, with the melancholy death preoccupations of an early adolescent, getting more and more details, and relating them to current interest in death and dying. He refers to eight or nine other techniques of joining which help when there was little or no "verbalized anxiety and the use of denial, projection, and all-encompassing repression was central."

Inpatient settings provide more complex situations, and the group method in turn must work differently in order to achieve the "genuine internalization of positive treatment goals by a majority of members" of the group (Lewis et al., 1970). One agency turned to a very forceful use of the group. The patients met four times a week and focused strongly on restrictions. When one member engaged in significantly deviant behavior—e.g., a suicidal attempt or physical assault—three requirements had to be met: (1) each member had to explore his own role in the deviance of his confrere; (2) everyone's feelings about the incident and its perpetration had to be expressed openly; and (3) the group then helped the patient by showing him alternative paths for handling his feelings. Working in a private intensive-care hospital, Masterson found psychoanalytic group therapy very "effective in reinforcing control of behavior and focusing the patient's consideration of therapy as an instrument to deal with his problems" (1972). They confronted behaviors in the group, thereby enhancing input that was dealt with much more intensively and deeply in the concomitant individual therapy.

In view of the opportunity they afford for more controlled conditions, residential treatment units have been used for specific studies in group therapy, such as behavioral contracting (Hauserman, Zweback, and Plotkin, 1972; Rawling and Gauran, 1973). Bardill (1972) used such a setting as a site for the exchange of positive reinforcements among preadolescent boys with severe concerns in basic trust, low self-esteem, and dependency conflicts. In contrast to this planned, specific behavioral modification approach is the work of Celia in Brazil. There a group club was used as a means for group interaction and the integration of individuals. According to the reports, the children formed their club, used its structure to face competitors, dramatized conflicts, and corrected fantasy by reality outreach (Celia, 1970). Osario (1970) utilized a similar technique with psychotic children in forming a therapeutic community or home. He believed this model involved the children more than a therapeutic schoolroom model. In time the therapeutic club, which incorproated group therapy as a part of its program, became the axis around which patients and team acted in the therapeutic task of reintegrating the child.

Lordi (1975) emphasizes new trends of consumer "rights," so he utilizes group methods in his inpatient adolescent therapeutic community. He sees it as a workshop in which the therapy team and adolescents meet "5 days a week to interact and to deal with overt and covert issues and agendas."

Social group homes resemble formal residential treatment units work homes (Tietz and Ramer, 1970). Since these children in these settings represent the consequences of psychological assaults, supportive group therapy offers them the opportunity to ventilate. In addition, this modality presents these children with an opportunity to enjoy sharing activities and developing skills.

Pregnant adolescents who plan to deliver derive benefit from a group experience, which, by definition, through circumstance, has a time-limited quality. The problem of pregnancy soon becomes involved with widening ranges of other factors and forces predominantly unknown to the young girl prior to this new experience. Essentially, several therapists (Black, 1972; Kaufman and Deutsch, 1967) report that medical management of these youngsters, who are more prone to difficulties in pregnancy, becomes easier. Effective programs reduce excessive weight gain and toxemia and increase the capacity to care for herself, the baby, and accordingly, subsequent pregnancies. Goldman, Murphy and Babikian (1973) involved eight poverty-level Puerto Rican and black females in twenty short-term, goal-directed group meetings. A control group and this group's dropouts demonstrated longer labors than the group members.

The Role of the Therapist

The traditional passive role of the therapist has come under attack increasingly (Phelan, 1974). Encounter therapy, for instance, incorporates several "active" techniques, such as environmental intervention, to foster a positive transference to the therapist, to motivate group members to attend sessions, and to stimulate positive, meaningful, and concerned encounters between the therapist and his group. Transactional analysis requires an active, intervening role for the group therapist, and the very nature of contractual techniques assures that he will state his expectations and premises in a manner that would ordinarily be proscribed by a classic psychoanalytic posture. Some argue that the therapist should in fact impress his individual tastes and personality upon the techniques he uses. There is increasing agreement that the therapist can and should use positive rewards and reinforcement, and many of the techniques outlined above are based upon this premise. Thus the therapist actively directs the group and may even be expected to provide it with a model (Spruiell, 1975).

Another aspect of the therapist's task is specificity of intervention. Therapists upholding the value of the specific, highly directed intervention maintain that it is not enough for them to project a benevolent, supportive, and permissive presence. One comparison found that specific intervention and direct rewards had a more effective impact on the achievement of children from a low socioeconomic area than did undirected "love and care."

Specific intervention on the part of the therapist necessarily involves the projection of his values and expectations upon the group; to the extent that he does this, as Azima cogently points out, it is his responsibility to be aware of his countertransference (1972).

Especially with the onslaught of growth centers and new roles for therapists in touching, communing, and confessing with their patients, self-disclosure by the leader becomes a serious topic. Self-disclosingness per se is of little value in promoting openness by patients or in ameliorating treatment results (Weiner and King, 1977). Lieberman's 1973 study shows that what is disclosed and under what circumstances are of greater importance. He found, for example, that self-disclosingness was useful when it conveyed personal interest and positive feelings and was part of a larger cognitive frame of reference. It was destructive when it conveyed negative feelings at a time when there was little support and no real cognitive frame of reference.

Leadership, preferably with male and female co-therapists, involves developing cohesiveness, identifying goals for the group, showing the group how to function, keeping the group task-oriented, serving as a model, and representing a value system. In carrying out these tasks, the leader may offer clarification of reality, analysis of transactions, brief educational input, empathic statements acknowledging his own feelings and those of members, and at times delineating the feeling states at hand in the group.

Preparation

Customarily, in office settings, the group meets once a week. Often mechanical problems, including travel to and from the group, confine the members to that pattern. Other settings, such as inpatient units, may hold meetings with greater frequency if indicated by therapeutic considerations. There is little data about office or clinic practice with groups that met more than once a week.

Simultaneous Practices

The major questions here involve parents, other caretakers, and sometimes siblings. Often the therapist and the appropriate school persons need to collaborate, especially when the child has a history of rebellions and acting-out behavior. Ideally, the patient's family should participate in the therapeutic process, even if only episodically (such as once monthly, or every two to three months). In reality, this often proves difficult. An alternative is to utilize parent group meetings at one-to-three-month intervals for the parents to compare notes and selves. (This assumes the father and/or mother is not in some type of formal therapy.) Family therapy, which includes the presence of the patient, also aids in the treatment.

Economic Factors

Obviously, in an office setting a group experience provides care at less cost than does individual therapy. Paraprofessional training programs suggest that these personnel can be utilized to offer even lower unit cost care than do the professionals. With the ever-increasing number of children needing help and with inflation and other economic factors disrupting the traditional pattern of providing care, more pursuit and use of group psychotherapy is in order for children and their families.

Follow-Up Patterns

As indicated above, the family system often has used the child as the scapegoat or as the emotional radar signal for its hidden interactional discomforts. Presumably, the child's therapy, often coupled with some form of family intervention, has altered the family's patterns enough that follow-up procedures can be instituted. Some therapists make clear to the child he is free to return to the group for a visit or to attend to other problems that might arise subsequently.

After children leave the group, it is wise to see them individually two or three times at intervals of perhaps three or four months to check on progress and any possible regressions. Interval histories from parents covering the original and associated problems over the same period also prove useful. In sum, the family knows that problems can reoccur or surface in other ways, so that the child and the parent remain vigilant, especially for the six to twelve months after the child terminates the group.

Evaluation

The results of group therapy with children are difficult to evaluate. Several reports using control groups show favorable results with nondirective play therapy, and with specific intervention group therapy for underachievers, and even for delinquents. Milieu therapy has resulted in striking improvement with ghetto children. It has also been a basic modality with childhood psychoses. Evaluating the results of group psychotherapy with children proves as difficult as assessing the outcome of their individual psychotherapy. Abramowitz (1976) reviewed empirical outcome research on children's activity, behavior modification, play and verbal groups and failed to find convincing evidence of effectiveness. At this point, impressionistically, it can be reported that children seem to feel unconditionally accepted by the therapist and the group members. The child gains the impression that "failures" are part of his development as a person. The child has obtained some inklings or more definitive insights into himself and his family's systems for handling life's stresses. He has experienced, sometimes with cognitive awareness, group cohesion and his own growth responses to it. Feelings of anxiety, inferiority, guilt, and insecurity find relief. Usually, years later he recalls the group and its happenings more than he recalls the therapist, often not even remembering the therapist's name. This finding emphasizes the overall value and productivity of the experiential nature of group psychotherapy.

References

Abramowitz, C.V. (1976) The effectiveness of group psychotherapy with children. *Arch. Gen. Psychiat.* 33.

Ackerman, N.W. (1955) Group psychotherapy with a mixed group of adolescents. *Int. J. Group Psychother.* 5:249.

Adams, J.D. (1976) Hospital play program: Helping children with serious illness. *Am. J. Orthopsychiat.* 46: 416.

Anderson, N., and R.T. Marrone. (1976) Group therapy for emotionally disturbed children: A key to affective education. *Am. J. Orthopsychiat.* 47(1):97–105.

Azima, F.J. (1972) Transference countertransference issues in group psychotherapy for adolescents. *Int. J. Psychother.* 1(4):52.

Bandura, A. (1969) Modeling and vicarious processes. In *Principles of Behavior Modification.* New York: Holt, Rinehart and Winston.

Barabasz, A.F. (1973) Group desensitization of test anxiety in elementary school. *J. Psychol.* 82:295.

Barcai, A., C. Umbarger, T. Pierce, et al. (1973) A comparison of three group approaches to underachieving children. *Am. J. Orthopsychiat.* 43:133.

Bardill, D.R. (1972) A behavior contracting based program of group treatment for early adolescents in a residential setting. *Int. J. Group Psychother.* 22:1.

Battin, R., and I.A. Kraft. (1968) Psycholinguistic evaluation of children referred for private consultation to a child psychiatrist. *J. Learning Disabil.* 1:600.

Bellucci, M.T. (1975) Treatment of latency age adopted children and parents. *Social Casework* 56:297–301.

Bender, L., and A.S. Waltman. (1936) Use of puppet shows as a psychotherapeutic method for behavior problems in children. *Am. J. Orthopsychiat.* 6:341.

Berkowitz, I., and M. Sugar. (1975) Indications and contraindications for adolescent group psychotherapy. In M. Sugar, ed., *The Adolescent in Group and Family Therapy.* New York: Brunner/Mazel.

Berkowitz, I. (1972) On growing a group: Some thoughts on structure, process and setting. in I. Berkowitz, ed., *Adolescents Grow in Groups: Experiences in Adolescent Group Psychotherapy.* New York: Brunner/Mazel.

Black, S. (1972) Group therapy for pregnant and nonpregnant adolescents. *Child Welfare* 51(8):516.

Brandes, N. (1971) Group psychotherapy for the adolescent. *Curr. Psychiat. Ther.* 11:18.

Brandt, D.E. (1973) A descriptive analysis of selected aspects of group therapy with severely delinquent boys. *J. Am. Acad. Child Psychiat.* 12:473.

Bratter, T. (1974) Reality therapy: A group psychotherapeutic approach with adolescent alcoholics. *Ann. N.Y. Acad. Sci.* 233:104.

Bratter, T. (1973) Treating alienated, unmotivated, drug-abusing adolescents. *Am. J. Psychother.* 27:585.

Celia, S.A. (1970) The club as an integrative factor in a therapeutic community for children. *Am. J. Orthopsychiat.* 40:130.

Cermak, S.A., F. Stein, and C. Abelson. (1973) Hyperactive children and an activity group therapy model. *Am. J. Occup. Ther.* 26(6):311.

Churchill, R.R. (1965) Social group work: A diagnostic tool in child guidance. *Am. J. Orthopsychiat.* 35:581.

Crowdes, N.E. (1975) Group therapy for preadolescent boys. *Am. J. Nursing* 75:92.

DeLara, L.E. (1969) Listening is a challenge: Group counseling in the school. *Ment. Hyg.* 53:600.

Duffy, J.H., and I.A. Kraft. (1966–67) Beginning and middle phase characteristics of group psychotherapy of early adolescent boys and girls. *J. Psychoanal. Groups* 11:23.

Egan, M.H. (1975) Dynamisms in activity discussion group therapy. *Int. J. Group Psychother.* 25(2):199.

Epstein, N. (1970 Brief group therapy in a child guidance clinic. *Social Work* 15(3):33.

Etters, L.E. (1975) Adolescent retardates in a therapy group. *Am. J. Nursing* 75:1174–1175.

Fishman, C.A., and D.B. Fishman. (1975) A group training program in behavior modification for mothers of children with birth defects. *Child Psychiat. Hum. Devel.* 6:3–14.

Flint, W., and C. Deloach. (1975) Parent involvement program model for handicapped children and their parents. *Except. Child* 41:556–557.

Gerstein, A.I. (1969) Variation in treatment technique in group activity therapy for children. *Am. J. Orthopsychiat.* 39:261.

Gersten, C. (1951) An experimental evaluation of group therapy with juvenile delinquents. *Int. J. Group Psychother.* 1:311.

Gibson, R.E. (1973) The ambassador and the system (electronic and otherwise). *Johns Hopkins Mag.* 24:2.

Ginott, H.G. (1961) *Group Psychotherapy with Children.* New York: McGraw-Hill.

Goldberg, A. (1972) On the incapacity to love: A psychotherapeutic approach to the problem in adolescence. *Arch. Gen. Psychiat.* 26:3.

Goldman, A.S., R.J. Murphy, and H.M. Babikian (1973) Group therapy in obstetric management of pregnant teenagers. *N.Y. State J. Med.* 73:407.

Gratton, L., and L. Pope. (1972) Group diagnosis and therapy for young school children. *Hosp. Comm. Psychiat.* 23:40.

Green, R., and M. Fuller. (1973) Group therapy with feminine boys and their parents. *Int. J. Group Psychother.* 23:54

Haizlip, T., C. McRee, and B.F. Corder. (1975) Issues in developing psychotherapy groups for preschool children in outpatient clinics. *Am. J. Psychiat.* 132(10):1061.

Hansen, J.C., T.M. Niland, and L.P. Zani. (1969) Model reinforcement in group counseling with elementary school children. *Personnel Guid. J.* 47:741.

Harris, M.B., and A.E. Trujillo. (1975) Improving study habits of junior high school students through self-management versus group discussion. *J. Counsel.* 225:513–517.

Hauserman, N., S. Zweback, and A. Plotkin. (1972) Use of concrete reinforcement to facilitate verbal initiations in adolescent group therapy. *J. Consult. Clin. Psychol.* 38(1):90.

Herrick, R.H., and C.M. Binger. (1974) Group psychotherapy for early adolescents—An adjunct to a comprehensive treatment program. *J.Am. Acad. Child Psychiat.* 13(1):110.

Hodgman, C.H., and W.H. Stewart. (1972) The adolescent screeing group. *Int. J. Group Psychother.* 22(1):177.

Hulse, W. (1960) Psychiatric aspects of group counseling of adolescents. *Psychiat. Quart.* 34(Suppl.):9.

Johnson, D.L., and S.R. Gold. (1971) An empirical approach to issue of selection and evaluation in group therapy. *Int. J. Group Psychother.* 21:456.

Josselyn, I.M. (1972) Adolescent group therapy: Why, when, and a caution. In I.H. Berkowitz, ed., *Adolescents Grow in Groups: Experiences in Adolescent Group Psychotherapy.* New York: Brunner/Mazel.

Kaufman, P.N., and A.L. Deutsch. (1967) Group therapy for pregnant unwed adolescents in the prenatal clinic of a general hospital. *Int. J. Group Psychother.* 17:309.

Kelley, J.B. (1974) Reaching out to parents of handicapped children—A group approach to an inner-city school. *J. School Health* 44:577–579.

Kernberg, P.F., and L.M. Ware. (1975) Understanding child development through group techniques and play. *Bull. Menninger Clinic* 39:409–419.

Kraft, I.A. (1961) Some special considerations in adolescent group psychotherapy. *Int. J. Group Psychother.* 11:196.

Kraft, I.A. (1968) An overview of group therapy with adolescents. *Int. J. Group Psychother.* 18:461.

Kraft, I.A., and W. Delaney. (1968) Movement communication with children in a psychoeducation program at a day hospital. *J. Am. Dance Ther. Assn.* 1:6.

Kraft, I.A., and J.W. Vick. (1973) Flexibility and variability of group psychotherapy with adolescent girls. In E. Schwartz and L. Wolberg, eds., *Group Therapy: An Overview.* New York: Intercontinental Medical Book Corp.

Laybourne, P.C., S. Shupe, and S.J. Sikkema. Open-ended brief group therapy on a pediatric ward (personal communication).

Leatherman, E.H., and S. Nehring. A unique camping program for adolescents (personal communication).

Lewis, J.M., J.T. Gassett, J.W. King, et al. (1970) Development of a protreatment group process among hospitalized adolescents. Timberlawn Foundation Report No. 40.

Lieberman, M.A., I.D. Yolom, and M.B. Miles. (1973) *Encounter Groups: First Facts.* New York: Basic Books.

Lilleskov, R.K., S. Harris, H. Hughson, et al. (1969) A therapeutic club for severely disturbed prepubertal boys. *Am. J. Orthopsychiat.* 34:262.

Lordi, W.M. (1975) Group psychotherapy in an adolescent therapeutic community. *Am. J. Orthopsychiat.* 45:224–225.

Lovell, L.M. (1973) The Yeovil Opportunity Group: A play group for multiply handicapped children. *Physiotherapy* 59(8):251.

Marshall, R.J. (1972) The treatment of resistances in psychotherapy of children and adolescents. *Psychother. Theory Res. Prac.* 9(2):143–148.

Marvitt, R.C., J. Lind, and D.G. McLaughlin. (1974) Use of videotape to induce attitude change in delinquent adolescents. *Am. J. Psychiat.* 131(9):996.

Masterson, J.F. (1972) *Treatment of the Borderline Adolescent: A Developmental Approach.* New York: Wiley.

Melnick, J., and A.R. Tims. (1974) Application of videotape equipment to group therapy. *Int. J. Group Psychother.* 24(2):202.

Melville, K. (1973) Changing the family game. *Sciences* 13:17.

Miller, A.H. (1973) The spontaneous use of poetry in an adolescent girls' group. *Int. J. Group Psychother.* 23:224.

Minde, K.K., and J.S. Werry. (1969) Intensive psychiatric teacher counseling in a low socioeconomic area: A controlled evaluation. *Am. J. Orthopsychiat.* 39:595.

Mumford, L. (1972) *Pyramids of Power.* New York: Harcourt, Brace, and Jovanovich.

Nielson, G.H. (1970) A project in parent education. *Can. J. Public Health* 61:210.

Olsson, P.A., and I. Myers. (1972) Nonverbal techniques in an adolescent group. *Int. J. Group Psychother.* 22:186.

Osario, L.C. (1970) Milieu therapy for child psychosis. *Am. J. Orthopsychiat.* 40:121.

Parker, L., P.W. Hogan, and I.A. Kraft. (1978) Short-term

family therapy: An intake catalyst for group treatment of adolescent girls. *Group Proc.*, 8:176–185.

Pasnau, R.O., L. Williams, and F.F. Tallman. (1971) Small activity group in the school. *Comm. Ment. Health J.* 7(4):303.

Pasnau, R.O., M. Meyer, L.J. Davis, et al. (1976) Coordinated group psychotherapy of children and parents. *Int. J. Group Psychother.* 26(1):89–103.

Patterson, G.R., and C. Anderson. (1964) Peers as social reinforcers. *Child Dev.* 35:951.

Peck, H.B., and V. Bellsmith. (1954) *Treatment of the Delinquent Adolescent.* New York: Family Service Association of America.

Phelan, J.R. (1974) Parent, teacher, or analyst: The adolescent—Group therapist's trilemna. *Int. J. Group Psychother.* 14(2):238.

Poole, A., and P. Ruck. (1972) Remedial play groups for the under-fives in a general hospital. *Physiother.* 58:132.

Pratt, S.J., et al. (1975) Behavior modification: Changing hyperactive behavior in a children's group. *Perspec. Psychiat. Care* 13:37–42.

Rachman, A.W. (1971) Encounter techniques in analytic group psychotherapy with adolescents. *Int. J. Group Psychother.* 21:319.

Rawling, E.I., and E.F. Gauran. (1973) Responders and nonresponders to an accelerated, time-limited group. *Perspec. Psychiat. Care* 11:65.

Rhodes, S.L. (1973) Short-term groups of latency-age children in a school setting. *Int. J. Group Psychother.* 23:204.

Richardson, C., and R.G. Meyer. (1972) Techniques in guided group interaction programs. *Child Welfare* 51(8):519.

Rinn, R.C., et al. (1975) Training parents of behaviorally disordered children in groups: A three-year program evaluation. *Behav. Ther.* 6:378–387.

Rizzo, A.E., A. Ossario, and L. Saxon. (1975) The organization of an adolescent unit in a state hospital: Problems and attempted solutions. In M. Sugar, ed., *The Adolescent in Group and Family Therapy.* New York: Brunner/Mazel.

Robinson, L. (1970) Role play with retarded adolescent girls: Teaching and therapy. *Ment. Retard.* 8(2):36.

Rose, S.D., (1972) *Treating Children in Groups.* London: Jossey-Bass.

Rosenthal, L. (1971) Some dynamics of resistance and therapeutic management in adolescent group therapy. *Psychoanal. Rev.* 58:353.

Sadock, B.J. (1975) Group psychotherapy. In A.M. Freedman, H.I. Kaplan, and B.J. Sadock, eds., *Comprehensive Textbook of Psychiatry II.* Baltimore: Williams & Wilkins.

Sands, R.M., R. Blank, B. Brandt, et al. (1973) Breaking the bands of tradition: Reassessment of group treatment of latency children in a community mental health center. *Am. J. Orthopsychiat.* 43:212.

Schacter, R.S. (1973) Kinetic psychotherapy in the treatment of children. *Am. J. Psychother.* 28(3):430.

Schaefer, J.W., H.S. Palkes, and M.A. Stewart. (1974) Group counseling for parents of hyperactive children. *Child Psychiat. Hum. Devel.* 5:89–94.

Schamess, G. (1976) Group treatment modalities for latency-age children. *Int. J. Group Psychother.* 26(4):455-473.

Schiffer, M. (1969) *The Therapeutic Play Group.* New York: Grune & Stratton.

Schulman, I. (1956) Delinquents. In S.R. Slavson, ed., *The Fields of Group Psychotherapy.* New York: International Universities Press.

Shapiro, Z., and I. Berkowitz. (1975) The impact of group experiences on adolescent development. In M. Sugar, ed., *The Adolescent in Group and Family Therapy.* New York: Brunner/Mazel.

Shere, E.S., and Y. Techman. (1971) Evaluation of group therapy with preadolescent girls: Assessment of therapeutic effects based on Rorschach records. *Int. J. Group Psychother.* 21:(1):99.

Singer, M. (1974) Comments and caveats regarding adolescent groups in a combined approach. *Int. J. Group Psychother.* 24(4):429.

Slavson, S.R. (1950) *Analytic Group Psychotherapy with Children, Adolescents, and Adults.* New York: Columbia University Press.

Slavson, S.R., and M. Schiffer. (1975) *Group Psychotherapies for Children.* New York: International Universities Press.

Soble, D., and J.J. Geller. (1964) A type of group psychotherapy for withdrawn adolescents. *Am. J. Dis. Child* 68:86.

Soo, E. (1974) The impact of activity group therapy upon a highly constricted child. *Int. J. Group Psychother.* 24(2):207.

Speers, R.W., and C. Lansing. (1965) *Group Therapy in Childhood Psychosis.* Chapel Hill: University of North Carolina Press.

Spruiell, V. (1975) Adolescent narcissism and group psychotherapy. In M. Sugar, ed., *The Adolescent in Group and Family Therapy.* New York: Brunner/Mazel.

Stamps, L.W. (1973) The effects of intervention techniques on children's fear of failure behavior. *J. Genet. Psycho.* 123:85.

Strunk, C., and L. Witkin. (1974) The transformation of a latency age girls' group from unstructured play to problem-focused discussion. *Int. J. Group Psychother.* 24(4):461.

Sugar, M. (1975) Group therapy for pubescent boys with absent fathers. In M. Sugar, ed., *The Adolescent in Group and Family Therapy.* New York: Brunner/Mazel.

Sugar, M. (1975) Office network therapy with adolescents. In M. Sugar, ed., *The Adolescent in Group and Family Therapy.* New York: Brunner/Mazel.

Sugar, M. (1975) The structure and setting of adolescent therapy groups. In M. Sugar, ed., *The Adolescent in Group and Family Therapy.* New York: Brunner/Mazel.

Thorpe, J.F., and B. Smith. (1952) Operational sequences in group therapy with young offenders. *Int. J. Group Psychother.* 2:24.

Tietz, W., and M. Ramer. (1970) Establishing a small group treatment home in the Mexican ghetto. *Am. J. Orthopsychiat.* 40:242.

VanScoy, H. (1972) Activity group therapy: A bridge between play and work. *Child Welfare* 51(8):528.

VanScoy, H. (1971) An activity group approach to seriously disturbed latency boys. *Child Welfare* 50(7):413.

Vick, J., and I.A. Kraft. (1973) Creative activities. In N.S. Brandes, ed., *Group Therapy for the Adolescent.* New York: Jason Aronson.

Weiner, M.F., and J.W. King. (1977) Self-disclosure by the therapist to the adolescent patient. In S.C. Feinstein and P. Giovaccitini, eds., *Adolescent Psychiatry.* New York: Jason Aronson.

Yalom, I.D. (1975) *The Theory and Practice of Group Psychotherapy,* 2nd ed. New York: Basic Books.

Treatment of Emotional Disorders in Children and Adolescents

CHAPTER 10

Psychodynamically Oriented Family Therapy

Rodney J. Shapiro

Current formulations about the family reflect divergent theoretical assumptions and emphasize different dimensions and levels of family functioning. The diversity of concepts is so great that even attempts to classify theories of family therapy show marked differences (Meissner, 1964; Beels and Ferber, 1969; Offer and Vanderstoep, 1975; Ritterman, 1977). Perhaps the only prevailing viewpoint that has general endorsement is that there is no one accepted theory of family therapy (Meissner, 1964; Bell, 1975).

It is also erroneous to view family therapy as a particular set of techniques. Just as there is a variety of theories, so there is a multiplicity of clinical practices, all of which fall under the general rubric of family therapy. Practitioners differ on issues of diagnosis, areas for intervention, techniques, and goals of treatment. From their survey of family therapists, the Group for the Advancement of Psychiatry (1970) concluded that family therapy is not a treatment method in the usual sense, in that there is no agreed-upon set of procedures.

In the light of this profusion of viewpoints and practices, can we justifiably define family therapy as a distinctive orientation? A number of writers have considered this question, and arrived at a similar conclusion. Despite the variety of ideas and practice in the field, a common assumption is shared by all family therapists. This is the notion that psychopathology resides in family systems rather than within individuals, and that any interventions designed to effect change in the family relationship system rather than an individual may be deemed family therapy (Bell, 1975; Foley, 1974; Minuchin, 1974b; Olson, 1970; Shapiro, 1976).

Family treatment of children and adolescents is virtually synonymous with family therapy per se, since the term "family" invariably denotes parents and offspring. A comprehensive survey of the entire field is not possible within the confines of a single chapter. I have therefore confined myself to a consideration of the most relevant areas of family therapy, and excluded many topics of interest not directly related to work with children and adolescents. Material on marital therapy has been omitted unless related to issues of parent-child relationships. Furthermore, the theories and treatment methods described in this chapter stem almost exclusively from studies of families in which presenting problems relate to children and adolescents rather than to adults.

The Development of Family Therapy

A number of writers have been struck by the serendipitous beginnings of family therapy. As early as 1949, John Bowlby noted that problems presented by a child often reflected tension between members of the family. Fortuitously, John Bell came across Bowlby's (1949) paper and mistakenly assumed that Bowlby in fact worked with whole families. This gave Bell the incentive to try what seemed like a radical maneuver, and he began attempting to involve whole families in the treatment of children and adolescents (Bell, 1975). Jackson and Weakland (1971) have described how they stumbled upon family treatment in the course of their research on schizophrenia.

In fact, though, no single individual or group can claim to have invented family therapy. The notion of working with whole families occurred independently to several clinicians and researchers during a short span of years in the 1950's (Olson, 1970). The concurrent and widespread indications of interest in the family point to the emergence of a *Zeitgeist* at that point in psychiatry that made possible a conceptual shift from the individual to the family unit. Antecedents of family therapy can be traced to the development of social psychiatry, major modifications in modern psychoanalytic thinking, and dissatisfaction with traditional child psychotherapy.

Sociologists were interested in the study of the family decades before the advent of family therapy (see, for example, Burgess, 1926), but their work had minimal impact on the mental health professions. It was the emergence of social psychiatry in recent years that provided a new perspective for research and clinical practice. Recognition was given to the significance of cultural forces and social settings in determining as well as ameliorating psychiatric disorders (Leighton, 1960; Spiegel, 1971). Interest was generated in studying social factors, particularly the social structure of the community, the effect of groups on individual behavior, and principles of communication (Ruesch, 1965). With a new awareness of the psychiatric implications of social organizations and social roles, the groundwork was prepared for the inevitable focus on the family as the primary social habitat of psychopathology.

A post-Freudian movement developed in reaction to the traditional focus on biological drive theory, and increasing emphasis was placed on the significance of social and cultural determinants of behavior (Horney, 1939; Fromm, 1941; Sullivan, 1953a). Analytic thinking progressively shifted to an interpersonal conceptualization of mental illness (Sullivan, 1953b) and the formulation of psychotherapy as a corrective interpersonal experience (Fromm-Reichmann, 1950). Erikson's (1950) developmental theory integrated individual maturational processes with the social and cultural environment, and his ideas strongly influenced theorists and clinicians. Interest in social roles and family structure fueled research and clinical studies related to the etiology of mental disorder in children. In the 1940's and 1950's an outpouring of research centered on the question of how family structure "causes" mental illness. Determinants of child pathology were sought in such factors as sibling order and rank, and the influence of specific parental personality traits. By far the greatest emphasis was on the "pathogenic" mother. Treatment of the mental patient was strongly influenced by studies such as David Levy's (1943) study of maternal overprotection, and Frieda Fromm-Reichmann's (1948) conceptualization of the "schizophrenogenic mother." Most psychodynamic approaches to mental disorder assumed the noxious influence of "bad" mothering to be the key predisposing factor for producing pathology in offspring.

Interest in the mother-child relation was based on a one-sided premise (the mother's effect on the child) rather than the interaction (the relationship) between the two. Nevertheless, these studies did represent a shift from the narrow intrapsychic view to a recognition of interpersonal determinants of child pathology. The focus on parent-child interaction was broadened to a family perspective with the spate of research studies on schizophrenia in the early 1950's. These investigations generated significant concepts of family functioning, and will be considered in a later section of this chapter.

The shift in theory from the individual child to the parent-child relationship to the family unit was paralleled by a similar movement in the practice of child psychotherapy. The first step occurred in the 1920's when the child guidance movement introduced the practice of including parents in the treatment of the child (Pattison, 1973). Care was then taken to avoid designating the parents as patients, even though they (usually only the mother) might receive counseling. The practice of child psychiatry has been influenced by this child guidance model, so that the separate treatment of parent and child is now commonplace. Primary importance is attached to treatment of the child, as reflected in the custom of assigning the therapist role to a psychiatrist, whereas the treatment of the parent is implicitly of secondary importance and hence assigned to a social worker or other "lower-status" helper.

Dissatisfaction with the traditional practice of child therapy inspired the consideration of alternative methods and led to experiments with family treatment. John Bell (1975) is generally regarded as one of the pioneering family therapists. He started working with whole families in an endeavor to provide more effective help for children than seemed possible with individual therapy. He was inspired to make this move by Bowlby's (1949) recognition of the family locus of problems presented to child guidance clinics.

Nathan Ackerman was also motivated by disenchantment with prevailing practices of child therapy. In one of his early papers, he pointed out the shortcomings of traditional child-parent tandem therapy as practiced in child guidance clinics (Ackerman, 1954). He noted that the separate treatment of the mother tends to reinforce two opposite trends. Either the mother uses the sessions to focus exclusively on the child rather than deal with her own problems, or else she focuses on herself only and lets the therapist take responsibility for the child. Ackerman noted that these were polar forms of resistance, and that such traditional treatment practices ignored the relationship between the mother and the child.

About the same time that Bell and Ackerman were putting their ideas into practice, other researchers and clinicians were independently stumbling upon the value of treating whole families. Olson (1970) succinctly describes the early work of such trailblazers as Bowen, Wynne, Boszormenyi-Nagy, and Don Jackson. As their writings were disseminated, the practice of family therapy developed into a major movement within the mental health professions.

The Influence of Systems Theory

The most singular theoretical assumption in family therapy is the formulation of the family as a system operating in accordance with the principles of general system theory. This theory, though based on biological principles, is particularly relevant for psychiatry (Bertalanffy, 1968).

Traditional psychiatry and psychology viewed the organism as a closed system—that is, a system considered to be isolated from its environment. System theory views the organism as essentially an open system—that is, a system that maintains itself in a constant exchange of matter with the environment; it is a continuous inflow and outflow process. By implication, the individual organism cannot be separated out of its environment, but has to be studied as part of a general context. A second crucial proposition of general system theory is the shift from the notion of linear causality to circular causality. Again, traditional psychiatric theory is based on an underlying assumption of linear causality—that is, a particular event gives rise to a particular consequence. A systems approach posits feedback processes to explain the maintenance of organismic functioning, in which an event A affects an event B, which in turn affects A, and so on, in circular fashion.

Several theorists adopted or modified principles of systems theory in order to develop a framework with which to understand family interaction and effect changes in family system (Jackson, 1965; Haley, 1959; Watzlawick, Beavin, and Jackson, 1967). One of the most significant derivations of system theory is the concept of family homeostasis (Jackson, 1957). The interacting dynamics of the family system tend toward the maintenance of a state of equilibrium. By implication, the system is resistant to changes that threaten to disrupt such equilibrium. This explains why attempts to change family members—for example, by means of psychotherapy—are resisted by the total family unit. To ensure the preservation of equilibrium, family interactions are monitored and modified by a constant flow of information, and this necessitates complex mechanisms of communication.

Communication Theories

Research on family communication stems from an initial project on general characteristics of communication that was directed by Gregory Bateson, and included Haley, Weakland, Jackson, and others (Weakland, 1976). This collaborative venture yielded many subsequent studies, with findings that have had great significance for the study and treatment of families.

A cardinal proposition is that a message cannot be interpreted in itself, but must always be related to the social context in which it is occurring—for example, the relationship between the communicators, the setting in which it occurs, and so on. Another significant theory is that all messages have two components—a quantity of information (report) and a directive (command) to the receiver (Watzlawick, Beavin, and Jackson, 1967). These ideas have important implications for clinical practice. In order to understand interactive processes, the therapist has to go beyond merely understanding the content (reports) of communication, and also detect the (often underlying) directive implications of the messages.

Perhaps the best-known concept to emerge out of this fruitful era of communication research, is what has become known as the double-bind theory. In studying families of schizophrenics, Bateson and his colleagues (1956) observed a typical pattern of communication in such families. The communicator (invariably a parent) would repeatedly send two concomitant messages to the identified patient. The first message is a negative injunction implying that a punishment will follow noncompliance with a particular demand. A second message (usually nonverbal) demands a response that conflicts with the first demand, yet also conveys the threat of punishment for noncompliance. A choice is forced upon the receiver by a third injunction that prevents the "victim" from avoiding the situation. The only possible responses to a double-bind predicament are necessarily irrational or a refusal to respond (withdrawal), both of which characterize schizophrenic interpersonal behavior. The original implication of the double bind as an etiological factor in schizophrenia was overly simplistic. Modifications of the concept have shifted to a view of the double bind as a significant interactional process that occurs widely and is not sufficient to account for schizophrenia (Bateson, 1972).

The double-bind hypothesis is valuable for the clinician who works with children and families, in that manifestations of such communication traps are frequent in disturbed families. Whether or not the double bind leads to or maintains severe psychopathology, there is no question but that it is a form of victimization, and an understanding of this process enables the therapist to intervene and rescue both parent and child from this repetitive mode of interaction.

Other premises arising from communication theory have had particular relevance for the treatment of families. One basic assumption is that all behaviors occurring in a social system are an outcome of, or function of, communicative interaction. In other words, behavior is communication, or communication is behavior (Watzlawick, Beavin, and Jackson, 1967; Weakland, 1976). It follows from this that "problems" have to be viewed as communications. A problem is some perceived behavior that arouses a negative reaction in the perceiver. The clinical implication of this view is that the therapist has to help the family reformulate problems from difficulties revealed by one person into interpersonal events related to two or more persons.

Therapists influenced by communications theory place significant emphasis on observable communication in working with families. They devote a great deal of attention to statements and actions as these occur in the sessions, rather than delving into individual thoughts, ideas, and feelings, particularly as these relate to past experiences. The family is observed in the here and now, and data is accumulated on patterns of interactive communication.

The communication group of therapists do not give credence to issues of diagnosis and individual psychopathology. It is considered irrelevant to ask, "What is wrong with this patient?" Instead, it is pertinent to ask: "What is going on in the interaction system of this family that produces the behavior that is seen as a problem?" Attempts to identify original causes or the roots of a problem are regarded as redundant and prone to error.

The Concept of Scapegoating

Perhaps the most widely accepted assumption in family therapy is that the emotionally disturbed child is a "scapegoat" in the family system. This viewpoint has been lucidly developed by Vogel and Bell (1968). Their central thesis is that in disturbed families the scapegoating of a particular child serves to unify and preserve the group. Conflict between the parental couple creates tension which is discharged by deflecting hostility or attributing emotional problems to the scapegoat. Vogel and Bell point out that the scapegoat in disturbed families generally tends to be a child or adolescent, because he or she is in a relatively powerless position compared to the parents and is young enough to mold for the role. It is also likely that a child will be chosen, because the continued functioning of a parent is more essential to the survival of the group than that of a child.

One of the thorny questions in family therapy is why a particular child becomes the scapegoat. Several writers have speculated on this, and the general consensus is that the determinants leading to selection of a particular scapegoat are complex and may include circumstantial factors. For example, a child may be selected merely by virtue of his physical appearance, some biological defect, sibling order, or simply being born at an inopportune period of family life. Any one of such circumstantial factors may elicit hostility and conflict in the parents, and therefore make the child susceptible for scapegoating.

Vogel and Bell point out that parents are inconsistent in relating to the scapegoat. They explicitly disapprove or complain about the child's behavior or problems, yet implicitly they encourage and reinforce a continuation of the child's difficulties.

Novak and van der Veen (1970) believe that the scapegoat theory put forth by Vogel and Bell is too one-sided. They reject the notion that the child is simply selected by the parents as a target for their problems, and argue that a more interactive process determines scapegoating. The selection of the particular child as a scapegoat is likely to depend not just on the parent's selection process but also on the personality of the child. For example, a child who is oriented toward emotionality, dependency, and personal involvement is more likely to become the focus of parent's problems. In fact, this argument is like the chicken and egg dilemma, since it could be equally well contended that the child became emotional, dependent, and involved because the parents selected him or her in the first place. As we shall presently see, though, the concept of one family member being identified as the locus of the problems, in order to maintain the unity of the group, is an underlying assumption in all theories of family therapy.

Family Studies of Schizophrenia

Over the past two decades a great deal of data has accrued from research and clinical studies of disturbed families, particularly families containing a schizophrenic member. Most of these investigations, conducted on families of adolescents and young adult patients, contributed a good deal to our knowledge of parent-offspring interaction and therefore have functional value for the therapist.

Wynne and his colleagues based their work on a psychodynamic view of schizophrenia, and attempted to identify a characteristic structure of roles in families that produce schizophrenics (Wynne et al., 1958; Ryckoff, Day, and Wynne, 1959). Wynne started with the premise that all humans have a fundamental need to relate to others, as well as a lifelong striving to develop a sense of personal identity. He identifies three forms of relating, each of which attempts to achieve a solution for the needs of both relating and identity. These three solutions are referred to as mutuality, nonmutuality, and pseudo-mutuality. Nonmutuality is characteristic of superficial institutionalized relationships (such as ephemeral business relations), but mutuality and pseudo-mutuality have particular significance in intimate relationships. Mutuality, as the term implies, describes relationships in which there is a mutual recognition of difference (divergence), and such relationships are prone to change and growth. In contrast, pseudo-mutuality is characterized by an intense need for fitting together at the cost of not permitting differentiation of the identities of the persons in the relationship. Pseudo-mutual relating is characteristic of families in which schizophrenic pathology develops. In such families, differentiation (divergence) is blocked by adherence to an inflexible organization of roles. Relationships are rigidly controlled, growth is stifled, and the threat of separation that might eventuate from individuation is thus averted.

In a series of carefully designed studies, Wynne and Singer tried to determine and quantify the relation between thought disorders in schizophrenic offspring and the communication styles of their parents (Wynne and Singer, 1963a, 1963b; Wynne, 1968; Singer and Wynne, 1965a, 1965b). Their collaboration has produced valuable insights into the subtle patterns of thought and communication in families with a psychotic member. Evidence from projective testing and observations of family interaction indicate that parents in these families show stylistic communication deviance, particularly in the areas of shared attention and meaning. The failure of these parents to establish and maintain shared foci of attention necessarily creates confusion and frustration in others with whom they transact. These findings fit compellingly with clinical impressions in treating severely disturbed families. My own experience, and familiarity with the work of many colleagues, points to a characteristic difficulty for the therapist in working with such families. The rigidity of defenses, the superficial level of interaction, the inability to pursue any one topic to a satisfactory conclusion, the resistance to expressing genuine autonomously conceived ideas and feelings, the ever-present pressures to conform to parental views—all these form a clinical composite that presents an enormous challenge to the therapist who hopes to make an impact on the system.

Lidz and his co-workers have also conducted extensive investigations on the families of young adult schizophrenics in order to determine what characteristics in such families seem pertinent to the production of a schizophrenic member. No single factor common to all these families seemed to account for the presence of schizophrenia; rather, all these families experienced a variety of dysfunctions in almost all areas of family life (Lidz, 1972). Thus the mothers of the patients all evidenced psychological disturbance, but to varying degrees and with very different types of psychopathology. Of extreme significance, however, was the finding that the husbands were equally disturbed, though again without one specific type of pathology (Lidz, Parker, and Cornelison, 1956).

Many of the families were described as being either schismatic or skewed (Lidz et al., 1957). Schismatic families were characterized by a state of constant strife between the parents. Each spouse undermined the worth of the other, and rendered ineffective their functioning as marital partners and as parents. In the families described as skewed, the marriage comprised an imbalance, in that one partner appeared to be strong and dominant while the other seemed weak, dependent, and helpless. This type of marriage is based on a trade-off. The dominant spouse's severe pathology goes unchallenged, and is even supported by the passive mate who can thus maintain a state of dependency. These families characteristically display a superficial appearance of harmony that is similar to the phenomenon of pseudo-mutuality as described by Wynne et al. (1958).

In studying the marital relationship in families generating a schizophrenic offspring, certain critical failures of parenting were noted by Lidz and his workers. These parents failed to maintain appropriate boundaries between themselves and their children, and this often led to incestuous problems and gender identity confusion. Parents typically seemed impervious to the emotional needs of their children, and their shared distortions of reality fostered irrationality in their children. Not surprisingly, siblings other than the identified patient are prone to become disturbed in this type of family milieu (Lidz et al., 1971). It was found that siblings of the same sex as the patient were more disturbed than opposite-sex siblings of the patient.

While Lidz's work is not remarkable for its scientific rigor (Olson, 1970), his finding did have significant impact on the development of family therapy. He influenced the direction of studying psychopathology in children by countering the simplistic notion of the pathogenic mother. He showed that there is no specific psychopathology in a mother that can easily explain the etiology of a severe disturbance like schizophrenia in a child. Not only was no one-to-one deficit to be found between mother and child, but he also brought into the picture the crucial role of the father as a source of influence, both in the parental relationship and in his relationship with the children. Lidz shifted from the influence of a single parent to the more complex effect of the marital relationship as the source of a pathology-producing milieu. Similarly, the exploration of the sibling subsystem extended our notion of psychopathology to encompass the whole family unit. This conception of shifting from the individual to the relationship system has become the hallmark of family therapy.

Bowen and his co-workers arranged for schizophrenics and their families to live together in a psychiatric ward. Over a period of four years, the study and treatment of such families produced a number of conclusions, some of which have strongly influenced the course of family therapy (Bowen, 1961, 1965, 1966).

The major concept in Bowen's theory is the "undifferentiated family ego mass," by which he means a quality of emotional oneness, as if the whole family comprises a single ego. Such families seem to present a fused cluster of egos, in which it is hard to distinguish the psychological attributes of one individual from another. Bowen sees a direct relationship between lack of differentiation of family members and severity of psychopathology. Consequently he stresses the importance of achieving greater differentiation in all family members as the primary goal of therapy.

Bowen, like his contemporary Theodore Lidz, relates the development of severe psychopathology in the child to a conflicted parental relationship rather than to a personality deficit in one or other parent. The parents create a climate of emotional fusion by triangulating a child into their relationship in order to defuse the tension between them. As the child becomes increasingly needed to stabilize the marital relationship, an intense interdependence develops between family members. The developmental progress of the child is impeded by strong opposition to any movement toward differentiation and separation from the family.

Bowen (1966) also observed that marital relationships in families of schizophrenics frequently reflect an "overadequate-inadequate" reciprocity. One of the spouses assumes a "sick" role (usually in addition to the triangulated child), manifesting a variety of emotional difficulties, while the other partner appears to function adequately. Bowen views this pattern as another means of diluting conflict between the couple, with the weaker spouse submitting to the stronger to avoid a continuation of hostilities. Whatever form the conflict takes, the relationship between parents of schizophrenics is invariably ungratifying and characterized by emotional distance. Bowen (1965) coined the term "emotional divorce" to define such marriages. The partners collude in maintaining constant emotional distance so that neither will feel threatened by the fusion and loss of self experienced in states of intimacy.

Although Bowen's ideas were generated by studying schizophrenics and their families, he asserts their validity for all forms of emotional dysfunction. The implicit assumption is that the characteristics of schizophrenic families differ in degree rather than kind from other types of disturbed families. For example, he proposes a continuum of differentiation, from ego fusion (extreme pathology) to relatively complete differentiation (Bowen, 1965). Most personal difficulties can therefore be attributable to an insufficient degree of ego autonomy, and family therapy (in Bowen's opinion) offers the most effective means to achieve greater differentiation of the self.

Bowen's ideas provide the groundwork for a methodology of treatment. The desired goal of greater differentiation is readily translatable into therapeutic strategy. The therapist guides each family member toward the adoption of an "I" position to the rest of the family. Each person's separateness is stressed, and encouragement is given to the expression of independent thoughts and opinions. The notion of interlocking triangles gives the therapist a perspective for understanding and modifying the family system. Interventions can be devised to obstruct habitual methods of interaction so that new forms of relating can be developed.

The major target of parental triangulation is the child, and Bowen therefore aborts this process by the early exclusion of the child from treatment sessions. The therapist can then focus on the parental relationship as the critical area for change. The risk is that the therapist may also become triangled. The skilled clinician actually utilizes the parents' attempts at triangulation by responding in ways that force them to resort to other (and healthier) means for resolving their conflicts. Since the therapist is vulnerable to becoming triangled by the parents, Bowen believes that the therapist needs to maintain a necessary stance of emotional detachment. In this respect Bowen differs markedly from many family therapists who prefer to plunge into an emotional involvement with the family.

In order for the parents to realize greater differentiation, they are directed by Bowen toward a careful exploration of their families of origin. Understanding the role that each parent had in his/her own family sheds light on the perpetuation of particular family dynamics. For example, the sibling position of a parent in the family of origin may explain the choice of particular sibling for scapegoating in the current family.

The importance of exploring the extended family derives from Bowen's idea that pathology in a specific child is the result of a multigenerational process of transmission (Bowen, 1966). Marriage partners are generally similar in their level of differentiation. If a child from such a union is triangled, he/she may reach adulthood as an even less differentiated person than either parent. Then that adult finds a mate of comparable immaturity, and a child of this union may become triangled and prone to severe psychopathology. In practical terms, the concept of generational transmission of disorder requires that the therapist examine the role of grandparents as part of the treatment of a child, preferably by actually including them in sessions where possible. The idea of exploring one's own family of origin is seminal in Bowen's methodology. He urges adult family members, as well as trainee therapists, to actually visit members of their extended families. They can thereby better understand and change their own role-determined behaviors in relation to their families so as to realize greater self differentiation and function more effectively.

Bridging Psychoanalytic and Family Concepts

A significant number of the pioneering family therapists were strongly influenced by their psychoanalytic training, despite their shift from an intrapsychic individual perspective to a family orientation. Among these are Ackerman, Bowen, Wynne, and Lidz. While they give priority to a social-system approach, these family therapists also resort to psychoanalytic concepts when exploring psychopathology or family relationships. On the other side of the fence, so to speak, a significant number of psychoanalysts give primary recognition to intrapsychic determinants, but also draw on family therapy concepts to facilitate their clinical work with children and adolescents (Ehrlich, 1973; Malone, 1974; Williams, 1975).

As both a child analyst and family therapist, Charles Kramer is in the unusual position of describing the advantages of family therapy while still maintaining the value of psychoanalysis. There is an unfortunate tendency for inidividual therapists (particularly analytically oriented practitioners) to dismiss family therapy as superficial, and conversely for family therapists to dismiss the vast storehouse of accumulated psychoanalytic knowledge. Kramer does much to bridge these two extremes. He has provided a carefully documented reappraisal of child analysis in the light of his own experience in working with many families (Kramer, 1968a, 1968b). He cites the major shortcomings of child therapy as stemming from the basic assumption of psychoanalytic theory that psychopathology (in the child) results from the internalization of earlier object relations, and that by implication current object relations are irrelevant for understanding or changing pathology. Because of this fundamental assumption, the literature in psychoanalytic therapy by and large ignores the significance of relationships such as those involving parents, siblings, and grandparents. Moreover, consideration is rarely given to the likelihood that current symptomatology is being maintained by the family system.

Kramer reflects a strong analytic bias in his practice of family therapy. Treatment is directed by therapist interpretations toward the goal of greater awareness in family members of preconscious fantasies, thoughts, and affect. He emphasizes family therapy as a method of treatment, but also upholds individual therapy as valuable, even as preferable to family therapy in some circumstances (such as with late adolescent patients). Because of his reliance on interpretation and insight, and his continued endorsement of individual psychotherapy, Kramer may be regarded as somewhat conservative by the more zealous advocates of family therapy. Yet his expertise as a child analyst lends him stature as a serious champion of family therapy. He has contributed significantly to the acceptance of family therapy as a treatment method for children and adolescents.

If some clinicians of analytic persuasion can endorse family therapy, it gains credibility or at least wins some recognition in psychoanalytic establishments. But the question as to whether family theory and psychoanalytic theory are compatible remains. A number of significant efforts have been made to integrate selected psychoanalytic ideas with current family theories. Neo-Freudian developments in object-relations theory have produced rich insights concerning interpersonal behavior (Fairbairn, 1953; Havens, 1973; Muir, 1975), and have particular relevance for family therapy. An outstanding example is the notion of projective identification, which has gained wide currency among marital and family therapists (Lloyd and Paulson, 1972; Stewart et al., 1975; Zinner, 1976). Projective identification was postulated as a defense mechanism by Melanie Klein (1946), who described it as a process in which parts of the self are split off and projected onto another, with consequent feelings of identification with that other person. Zinner (1976) has emphasized the interactional component of this defense mechanism. He postulates that projective identification can be maintained only if there is willing collusion between the subject and object, so that the object repeatedly manifests those attributes that the subject has projected onto him or her. While this process is frequently characteristic of marital interaction, it also extends to relationships with children. It is common for a scapegoated child or adolescent to be the repository of projected disavowed attributes of one or other parent. Zinner and Shapiro studied families of disturbed adolescents and describe parental views of the offspring as "defensive delineations" (Shapiro, 1968; Zinner and Shapiro, 1972). They discovered that the adolescent patients felt bound to behave in ways that actually supported their parent's distorted perceptions of them.

Boszormenyi-Nagy has developed a conceptual framework designed to bridge individual psychodynamic and family theory (Boszormenyi-Nagy, 1972; Boszormenyi-Nagy and Spark, 1973). A key aspect of his theory is that family members are bound by ties of loyalty and obligation. In place of the usual homeostatic view of family interaction, Nagy proposes a more complex and subtle mechanism of reciprocal obligations and ties of loyalty, based on ethical principles of duty, fairness, and justice. Failure to comply with obligations creates guilt feelings, and guilt-laden loyalty issues are often explanatory of otherwise seemingly irrational behavior.

Boszormenyi-Nagy's formulations have not been widely adopted because of their complexity and the difficulty which many therapists experience in translating the dynamics of families they see into such complicated and obscure terminology. Nevertheless, the concept of loyalty does have practical implications of great value for the therapist. One overriding implication is that the symptom presented by one family member can be understood as a component of the family loyalty system. In other words, the symptomatic member balances his ledger of obligation to his family by supporting the regressive needs of all the family members through his symptomatic behavior. A major consequence for therapy is that the patient becomes increasingly guilty should he undergo symptomatic improvement. In other words, to get "better" is to be disloyal and harmful to his family. This line of conjecture fits the common observation that the improvement of one family member in psychotherapy is resisted and often sabotaged by the rest of the family.

Boszormenyi-Nagy's loyalty concept also provides a better understanding of the multigenerational family system. Each parent in a nuclear family may be carrying a legacy of obligations and loyalty ties to his/her family of origin that conflicts with a full emotional commitment to the current nuclear family. Often the spouse and children are utilized in ways to help achieve resolution of obligations to the family of origin. For example, if a spouse has "failed" to gratify some vicarious ambition for his or her parent, this demand may then be placed on one of the children in the new family so as to help settle the account with the grandparent generation.

An important component of Boszormenyi-Nagy's clinical work with families is the goal he sets of helping family members become aware of the network of obligations and loyalty bonds within the nuclear family and between generations. Normative functioning is possible as one obtains an appropriate balance of loyalty to oneself as well as to one's family. The therapist thus makes it possible for the individual to compromise between needs for autonomy and needs for relatedness.

Helm Stierlin has produced an extensive body of literature directed primarily toward an integration of family systems theory and psychoanalytic concepts of relationships. His theoretical formulations have come out of intensive clinical observations and treatment of adolescents and their parents (Stierlin, 1974, 1975a, 1975b). A central theme in his writings is the experience of adolescents separating from their families, a universal phenomenon that graphically reveals characteristic modes of interaction between parents and adolescents. Stierlin sees separation as the core developmental task for both the adolescent and his family (1975a). His analysis of the different relational patterns between parents and children was based on studies of runaway adolescents. Stierlin distinguished different types of runaways (abortive, casual, and crisis), all of whom are attempting to resolve a family difficulty in allowing a normative process of separation. The type of runaway attempt reflects a characteristic mode of parent-child interaction, which in turn reflects characteristic modes of husband-wife interaction.

Stierlin distinguishes three transactional modes of parent-child relationships: the binding, the delegating, and the expelling modes. He then relates these modes to the quality of the parental relationship. A centripetal type of marital relationship characterizes partners who are glued to each other and fearful of any separation; a centrifugal relationship is one in which the partners are moving apart from one another, and in which there is an uprooted quality of relationship. Most parents of adolescents choose one or other of these modes in order to resolve the developmental problem of middle-age years.

The transactional modes between adolescents and parents reflect the relative dominance of either centripetal or centrifugal relationship between the parents. When centripetal forces dominate, the characteristic mode of transaction is "binding," in which case the whole family is bound together. This mode of transaction is typical of nonrunaways or only abortive attempts at running away. When centrifugal forces dominate, they result in an expelling mode of interaction, usually reflected by a casual runaway. When both centripetal and centrifugal forces are strong this produces a mode of "delegating," in which the adolescent is sent out on a "long leash" as a delegate for the parents' vicarious needs. Such runaways are regarded as crisis runaways.

Stierlin's analysis of runaway behavior is ingenious, though perhaps somewhat too facile and categorical in light of the impressionistic nature of the studies from which it derives. Nevertheless, his formulations have appeal for therapists who value both an individual and family orientation. By extending intrapsychic individual conflicts into a family interaction model, he has demonstrated that there is probably an artificial boundary between individual and group dynamics.

Despite his philosophical proclivities, Stierlin is also an excellent and pragmatic clinician. He gives valuable suggestions for treating adolescents and their families (1975b). For example, he cautions the family therapist about typical countertransference traps that arise in the course of therapy. He points out that most therapists are tempted to side with either the adolescent or the parents. A therapist may easily sympathize with an adolescent who is perceived as a victim of unsympathetic parents. It has to be remembered that not only is the adolescent victimized by the parents, but that he or she also victimizes the parents. As a scapegoat for the parents, the adolescent is in a strategic position to control the parents through guilt, since his problems represent constant proof of their failure. By siding with the adolescent, the therapist increases parental guilt and hostility, and also supports more acting out on the part of the adolescent. Conversely, many older therapists tend to side with the victimized parents, whom they see as being bullied and manipulated by the adolescent. This may result in encouraging the parents to be less compassionate and more victimizing, and the therapist consequently loses a working alliance with the adolescent. Finally, Stierlin cautions against the frequent tendency of therapists to present themselves as examples of effective parenting. This usually stems from the competitive needs of the therapist and is counterproductive. The parents' already impaired confidence is further diminished, and their effectiveness as parents is lessened.

Structural Family Therapy

The work of Salvador Minuchin and his colleagues has had far-reaching influence in the field of family therapy, and has also had considerable impact on child psychiatry, particularly with regard to the treatment of psychosomatic disorders in children and adolescents. Minuchin's thinking can be seen as a development of the sociological framework proposed by John Bell (1975). Man is viewed as always functioning in terms of a social context, and an understanding of the overall context is a prerequisite for understanding and modifying individual behaviors.

Minuchin's method of treatment is known as structural family therapy, and it is based on the concept of changing the structure of a family system. Family structure is the total system of interactional patterns that operate between members of a family, and these patterns reflect the underlying rules of how each family member is expected to relate with every other member (Minuchin, 1974a). Some transactional patterns are relatively constant for all families, since they are based on universal rules of family organization, such as the power hierarchy that differentiates parents from children. However, much more important from the therapy point of view is the notion that each family has its own idiosyncratic structural system. Patterns of mutual expectations are developed in the course of the myriad events and relationship negotiations that make up a family's history. Each family has its own unique developmental history, and the coalitions and splits that prevail at any period of time would be reflected in particular patterns of communication (Minuchin, 1974a; Camp, 1973).

Minuchin's approach is based on the concept of changing the structural organization of the family, rather than any one individual, on the assumption that a change of family structure forces a change in the position of each family member in relation to other family members, and the consequent alteration of interaction pattern modifies symptoms or problems.

The notion of family subsystems and their boundaries plays a central role in Minuchin's methodology. Every family adopts a system of decentralization of functioning. Various functions are differentiated and carried out through the subsystems comprising the total unit. Subsystems can be regarded as individual family members, dyads (parental couple, or parent-child), generation or sex subsystems, and so on. A normatively functioning family unit is one in which the subsystems function collaboratively, but without undue interference between them. It follows, then, that clear-cut boundaries are imperative between subsystems in order to make such functioning possible. When families are not functioning adequately, the boundaries between the subsystems are either inappropriately diffuse or inappropriately rigid. Diffuse boundaries prevent clear differentiation and autonomous functioning of subsystems, with a consequent confusion of what is expected from which family member. When the boundaries are overly rigid, there is a notable lack of communication and cooperation between subsystems.

The operation of diffuse or rigid boundaries gives rise to family transactional styles that Minuchin terms enmeshed and disengaged family systems. Families cannot be categorized simply on the basis of being either enmeshed or disengaged, since most families have subsystems that may be one or other at different points. For example, a father may take a disengaged position at a certain period of family life, while his wife and children are overly enmeshed as a subsystem. At a later point the parents may move closer and become enmeshed, and the mother and children may disengage. Nevertheless, it is instructive to place different areas of a family system on the continuum from disengaged to enmeshed, in order to locate sources of greatest difficulty. A tendency to either extreme of the continuum denotes a dysfunctional area of family structure, since a family is unable to effectively adapt to internal or external sources of stress if the subsystems are inefficient (Minuchin, 1974a, 1974b).

Minuchin has provided family therapists with a lucid methodology of treatment that is logically derived from his conception of family structure (Minuchin et al., 1967; Minuchin, 1974a, 1974b). He stresses the point that the therapist becomes part of the family structure, and his behavior can therefore be used to promote change in the overall system. Four phases of therapy are described. The initial phase is concerned with making an accurate assessment of the structure of a family (diagnosis). The next step involves a determination of the goals of treatment (what aspects of the structure need to be changed). The therapist tests out and selects the most effective strategies for a particular family, which he then utilizes for ongoing treatment. The final phase is an evaluation of the results of trying these strategies.

Many of Minuchin's techniques have been popularized in the frequent demonstrations of structural family therapy given by him and his colleagues. Typical examples include methods of "joining" a particular family member, restructuring the seating arrangement and interactional patterns in order to modify existing boundary systems, and skillfully getting the family to relabel symptoms to transform them into interpersonal issues. These strategies are fascinating to observe, particularly since the effects of their deployment are readily apparent when observing videotapes of the therapy in process. Perhaps the most compelling evidence of the effectiveness of Minuchin's methodology is the high degree of success that he and his colleagues appear to be having with the application of structural family therapy to severe psychosomatic disorders in children and adolescents (Minuchin et al., 1975; Rosman, Minuchin, and Liebman, 1975; Liebman, Minuchin, and Baker, 1974).

While Minuchin's methodology of treatment is generally regarded as sophisticated and creative, his personal style of therapy tends to incur the displeasure of psychoanalytically trained psychotherapists. His charismatic personality is used to full effect to make impact on families, and his methods of joining members may seem disconcertingly contrived to less flamboyant therapists. For example, Minuchin often introduces an issue to explore during a session because *he* is convinced of its importance, rather than allowing the family time to interact and bring current concerns to the surface. Other less forceful therapists are likely to generate resistance by imposing directions on the family, particularly if they are not in tune with the real issues concerning a family at a particular point in time. Nevertheless, the most enduring value of Minuchin's work is not his style of therapy, but rather the principles of structural family therapy that provide therapists with a framework for evaluating and treating families. Structural family therapy is gaining increasing numbers of adherents who attest to its effectiveness as a method of treatment.

General Treatment Principles

As we have seen, several of the major family theorists have provided methodologies of treatment based on their concepts. Bowen and Minuchin are particularly noteworthy as contributors to the development of treatment methods. There are also several family therapists, known more for their clinical skills than their conceptual viewpoints, who have significantly influenced the practice of family therapy. Such therapists include John Bell (1975), who offers us details of his practice right down to such matters as how he sets up his office for interviews. Satir (1967) also provides valuable details of her work, although her success with families may derive as much from the impact of her unique personality as from her technical procedures.

Bell and Satir are particularly useful for learners, since few family therapists explicate clinical techniques in such detail, particularly in relation to work with children in families. A notable exception is a brief but well-documented guide for family therapists authored by John Sonne (1973). Sonne's approach seems to derive from fundamental principles of individual psychotherapy. For example, he recommends that the therapist not provide much structure to the family in order to better observe patterns of behavior without contamination by excessive therapist activity. This posture of the therapist resembles the psychoanalyst's exercise of restraint. Another practice recommended by Sonne, also based on long tradition, is to specify an initial period of interviews (usually three) as evaluational consultation family interviews that lead to a disposition for treatment. Because of such proposals, Sonne may be viewed as a conservative family therapist. Yet novices would do well to assimilate such carefully thought out methods based on tried and true principles of psychotherapy. Sonne's work is a welcome antidote to some of the facile and idiosyncratic practices that too often pass for how-to-do-family-therapy training courses.

In an earlier publication, Sonne and his colleagues (1962) explored the phenomenon of the absent-member in family therapy with families containing a schizophrenic member. It is a common occurence for one or more members of a family either not to participate at all or to drop out at some point in family treatment. Such events are often passed off as insignificant by the family, and all to often overlooked by the therapist. Sonne and his colleagues found that the absence of a family member is a critical situation in treatment, in that it represents a major form of resistance to change.

While the absent family member often appears to be the healthiest family member, he or she is in fact participating in the maintenance of family pathology. While these observations were made on families with schizophrenics, it seems likely that the absent-member maneuver is a form of resistance common to many families in treatment.

Carl Whitaker is perhaps the most admired and influential clinician in the field of family therapy. Demonstrations of his work (live and videotaped) leave a deep impression on viewers. He has a rare facility for unsettling entrenched family defenses, for establishing rapport with difficult patients, and for detecting the underlying core issue in a family system. And yet Whitaker's approach to families has not been formulated into a particular method of therapy that can be explained and taught. On several occasions I have observed Whitaker work with difficult cases, and shared astonishment and admiration with my colleagues when he surprised the family (as well as ourselves) with an intervention that suddenly seemed to shift the direction of the interview into an unusually productive area. The effects of the intervention were always apparent, but the rationale for the particular intervention was usually obscure.

Whitaker is an inspiring therapist, but virtually impossible to imitate. Even those trainees who work directly with him frequently complain that he is unpredictable and hard to understand (Napier and Whitaker, 1972). In fact, the reason that it is impossible to translate Whitaker's therapy into structured methodology is that he follows no consistent system or method. He seems to rely on his preconscious associations to the emotional climate of the family as the route to the underlying dynamics. This approach is heavily rooted in what is commonly dubbed "the use of self." Not only does he intervene and react with little conscious inhibition, but he also readily shares personal fantasies in order to facilitate movement in the sessions. His work is rendered even more cryptic by the fact that he deliberately attempts to confuse families in order to unsettle their habitual styles of behavior (Whitaker, 1976a, 1976b). A favorite device of Whitaker's is to voice what seems to be obscure, irrelevant, or even outrageous comments so that the family is unsure whether he is rambling, somewhat crazy, or putting them on. The apparent irrationality of his utterances throws the family off guard; the covert content of the message can then penetrate because of their momentary lapse in defensiveness.

Although Whitaker's style is highly personal and idiosyncratic, he also advocates clear-cut principles of treatment that have generalizable validity for most forms of family therapy. These principles of treatment have to do with what he refers to as the structure of the treatment session (Napier and Whitaker, 1972). It is essential that the therapist lay down the ground rules for the session, particularly regarding membership of family members. Should the family resist by not turning up with all the members he asked for, he will simply not meet with them. He also determines whether or not to work with a co-therapist as part of the treatment structure. On the other hand, he does not decide the initial direction of a session, but rather leaves it to the family to start talking, and he senses what the issues are and responds accordingly.

Whitaker (1976b) aptly describes family therapy as a political process. He refers here to the task of establishing a relationship with the family, and thereby gain a means of access in order to produce change. One of the key factors in gaining a relationship with a family is immediately to succeed in forming an alliance with the father, since in many families it is the father who is the most resistant to treatment.

Whitaker strongly endorses the use of co-therapy. For his style of working co-therapy has particular value, in that one therapist can allow himself to become emotionally involved while the other can rescue him when needed. The relationship of co-therapists is complex and can foster psychological growth in trainees. He also sees value in co-therapy serving as a model relationship for families. Furthermore, having a co-therapist makes it easier to terminate appropriately with a family. A mutual rewarding relationship between the therapists prevents either one from establishing an excessive emotional involvement with the family, and this reduces the difficulty of separating when termination is necessary.

Whitaker's work with families containing young children is particularly illuminating. He is one of the few family therapists who encourages the inclusion of young children on a continued basis, and who works directly with them in order to produce changes in the family system. He lacks the inhibitions that most therapists have in discussing certain topics in front of young children. On the contrary, Whitaker asserts that children can tolerate discussion of any topic without dramatic repercussions as long as the therapist is trying to be helpful rather than simply provocative (Whitaker, 1976a). Whitaker has a gift for establishing facilitating relationships with children of all ages. This is because he is not afraid to allow himself to be childlike, and his interactions with young children frequently serve to reveal the unconscious concerns of the parents.

Many family therapists seem to have difficulty in relating to young children. They typically avoid the problem either by never including children on the basis of their being too young, or by quickly excluding them after one or two sessions with the justification that change will be better effected working directly with the marital pair. From numerous discussions that I have had with a wide range of family therapists, I have come to the conclusion that few family therapists know quite what to do when young children are present. Whitaker's work is of particular value in that his methods of relating to young children are learnable, even though his flair for relating to children stems in part from his personality style. For example, he makes it a point of asking children many questions that are relevant to their particular concerns. He may talk with a two-year-old about a doll, teddy bear, or security blanket, and a five-year-old about bad dreams, cuddling with Mommy, or feelings about Grandpa. Many family therapists, particularly if they have not been intensively trained in child therapy, are unaware of the concerns that children have at different ages. Whitaker teaches us that children are responsive when related to appropriately, and that they can provide rich material for working therapeutically with the whole family.

Issues of Family Assessment and Diagnosis

It is axiomatic that one cannot solve a problem unless one has some understanding or definition of the problem in the first place. It is therefore difficult to refute the necessity for a diagnosis of the problems presented by a family in order to help them effectively. While few family therapists would object to the need for evaluation, there is considerable confusion as to what evaluation means in family therapy.

It is questionable whether we can in fact utilize the notion of diagnosis as traditionally conceived in general psychiatry. Framo (1970) observes that the premises of family therapy entail a view of the total context of a family, so that it makes little sense to use existing classifications of individual diagnosis for evaluating family systems. However, it has become commonplace for family therapists to characterize families according to the diagnosis of an individual patient, particularly when the patient is an adolescent. This practice, criticized by Framo (1970) as crude and misleading, cannot be excused on the grounds of notational simplicity (abbreviating "family containing a schizophrenic" to "schizophrenic family"), since even the best-known family researchers conceptualize whole families as schizophrenic or delinquent or psychosomatic on the basis of a diagnosis made on one child or adolescent. What this situation seems to present, in my opinion, is marked ambivalence among family therapists toward the notion of diagnosis. While there is an appropriate rejection of traditional nosological categories the need for diagnosis persists, and with no satisfactory substitute available the temptation is to employ existing diagnostic labels.

Nathan Ackerman (1950, 1958), gave considerable thought to the thorny question of diagnosis, and his approach is perhaps most representative of those family therapists who do attempt thorough evaluations of families containing children or adolescents. Ackerman recognized that traditional adult categories of diagnosis are inappropriate for children, particularly preschool children, because of the incomplete personality development of the children, as well as for adolescence, a period marked by instability and change. While he stressed the importance of evaluating the child in the context of the family, he also gave credence to the importance of exploring and noting characteristics of the identified child and adolescent patient as well. He proposes four broad categories of evaluation for children or adolescents and their families: the organization of the child's personality here and now; the child's relationship with other family members; developmental and clinical history of the child; and the psychological characteristics of the family as a group.

The task of child diagnosis is often dealt with by simply allowing the passage of time to confirm whether or not a particular problem is a transient phenomenon. Adolescents represent a more challenging diagnostic picture in that they have already developed complex personality organizations. Furthermore, the period of adolescence is relatively extensive, roughly from 12 to 21 years (Werkman, 1974). Generally, it is useful to subdivide the period of adolescence into two or more developmental phases (Werkman, 1974; Everett, 1976). The developmental task of early adolescence (13 to 16 years) is the need for the adolescent to achieve a sense of autonomy in the milieu of family bonds and peer pressures. The difficulties of this task is exacerbated by the turmoil caused by the sudden onset of puberty and psychosexual impulses. Later adolescence (17 through 21 years) is usually concerned with a further phase of growing autonomy, reflected primarily in the development of heterosexual attachment and disengagement from parental dependency. In this phase, the college social matrix often achieves unusual significance for late adolescents experiencing their first major separation from home (Sobel, 1968).

Some clinicians tend to overlook the diagnostic significance of the family when the patient is a late adolescent. What is often not appreciated is the fact that parents are affected, as much as the teenager, by the changes inherent in adolescence. Brown (1970) has described how the conflicts of adolescents usually revive latent parental conflicts, and these parental difficulties often become masked by scapegoating of the adolescent. The adolescent does not develop in a vacuum; the develomental task of adolescence is one that is shared by both the teenager and the family. It therefore makes sense to adopt the viewpoint that adolescence is a development task for the whole family.

While individual-oriented clinicians often neglect the family dimension, many family therapists are culpable of neglecting individual evaluations. Beginning family therapists, in particular, may not detect significant diagnostic clues in individuals. I have seen more than one such therapist completely miss signs of organic deficit, retardation, and psychosis. One does not abandon a family perspective if one utilizes existing guidelines for determining important data about disorders reflected by a child or adolescent (Lourie and Rieger, 1974; Werkman, 1974). Some skillful attention to individual diagnosis also has preventive value—for example, in detecting severe psychopathology or potential psychopathology in one or more siblings.

By and large, most family therapists adopt a developmental approach to understanding the family as a whole, as well as the identified patient in particular. The reader can refer to various sources for examples of such approaches (Ackerman, 1958, 1966; Satir, 1967; Bell, 1975). An excellent review of various methods for classifying families has been compiled by Fisher (1977).

Indications for Family Therapy

Confirmed family therapists do not characteristically think in terms of whether or not family therapy is appropriate, but rather consider whether there is any possible reason why family therapy should not be appropriate (Whitaker, 1975). The individual therapist who is sympathetic to family therapy would regard the latter as one optional modality among several. The issue is complicated by the developmental characteristics of children and adolescents.

For children, the problem of age and maturity is significant. If a young child is the identified patient, the therapist will often suggest play therapy in addition to family treatment, or family treatment without including the child. As we have seen, Whitaker (1976a) is one of few therapists who encourages the inclusion of young children in family treatment. Even well-known family therapists such as Bell (1975) and Satir (1967) exclude children from family therapy if they are too young. Reasons given for excluding young children are that they cannot comprehend a verbal form of treament and that they are unable to tolerate the inactivity and attention required for a full hour session. However, most family therapists tend to include the identified patient and siblings, no matter how young, for at least several initial meetings, and then may continue without the youngest children. Including the children for at least some sessions is important because it provides the therapist with first-hand observation of parent-child interaction.

More problematic is the issue of separate treatment (instead of or in addition to family therapy) for the adolescent identified patient. Many family-oriented clinicians contend that, despite its effectiveness, family therapy should not be the only method of treatment for adolescents (Solow and Cooper, 1975; Everett, 1976). The reason for advocating separate treatment is that adolescents are in the process of individuation and therefore need an independent relationship to facilitate their growth.

Williams (1975) has carefully considered the notion that disturbed adolescents, who need help in resolving ambivalent ties, require a one-to-one relationship with an adult outside of the family. He believes, however, that such one-to-one therapy would be neutralized by family resistance, and he gives cogent reasons why family therapy is the most appropriate form of overall treatment. The major conflicts of adolescents are invariably reflected in the whole family rather than the patient alone. The ambivalence concerning independence is a problem within all members of the family. Parents and siblings are just as threatened as the adolescent by the implications of object loss and separation inherent in achieving independence. Similarly, the recrudescence of oedipal conflict arouses anxiety about erotization of the parent-child relationship in both the adolescent and the parents. Finally, an important task for the adolescent is the integration of the rage that he experiences. Individual therapy precludes direct expression of anger that the adolescent feels toward his family, whereas family therapy can successfully allow the adolescent and family to "fight" and experience a safe resolution of the conflicts and anger.

Engaging with Children and Adolescents

Family therapists are disinclined to include young children in family meetings (Zilbach, Bergel, and Gass, 1972). We have noted Whitaker's insistence on the value of including even young children, and he has demonstrated the means for engaging verbally with them. Not every therapist is able to adopt Whitaker's methods. However, there are other helpful strategies for engaging young children that are easy to employ in family diagnostic and treatment sessions.

Orgun (1973) suggests that since children under ten years of age are uncomfortable in the office setting, the early diagnostic interviews be done in a playroom setting. He uses the child's play activity as a starting point for interpretation, and this leads toward play activity as a form of communication with family members. The most natural setting, of course, is the child's home, and home visits are frequently employed and are well suited to family observation and therapy (Behrens and Ackerman, 1956; Friedman, 1962).

Several workers have employed art and drawing for evaluation purposes, and these techniques are particularly attractive and engaging for children as well as family members (Bing, 1970; Rubin and Magnussen, 1974). Another method, adopted for individual child play therapy, is the use of puppet play for evaluating families with children between 5 and 12 years of age (Irwin and Malloy, 1975). The use of art as a facilitator in the actual therapy process also holds much promise, particularly in terms of opening up focal areas of significant conflict (Kwiatkowska, 1967).

It is obvious to most family therapists that inclusion of the young child is important for at least evaluation purposes. However, it is also valuable to include the child in at least some of the ongoing therapy sessions. Guttman (1975) correctly points out that the child may better help the therapist understand the family system. For example, the child often "acts out" a family problem during a session. Bowen (1966) excludes the child early in the treatment process in order to subvert the tendency of parents to triangle the child into their conflicts. Yet it could be argued that this is all the more reason to include the child in treatment. When the parents attempt to triangle the child into their conflicts, the therapist can intervene effectively because of the here-and-now revelation of this family defense.

Children are apt to present management problems. Satir (1967) offers some helpful suggestions for managing and yet including the children during the treatment process. She stresses the importance of the therapists making explicit some simple rules so that the family and children are aware of these. These may include rules against damaging of furniture, talking out of turn, numbers of trips to the toilet, and so on.

In establishing a therapeutic alliance with the adolescent, the therapist has to avoid the trap of siding with him/her against the parents. Such an eventuality would diminish the respect of the adolescent for the therapist, and would antagonize the parents, with the likely result that family treatment becomes impossible. Stierlin (1975b) has cautioned therapists to avoid the polar positions of siding either with the adolescent against the parents or with the parents against the adolescent.

In certain respects the adolescent has an ambiguous role in the family treatment session. On the one hand, he is striving to see himself as separate from the rest of the family and many of his actions are designed to prove this, but on the other hand his distress is overwhelming evidence of how emotionally involved he is with the family. The adolescent is in transition between childhood and adulthood, and this ambiguous role is also reflected in the family sessions. Some of his behaviors and reactions may appear strikingly immature, yet the adolescent yearns to be regarded as an adult member of the family. The therapist has to be sensitive to the confusion and ambivalence experienced by the adolescent and therefore adopt a flexible stance in relating to him or her. In my own experience, the one quality of the therapist that is of most value to the adolescent is that of fairness. Adolescents are intimidated by judgmental authority figures, but this does not mean that the therapist should appear as a "buddy" either. What most adolescents want from the therapist—and basically what they want from their families—is an attitude of nonjudgmental fairness. Since the therapist is not emotionally embroiled in the family, he is in the best position to provide this balance.

Membership Requirements for Treatment

A common question that crops up in training family therapists is whether to include all the siblings of the identified patient, and whether to include extended family members when available. To omit siblings, at least from the initial sessions, is a major error. The identified patient has a complex relationship with his siblings that reveals much about the family system (Bank and Kahn, 1975). The most compelling argument for including siblings, however, is the unique advantage of family therapy as a preventive treatment method. Meissner (1970) has reviewed evidence that the nonsymptomatic siblings of severely disturbed children may frequently mask severe underlying disturbances.

Extended family members are seldom invited for family meetings, since they rarely live in the same household as the nuclear family. Generally, the extended family members most significant are the grandparents, since the marriage partners in disturbed families are inevitably still engaged in unresolved difficulties with their own families of origin. The concept of a multi-generational transmission of behavior patterns has been proposed and clinically demonstrated (Mendell and Fisher, 1956; Bowen, 1966; Mendell, Cleveland, and Fisher, 1968). Particular areas of struggle persist as themes from generation to generation. The pathology manifested in the identified patient is a difficulty that has been running through that family for several generations. Including the grandparents can therefore be helpful in understanding and treating the characteristic difficulties of a family.

The roles of fathers in family therapy is a problematic issue. There is no question that it is as crucial to include fathers as it is to include any other family members in evaluation and treatment. Pioneering studies in the fifties made us aware of the significant role of fathers in contributing to schizophrenic pathology in children and adolescents (Lidz, Parker, and Cornelison, 1956), and subsequent studies have confirmed the influence of fathers in contributing to a wide range of child disturbances (Lynn, 1974; L'Abate, 1975). Not only are fathers instrumental in determining the nature of family dysfunction, but they are also significant as sources of resistance to treatment (Whitaker, 1976b). Forest (1969) studied the experience of several family therapists, and concluded that the father is the most difficult of all family members to engage in the treatment process. This impression was corroborated in subsequent research (Shapiro and Budman, 1973; Slipp, Ellis, and Kressel, 1974). Recently a large number of family therapists were respondents to a questionnaire clearly demonstrating that fathers offered the most resistance to family therapists (Berg and Rosenblum, 1977).

It is beyond the scope of this section to examine the complex causes of resistance in fathers, particularly since many of these relate to broader issues of the social role of adult males in society. However, it is important to also caution the reader against the fallacy of blaming the father alone for a family's resistance to treatment. From my own experience, it is clear that families will influence a father's resistance depending upon their own needs. For example, if a wife and children are positive in their motivation for treatment, it is rare for a father to take a totally oppositional stance; however, if a mother is ambivalent, she will often use the father's more apparent resistance as an excuse for not coming in.

Problems Treated by Family Therapists

Historically, family therapy is most clearly associated with the study of schizophrenic offspring and their parents, yet we lack any firm evidence of its efficiency as a treatment method for psychotic disorders. However, a number of other childhood disorders that have proved inappropriate for or resistant to individual therapy have been tackled with varying degrees of success by family therapists.

Perhaps the most outstanding contribution of family therapy has been in the area of childhood psychosomatic difficulties. Minuchin and his colleagues have developed a conceptual model that makes the nature of such disturbances explicable in a family context, and provides a framework for effective treatment (Minuchin et al., 1975; Rosman, Minuchin, and Liebman, 1975). The theory holds that characteristic family interaction patterns can provide continual reinforcement for a psychosomatic illness. The thrust of structural family therapy is to alter the structural organization of the family so that the child cannot be triangulated by the parents as a solution for their own interpersonal conflicts. The structural approach has been used mainly for the treatment of anorexia nervosa (Barcai, 1971; Aponte and Hoffman, 1973; Wold, 1973; Rosman, Minuchin, and Liebman, 1975), but it is being extended to other severe psychosomatic illnesses such as intractable asthma (Liebman, Minuchin, and Baker, 1974).

In their classic study of antisocial behavior in children, Johnson and Szurek (1952) anticipated some of the key concepts of family therapy. They noted, for example, how the parents of these children tended to condone the very behavior that they were strongly condemning. Even more striking was their conception of scapegoating, proposed years before it became known through family theory. Johnson and Szurek's work facilitated the conceptual shift from the intrapsychic dynamics of the child to the more complex perspective of dysfunctional behavior as a function of parent-child interaction. Consequently, even dedicated psychoanalysts have come to acknowledge the crucial role of the parents in understanding behavioral difficulties in children, and to some extent may even include the family or parents in the treatment process (Reiner and Kaufman, 1960).

Family therapy is particularly well suited to the treatment of behavioral disorders, since the inclusion of the parents makes the reinforcing factors as well as the potential solution directly accessible to the therapist. Thus Safer (1966) was able to treat lower socioeconomic class aggressive children, a group typically unable to tolerate psychotherapy, through direct involvement of their families. His approach was based on providing structure and direction to the family rather than reflecting feelings or insights, and he claims he achieved a 40% improvement rate. Speck (1971) offers some practical guidelines for working with families of acting-out children. An important part of his therapeutic goal is to help the parents achieve more executive control over the child. He points out that such children are usually "parentified" and therefore able to control the parents.

Friedman, Sonne, and Speck (1971) have assembled several studies on sexual acting-out teenagers that demonstrate a clear relationship between the deviant behavior and family dynamics. Other studies have increased our understanding of the family dynamics that create a disposition toward incest, and family therapy seems to offer the most appropriate format for treatment of these problems (Machotka, Pittman, and Flomenhaft, 1967; Eist and Mandell, 1968; Gutheil and Avery, 1977).

Certain categories of child and adolescent problems are particularly resistant to traditional forms of psychotherapy. Deaf patients are rarely seen in individual therapy because of their resistance to this mode of treatment. Shapiro and Harris (1976) described the successful treatment of an extremely resistant deaf female adolescent and her family, and in reviewing a number of similar cases, concluded that family therapy offers a hopeful approach for problems of deaf children and adults.

A family approach also facilitates treatment of infants or very young children presenting severe psychological problems. For example, Palazzoli and co-workers (1974) employed family therapy to treat a two-year-old girl with symptoms of anorexia nervosa. Children who are too handicapped or incapacitated to engage meaningfully in verbal individual treatment can be helped by a family approach that helps the parents deal more effectively with these children. This approach has been employed with families of mentally retarded children, and children with severe physical handicaps and organic deficits (O'Connor and Stachowiak, 1971; Hall and Taylor, 1971; Gayton and Walker, 1974).

Varieties of Family Treatment

Family therapy is generally understood to mean a therapist (or co-therapists) working with a whole family, or subdivisions (such as parents) of a family. However, there are several important variations of family therapy that merit consideration.

Multiple family therapy has been promoted by Laqueur and his collaborators (1971, 1976) and has achieved wide recognition. The procedure in multiple family therapy involves bringing together several families, or parts of families, at the same time. There are no fixed rules as to the number of families required, membership from each family, or number of therapists. The idea, very simply, is to utilize a format much like group therapy, in which families share feelings, attitudes, and information, and provide feedback to each other. Multiple family therapy seems particularly useful for families that have difficulty in relating to institutionalized authority figures. It has been shown that culturally disadvantaged families and socially deviant adolescents, who typically resist psychotherapists, respond readily to this treatment approach (Bartlett, 1975). Multiple family therapy has also been used to good effect with schizophrenic adolescents and young adults and their families (Laqueur, LaBurt, and Morong, 1971). This approach has less enforced intimacy than individual therapy, and to some extent family therapy, and it is therefore probably experienced as less threatening by psychotic individuals and their families. One disadvantage is created by the increased complexities of having several family systems interacting at the same time. It requires considerable sensitivity and knowledge of group dynamics to detect the significant themes common to all the families during a particular session. From what I have observed, therapists appear to have less command of structuring the treatment process in multiple family therapy than in other forms of family therapy.

Network therapy is also well known,but less widely practiced than multiple family therapy. In network therapy, an attempt is made to get together all members of the social networks to which an identified patient belongs, including friends, extended family, neighbors, and so on. This method, developed by Speck and others, is based on the assumption that psychopathology derives from disruptions in the broader social network of the particular patient and his family (Speck and Rueveni, 1969; Speck and Attneave, 1971). It is not possible to state how effective this approach is, and the logistics of bringing in and working with large numbers of persons seems to discourage many attempts to utilize network therapy.

Multiple impact psychotherapy is a procedure devised by MacGregor (1962). As the name implies, multiple impact therapy involves multiple therapeutic interventions with a family. MacGregor used a team of professionals, each of whom worked with various family members. Sessions were held for individuals, dyads, the whole family, and full team-family gatherings. Intensively continuous therapy was employed with each family over a period of several days. The concept behind multiple impact therapy is that powerful continuous interventions at a point of crisis (when a patient is presented as symptomatic) are most likely to influence the family system to alter its usual defensive modes of interaction.

Techniques based on behavior therapy have been applied with increasing frequency to family situations. The behaviorist accepts the specific problems presented by family members (invariably the parents) and will aim at modification of these presenting problems. This approach clearly avoids theoretical family therapy constructs of interaction, and focuses on a technique of treatment rather than a theory of family organization (Fisher, 1976).

The identified patient is usually a child or adolescent brought to the attention of the therapist by parents who are anxious about or displeased with behavior regarded as strange or annoying (Hawkins et al., 1966; Patterson and Brodsky, 1966; Patterson et al., 1967). One popular method of behavior treatment is to "train" the parents in techniques of operant conditioning and other behavioral techniques so that they can "treat" the child in the home environment (Wagner, 1973). Sometimes other important adult figures in the child's life are also utilized as behavior therapists, most typically the child's teacher (Patterson, 1976).

Behavior therapy with families is essentially an unchanged methodology based on behavior therapy with individuals. It has simply been applied to members of families, thereby introducing the term "family" and the consequent confusion as to whether or not this constitutes family therapy. The situation is not very different from that of traditional parent counseling. The typical guidance model consists of individual treatment of the child, with some counseling for the mother or parents, and yet this procedure is sometimes incorrectly referred to as family treatment. As noted earlier, the basic assumption in family therapy is that the task is to alter the organization of the family system, not modify the behavior of only one individual member.

As a family therapist, I cannot help but have reservations about the wisdom of applying behavioral techniques to one member of a family. It is not simply the possibility that the behavior therapist misses the subtle relationship issues in the family, but the real possibility that he may bring about a semblance of conflict resolution at the cost of increased scapegoating of the identified patient. The behavior therapist accepts the scapegoated patient's behavior as deviant. Patterson (1976), one of the leading figures in the field, states quite explicitly that he advocates training parents and teachers to employ behavioral techniques in order to reduce "deviant" behavior in the child. The family therapist, on the other hand, views the child's behavior as a reflection of a dysfunctioning system, and therefore (paradoxically) adaptive in terms of the particular family structure.

An Assessment of Family Theory

As noted earlier, family therapy lacks a uniform and generally acceptable body of theory. By and large, the field is divided between two conceptual trends. On the one hand, there is a communality of ideas among those who give priority to a systems model of family theory; on the other hand, there are those who give weight to theories of individual psychodynamics as well as systems theory.

The first group comprises family therapists known for their advocacy of communications theory. These include Haley, Jackson, Weakland, and Satir. In their conceptualizing and treatment methods, they maintain a focus on the system rather than the individual. They maintain that family therapy should be confined to observable here-and-now processes, and tend to discount inferences about unconscious determinants, covert feelings and thoughts, and historical causality. The drawback with this model is that it achieves relative purity of purpose at the expense of sufficient depth to account adequately for the profound complexities of human relationships. This is reminiscent of the simplistic thinking of early behavior therapists, who also brashly denounced psychodynamic tradition and restricted themselves to a rigid model of psychotherapy.

On the other hand, attempts to integrate family systems concepts with major psychoanalytic insights is still very much in an uncertain stage of development. While theorists such as Boszormenyi-Nagy, Stierlin, Wynne, Lidz, and Bowen are mindful of the need to understand and formulate the complexities inherent in family interaction, they have done so at the cost of generating overly obscure terminology that is more impressionistic than precise. One consequence of this lack of precision has been the proliferation of a host of ideas, many of which seem similar or overlap with each other (Meissner, 1964; Olson, 1970). Thus Bowen's (1966) formulation of an "undifferentiated family ego mass" overlaps to some degree with such concepts as Stierlin's (1974) "binding" mode of interaction and Minuchin's (1974a) concept of "enmeshment". Further examples are Lidz's notion of marital "schism and skew" (Lidz et al., 1957), which is somewhat similar to Bowen's (1961) "overadequate-inadequate reciprocity" and Wynne's (1961) analysis of "alignments and splits" in the family. "Emotional divorce" (Bowen, 1965), "pseudo-mutuality" (Wynne, 1958), and a "centrifugal" mode of interaction (Stierlin, 1974) all refer to manifestations of emotional distance in families.

Clearly there is a need to reduce this conceptual confusion and fragmentation. Instead of adding new terms to the pool of family theory, theorists would do better to clearly define and reduce the number of existing concepts. Already there is some indication that this is beginning to occur (Klugman, 1976).

Another unfortunate trend in the family field has been the cavalier practice of proposing as theories what are in fact no more than impressions, observations, or hypotheses. Olson (1970) has analyzed a number of the best-known concepts and shows that they do not warrant being called theories. As an example, he demonstrates that the double bind is a hypothesis rather than a theory. Bowen himself admits that one of his cardinal ideas,the "undifferentiated family ego mass," is more clinically utilitarian rather than accurate (Bowen, 1966).

A controversial issue in family theory relates to the derivation of most prevailing concepts. The pioneering work of virtually all the major family theorists was done on an extreme sample of the population—namely, schizophrenics and their families—and the findings may not have applicability to the general area of psychopathology. Yet therapists like Bowen extend their concepts to all forms of family dysfunction. Furthermore, most practicing family therapists utilize existing concepts simply because there are few satisfactory terms available other than those derived from studies of psychotic families.

While many of the family concepts are imprecise, and not scientifically verified, they do have the ring of phenomenological truth. Most family therapists can attest to the common experience of calling to mind a well-known family concept that seems just right to describe a particular event during treatment of a family. Trying to explain terms like "pseudomutuality" or "enmeshment" to a non-family therapist is a difficult exercise in communication. However, such terms have a compelling validity when one actually observes a family interacting in a pseudo-mutual fashion, or when family members answer for each other and say much the same thing, the observer begins to experience a sense of "enmeshment." In other words, these family theorists have put into words events that are hard to define but really do occur. It is for this reason that these concepts are in common use and survive, despite their lack of precision. Clearly we are still in a phase of observation and description in studying families. What seems to be required now is a more disciplined research methodology and an insistence on unambiguous operational definitions of family process. The work of Wynne and Singer (1963a) on communication deviance represents one of the few endeavors of striving for greater methodological precision, and hopefully their example will provide an incentive for others to follow.

Concluding Comments

It is reasonable to expect that if family therapy is to have some enduring impact on the broad field of psychiatry, this is most likely to occur in the area of child and adolescent psychiatry. As we have noted, family therapy developed out of attempts to better understand and treat disturbances in children. On a pragmatic level, too, it is more feasible to utilize family treatment for children or adolescents rather than for adult patients. It seems logical to invite parents to participate in the treatment of a child. However, it is more difficult to persuade an adult identified patient that a spouse and children should be involved in the therapy. This patient's resistance will likely be matched by family members wondering what they have to do with his/her treatment.

Since family therapy seems most closely allied to the area of child psychiatry, it is fitting to conclude with some reflections on the state of this relationship. Understanding individual behavior in a context of relationship systems is basic to family theory, but is also having impact on traditional analytic thinking. Judd Marmor (1968, p. 4), goes so far as to state that the systems approach is revolutionizing psychoanalytic thought. An increasing number of traditional journals in child and adolescent psychiatry are also reflecting interest in notions derived from family studies and therapy.

Family therapy is currently experiencing a tidal wave of popularity at psychiatric conferences and workshops throughout the country. It is also impossible to work in any progressive mental health institution without at least some contact with family therapy techniques and formulations.

Despite the marked visibility of family therapy, and its theoretical significance, it is also true to say that family therapy has not been welcomed in traditional training institutions, particularly in child psychiatry (Group for the Advancement of Psychiatry, 1970; McDermott and Char, 1974; Shapiro, 1976). Child psychiatrists reflect a continuum of attitudes toward family therapy ranging from some concessions of its merits to outright opposition. There is a general agreement, though, that family therapy and child psychiatry are currently dichotomized.

Malone (1974) recognizes the gulf between the two fields and acknowledges that most analysts and child psychiatrists oppose family therapy, and that the majority of family therapists reject analytically oriented child psychiatry. Kramer (1968a; 1968b) is one of the few clinicians who can claim to straddle both camps. McDermott and Char (1974) portray a situation of "undeclared war" between child and family therapy. They attack family therapy in no uncertain terms, pointing out what they regard as its major flaws. One of their strong objections is that the family therapy movement seems to have become "antimedical."

On the other hand, most family therapists are critical of the individual intrapsychic model of child psychiatry. Thus Whitaker (1975) states flatly that in working with adolescents there are no contraindications at all for family therapy, and he cannot see the wisdom of individual therapy under any circumstances. Montalvo and Haley (1973) ironically describe a few positive features of individual child therapy, but explain these as being due to the fact that individual child therapy actually influences the family system in minor ways, though without the awareness of the therapist and family.

While serious advocates of family therapy and individual (particularly psychoanalytic) therapy are in opposition, a large number of practitioners from both areas tend to subscribe to compromise positions. We have seen that Nathan Ackerman valued traditional psychoanalytic and developmental concepts for evaluation of the child and adolescent and family. Many other pioneers of family therapy, such as Lidz, Wynne, and Boszormenyi-Nagy, utilized psychoanalytic as well as family constructs in their theories, as we have already noted. Nevertheless, they give clear priority to family therapy as their choice of treatment.

A number of individual therapists are supportive of family therapy. Williams (1975) subscribes to the value of family therapy for the treatment of adolescents, but he carefully cites conditions in which it is most appropriate, and by implication suggests that there are situations in which it is not appropriate. Since his point of view corresponds most closely with the mainstream of individual therapists friendly to the family approach, it is as well to indicate in brief what he regards as definite indications for utilizing family therapy with adolescents. He declares that for assessment purposes, it is always good to have family interviews in order to enhance the understanding of adolescents. He believes that family therapy can be used intermittently in the course of individual therapy in order to overcome points of resistance. Again, when an adolescent in individual therapy is in a state of crisis, a family meeting can be helpful. He also advocates family interviews as definitely helpful while an adolescent is hospitalized. Finally, he suggests that in cases of emotional enmeshment of the adolescent and family, family therapy is desirable.

In like fashion, Ehrlich (1973) posits a definitive psychoanalytic approach to the practice of child psychiatry, but does indicate the possibility of family therapy proving useful as an adjunctive therapeutic procedure under certain circumstances. Similarly, Reiner and Kaufman (1960) present a psychoanalytic diagnostic and treatment approach for delinquents, but concede the usefulness of family treatment in order to influence the negative effects of parental psychopathology on the delinquents. Perhaps the most representative of the traditionally trained child psychiatrist relatively receptive to family therapy, is the position of Spotnitz (1975). He attempts to distinguish the usefulness of several modes of therapy for different types of disturbances in adolescents. For example, he suggests that individual therapy is best indicated for the emotionally overreactive adolescent; group therapy is best for the narcissistic, schizophrenic, and drug-prone teenager; and family therapy can be used as part of a combination of treatment modes (individual, group, and family) for severe behavior disorders, character disturbances, and cases of schizophrenia. Spotnitz views family therapy as valuable, but as only one of an assortment of possible techniques that can be used separately or in combination with adolescents.

It is not uncommon for individual therapists to acknowledge some value in family therapy but also warn of difficulties or dangers with this approach. Thus Augenbraun and Tasem (1966) believe that family therapy is an ill-considered treatment for extremely disturbed children, and that at best it should be used to pave the way to individual therapy for the child. Guttman (1973) also argues that patients (particularly young adult psychotics) may be too anxious to tolerate a family therapy approach. This position is stated with conviction, despite a notable lack of data to support this point of view.

From this brief survey, it is clear that a dichotomy does exist between family therapy and child and adolescent psychiatry. However, the signs of accommodation are present and bode well for the future. It would be premature to adopt an either/or position at this stage of psychiatric development. An integration of the rich heritage of psychodynamic psychiatry with the newer dimension of family therapy has not yet been achieved, but this clearly is the challenge that is at hand and offers to yield the best of both worlds.

References

Ackerman, N.W. (1958) *The Psychodynamics of Family Life.* New York: Basic Books.

Ackerman, N.W. (1954) Interpersonal disturbances in the family: Some unresolved problems in psychotherapy. *Psychiatry* 17:359–368.

Ackerman, N.W. (1966) *Treating the Troubled Family.* New York: Basic Books.

Ackerman, N.W., and R. Sobel. (1950) Family diagnosis: An approach to the preschool child. *Am. J. Orthopsychiat.* 20:744–753.

Ackerman, N.W., and M.L. Behrens. (1974) Family diagnosis and clincial process. In S. Arieti, ed., *American Handbook of Psychiatry,* Vol. II. New York: Basic Books, pp. 37–50.

Aponte, H., and L. Hoffman (1973) The open door: A structural approach to a family with an anorectic child. *Fam. Proc.* 12:1–44.

Augenbraun, B., and M. Tasem. (1966) Differential techniques in family interviewing with both parents and preschool child. *J. Am. Acad. Child Psychiat.* 5:721–730.

Bank, S. and M.D. Kahn. (1975) Sisterhood-brotherhood is powerful: Sibling sub-systems and family therapy. *Fam. Proc.* 14:311–337.

Barcai, A. (1971) Family therapy in the treatment of anorexia nervosa. *Am. J. Psychiat.* 128:66–70.

Bartlett, D. (1975) The use of multiple family therapy groups with adolescent drug addicts. In M. Sugar, ed., *The Adolescent in Group and Family Therapy.* New York: Brunner/Mazel, pp. 262–282.

Bateson, G. (1972) *Steps to an Ecology of Mind.* New York: Ballantine, pp. 271–278.

Bateson, G., D.D. Jackson, J. Haley, and J.H. Weakland. (1956) Toward a theory of schizophrenia. *Behav. Sci.* 1:251–264.

Beels, C.C., and A. Ferber. (1969) Family therapy: A view. *Fam. Proc.* 8:280–318.

Behrens, M.L., and N.W. Ackerman (1956) The home visit as an aid in family diagnosis and therapy. *Social Casework* 37:11–19.

Bell, J.E. (1975) *Family Therapy.* New York: Jason Aronson.

Berg, B., and N. Rosenblum. (1977) Fathers in family therapy: A survey of family therapists. *J. Marr. Fam. Counsel.* 3:85–91.

Bertalanffy, L. von. (1968) *General System Theory.* New York: George Braziller.

Bing, E. (1970) The conjoint family drawing. *Fam. Proc.* 9:173–194.

Boszormenyi-Nagy, I. (1972) Loyalty implications of the transference model in psychotherapy. *Arch. Gen. Psychiat.* 27:374–380.

Boszormenyi-Nagy, I., and G.M. Spark. (1973) *Invisible Loyalties.* New York: Harper & Row.

Bowen, M. (1961) Family psychotherapy. *Am. J. Orthopsychiat.* 31:40–60.

Bowen, M. (1965) Family psychotherapy with schizophrenia in the hospital and in private practice. In I. Boszormenyi-Nagy and J.L. Framo, eds., *Intensive Family Therapy.* New York: Harper & Row, pp. 213–243.

Bowen, M. (1966) The use of family theory in clinical practice. *Comp. Psychiat.* 7:345–374.

Bowlby, J. (1949) The study and reduction of group tensions in the family. *Hum. Relat.* 2:123–128.

Brown, S.L. (1970) Family therapy for adolescents. *Psychiat. Opin.* 7:1

Burgess, E.W. (1926) The family as a unity of interacting personalities. *Family* 7:3–9.

Camp, H. (1973) Structural family therapy: An outsider's perspective. *Fam. Proc.* 12:269–277.

Ehrlich, F.M. (1973) Family therapy and training in child psychiatry. *J. Am. Acad. Child Psychiat.* 12:461–472.

Eist, H.I., and A.U. Mandell, (1968) Family treatment of ongoing incest behavior. *Fam. Proc.* 7:216–232.

Erikson, E.H. (1950) *Childhood and Society.* New York: Norton.

Everett, C.A. (1976) Family assessment and intervention for early adolescent problems. *J. Marr. Fam. Counsel.* 2:155–165.

Fairbairn, W.R.D. (1952) *An Object-Relations Theory of the Personality.* New York: Basic Books.

Fisher, L. (1976) Dimensions of family assessment: a critical review. *J. Marr. Fam. Counsel.* 2:367–382.

Fisher, L. (1977) On the classification of families. *Arch. Gen. Psychiat.* 34:424–433.

Foley, V.D. (1974) *An Introduction to Family Therapy.* New York: Grune & Stratton.

Forest, T. (1969) Treatment of the father in family therapy. *Fam. Proc.* 8:106–118.

Framo, J.L. (1970) Symptoms from a family transactional viewpoint. In N.W. Ackerman, ed., *Family Therapy in Transition.* The International Psychiatry Clinics, Vol. 7, No. 4. Boston: Little, Brown, pp. 125–171.

Friedman, A.S. (1962) Family therapy as conducted in the home. *Fam. Proc.* 1:132–140.

Friedman, A.S., J.C. Sonne, and R.V. Speck, eds. (1971) *Therapy with Families of Sexually Acting-Out Girls.* New York: Springer.

Fromm, E. (1941) *Escape from Freedom.* New York: Rinehart & Company.

Fromm-Reichmann, F. (1948) Notes on the development of treatment of schizophrenics by psychoanalytic psychotherapy. *Psychiatry* 11:267–277.

Fromm-Reichmann, F. (1950) *Principles of Intensive Psychotherapy.* Chicago: University of Chicago Press.

Gayton, W.F., and L.J. Walker, (1974) Family management of Down's syndrome during the early years. *Am. Fam. Physician* 9:160–164.

Group for the Advancement of Psychiatry. (1970) *The Field of Family Therapy.* Vol. 7, Report No. 78. New York.

Gutheil, T.G., and N.C. Avery. (1977) Multiple overt incest as family defense against loss. *Fam. Proc.* 16:105–116.

Guttman, H.A. (1973) A contraindication for family therapy. *Arch. Gen. Psychiatry* 29:352–355.

Guttman, H.A. (1975) The child's participation in conjoint family therapy. *J. Am. Acad. Child Psychiat.* 14:490–499.

Haley, J. (1959) The family of the schizophrenic: A model system. *J. Nerv. Ment. Dis.* 129:357–374.

Hall, J., and K. Taylor. (1971) The emergence of Eric: Cotherapy in the treatment of a family with a disabled child. *Fam. Proc.* 10:85–96.

Havens, L.L. (1973) *Approaches to the Mind.* Boston: Little, Brown.

Hawkins, R.P., R.F. Peterson, E. Schweid, and S.W. Bijou. (1966) Behavior therapy in the home: Amelioration of problem parent-child relations with the parent in a therapeutic role. *J. Exper. Child. Psychol.* 4:99–107.

Horney, K. (1939) *New Ways in Psychoanalysis* New York: Norton.

Irwin, E.C., and E.S. Malloy. (1975) Family puppet interview. *Fam. Proc.* 14:179–191.

Jackson, D.D. (1957) The question of family homeostasis. *Psychiat. Quart.*, Supp. 31:79–90.

Jackson, D.D. (1965) The study of the family. *Fam. Proc.* 4:1–20.

Jackson, D.D, and J.H. Weakland. (1971) Conjoint family therapy: Some considerations on theory, technique, and results. In J. Haley, ed., *Changing Families.* New York: Grune & Stratton, pp. 13–35.

Johnson, A.M., and S. A. Szurek, (1952) The genesis of anti-social acting out in children and adults. *Psychoanal. Quart.* 21:322–343.

Klein, M. (1946) Notes on some schizoid mechanisms. *Int. J. Psychoanal.* 27:99–110.

Klugman, J. (1976) "Enmeshment" and "fusion." *Fam. Proc.* 15:321–323.

Kramer, C.H. (1968a) *Psychoanalytically Oriented Family Therapy.* Chicago: Family Institute of Chicago.

Kramer, C.H. (1968b) *The Relationships Between Child and Family Psychopathology.* Chicago: Family Institute of Chicago.

Kwiatkowska, H. (1967) Family art therapy. *Fam. Proc.* 6:37–55.

L'Abate, L. (1975) Pathogenic role rigidity in fathers: Some observations. *J. Marr. Fam. Counsel.* 1:69–79.

Laqueur, H.P. (1976) Multiple family therapy. In P.J. Guerin, ed., *Family Therapy.* New York: Gardner Press, pp.405–416.

Laqueur, H.P., H.A. LaBurt, and E. Morong. (1971) Multiple family therapy: Further developments. In J. Haley, ed., *Changing Families.* New York: Grune & Stratton, pp. 82–95.

Leighton, A.H. (1960) *An Introduction to Social Psychiatry.* Springfield, Ill.: Charles C Thomas.

Levy, D.M. (1943) *Maternal Overprotection.* New York: Columbia University Press.

Lidz, T. (1972) The influence of family studies on the treatment of schizophrenia. In C.J. Sager and H.S. Kaplan, eds., *Progress in Group and Family Therapy.* New York: Brunner/Mazel, pp. 616–635.

Lidz, T., B. Parker, and A.R. Cornelison. (1956) The role of the father in the family environment of the schizophrenic patient. *Am. J. Psychiat.* 113:126–132.

Lidz, T., A.R. Cornelison, S. Fleck, and D. Terry. (1957) The intrafamilial environment of schizophrenic patients: II. Marital schism and marital skew. *Am. J. Psychiat.* 114:241–248.

Lidz, T., S. Fleck, Y.O. Alanen, and A.R. Cornelison. (1971) Schizophrenic patients and their siblings. In J.G. Howells, ed., *Theory and Practice of Family Psychiatry.* New York: Brunner/Mazel, pp. 782–806.

Liebman, R., S. Minuchin, and L. Baker. (1974) The use

of structural family therapy in the treatment of intractable asthma. *Am. J. Psychiat.* 131:535–540.

Lloyd, R.A., and I. Paulson. (1972) Projective identification in the marital relationship as a resistance in psychotherapy. *Arch. Gen. Psychiat.* 27:410–413.

Lourie, R.S., and R.E. Rieger. (1974) Psychiatric and psychological examination of children. In A. Arieti, ed., *American Handbook of Psychiatry,* Vol. II. New York: Basic Books, pp. 3–36.

Lynn, D.B. (1974) *The Father: His Role in Child Development.* Monterey, Calif.: Brooks/Cole.

McDermott, J.F., and W.F. Char. (1974) The undeclared war between child and family therapy. *J. Am. Acad. Child Psychiat.* 13:422–436.

MacGregor, R. (1962) Multiple impact psychotherapy with families. *Fam. Proc.* 1:15–29.

Machotka, P., F.S. Pittman, and K. Flomenhaft. (1967) Incest as a family affair. *Fam. Proc.* 6:98–116.

Malone, C.A. (1974) Observations on the role of family therapy in child psychiatry training. *J. Am. Acad. Child Psychiat.* 13:437–458.

Marmor, J. (1968) *Modern Psychoanalysis.* New York: Basic Books.

Meissner, W.W. (1964) Thinking about the family—Psychiatric aspects. *Fam. Proc.* 3:1–40.

Meissner, W.W. (1970) Sibling relations in the schizophrenic family. *Fam. Proc.* 9:1–25.

Mendell, D., and S. Fisher. (1956) An approach to neurotic behavior in terms of a three-generation family model. *J. Nerv. Ment. Dis.* 123:171–180.

Mendell, D., S.E. Cleveland, and S. Fisher. (1968) A five-generation family theme. *Fam. Proc.* 7:126–132.

Minuchin, S. (1974a) *Families and Family Therapy.* Cambridge, Mass.: Harvard University Press.

Minuchin, S. (1974b) Structural family therapy. In S. Arieti, ed., *American Handbook of Psychiatry,* Vol. II. New York: Basic Books, pp. 178–192.

Minuchin, S., B. Montalvo, B.G. Guerney, B.L. Rosman, and F. Schumer. (1967) *Families of the Slums.* New York: Basic Books.

Minuchin, S., L. Baker, B.L. Rosman, R. Liebman, L. Milman and T.C. Todd. (1975) A conceptual model of psychosomatic illness in children. *Arch. Gen. Psychiat.* 32:1031–1038.

Montalvo, B., and J. Haley. (1973) In defense of child therapy. *Fam. Proc.* 12:227-244.

Muir, R. (1975) The family and the problem of internalization. *Brit. J. Med. Psychol.* 48:267–272.

Napier, A., and C. Whitaker. (1972) A conversation about co-therapy. In A. Ferber, M. Mendelsohn, and A. Napier, eds., *The Book of Family Therapy.* New York: Science House, pp. 480–506.

Novak, A.L., and F. van der Veen. (1970) Family concepts and emotional disturbance in the families of disturbed adolescents with normal siblings. *Fam. Proc.* 9:157–171.

O'Conner, W.A., and J. Stachowiak. (1971) Patterns of interaction in families with low adjusted, high adjusted, and mentally retarded members. *Fam. Proc.* 10:229–241.

Offer, D., and E. Vanderstoep. (1975) Indications and contraindications for family therapy. In M. Sugar, ed., *The Adolescent in Group and Family Therapy.* New York: Brunner/Mazel, pp. 145–160.

Olson, D.H. (1970) Marital and family therapy: Integrative review and critique. *J. Marr. Fam.* 32:501–538.

Orgun, I.N. (1973) Playroom setting for diagnostic family interviews. *Am. J. Psychiat.* 130:540–542.

Palazzoli, M.S., L. Boscolo, E.F. Cecchin, and G. Prata. (1974) The treatment of children through brief therapy of their parents. *Fam. Proc.* 13:429–442.

Patterson, G.R. (1976) Parents and teachers as change agents: A social learning approach. In D.H.L. Olson, ed., *Treating Relationships.* Lake Mills, Iowa: Graphic Publishing, pp. 189–216.

Patterson, G.R., and G. Brodsky. (1966) A behavior modification program for a child with multiple problem behaviors. *J. Child Psychol. Psychiat.* 7:277–295.

Patterson, G.R., S. McNeal, N. Hawkins, and R. Phelps. (1967) Reprogramming the social environment. *J. Child Psychol. Psychiat.* 8:181–195.

Pattison, E.M. (1973) Social system psychotherapy. *Am. J. Psychother.* 17:396–409.

Reiner, B.S., and I. Kaufman. (1960) *Character Disorders in Parents of Delinquents.* New York: Family Service Association of America.

Ritterman, M.K. (1977) Paradigmatic classification of family therapy theories. *Fam. Proc.* 16:29–48.

Rosman, B.L., S. Minuchin, and R. Liebman. (1975) Family lunch session: An introduction to family therapy in anorexia nervosa. *Am. J. Orthopsychiat.* 45:846–853.

Rubin, J.A., and M.G. Magnussen. (1974) A family art evaluation. *Fam. Proc.* 13:185–200.

Ruesch, J. (1965) Social psychiatry. *Arch. Gen. Psychiat.* 12:501–509.

Ryckoff, I., J. Day, and L.C. Wynne. (1959) Maintenance of stereotyped roles in the families of schizophrenics. *Arch. Gen. Psychiat.* 1:93–98.

Safer, D.J. (1966) Family therapy for children with behavior disorders. *Fam. Proc.* 5:243–255.

Satir, V. (1967) *Conjoint Family Therapy.* Palo Alto, Calif.: Science and Behavior Books.

Shapiro, R.L. (1968) Action and family interaction in adolescence. In J. Marmor, ed., *Modern Psychoanalysis.* New York: Basic Books, pp. 454–475.

Shapiro, R.J. (1976) Developing family therapy as a viable orientation in traditional training institutions. In R.W. Manderscheid and F.E. Manderscheid, eds., *Systems Science and the Future of Health.* Washington, D.C.: Groome Center and Society for General Systems Research, pp. 123–127.

Shapiro, R.J., and S.H. Budman. (1973) Defection, termination, and continuation in family and individual therapy. *Fam. Proc.* 12:55–67.

Shapiro, R.J., and R.I. Harris. (1976) Family therapy in treatment of the deaf: A case report. *Fam. Proc.* 15:83–96.

Singer, M.T., and L.C. Wynne. (1965a) Thought disorder and family relations of schizophrencis: III. Methodology using projective techniques. *Arch. Gen. Psychiat.* 12:187–200.

Singer, M.T., and L.C. Wynne. (1965b) Thought disorder and family relations of schizophrencis: IV. Results and implications. *Arch. Gen. Psychiat.* 12:201–212.

Slipp, S., S. Ellis, and K. Kressel. (1974) Factors associated with engagement in family therapy. *Fam. Proc.* 13:413–427.

Sobel, R. (1968) Special problems of late adolescence and the college years. In J. Marmor, ed., *Modern Psychoanalysis.* New York: Basic Books, pp. 476–491.

Solow, R.A., and B.M. Cooper (1975) Co-therapists as advocates in family therapy with crisis-provoking adolescents. In M. Sugar, ed., *The Adolescent in Group and Family Therapy.* New York: Brunner/Mazel, pp. 248–261.

Sonne, J.C. (1973) *A Primer for Family Therapists.* New Jersey: Thursday Press.

Sonne, J.C., R.V. Speck, and J.E. Jungreis. (1962) The absent-member maneuver as a resistance in family therapy of schizophrenia. *Fam. Proc.* 1:44–62.

Speck, R.V. (1971) Some techniques useful with acting-out families. In A.S. Friedman, J.C. Sonne, and R.V. Speck, eds., *Therapy with Families of Sexually Acting-Out Girls.* New York: Springer, pp. 118–123.

Speck, R.V., and U. Rueveni. (1969) Network therapy—A developing concept. *Fam. Proc.* 8:182–191.

Speck, R.V., and C.L. Attneave. (1971) Social network intervention. In J. Haley, ed., *Changing Families.* New York: Grune & Stratton, pp. 312–332.

Spiegel, J. (1971) *Transactions.* New York: Science House.

Spotnitz, H. (1975) Object-oriented approaches to severely disturbed adolescents. In M. Sugar, ed., *The Adolescent in Group and Family Therapy.* New York: Brunner/Mazel, pp. 216–230.

Stewart, R.H., T.C. Peters, S. Marsh, and M.J. Peters. (1975) An object-relations approach to psychotherpy with marital couples, families, and children. *Fam. Proc.* 14:161–178.

Stierlin, H. (1974) *Separating Parents and Adolescents.* New York: Quadrangle/New York Times Book Co.

Stierlin, H. (1975a) Family therapy with adolescents and the process of intergenerational reconciliation. In M. Sugar, ed., *The Adolescent in Group and Family Therapy.* New York: Brunner/Mazel, pp. 194–204.

Stierlin, H. (1975b) Countertransference in family therapy with adolescents. In M. Sugar, ed., *The Adolescent in Group and Family Therapy.* New York: Brunner/Mazel, pp. 161–177.

Sullivan, H.S. (1953a) *Conceptions of Modern Psychiatry.* New York: Norton.

Sullivan, H.S. (1953b) *The Interpersonal Theory of Psychiatry.* New York: Norton.

Vogel, E.F., and N.W. Bell. (1968) The emotionally disturbed child as the family scapegoat. In G. Handel, ed., *The Psychosocial Interior of the Family.* Chicago: Aldine, pp. 424–442.

Wagner, M.K. (1973) Parent therapists: An operant conditioning method. In H.H. Barten and S.S. Barten, eds., *Children and Their Parents in Brief Therapy.* New York: Behavioral Publications, pp. 292–298.

Watzlawick, P., J.H. Beavin, and D.D. Jackson. (1967) *Pragmatics of Human Communications.* New York: Norton.

Weakland, J. (1976) Communication theory and clinical change. In P.J. Guerin, ed., *Family Therapy.* New York: Gardner Press, pp. 111–128.

Werkman, S.L. (1974) Psychiatric disorders of adolescence. In S. Arieti, ed., *American Handbook of Psychiatry,* Vol. II. New York: Basic Books, pp. 223–233.

Whitaker, C.A. (1975) The symptomatic adolescent. In M. Sugar, ed., *The Adolescent in Group and Family Therapy.* New York: Brunner/Mazel, pp. 205–215.

Whitaker, C.A. (1976a) Symbolic sex in family therapy. In G.P. Sholevar, ed., *Changing Sexual Values and the Family.* Springfield, Ill.: Charles C Thomas, pp. 136–143.

Whitaker, C.A. (1976b) Third Nathan Ackerman Memorial Address (1973): The technique of family therapy. In G.P. Sholevar, ed., *Changing Sexual Values and the Family.* Springfield, Ill.: Charles C Thomas, pp. 144–157.

Williams, F.S. (1975) Family therapy: Its role in adolescent psychiatry. In M. Sugar, ed., *The Adolescent in Group and Family Therapy.* New York: Brunner/Mazel, pp. 178–193.

Wold, P. (1973) Family structure in three cases of anorexia nervosa: The role of the father. *Am. J. Psychiat.* 130:1394–1397.

Wynne, L. (1961) The study of intrafamilial alignments and splits in exploratory family therapy. In N. Ackerman, F.L. Beatman, and S.H. Sherman, eds., *Exploring the Base for Family Therapy.* New York: Family Service Association of America, pp. 95–115.

Wynne, L.C. (1968) Methodological and conceptual issues in the study of schizophrenics and their families. *J. Psychiat. Res.* 6:185–199.

Wynne, L.C., I.M. Ryckoff, J. Day, and S.I. Hirsch. (1958) Pseudo-mutuality in the family relations of schizophrenics. *Psychiatry* 21:205–220.

Wynne, L.C. and M.T. Singer (1963a) Thought disorder and family relation of schizophrenia: I. A research strategy. *Arch. Gen. Psychiat.* 9:191–198.

Wynne, L.C. and M.T. Singer. (1963b) Thought disorder and family relations of schizophrenics: II. A classification of forms of thinking. *Arch. Gen. Psychiat.* 9:199–206.

Zilbach, J.J., E. Bergel, and C. Gass. (1972) The role of the young child in family therapy. In C.J. Sager and H.S. Kaplan, eds., *Progress in Group and Family Therapy.* New York: Brunner/Mazel, pp. 385–399.

Zinner, J. (1976) The implications of projective identification for marital interaction. In H. Grunebaum and J. Christ, eds., *Contemporary Marriage: Structure, Dynamics, and Therapy.* Boston: Little, Brown, pp. 293–308.

Zinner, J., and R. Shapiro. (1972) Projective identification as a mode of perception and behavior in families of adolescents. *Int. J. Psychoanal.* 53:523–530.

Treatment of Emotional Disorders in Children and Adolescents

CHAPTER 11

Family Therapy: Systems Approaches

M. Duncan Stanton

Introduction

It is rare for symptomatic behavior to develop in a vacuum. Instead, there are nearly always other individuals involved in the process, usually "significant others" such as parents, siblings, and peers. The conglomerate of the symptomatic person and these significant others forms a system—an interpersonal system. Such a system is *nonsummative* in that it is more than the sum of each of the individual personalities, but also includes their interactions (Olson, 1970). The actors in the system are to a greater or lesser degree interdependent. Actions by one or more of them affect the others. Some actions may change the system permanently, while others result in only temporary alteration. The extent to which this happens depends in part on the power vested in the particular person(s) taking the action—power deriving from at least three sources: (a) external systems (e.g., society); (b) history of the particular family system (e.g., a predominantly patriarchal vs. matriarchal tradition); and (c) the needs of the family system for survival and maintenance at a particular time (e.g., one member is more able to provide food or laughter, and is at that point more powerful). In general, parents have more power than their offspring, and older children more than younger. Whatever the power distribution, however, the family can be regarded as an interpersonal system that is in many ways analogous to other cybernetic systems. It is of the nonlinear type (e.g., the relationship between A and B is cyclic rather than A *causing* B), with complex interlocking feedback mechanisms and patterns of behavior that repeat themselves in sequence. If one observes a given family long enough, such sequences can be observed and particular phases within a sequence can even be predicted before they reoccur. As a hypothetical example, two parents may get into an argument, their daughter cries, the parents stop arguing and shift focus to the child, soon one parent disengages from spouse and child while the other stays involved with the child, the child eventually stops crying, the parents may not talk for some time, they reengage later, another argument ensues, and the pattern repeats itself. As with this example, then, "symptoms" can be viewed simply as particular types of behaviors functioning as homeostatic mechanisms that regulate family transactions (Jackson, 1965; Minuchin et al., 1975). From this perspective, a person's problems cannot be considered apart from the *context* in which they occur and the *functions* which they serve. Further, an individual cannot be expected to change unless his family system changes (Haley, 1962); "insight" per se is not necessary. Such a view is radically different from and discontinous with individually or intrapsychically oriented cause-and-effect explanations of dysfunctional behavior. It is a new orientation to human dilemmas (Haley, 1969).

This chapter will attempt to present the theoretical and operational facets of several approaches to therapy that generally subscribe to the above model of child and adolescent dysfunctioning. These are the (a) strategic, (b) structural and (c) triadic-based "go-between" modes.[1] They fall under the rubric of what Madanes and Haley (1977) have defined as the family "communication" therapies, but for the sake of brevity and convention will henceforth be referred to as "systems" approaches. The intergenerational family systems theory of Murray Bowen will not be dealt with; it is covered elsewhere in this volume. However, it would be a gross disservice not to recognize the importance of Bowen's work for the other schools. Although the content of his formulations is often psychoanalytic, there has been no more influential and seminal thinker in the field. All systems approaches owe him a debt for his ideas on such matters as the transmission of symptoms across generations, interpersonal triangulation, marital and family fusion and differentiation, family reciprocity, hospitalization of whole families, and the notion that shifts in the behavior of at least one member serve to change the total family system.

At the outset it should be stated that there is no way that a chapter of this type can do justice to these various schools. It is particularly hard to present the intricacies, complexities, specific techniques, and richness of their work. We must necessarily be superficial—skimming the surface. For a more intimate understanding, the reader is referred to the literature referenced herein, or to the many excellent narrated videotapes and films distributed by the proponents. A better alternative would be to enroll in one or more of the numerous workshops conducted by each school.[2] Of course the best way to learn is actually to try the treatment of interest in an actual clinical situation—preferably with qualified supervision.

History

In the late 1940's and early 1950's, a number of people such as Nathan Ackerman, John Elderkin Bell, and Murray Bowen were developing techniques for treating emotional problems within the family. The approaches discussed in this chapter also had their historical antecedents during this period, particularly with a 1952 communications project launched in Palo Alto, California, by Gregory Bateson which also included Jay Haley, John Weakland, and William Fry. Concomitantly, Don D. Jackson was starting to work with schizophrenics and their families at the Palo Alto VA Hospital and was developing the concept of family homeostasis. He joined the Bateson project as a consultant in 1954. From this collaboration came the important work which led to the double-bind theory of schizophrenia (Bateson et al., 1956). While the double bind was originally associated with the early life experience of the schizophrenic, the Palo Alto group eventually determined that it also applied to *current* situations—i.e., schizophrenic behavior was a response to a present situation existing in the family (Haley, 1972). These revelations, tied together with (a) communications and cybernetic systems theory and (b) studies (by Haley and Weakland) of Milton Erickson's hypnotic and therapeutic techniques, formed the basis for the therapeutic work that developed later—i.e., the strategic approach. Haley's (1963) influential book *Strategies of Psychotherapy*, which deals with the maneuverings of therapist and patient during individual treatment, also stems from this period.

In 1959, Jackson formed the Mental Research Institute (MRI) and brought Virginia Satir aboard. They were joined by Haley in 1962. Subsequent to Jackson's death in 1968, several others have served as director of MRI, including John Elderkin Bell and the present director, Jules Riskin. The MRI strategic therapy work has primarily been carried on by Weakland, Paul Watzlawick, Richard Fisch, and Arthur Bodin.

Mara Selvini Palazzoli had been working from a psychoanalytic perspective with anorexia nervosa cases in Italy in the 1960's, with particular interest in the mother-child dyad. Her studies began to expand to include the total familial context as it related to the symptom, and she eventually started treating whole families (1970; 1978). In 1967 she established the Institute for Family Studies in Milan. She was influenced early on by the studies of Lyman Wynne and Margaret T. Singer on communication patterns within families with a schizophrenic member. Later figures of importance included Bateson, Haley, Watzlawick, and others. In 1971 the institute was reorganized to include its present four members—Luigi Boscolo, Gianfranco Cecchin, Giuiana Prata, and Selvini. The group began its work with families in which a young member displayed schizophrenic patterns in 1972.

In 1967 Haley left Palo Alto to join Salvador Minuchin and Braulio Montalvo at the Philadelphia Child Guidance Clinic. Minuchin and Montalvo had arrived there in 1965 from the Wiltwyck School for Boys in New York. At Wiltwyck, they and other associates had been developing techniques for treating delinquent boys and their families, most of whom were black or Puerto Rican (Minuchin et al., 1967). (Guerin [1976] feels that this work was partly influenced by the psychoanalytically oriented family approach of Nathan Ackerman, although some people think Ackerman was psychoanalytic primarily in terminology, but more structural in his actual therapeutic operations.) In Philadelphia, these people worked with other staff to transform a traditional child guidance clinic into a family-oriented treatment center. They also collaborated in the development of what came to be known as structural family therapy and established a program to train poor and black people to treat families. In the early and mid-1970's, Minuchin devoted much of his time to the family treatment of psychosomatic disorders, while Haley rekindled his interest in the family therapy of youthful schizophrenics. In 1976, Haley left for Washington, D.C., to join the faculty of the University of Maryland Medical School and establish his own family therapy institute in conjunction with his wife, Cloé Madanes.

Gerald Zuk was working with the mentally retarded in the late 1950's and became interested in the family reactions to such children. In 1961, he joined the staff of the Eastern Pennsylvania Psychiatric Institute in Philadelphia, where he remains to this day. In 1964, he organized the first national meeting of experienced family therapists. He collaborated with the psychodynamically oriented family therapy people at EPPI, such as Ivan Boszormenyi-Nagy, David Rubinstein, and James Framo, but began to shift more toward a systems approach as time went on. Much of his early work was with schizophrenics. His writings on a triadic-based, go-between therapy emerged in the late 1960's.

Strategic Family Therapy

Haley (1973b) has defined strategic therapy as that in which the clinician initiates what happens during treatment and designs a particular approach for each problem. Strategic therapists take responsibility for directly influencing people. They want to enhance their power and influence over the interpersonal system at hand in order to bring about change. In fact, they are not as concerned about family theory as they are with the theory and means for inducing change. Prominent figures subscribing to this approach are (a) the Mental Research Institute group, including Weakland, Watzlawick, Fisch, and Bodin; (b) Jay Haley; (c) Mara Selvini Palazzoli and associates in Italy; (d) Milton Erickson; and (e) Richard Rabkin. Since the purpose in this chapter is to cover family treatment, the latter two will not be discussed; although they see families and couples as the situation demands, the preponderance of their work is with individuals. However, Erickson's influence (especially on Haley and Weakland) as an originator of strategic therapy cannot be overestimated; Haley feels that almost all the therapeutic ideas applied in the approach had their origins in his work in some form.[3] (The reader is referred to Haley's [1967, 1973b] books on Erickson and to Rabkin's [1977] recent book for a more complete understanding of their techniques.) In the present context, we will restrict discussion to strategic therapies which are undertaken primarily within a family systems framework.

Theoretical Contributions

Some of the important concepts for this approach have been mentioned earlier, such as family homeostasis, the double bind, nonlinearity of the family system, existence of repetitive behavioral sequences, necessity of viewing symptoms within their context, and the need for family system changes as a precursor for or concomitant of individual change. In addition, strategic family therapists see symptoms as the resultants or concomitants of misguided attempts at changing an existing difficulty (Watzlawick, Weakland, and Fisch, 1974). However, such symptoms usually succeed only in making things worse—for example, in the case of the depressed person whose family frantically tries and tries to cheer him up and he only gets more and more depressed; thus the attempt to alleviate the problem actually exacerbates it. Further, individual problems are considered manifestations of disturbances in the family. A symptom is regarded as a communicative act that serves as a sort of contract between two or more members and has a function within the interpersonal network. It is a label for a sequence of behaviors within a social organization (Haley, 1976). A symptom usually appears when a person is "in an impossible situation and is trying to break out of it" (Haley, 1973b, p. 44). He is locked into a sequence or pattern with the rest of his family or significant others and cannot see a way to alter it through non-symptomatic means.

Some of the other major concepts and theoretical constructs developed by proponents of this approach (reviewed in more detail elsewhere by Stanton, 1980) are presented below.

Life cycle

Haley (1973b) and Erickson, endorsed by Weakland et al. (1974), have stressed the importance of the family developmental process as a framework for explaining symptomatology. All families undergo normal transitional steps or stages over time, such as birth of the first child, child first attending school, children leaving home, death of a parent/spouse, and so forth. These are crisis points, which, although sometimes tough to get through, are usually weathered by most families without inordinate difficulty. Symptomatic families, however, develop problems because they are not able to adjust to the transition. They become "stuck" at a particular point. As a prime example, Haley cites the difficulty that families of schizophrenic young people have in allowing them to leave home. The "problem" is not the child, then, but rather the crisis stage the family has entered. It thus makes more sense to talk of families in relation to where they are developmentally than to try to define a family typology or a family symptomat logy.

Triads

Since the 1950's a number of family therapists have identified the triangle as the basic building block of any emotional (interpersonal) system (Madanes and Haley, 1977). When tension between members of a two-person system become high, a third person is brought into the picture. An emotional system—e.g., a family—is composed of a "series of interlocking triangles" (Bowen, 1966). Haley (1971b; 1973a) has stressed the importance of the triangle or triad for conceptualizing problems and their treatment. Specifically, he notes that most child problems include a triangle consisting of an overinvolved parent-child dyad (a cross-generational coalition) and a peripheral parent. When a child displays symptoms, the therapist should assume that at least two adults are involved in the problem and the child is both a participant and a communication vehicle between them. In single-parent families, a grandparent may be involved—a three-generational problem.

Conflicts can cut across several levels in the familial hierarchy. Haley typifies the psychotic family as one in which grandparents cross generational lines, parents are in conflict over a child, and a parental child saves the "problem" child from the parents. Haley posits that "an individual is more disturbed in direct proportion to the number of malfunctioning hierarchies in which he is embedded" (1976, p. 117).

Theory of Change

A basic tenet of strategic family therapy is that therapeutic change comes about through the "interactional processes set off when a therapist intervenes actively and directively in particular ways in a family system" (Haley, 1971a, p. 7). The therapist works to substitute new behavior patterns or sequences for the vicious positive feedback circles already existing (Weakland et al., 1974). The MRI group has defined two kinds of change. *First-order* change is the allowable sort of moving about within an unchanging system in a way which makes no difference to the group or family. *Second-order* change is a shift that actually alters the system. An example of the first might be a son living at home and failing in school who quits his education and gets fired from a series of jobs; his incompetence remains constant, and he is still deemed unable to take care of himself, albeit in a different field of endeavor. However, if he leaves home, gets married, or becomes successful in a respected occupation, these could be examples of second-order change, for the system itself and his role in it have changed. To be successful, therapy must bring about second-order change (Watzlawick, et al., 1974).

Applicability

Strategic therapists, since they assume treatment for any behavioral problem or dysfunction must in some ways be tailored to the people and situation involved, would probably take the position that their approach is not limited to any particular symptoms. Of course, much of the earlier work was done with schizophrenics (and Haley has continued this as a major interest), but succeeding years have seen a plethora of problems dealt with by strategic family therapists. The MRI group, Haley, Selvini, and others have worked with cases ranging widely in age, ethnicity, socioeconomic status, and chronicity. The following is a sampler of some of the disorders which have been treated and written about from the strategic viewpoint:

aging, alcoholism, anorexia and eating disorders, anxiety, behavior problems, crying, delinquency, depression, drug addiction, encopresis, identity crises, marital problems, obsessive-compulsive behavior, obsessive thoughts, pain, phobia, schizophrenia, school problems, sexual problems, sleep disturbance, temper tantrums, and work problems (Alexander and Parsons, 1973; Haley, 1973b, 1976, 1979; Hare-Mustin, 1975, 1976; Klein, Alexander, and Parsons, 1977; Parsons and Alexander, 1973; Selvini Palazzoli et al., 1974, 1978; Solyom et al., 1972; Stanton and Todd, 1979; Weakland et al., 1974). In addition, Weakland (1977) has suggested that this approach to therapy has been unnecessarily overlooked in the treatment of physical illness and disease. In short, that a particular problem has not been treated strategically is not so much a function of inappropriateness as that it simply has not been tried.

Methods

This section will include aspects of treatment which apply generally to all the strategic family therapists, followed by discussion of techniques that particular proponents emphasize or use more exclusively. To begin with, strategic therapists are concerned with techniques that *work*, no matter how illogical they might appear. They care less about "family dynamics" than about how their interventions can bring about beneficial change in the people involved, with due consideration for their individual personalities. Strategic therapists are also pragmatic and symptom-focused. Their approach is essentially a behaviorally oriented, "black box" one in which "insight" or "awareness" are not considered necessary or important for change to occur. Understanding one's motivations is of little value if one doesn't *do* something about one's problems. Perceptions and subjective "feelings" are seen more as dependent than independent variables, since they change with changes in interpersonal relationships. Because repetitive sequences in families exist in the present—i.e., they are being maintained by the ongoing current behavior of the family or people in the system—altering them requires intervention in the existent process rather than harking back to past events. The therapist must find ways to stop the family's "game without end." This cannot be done unless the therapist takes deliberate action to alter it—being thoughtful and reflective and merely sitting back and making interpretations will generally not work. Nor should the therapist simply try to make the family "aware" of the cycle by pointing it out to them, as this will usually engender more resistance. All aspects of the repetitive sequence may not have to be shifted, but only enough of them to cause the symptom to disappear (Hoffman, 1976).

Diagnosis in strategic therapy is done by making an intervention—a therapeutic act—and observing how the system, i.e., the family members, respond to it. For example, the therapist may want to see if a father and his son can relate comfortably in the presence of the mother, so he requests that the two males discuss some matter together. If the mother interferes in this dialogue, the therapist has clarified a problem area. By pushing a little harder and concurrently supporting the mother, the rigidity of the system can be tested further. This sort of diagnosis is different from the conventional kind, and is geared directly to the treatment effort. In a sense, every therapeutic intervention has diagnostic value, while every diagnostic move has therapeutic potential. Further, the use of conventional diagnostic labels can actually hamper treatment, because they place the therapist in the position of supporting (a) the identified patient as the problem (rather than the relationships within the system) and (b) the idea that the identified patient or the symptom is immutable. "Buying into" the system and the family's view can crystallize a problem and make it chronic (Haley, 1976).

From the above, the reader should not be misled into thinking that treatment quickly changes direction toward, say, problems of other members, such as between parents. For the most part, strategic therapists keep the focus on the identified patient and his problem. If other problems are presented, the tendency is to put off dealing with them until the presenting problem is handled. At that time, a recontracting can be undertaken to deal with additional problems. Haley, in particular, holds to this principle.

First contact with the family is generally taken through several stages by the strategic therapist. Following a "social" stage, the therapist inquires about the problem—solicits information. In the next phase, the family members are asked to talk to each other, eventually leading to a stage where goals are set and desired changes clarified (see Haley's [1976] excellent chapter on the initial interview for further details of this process). Unlike most other family therapy approaches (Madanes and Haley, 1977), the idea here is to go with the problem as defined by the family, again, even if focus remains on the identified patient. This maximizes the family's motivation for change and increases leverage toward that end. Strategic therapists are very wary of getting caught in overt power struggles. Thus they will employ skill and maneuvering to get covert control, but do so in the service of the situation as defined by the family. They accept what the family offers, since that is what it is ready to work on, and then may use implicit or indirect ways of turning the family's investment to positive use (Weakland et al., 1974). Further, the problem to be changed must be put in solvable form. It should be something that can be objectively agreed upon—e.g., counted, observed, or measured—so that one can assess if it has actually been influenced.

Just as dynamic therapy is largely based upon interpretations, the main therapeutic tools of strategic therapy are tasks and directives. *This emphasis on directives is the cornerstone of the strategic approach.* Much of the discussion that takes place early in a session is aimed at providing information necessary for the therapist to arrive at a directive or task. Subsequent interaction might then center on either how to carry the directive out or on actually performing the task in the session. Haley (1976) notes that the best task is "one that uses the presenting problem to make a structural change in the family" (p. 77). Further, a task is usually designed to be carried out between sessions as a means of using time more fully and generalizing what transpires in the session to the outside world. Per the example above, this might involve arranging for father and son to spend at least half an hour together during the upcoming week. Hoffman (1976) notes that if the problem behavior is a chronically pervasive one (e.g., a psychosomatic or communicational disorder), a more effective tack to take may be to focus on the *management* of the problem rather than the problem itself. This usually flushes out parental disagreement, so the task becomes one of getting the parents together so they can make the child behave appropriately despite his "illness."

Strategic *family* therapists tend to involve all systems of import in the treatment process, in addition to the immediate family. This could include grandparents, the school, the work situation, or whatever. They don't as a rule recommend seeing a client alone in therapy because this requires that the therapist be able to estimate from talking to the individual what his situation is and what effect interventions will have on those not present; it is felt that the average therapist does not usually have this skill and if he can avoid working at such a handicap, he should (Haley, 1976). However, this is not a hard and fast rule, and strategic therapists (especially the MRI group) will see individuals, parents, or couples alone as the situation demands.

Strategic therapists are also not prone to engage in co-therapy as it is usually practiced, although they routinely work with one or more colleagues observing sessions from adjoining rooms; these colleagues may help out at times and even enter the room and take sides on an issue as a way of facilitating a change in the process (see Weakland et al., 1974, for further clarification).

In a sense, much of what goes on in strategic therapy is to make explicit what has been implicit within the family. For example, if it is found that a parent has been surreptitiously providing a drug-abusing child with drugs, a strategic therapist might attempt to negotiate a contract as to (a) how much drug use is allowed, (b) when, and (c) who should dole out the chemicals—just so long as it is aboveboard and agreed upon; this would essentially be a paradoxical move meant to stop the parent(s) from abetting the drug-taking of their offspring.

Strategic therapists may make interpretations, but they are rarely done to bring about "understanding" as much as to shift views of reality—to "relabel." They are directed more at process than content. For example, in the aforementioned situation with father-son antagonism, the therapist could state that since the father had not practiced talking with his own father, he didn't know how to pass this kind of behavior on to his son; he had had no model to learn from. In this case, the veracity of the interpretation is not as important as the change it is designed to bring about: that is to say, it can be used as a means to facilitate father and son talking together by (a) removing blame from father, (b) giving him a nonaccusatory reason for the difficulty he is having, (c) empathizing with him, and (d) indicating that the present problem is just a matter of practice—the implication being that change is possible and may not even be that hard to effect.

The tendency of people who practice this treatment is to ascribe positive motives to clients. This is primarily because blaming and negative terms tend to mobilize resistance, as family members muster their energies to disown the pejorative label. For example, "hostile" behavior might be relabeled as "concerned interest" (Weakland et al., 1974). Such an approach also has a paradoxical flavor, as the family finds that its efforts to fight are redefined (Haley, 1963). Another facet of this tack is that simply defining problems as interactional or familial stumbling blocks serves to have them viewed as *shared*, rather than loading the blame on one or two particular people—this is a "we're all in this together" phenomenon (Weakland, 1977).

No chapter dealing with strategic therapy would be complete without a discussion of the technique of paradoxical instruction (Erickson, in Haley, 1967, 1973b; Frankl, 1960; Haley, 1963, 1976; Hare-Mustin, 1976; Watzlawick, Beavin, and Jackson, 1967; Watzlawick, Weakland, and Fisch, 1974; Weakland et al., 1974). To quote Hare-Mustin: "Paradoxical tasks are those which appear absurd because they exhibit an apparently contradictory nature, such as requiring clients to do what in fact they have been doing, rather than requiring that they change, which is what everyone else is demanding" (1976, p. 128). This has sometimes been called "prescribing the symptom." It is partly based on the assumption that there is great resistance to change within a family and a therapist entering their context is put under considerable pressure to adopt their ways of interacting and communicating. Succumbing to this pull will render the therapist ineffective. In addition, the family resists the therapist's efforts to make them change. If, however, the therapist tells them to do what they are already doing, they are in a bind. Should they follow his instructions and continue the prescribed behavior? They are thus doing his bidding and therefore giving him undue power; he gains control by making the symptom occur at his direction. If they resist the paradoxical instruction, and therefore the therapist, they are moving towards "improvement" (and in the long run also doing his bidding). The confusion that occurs as to how to resist leads to new patterns and perceptions and thus to change—at the very least it can help to achieve a certain amount of detachment from the disturbing behavior (Hare-Mustin, 1976). In this way a directive that appears on the surface to be in opposition to the goals being sought actually serves to move toward them. It is often couched to the family in terms of "getting control" of the symptom—e.g., "If you can turn this symptom on when you try, you will be able to control it, instead of it controlling you." The paradoxical directive can be given to the whole family or to certain members. For example, one could ask a boy who gets stomachaches when his parents leave him alone to try to get sick at a particular time, while instructing the parents to go outside the house together for at least ten minutes at that same time. An alternative approach is to instruct a rapidly improved client to have a relapse—once again to "get control"; this move "anticipates that in some patients improvement may increase apprehension about change and meets this danger by paradoxically redefining any relapse that might occur as a step forward rather than backward" (Weakland et al., 1974, p. 160). Finally, Haley (1976) has outlined eight stages in undertaking a paradoxical intervention: (1) a client-therapist relationship defined as one to bring about change; (2) a clearly defined problem; (3) clearly defined goals; (4) the therapist offers a plan, usually with rationale; (5) the therapist gracefully disqualifies the current authority on the problem—e.g., spouse or parent; (6) a paradoxical directive is given; (7) the response is observed and the therapist continues to encourage the (usual) behavior—no "rebellious improvement" is allowed; (8) the therapist should avoid taking credit for any beneficial change that occurs, such as symptom elimination, and may even display puzzlement over the improvement. He has stated (1963) that the basic rule seems to be "to encourage the symptom in such a way that the patient cannot continue to utilize it" (p. 55). Sometimes this can be done by making the cure more troublesome than the symptom itself, such as by prescribing an increase in the frequency or intensity with which the symptom is to occur.

The Brief Therapy Center Approach

Since 1967 the MRI group has been developing a brief treatment (ten-session) model for treating a multitude of problems (Weakland et al., 1974). The MRI approach employs all the methods discussed so far in this section. In addition, there are aspects of this innovative program that deserve to be mentioned. People are viewed as developing "problems" in two ways: either they treat an ordinary difficulty as a problem, or they "treat an ordinary (or worse) difficulty as no problem at all—that is, by either overemphasis or underemphasis of difficulties in living" (p. 148). The therapy approach that the MRI group uses is in some ways low-key, even if it is strategic. For instance, they feel that behavioral instructions that are carefully framed and made indirect, implicit, or apparently insignificant are more effective; they tend, therefore, to suggest a change rather than order it. In this way they differ from Haley, who at times may be more forceful in giving directives. They also tend to proceed in a step-by-step approach to eliminating a symptom, looking for minor, progressive changes rather than sweeping ones—they prefer to "think small" because in their experience it tends to work better. Paradoxical instructions are a mainstay of the method and are considered the "most important single class of interventions" in their treatment.

The (Milan) Institute for Family Study Approach

This group has developed a kind of "long, brief" family therapy for treating such problems as anorexia, encopresis, and in particular, families in schizophrenic transaction. Cases are seen by a heterosexual team of co-therapists, and observed concomitantly by another, similar team. Ten, and sometimes up to twenty, sessions are usually involved, normally spaced one month apart from each other. (This interval was instituted because many of the families had to travel hundreds of miles for treatment, and also because it actually seemed to work better—a kind of "incubation" period between sessions proved more effective.) The first session includes all members of an immediate family living together, as do most succeeding sessions. Sessions follow a more or less standard format including (a) information giving and discussions that allow observation (without comment) of the family's transactional style; (b) discussion of the session in a separate room by the co-therapists and observers; (c) rejoining the family by the therapists in order to make a brief comment and a (usually paradoxical) prescription; (d) a post-session team discussion of the family's reaction to the comment or prescription, along with formulation and writing of a synopsis of the session.

More important than the simple mechanics of this approach, however, are at least two techniques which are their trademarks. The first of these is *positive connotation*. The idea here is that all symptoms are highly adaptive for the family and should be connotated positively. In a sense, everything that everybody does is for good reason and is understandable; this orientation is not unlike that developed separately by Boszormenyi-Nagy and Spark (1973) and Stanton and Todd (1979). Criticism is never voiced because it simply mobilizes the family to make negative or depressive maneuvers which render the therapist impotent. Selvini Palazzoli et al. (1974) note that through positive connotation "we implicitly declare ourselves as allies of the family's striving for homeostasis, and we do this at the moment that the family feels it is most threatened. By thus strengthening the homeostatic tendency, we gain influence over the ability to change that is inherent in every living system." (p. 441). In other words, total acceptance of the family system by the therapists enables them to be accepted in the family game—a necessary step toward changing the game through paradox (Selvini Palazzoli et al., 1978).

Perhaps the most distinctive and creative feature of the Milan group's approach is its handling of paradoxical instruction. They have carried this technique to new heights. Rather than limiting themselves to directives pertaining primarily to the symptom or the identified patient, they try to give prescriptions which include *the whole family system*. For example, they might direct all members to continue the specific symptom-related behavior patterns they have heretofore engaged in. Granting that the family may resist exhortations to do something different—to change—Selvini and associates turn this resistance back on itself. It is hard, in such a brief presentation, to capture the dramatic, even startling, directives they come up with. One such might be to have the children become parents to their parents. Another might be for the therapists to publicly prescribe for themselves the task of doing their utmost to become, for a parent of the identified patient, the (grand)parents that had disappointed him in early life; but this time they will avoid the (grand)parents' mistakes. Or the therapists might declare total impotence, having "no idea what to do." This is a way of forcing the family to do something, anything, different, in order to retain their adversaries (the therapists) and keep the game going. Such interventions are based on hypotheses about the function of a problem in a family and are made in order to test these hypotheses. The family's reaction then become the litmus whereby a given hypothesis is confirmed or not. Often this is a trial-and-error process, as all interventions of this sort cannot be expected to hit home every time. Selvini Palazzoli et al. (1974, 1978) emphasize, in addition, that each family is different, so that the prescription will vary from case to case and must be appropriately tailored. They found it rarely helpful to try to transpose to later situations prescriptions which had been successful with earlier cases.

The question does arise as to how widely applicable is the approach of the Milan group. In addition to being able to maintain a creative, simpatico, relatively noncompetitive therapeutic team—in itself no mean achievement—they have operated in a therapeutic context that has distinctive features. Many of the families travel great distances to be treated by not one, but four, prestigious psychiatrists, providing the latter with a certain amount of built-in clout and power. Also, the respect and status accorded the "doctor" may be greater in Italy than in many other countries.[4]

Haley's approach

Again, the general material presented earlier applies to the therapy that Jay Haley performs and supervises. There are, however, certain principles and treatment situations to which he has given particular attention and emphasis, and some of these will be briefly covered here.

Haley was one of the first to clarify the means by which conventional mental health institutions were not providing effective treatment. This arose from his early experience with schizophrenics in which identified patients would improve in the hospital, return home, and suffer rapid relapse. He noted that the hospital served to perpetuate a pattern that interfered with effective cure. If the identified patient improved while out of the hospital, a crisis occurred in the family, the person was rehospitalized and stabilized, and change could not come about (Haley, 1970, 1971a). Over the years subsequent to this early exposure, Haley has worked with the families of severely disturbed young people and through trial and error has been developing a model for treating them. Much of the problem revolves around the person (a) leaving home, or being allowed to do so, and (b) becoming competent and individuated (Haley, 1973b; Hoffman, 1976). He notes that these parents often display a terror of separation. An important principle is for the therapist to have maximum administrative control of the case, including medications, rehospitalizations, etc. The general therapeutic strategy is to be fairly authoritarian and less exploratory, especially at the beginning of treatment, since this is usually a time of family crisis (Haley, 1976). He particularly wants to get the parents to hold together and be firm about their offspring's behavior—to weather a crisis together—so that the change will "take hold." He warns therapists against dealing with the parents' relationship and marriage per se until improvement is brought about in the child, since "rushing to the marriage as a problem can make therapy more difficult later" (1976, p. 141). At this writing, Haley is preparing a book (1979) that will clarify this treatment model, although some of the material has already been presented via edited videotapes.

In his recent book, *Problem-Solving Therapy*, Haley (1976) discusses the stages that therapy goes through. These may involve several shifts. For example, it is sometimes better in a single-parent family to deal with the grandmother first and then the mother, before the child's problem can be confronted. An important concept also is that intermediate stages may have to be as aberrant as the presenting stage, before a "normal" adaptation can be achieved. For instance, if a father and daughter are too involved with each other and the mother is peripheral, an intermediate step might be to try to get mother and daughter to spend an inordinate amount of time together, while partially excluding father, before finally shifting to a point where the involvement of each parent with the child is roughly equivalent. This is going from one problem stage to another problem stage before heading for a "normal" stage. In other words, the therapist may not be able to go directly from the problem at the outset to a "cure" arrangement at the end.

One of the earlier dictates of family treatment was to "spread the problem" among the children in the family, often by noting that the siblings have problems too. Haley cautions against this because he feels it only succeeds in making the parents feel worse. They may end up by increasing their attack upon the problem child because he has caused them to be put in a situation in which they are accused of being even *more* "awful" for fostering a *second* problem child.

Behaviorally oriented therapists and others have decried for years the notion of symptom substitution—i.e., the idea that if you remove one symptom, another will pop up in its place. Haley agrees with them on this, but rephrases it. He sees the issue as one of symptom salience. People may come in with several problems, but choose to work on the most bothersome first (or they may have several but only *mention* the one). If that problem is eliminated, they may request to deal with the second priority problem, etc., until all are attenuated or eliminated.

Outcome

Despite the widespread attention and application that strategic therapy has received, there is not a great deal of therapy outcome research specifically on this approach. The family crisis therapy of Langsley, Machotka, and Flomenhaft (1971), did use many techniques similar to those of the MRI Brief Therapy Center. Their results from an 18-month follow-up showed that family crisis therapy as an alternative to hospitalization cut in half the number of days patients spent in the hospital compared to controls who were hospitalized according to standard procedures; the cost was also one-sixth as much. In one of the best studies in the literature, Alexander and Parsons (1973; Parsons and Alexander, 1973) compared a behaviorally oriented family therapy based on systems theory (Haley, 1971b; Watzlawick, Weakland, and Fisch, 1967) with three other approaches to treating delinquency: a client-centered family approach, an eclectic-dynamic approach, and a no-treatment control group. Results for the systems treatment were markedly superior to the other groups—recidivism was cut in half; the remaining three treatment conditions did not differ significantly from each other. Equally important, a three-year follow-up (Klein, Alexander, and Parsons, 1977) showed that incidence of problems in siblings was significantly lower for the family systems treatment—a clear-cut case of primary prevention. In another study, the MRI group (Weakland et al., 1974) performed short-term follow-ups on 97 of their cases drawn from a broad spectrum of problems or disorders and found approximately three-quarters (72%) of them were either successful (40%) or significantly improved (32%). These results are higher than the gross improvement rates of 61–65% noted for non-family individual therapy (Bergin, 1971), and are more striking when one considers that no cases went for more than ten sessions. However, the lack of control or comparison groups does limit the conclusions that can be drawn, and it is also difficult to accept without reservation their allusion that the success rate for schizophrenics was as high as for, say, work problems. In a study of the effectiveness of family therapy with drug addicts (Stanton, 1978; Stanton and Todd, 1979; Stanton et al., 1980), family treatment more than doubled the number of days free from drugs compared with a standard methadone program; this study used a combination of Haley's approach to treatment with Minuchin's structural approach, although the emphasis was on the former. Finally, Haley is gathering outcome data on his work with youthful schizophrenics, but although the data look promising, it is not clear when they will be published.

Structural Family Therapy

The structural approach to family treatment grew out of the earlier work of Minuchin, Montalvo, and others at Wiltwyck plus Haley's later collaboration when all of them were in Philadelphia. In recent years, structural therapy has gathered a considerable following, due primarily to the great many workshops, presentations, and training videotapes sponsored or developed by its proponents, and also to the publication of Minuchin's (1974a) foundational book, *Families and Family Therapy*. In the structural viewpoint the family is seen as an open, sociocultural system in transformation—i.e., it progresses through developmental stages (as discussed earlier). The structural therapist regards an individual within his social context—as he interacts with his environment. Thus changing the structure or organization of the context changes the positions of the members within it and consequently alters their experience. Their complementary demands are modified.

Theoretical Contributions

The focus in structural therapy is less on theory of change than on theory of family. The structural model per se is not particularly complex, theoretically. The most primary concept is that of *boundaries*, whether between individuals or groups of individuals within a family. Of particular import are the boundaries between family subsystems—these boundaries are the "rules defining who participates and how" (Minuchin, 1974a, p. 53). Most problems arise when the boundaries that define intergenerational subsystems are stronger than those which define generational subsystems. An example of this is when the boundary separating a parent-child dyad from a dyad formed by the other parent and a second child is more solid than the boundary separating the two parents from the children; the coalitions in this case are one parent-child subsystem versus another parent-child subsystem. Just as often, only one child could be involved and the system could be stuck in a "rigid triad," where the child detours or deflects parental conflicts.

A central concept in structural therapy is the continuum of *enmeshment-disengagement*. These are the extremes of boundary functioning within families. The enmeshed family is overly tight, and children are allowed little or no autonomy. If the integrity or "closeness" of the system is threatened, the enmeshed family responds rapidly and defensively. Further, behavior change or reaction to stress in one member reverberates throughout the system. The heightened sense of belonging in these families comes at the cost of individual independence (Minuchin, 1974a).

In disengaged families, members may function autonomously, but there is little loyalty and a distorted sense of independence. They cannot request support when needed, and lack a capacity for interdependence. In such families, parents abdicate their authority and other members tend to operate within their own, separate little domains, relative to the rest of the family. Stresses in one member do not readily affect the others (Minuchin, 1974a).

Some of the most important work to come out of the structural camp is in the area of psychosomatic illness in children and adolescents (Minuchin et al., 1975, 1978). An open systems (multiple feedback) model has been developed in which the symptom is seen to serve a function in maintaining dysfunctional patterns within the family. It is a nonspecific model in that different symptoms (asthma, anorexia nervosa, and labile diabetes mellitus) can arise in similar family systems, thus implying that treatment goals for these families will be similar; despite the specific kind of symptom, most will require a similar kind of restructuring. Five characterisitics are noted for these families: (a) they are very enmeshed; (b) they tend to be overprotective; (c) a good deal of rigidity and resistance to change is common; (d) there is considerable avoidance of overt conflict within the family; and (e) the identified patient is involved in parental conflict (Liebman et al., 1976). Minuchin et al. (1975) state that three conditions are necessary (but not independently sufficient) for development and maintenance of such disorders in children: (1) a family organization that encourages somatization; (2) the child is involved in parental conflict; and (3) a preexistent condition of physiological vulnerability. A striking example of how the psychosomatic child responds to stresses affecting the family and becomes a conflict-detouring mechanism has been presented by Minuchin (1974a) and Minuchin, Rosman, and Baker (1978). Plasma-free fatty acid (FFA) levels (which indicate emotional arousal) were monitored for all members of a family while the children observed their parents in a stressful situation. The children watched through a one-way mirror and later entered the room. When the children were in the room the parents' FFA levels dropped, while the children's levels increased. The identified patient's level stayed high for a prolonged period. In an analysis of this and eight other cases, Rosman[5] obtained a correlation of −.92 between FFA levels for the most labile parent and the identified patient. This evidence supports the notion of the function of the symptom within the family and also underscores the idea of a family being more than its parts—the process extends across physical boundaries and makes the family a physiologically interdependent system.

Applicability

In the structural approach, the person is viewed as interacting with his context—both affecting it and being affected by it. Thus the structural framework applies to most human "emotional" problems. Some writers have criticized this approach as being too crisis-oriented, active, and confronting to be applied with, say, intellectualizing upper-middle-class families. This idea appears to be based in part on the various videotapes and films that have been produced on structural therapy; most of them are with lower- or working-class families or with families who are severely dysfunctional. However, it has always been a structural tenet that the principles and techniques must be modified in their presentation in order to adapt to family style and values. Minuchin (1974a) has noted that for therapy to succeed the therapist has to be able "to enter the system in ways that are syntonic with it. He must accommodate to the family, and intervene in a manner that the particular family can accept" (p. 125). This writer has observed many structural therapists—inluding Minuchin—working with intellectualizing families and has concluded that the criticism derives primarily from lack of information and is really not well founded. In other words, structural therapists treat people at all economic levels and from all ethnic groups, despite their development of techniques with poor and minority families. Some of the disorders which structural therapists have treated and written about are: anorexia nervosa, asthma, behavior problems, delinquency, diabetes, drug addiction, elective mutism, encopresis, hyperactivity, mental retardation, minimal cerebral dysfunction, problems of the poor, preschool problems, psychogenic pain, schizophrenia, school avoidance, and school problems (Andolfi, 1978; Aponte, 1976a, 1976b; Aponte and Hoffman, 1973; Baker et al., 1975; Berger, 1974, 1976; Combrinck-Graham, 1974; Fishman, Scott, and Betof, 1977; Jemail and Combrinck-Graham, 1977, Liebman et al., 1974a, 1974b, 1974c, 1976a, 1976b; Minuchin, 1974a; Minuchin et al., 1967, 1975; Moskowitz, 1976; Rosenberg, 1978; Rosenberg and Lindblad, 1978; Rosman et al., 1975, 1976; Stanton, 1978; Stanton and Todd, 1979; Stanton et al., 1980;

Umbarger and Hare, 1973). However, there has not been much structural writing, theory, or clinical work in the areas of either schizophrenia or marital therapy; it has also, for the most part, been aimed more at children and adolescents than adults.

Methods

To avoid redundance, it should be noted that both the structural and strategic schools subscribe to the following (previously discussed) aspects or methods of treatment: emphasis on the present rather than the past, pragmatic view of treatment, symptoms seen in context, symptoms are both system-maintained and system-maintaining, therapist should be active, repetitive behavioral sequences are to be changed, the family life cycle and developmental stage are important, diagnosis is obtained through intervention, use of task assignment, and use (or not) of interpretation. Both approaches hold to an implicit faith that people can be educated and can change if treatment brings about a new experience for them; in other words, new and alternative ways can be learned. Except in cases with life-threatening potential such as anorexia, structural therapists are not as symptom-focused as strategic therapists, but they are much more symptom-oriented than psychodynamic therapists. They also see therapy as progressing through the kinds of stages discussed earlier for Haley (1976). They tend to devote a considerable amount of energy to "joining" parents positively and reducing parental guilt over the child's problem; this is because blaming parents only ignites them to battle against the therapist and thus directly undermines beneficial change. Structural therapists may not be as specific as strategic therapists, but they do want to negotiate a therapeutic contract on the nature of the problem and the goals for change (Minuchin, 1974a).

In structural family therapy the tendency is often to move in fast to break up family dysfunctional patterns. The diagnostic process involves joining and knowing a family—accepting and learning its style in a sort of blending experience. The therapist accommodates and adapts, thus gaining a subjective knowledge of the transactional patterns. From there he can probe for flexibility and change, with an eye toward transforming the system. He may join certain subsystems in order to strengthen them (e.g., getting a browbeaten wife and daughter to speak up by asserting that "the women in this family have some important things to say"). Reactions to such restructuring help to give the therapist a more complete picture. Throughout he is trying to stay both within and without the system. He accommodates, but retains enough independence both to resist the family's pull and to challenge it at various points. His diagnosis will less likely be a single term than a sentence that implies a direction for treatment—e.g., "the girl's encopresis is covertly supported by father to keep mother busy so that she isn't always cleaning up after *him*."

This approach *focuses on the family hierarchy*, with parents expected to be in charge of their offspring; the family is not seen as an organization of equals. This emphasis distinguishes it from the other approaches, and leads to a therapy aimed at (a) differentiating subsystems within enmeshed families, or (b) increasing the flow among subsystems when families are disengaged (Madanes and Haley, 1977).

More emphasis is placed on nonverbal than verbal behavior in structural therapy. Patterns such as "who speaks to whom" are important to identify, despite the content of the message. Also, the therapist uses many nonverbal techniques, particularly to establish boundaries. These could include separating parents from children by chair placement, seating oneself between an intrusive parent and another dyad, asking a family member to watch from an observation room, etc. Boundaries can also be made more permeable by getting disengaged members of subsystems to relate differently. The therapist might ask a member to "see if you can get your father to talk to you." If it doesn't work, the therapist could press again with "The way you are going about it isn't working. Can you try a different way, a way so that he might be able to hear you better?" The point here is that the content of the dyadic communication is less important than the process whereby disengaged entities are reengaged, consequently altering the structure of the family at that point.

Structural therapists think to a great extent in visual, spatial terms. Conceptualizing a treatment plan usually involves a sort of map with symbols for diffuse, clear, and rigid boundaries, affiliations, overinvolvement, conflict, coalitions, and detouring. While a given map depicts only a momentary status of a family, it can help the therapist to diagnose and also define what interventions are to be made. A typical sequence of maps would show at least three stages: present status, status expected after first structural intervention, and final status for the treatment or for a particular session. A therapist may enter a session with such a schema in mind. Unlike the MRI group, structural therapists consciously try to revise relationships during sessions, while the family is sitting in the room (Hoffman, 1976). They also want to make an event such as a marital battle "live" again, perhaps by reenacting it rather than talking about it. Further, Minuchin usually refuses to let a family member talk about members who are present in a session—he does not like people to speak for or about others in a way that squelches individuality.

There is an essential aspect of structural therapy that differentiates it from the strategic kind, especially that practiced at MRI. (Haley falls in a position midway between the two.) In a sense, it relates to the ways in which theory dictates, and is also consistent with, practice. The strategic therapist highlights the symptom and what goes on outside the treatment setting. He is concerned with the behavioral sequences that occur, without special note (theoretically) as to either their origin within, or the way they delineate, the family structure. He can even be somewhat personally "distant" in a session and still be consistent with his theory. In contrast, the structural therapist must *use himself* within the session to be theoretically consistent. This is because practically anything that is said or done by a family member has a structural message—i.e., it identifies a structural "rule. "Nearly every statement carries a message of agreement or disagreement and is directed toward a person or persons; it thus denotes closeness or distance and defines some sort of subsystem boundary. A mother telling her daughter to leave her younger brother alone might imply mother-daughter distance and mother-son closeness. A father's disagreement with a therapist's suggestion that he spend more time with his family could be seen as an indication of distance between father and the other members, and also distance from the therapist who has momentarily sided with the rest of the group. Thus it is incumbent upon the structural therapist not only to note the "who-to-whom" aspect of messages, but also to increase intensity, change seating positions, and make other moves that challenge or restructure the family. He cannot sit back indefinitely, letting the structure unfold and reinforce itself, and still accomplish his purported objectives. He *must* intervene directly, within the session, in accordance with his theory. If he did not take such actions, the family structure, as manifested both by the order and the intended target(s) of its sequential behaviors, would remain unchanged.[6]

It should be understood that the structural therapist is not trying to wrench family members apart and make each stand emotionally naked and alone. The whole idea of restructuring is to shift supports around, recognizing that people will not move to the unknown in a situation of danger. The healing potential of the family is assumed, and supports are provided to facilitate movement (Minuchin, 1974a). For example, working directly to separate an unmarried, overinvolved mother and her son will usually not succeed unless she can get support from other quarters, such as from her own siblings, friends, boyfriends, work associates, and so forth; in this case the first step might be to bolster these natural supports before attending to the mother-son enmeshment.

Minuchin (1974a, 1974b) defines the goal of therapy as inducing a "more adequate family organization" of the sort that will maximize the growth potential in each of its members. He notes that people will change for three reasons. First, their perception of reality has been challenged. Second, alternative possibilities are presented that make sense to them. Third, once alternative transactional patterns have been tried out, new relationships appear which themselves become self-reinforcing.

Structural therapists for the most part deal with those members of a family who live within a household or have regular contact with the immediate family. Rarely, for instance, are grandparents brought to treatement if they live some distance away or are not in touch. The general idea is to involve in treatment those interpersonal systems that have regular or daily impact on the problem. This would probably include schoolteachers, counselors, and principals if the presenting problems were school-related (Aponte, 1976a).

Compared with other psychotherapies, structural family therapy tends, like strategic therapy, to be brief. Six months of regular treatment is considered to be somewhat lengthy. In this approach, the preference is to bring a family to a level of "health" and then stand ready to be called in the future, if necessary. Such a model is seen to combine the advantages of short- and long-term therapy (Minuchin, 1974b).

The structural group does not limit its members to any one profession. Indeed, they have intensively trained hundreds of people from various fields (Flomenhaft and Carter, 1977). As mentioned earlier, they also established a program for training poor people from minority groups to become therapists (Haley, 1972). What they do prefer, however, is a person who is unafraid to take action and not desirous of a co-therapist (since co-therapy per se is rarely practiced). The people who have most difficulty in learning this approach are those who come from an individually and psychoanalytically oriented background. The system for training that has been developed is highly teachable and is supplemented by videotapes and films. In 1974, the Center for Family Therapy Training was established at the Philadelphia Child Guidance Clinic under the direction of Salvador Minuchin. Training people to be family therapists has been a major activity of Minuchin and a number of his colleagues over the past several years.

Outcome

The major outcome research done on a structural model has been with psychosomatic problems (anorexia, asthma, diabetes) and drug addiction. Considering the usual rates of 40–60% improvement on follow-up for anorectics, the structural therapy rate of 86% complete recovery from both the anorexia and its psychosocial components (follow-ups ranged from 1½ to 7 years) is quite striking (Minuchin, Rosman, and Baker, 1978; Rosman et al., 1976). Another study mentioned earlier combined the Haley and structural approaches in dealing with drug addiction. In a six-month post-treatment follow-up of the addicts, those engaged in family therapy had twice the average number of days free from heroin and opiates compared to regular methadone treatment—i.e., 80% versus 36% (Stanton, 1978). Gurman and Kniskern (1978) have reviewed over 200 outcome studies of family and marital therapy. They state that of the nonbehavioral marital-family studies, the "most impressive results" have emerged with structural family therapy. Despite lack of control groups for the psychosomatic research, they note that the "seriousness, even life-threatening nature, of the psychosomatic disorders studied in the uncontrolled investigations and the use of highly objective change measures (e.g., weight gain, blood sugar levels, respiratory functioning) constitute, to us, compelling evidence of major clinical changes in conditions universally acknowledged to have extremely poor prognoses untreated or treated by standard medical regimens" (p. 832).

Triadic-based, "Go-between" Family Therapy

This is the approach primarily developed by Gerald Zuk and will hereafter be referred to as "go-between" therapy. There is some difficulty in classifying this approach relative to the strategic and structural models. It is not at the level of a "school," but is more the personal brand of therapy of a skilled, innovative, systems-oriented clinician who has been active in the field for many years. It is also not a subset of the other schools, but in many ways falls in a position between them. Its inclusion here is mainly to provide a more well-rounded picture of family systems therapies.

There are a number of basic similarities between go-between therapy and other systems approaches. Like the strategic and to some extent the structural models, it (a) focuses on the sources of leverage and power in the family, (b) is conceptualized in positive and negative feedback terms, (c) devalues insight as explanatory of change, and (d) emphasizes the forms of negotiation that occur in family therapy both between therapist and family and within the family itself (Zuk, 1971). Again, such notions as "transference" and subjective "feelings" are not given primary attention.

Theoretical Contributions

Zuk has introduced a number of concepts to the family therapy field. Since the mid-sixties, he has stressed the importance of a triadic (versus dyadic) view of families and their treatment, noting that most previous approaches had limited their views to collections of dyads such as mother-child, father-child, father-mother, etc. Zuk notes the great difference between two-person and three-person relationships, as the dyad (or even a series of dyads) excludes the effect of the third party on the relationship between the first and second (Zuk, 1966, 1971). On this point his thinking is in harmony with a number of others in the field such as Bowen, Haley, Minuchin, and Satir. Zuk has set for himself the task of defining rules and relationships governing systems of more than two people.

Pathogenic Relating

This refers to a kind of process that goes on within a family. It is identified by the therapist in an interview. The extent to which it exists is judged by the therapist from his observation of "tension-producing, malevolent, intimidating patterns of family members toward each other and the therapist" (Zuk, 1975, p. 15). Pathogenic relating is a destructive process and includes such interactions as the silencing of a member by the family ("silencing strategies"), threats of physical violence, selective inattention, scapegoating, unfair or inappropriate labeling, myths or rituals of uncertain origin and accuracy, and shared family efforts at creating distraction (Zuk, 1971). The therapist decides the severity or level of pathogenic relating based upon his experience.

Go-between Process

This is the process by which the therapist takes and trades the roles of mediator, side-taker, and celebrant in family treatment. Alternatively, family members can conduct a kind of go-between process of their own as a means of resisting the therapist's interventions. There are four steps in the process: (a) identification of an issue by therapist or family member on which there are at least two sides or opponents; (b) intensification of conflict and movement by therapist or family member into a go-between role; (c) efforts by go-between and other principals to define and delimit their respective roles or positions; (d) reduction of the "conflict associated with a change in the positions of principals or with a redefinition of the conflict, or both" (Zuk, 1971, p. 47).

"Continuity" and "Discontinuity" Values

Zuk has given considerable emphasis to the importance of family and therapist values in the therapeutic process. He defines a continuity-discontinuity dichotomy that pervades family systems. To quote:

> "Continuity" values are those that stress the goodness of human interconnectedness, caretaking and nurturance. They emphasize the wholeness and indivisibility of human experience, and stress the essential quality of people. "Discontinuity" values are those that stress the goodness of rationality, of orderliness and efficiency, of adherence to rules and regulations, of analytic procedures. (Zuk, 1978, p. 18)

Zuk notes that wives and children tend toward continuity values, while husbands and society (or neighborhoods) lean toward the discontinuity side. Conflicts among any of these subsystems are usually drawn along the line between the two types; an impasse is reached in which those advocating one value attempt to subjugate proponents of the other, leading to pathogenic relating.

Therapist as Celebrant

This is one of Zuk's more recent concepts. Like a judge, priest, or civic official, Zuk notes that the therapist is often called upon "to officiate at or 'celebrate' an event that has been deemed important by the family, such as a death or a birth, a separation or reconciliation, a runaway or return from runaway of a family member, a hospitalization or release from hospitalization, a loss or recovery of a job. As celebrant the therapist confirms and signifies that the event did indeed occur" (1975, p. 13). Thus he seals and labels a change—gives it his stamp. His input serves as testimony to whether a change is important or not. He can use this role to expand a family's narrow definition of a problem, thus employing his influence in effecting beneficial change.

Applicability

Although this approach was developed in its earlier years through work with schizophrenics and mentally retarded children, its proponents have treated a fairly wide range of disorders. Some of the other problems which have been dealt with and written about are adolescent drug use, behavior problems, childhood emotional disturbances, marital difficulties, school problems and truancy, and suicidal gestures (Garrigan and Bambrick, 1975, 1977a; Zuk, 1971, 1975). Zuk feels the primary contraindication for family treatment is when a family has a fixed attitude that the therapist is serving as an agent of some other person or institution such that therapy has a disciplinary function. Zuk also doubts the value of family treatment extending beyond fifteen months. Finally, Zuk (1971) has expressed reservations about the effectiveness of this kind of treatment for many lower-class families.

Methods

In the go-between approach, change is defined as either an input into or an outcome of a process of *negotiation* "in which the therapist takes an active role in actually defining the change he wishes for the patient(s)" (Zuk, 1971, p. 10). Change arises out of the various contests between therapist and family. The therapist not only serves as a "releaser" of change but also as a "fashioner" of it.

The goal of this therapy is to shift the balance of

pathogenic relating among family members so that new, more productive forms of interpersonal relating become possible (Zuk, 1966, 1971). The therapist wants to alter the kinds of "vicious, repetitive patterns" that occur in dysfunctional families. Although Zuk himself is not particularly symptom-focused, others who use this approach, such as Garrigan and Bambrick (1977b), stress the goal of symptom reduction.

A major initial goal in treatment is to get a commitment from the family to be treated on the therapist's terms. Usually, Zuk states to a family that he will need three or four sessions to make an "evaluation" of the problem in order to determine the best way to alleviate it. He tries to exact a contract from the family on this. The degree of resistance encountered in making this contract is used by the therapist as a prognostic sign. This engagement period is a pivotal one in therapy. Zuk also notes that short-term approaches seem to work better because this is the time frame that the majority of families are willing to accept; an interminable contract is less effective, because families are less liable to agree to it (Zuk, 1976).

The therapist begins treatment with the goal of first assessing what is "wrong" with the family—i.e., the nature of its pathogenic relating—and then to communicate this (tactfully, in most cases) to them. They are not expected to accept his communication without testing. However, the testing itself is a first step. This engagement process, like termination, is one of a series of "critical events" that occur in family therapy.

Go-between treatment is a "clinical application of the concepts of coalition or alliance, mediation and side-taking" (Zuk, 1971, p. 14). It focuses on the here and now rather than the past. Co-therapy is rarely used. A number of tactics and strategies are used to intervene and reduce or undercut family resistance. The role of go-between played by therapist is not synonymous with the go-between *process* but is one step within it. The first move is to catalyze conflict, followed by the second step of therapist moving into a go-between role. The therapist selects an issue or issues to be struggled over or negotiated, and he takes the mediator role. In the third step, the therapist switches from the role of go-between to that of side-taker and sides judiciously with one, then the other. As in Bowenian therapy, he may make an open alliance with one member in order to disrupt the existing homeostatic balance. During this discussion, he sets limits or rules out certain behaviors, while evolving toward the point where he can introduce initiatives or alternatives that had not occurred to the principals in the conflict. Thus he is constantly structuring and directing the treatment process.

The therapist must remain flexible and unpredictable in go-between therapy to avoid feeding into the pathogenic process or being sidetracked from his attempts to produce change. At times he can be active and intrusive, at others inactive and passive. He can take sides or refuse to do so, selectively supporting members holding either continuity or discontinuity values. Interpretations might be used for their content or validity, or à la Haley (1963), as maneuvers to keep in a one-up position vis-à-vis the family. Sometimes informing a family of intent to terminate because of lack of progress can mobilize them to work harder to change. Behavioral assignments can also be used to allow generalization outside the treatment setting, although they are not accorded as much emphasis as that given by, say, strategic therapists.

What does it take to become a family therapist oriented in the go-between method? Zuk has emphasized that the therapist's values—the extent to which they are rigidly held and also are dissonant with the family's values—are a key to success or failure. He has called for closer scrutiny of therapist characteristics. More specifically, the most systematic attempt to answer questions about go-between therapists has been made by Garrigan and Bambrick (1977b). They undertook a four-year project to train male and female counseling psychology doctoral students in a short-term go-between therapy model. The results were generally positive (with no reported differences between the sexes). They estimate that 150 hours of training can enable such trainees to learn elements of the system and apply them effectively in the family treatment of emotionally disturbed children. However, they believe three years of intensive post-master's or doctorate training are necessary to function fully, independently, and effectively as a family therapist.

Outcome

Very little outcome research has emerged utilizing the go-between model. The primary studies in the field have been done by Garrigan and Bambrick (1975; 1977a; 1979). In one study, patients were 28 white, middle-class boys and girls, ages 11 to 17, from intact families who were enrolled in a class for the emotionally disturbed; none had evidence of psychoses, mental deficiency, hearing loss, or language disorder. Half the group was involved in brief therapy (10 to 15 sessions), and the other half (controls) had parent group discussions and seminars made available to them. All cases were involved in an ongoing process of educational and psychological treatment, and the family therapies were offered as an additional therapeutic element. The therapists were predoctoral counseling students. One- to two-year follow-ups were obtained in 85% of the cases. The major findings were that the family therapy group showed significantly more improvement in the identified patient's symptoms in the classroom and home, plus perceived improvement in their parents' marital relationship.

In a second study (Garrigan and Bambrick, 1979), the same procedures, in the same setting, were followed as in the first, except that all the 24 identified patients were oldest male siblings and one-third came from single-parent/mother families. Effectiveness of family therapy was not as pronounced in this second study, compared with the first; some classroom symptoms decreased, as did schizoid withdrawal. Overall results seemed to be affected by family structure, as less success was obtained with single-parent families. In fact, an interaction occurred in which mothers of intact families treated with family therapy perceived symptom reduction, while single-parent mothers perceived an increase in their sons' symptoms following treatment.

These two studies are part of a six-year research program. As of this writing, the total number of families involved has reached 70—35 controls and 35 experimentals.[7] Garrigan and Bambrick have used a good experimental design and a number of valid, reliable measures. Unfortunately, they did not report the extent to which the controls actually engaged in the parents' groups and seminars, so it is not clear whether they were no-treatment groups, alternative-treatment groups, or a combination of the two. Nonetheless, Zuk (1976) feels these are among the most objective studies in the literature, partly due to replication of results with different samples, and partly because, although they tested his treatment model, they were not done by him or at his institution.[8]

Comparisons

Throughout this chapter differences and similarities among the various systems groups have been noted where appropriate. In this section a few more will be discussed. Comparisons with other family therapy approaches, such as the psychodynamic and behavioral, are presented elsewhere in this volume and will not be covered.

Since the systems groups hold many similar views on symptoms, change, and treatment, and since most of them have observed each other's work, it is not surprising that considerable blurring has occurred among them, especially in their techniques. Sometimes they give different names to similar events. Sometimes they differ only in emphasis. For instance, Zuk makes many moves in treatment, such as fortifying generational boundaries, moving people's chairs, and supporting weaker family members, which could clearly be viewed as structural. Structural and strategic therapists both attempt to unbalance a system by joining with a family member on a conflictual point—an example of the go-between role. Minuchin does not write much about repetitive behavior cycles, but he is keenly attuned to them and often intervenes accordingly (Hoffman, 1976). The MRI and Milan groups do not talk about changing family structures, but their operations reveal this cognizance; for instance, deciding which family member(s) should undertake a task and which should not be involved in it is, in and of itself, a structural decision. In addition, Haley sometimes talks in terms that do not often get into his writings, such as discussing the "terror of separation" observed in schizophrenic families, or the inability of a family to let a member be more than a "ghost" or become a "whole person." Finally, when a structural therapist makes a move to obtain a "natural support" for a parent—e.g., obtaining a boyfriend for a single mother who is overinvolved with her son—there is an implicit assumption of "need" in that person that has to be *met*—perhaps in a different way, but nevertheless met—rather than ignored, reduced or eliminated.

Focus on the symptom or presenting problem differs among the groups. Haley and the MRI group are symptom-oriented, while Minuchin and Zuk tend to deemphasize the symptom. It should be noted, however, that when the structural group that undertook the psychosomatic work was faced with the life-threatening symptoms of anorexia and at the same time was under the scrutinizing eye of rigorous research, the symptom became a much more acceptable, or even inescapable, focal point.

Summary and Conclusions

Family approaches to treating symptomatic behavior in children and adolescents have gained considerable popularity and momentum in recent years. This is partly due to the scarcity of impressive outcome results in traditional child therapy and the growing recognition of the importance of fathers in the treatment of their children (Levitt, 1971; Gurman and Kniskern, 1978). Also, many of the processes that occur in child therapy can be interpreted as systems interventions (Montalvo and Haley, 1973), and once this is recognized, the transition to a treatment that includes the family directly is much easier to make.

Within the family therapy field there has been an ongoing struggle between two major camps—the psychoanalytically or psychodynamically oriented group and the systems group. At this time it seems fair to say that the systems group holds the center of the stage and has been there pretty much since the death in 1971 of Nathan Ackerman, the most "creative and zealous" proponent of the psychoanalytic approach (Guerin, 1976). In the author's opinion, there are at least three reasons for this development. First, it coincides both with the growing popularity of systems thinking within the mental health fields in general and with the increasing unpopularity of psychoanalysis and other prolonged and expensive therapies. Second, the systems groups may have devoted greater effort to training therapists at all levels and have developed more teachable techniques and more and better training aids, such as films and videotapes. Third, even though treatment outcome and efficacy data are not plentiful even among systems groups, the psychodynamically oriented people have shown an almost total lack of vigor in this respect—particularly in the child and adolescent area. As a result, their credibility, especially among younger professionals, has suffered.

On the other hand, the systems groups often tend to ignore the work of other schools and may possibly be handicapping themselves unnecessarily. For example, the formulations of Boszormenyi-Nagy and Spark (1973) on family loyalties and balances across generations are intriguing and appear to have great theoretical potential. While their therapeutic methods have not yet, in this writer's opinion, shown demonstrable efficacy, the theory might be helpful to systems therapists. First of all, the idea of loyalty to one's family "makes sense" to clients and can be used by the therapist as a way of joining and communicating with a family. The notion that offspring often feel they have to pay back a debt to their parents in order to be free and autonomous could readily be adapted in therapy tasks; it gives some idea of where leverage can be placed and how structures could be approached. In short, here is a theory with apparent validity, at least at some level, and its possible applications for systems therapists have gone unnoticed and unexplored. Since they have to an extent synthesized communications theory, paradox, boundaries, family characteristics, and structural concepts such as triangulation (Guerin, 1976), perhaps the structural people are the ones to bridge the gap.

A point as to who gets credit for a child's improvement deserves emphasis. The author has observed the work of many family therapists from different camps and has only heard this topic clearly stressed by strategic and structural therapists. The idea is that the more a child's *parents* feel responsible for helping him improve, the greater are the chances that the positive effects of treatment will *last*. If the parents and family feel overly indebted to the therapist, they will see themselves as less competent to cope effectively with new situations or future symptom-provoking events. On the other hand, a sense of accomplishment in having helped and corrected the original problem will prompt them to feel more confident in handling future difficulties. Thus the therapist wants to underscore to them the extent to which their efforts, ideas, and commitment really did "turn things around." If a family terminates a successful treatment feeling that it, rather than the therapist, was responsible for beneficial change, the chances for long-term success are increased.

New Directions

It seems fitting at this juncture to prognosticate on the future of systems approaches to family therapy. A number of recent developments give clues to where the field is heading. Some of what, in the writer's view, are the most promising will be highlighted.

It is predicted that Haley's (1979) work with severely disturbed young people will become the treatment model of choice. The reader can look forward to its publication.

The work of the MRI group is just now beginning to have the influence it deserves. As it is refined, a more complete cataloguing of specific treatments for particular problems will probably emerge.

The brief therapy work of Selvini Palazzoli and associates is worth watching. This group was one of the first to recognize the importance of the family in anorexia nervosa and has since taken off in new directions, particularly in the use of paradox as a therapeutic tool. They have a flair for the innovative and we can expect many good things yet to come.

The go-between approach has not gathered a very large following to date—partly due to a need for a more comprehensive theory. However, the training model presented by Garrigan and Bambrick in collaboration with Zuk shows promise. With a few more strong proponents, it should be on its way.

The psychosomatic work of Minuchin and associates has gained widespread acceptance. The family therapy training center he has established with Marianne Walters, Stephen Greenstein, and others has been lauded as "the most influential in the world" (Bloch, 1976). Nonetheless, Minuchin has diverted even more of his energies to the task of how best to train competent, effective therapists. We can anticipate that the programmatic and supervisory models to be developed will become an example for others to follow.

Mental retardation as a field has received slight notice from family therapists. This is unfortunate because the level of adaptation and autonomy that a retarded person reaches as an adult is contingent upon the ways in which his family responds to his handicap. A clinical program developed by Samuel Scott, Charles Fishman, Nila Betof, and associates (see Fishman, Scott, and Betof, 1977) has been addressing such issues for several years, and their work is now reaching fruition.

The family approach to drug and alcohol problems has been gaining momentum. Although marital treatment for alcoholism is hardly a new approach, the systems-oriented family-marital treatment model being developed by Berenson (1976) is a leap forward; much will be heard of it in the future. In the drug addiction area, certain structural/strategic work (Stanton, 1978; Stanton et al., 1978, 1980) is showing encouraging results in a field that is replete with clinical and theoretical papers but has been without cohesive, tested models of family therapy.

Notes

1. It should be noted at the outset that this writer has had more intensive and direct experience with the structural and Haley approaches than with the other family systems approaches discussed in this chapter.
2. For material on workshops and film or videotape rentals, the following names and addresses should be helpful.

   Strategic Family Therapy:

   Family Therapy Institute (Haley)
   4602 North Park Avenue
   Chevy Chase, Maryland 20015

   Brief Therapy Center
   (Bodin, Fisch, Watzlawick, & Weakland)
   Mental Research Institute
   555 Middlefield Road
   Palo Alto, California 94301

   Structural Family Therapy (Minuchin and associates):

   For films and videotape rentals, write the Video Department, and for workshops, write:

   Center for Family Therapy Training
   Philadelphia Child Guidance Clinic
   34th Street and Civic Center Boulevard
   Philadelphia, Pa. 19104

   Triadic-Based Go-Between Family Therapy:

   Gerald Zuk, Ph.D.
   Family Psychiatry Department
   Eastern Pennsylvania Psychiatric Institute
   Henry and Abbottsford Roads
   Philadelphia, Pa. 19129
3. J. Haley, personal communication, August 1978.
4. These last two points have been made to the author by Avner Barcai in a personal communication, July 1978.
5. B. Rosman, personal communication, September 1977.
6. Credit for most of the points in this paragraph goes to Stephen Greenstein, in a personal communication with the author, August 1978.
7. A. Bambrick, personal communication, August 1978.
8. G. Zuk, personal communication, July 1978.

Acknowledgments

The author would like to express appreciation to the following for their helpful comments on an earlier version of this manuscript: Stephen Greenstein, Ph.D., Jay Haley, M.A., Lynn Hoffman, M.S.W., A.C.S.W., Cloe Madanes, Ph.D., Salvador Minuchin, M.D., Braulio Montalvo, M.A., Paul Watzlawick, Ph.D., John H. Weakland, Gerald Zuk, Ph.D. Of course, responsibility for the final product is solely that of the author.

References

Alexander, J.F., and B.V. Parsons. (1973) Short-term behavioral intervention with delinquent families: Impact on family process and recidivism. *J. Abnorm. Psychol.* 81:219–225.

Andolfi, M. (1978) A structural approach to a family with an encopretic child. *J. Marr. Fam. Counsel.* 4:25–29.

Aponte, H.J. (1976a) The family-school interview: An eco-structural approach. *Fam. Proc.* 15:303–311.

Aponte, H.J. (1976b) "Underorganization" in the poor family. In P. Guerin, ed., *Family Therapy: Theory and Practice.* New York: Gardner Press.

Aponte, H.J., and L. Hoffman. (1973) The open door: A structural approach to a family with an anorectic child. *Fam. Proc.* 12:1-44.

Baker, L., S. Minuchin, L. Milman, R. Liebman, and T.C. Todd. (1975) Psychosomatic aspects of juvenile diabetes millitus: A progress report. In *Modern Problems in Pediatrics*, Vol. 12. White Plains, N.Y.: S. Karger.

Bateson, G., D.D. Jackson, J. Haley, and J. Weakland. (1956) Toward a theory of schizophrenia. *Behav. Sci.* 1:251-264.

Beels, C.C., and A. Ferber. (1969) Family therapy: A view. *Fam. Proc.* 8:280-318.

Berenson, D. (1976) Alcohol and the family system. In P.J. Guerin, ed., *Family Therapy: Theory and Practice.* New York: Gardner Press.

Berger, H. (1974) Somatic pain and school avoidance. *Clin. Pediat.* 13:819-826.

Berger, H. (1976) Minimal cerebral dysfunction: How families affect children with MCD. *Philadelphia Child Guid. Clin. Dig.* 1:1.

Bergin, A.E. (1971) The evaluation of therapeutic outcomes. In A.E. Bergin and S.L. Garfield, eds., *Handbook of Psychotherapy and Behavior Change.* New York: Wiley.

Bloch, D.A. (1976) Notes and comment: Aponte appointment—Medical divergence. *Fam. Proc.* 15:168.

Boszormenyi-Nagy, I., and G.M. Spark. (1973) *Invisible Loyalties.* New York: Harper & Row.

Bowen, M. (1966) The use of family theory in clinical practice. *Comprehen. Psychiat.* 7:345-374.

Combrinck-Graham, L. (1974) Structural family therapy in psychosomatic illness. *Clin. Pediat.* 13:827-833.

Fishman, C., S. Scott, and N. Betof. (1977) A hall of mirrors: A structural approach to the problems of the mentally retarded. *Ment. Retard.* 15:24.

Flomenhaft, K., and R.E. Carter. (1977) Family therapy training: Program and outcome. *Fam. Proc.* 16:211-218.

Frankl, V. (1960) Paradoxical intention. *Am. J. Psychother.* 14:520-535.

Garrigan, J.J., and A.F. Bambrick. (1975) Short-term family therapy with emotionally disturbed children. *J. Marr. Fam. Counsel.* 1:379-385.

Garrigan, J.J., and A.F. Bambrick. (1977a) Family therapy for disturbed children: Some experimental results in special education. *J. Marr. Fam. Counsel.* 3:83-93.

Garrigan, J.J., and A.F. Bambrick. (1977b) Introducing novice therapists to "go-between" techniques of family therapy. *Fam. Proc.* 16:237-246.

Garrigan, J.J., and A.F. Bambrick. (1979) New findings in research on go-between process. *Int. J. Fam. Ther.* 1:76-85.

Guerin, P.J. (1976) Family therapy: The first 25 years. In P.J. Guerin, ed., *Family Therapy: Theory and Practice.* New York: Gardner Press, pp. 1-22 .

Gurman, A.S., and D.P. Kniskern. (1978) Research on marital and family therapy: Progress, perspective and prospect. In S.L. Garfield and A.E. Bergin, eds., *Handbook of Psychotherapy and Behavior Change: An Empirical Analysis,* 2nd ed. New York: Wiley.

Haley, J. (1962) Whither family therapy. *Fam. Proc.* 1:69-100.

Haley, J. (1963) *Strategies of Psychotherapy.* New York: Grune & Stratton.

Haley, J., ed. (1967) *Advanced Techniques of Hypnosis and Therapy: Selected Papers of Milton H. Erickson.* New York: Grune & Stratton.

Haley, J. (1969) An editor's farewell. *Fam. Proc.* 8:149-158.

Haley, J. (1970) Approaches to family therapy. *Int. J. Psychiat.* 9:233-242.

Haley, J. (1971a) A review of the family therapy field. In J. Haley, ed., *Changing Families.* New York: Grune & Stratton, pp. 1-12.

Haley, J. (1971b) Family therapy: A radical change. In J. Haley, ed., *Changing Families.* New York: Grune & Stratton, pp. 272-284.

Haley, J. (1972) We're in family therapy. In A. Ferber, M. Mendelsohn, and A. Napier, eds., *The Book of Family Therapy.* New York: Science House, pp. 113-122.

Haley, J. (1973a) Strategic therapy when a child is presented as the problem. *J. Am. Acad. Child Psychiat.* 12:641-659.

Haley, J. (1973b) *Uncommon Therapy.* New York: Norton.

Haley, J. (1976) *Problem-Solving Therapy.* San Francisco: Jossey-Bass.

Haley, J. (1979) *Leaving Home: Therapy with Disturbed Young People.* New York: McGraw-Hill.

Hare-Mustin, R. (1975) Treatment of temper tantrums by a paradoxical intervention. *Fam. Proc.* 14:481-485.

Hare-Mustin, R. (1976) Paradoxical tasks in family therapy: Who can resist? *Psychother. Theory Res. Prac.* 13:128-130.

Hoffman, L. (1976) Breaking the homeostatic cycle. In P. Guerin, ed., *Family Therapy: Theory and Practice.* New York: Gardner Press.

Jackson, D.D. (1965) The study of the family. *Fam. Proc.* 4:1-20.

Jemail, J., and L. Combrinck-Graham. (1977) A therapeutic preschool as an adjunct to family therapy. *Philadelphia Child Guid. Clin. Dig.* 8:1.

Klein, N.C., J.F. Alexander, and B.V. Parsons. (1977) Impact of family systems intervention on recidivism and sibling delinquency: A model of primary prevention and program evaluation. *J. Consult. Clin. Psychol.* 45:469-474.

Langsley, D.G., P. Machotka, and K. Flomenhaft. (1971) Avoiding mental hospital admission: A follow-up study. *Am. J. Psychiat.* 127:1391-1394.

Levitt, E.E.. (1971) Research on psychotherapy with children. In A.E. Bergin and S.L. Garfield, eds., *Handbook of Psychotherapy and Behavior Change.* New York: Wiley.

Liebman, R., S. Minuchin, and L. Baker. (1974a) An integrated treatment program for anorexia nervosa. *Am. J. Psychiat.* 131:432-436.

Liebman, R., S. Minuchin, and L. Baker. (1974b) The role of the family in the treatment of anorexia nervosa. *J. Am. Acad. Child Psychiat.* 13:264-274.

Liebman, R., S. Minuchin, and L. Baker. (1974c) The use of structural family therapy in the treatment of intractable asthma. *Am. J. Psychiat.* 131:535–540.

Liebman, R., P. Honig, and H. Berger. (1976a) An integrated treatment program for psychogenic pain. *Fam. Proc.* 15:397–406.

Liebman, R., S. Minuchin, L. Baker, and B. Rosman. (1976b) The role of the family in the treatment of chronic asthma. In P. Guerin, ed., *Family Therapy: Theory and Practice.* New York: Gardner Press.

Madanes, C., and J. Haley. (1977) Dimensions of family therapy. *J. Nerv. Ment. Dis.* 165:88–98.

Minuchin, S. (1974a) *Families and Family Therapy.* Cambridge, Mass.: Harvard University Press.

Minuchin, S. (1974b) Structural family therapy. In G. Caplan, ed., *American Handbook of Psychiatry,* rev. ed., Vol. 2. New York: Basic Books.

Minuchin, S., B. Montalvo, B.G. Guerney, B.L. Rosman, and F. Schumer. (1967) *Families of the Slums.* New York: Basic Books.

Minuchin, S., L. Baker, B.L. Rosman, R. Liebman, L. Milman, and T.C. Todd. (1975) A conceptual model of psychosomatic illness in children. *Arch. Gen. Psychiat.* 32:1031–1038.

Minuchin, S., B. Rosman, and L. Baker. (1978) *Psychosomatic Families: Anorexia Nervosa in Context.* Cambridge, Mass.: Harvard University Press.

Montalvo, B., and J. Haley. (1973) In defense of child therapy. *Fam. Proc.* 12:227–244.

Moskowitz, L. (1976) Treatment of the child with school-related problems. *Philadelphia Child Guid. Clin. Dig.* 5:1.

Olson, D.H. (1970) Marital and family therapy: Integrative review and critique. *J. Marr. Fam.* 32:501–538.

Parsons, B.V., and J.F. Alexander. (1973) Short-term family intervention: A therapy outcome study. *J. Consult. Clin. Psychol.* 41:195–201.

Rabkin, R. (1977) *Strategic Psychotherapy.* New York: Basic Books.

Rosenberg, J.B. (1978) Two is better than one: Use of behavioral techniques within a structural family therapy model. *J. Marr. Fam. Counsel.* 4:31–39.

Rosenberg, J.B., and M. Lindblad. (1978) Behavior therapy in a family context: Treating elective mutism. *Fam. Proc.* 17:77–82.

Rosman, B.L., S. Minuchin, and R. Liebman. (1975) Family lunch session: An introduction to family therapy in anorexia nervosa. *Am. J. Orthopsychiat.* 45:846–853.

Rosman, B., S. Minuchin, R. Liebman, and L. Baker. (1976) Input and outcome of family therapy in anorexia nervosa. In J.L. Claghorn, ed., *Successful Psychotherapy.* New York: Brunner/Mazel.

Selvini Palazzoli, M. (1979) The families of patients with anorexia nervosa. In E.J. Anthony and C. Koupernik, eds., *The Child and His Family.* New York: Wiley.

Selvini Palazzoli, M. (1978) *Self-Starvation: From Individual to Family Therapy in the Treatment of Anorexia Nervosa.* New York: Jason Aronson, Inc.

Selvini Palazzoli, M., L. Boscolo, G.F. Cecchin, and G. Prata. (1974) The treatment of children through brief therapy of their parents. *Fam. Proc.* 13:429–442.

Selvini Palazzoli, M., L. Boscolo, G.F. Cecchin, and G. Prata. (1977) Family rituals: A powerful tool in family therapy. *Fam. Proc.* 16:445–453.

Selvini Palazzoli, M., L. Boscolo, G. Cecchin, and G. Prata. (1978) *Paradox and Counterparadox: A New Model in the Therapy of the Family in Schizophrenic Transaction.* New York: Jason Aronson.

Solyom, L., J. Garza-Perez, B. L. Ledwidge, and C. Solyom. (1972) Paradoxical intention in the treatment of obsessive thoughts: a pilot study. *Comp. Psychiat.* 13:291–297.

Stanton, M.D. (1978) Some outcome results and aspects of structural family therapy with drug addicts. In D. Smith, S. Anderson, M. Buxton, T. Chung, N. Gottlieb, and W. Harvey, eds., *A Multicultural View of Drug Abuse: Selected Proceedings of the National Drug Abuse Conference—1977.* Cambridge, Mass.: Schenkman.

Stanton, M.D. (1980) Strategic approaches to family therapy. In A.S. Gurmon and D.P. Kniskern, eds., *Handbook of Family Therapy.* New York: Brunner/Mazel, in press.

Stanton, M.D., and T.C. Todd. (1979) Structural family therapy with drug addicts. In E. Kaufman and P. Kaufmann, eds., *The Family Therapy of Drug and Alcohol Abuse.* New York: Gardner Press.

Stanton, M.D., T.C. Todd, D.B. Heard, S. Kirschner, J.I. Kleiman, D.T. Mowatt, P. Riley, S.M. Scott, and J.M. Van Deusen. (1978) Heroin addiction as a family phenomenon: A new conceptual model. *Am. J. Drug Alcohol Abuse* 5:125–150.

Stanton, M.D., T.Ç. Todd, and associates. (1980) *The Family Therapy of Drug Addiction.* To be published.

Umbarger, C., and R. Hare. (1973) A structural approach to patient and therapist disengagement from a schizophrenic family. *Am. J. Psychother.* 27:274–284.

Watzlawick, P., J.H. Beavin, and D.D. Jackson. (1967) *Pragmatics of Human Communication.* New York: Norton.

Watzlawick, P., J. Weakland, and R. Fisch. (1974) *Change: Principles of Problem Formation and Problem Resolution.* New York: Norton.

Weakland, J.H. (1977) "Family somatics": A neglected edge. *Fam. Proc.* 16:263–272.

Weakland, J., R. Fisch, P. Watzlawick, and A.M. Bodin. (1974) Brief therapy: Focused problem resolution. *Fam. Proc.* 13:141–168.

Zuk, G.H. (1966) The go-between process in family therapy. *Fam. Proc.* 5:162–178.

Zuk, G.H. (1971) *Family Therapy: A Triadic-Based Approach.* New York: Behavioral Publications.

Zuk, G.H. (1975) *Process and Practice in Family Therapy.* Haverford, Pa.: Psychiatry and Behavioral Science Books.

Zuk, G.H. (1976) Family therapy: Clinical hodgepodge or clinical science? *J. Marr. Fam. Counsel.* 2:299–303.

Zuk, G.H. (1978) Value conflict in today's family. *Marr. Fam. Living* 60:18–20.

Treatment of Emotional Disorders in Children and Adolescents

CHAPTER 12

Families of Institutionalized Children

G. Pirooz Sholevar

Introduction

In spite of significant developments in the field of family therapy in the past twenty-five years, the phenomenon of institutionalization of children has not been examined from the viewpoint of family systems theory. The institutionalized child usually is considered to be a disturbed youngster suffering from severe individual psychopathology rather than manifesting the dysfunctions of his family system. It is time that family therapists extend the insights gained from treatment of whole families into the phenomenon of institutionalization, since such a large number of children are institutionalized throughout the country. There are 70,000 children in psychiatric hospitals, 10,000 children in residential treatment centers, 44,000 children in correctional facilities, 80,000 in institutions for dependent and neglected children and 200,000 children in foster care (Lourie and Lourie, 1971).

One possible reason for this lack of attention by family therapists to the phenomenon of institutionalization is their dislike for an event that disrupts the integrity of the family unit. Family therapists have generally encouraged families to reabsorb an institutionalized family member. In fact, one of the most exciting studies in the family therapy field is a research project that has successfully prevented psychiatric hospitalization of adult patients (Langsley and Kaplan, 1968).

The purpose of this chapter is to examine the relationships within families who institutionalize their children with the hope of uncovering the familial forces that tend to extrude a family member as a way of gaining family equilibrium. From a family systems perspective, a symptom such as aggressive, suicidal, or psychotic behavior is seen as a manifestation of the family system dysfunction rather than the result of the individual pathology (Ackerman, 1958; Haley, 1963; Sholevar, 1970). From this point of view, a symptomatic child is one manifestation of the conflicts of the family group whose relationships with one another reciprocally influence the adaptive and nonadaptive behavior of each family member. This perspective does not deny the importance of individual dynamics in understanding the phenomenon of institutionalization but such considerations are beyond the scope of this chapter and are well illustrated in the excellent chapters by Rinsley and Petti (see chapters 12 and 13).

The data for this study are taken from approximately sixty Black and Caucasian families from middle- and lower-class families. Some families were intact, while others had broken. Each family had a child in a facility such as a short-term psychiatric inpatient unit, a long-term psychiatric hospital, a residential treatment center, a day treatment center or outpatient clinic. The variety of individual symptoms resulting in institutionalization included runaway behavior, aggressive and unmanageable behavior, stealing, delinquent behavior, suicidal behavior, psychotic reaction or fecal soiling (encopresis). The data were collected in conjoint family sessions including parents and the institutionalized child all of the time, siblings some of the time, and extended family members and friends occasionally.

Characteristics of Families of Institutionalized Children

Many signs of disturbed behavior and relationships were observed in the nuclear and extended families of institutionalized children. Emotional disturbance and dysfunctional relationships were in no way limited to the institutionalized child. A description of the behavioral and relational characteristics of the institutionalized children, their family members, and their family system follows.

The Parents

The parents of institutionalized children, operating in a disordered family system, manifested profound degrees of emotional disturbance. They suffered from severe overt or covert marital problems, were in conflict with members of their families of origin, were socially isolated, and frequently showed other symptomatic behaviors.

Even with intact marriages, the marriages in this group of sixty families were all unsatisfactory, as none of the basic needs of the marital partners—such as companionship, nurturance, protection, trust, sexuality, etc.—was met. The ways of dealing with marital disharmony were varied. Some couples presented a façade of a united front although they were actually emotionally divorced. Some engaged in open conflict. Initially, many parents appeared united but helpless in dealing with their problem child. The seemingly desired reduction in the child's symptoms or his removal from home usually brought any apparent harmony to an end and resulted in the surfacing of underlying marital discord.

Physical distancing and avoidance were employed frequently by the couple to avoid open fighting. Some of the emotionally divorced parents spent almost all of their free time away from home in bars, in churches, at golf courses, or attending to hobbies. Where parents would not criticize each other's behavior, they often selected one of their children as the agent for attacking their marital partner. A child also could be used as a repository of the negative feelings for the spouse. Here, the negative feelings were denied on the marital level but projected onto the child, where it met with parental overreaction. In the families where marital conflict was open and continuous, the parents fought with each other over trivia rather than face the underlying conflicts in their relationships. In such chronically unstable families, the actual issues between the couple remained hidden and unspoken while both the parents tried to outmaneuver and manipulate the other.

Sexual satisfaction between the parents was almost nonexistent, and sexual relationships were often characterized by the woman's withholding sex in an attempt to control or punish the man for allegedly or in fact treating her poorly. The men distrusted women and demanded sexual satisfaction in an impulsive manner; they became infuriated when they were denied sexually. In anger and disappointment, the men resorted to actions such as drinking or infidelity to discharge the sexual and hostile urges they felt toward their frequently rejecting wives, on whom they were very dependent. Other times, it would be the women who entertained other men in an attempt to humiliate, reject, and get even with their husbands. Sometimes the women tried to transform their fear and hatred of sex (i.e., men) into love of God and immersed themselves in church functions.

The sexual life of single mothers was practically nonexistent. Although some women craved affection from men, they avoided them, as they did not consider themselves sexual or attractive and felt inferior to men. They tended to believe a woman's life was one of continual suffering, while men reaped all the pleasures. This belief was reinforced by their experience to which they unwittingly contributed: as soon as they made demands on their husbands, the husbands had deserted. The negative attitude of the women toward men was a significant contribution to the development of both symptomatic behaviors and institutionalization of boys in a much higher number than girls in the family. The resentment of the mothers toward their deserting, irresponsible, and periodically violent men was transferred to their male children. The children were kept immature partly in order to prevent them from growing up into dangerous or disappointing men like their fathers. Thus it was not unusual to find the regressive symptom of fecal soiling in some of the institutionalized children.

One of the most frequent symptoms in mothers of institutionalized children was *depression*. The depression of such mothers manifested itself by the lack of ability to invest emotionally in any aspect of their lives, most particularly in their children and men. Underlying the depression was a tremendous amount of anger as they perceived themselves as victims of their children, their husbands, and their own parents. They often felt mistreated, abused, and taken advantage of by everyone. They had no interests or hobbies and spent much of their time being inactive. The only exception to this mode of existence was active religious involvement, but on closer examination, the women's religiosity proved to be actually the means of symptomatically avoiding their marital partners and their children via a defensive homeostatic substitution.

There were very few attempts by mothers to remedy the unsatisfactory condition of their lives. Any corrective attempts were infrequent and often impulsive, resulting in the breakup of the relationship, self-injury, or of such a long-term nature that they were unrealistic.

The parents of institutionalized children exhibited an enormous amount of *anger* and *mistrust* to anybody involved with the family in a helping capacity. They mistrusted and attempted to manipulate mental health services, the juvenile court system, and social welfare agencies. The public school system was the most commonly mistrusted and scapegoated.

A frequent finding was the *history of institutionalization* in childhood of one or both parents of an institutionalized child. Institutionalization usually occurred before the parent was ten years old. It often was vividly yet incompletely relived in the initial family sessions. The parents reported their own past insitutionalization with no significant anger or bitterness toward their own neglectful or rejecting parents. Almost uniformly, the parents justified the action of their own parents by incriminating themselves with a detailed account of their own faults. The devalued image the parents had of themselves was projected later onto their children. Therefore, the parents viewed their institutionalized child as well as themselves as "bad," "possessed," or "cursed." At no time was the institutionalized child really seen as a "sick" person who could be changed by treatment. He was seen as an "evil" being who had to be "put away," "punished," or "exorcised."

The Institutionalized Child

The institutionalized child manifested a wide range of symptoms and deficiencies in ego functioning, such as difficulties in controlling impulses and aggression, in identity formation, in learning behavior, in reality testing, in establishing autonomy, and in relationships with peers and adults. The most common deficiency in the institutionalized child, however, was the inability to regulate his *self-esteem*. One of the primary reasons for his very low self-esteem was his identification with the devalued parental image, via projective identification, projected onto him by his parents. This collusive acceptance of the projective identification left him feeling worthless, "evil," and "bad." A second reason for low self-esteem was the continuous exploitation of the child by the parents in their marital conflicts. In comparison to the impact of extremely low and unstable self-esteem, the other deficiencies in ego functioning seemed much less significant.

The institutionalized child usually was clever, curious, and demanded an explanation when limits were placed on his behavior; he was often capable of attracting the attention of a member of the extended family, a community member, or someone on the school staff due to a sense of humor, good sports ability, brightness, or some other kind of talent. In fact, it was unusual to encounter an institutionalized child who was not attractive in some way.

The institutionalized child was often involved in a collusive relationship with one or more adult members of his family, resulting in his dysfunctional behavior and diffusion of his identity. Constant role assignment and triangulation (Bowen, 1972) by his parents resulted in loss of his autonomy. He viewed himself only as a receiver of interactions rather than as an independent person in relation to other people. Triangulation also crippled his capacity to participate in age-appropriate activities such as making friends or going to school.

One interesting and common quality of the institutionalized child was his ability to exhibit affectionate behavior. This was probably the result of the collusive relationship with one or both parents which had brought with it intermittent closeness. The ability to be affectionate and loving was alternated with an abrupt emergence of aggressive and destructive behavior. The younger siblings were often the target of the rapidly alternating affectionate and aggressive behavior.

The institutionalized child needed to be the center of attention and reacted violently when he was not. He had to be in constant contact with the teacher or the group leader; this appeared to be related to his having been used constantly in family situations by one parent against the other parent (coalition) to the point that his self-esteem and identity depended on assigned roles. Lack of role assignment was accompanied by a tremendous drop in his already low self-esteem to the point of panic. At such points, he was driven into impulsive and aggressive behavior. Related to the collusive relationship was the child's feelings of omnipotence and being special. Although the behavior of the child was tolerated at home for a long time, he was eventually penalized when he carried out his assigned family role in a way that brought the family into conflict with the community, necessitating his removal from the neighborhood and home.

The Siblings

The siblings of the institutionalized children were affected by their family's dysfunctions in many different ways. Some were institutionalized, while others withdrew from the family system; whichever pathway they chose, few escaped the family pathology.

When one child came to be institutionalized, another sibling often became the triangulated or scapegoated child and would become symptomatic. The family then attempted to extrude the second member as well. At other times, the family would request institutionalization for two or more siblings at the same time. If one child was institutionalized and showed some improvement and if the family had developed a good working relationship with the institution, other children would then be offered to the institution for improvement—the institution was incorporated into the family system. This request at times was an abuse of the institution, such as a mother's asking for admission of her five children so she could return to school.

Another striking finding was the large number of siblings who were concomitantly in different institutions. Frequently the other institutions involved were of a dissimilar category; this was because the presenting problems in the cases of multiple insitutionalizations were different. For example, one sibling might be in a hospital while other siblings were in correctional facilities or group homes.

The emotional status of the sibling group was of great interest. The institutionalized child frequently was not the most disturbed member of the family group. Often there was a child who exhibited withdrawn, mute, or bizarre behavior in contrast to that of the institutionalized child. However, the aggressive or destructive behavior of the institutionalized child was more troublesome to the school and community.

Sometimes the withdrawal was only from the family system, and these children tended to be relatively successful. For example, some siblings spent many hours per day in sports activities, which kept them outside of the house and away from unhealthy interactions of the disturbed family system. Early marriage and/or pregnancy and early work histories were other ways of escape taken by siblings. In such cases, the "well sibling" occupied a marginal position within the family and attempted to find acceptance outside of the home. The "well siblings" were often incapable of developing close relationships, and their vulnerability to demands of intimate relationships has been described by other family therapists (Jackson, 1967; Haley, 1963). "Healthy siblings" were almost never totally free and mobile in their own families. They were fearful of any confrontations with their parents, and frequently acted sadistically toward the institutionalized child.

The Family Unit

The family of the institutionalized child suffered from multigenerational family dysfunction. Relationships between the three generations were overtly or covertly conflictual or the members of different generations were "emotionally cut off" from each other because of longstanding relational conflicts. The presence of multiple symptomatic behavior in many of the members of the extended family of the institutionalized child was also suggestive of a three-generational family dysfunction.

In the families of institutionalized children, it was found that a number of the parents—particularly the mothers—were not reared by their own mothers but were raised in institutions or by their grandparents. The relationship with the grandparents often was severed around the age of adolescence or deteriorated into a hostile one that left the mothers isolated or involved in a hostile, dependent relationship with both their grandparents and their own parents. These mothers felt rejected and worthless but strongly repressed their rage toward their own mothers while at the same time identifying with them (identification with the aggressor—A. Freud, 1954). They handled their subsequent relational conflicts by projecting all blame or unacceptable qualities onto their spouses and children.

In many cases, it appeared that the mothers were

repeating their own past by extruding their child from the family unit and placing him in an institution. An ego-syntonic, three-generational projective mechanism appeared to be operative in such cases. The identified patients dutifully played their parts in facilitating this mechanism. In some families where the mothers were more adequately cared for as children by their grandmothers—due to the absence or negligence of their own mothers—the institutionalization of their child appeared to be a repetition of the same act. The only difference was that here the institution was looked upon as a kind grandmother and was thought to be a beneficent place rather than a punitive one.

In summary, many of the behavioral symptoms presented by the institutionalized child were a result of family dysfunctions—often of a multigenerational nature. The disturbed behavior of the institutionalized child reflected some of the deeper relational conflicts within the family and served a homeostatic function by allowing the adults to deny their conflicts and appear united in dealing with the institutionalized child. Some family structures were seen more commonly in combination with particular symptoms and will be described below.

Runaway Reaction

Runaway children were admitted frequently to institutions. Stierlin's "delegate mode" of runaway behavior (1973) was a common finding; the runaway child, usually an adolescent girl, would become extremely active sexually in the community but in a way that would appear to gratify the parents. It was as if the "id" of the parents was delegated to and operated through the child, who was making up for the parental lack of sexual gratification. Casual runaway behavior in families with an expelling interactional mode was also seen frequently. Much of this type of runaway behavior that resulted in institutionalization was of a prolonged nature after the children had maintained themselves in the community for at least one to two months without being arrested by the police. Our sample did not include any children with "abortive" runaway behavior.

Sexual Aberrations and Incest

Symptoms of a sexual nature were often found in adolescents. Sexual acting out and confused sexual identity related to familial dysfunction were frequent symptoms in families where parents had severe sexual problems. For example, a bisexual adolescent girl with a severely confused sexual identity was found to be the victim of an active incestuous relationship with her stepfather at home. This girl was driven by tremendously strong heterosexual and homosexual desires.

Incestuous families were often discovered incidentally when other behavioral problems manifested themselves in the families. For example, one family brought their chronically suicidal and sexually confused adolescent daughter for treatment. The absence of generational boundaries in this family, the lack of a sexual relationship between the parents, the rejecting attitude of the mother toward her husband and daughter, together with the impulsivity of the father, made the therapist suspicious of an incestuous family relationship. Explorations in this area met with defensiveness on the part of the family. A year later, however, the mother initiated legal action, petitioning for a divorce from her husband on the grounds of his incestuous relationship with her daughter. We found these family characteristics present frequently in incestuous families (Sholevar, 1975). It also supported our previous conviction that incestuous behavior was much more common than acknowledged and only surfaced when it was complicated by a pregnancy of the daughter or when the parents wished to use it as grounds for divorce.

Suicide

Suicidal behavior often was a reason for institutionalizing a child and was a symptom present in different intensities among each generation of the family group. Along with suicidal behavior, death and murderous wishes were commonly present in suicidal families and directed at either the symptomatic child or the mother of such a child. Repeated suicidal attempts were not uncommon findings in parents, particularly the mothers of an institutionalized child. However, a review of the communications of the family members revealed that the death wishes toward the suicidal person significantly outweighed actual suicidal expressions.

Suicidal families were found to be shame-ridden and highly sensitive to the opinion of people outside of the family—a characteristic that preceded the suicidal act. Following the suicide, the families isolated themselves from the community and did not allow outsiders entry into their family life. At such times, if a family therapist saw the family for other reasons (i.e., symptoms in another member), he found the family "protective shell" (Wynne et al., 1958; Wynne, 1965) almost impenetrable.

Marital Dissatisfaction

The aggressive, unsocialized children in the institutions were usually the product of families where the wives constantly complained of their unsatisfactory lives, while the husbands reacted to the same conditions by withdrawing from the family unit. The mothers frequently were depreciated, neglected, abused, and punished during their childhoods by their unhappy, complaining, and insensitive parents. They later succeeded in establishing similar relationships with their husbands and sons in such a way that their husbands became their new punishers, then passed the role to the "symptomatic" children when the husbands left. The fathers welcomed the aggressivity of the sons as a means of punishing their depriving wives as well as vicariously experiencing their own shaky masculinity. The image of the male as a devalued, dangerous, and impulsive figure was a common finding in the families of aggressive, unsocialized children.

Disciplinary Difficulties and Fire-Setting

In some families of aggressive, unsocialized children, the parents operated as if to prove themselves incapable of controlling or directing their children. At times, there seemed to be a competition between the parents to prove themselves *the least* capable one in managing their children. The institutionalized children in such families were wild from an early age and exhibited other symptoms such as sleeping disorders, etc. They were found also to be in strong collusive relationships with both parents —particularly the mother.

Fire-setting children came from similar familial backgrounds. The mothers in the families were distinctly depressed, overtly rejecting, and neglectful. They showed confusion in their sexual identities and had an "anti-men" attitude that resulted in either very unstable marriages or marital breakups; one mother was a homosexual. Often the mothers' hostile feelings toward men resulted in their holding their sons accountable for the negative past behavior of the fathers. Reality testing was adequate in fire-setters, and their actions appeared to be motivated primarily by rage reactions toward their parents. Although fire-setting was present more often in boys, our sample included a number of adolescent fire-setting girls.

Psychotic Reaction

Children presenting with chronic psychotic reactions were found to have stable and seemingly satisfactory families. Actually, the couples in the families were often hiding a tremendous degree of marital dissatisfaction characteristic of stable-unsatisfactory families (Jackson, 1967). The children developed chronic psychotic reactions as a result of becoming repositories for the covert resentments the parents had toward each other. In such cases, all these negative feelings were denied on the marital level and actively searched for in the children. Children with acute psychoses were commonly from unstable-unsatisfactory families.

Encopresis

Our sample included some institutionalized children with the symptom of encopresis. Encopretic children were restricted and infantile in their personalities. They were generally the product of depressed and hostile parents who usually were rejected by their own parents. The father was absent in all but one of the encopretic families in this study (see "Persistent Encopresis in Adolescence," this volume).

Theoretical Considerations

Observation of significantly disturbed behavior and relationships in all members of the nuclear family of institutionalized children suggested that there was a disturbance in the whole family system (see chapters 10 and 11 for a general theoretical description of family therapy). The parents, as well as the siblings, exhibited significantly disturbed behavior; in fact some of the siblings or parents were actually the most disturbed members of the family. Maital relationships were poor, as the parents were unable to deal with their conflicts in an open, sustained, and effective manner; instead, they denied their conflicts or broke up the relationship. One of their children—usually the institutionalized child—was chosen by one parent to form a coalition against the other parent in order to lower the marital tension. The development of the child was severely disturbed as a result of this parental exploitation.

Significant disturbances were observed in the relationships with the parental families of origin. Grandparents showed different degrees of dysfunction, too. The conflict between the parents and their families of origin were observed whenever they interacted, and at times the relationship was broken off due to the severity and prolonged nature of the conflicts. The grandparents were disapproving or hositile to the parents and at times were legal petitioners against the parents on behalf of the children. Despite this apparent concern, the children were not nurtured by the grandparents either, and primarily were exploited by the grandparents against the parents. This, together with the frequent occurrence of disturbed behavior on all levels of the families of origin, pointed toward a *three-generational conflict and disturbance* in the family system. As a result, we were compelled to view the institutionalization phenomenon as a clinically observable familial dysfunction involving at least the members of three or more generations where each person avoided facing differences with the members of his own generation. The grandparents denied their conflicts and projected them onto the parents. The parents of the institutionalized child in turn completed the process of projection by extending it onto their children. This phenomenon is similar to transmission of symptoms across generations (Bowen, 1966, 1972).

The parents, exploited by their families of origin, had no chance to develop self-esteem or to differentiate themselves sufficiently from their families of origin. They were unable to recognize their assets and needs or to gain satisfaction through their own actions. The exploitative nature of their parents' interaction with them left them with a distorted inner representational world in which their internalized "objects" were frustrating and neglectful and they felt worthless and helpless. They made their children the targets of their projective identification, projection, and blaming so that the children ended up being exploited, undifferentiated, and poorly individuated. Often, the role assigned to the child was part of the unconscious fantasy shared by the whole family and maintained the distorted mental images held by the family members. The family members, however, were not cognizant of the shared fantasies that motivated their actions and reactions.

The institutionalized child was an active component of the multigenerational conflicts. He was involved closely with the dysfunctional operations of the family system and enjoyed his participation in it. Often, when the father left, the child undertook the role vacated by him in the nuclear family, which often corresponded with the mother's past conflictual relationships. The child then acted as the *punisher* for the mother. It is ironic to note that the institutionalized child would eventually mobilize social systems against the deficiencies of the family, in this way having a corrective role toward his family's dysfunction.

The assigned behavior in an institutionalized child, although adaptive within a dysfunctional family system, left him unprepared and incapable of participation in other systems outside of the family. His position in the family seemed also to make him susceptible to triangulation and scapegoating outside of the family. The eventual reaction by the community—together with the further scapegoating by the family—resulted in the institutionalization of the child.

In summary, an extensive and severe degree of family relational disturbance, involving at least three generations and interfering with differentiation and regulation of self-esteem in family members, appears necessary in order to produce a behavioral disorder severe enough to require institutionalization of a family member.

Treatment of Families with an Institutionalized Child

Treating a family with an institutionalized child is a long, difficult process and requires the correction of the underlying dysfunction of the nuclear and extended family system. This will allow the establishment of family equilibrium without the need to institutionalize a child. There are distinct therapeutic considerations in working with families of institutionalized children according to the stage and degree of completion of the institutionalizing process. If the family starts in treatment prior to the institutionalization of a child, the worthiest goal in working with them is a strong attempt to prevent institutionalization altogether. Nevertheless, it should be kept in mind that institutionalization cannot be prevented in all families, and even in cases where institutionalization occurs, the family therapist has an important therapeutic role to fulfill.

When working with families that request institutionalization of their children, one should be aware of the families' rigidity and deal with it early and in an effective way. The tendency of families to ignore and bypass mental health services and their recommendations is a strong one. While in treatment they continue to push for institutionalizing their child through other routes, such as family court. Assessment of the total family system in conjoint family sessions is essential, and the inclusion of the extended family members is extremely valuable in undermining the institutionalization process. The conflicts between the parents or between parents and other adults in the family need to be explored in order to disengage the child from active involvement in the parental conflicts.

Once the child is institutionalized, it is important to prevent his parents from taking him home early in order to re-engage him in the family conflicts. A pattern of frequent and interrupted institutionalization usually results in the ineffectiveness of family therapy, as well as in the residential treatment of the child. To prevent sabotaging of the therapeutic intervention, it is helpful to continue the child's stay in the institution until the parents have started to work directly with each other. The goal of uncovering the conflicts between the adult family members can be achieved only by careful assessment and selection of strategies. Injudicious choices of strategies threaten the family homeostasis and heighten the scapegoating of the child. In cases where exploitation of the child by his family is great, it is helpful to involve family court in treatment to maximize family cooperation. The legal pressures on the family should not be released before the family cooperates fully with the treatment.

In a residential treatment center, the family often views the therapist as an intrusive outsider who is attempting to undermine the most prominent defense of the family by unearthing the general family dysfunctions. The therapist is considered a person to be defended against and who should be kept ignorant of what is going on within the family. Because of the family's rigidity, members cannot visualize a way of relating that is different from their customary way and perceive the therapist as a person who is attempting to undermine their family unit. On the other hand, milieu staff are privy to family information as they frequently observe spontaneous family interactions on the unit. It is therefore important that the family therapist in a residential program does not function as "the person" who treats the family but as the final pathway for the flow of information about the family. In this way, the total staff communicates all pertinent family information to the family therapist, who utilizes the family data in the finalized treatment plan. The regular sharing of information enables the milieu staff to deal with difficult family interactions in a knowledgeable fashion and take the necessary immediate action, as when a crucial absentee family member "sneaks" onto the unit for a visit.

It is essential for the family therapist to recognize the multigenerational nature of the institutionalization phenomenon and explore the relationships between the members of all three generations. Using such data enables the therapist to point out the repetition of family history in which the parents (often the mother) and child are continuing conflicted relationships that originated between the mother and her own parents. The conflicted family relationships often extend and repeat themselves between the family members and the residential treatment staff, too.

The concept of "permeability and impermeability" of the "family protective shell" (Wynne et al., 1958; Wynne, 1965) is a significant one and should be kept in mind in the treatment of the family. The family is most open to therapeutic intervention at the outbreak of serious symptoms, such as suicidal or runaway behavior. At these times—often in the very first family session—the family may reveal readily its dysfunctional patterns and make it possible to define the problem in family terms rather than as an individual problem. It is important to utilize fully this initial opportunity, since the possibility may not appear again due to the reemergence of family defenses.

Families of institutionalized children are masterful when it comes to power maneuvers. They often insist—openly or subtly—on the exclusion of some family members from the outset of treatment. This maneuver makes the recognition of family members who play significnt roles in conflicts, or who can be important resources, difficult. They exaggerate the presenting symptom of the institutionalized child greatly, such as reporting significant fire-setting behavior when the child only has shown an interest in watching a match burn to its end, and they minimize the disorders of other family members. An attempt in the initial sessions to point out the skewed nature of such complaints usually results in strong protest by the family and an effort to intimidate the therapist and discredit his observations. It is crucial that the therapist does not become intimidated by the family and continues on to point out the family's patterns, since the therapist's firm stand sets the tone and direction of the treatment from the outset. These defensive patterns are part of the rigidity of the family system and need to be addressed early in the treatment.

An important characteristic of the families of institutionalized children is their tendency to deny their conflicts as soon as a temporary compromise is reached. It is important to help the family members develop a long-term view of their lives rather than continue on with their circumscribed and temporary perspective. Often the family loses motivation for treatment, especially during times of temporary relief. At such points, the therapist should attempt to maintain at least minimum contact with the family. With the realization that they may have only experienced a short respite from their symptoms, the family can recommence its work of resolving its conflicts when the problems resurface.

Self-deprivation is usually a well-established pattern in the families of institutionalized children, and altering the attitude of the family members to seek satisfaction and success often appears to be an impossible task. In single-parent and isolated families, the achievement of this goal requires finding other sources of nurturance and assistance for the families in addition to the resolution of family conflicts. Part of the therapeutic task is the encouragement and planning with the family for activities that can lead to gratification, such as getting a job, making new friends, and relating to members of the opposite sex. When the parents become involved in their own lives, it helps them to establish an appropriate distance from their children. Their self-definition and self-esteem become less dependent on their overinvolvement with their children and this usually provides the children with more room for development into autonomous individuals. It should be kept in mind that the secondary support groups for inner-city families are not necessarily the ones related to them by blood ties or kinship. An attempt should be made to mobilize all possible sources for family support in the extended families or in the community.

The ultimate goal of working with the family of an institutionalized child is to help the parent(s) to achieve maturity so that they are able to perceive their own needs and actively attempt to satisfy them through their marital partner and other adults without exploiting, triangulating, or overinvolving their child. They need to develop the capacity to deal with the members of their families of origin as adults relating to adults, rather than immature children making up for past disappointments or by discharging their long-suppressed rage on inappropriate targets. Lastly, mastery of a variety of direct interventional strategies as well as nondirective and insight-producing techniques are necessary in treatment to goad the institutionalizing family into change.

Summary

The exploration of family dynamics resulting in institutionalization of children and adolescents is a promising but neglected area for the family therapist. Data from conjoint family sessions of children in a variety of residential programs are presented which illustrate some of these dynamics. Information about the extended families is included whenever possible. An examination of the behavior of the parents and the family systems of the "institutionalized child" and his "well siblings" reveal significant degrees of disturbance in all members of such nuclear families. Further exploration of the relationships of the parents with their families of origin also reveals significant relational and behavioral disturbance.

In this chapter, several family patterns are presented and correlated with the institutionalized child's behavior. It is suggested that the institutionalization phenomenon is the end result of a three-generational family conflict where dissatisfaction is denied on the level of prior generations and projected onto the child. The family then attempts to institutionalize a child or several children as a way of gaining family equilibrium. The "institutionalized child" is the child who is most actively involved in a collusive relationship with one (or both) of the parents against the other parent or the grandparents. The immediate goals of family therapy are chosen according to the degree of completion of the "institutionalization process" within the family, while the ultimate goal remains the creation of a more effectively functioning family group. Some strategies for intervention are recommended.

Acknowledgement

The valuable editorial assistance of Ms. Marilyn Luber is acknowledged.

References

Ackerman, N.W. (1958) *Psychodynamics of Family Life*. New York: Basic Books.

Ackerman, N.W. (1966) *Treating the Troubled Family*. New York: Basic Books.

Boszormenyi-Nagy, I., and J.L. Framo. (1965) *Intensive*

Family Therapy. New York: Hoeber Medical Div., Harper & Row.

Bowen, M. (1966) The use of family theory in clinical practice. *Comp. Psychiat.* 7:345–374.

Bowen, M. (1972) Toward the differentiation of self in one's own family. In J. Framo, ed., *Family Interaction*. New York: Springer.

Freud, A. (1954) *The Ego and Mechanism of Defense*. New York: International University Press.

Haley, J. (1963) *Strategies of Psychotherapy*. New York: Grune & Stratton.

Jackson, D. (1967) *Pragmatics of Human Communication*. In P. Watzlawick, J. Beaven, and D. Jackson, New York: Norton.

Langsley, D.G., and D.M. Kaplan. (1968) *The Treatment of Families in Crisis*. New York: Grune & Stratton.

Lourie, N., and B. Lourie. (1971) A non-categorical approach to the treatment programs for children and youth. In S. Chess and A. Thomas, eds., *Annual Progress in Child Psychiatry and Child Development*. New York: Brunner/Mazel.

Sholevar, P.G. (1970) Family therapy. *J. Albert Einstein Med. Center* 18(2):61–66.

Sholevar, P.G. (1975) A family therapist looks at the problem of incest. *Bull. Am. Acad. Psychiat. Law* 3(1):25–31.

Stierlin, H. (1973) A family perspective on adolescent runaways. *Arch. Gen. Psychiat.* 29:56–72.

Wynne, L.C., I. Ryckoff, J. Day, and S.I. Hirsch. (1958) Pseudomutuality in the family relations of schizophrenics. *Psychiatry* 21:205–220.

Wynne, L.C. (1965) Some indications and contraindications for exploratory family therapy. In I. Boszormenyi-Nagy and J.L. Framo, eds., *Intensive Family Therapy*. New York: Hoeber Medical Div., Harper & Row.

CHAPTER 13

Principles of Therapeutic Milieu with Children

Donald B. Rinsley

Introduction

As here defined, the term "therapeutic milieu" has reference to a psychiatric hospital, inpatient or residential service, center or facility comprised of a multidisciplinary professional and paraprofessional staff whose efforts are devoted to the diagnosis and full-time treatment of preadolescent and adolescent children suffering from major mental disorder. The phrase "major mental disorder" is taken to include the psychoses and borderline conditions irrespective of their presenting symptomatology. Not included are those children who are primarily mentally retarded or brain-injured, with or without major "functional" disorder and symptomatology, who require other specialized residential settings, the characteristics of which will not be discussed here.

The salient functions of a full-time residential or inpatient service devoted to psychotic and borderline children are several, including:

1. Detailed individual case study, including definitive psychiatric evaluation and assessment; thorough cognitive-intellectual, thematic, projective, and achievement test study; and comprehensive historical and psychosocial assessment and evaluation of the individual child and of the child's family.

2. Based upon such study, selection of those child patients who require and can most benefit from intensive treatment within the particular setting to which they may be admitted (Szurek et al., 1971).

3. Selection and application of therapeutic modalities, comprehensively including the milieu, individual, group and family therapies, pharmacotherapy, occupational and recreational therapies, and special education (residential school) as aspects of an individualized program directed toward *both* short-term symptomatic remission *and* the inception of lasting, healthy personality change.

4. Treatment of the family as integral to the inpatient process with the child, oriented toward the amelioration and remodeling of pathogenic familial relationships and interactions.

As will be noted from the foregoing, the residential milieu is per se neither a foster placement facility, boarding home, "school," nor correctional institution, nor is it simply a harbor, haven, or asylum for "troubled" children, although it may serve any or all of these functions from time to time. If a given residential milieu is to be genuinely therapeutic in the sense above noted, it will possess a number of fundamental characteristics, among which are the following:

It will be staffed by adequate numbers of trained personnel who basically like children and like to work with them, who are empathic with the general needs of the young and to the particular needs of those with serious mental illness.

Its staff will be selected from applicants who are, so far as may be determined, mature adults who are free of significant or disabling psychological problems, able constructively to utilize in-service supervision and training, and able to cope constructively with the emotional buffetings to which their work with seriously disturbed children will inevitably and repeatedly subject them.

It will present to the inpatient child and adolescent an environment that is essentially devoid of the multiple-binding communications, pseudo-intimacy, pseudo-hostility, and the sorts of age, gender, role, and intergenerational blurring and confusion that typify the families of children with major psychopathology.

Hence, along with carefully monitored and titrated opportunities for individual growth and identity consolidation, it will provide appropriately graded "external" controls for "raw" instinctual expression as basic to the environmental safety, stability, and predictability that all children require if they are progressively to socialize, and that seriously mentally ill children require in even greater measure if they are to recover. A genuinely therapeutic milieu will begin vigorously to provide the essentials of adequate parenting from the moment the child is admitted into residence; its staff will, as it were, take charge from the beginning and will maintain their role *in loco parentis* throughout the subsequent course of the child's residential treatment.

Its staff will be prepared and able both to confront and to interpret the child's symptomatic behavior; the latter, whether active or passive, actively resistive or aversive, always conveys significant meaning in terms of transference to the staff and the physical features and structure of the milieu (Rinsley and Inge, 1961; Rinsley, 1974a) and thereby provides important insights into the child's prior overdetermined preadmission experiences and conflicts. Its confrontation, clarification, and interpretation directly within the milieu are essential if the meaning of such behavior is to be understood and the child helped to translate it into consensual secondary-process communication.

To be therapeutically effective, it must be able to function with a high degree of programmatic autonomy. If a "free-standing" facility, it must evolve its own coherent administrative operations, in-service training, supervisory structure, and ongoing continuing education program conducted by the staff professionals who are charged with carrying out its clinical mission; if the facility is a part, division, or section of a larger health care organization, such as a public or private mental hospital, it must enjoy considerable freedom from bureaucratic and political intrusions and administrative policies which would undermine its uniqueness and impose upon it organizational practices that have nothing to do with the treatment of sick children. Most important, the facility will operate most effectively and therapeutically when it is able to "match" its clinical program to the needs of its patients; admission must therefore be selective and not determined by political or bureaucratic and administrative expediency, a sad fate of some residential programs funded (hence, controlled) by urban, county, state, and federal agencies.

Finally, experience teaches that a therapeutic milieu for children and adolescents cannot co-function adequately as a therapeutic milieu for adults. Inpatient children should reside in a milieu designed for and operated in accordance with their particular needs, and not in adult wards or facilities. As the core of treatment centers upon the process of identification, the adult role models offered to inpatient children should not be those provided by disturbed and distracted adults, but rather by mature, healthy care-providers. Again, except for adult-supervised recreational activities, it is wise not to "mix" populations of preadolescent or latency age children with those of adolescents.

A major indicator of immaturity—namely, low levels of frustration tolerance—is typical for children in general and especially characterizes a majority of those who suffer from major mental disorder. Such children communicate their inner suffering in large measure by means of maladaptive behavior aimed at both mitigating their felt internal disequilibrium and attracting and warding off others', particularly adults', attention to and awareness of it. Such behavior, appropriately termed *symptomatic*, conveys near-intolerable and disruptive degrees of anxiety, guilt, and depression which have in significant measure impaired the ego's synthetic and perceptual functions (Rinsley, 1971a). As Hendrickson and co-workers (1959a, 1959b) have pointed out in the case of hospitalized adolescents, symptomatic behavior must be brought under firm control as quickly as possible for the avowed purpose of assisting the child toward beginning to translate it into progressively more meaningful consensual communication, thereby to reduce disruptive degrees of anxiety and to restore a measure of self-esteem that has been further impaired as a result of the child's inevitable and sensitive awareness of the pejorative effect of his behavior on others and on his relationships.

Historical Considerations

The history of inpatient psychiatric and residential care and treatment of preadolescent and adolescent children has been reviewed by Beskind (1962) and more recently by Barker (1974). They note that the earliest specialized residential facilities for children were opened in the 1920's in the United States, and that by the middle 1930's a considerable body of knowledge of inpatient or residential diagnostic and therapeutic practice had been developed. Among these pioneering residential facilities are mentioned the mixed adult-child program at the Allentown State Hospital (Klopp, 1932); the Children's Service of the New York State Psychiatric Institute (Potter, 1934a, 1934b); the children's psychiatric ward at Bellevue Hospital in New York (Bender, 1937); the Emma Pendleton Bradley Home (now, Hospital) at East Providence, Rhode Island (Bradley, 1936); the adolescent unit for boys at Bellevue Hospital (Curran, 1939) and the Hawthorne Cedar Knolls School in New York, which had opened in 1906 to receive and treat "disturbed" delinquent youths (Alt, 1960).

The two decades following World War II witnessed the opening of increasing numbers of specialized psychiatric and residential services for children and youth, with concomitant burgeoning of literature devoted to an increasing variety of approaches to and techniques for the understanding and treatment of disturbed juveniles. Expanding attention was now devoted to the subject of "therapeutic milieu," with a variety of points of view expressed in the work of such writers as Robinson (1947), Krug, Hayward, and Crumpacker (1952), Redl and Wineman (1951, 1952), Bettelheim and Sylvester (1952), Bettelheim (1950), Noshpitz (1962), Hendrickson et al. (1959a, 1959b), Rinsley 1963, 1965, 1967a, 1967b), and others (Reid and Hagan, 1952). In Great Britain, the number of full-time and combined day and full-time inpatient services for youth had increased from 11 in 1957 to 50 in 1970 (Wardle, 1970) and by the latter date, psychiatric inpatient programs had attained a high level of theoretical and practical sophistication, and of therapeutic expertise and comprehensiveness.

The evolution of the concept of therapeutic milieu in the case of children is inextricably related to the pristine concept of psychoanalytic hospital (sanitarium) treatment set forth by Simmel (1929). Simmel originally viewed the psychoanalytic hospital as a harbor or haven, a supportive environment within which the otherwise arduous work of analytic treatment could be carried out by and with those patients lacking sufficient ego strength to utilize the analytic process within the outpatient consulting room. His pioneering work was in turn taken up by the Menningers in the 1930's and 40's (Menninger, 1936, 1937), who proceeded to develop the inpatient milieu as an increasingly comprehensive therapeutic instrumentality directed toward conscious and unconscious, and derivative interpersonal processes. This view of the inpatient or residential environment as itself the major instrumentality of treatment found further expression in the work of Bettelheim and his colleagues with autistic children at the Orthogenic School in Chicago (1950, 1952), Redl and his colleagues in the case of "ego-deficient" youngsters (Redl and Wineman, 1951, 1952), and Hendrickson et al. (1959a, 1959b), Noshpitz (1962), Masterson (1972), and Rinsley (1974a) in the case of adolescents with major psychopathology (Adilman, 1973).

Criteria for Admission into Residence

Admission of a preadolescent or adolescent child into full-time inpatient or residential treatment is and should be a highly selective procedure based upon as thorough knowledge as possible of the preadmission situation of the child, the family, and their wider social environment (Szurek et al., 1971). Ideally, the child and the responsible parents or guardians should receive planned preparation for the admission in order to assist them in beginning to work through the anticipated separation and in recognizing and communicating the numerous regressive, anxiety-producing fantasies they harbor regarding themselves and the staff and environment of the residential setting (Rinsley and Hall, 1962). While unheralded or "emergency" admission of children into residence may in some cases appear unavoidable, the child's and the parents' early resistances are usually enhanced thereby, especially if the admission is engendered by a third party, such as by court order.

Potter's original criteria for inpatient treatment of children included the following (1934a, 1934b):

1. Those cases in which the child's behavior or conduct was so disruptive as to preclude outpatient treatment.
2. Those cases in which severe neurotic or psychotic disorder precluded adjustment at home or at school, and for whom intensive and extensive psychotherapy was needed.
3. Those cases in which the home situation was so difficult or disturbed as to necessitate admission to relieve family tensions.
4. A smaller number of cases for whom a period of inpatient treatment was required prior to later placement of the child in foster-type care.

Wardle's criteria, "sufficient in themselves to justify admission," include the following (1974):

1. The child's behavior endangers himself or others or is unacceptable in a nonpsychiatric setting because of its bizarreness or its failure to respond to ordinary social measures.

2. Behavior appears irrational or bizarre, psychiatric symptoms are clearly in evidence, *and* diagnostic investigation and treatment are impossible in the present social setting and in less than a full-time residential one.

3. The child's behavior displays progressive deterioration such that failure to admit will permit ongoing worsening of and damage to the child's interpersonal relationships such that rehabilitation will become difficult or impossible.

4. Essential diagnostic investigation and treatment can only be carried out in an inpatient setting.

In addition, Wardle cites several "relative" criteria for admission, among which are failure of outpatient treatment to engender improvement, and importantly, the presence of a social (including, home) environment which is "causing the persistence of symptoms."

Easson's criteria for inpatient treatment (1969), while specifically concerned with adolescents, may as well be applied in the case of younger children. The criteria he sets forth amount, in effect, to a generalization concerning drive and impulse control; thus, the inpatient child candidate "lacks sufficient strength to control . . . drives and impulses," cannot channel the latter in the service of mastery and growth, and is unable to utilize relationships with others in the home, the school, and the wider social environment in the service of ongoing psychosocial development. Easson comments: "A profound deficit in ego strength should be present before hospitalization is considered."

Szurek et al. (1971) comment that the vast majority of inpatient children admitted to their service suffer from psychotic illness, and that admission into full-time inpatient treatment occurs only after outpatient evaluation and therapy indicate its necessity.

The "deficit in ego strength" to which Easson makes reference comprises the following major components (Rinsley, 1971a, 1974a):

Failure of normal repression.

Persistence of primitive mechanisms of defense, with reliance upon projection, introjection, regression, and denial.

Predominance of anxiety of the instinctual type.

Impairment of the ego's synthetic function, leading to disruption of self-environment relations and dissemblement of perceptual, cognitive-ideational, affective, and motoric functions.

Lack or deficiency of "basic trust."

Pervasive impairment of object relations with related impairment of phase-specific development (Rosenfeld and Sprince, 1963).

Persistence of primary narcissism, with various degrees of persistent infantile-megalomania.

Persistence of primary process thinking, transitivism, and gestural and word magic.

Failure of sublimation of "raw" instinctual impulses.

Various degrees of impairment, including abject failure, of self-object differentiation (Masterson and Rinsley, 1975; Rinsley, 1977a, 1977b).

It will be evident, from the above considerations, that the child who is found, on adequate clinical study, to require full-time residential or inpatient treatment is also found to be suffering from major psychopathology, the more specific nature of which will now be discussed.

The Patient Population: General Characteristics

The psychopathology of inpatient preadolescent and adolescent children is discovered almost invariably to fall into two major diagnostic categories—viz., psychosis (schizophrenia) and borderline disorder (Ekstein, 1966; Masterson, 1972, 1973, 1974, 1975; Rinsley, 1977a, 1977b). The former in turn comprises two groups of severely disturbed children—viz., a process-nuclear group we have termed, after Fliess (1961), autistic-presymbiotic (presymbiotic), and a less prognostically ominous group of more "reactive" cases we have termed symbiotic (Rinsley, 1971b); an understanding of both groups is in turn predicated upon an understanding of the mother-child relationship through the fourth year of postnatal life.

The Autistic-Presymbiotic Group

Included in this group of children are those candidates for inpatient treatment who have variously been diagnosed as suffering from "nonremitting schizophrenia" and "infantile psychosis" (Reiser, 1963; Kolvin et al., 1971), "pseudo-defective" schizophrenia (Bender, 1947, 1956), "nuclear" or "process" schizophrenia, and some cases of early infantile autism (Kanner, 1943, 1949, 1972). They appear never to have emerged from the stage of normal autism (Mahler, Pine, and Bergman, 1975), hence have never achieved, much less separated from, the normal mother-infant symbiosis, which reaches its peak between three and five months postnatally (Mahler, Pine, and Bergman, 1975; Rinsley, 1974a, 1974b).

Failure of normal infantile imprinting in these children gives rise to a variety of ensuing somatic and physical developmental signs (difficulties with equilibrium, gait, and station; labyrinthine function; linguistic articulation; visual-motor integration; neuromuscular coordination), intellectual pseudo-retardation, pervasive inability to relate to others, and persistence of magic-omnipotence and infantile megalomania. Failure of primary identification in these children underlies their failure of development of the infantile stimulus barrier with arrest at the auto-erotic stage of development (the infantile pre-object, Spitz, 1971) such that erogenous zones pursue independent pleasure gain and normal developmental phase specificity is essentially nonexistent (Freud, 1905, 1914; Fliess, 1961). Failure of development of object permanency (Piaget, 1937) and of object constancy (Fraiberg, 1969) continues *pari passu* arrest at archaic sensori-motor levels of cognitive growth.

Autistic-presymbiotic children function on the level of part-object relations; their pervasive developmental arrest is based upon their almost total inability to have differentiated self- from object-representations (Jacobson, 1954, 1964; Rinsley, 1977a) with ensuing persistence of a fundamentally transitivistic perception of the self and the object world.

The relatively early onset of symptomatology in these cases parallels a sweeping failure of normal learning and coping; the child has remained profoundly unsocialized, and school failure is in early evidence. Indeed, many of these children are diagnosed as suffering from mental retardation or from some otherwise unspecified variety of encephalopathy, and as a result, some find their way into institutions for the retarded and brain-injured. Their psychopathology may ultimately be traced to, and seen to result from, *developmental arrest or fixation at the phase of pervasive lack of self-object differentiation.*

The histories of these inpatient children are replete with very early, ongoing, and repetitive psychological and physical rejections and abandonments, disruptions and losses of parent-child ties, early childhood depersonifications, and psychological and physical batterings (Rinsley, 1971b). They tend to come from fragmented pseudo-families as exemplified by parental separations and divorces and episodes of interpersonal and familial violence. Exceptions to these generalizations are many cases of early infantile autism, the etiology of which remains a matter of controversy, and cases of childhood schizophrenia whom Goldfarb (1961, 1964) classifies within his "organic group."

The Symbiotic-Borderline Group

Included in this group of candidates for inpatient or residential treatment are children who regularly receive a wide variety of clinical diagnoses, and who present with an even wider range of symptomatology. In contrast to the foregoing group, the symbiotic-borderline group displays symptomatic developmental arrest based upon *failure of separation-individuation* (Mahler, 1952, 1971, 1972, 1974, 1975; Masterson and Rinsley, 1975; Rinsley, 1977a, 1977b). These children have indeed achieved the elements of a need-satisfying mother-infant symbiosis, and their psychopathology is a reflection of their inability to have desymbiotized, as it were.

The Symbiotic Psychotic Subgroup

The protean symptomatology of this subgroup of psychotic children has been described by Mahler (1952) and it is noted to persist, in the absence of treatment, throughout the preschool and latency years and on into adolescence. Pervasive disruptions and distortions of bodily boundaries and image, pan-anxiety, fluctuating hyperactivity and withdrawal, frightening sensory-perceptual distortions, often dramatic refusion and reunion fantasies and delusions and sweeping cognitive, reality-adaptive, and coping failure typify these children. Their developmental failure appears to be derived from arrest or fixation which occurs during the symbiotic phase or the ensuing differentiation and practicing subphases of separation-individuation (3 to 15 months postnatally), although, as in Mahler's original cases, florid psychotic symptomatology may not appear until ages 3 to 4 years. As in the case of autistic-presymbiotic children, *the clinical picture is reflective of developmental arrest or fixation during the period prior to the achievement of a significant degree of self-object differentiation*, but with the occurrence of desperate efforts toward it by means of "transitional mechanisms," especially of the paranoid and hysterical types as described by Fairbairn (1941). Clinical and projective-thematic test study of these children during the latency years establishes the psychotic diagnosis; during adolescence, the presence of classical schizophrenic thought disorder (Bleuler, 1950) is confirmatory.

The Borderline Subgroup

Until recently, children classifiable in this subgroup comprised diagnostic and prognostic puzzles. Depending upon their predominant symptomatology—i.e., whether autoplastic or alloplastic—they received such nosologic labels as: "severe neurosis"; "ego defect and developmental arrest" and "superego defect" (Easson, 1969); character disorder or character neurosis; pseudo-psychopathic schizophrenia (Bender, 1959); "adjustment reaction" of childhood or adolescence; "delinquency"; various "conduct" and "behavior" disorders and the like. The borderline individual, particularly the borderline child, had been considered by some to be suffering from psychopathology indistinguishable from that of psychotic, particularly schizophrenic disorder (Rinsley, 1977a).

The etiology of borderline psychopathology, including the developmental arrest which underlies it, has since been clarified by Masterson (1972, 1975, 1976), by Masterson and Rinsley (1975), and by Rinsley (1977a, 1977b) and others (Carter and Rinsley, 1977). It may be described as a particular defect in object relations based upon a particular form of "push-pull" mother-infant relationship that results in *a condition of partial self-object differentiation which results from developmental arrest or fixation which occurs no later than the rapprochement subphase of separation-individuation* (16–26 months postnatally). Hence, like the symbiotic psychotic child, the borderline child remains locked in an unresolved mother-infant tie from which, unlike the former, a partial separation has been made. Reliance upon "transitional" mechanisms is readily discerned clinically, even as their appearance is not quite so florid as in the case of the symbiotic psychotic child.

The Patient Population: Family Characteristics

It is now well established that the families of seriously disturbed children are the loci of, and are regularly discovered to harbor, serious psychopathology. It may be said that the full-time inpatient child, the "identified patient," represents the tip of the iceberg, as it were, of family pathology whether that pathology has been *a priori* etiologic for the child's illness or whether it reflects an otherwise healthy family's miscarried efforts to organize itself around and cope with a disturbed and disturbing offspring or sibling.

Experience with the families of inpatient children confirms their close similarity to the pathogenic families described in the work of Bateson, Lidz, and Wynne et al. (Mishler and Waxler, 1968). Bateson's concept of the "double bind" refers to a learning context in which the growing child is repeatedly subjected to incongruent, mutually exclusive imperatives from which no escape is possible and concerning which no further discussion ("metacommunication") can be developed, the ongoing so-called Catch-22 situation; the result is to force the child to deny significant aspects of his self and his experience. Lidz's contributions concern families characterized by blurring or obfuscation of age, gender, and generation roles, by barely inhibited murderous and incestuous fantasies, and by patterns of irrational thinking and of distorted perception of the extrafamilial world that are taught to the growing children. The contributions of Wynne and his colleagues center upon families characterized by excessively rigid or loose and ambiguous role structures, by "pseudo-mutuality" which conceals an absence of genuine role complementarity, by fragmented and disjointed communication and interaction, and by irrational shifts of attentive focus; the child conforms to the family nexus as a result of pressures to maintain the pseudomutual façade and to deny the basic meaninglessness of the family's relationships, and the imposition of family sanctions effectively isolates him from extrafamilial sources of socialization (the "rubber fence" phenomenon).

Zentner and Aponte (1970) apply the phrase "amorphous family nexus" to such pathogenic families. They refer to them as "families with a primitive, poorly differentiated and too broadly encompassing nexus. The individuals in these families have no meaningful self-image outside of the family nexus. Within this nexus, they do not clearly differentiate themselves from other members."

The deleterious effects that accrue as a result of growing up in such families are seen to result, in effect, from defective parenting. Winnicott (1949, 1951, 1960) has made reference to such parenting in terms of failure of what he terms "good-enough mothering," by which he means a mode of mother-child interaction in which the mother recognizes and satisfies the growing child's needs only as they are perceived as pseudo-complementary reflections of her own needs. More generally, such pathogenic parent-child interactions may be viewed as examples of *depersonification* (*appersonation*) of the child, who is thereby perceived and dealt with by the parent as something or someone other than what in fact he really is (Rinsley, 1971b); there is no genuine "goodness of fit" between parent and child, with the result that growing up leads to progressive distortion of the child's self-identity.

In the case of autistic-presymbiotic children, depersonification is found to have extended from very early infancy. The mothers of these children are "perplexed" (Goldfarb, 1961, 1964), and the neonate is perceived and dealt with as a transitional or fetishlike object or as a frightening persecutory figure, or in some instances, its very existence is denied. In many cases, such pervasive depersonification reflects the mother's own profound psychopathology; in some, it reflects the anxiety and confusion experienced by the otherwise healthy mother of an innately underresponsive, bizarre, or monstrous infant.

In the case of symbiotic-borderline children, parental pathology is almost invariably found to be related to the unfolding course of the child's symptomatology. Common to both the symbiotic psychotic and borderline cases is arrest or failure of separation-individuation, characterized by persistent separation anxiety, which in the former cases is of the instinctual type and in the latter cases becomes partly structuralized in the form of abandonment depression (Masterson and Rinsley, 1975). Thus among symbiotic psychotic children, the separation anxiety is conveyed in pervasive terror of self-extinguishment, with near-total effacement of what little in the way of a self-object boundary has indeed developed, sweeping refusion-reunion fantasies, and frenetic efforts toward restitution. Among borderline children, the separation anxiety leads to the formation of a particular kind of internal object relations, based in turn upon the mother's acceptance and reinforcement of the child's passive-regressive and dependent behavior and her threat of withdrawal of libidinal supplies in the face of the child's efforts toward separation-individuation (Masterson, 1975, 1976; Masterson and Rinsley, 1975; Rinsley, 1977a; Carter and Rinsley, 1977). Diagnostic differentiation between the symbiotic psychotic and borderline syndromes is not rarely difficult, particularly during latency and in early adolescence. From a natural historical standpoint, with no or inadequate treatment, the former regularly eventuates in unipolar-bipolar psychotic, schizo-affective, and other schizophrenic disorders of later life, while the latter later emerge as borderline personalities (Grinker, Werble, and Drye, 1968; Kernberg, 1975; Masterson, 1976).

The Therapeutic Milieu

General Considerations

As noted before, a therapeutic milieu for seriously mentally ill children must meet two fundamental needs, one of which is expressed by *all* children, whether well or ill, the other of which is expressed in repetitive, ongoing fashion by the latter. The first of these, termed *ego support* (Noshpitz, 1962), consists essentially in providing the fundamentals of adequate parenting per se, thereby to attempt to "make good" the deficient, destructive pseudo-parenting to which the sick child has long been exposed, hence comprises efforts toward undoing the effects of the child's long-standing depersonification. Ego support is provided by age- and ability-appropriate occupational, recreational, and educational activities and programs that function as components of the overall individualized treatment plan; such activities and programs are articulated and effected by carefully selected adult staff members with demonstrated expertise in their respective fields of work, who are themselves psychologically healthy, who enjoy children, and who are not put off by the symptomatic behavior of those with serious mental disorder.

The second need, termed *ego interpretation* (Noshpitz, 1962), refers to the more directly diagnostic-therapeutic features of the milieu, involving the full use of technical knowledge and procedures for exploring, uncovering, understanding, and ultimately altering the child's psychopathology and that of the family within which it originated. It is in respect to this area of inpatient work that the interdisciplinary team of child psychiatrist and psychoanalyst, clinical child psychologist, and psychiatric social worker–family therapist have their most significant impact upon the inpatient child.

It must be noted that many otherwise well-intended and well-staffed residential facilities for disturbed children are oriented toward meeting the former need, and significantly if not totally neglect the latter (Rinsley, 1963). The fact is that such children will not simply "grow out of it" (Masterson, 1967), that for them "love is not enough." These considerations are of particular importance in view of the recent and current emphasis upon children's rights and the right to treatment.

Inability or failure to provide in-depth (ego-interpretive) treatment within the inpatient milieu results from an amalgam of staff countertransference resistances toward the enormously regressive "pull" of the seriously mentally ill child and finds expression in a variety of ways. One of these involves the common practice of euphemistic underdiagnosis of the severity of the child's psychopathology, which finds rationalized expression in staff reluctance or inability to confront and control the maladaptive, symptomatic behavior that expresses it; the last in turn precludes exposure and interpretation of the child's underlying conflicts and he remains essentially unchanged. Again, staff failure to "take charge" may also reflect their unconscious projective identification with, hence their equally unconscious need to provoke or stimulate, the child's symptomatic "acting out" (Johnson, 1949; Johnson and Szurek, 1952), of particular importance in the case of the hospitalized adolescent. Thus, one witnesses the excessively, even egregiously overpermissive milieu, which like the so-called open classroom eschews disciplined child care and guidance and confers opportunities for adultomorphic decision-making and responsibilities upon sick children who are totally incapable of assuming them. Again, there is the milieu in which the prime goal is to keep the child "active," such that he is literally pushed into all sorts of occupational and recreational-athletic activities to keep him busy, including picnics, hikes, camp-outs, etc., by means of which attention to and awareness of the child's psychopathology is effectively warded off. Finally and all too commonly, there is the inpatient milieu which, having underdiagnosed the child and the family, proceeds toward premature discharge in the wake of any degree of overt symptomatic or behavioral "improvement," an increasingly frequent phenomenon as various private and public third-party insurers and underwriters have come to dictate wholly inadequate and misguided time-limited and statistically and financially based "standards" for residential care and treatment.

The basic functions of the therapeutic inpatient milieu for preadolescent and adolescent children may be enumerated as follows (Rinsley, 1971a):

1. Removal of the child from the pathogenic family nexus and from the wider social environment, the demands and expectations of which have overwhelmed him.

2. Shelter and protection, including interpersonal, pharmacological, and physical modalities to limit and titrate incident stimuli, hence to minimize the occurrence of further trauma to the already traumatized ego.

3. Appropriate and consistent, hence predictable, "external" controls to catalyze the translation of communications conveyed by symptomatic verbal and nonverbal behavior into consensual secondary-process language.

4. Opportunities for controlled therapeutic regression with emergence of transference material which in turn reveals the spectrum of the child's overdetermined coping efforts and responses, including those which convey his resistances to treatment (v. inf.).

5. Detection, recognition, clarification, confrontation, and interpretation of the child's and the family's manifold of mutually depersonifying communications and relationships.

6. Promotion of the child's identification with healthy, empathic adult caretakers and the use of appropriate peer-group interactions to provide carefully monitored opportunities for enhanced reality testing and for the acquisition of age- and ability-appropriate cognitive-intellectual and psychosocial skills.

The Course of Treatment: The Three "Phases"

Extensive experience with the intensive full-time inpatient treatment of adolescents led Rinsley (1965, 1971a, 1974a) and Masterson (1971, 1972) to conclude that the course of treatment of a child in residence proceeds through three distinguishable stages or phases; they termed these phases, respectively: *resistance, definitive* (*introjective*) and *resolution* (Rinsley), and *testing*, *working-through* and *separation* (Masterson); the triphasic course of treatment may be confirmed in the case of younger, preadolescent children as well. As will be further elaborated below, recognition of these phases conveys to the therapeutic staff a more thorough understanding of any particular example or manifestation of patient behavior. Thus, for example, elopement or running away during the resistance (testing) phase almost always communicates the need to avoid, evade, or preclude the impact of treatment, hence must so far as possible be prevented; during the resolution (separation) phase, however, running away often represents a positive effort toward individuation, and while not as such condoned by the staff, does not call for significant negative sanctions.

The Resistance (Testing) Phase

Irrespective of the particular route by which the child and the parental figures entered the combined inpatient-family treatment process, and whether such entrance was voluntary or involuntary, they quickly begin to resist the treatment. Analysis of such resistance inevitably reveals a welter of underlying primitive, often fearsome fantasies which center upon the anticipated dire effects of separation and loss and of exposure of the mutually depersonifying features of the pathogenic family nexus (Rinsley, 1965, 1971b, 1974a; Rinsley and Inge, 1961; Rinsley and Hall, 1962). During this phase, the child's resistance maneuvers are seen to resemble the behavior of separated infants during what Bowlby (1960a, 1960b, 1961) has termed the stage of protest. They are manifested in a wide variety of ways, ranging from adroit dissimulation with pseudo-compliance ("There's nothing wrong with me—I'm okay."), which is common among late latency and adolescent inpatients, through gross negativism and withdrawal ("I can make you go away, disappear, then you won't bother me and I can't hurt you . . . ") to gross rebelliousness and destructiveness ("I'll create such an uproar that you'll get rid of me . . . ") and efforts to run away.

In symbiotic cases, resistance behavior is oriented toward warding off staff attention to and awareness of the child's powerful refusion-reunion fantasies and, as manifested in the family therapy process, toward maintaining in concealment the nexus of depersonifying communications and interactions and the secondary gains associated with them and with the patient's ongoing symptomatology. In presymbiotic cases, resistance behavior is directed toward self-preservation at any cost, including precluding staff knowledge of the terrifying part-object content of the child's autistic pseudocommunity and of the child's associated efforts to extinguish (scotomatize) and, alternatively, to make restitutive restoration of staff figures (Dewdney, 1973).

In the case of the symbiotic-borderline child, the resistance phase usually occupies no less than a period of one year in residence; in the case of the presymbiotic child, periods of up to several years of residence are usually required before the resistance phase comes to a close.

The Definitive (Working-Through) Phase

The second, definitive or working-through phase of treatment has its inception as the preceding resistances proceed to fall away in the wake of the child's and the family's growing trust in the treatment staff and program. For the child, this means giving up, as it were, his core of infantile megalomania and of "bad" internal representations to the staff and gradually replacing them with "good" representations based upon positive identifications, and the child's and the family's increasing comfort with their and the staff's exposure of and insight into their pathogenic nexus. The early part of this phase is often a time of notable storm and stress for all concerned; the remodeling of the family nexus is understandably very upsetting, particularly as the child's "giving up" (externalization) of his "bad" core representations signifies the inception of the depressive working-through which Fairbairn (1941, 1951) has characterized in terms of his stage of transitional "quasi-independence." Thus the child will appear to be regressing and disorganizing, the parents' anxiety will mount substantially and they will not rarely make a strong effort to terminate the whole proceeding by attempting to remove the child from residence against advice, in some cases necessitating resort to legal means to keep the child in treatment. When this stormy period has been successfully traversed, the latter part of the definitive phase witnesses the appearance of the onset of the child's separation-individuation and of the parents' growing satisfaction with their child's efforts and improvement.

In the case of the symbiotic-borderline child, the definitive phase of treatment ordinarily occupies another 12 to 24 months of intensive work. In the case of those presymbiotic children who have successfully worked through their prolonged antecedent resistance phase, a similar period of good progress may be expected to characterize their definitive treatment phase.

The Resolution (Separation) Phase

This third and final phase of treatment witnesses the consolidation of the work of the antecedent definitive phase, the completion of depressive working-through, and the ensuing attainment of whole-object relations (Klein, 1932, 1935, 1940, 1946). During this period, closely supervised parent-child visits undergo relaxation, the child receives progressively expanded privileges with the assumption of increasing responsibility for himself, and the frequency and length of off-grounds passes and home visits are increased. By this time, substantial resolution of the pathologic family nexus has signalled the parents' enhanced readiness to assume the roles of healthy parents and the responsibilities of adequate parenting. Several more months of "separation work" are ordinarily required as the child becomes prepared to depart the residential environment and the parents become prepared to "reacquire" him.

Basic Goals of Treatment

For the presymbiotic child, the inpatient setting provides a highly protective, maximally predictable environment organized around and in support of the individual psychotherapeutic process. In decreasing degree as the child progresses, the milieu functions to monitor and limit incident stimuli and stress, including peer-competitive experiences, thereby to husband the child's few ego functions and resources and to promote positive introjections which will eventually serve as core ego nuclei to catalyze the formation of the patient-therapist symbiosis. The chief task and goal of the resistance phase of treatment in the case of the presymbiotic child becomes the eventual working through of the rapidly evolving, prolonged "transference psychosis" which is based upon enormously primitive, archaic experiences resulting from early object loss. The ongoing work of the ensuing definitive and resolution phases comprises further resolution of the symbiosis, with eventual desymbiotization and significant progress toward separation-individuation. The basic course of inpatient treatment may thus be diagrammed as in Figure 1 (Rinsley, 1974a).

In the case of the symbiotic-borderline child, the chief task and goal of the resistance phase of treatment comprises recognition, exposure, confrontation, and beginning interpretive resolution of the symbiotic mother-infant tie, the "tie that binds." A major part of this work centers upon the child's fantasies of reunion with the maternal part-object and of megalomanic control of other family members. As it proceeds, treatment focuses increasingly upon progressive resocialization, including expanded peer-competitive experiences and increasing responsibility, as tolerated. While often helpful in carefully selected cases, individual psychotherapy is not essential for the symbiotic-borderline child in residence, particularly during the resistance phase when it is likely to become enmeshed in the child's staff-splitting resistance maneuvers; rather, considerable in-depth work can be accomplished with the ward or team psychiatrist directly within the child's living area, a more extended concept of the idea of the "life space interview" originally developed by Redl (1959). The basic course of inpatient treatment may thus be diagrammed as in Figure 2 (Rinsley, 1974a).

Specific Characteristics of the Milieu

The healthy, growth-promoting family possesses several essential characteristics that catalyze the optimal maturation and development of its children. Such a family is biparental—that is, it begins and endures with both mother-surrogate and father-surrogate; it provides a basic domicile, including adequate physical shelter and diet; it functions in accordance with definitive, consensually validated and appropriately flexible personal-interpersonal, age, intergenerational, and gender-specific roles—hence it appropriately *personifies* its members; it provides consistent, predictable age- and ability-graded controls and discipline, progressively to curb and redirect the children's egocentricity and infantile-grandiosity—hence to promote intra-familial, and later, extra-familial socialization; it offers to all its members, particularly the children, appropriate opportunities for constructive play and a "positive learning environment" that effectively reinforces the child's innate curiosity and

Figure 1

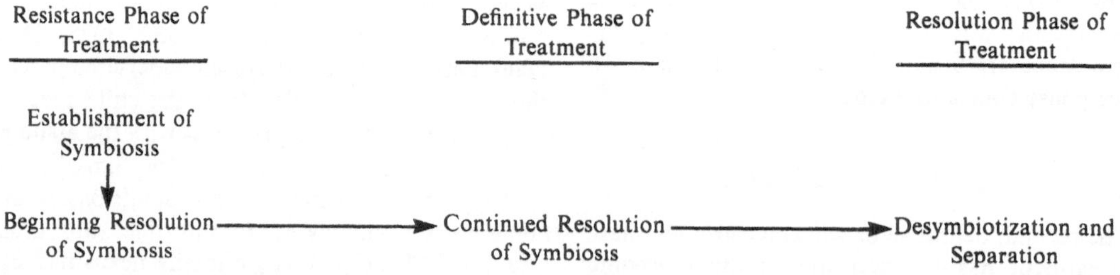

avidity for knowledge of himself and the world he lives in and which provides fundamental back-up for the school's primary task of imparting literate cognitive skills; it reinforces the child's innate drive toward separation-individuation and increasing autonomy while it concomitantly provides the necessary means for the satisfaction of his dependency needs.

Although the inpatient or residential milieu is certainly not a nuclear family, the extent to which its ego-supportive functions approximate those of the healthy family will in turn determine the effectiveness of its primary function of rehabilitative treatment and cure of the mentally ill child. Because the inpatient child is a sick child, however, the distinction between the therapeutic milieu's ego-supportive (i.e., basic child rearing) and ego-interpretive functions and modalities is ultimately artificial: all staff members in fact and in varying degrees perform both functions in a comprehensive, shared effort to understand the how and the why of the child's illness.

The Diagnostic Process

Although, under optimal circumstances, the staff has acquired significant preadmission knowledge of the child and the family, the in-depth diagnostic process begins at the point of the child's actual admission into residence. The diagnostic team comprises the psychiatrist, who performs the comprehensive mental status examination utilizing verbal and nonverbal (i.e., play) interviews and is responsible for the physical, neurological, laboratory, roentgenologic, and other special examinations and studies as indicated; the clinical psychologist, who administers normative-cognitive, thematic, projective, and other special (i.e., achievement) tests; and the psychiatric social worker, who conducts the in-depth family study. In some settings, the trained special educator serves as a diagnostic team member who assembles the relevant prior academic records and information, including previous grade placement data, and who administers special tests, such as the Wide Range Achievement Test, to determine prior and current educational achievement and potential. In addition to the above, other primary and adjunctive staff members who have been in daily or frequent contact with the child following the latter's admission provide the diagnostic team with significant information and inferences concerning the child, based upon their own observations of his day-to-day behavior within the milieu.

The diagnostic process will usually require no less than two or more weeks to be completed, following which a comprehensive diagnostic conference is convened, attended by all staff members with current or future responsibility for the child. At the conference, the diagnostic team presents the assembled data and findings, a final diagnosis is developed, and an individualized therapeutic plan is formulated.

Structure of the Residence

As previously noted, children suffering from major psychopathology should not be domiciled with inpatient or hospitalized adults; by the same token, intensive treatment is best addressed to the preadolescent and adolescent child within his respective peer groups, so younger children and adolescents are best not co-domiciled; again, the needs of early and middle adolescents differ significantly from those of chronologically late adolescents and young adults, hence it is best that they reside in wards or units specialized for them.

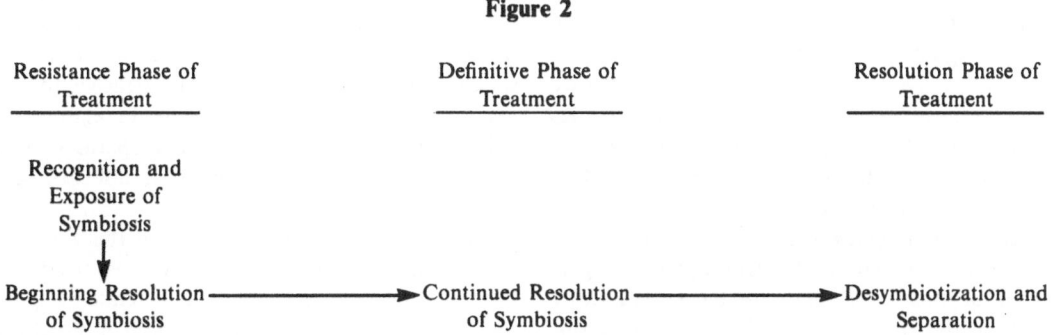

Figure 2

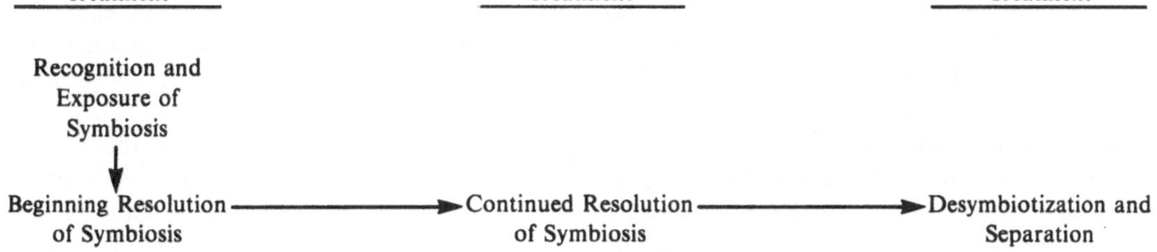

Although many residential facilities of necessity admit both presymbiotic and symbiotic-borderline children into co-residence, their therapeutic needs and the individualized programs developed for them differ widely, particularly during the resistance phase of treatment. Ideally, therefore, they are best not treated together.

The maximum patient population resident in any given ward or inpatient or residential unit should not exceed 15 children. Thus a facility staffed and budgeted for 60 inpatients should have four wards or units; for 30 inpatients, two such wards or units. Some facilities utilize coeducational units, while others separate the sexes within the primary domicile but provide for mixed off-ward or off-unit occupational, recreational, and educational classes and activities.

Of notable importance for the treatment of seriously ill youngsters is the concept of the self-contained milieu. To minimize excessive, traumatogenic stimulation, to minimize the expenditure of time and energy by both the staff and the patients, and to facilitate the close supervision the latter require, especially during the resistance and early definitive phases of treatment, all of-ward or off-unit therapeutic and ancillary services and activities, including the dining area, should be readily accessible within one building and within short travel distances, and outside playground areas should be located close by. Conversely, widespread, far-flung cottage-type facilities with long distances separating scheduled activities prove inimical to the intensive treatment and careful management which these children require.

Controversy regarding the role and significance of the closed (locked) ward or unit as over against the semi-open or open ward or unit continues to be one of the bugbears of institutional administration and practice. It is generally agreed that children should be *locked out* of and away from certain places and situations and *not locked in*, as it were (Robinson et al., 1957); of equal importance is the use of the closed setting to lock out unauthorized intruders. The significance and importance of the closed setting has been earlier pointed out by Ryan (1962) and in the case of hospitalized children by Rinsley (1963, 1971a, 1974a). Such a setting provides protection and security, symbolizes for the disturbed child the staff's much-needed control, fosters therapeutic degrees of regression, and inhibits or precludes running away. In the case of psychotic and borderline children, the semi-open setting is reserved for those youngsters who have successfully carried out the arduous work of the resistance and early definitive phases, hence are ready to assume increased responsibility for themselves within a context of decreasing degrees of staff supervision.

Physical Features of the Residence

Standards regarding the physical environment within inpatient or residential facilities have been set forth in *Standards for Psychiatric Facilities Serving Children and Adolescents* (American Psychiatric Association, 1971) and in the *Accreditation Manual for Psychiatric Facilities Serving Children and Adolescents* (Joint Commission on Accreditation of Hospitals, 1974), to which the reader is referred.

Administrative Structure and Staffing

As Noshpitz (1975) has pointed out, there is considerable variation among children's residential-inpatient facilities in respect to patterns and philosophies of administration. He distinguishes three major administrative formats, however, which he terms, respectively, *team-oriented*, *authority-oriented*, and *therapist-dominated* (a better term for the last would be *therapist-centered*).

The *team-oriented* format emphasizes intensive staff communication and collaboration centering upon understanding and coping with the details of the child's daily interactions and behavior; the team leader may be specifically designated or may "emerge" from any of the various professional disciplines depending upon whether the facility is of the "hospital type," the "casework type" or some other type. The *authority-oriented* format centers upon the single dominant leader or chief who meets with the various therapeutic teams, explains patient behavior, interprets countertransference, and formulates the treatment plans. The *therapist-centered* format is focused upon the child's individual therapist, who provides direction for the therapeutic team, leaving the everyday details of ward or unit administration to someone else. Irrespective of the particular administrative format, the individual who is ultimately in charge will depend upon whether the facility operates in accordance with the so-called medical model or some other (i.e., casework) model.

Of the three major formats, the therapist-centered is the least suited to the intensive residential treatment of very sick children; it tends to spawn multiple clinical-administrative splits and dichotomies that the child finds easy to exploit during the resistance and early definitive phases of treatment.

The Closed Ward or Unit. The closed ward or unit, which frequently also serves as the admissions area for new patients, requires a relatively high staff: patient ratio to provide intensive around-the-clock attention to and interaction with the patients. Ideally, each closed area will have a therapeutic team throughout the morning and at least part of the afternoon shifts, comprised of the psychiatrist, the psychiatric nurse, and several trained child care workers (CCW's). During these shift periods, the team will have no fewer than two CCW's, who, together with the psychiatrist and the nurse, will provide a staff: patient ratio of close to 1:4 for a 15-bed ward or unit. For the remainder of the 24-hour period—i.e., part of the afternoon and throughout the night shifts—two to three CCW's (ratios 1:7 to 1:5) with an on-call nurse are recommended.

The Semi-Open ("Open") Ward or Unit. The semi-open ward or unit will usually be locked during the hours of darkness and unlocked during the hours of daylight. To attain semi-open ward or unit status, the patient will have progressed in treatment to the point at which he is able to respond quickly to verbal (nonphysical) controls, does not require major or long-term restrictions, and does not ordinarily constitute an elopement risk. Such a ward or unit will usually function therapeutically with the psychiatrist and the nurse plus at least one CCW on duty during the morning and part of the afternoon shifts (ratio 1:5) and with one or two CCW's (ratios 1:15 to 1:7) at other times.

It is recognized that the on-ward or on-unit staffing patterns of many excellent inpatient facilities for children and adolescents will differ from those cited here, and that the professional and paraprofessional staffing of the various treatment teams will differ in accordance with the particular "model" with which the facility operates. Further statements and recommendations regarding accepted general staffing will be found in the aforementioned *Standards* and *Accreditation* manuals.

Off-Ward or Off-Unit (Adjunctive) Staff. The adjunctive staff of the residential or inpatient facility comprise full-time occupational therapists, recreational therapists, and special educators (teachers), the roles and functions of whom are discussed in some detail by Robinson et al (1957); what follows will serve to complement that discussion.

Because the core purpose of the therapeutic milieu is diagnostic and therapeutic, all adjunctive work addressed to the child should articulate closely with, and in fact serve as component of, the child's individualized treatment plan. Occupational and recreational therapies and residential school, while specific unto themselves and carried out by trained professional staff, do not serve the patient as ends in themselves but rather as they articulate with the patient's therapeutic needs and his capacities and limitations. How and at what point in the course of treatment they are prescribed for the child and the specifics of the tasks they address to him are thus highly individualized considerations.

The occupational therapy (OT) area should be cheerful but not overly stimulating, fully equipped and staffed by trained OT's experienced in work with disturbed children. The sessions or classes may be intensive 1:1 patient-therapist interactions, as in the case of presymbiotic children, or larger-ratio classes not exceeding six patients with one therapist. OT, sometimes called a small-muscle-group activity, works with tasks, materials, and projects of highly symbolic significance; OT, akin to play therapy, reveals and allows interpretation of unconscious, preconscious, and conscious material of great importance in helping the patient directly as well as for the on-ward or on-unit treatment team's understanding of the patient at any given point during his treatment.

Recreational therapy (RT) comprises a range of indoor and outdoor activities utilizing "small" and "large" muscle groups, ranging from the intensive 1:1 session or "class" employing sedentary games to peer-competitive sports, hikes, camping, and the like. Here again, the specific RT prescription will reflect such considerations as the presymbiotic child's need for stimulus-limited, controlled play and the symbiotic child's need for peer-competitive group games and sports to redirect infantile-grandiosity and to enhance desymbiotization and socialization.

Residential (academic) school has been discussed and described in detail by Morrow et al. (1972) and Rinsley (1974b). Dunn's (1963) view that attending school is the child's "occupation" must be tempered in light of the fact that "getting well" becomes the sick child's primary task and the fact that school failure or retardation is one of the most sensitive indicators of significant childhood psychopathology. Residential school is accordingly viewed as a definitive adjunct to intensive inpatient treatment; it is prescribed in accordance with the individualized treatment plan, and in a minority of cases withheld until the child is able to utilize it in the service of acquiring and consolidating literate cognitive skills. Depending upon the age, abilities and psychopathology of the inpatient population, the school will provide curricula ranging from basic core subjects through senior high school courses. Ratios will vary from that of the intensive, primarily therapeutic 1:1 class for the presymbiotic child through a maximum 1:6 higher-ratio, primarily academic class. Increasingly in inpatient facilities, classes and teachers are accredited through local and state school boards and boards of education so that credits earned while in residence may be applied toward graduation when the child is discharged and reenrolls in regular school.

Individual and Group Psychotherapies

The role and significance of individual psychotherapy in residential treatment have been discussed by Greenwood (1955) and by Robinson et al. (1957) and more recently reviewed by Hersov (1974). In the formal sense, individual psychotherapy (and of course psychoanalysis) comprise scheduled 1:1 patient-therapist interactions which, within the inpatient setting, are sequestered away from the mainstream of the milieu, usually but not invariably in the therapist's office; individual psychotherapy sessions may also occur elsewhere, such as in the child's room on the ward or unit if the child is too disturbed to leave it. As in the case of any other therapeutic activity, individual psychotherapy is prescribed and functions optimally within the context of the child's individualized treatment plan. For the presymbiotic child, as noted before, individual psychotherapy is prescribed and started very early in the child's residential experience. For the symbiotic child, it is in many cases best delayed until the child has "engaged with" the milieu, hence has in significant measure worked through the resistance phase of treatment. It should be understood, of course, that in an intensive inpatient setting, the nonscheduled, daily in-depth interactions between the child and the residential psychiatrist or other team leader in effect constitutes individual therapy insofar as they comprise an ongoing process that addresses itself to genetic-dynamic and transference issues.

Group psychotherapy is effectively utilized within the residential setting, and is of particular importance in the case of adolescents (Berkovitz, 1972). The group therapeutic method may be used in accordance with a variety of theoretical approaches, and again should be prescribed as a component of the individualized treatment plan. Group therapy should be avoided in the case of presymbiotic children until much of the definitive phase of treatment has been worked through, while scheduled on-ward or on-unit meetings may be initiated earlier in the case of symbiotic children whose desymbiotization-socialization work begins as an integral feature of the resistance phase.

Experience teaches that it is wise to avoid the use of "outside" visiting or attending physicians and other professionals for psychotherapeutic or other work with inpatient children (Rinsley, 1974a). As in the case of other professionals, the therapist or worker should be a full-time staff member in intimate daily contact and communication with the patient and the treatment team in order to minimize the splitting maneuvers of which seriously disturbed children are eminently capable (Rinsley and Inge, 1961; Szurek et al., 1971; Rinsley, 1972).

Treatment of the Family

The contemporary practice of family therapy in inpatient or residential treatment varies between the extremes of admission of entire families into residence (Weddell, 1961) to the extended, virtual exclusion of parents and other family members after admission of the child (Kahan, 1971). In actual fact, neither extreme represents optimal care and treatment. As Hersov (1974) points out, the traditional child guidance–type casework model has in various centers given way to the use of family therapy, including conjoint techniques based upon psychodynamic principles.

In the case of intensive inpatient treatment of presymbiotic and symbiotic children, remodeling of the disturbed family nexus is essential in most cases for optimal results with the "designated" child patient, and so far as possible, full participation of parents and, when indicated, other family members should constitute a requirement before any child is admitted into full residence. It is understood, of course, that a majority of children admitted into full-time inpatient or residential treatment will expect, and will be expected, to return to the family; should the latter continue pathogenic, the results can well be catastrophic.

While family therapy may be conducted by any qualified process-trained professional, it is often best carried out in the hands of a trained psychiatric social worker who functions in close collaboration with other therapeutic staff and who is knowledgeable in and in touch with the wider psychosocial aspects of the individual case. An essential feature of family therapy comprises early, ongoing, and in-depth resistance work (Rinsley and Hall, 1962) directed toward uncovering the specifics of the family's pathology, including the depersonification of the child (v. sup.), significant resolution of which heralds the beginning of the family's trust in the facility and its staff and of resolution of the so-called loyalty problem; thus the parents begin to communicate to their child that he is in effect free to repose *his* trust in the staff, to share with them the "family secrets." With these, the definitive phase of treatment has indeed begun.

A major responsibility of the family therapist has to do with careful monitoring and control of patient-family communications and interactions during the resistance and early definitive phases of treatment, to preclude reabsorption of the child in the family's nexus of pathological relationships. Family visits are always supervised until sufficient progress has occurred such that resurgence of the family's and the child's interdigitated pathology does not occur. When this has proven effective, unsupervised intramural, on-grounds, off-grounds and home visits naturally follow.

A Comment on "Institutionalization"

Within recent years, and especially during the decade of the 1960's, full-time psychiatric inpatient and residential treatment has come under increasing public scrutiny, and from a number of quarters, under assault. Several sources of the ensuing controversy over "institutional" treatment may be readily identified. One major source has been individuals and groups concerned with the civil-constitutional rights of hospitalized mental patients, centering especially upon involuntary civil commitment and buttressed by a host of judicial rulings and decisions aimed at guaranteeing the patient's right to treatment. Their concern has been with the nontherapeutic, custodial warehousing of the mentally ill as a form of incarceration without the constitutional protection of due process of law, and they have wrought numerous and sweeping changes in the laws governing and the procedures concerning the involuntary hospitalization of both mentally ill adults and children.

Along with these concerned lay and professional individuals and groups have come others who adopt the extreme views that mental illness is a myth (Szasz, 1974), that inpatient facilities, especially state institutions, are in reality political prisons, and that any and all forms of inpatient, residential or hospital treatment of the mentally ill are per se ineffective, detrimental, and destructive.

A third source has comprised the burgeoning number of public and private third-party cost insurers and underwriters called upon to fund inpatient care and treatment, and who have increasingly managed to influence it. Along with the general untoward effects of economic inflation, the increasingly burdensome systems and procedures of accountability that the courts and the cost underwriters have demanded and established to monitor the provision of health care have, as expected, added substantially to its costs. Again, as expected, the emphasis has been placed on short-term, revolving-door programs directed toward minimal cost expenditure (Rinsley, 1963).

A fourth source has been the community mental health approach, which reached a peak in the 1960's and which continues to have enormous impact on the entire health field. Thus, the emphasis toward getting the patient back into the community, where he will presumably again become productive; the result has been the near-wholesale dumping of the seriously mentally ill from hospital facilities into "outpatient" and foster home-type facilities. Within such a context, long-term inpatient or residential care and treatment have been looked upon with suspicion, and as expected, clinically excellent inpatient programs and diagnostically and therapeutically deficient facilities have willy-nilly been lumped together.

There is accumulating evidence of growing public and legislative awareness of the pejorative effects of rampant anti-institutionalism and of the need for excellent institutional treatment for the very sick, including very sick children and youth.

References

Accreditation Manual for Psychiatric Facilities Serving Children and Adolescents. (1974) Accreditation Council for Psychiatric Facilities. Chicago: Joint Commission on Accreditation of Hospitals.

Adilman, P.H. (1973) Some concepts of adolescent residential treatment. *Adolescence* 8:547–568.

Alt, H. (1960) *Residential Treatment for the Disturbed Child.* New York: International Universities Press.

Barker, P. (1974) *The Residential Psychiatric Treatment of Children.* New York: Wiley.

Bender, L. (1937) Group activities on a children's ward as methods of psychotherapy. *Am. J. Orthopsychiat.* 17:40–57.

Bender, L. (1947) Childhood schizophrenia: Clinical study of 100 schizophrenic children. *Am. J. Orthopsychiat.* 17:40–56.

Bender, L. (1956) Schizophrenia in childhood: Its recognition, description, and treatment. *Am. J. Orthopsychiat.* 26:499–506.

Bender, L. (1959) The concept of pseudopsychopathic schizophrenia in adolescents. *Am. J. Orthopsychiat.* 29:491–512.

Berkovitz, I.H. (1972) *Adolescents Grow in Groups: Experiences in Adolescent Group Psychotherapy.* New York: Brunner/Mazel.

Beskind, H. (1962) Psychiatric inpatient treatment of adolescents: A review of clinical experience. *Comprehen. Psychiat.* 3:354–369.

Bettelheim, B. (1950) *Love Is Not Enough.* Glencoe, Ill.: Free Press.

Bettelheim, B., and E. Sylvester. (1952) A therapeutic milieu. *Am. J. Orthopsychiat.* 22:314–334.

Bleuler, E. (1950) *Dementia Praecox or The Group of Schizophrenias.* New York: International Universities Press.

Bowlby, J. (1960a) Separation anxiety. *Int. J. Psycho-Anal.* 41:89–113.

Bowlby, J. (1960b) Grief and mourning in infancy and early childhood. *Psychoanal. Study Child* 15:9–52.

Bowlby, J. (1961) Processes of mourning. *Int. J. Psycho-Anal.* 42:317–340.

Bradley, C. (1936) A children's hospital for neurological and behavior disorders. *J.A.M.A.* 107:650–652.

Carter, L., and D.B. Rinsley. (1977) Vicissitudes of "empathy" in a borderline adolescent. *Int. Rev. Psychoanal.* 4:317–326.

Curran, F.J. (1939) Organization of a ward for adolescents in Bellevue Psychiatric Hospital. *Am. J. Psychiat.* 95:1365–1388.

Dewdney, D. (1973) A specific distortion of the human facial percept in childhood schizophrenia. *Psychiat. Quart.* 47:82–94.

Dunn, L.M. (1963) *Exceptional Children in the Schools.* New York: Holt, Rinehart and Winston.

Easson, W.M. (1969) *The Severely Disturbed Adolescent: Inpatient, Residential and Hospital Treatment.* New York: International Universities Press.

Ekstein, R. (1966) *Children of Time and Space, of Action and Impulse.* New York: Appleton-Century-Crofts.

Fairbairn, W.R.D. (1941) A revised psychopathology of the psychoses and psychoneuroses. In *An Object-Relations Theory of the Personality.* New York: Basic Books, pp. 28–58 (1954).

Fairbairn, W.R.D. (1951) A synopsis of the development of the author's views regarding the structure of the personality. In *An Object-Relations Theory of the Personality.* New York: Basic Books, pp. 162–179 (1954).

Fliess, R. (1961) On the mother-child unit: Its disturbances and their consequences for the ego of the neurotic adult. In *Ego and Body Ego: Contributions to Their Psychoanalytic Psychology.* New York: Schulte.

Fraiberg, S. (1969) Libidinal object constancy and mental representation. *Psychoanal. Sudy Child* 24:9–47.

Freud, S. (1905) Three essays on the theory of sexuality. *Standard Edition* 7:125–245. London: Hogarth Press (1957).

Freud, S. (1914) On narcissism: An introduction. *Standard Edition* 14:69–102. London: Hogarth Press (1957).

Goldfarb, W. (1961) *Childhood Schizophrenia.* Cambridge, Mass.: Harvard University Press.

Goldfarb, W. (1964) An investigation of childhood schizophrenia: A retrospective view. In S.I. Harrison and J.F. McDermott, eds., *Childhood Psychopathology: An Anthology of Basic Readings.* New York: International Universities Press, pp. 688–709 (1972).

Greenwood, E.D. (1955) The role of psychotherapy in residential treatment. *Am. J. Orthopsychiat.* 25:692-698.

Grinker, R.R., B. Werble, and R.C. Drye. (1968) *The Borderline Syndrome: A Behavioral Study of Ego Functions.* New York: Basic Books.

Hendrickson, W.J., and D.J. Holmes. (1959a) Control of behavior as a crucial factor in intensive psychiatric treatment in an all-adolescent ward. *Am. J. Psychiat.* 115:969–973.

Hendrickson, W.J., D.J. Holmes, and R.W. Waggoner. (1959b) Psychotherapy with hospitalized adolescents. *Am. J. Psychiat.* 116:527–532.

Hersov, L.A. (1974) Neurotic disorders with special reference to school refusal. In P. Barker, ed., *The Residential Psychiatric Treatment of Children.* New York: Wiley.

Jacobson, E. (1954) Contribution to the metapsychology of psychotic identifications. *J. Am. Psychoanal. Assn.* 2:239–262.

Jacobson, E. (1964) *The Self and the Object World.* New York: International Universities Press.

Johnson, A.M. (1949) Sanctions for superego lacunae of adolescents. In K.R. Eissler, ed., *Searchlights on Delinquency: New Psychoanalytic Studies.* New York: International Universities Press, pp. 225–245.

Johnson, A.M., and S.A. Szurek. (1952) The genesis of antisocial acting out in children and adults. *Psychoanal. Quart.* 21:323–343.

Kahan, V.L. (1971) *Mental Illness in Childhood: A Study of Residential Treatment.* London: Tavistock.

Kanner, L. (1943) Autistic disturbances of affective contact. *Nervous Child* 2:217–250.

Kanner, L. (1949) Problems of nosology and psychodynamics of early infantile autism. *Am. J. Orthopsychiat.* 19:416–426.

Kanner, L. (1972) *Child Psychiatry,* 4th ed. Springfield, Ill.: Charles C Thomas.

Kernberg, O.F. (1975) *Borderline Conditions and Pathological Narcissim.* New York: Jason Aronson.

Klein, M. (1932) *The Psycho-Analysis of Children.* London: Hogarth Press. (Delacorte Press/Seymour Lawrence, 1975)

Klein, M. (1935) A contribution to the psychogenesis of manic-depressive states. In *Melanie Klein: Love, Guilt and Reparation and Other Works, 1921–1945.* London: Hogarth Press (Delacorte Press/Seymour Lawrence, pp. 262–289, 1975).

Klein, M. (1940) Mourning and its relation to manic-depressive states. In *Melanie Klein: Love, Guilt and Reparation and Other Works, 1921–1945.* London: Hogarth Press (Delacorte Press/Seymour Lawrence, pp. 344–369, 1975).

Klein, M. (1946) Notes on some schizoid mechanisms: In *Melanie Klein: Envy and Gratitude and Other Works, 1946-1963.* London: Hogarth Press (Delacorte Press/ Seymour Lawrence, pp. 1–24, 1975).

Klopp, H.I. (1932) The Children's Institute of the Allentown State Hospital. *Am. J. Psychiat.* 88:1108–1118.

Kolvin, I., et al. (1971) Studies in childhood psychoses, I-VI. *Brit. J. Psychiat.* 118:381–419.

Krug, O., H. Hayward, and B. Crumpacker. (1952) Intensive residential treatment of a nine-year-old girl with an aggressive behavior disorder, petit mal epilepsy and enuresis. *Am. J. Orthopsychiat.* 22:405–427.

Mahler, M.S. (1952) On child psychosis and schizophrenia: Autistic and symbiotic infantile psychoses. *Psychoanal. Study Child* 7:286–305.

Mahler, M.S. (1971) A study of the separation-individuation process and its possible application to borderline phenomena in the psychoanalytic situation. *Psychoanal. Study Child* 26:403–424.

Mahler, M.S. (1972) On the first three subphases of the separation-individuation process. *Int. J. Psycho-Anal.* 53:333–338.

Mahler, M.S. (1974) Symbiosis and individuation: The Psychological birth of the human infant. *Psychoanal. Study Child* 29:89–106.

Mahler, M.S., F. Pine, and A. Bergman (1975) *The Psychological Birth of the Human Infant: Symbiosis and Individuation.* New York: Basic Books.

Masterson, J.F. (1967) The symptomatic adolescent five years later: He didn't grow out of it. *Am. J. Psychiat.* 123:1338–1345.

Masterson, J.F. (1972) *Treatment of the Borderline Adolescent: A Developmental Approach.* New York: Wiley-Interscience.

Masterson, J.F. (1973) The borderline adolescent. In S.C. Feinstein and P.L. Giovacchini, eds., *Adolescent Psychiatry,* Vol. 2. New York: Basic Books, pp. 240–268.

Masterson, J.F. (1974) Intensive psychotherapy of the adolescent with a borderline syndrome. In S. Arieti, ed., *American Handbook of Psychiatry,* rev. ed., Vol. II. New York: Basic Books, pp. 250–263.

Masterson, J.F. (1975) The splitting defense mechanism of the borderline adolescent: Developmental and clinical aspects. In J.E. Mack, ed., *Borderline States in Psychiatry.* New York: Grune & Stratton.

Masterson, J.F. (1976) *Psychotherapy of the Borderline Adult: A Developmental Approach.* New York: Brunner/Mazel.

Masterson, J.F., and D.B. Rinsley. (1975) The borderline syndrome: The role of the mother in the genesis and psychic structure of the borderline personality. *Int. J. Psycho-Anal.* 56:163–177.

Menninger, W.C. (1936) Psychiatric hospital treatment designed to meet unconscious needs. *Am. J. Psychiat.* 93:347–360.

Menninger, W.C. (1937) Psychoanalytic principles applied to the treatment of hospitalized patients. *Bull. Menninger Clinic* 1:35–43.

Mishler, E.G., and N.E. Waxler. (1968) *Family Processes and Schizophrenia.* New York: Science House.

Morrow, J.T., et al. (1972) The educational component of residential treatment centers. In *From Chaos to Order: A Collective View of the Residential Treatment of Children.* New York: Child Welfare League of America.

Noshpitz, J.D. (1962) Notes on the theory of residential treatment. *J. Am. Acad. Child Psychiat.* 1:284–296.

Noshpitz, J.D. (1975) Residential treatment of emotionally disturbed children. In S. Arieti, ed., *American Handbook of Psychiatry,* rev. ed., Vol. V. New York: Basic Books, pp. 634–651.

Piaget, J. (1937) *The Construction of Reality in the Child.* New York: Basic Books (1954).

Potter, H.W. (1934a) A service for children in a psychiatric hospital. *Psychiat. Quart.* 8:16–31.

Potter, H.W. (1934b) The treatment of problem children in a psychiatric hospital. *Am. J. Psychiat.* 91:869–880.

Redl, F. (1959) Life space interview techniques. *Am J. Orthopsychiat.* 29:1–18.

Redl, F., and D. Wineman. (1951) *Children Who Hate.* Glencoe, Ill,: Free Press.

Redl, F., and D. Wineman. (1952) *Controls from Within.* Glencoe, Ill.: Free Press.

Reid, J.H., and H.R. Hagan. (1952) *Residential Treatment of Emotionally Disturbed Children.* New York: Child Welfare League of America.

Reiser, D.E. (1963) Psychosis of infancy and early childhood, as manifested by children with atypical development. *New. Eng. J. Med.* 259:790–798, 844–850.

Rinsley, D.B. (1963) Psychiatric hospital treatment with special reference to children. *Arch. Gen. Psychiat.* 9:489–496.

Rinsley, D.B. (1965) Intensive psychiatric hospital treatment of adolescents: An object-relations view. *Psychiat. Quart.* 39:405–429.

Rinsley, D.B. (1967a) Intensive residential treatment of the adolescent. *Psychiat. Quart.* 41:134–143.

Rinsley, D.B. (1967b) The adolescent in residential treatment: Some criticl reflections. *Adolescence* 2:83–95.

Rinsley, D.B. (1971a) The Fifth Annual Edward A. Strecker Memorial Lecture: Theory and practice of intensive residential treatment of adolescents. In S.C. Feinstein, P.L. Giovacchini, and A.A. Miller, eds., *Adolescent Psychiatry,* Vol. 1. New York: Basic Books, pp. 479–509.

Rinsley, D.B. (1971b) The adolescent inpatient: Patterns of depersonification. *Psychiat. Quart.* 45:3–22.

Rinsley, D.B. (1972) A contribution to the nosology and dynamics of adolescent schizophrenia. *Psychiat. Quart.* 46:159–186.

Rinsley, D.B. (1974a) Residential treatment of adolescents. In S. Arieti, ed., *American Handbook of Psychiatry,* rev. ed., Vol. II. New York: Basic Books, pp. 353–366.

Rinsley, D.B. (1974b) Special education for adolescents in residential psychiatric treatment. In S.C. Feinstein and P.L. Giovacchini, eds., *Adolescent Psychiatry,* Vol. 3. New York: Basic Books, pp. 394–418.

Rinsley, D.B. (1977a) An object relations view of borderline personality. In P. Hartocollis, ed., *Borderline Dis-*

orders: The Concept, The Syndrome, The Patient. New York: International Universities Press, pp. 47–70.

Rinsley, D.B. (1977b) Borderline psychopathology: A review of etiology, dynamics and treatment. *Int. Rev. Psycho-Anal.* 5:45–54.

Rinsley, D.B., and D.D. Hall. (1962) Psychiatric hospital treatment of adolescents: Parental resistances as expressed in casework metaphor. *Arch. Gen. Psychiat.* 7:286–294.

Rinsley, D.B., and G.P. Inge, III. (1961) Psychiatric hospital treatment of adolescents: Verbal and nonverbal resistance to treatment. *Bull. Menninger Clinic* 25:249–263.

Robinson, J.F. (1947) Resident psychiatric treatment of children. *Am. J. Orthopsychiat.* 17:484–487.

Robinson, J.F., et al. (1957) *Psychiatric Inpatient Treatment of Children.* Washington, D.C.: American Psychiatric Association.

Rosenfeld, S., and M.P. Sprince. (1963) An attempt to formulate the meaning of the concept "borderline." *Psychoanal. Study Child* 18:603–635.

Ryan, J.H. (1962) The therapeutic value of the closed ward. *J. Nerv. Ment. Dis.* 134:256–262.

Simmel, E. (1929) Psycho-analytic treatment in a sanitarium. *Int. J. Psycho-Anal.* 10:70–89.

Spitz, R. (1971) *The First Year of Life: A Psychoanalytic Study of Normal and Deviant Development of Object Relations.* New York: International Universities Press.

Standards for Psychiatric Facilities Serving Children and Adolescents. (1971) Washington, D.C.: American Psychiatric Association.

Szasz, T.S. (1974) *The Myth of Mental Illness, rev. ed. New York: Harper & Row.*

Szurek, S.A., et al. (1971) Inpatient Care for the Psychotic Child. The Langley Porter Child Psychiatry Series, Vol. 5. Palo Alto: Science and Behavior Books.

Wardle, C.J. (1970) Report on investigation into recruitment and training for nursing staff of inpatient units for children and adolescents. Submitted to the Royal Medico-Psychological Association, London.

Wardle, C.J. (1974) Residential care of children with conduct disorders. In P. Barker, ed., *The Residential Psychiatric Treatment of Children.* New York: Wiley, pp. 48–104.

Weddell, D. (1961) Family centered nursing. *Int. Nursing Rev.* 8:20–25.

Winnicott, D.W. (1949) Mind and its relation to the psyche-soma. In *Collected Papers: Through Paediatrics to Psycho-Analysis.* New York: Basic Books (1958).

Winnicott, D.W. (1951) Transitional objects and transitional phenomena. In *Collected Papers: Through Paediatrics to Psycho-Analysis.* New York: Basic Books (1958).

Winnicott, D.W. (1960) Ego distortion in terms of true and false self. In *The Maturational Processes and the Facilitating Environment.* New York: International Universities Press (1965).

Zentner, E.B., and H.J. Aponte. (1970) The amorphous family nexus. *Psychiat. Quart.* 44:91–113.

CHAPTER 14

Residential and Inpatient Treatment

Theodore A. Petti

Introduction

A wide array of residential and hospital treatment facilities for children and adolescents exists. This includes short-term university-based inpatient units; short-term and intermediate units in psychiatric county and state hospitals; residential treatment centers; therapeutic group homes; boarding schools; residences; and juvenile detention centers. We will be limiting ourselves to short-term and intermediate psychiatric hospital and residential treatment centers. Robinson et al. (1957) define an inpatient psychiatric service for children as "a medical institution or unit of a medical institution; its function is the diagnosis and treatment in residence of children with psychiatric disorders. It provides round-the-clock treatment for children whose needs make such a regime the treatment of choice. . . ."

The short-term inpatient hospital unit as a form of residential treatment is meant to describe a university or university-affiliated service with a limited number of inpatient beds for 24-hour care provided during a 4- to 12-week period within a highly structured setting. It has high-quality clinical, educational, and research objectives, is directed by a child psychiatrist, and is dedicated to a team approach. An intermediate-length unit can be composed of a government, university or private program, not necessarily directed by a psychiatrist, but with psychiatric consultation and a goal of treating and returning the youngster back to the community within a period of three years or less. There is no typical residential treatment center and no general agreement as to what defines a residential treatment center (American Association for Children's Residential Centers, 1972; Evangelakis, 1974). Residential treatment for the chronically and severely psychotic or brain-damaged whose prognosis for future functioning in the community is minimal and where predominantly custodial care must be provided are deliberately excluded from this presentation, as are facilities for juvenile delinquents, for infants and children under six, or those specific for the mentally retarded. However, the principles enumerated in this chapter can be generalized to varying degrees for such specialized facilities.

History

The residential treatment of children and adolescents has evolved with the changes in our culture and the needs of our society. The roots of residential treatment can be traced to the common desire to help children. Orphanages, facilities for the retarded and defective, the delinquent, the emotionally disturbed, and boarding schools all have played a role in our present diverse concept of residential treatment. The first orphanage in the United States was founded in 1729 (Lewis and Solnit, 1975; Marks, 1973), and the New York House of Refuge was established in 1825 (Kahn, 1963). Dr. Howe's School for Defectives, founded in 1848 at the Perkins Institute in Boston, is felt to be the first institutional setting for retarded, disturbed children in the country (Kanner, 1964). Wolfensberger contends that institutions circa 1850 were expressly created to help a number of deviant groups in the United States become less so. The goal was to bring them together in one place so that expert and intensive attention could be used to educate them, and by a combination of decreasing his intellectual impairment and increasing more socially adaptive skills, the impaired individual could learn to function at a minimally acceptable level in society. The education "was to consist mostly of the transformation of poorly socialized, perhaps speechless, and uncontrolled children into children who could stand and walk normally, have some speech, eat in an orderly manner, and engage in some kind of meaningful work" (Wolfensberger, 1974). Hospital units for emotionally disturbed children began in the early 1920's initially for those suffering from the sequellae of epidemic encephalitis: the children's ward of the psychiatric division of Bellevue Hospital, New York; and the Franklin School of Philadelphia (Robinson et al., 1957). In his seminal work, *Wayward Youth* (1925) August Eichhorn was the first to use psychoanalytic principles in the residential treatment of so-called delinquent adolescents. The adolescent inpatient boy's unit at Bellevue Hospital in New York (Curran, 1939) was the first such facility for boys 12 to 16 years created expressly to segregate and deal with the unique problems of that age.

Sonis (1967) noted two patterns in the development of residential treatment centers. The group descended from orphanages, child care institutions and group foster homes, developed a focus emanating from the relation of disturbed behavior to the child's experience of past neglect, and has had, as a group, to move beyond the concept of love as the universal cure. Those centers evolving from the medical model needed to struggle with the need to move beyond the psychodynamics of the individual child and to use the milieu as a constructive force. Recent reviews (Barker, 1974; Rinsley, Chapter 12) have described the history of hospital and residential treatment of disturbed youth and helped place the evolution of such units into a better perspective.

Theoretical Considerations

Providing short-term intensive therapeutic and diagnostic services or therapeutic intermediate-length care in the late 1970's is costly and should be utilized in the most efficient manner. The concept of adequate secondary prevention, as enumerated by Petti (1977a), is the cornerstone for a rational and progressive use of these valuable resources. At a time when programs for care of acutely disturbed children are losing their funding or being restricted in their staffing and bed capacity (Sackin and Meyer, 1976), there needs to be movement toward expanding such services. If we value our most precious natural resource, our youth, then we must demand that every emotionally disturbed child have access to a sufficiently comprehensive evaluation in the least restricted setting that can provide the adequate services and planning necessary for the individual youth to function at least at a minimal level conducive to future growth and development. This commits society to preventing the downward spiral of moderately to severely disturbed children so poignantly described in *Deviant Children Grown Up* (Robins, 1966).

Many professional as well as lay persons view hospitalization of a child as the last resort: an alternative to be effected only when the family, school, and community can no longer tolerate the misfit; when psychotherapeutic or other interventions, no matter how well or poorly conceived, have been shown to be absolute failures; or when the child is so suicidal, destructive, or out of contact with reality that little else can be done. The decision which should be measured and deliberate to hospitalize or place the child in a residential center (Robinson et al., 1957) is frequently made in haste and often in the state of extremis.

The acute-care inpatient unit must maintain its traditional role of accepting children with acute psychiatric disorders who require a highly structured environment for both evaluation and treatment and serve as a resource for the diagnostic evaluation of children for whom outpatient facilities are inadequate. But more importantly, for children from moderately intact natural or foster homes, where the child continues to be troubled or trouble occurs even with psychotherapy and environmental manipulation, a brief hospitalization can be growth-enhancing rather than regressive or retarding.

The short-term university inpatient unit should also be a catalyst to the development of new and creative services for disturbed children, for the whole spectrum from implementation and evaluation of various treatment modalities to the support of innovative community programs. It should have its roots in the scientific rigor of clinical medicine and psychology and rest on a foundation steeped in humanitarian principles (Conners, 1977). Such a unit must be open to the needs of the region it serves, a resource for training the whole range of mental health providers to youth, and be responsible for creating an environment that will facilitate appropriate care for each child.

Who to Admit and Why

Consideration of who to admit and why is a crucial theoretical and practical issue. The types of children, problems or diagnoses, degree of psychopathologic severity, and preadmission environmental situations are so diverse in the age range of 6 to 14 years and 12 to 17 years that no one unit can handle them all, or at least all at the same time. D'Amato (1969) asserts that admission for residential treatment should be effected only for those children who need the totality of separation from their former ties in the community, special education and psychiatric treatment. The factors calling for separation include: the existence of a dangerous and destructive situation; allowance for better diagnosis; the child's need for new adaptive behaviors; and the pressing need to relieve existing pressures and allow for a restoration of family living.

Children with behavior so disturbed that other forms of treatment or care would be difficult or impossible to effect, the need for short-term removal of a child from adverse conditions, and the need for more accurate diagnosis are generally acceptable admission criteria. However, numerous workers have decried the inconsistencies in terminology and in application of criteria for residential placement (Sackin and Meyer, 1976; Maluccio and Marlow, 1972). Diagnostic labels are usually not helpful in designating the appropriateness for short term or intermediate length care. However, a recent publication has compiled the diagnoses of children and adolescents that would require admisssion for acute and intermediate care, delineated the reasons for admission, and ascribed the duration of expected length of stay and justifiable criteria for extension (Silver, 1976).

Barker (1976) argues against admitting children who have no home or a home that will remain unstable, and refers to the work of others to buttress this point (Barker, 1974). Ney and Mills (1976) will not accept a child in their intensive program who does not belong to an intact family unless those who will care for him/her post discharge will be actively involved with their staff during the hospitalization. Shaw and Lucas (1970) argue against the admission of the retarded, the psychopathic (those who lack the ability to establish a relationship), and the severely psychotic.

Contraindications to admission listed by Wardle (1974) include evidence that home and community relationships could suffer as a consequence of admission; the child's conviction that he is being put away or punished cannot be altered; or the child's antisocial behavior is specifically limited to stealing and has its roots in deprivation or neglect. Kester (1966) sees such family dynamics as relief at hospitalization and anticipated relinquishing of responsibility, parental opposition vigorously maintained in families that may need the child's presence to preserve a tenuous situation, and lack of motivation for family casework as relative contraindications to placement.

In summary, short-term hospitalization is appropriate for any child or adolescent who is in an acute state of crisis that demands a structured setting for its resolution, who is failing to benefit from existing treatments and requires a new approach which cannot be successfully initiated from an outpatient setting, or who needs an evaluation that circumstances demand be completed in a highly structured setting where degree of parental involvement can be flexibly managed.

Children who are homeless, residing in a youth shelter or a foster home where they are being rejected, or in a natural home that is falling apart, or those with brain damage or functional retardation are extremely difficult to manage, but they can benefit from short-term hospitalization if effective post discharge planning is instituted at or prior to hospitalization.

This excludes from short-term care the severely disturbed very young autistic, retarded, or brain-damaged child for whom a good diagnostic evaluation and realistic plans for longer-term residential placement can or have been completed on an outpatient basis; it also excludes the older aggressive, frequently institutionalized youth with chronic problems for whom long-term highly structured placement is the treatment of choice. It is not appropriate to use such a facility as an interim placement between a deteriorating home and longer-term placement, as a brief respite for harried parents and children on a repeated crisis basis (Sackin and Meyer, 1976), or as a shelter or a home for young delinquents.

The hue and cry regarding institutionalization of youth has mainly stemmed from unfortunate experiences with custodial-like state facilities, particularly those treating delinquent adolescents, chronic psychotic or brain-damaged children, and the mentally retarded (Weiss and Pizer, 1970).

Intermediate hospitalization or residential placement can be beneficially utilized for many of the children appropriate for short-term care, except for many of the transient situational reactions, school phobic and other reactions that generally respond to the short-term stay. Youth who require one or two years separation from their families or who need a length of time to be free of the intense involvement of foster home placement, those who may be delinquent or predelinquent with the capacity to establish a relationship and do experience anxiety or depression all would be appropriate for such a setting.

As noted by Weintrob, (1975), the acutely suicidal, homicidal, destructive, assaultive youth would be better treated in a highly structured and secure inpatient setting. Those who remain actively suicidal, disorganized, threatening, and assaultive need intermediate or long-term hospitalization. He argues for selective use of intermediate and long-term placement while asserting that a large group of adolescents could benefit from a 1- to 3-month hospitalization followed by referral to longer-term care at a residential treatment center "so that they can consolidate their newly won gains, and continue to grow and develop in a less protected, less specialized setting."

Children who fall into the triad of brain-damaged, psychotic, and retarded need special facilities that are more custodially oriented toward their basic human needs and perhaps should not be designated as therapeutic. This is especially true for the older youth who has never advanced beyond the infant stage of development. Youthful hard-core delinquents need specialized programs that fall under the rubric of residential care, but often not that of a center which takes a mixture of troubled children. There are exceptions to this rule (Alt, 1960).

Regardless of the criteria for inclusion or exclusion from a residential treatment setting, an almost inherent force seems to operate, generated by the staff and at times the children themselves, to exclude from the setting the more severely disturbed, regressed, or assaultive child in favor of the more easily treated child who will almost certainly guarantee success by any measure (Hobbs, 1975). A unit does need to have control over its own admissions (Barker, 1974) to assure that too many of certain types of children are not all resident at the same time while assuring sufficient homogeneity to form a milieu. But society must not allow such facilities to shirk their responsibilities to service the more severely disturbed children.

Patient's Rights

Once residential placement is considered, the fundamental issue involving basic rights becomes of importance. "Systems, rules, and laws in themselves will never adequately protect childrens' rights or fulfill childrens' needs. . . . children must rely on adults to speak for them" (Thies, 1976). Children's rights within any institution will ultimately depend on the adults in that setting. The trend toward institutionalization and custodial care that is so abhorred began with the very optimistic early workers in the mental health/mental retardation forefront of the late 1800's. Wolfensberger (1974) traces the later dangerous trends of isolation, enlargement, and economization to early paternalistic endeavors with the retarded. Similar trends seem to exist for the delinquent and the psychotic.

Much of the designated abuse encountered within the psychiatric setting, aside from the institutions for the retarded, delinquent, and chronically psychotic, stem from the large state hospitals (Hobbs, 1975). The decision in the celebrated case of *Bartley vs. Kremens*, heard by United States District Court for the Eastern District of Pennsylvania, asserted that minors are entitled to the protection of legal due process that may not be waived by the child's parents and are comparable to those of adults who have been involuntarily committed for hospitalization (*Bartley vs. Kremens*, 1975). This would include an unbiased hearing within 72 hours of admission, another hearing within two weeks to determine continued need for hospitalization, and appointed legal counsel to advise them of their rights. An appeal is presently before the Supreme Court, but repercussions, both positive and negative, have spread from coast to coast.

As a result of mounting pressures, many emanating from the *Bartley vs. Kremens* decision, a new mental health law went into effect in the state of Pennsylvania on September 7, 1976. Some states have passed similar legislation and others are likely to move in this direction (Beyer and Wilson, 1976). Under the new law, any person 14 years of age or older may admit himself to a psychiatric facility. Persons under 14 may be voluntarily admitted by their parents, guardian, or persons standing in loco parentis. Upon the voluntary or involuntary admission to a psychiatric facility, the parents of the under-14 child must be given and sign a written statement relating to the child's rights. The child over 14 must also be given the same opportunity. A person cannot be accepted for voluntary institutional treatment unless they or their guardians (for those under 14) have had a thorough explanation of the findings of the preliminary evaluation—specific psychopathology, proposed treatment, the types of diagnostic or therapeutic procedures in which a child may be involved and the restraints, restrictions, or medications to which the child may be subject.

The child over 14 and parents of the under 14 must be offered the opportunity to participate in the development of a treatment plan for the child that must be formulated within 72 hours. The child may withdraw or be withdrawn (for the under 14) from treatment at any time, though a request to agree to remain in the institutional setting for a specified period of up to 72 hours after requested termination of the hospitalization can be made. At admission they are asked to specify this period of time. The concept is novel yet loaded with problems, especially regarding children over 14.

Any parent, guardian, or interested person can object to the voluntary examination and treatment of the child and can file an objection in writing with the director of the facility, judge or mental health review officer. Then a hearing must be held within 72 hours by a court officer who shall determine whether the voluntary treatment is in the best interest of the child and is the least restrictive alternative available. The court appoints an attorney to represent the minor for the scheduled hearing. A controversial aspect of the law requires registry of any child or adult admitted voluntarily or involuntarily to a psychiatric facility.

Interestingly, the appointed guardian of these rights, the court, historically has been one of the chief abusers of the inappropriate use of psychiatric facilities. Though more a problem with the commitment of adolescents than children, the court has been guilty of referring children with numerous social and nonpsychiatric medical problems for psychiatric evaluation. This abuse has decreased.

The new law also creates a problem for the provision of services to the troubled child from a family in the throes of separation or divorce. Often a combination of functional and organic difficulties so clouds the issues that psychiatric inpatient intervention either of a preventive nature or for more intense diagnosis and treatment is indicated. One parent may object, usually the parent without custody, blaming the other and then interceding in interrupting the evaluation or the therapy. Or the parent with custody may be so intimidated by the possibility of the spouse interjecting criticism, blame, and condemnation that although a psychiatric hospitalization may be indicated and strongly advised, the parent with custody feels at a loss to effect this change and fears a legal battle. Visitation rights in such instances are also fraught with almost insolvable problems.

The other issue of course is what happens to the child or adolescent once hospitalization or residential treatment is effected. The Joint Commission on Accreditation of Hospitals (1974), for facilities servicing children and adolescents, has set stringent and demanding criteria regarding the rights of youth to treatment. This decreases the bind placed on the program director between choosing necessary services for the youth against the needs of the institution and staff. Thies (1976) sees a struggle between the institution and the child and enumerates the "rights to privacy, freedom of expression, choice of activities, protection from adults and peers, possession of personal items, communication with others, freedom of movement, and especially the right to treatment. . . ." as encroached upon by administrative rather than treatment decisions.

These issues are not peculiar to residential treatment (Koocher, 1976). In a society with great but limited wealth, where do we set our priorities? Is youth our number one asset, and if so, how much are we willing to underwrite services and needed research in order to assure adequate nurturing? How do we lessen the strength of the "hidden agendas" that Thies (1976) describes: the choice between survival of the program versus needs of the child for treatment; allowing the child some freedom to act up without decreasing overall services; providing each child the care he needs without depriving other children of their services?

Continuity of Services

The right to treatment in the least restrictive setting is a vital feature of delivery of mental health service. Planning for discharge should be a crucial element in the hospitalization of any child and especially for the child from a chaotic environment. Such planning should begin at or prior to the admission and must take into consideration the totality of experiences that will be beneficial and growth-enhancing at discharge. This of course includes appropriate changes for the family, foster or group home personnel, redefining the life space for the child, appropriate school placement, therapy if indicated, knowledge of the social skills necessary to succeed in the community setting, dealing with potential future problems in the environment and allotting time to help resolve issues of separation from the unit. From their review of the literature, Maluccio and Marlow (1972) conclude that the eventual outcome for the child is more significantly related to the supports and services provided for the child and family after residential care than any other set of factors. Barker (1974) notes that the short-term hospitalization is but a fraction of that individual's whole life in terms of time, but can and should play a major positive influence for shaping that life. The same is true for intermediate placement. What happens to the child immediately after placement is the initial variable determining whether the child will continue to consolidate his growth or fall prey to a hostile or nonnurturing environment. Having a definite date for discharge in mind also helps decrease the anxiety of the child and his caregivers and provides a boundary for both the acute hospitalization and the intermediate placement.

A major difference between the institutionalized and noninstitutionalized disturbed and disturbing child has been the ability of the latter child's immediate caregivers to accommodate, adaptively or pathologically, to his/her behavior (Sackin and Meyer, 1976). The home is a major environmental set of pressures exerted on the child's growth and development. Most workers expect the child ultimately to return to a home. It is the responsibility of the treatment unit to make an accurate assessment of the home situation, to identify the strengths and weaknesses, both potential and real, to determine the interaction of factors resulting in the disharmony, and to devise an approach which will ultimately allow a constructive disposition back into the community.

Approaches to achieving these goals vary with regard to institutional and philosophical tenets. Some programs require that the parents be seen as a family (Orvin, 1974), and some will advocate hospitalization of the whole family (Abroms, Fellner, and Whitaker, 1971); others require once- or twice-weekly sessions with the parents with or without the child. Programs serving a large region might see the family members regularly but infrequently, while insisting that the family be seen frequently in their community (American Association for Children's Residential Centers, 1972), and that regular communication be maintained between the local community resource and the hospital staff. Ney and Mills (1976) report a time-limited program directed toward an hypothesized disturbance within the family, which, through a variety of therapeutic modalities, strives to "initiate positive behavioral and psychological changes in the child and to provide the parents with the techniques they require to feel more successful at parenting." Many programs utilize a variety of these approaches to achieve the stated goals. It has become evident that many families require more than insight into the problems of the home (Taylor and Alpert, 1973), and the teaching of assertion and specific behavioral approaches for interacting with the child have begun to be incorporated into the inpatient work with parents.

The other equally as important aspect of family work is the need to consider the parent's reaction to the separation resulting from hospitalization (Mandelbaum, 1962; American Association for Children's Residential Centers, 1972). When the decision for hospitalization or placement in a longer-term facility is made as an act of capitulation, the feeling that all else has failed and no other choice was possible, one of several things happens. The parents may become extremely guilty and remorseful for inflicting this cruel penalty (this is especially true if they felt coerced by the school or a helping agency to that position) and may push for rapid discharge. They may feel that they have done all that is humanly possible, the child is just so "bad" or unmanageable that they, psychologically at least, give up all feelings of responsibility or involvement. They may be so ambivalent about the hospitalization that they convey this to the child, which in turn results in a series of rapid mood and behavioral shifts. The parents need to be apprised of all that is happening with the child from the decision to hospitalize through discharge and be active participants in all planning (Taylor and Alpert, 1973). Failure to involve the parents is a common factor in the failure of intermediate hospital and residential placement.

In a well-planned and implemented decision for admission, the problems of separation are present but more readily defined and workable. The parents should have less difficulty and be able to handle the short-term hospitalization and assist and implement the program for both the present and follow-up care. All these factors must be considered in planning for both admission and discharge from the hospital and determining whether the family has the resources and motivation to readmit the child to their home.

The Role of Education and the Classroom

School is the other major environmental stress for the child and often is a setting associated with failure or frustration. Learning and academic achievement are basic tasks of youth. Difficulties in the acquisition of the necessary skills to complete these tasks or emotional blocks to the effective use of native intellect and acquired skills are almost universally found in children requiring residential treatment. Most have a history of behavioral problems, to some degree related to school. Emphasis on the more traditional passive acquisition of facts and cognitive operations in learning have not been successful. The American Association for Children's Residential Centers (1972) relate impairment in the capacity to learn as predating school and secondary to early disturbances in personality development. Equally important and perhaps primary factors for many of these children are the specific developmental delays or perceptual blocks to their ability to learn. Prior to getting the child turned on to school, some very basic steps must be taken.

A very thorough psychoeducational assessment of the child's cognitive levels of intellectual functioning, achievement levels, language development, perceptual-motor and intermodal skills must be pursued, and a prescription to deal with the specific child and his assets and liabilities must be formulated prior to requesting "work" from the child in the classroom. The task is then to help the child tap his developmental thrust to learn in a manner that will be self-sustaining over time and allow maintenance of this basic motivation (Copeland, 1974). Simultaneously, the need to develop the behavioral skills necessary for functioning in the structured setting of a classroom must be achieved, and the possible conflicts experienced by the child regarding the acquisition of knowledge must be addressed. Development of realistic goals both within the residential unit and for the future must be pursued (Solow, 1974; Forness and Langdon, 1974).

It is imperative that prior experiences in school be considered in overall planning, that previous school data regarding past behavior and performance be obtained, and a liaison established with the school setting where the child will be enrolled so that a viable program that begins in the residential setting can be coordinated into a smooth transition to the community (Nichtern, 1974).

The school is not an isolated component in the hospital setting (Evangelakis, 1974) and must be integrated into the overall care plan for the child. The teachers or special educators should have considerable input into diagnostic, therapeutic, and dispositional procedures (King, 1974; Alt, 1960; Petti, 1977a). They should be at the forefront of developing, evaluating, or implementing new methods of teaching and assessment, and training students in both traditional and innovative methodologies and in providing guidance for nonschool activities (Krueger, 1977).

The Therapeutic Milieu

Thus far, the theoretical underpinnings of a therapeutic institution have been described. All is for nought without a therapeutic milieu within which it can all take place. This concept is considered in great detail in Chapter 12 by Rinsley. It is crucial that a therapeutic milieu be established if the goals of hospitalization or residential care are to be accomplished. A constant form of negative pressure exerts itself in terms of providing for the needs of the staff rather than for those of the children (Hobbs, 1975); this issue must be addressed and resolved repeatedly to allow maintenance of the growth enhancing environment.

A succinct ascribable statement regarding this concept has been formulated by the American Association for Children's Residential Centers (1972):

> An environment that is therapeutic can be the consequence only of a conscious and planned use of time, space, people, and interpersonal relationships. In respect to the magnitude of the tasks expected of them, basic elements of a therapeutic milieu may at first seem remarkably few in number and disconcertingly simple in concept. There are three: people, things, and culture-ways. Melding these elements by intent rather than accident, while allowing for improvisation; using them knowingly rather than innocently; applying them differentially in the service now of individualization and then of system maintenance, calls for high levels of professional sophistication and craftsmanship.

Most workers (D'Amato, 1969; Evangelakis, 1974) cite the presence of stability, flexibility of staff and program, cohesiveness of staff, goal-directedness, and openness as necessary conditions for effective operation. Both hospitalization (Orvin, 1974) and residential treatment (American Association for

Children's Residential Centers, 1972) are considered habilitative rather than rehabilitative. All therapeutic goals are direcly dependent upon the therapeutic milieu for their successful completion. Models for hospital and residential care have been reviewed (Barker, 1974; Orvin, 1974), and all have a setting in which they can be most effective. Rinsley cites these various models and provides an in-depth view (Rinsley, Chapter 12).

It is imperative given the short period of involvement with the child that maximum benefit be derived from that experience and for the workers involved. Every individual involved with direct patient care must not only serve as a consistent, flexible person for the child and his/her parents, but must also of necessity function as a reliable observer and collector of clinical data so that cogent and relevant clinical decisions can be formulated and implemented. In an institution devoted to training, each of those individuals must also serve as a role model, teacher and supervisor, for students and trainees. The requirement for noncustodial oriented personnel is perhaps more compelling for an acute-care facility than for longer-term placements. However, it is becoming more clear that professionalization of child care staff will be more of an imperative for all child therapeutic services in the future (Foster et al., 1972). The children will receive what we as a society are willing to pay for!

The unionization of nonprofessional and professional staff is now becoming a regular occurrence for residential facilities. On the positive side, this means an upgrading, at least in salaries, benefits, and possible working conditions for the child care workers. It is an impetus to upgrading the positions and a potential force for movement away from custodial care. The negative aspects are the adversary role artificially created between those making administratively clinical decisions and those making the on-line clinical decision. The system becomes rigid regarding flexibility of hours, duties, etc., with a potentially regressive move toward more, rather than less, institutionalization of these vital children's services. The program director is frequently caught between his own needs to be open with his staff and the concepts of unfair practices and "grievable behaviors" regarding the discussion of some basic clinical issues. The unions paradoxically become a force for stagnation. The flexibility of a program can be drastically curtailed if union leadership has a hidden agenda for maintaining the status quo. On the other hand, a progressive union has and can provide a positive form of leadership in assuring quality programming, growth, and the opportunity to develop for its members while protecting their reasonable interests.

Accountability

With increasing services and rising personnel and overhead costs for residential programs, greater pressures can be expected from various third-party payers for some degree of accountability (Herstein, 1975). Moreover, with the relative paucity of short-term hospital beds and openings in residential centers compared to the overall need, it behooves such facilities to monitor objectively the child's course in the residential setting and after discharge. Maluccio and Marlow (1972) note the dearth of such endeavors and conclude from their review that "there is no conclusive evidence on the effectiveness of residential treatment." It is imperative for the residential unit to assess progress and outcome of treatment from a multifaceted approach (Conners and Delamater, 1976). This includes both global assessment and individual item analysis, monitoring of short- and long-term goals, evaluation of changes in the family, behavioral and achievement progress in school, and changes in behavior and attitude necessary for successful community placement. Systematic direct observation of behaviors for clinical, training, and research goals should be a prerequisite for certification of a short-term unit. "It [direct observation] is an inescapable requirement in any child-oriented work . . ." (D'Amato, 1969). The difficulties inherent in such an evaluation are enumerated by Herstein (1975), who notes that "evaluation methods should be geared to specific clients, goals, goal attainments, periods of time and treatment modalities."

This of course is more critical for the short-term diagnostic and treatment unit than the longer-term facility. Attempts have been made in the past to incorporate such a system in the longer-term facilities, but have suffered from methodological flaws (Shaw and Lucas, 1970). More recently, Davis (1976) describes the evolving system at Children's Village, a residential treatment center for boys, and discusses how the data can be utilized for assessing changes in the organization, impact of particular types of treatments for certain types of children as well as for agency-wide planning. He also relates how such data when fed back to the staff can enhance the efficacy of treatment. Millman and Schaefer (1975) elaborate on how such a system of data collecting and feedback can enhance the efficiency in responding to the needs of small groups of children and the need for computer technology (Pancost and Millman, 1975) to deal in a meaningful manner with the complex, voluminous data. Similar programs with systematic collection of data and feedback to the staff has been described for a research unit for disturbed children (Monkman, 1972) and for a clinical residential unit for adolescent girls (Johnson et al., 1976).

The Program

The Nonhuman Environment

The following section will consider the components of a residential unit: setting, physical facilities, staff composition, back-up service, and daily functioning. The variability in such features between residential programs is as great as the variety of children they serve and purposes they have established. Theoretical and actual detailed descriptions of such programs are available (Robinson et al., 1957; Reid and Hagan, 1952; Monkman, 1972; Taylor and Alpert, 1973; Evangelakis, 1974; Barker, 1974; Rees, 1974; Rinsley, this book; Alt, 1960; Rogers, 1965; Garber, 1972; Allerhand, Weber, and Haug, 1966; Ahnsjo, 1969).

A short-term unit will serve as an example of residential placement and depict one approach to meeting the objectives described earlier. There is no unique setting peculiar to such a unit, and much depends on specific objectives, population served, location of related services, etc. It is important that it be accessible to the families of children it serves. Location in or proximal to an urban area is more favorable than in an isolated rural area; most community agencies, ancillary services, and children referred to such centers come from urban areas. Detailed accounts of the various factors that should help determine the setting are available (Robinson et al., 1957; Barker, 1974; Joint Commission on Accreditation of Hospitals, 1974). "The nonhuman environment—architecture, building layout, space, trees, landscaping, color and decorating artifacts—is also of strategic therapeutic importance" (American Association for Children's Residential Centers, 1972).

Such units can exist in a variety of settings. In Pittsburgh and many other large urban areas, the child and adolescent units are located within psychiatric hospitals. Space apportioned for sleeping quarters and corridors have minimal state requirements for size. A lounge area is necessary to provide living space for the children and an easily observable area for the staff collection of behavioral data. An area for family-style eating can be located on or off the unit. It should have a definite structure with tables arranged so that small groups of children and staff can be seated together. Colors are noninstitutional, and the children are encouraged to personalize their rooms with posters, artwork, projects completed in O.T. or school, snapshots, and other objects from home. The unit should have warm and pleasing architectural features with adequate lighting.

Rooms for play therapy, interviewing parents or patients and for one-to-one remedial reading or teaching are necessary as is a room set up for videotaping with the capacity for rapid feedback to child, therapist, or parents. A group snack area should also be provided, particularly if eating facilities are located elsewhere.

An area for staff to convene for conferences and for small treatment, team, or problem-oriented groups, an area for the medical records secretary, ward clerk, and program secretaries should be sufficiently isolated to allow for pleasant, nondistracting working conditions. A treatment examining room with medicine cabinet, first-aid equipment, and emergency cart should be present in any residential treatment facility. Office space for professional staff to prepare materials and formulate care plans is crucial. Certain members of the team—social workers, head nurse, psychologist, and director—need private rooms with phones due to the nature of their functions. Cubicles that afford privacy should be provided for the educators, research assistants, and trainees.

Classrooms should maximally accommodate 6 to 8 children. For 9 or more children, two classrooms are essential. One can be arranged in a manner similar to that of a nonhospital school with individual desks, study carrels, and learning centers. Seating arrangements should be regular to assist in establishing consistency of expectations. The learning centers consist of visual-auditory-kinesthetic equipment such as language masters, tape recorders, statistiscope, tachistoscope, form felt boards and chalk boards, abacus, counting sticks, sandpaper alphabet, and raised number clocks. An observation room for viewing the teaching and for collecting observation data is a necessity. Sufficient space should be allotted to permit the teacher, teaching assistants, or trainees to move freely and to be readily accessible to the children. The wall space should provide a listing of expected behaviors that are presented in positive terms, posters and materials to orient the child to the wider world, and opportunities to display completed work.

The second classroom can be similar to the first or be designed as a group room. Tables are utilized rather than desks to allow more flexible seating arrangements, peer tutoring, and individual or small-group instruction to occur. Activities such as flash-card review, spelling bees, phonetic review of words, math games, work at the blackboard, oral reading, verbal and written language review, and fine motor/gross motor games should be available. Both classrooms should provide the child with a sense of positive achievement, positive expectations, and positive consequation of appropriate and adaptive behaviors. A system should be available to signal the teacher regarding completion of the work, or difficulty in the assignment contingency that would normally result in a striving for the adult's attention—e.g. a system of red flag/ green flag to signal such a need has been developed to ameliorate these problems (Trapasso, 1977).

Other essential facilities include a gym area that is sufficiently large to allow for kickball, basketball, and indoor baseball; an area for occupational and recreational therapy including facilities for weaving, woodworking, pottery, artwork as well as ping-pong, pool, and dancing. Provision must be made for getting out into the community—for plays, social events, museums, and special programs. Facilities in urban settings must offer the opportunity to go to parks and beaches. Swimming is a cherished event. A van or small bus is useful. An outdoor patio area and greenhouse are welcome additions to most facilities.

The Staff

It is people that allow a program to function. The ideal grouping of ward staff would provide the greatest degree of growth with the least amount of regression and pain (for both patients and staff). The problem ensues when balancing the ideal versus the reality of limited funding. For a 12-bed unit, which can also serve one or two day patients and is committed to providing optimal clinical care, meaningful quality research, and training while maintaining a rewarding enough working environment to retain competent and motivated staff, the following staffing requirement is practical, though costly.

The director of a child or adolescent hospital unit should preferably be a child psychiatrist or a general psychiatrist with special training in adolescent work. A psychiatrist has the needed credentials to move within the hospital setting, has had rigorous training, and is steeped in the medical ethic. Such facilities have functioned in a highly accredited manner directed by nonmedical personnel (e.g. psychologists, social workers, and nurses) with the consultation of trained psychiatrists. Few directors can meet the qualifications set for the "power parent," the individual who must be a strong integrator for the interdisciplinary approach, a leader for the staff, and a persuasive interpreter of the program to other components of the mental health system and the community as a whole. "The qualities of foresight, compassion, courage, patience, militancy, and judgment must be outstanding parts of his personality" (Mayer, 1958). He must not take himself so seriously that he loses sight of his need to help the children, the staff, the trainees, and him/herself to grow. It should be a person who can accept criticism without perceiving an attack and whose use of power is tempered by a sense of responsibility. Empire-building is self-defeating and destructive to programming for growth (Grace, 1974). The individual must be as at ease with children and parents as with staff and trainees, should be accessible without fostering dependence, and should be willing to serve as a positive role model. The director must be flexible, be adaptable to rapidly changing situations, be empathic to the needs of others and be firm and decisive when needed. He must know the children, have regular contact with them, and be an active participant in their care. Prior administrative experience in formulating and implementing meaningful policies and decisions should be required.

An assistant director is necessary for smooth functioning of a complex unit. Training in child or adolescent psychiatry is not as necessary for this position, which predominantly coordinates the therapeutic interventions, data collection, assists in the supervision of staff and trainees, coordinates in-service training, and assists the director in implementing the ward policies. The individual must share similar views regarding evaluation and treatment, be assertive and capable of supporting those views, yet feel free to express divergent opinions in an appropriate manner. A clinical psychologist, research social worker, or nurse clinician with research training who has a background in working with children or adolescents would be suited for such a position.

A head nurse, preferably with a baccalaureate degree, experience as a staff nurse, special orientation to children with administrative and interpersonal skills is a key factor in the functioning of a unit. This person, traditionally female, interfaces with all levels of staffing and must be adroit at the implementation of principles and directives into concrete tasks set by the staff. The role is arduous, since the program director sets expectations for performance and changes in policy and the staff seek her aid in reducing the level of change, altering workloads, etc., while fellow professionals (teachers, occupational therapists, researchers, trainees) make other requests. The person must be goal-oriented yet flexible, have a sense of humor, be able to tolerate constantly being in the hot seat, be supportive of young nursing staff, and serve as a positive role model and "mother" for the unit (that might be a problem should that position be filled by a male). In many respects, that individual must have many of the attributes of the director, since the relationship with nursing and administrative personnel is very similar to the director's. The person must share the overall programatic philosophy of the director and be able to work cooperatively and enjoy open communication with that person. The capability to delegate and use authority in an equitable manner is a critical asset.

The head nurse coordinates, guides, and directs the nursing regimen for the ward and oversees the maintenance of nursing functioning, care plans, and progress notes. Assessment of nursing staff function, and suggestion or implementation of program changes that encourage smoother, more efficient and effective operation of the unit are routine responsibilities. He/she also conducts regular conferences to improve patient care and promote staff development, is actively involved in research protocols and in work with parents.

The child psychiatrist or psychologist who functions as the primary therapist can be a staff person or a trainee who is closely supervised by the director or assistant director. The therapist is responsible for integrating the various facets of the individual case and in developing the care plan, overseeing the medical care (psychiatrist), and serving as the child's advocate. The primary task is to understand how this may be used to assist the child toward healthier growth and development in the future. Training and experience in child development, group and individual dynamics and a positive regard for children are essential.

The senior social worker is the main liaison between the referring agencies, the parents, and the unit, is an integral member of the therapeutic team and assumes a variety of responsibilities ranging from intensive work with parents, supervising dispositional planning, doing the initial screening of referrals, supervising and coordinating family work and formally and informally offering supervision and support to trainees and staff. This person, who should have A.C.S.W. certification and prior experience in working with families of disturbed children, participates in all staffings or supervises those who represent the family work component. The senior social worker must have a solid fund of knowledge and understanding of psychopathology, family dynamics, systems theories, social and psychological factors related to dysfunction in children and families, group dynamics and process, and of the mental health care delivery system within the region of service commitment. This person must meet all the requirements for a senior social worker in any of the other treatment modalities for children plus be flexible in approach, be able to work in a true team setting, and be tolerant of ambiguity, constantly changing priorities, procedures and staff.

A second social worker or case aide with at least a baccalaureate degree in social work is necessary for an acute-care facility serving more than 10 children. This worker must be highly motivated, be able to work with families and work in a team setting. He/she would share responsibility for the family work, participation in advisory groups for ward policy, and in follow-up evaluations of children discharged form the hospital. Such a person would also be required in an intermediate or residential setting, since so much family work and planning is necessary to help the child make the transition to the community.

The school psychologist is another key member in the short term unit. A master's degree in educational psychology, a commitment to helping learning-disabled children and children with psychological blocks to learning, a high energy level and motivation to develop and evaluate innovative approaches to assessment and treatment of such disorders are necessary qualifications. It is essential that this individual have a solid grounding in both traditional and contemporary approaches to school-related disorders, familiarity with the most recent literature, and a genuine thrust to learn. He/she must have a good working knowledge of the educational system and its functioning at all levels, experience in the classroom, and the facility to communicate meaningfully with teachers and consultants in the fields of language and speech, reading, child care/child development, special education, and other related specialties.

This job is a combination of multiple integrating functions: the psychometric multifaceted evaluation of cognitive, achievement and intellectual functioning of the child; development of an individualized teaching prescription for each child which is extended to games, activities, and trips during nonschool times; supervising the collection of data regarding preadmission functioning; supervising the implementation of the psychoeducational prescription; supervising the continuing education of the teaching staff, assistants and trainees; supervising the smooth transition to the community or residential school; supervising the follow-up to ascertain how the child is functioning after a month, three months, six months, and one year; and assist in coordinating programs involving the overall milieu, the classroom and leisure time. Such a role in the longer-term units may not have the same order of importance since assessments would be less frequent, the educational component would generally be larger requiring a master teacher or principal, and many of the nonschool-related activities would be coordinated by clinical psychologists.

The teacher, preferably one teacher and one educational aide or assistant for six children, should be certified at the master's or bachelor's level in special education of learning-disabled and emotionally disturbed children. The personal qualities of flexibility, humor, high energy level and good interpersonal skills as well as high motivation to help children and participate in innovative programs and their assessment are crucial. The teachers must be willing and able to move out of the sheltered environment of the classroom and into the ward and its extensions to help implement the individualized psychoeducational prescription for each child. The teachers and teacher's aides must also be physically able to participate in gym, recreational and sports activities and to work with other professionals in making institutional care a meaningful activity. In longer-term facilities, teachers with special skills in horticulture, physical, educational, occupational, vocational, and recreational therapy are needed.

The nurses and child care workers as a group have the most sustained relationship with the children regarding duration and intensity of interaction. Their backgrounds, experiences, and training are quite different. Nurses need to be registered and should have some experience with children. Like physicians, they are trained in the medical tradition and are oriented to treating disease. They oversee the implementation of care plans, and their role is continuing to evolve from carrying out the doctors' orders to formulating care plan objectives, involvement with research, systematic collection of clinical data, and participating in the classroom, while maintaining their traditional role of giving medication, preparing children for procedures, overseeing activities of daily living and performing such procedures as first aid, audiograms, and escorting children for procedures. The ability to lead and supervise other personnel and grounding in the medical tradition in part distinguishes their role from the child care worker. The nurse's role is more important in the hospital than in the residential treatment center.

The child care worker should be a professional or preprofessional person who has had solid training in normal and abnormal child development, is motivated to learn more about the development and care of disturbed children, and who can provide an adequate role model for the children, students, and trainees. The requirement of a baccalaureate degree in child care/child development or a degree in a related field with experience is essential to assure quality. The child care worker's role has increased importance in a nonhospital, longer-term setting.

Both nurses and child care workers are on the front line in the delivery of mental health care in the institutional setting. Both need to have the experience or training necessary to allow them to have a level of reasonable expectancy commensurate with the child's psychosocial and cognitive ability; they must be able to work constructively with the child in the structured school and relatively unstructured leisure-time settings. As the primary providers of care, they must be aware of and empathic to the needs of the child, be knowledgeable objective observers and collectors of clinical data, demonstrate the ability to form constructively meaningful relations with the children and act as a catalyst in assisting the children to interact with one another in an adaptive and positive manner. They must be motivated and able to provide ongoing treatment through the media of the milieu, contribute to ward policy-making, and interpret the child's behavior to parenting adults and assist them in accepting and helping to change their child's behavior.

The attributes and qualities essential for all staff that have direct and primary care responsibilities—teachers, nurses, child care workers—include the following: the maturity to accept fully the concept that the program exists to help the child, not to provide for the staff's needs; a clear sense of their own individual identity and of their professional identity as members of a helping profession; competency and skill in implementing a comprehensive care plan; a genuine positive regard for children; ability to empathize with a child or fellow staff member's needs without becoming overinvolved in a nontherapeutic manner; emotional stability; flexibility, adaptability; ability to set firm, consistent nonpunitive limits; ability to accept constructive criticism and a desire to grow within the program; honesty tempered by tactfulness; ability to work toward a cohesive integration of individual, group, and program goals; ability to serve as a positive role model; leadership capabilities and good interpersonal skills; physical fitness sufficient to be involved in all activities; ability to work with parents; and self-control over the natural proclivity to overpossessiveness. Such an individual must also be capable and motivated to serve as a child advocate and constructively challenge the system and to be curious and involved in attempts to learn more about childhood disorders and their treatment. The qualifications are of course idealized, and it is the rare person who can meet all of them; however, the goal should be to recruit personnel who at least have the potential to meet these criteria and who are unlikely to get burned out in the process of working on an intensive care unit or in a more residential center.

Those employed in acute care facilities must be self-starters who can tolerate repeated frustrations and rapid turnover of children and staff and can make rapid professional decisions. Those employed in the intermediate and long-term facilities have less need for those attributes and a greater need for group management skills and a tolerance for less structure. More detailed descriptions of the attributes, qualities, and qualifications for such workers abound in the literature (Adler, 1976, Mayer, 1958; Brown et al., 1974; American Association for Children's Residential Centers, 1972; Barker, 1974; Foster et al., 1972). For a 12-bed unit, a minimum of 8 nurses, 8 child care workers and 4 members of the teaching staff are required. Fewer personnel would be required for the longer-term facilities.

Support Facilities

Support facilities are critical for the short-term unit and important for the longer-term facilities. The back-up of a comprehensive university medical center is essential for the functioning of a unit described above. This includes: radiologic services (for computerized axial tomography, chest and skull x-rays, and brain scans); a full complement of pediatric services (emergency room; complete ophthalmologic, audiologic, and dental departments; and specialized clinics); sophisticated laboratory facilities (special diagnostic studies, serum drug levels for anticonvulsant and psychopharmacologic agents, EEGs, all-night sleep EEGs, psychophysiologic studies, etc.); education facilities and expertise in related fields (special education, psychology, language and speech, child care and child development, art therapy, etc.), and the resources of a broad-based department of psychiatry and child psychiatry. Board certified pediatricians should be on 24-hour call and be routinely involved in seeing the children or adolescents.

Nature of the Interventions

Different psychiatric units are structured along the prevalent philosophical lines of the director and are determined by their designated functions. A unit that is designed for evaluation and intensive short-term treatment might use the following approaches in terms of general categories:

- Preadmission evaluation
- Admission procedures
- Intake conference
- The first two weeks
- Diagnostic conference
- The second two weeks
- Treatment conference
- Time to discharge
- Disposition conference
- Follow-up
- Community relations

Preadmission Evaluation

A clear definition of inclusion and exclusion criteria must be available for referral agencies with guidelines regarding intake and screening procedures. The social worker should be the person who receives the referral material, matches the clinical picture presented with set admission criteria, consults with the director about the appropriateness of placement, and promptly gives a response. In cases involving special management problems, other members of the team—psychologist and head nurse—are involved in the decision. A preadmission evaluation of the child that would consist of a psychiatric, psychologic, and psychosocial assessment is ideal so that early formulation of target behaviors and specific interventions can be accomplished (Ney and Mills, 1976). The child and his care givers should have the opportunity to visit the unit to help ameliorate the anticipatory anxiety. Release of information from previous professional involvements should be obtained so that pertinent past and present history can be assembled.

A financial assessment is obtained to determine any limitations so that prompt additional funding can be sought. The primary therapist presents the parent or guardian with a written statement related to the child's rights, a thorough explanation of the preliminary examination, the proposed treatment, type of diagnostic or therapeutic procedures to expect, the restraints or restrictions that might occur (e.g., time out from reinforcement; need for a quiet room; possibility of locked seclusion for uncontrolled behavior; locked ward setting) and describes general ward policy. The caregivers are urged to give 72 hours notice prior to removal of the child from the program and are asked to sign a waiver requesting a copy of the form not be sent to the local mental health unit if they prefer privacy of information. They also are informed that the child may be involved in a research protocol, and their permission with informed consent might be requested, though this is generally not a condition of admission.

Admission Procedures

The child is escorted to the unit, meets the other children, is introduced to the ward policy, gets settled in his room, has a physical exam by a psychiatrist or pediatrician; vital signs are taken by a nurse, and a determination of preferences regarding foods, activities, etc., is made. The mother is seen by a staff nurse to obtain a detailed nursing history and by the social worker for a more intensive psychosocial history. Both mother and father should complete some standardized form indicating problematic behaviors—e.g. the Deviant Behavior Inventory (Novick et al., 1966), which gives a detailed assessment of deviant behavior, or the Langner Scales which provide similar material (Langner et al., 1976). The parents are given a brochure describing the unit, scheduling, telephone numbers, visiting hours and regulations, and routine appointments are set up with the social worker.

The child is observed during designated times by the child care workers and nurses who score standardized inventories—e.g., Children's Behavior Inventory (CBI) of Burdock and Hardesty (1964); direct observations of target behaviors (Conners and Delamater, 1976); or specialized scales—e.g., the Scale of School Age Depression (SoSAD), since so many of these children are depressed (Petti, 1977b). Reliability observations are done by research aides or specially trained child care staff.

Intake Conference

Within 72 hours, a conference is held and attended by the team: a staff psychiatrist, the primary therapist, educational staff, nursing staff, social workers, and trainees. There is a review of materials available on admission and assessment of what procedures need to be completed before the diagnostic conference, collaboration of the interdisciplinary team for a more rapid complete assessment, development of detailed initial care plans involving target behaviors for observation and intervention and delineation of work anticipated with the family, in the school, and with outside agencies. Dates are set for future conferences, accountability is established regarding treatment and areas of responsibility, and long- and short-term goals and expected length of time for achievement of these goals are stipulated.

The First Two Weeks

During this period of time a child's behavioral and social skills are assessed by a psychologist and ward personnel. The psychoeducational battery is completed to determine specific learning disabilities that are present, and then to write a psychoeducational prescription according to the specific strengths and needs of the child. The test battery might profitably consist of the WISC-R, WRAT, Bender-Gestalt, Beery DVMI, Siverolli, Wepman, Boehm Test of Basic Concepts (between K and 2nd grade), Draw a Person, and Key Math Tests. Optional studies diagnostically indicated include the Peabody Picture Vocabulary Test, Frostig Developmental Test of Visual Perception, Doren Test of Word Recognition, and Slingerland Tests for Language Disability. A nurse completes an audiogram and further audiologic examination would require more specialized expertise. The school psychologist, in conjunction with the teachers, develops an individualized prescription that is monitored from week to week regarding its utility. In the classroom the teaching plan is updated daily in conjunction with the prescription. This can be done weekly in an intermediate setting.

On the unit the various observational measures are collected, staff develop subjective opinions concerning the assets and liabilities of each child, parent interactions are observed following the first week of admission, activities of daily living are assessed, and the staff actively encourages appropriate peer interactions and group involvement. The family worker continues to collect past data regarding both the family and the child and begins moving in the direction of dealing with current and future problems. The family is assessed for its needs for parent effectiveness training and behavioral skills in helping their child interact in a more socially appropriate manner and allowing the maximum amount of growth and development within the home setting. If such training is needed, an assessment interview with a therapist(s) is conducted and a contract established between the parent, the child, and the therapist regarding specific interventions. This is conducted using a model similar to that employed by Hanf (1970), and modified by Forehand and co-workers (Forehand and King, 1977), which uses videotaping and videotape feedback for both the child and the parent.

A prescribed schedule that is available to the children and staff provides a framework of consistency. Evangelakis (1974) and Wardle (1974) provide examples of scheduling which allots reasonable time for eating, school and leisure time, planned recreational activities, group activities, and individual or group psychotherapy.

Eating is done as family-style breakfast, lunch, or dinner where the children help staff set up for the whole group and may assist the care workers to serve. Class sessions are 45 minutes to an hour in duration and alternate between two classrooms, gym, occupational therapy, creative dramatics, swimming, the library, and other activities. Completing a comprehensive psychoeducational assessment, turning the child back on to school, and teaching the child the basic social behaviors and learning skills necessary for successful participation in the school setting are major interventions for the short-term unit. The longer-term units should have a stronger remedial function, though both processes are interdependent.

The child also begins his/her involvement with the primary therapist and child care worker. The form of this intervention is dependent on the needs of the child and the theoretical orientation of the therapist (Rinsley, Chapter 12; American Association for Children's Residential Centers, 1972). In dynamically oriented therapy, the goal for the short-term stay is to derive an understanding of the psychodynamics, provide support, and when indicated, help prepare the child for a longer-term therapeutic relationship; that for the longer-term unit is for developing a relationship similar to that of the outpatient or day hospital facility. Behavioral approaches are similar to those used in other settings and include overcorrection (Calpin and Hertweck, 1977), social skills training (Bornstein, Bellack, and Hersen, 1977; Bornstein, 1976; Petti et al., 1977c), response cost and contingent reinforcement (Monkman, 1972), and the use of biofeedback (Delamater et al., 1977). The correct selection of appropriate behavioral techniques is well researched and should follow available data (O'Leary and Wilson, 1975).

Diagnostic Conference

Ward observations are discussed by the child's nurse and child care worker, who detail the child's level of functioning, quality of peer interactions, relationship to staff, and effects of interventions and are followed by presentation of systematically collected observational data. Feedback by a research assistant detailing the staff's response to the child's adaptive and nonadaptive behavior is important in order to maintain behaviorally sound staff reactions (Conners and Delamater, 1976). Psychoeducational projective data and the complete psychosocial history are presented followed by the medical and psychiatric assessments. A diagnosis is formulated, the dynamics are discussed and the care plan, short- and long-term goals are reassessed and updated. Generally at this time, the indications for psychopharmacologic, biofeedback, specific behavioral, or other intervention are discussed for implementation. Plans for disposition and discharge date become more concrete. Involved professionals from the community are requested to attend and participate in all the conferences.

The Second Two Weeks

Implementation of the care plan, intensive therapy, outings with the family, and a dialogue with agencies and personnel who will be involved with the child in terms of return to the community or active seeking for other placement continue or are initiated during this period. Social skills achievement are assessed by ward evaluations and in creative dramatics. Specific therapeutic interventions and movement in the school setting concerning development of better learning skills are constantly monitored and the care plan interventions revised as needed.

Treatment Conference

Update of the situation. Discharge date set. Revision of care plan and evaluation of success in achievement of short- and long-term goals.

Time to Discharge

Continue to implement care plan. Prepare child, family, and the community for discharge.

Disposition Conference

Summarize the hospital stay. Assess degree of success in achieving long and short term goals. Define the prognosis, set a date for follow-up at six months and 12 months, and redefine long- and short-term goals. Assign responsibility for assuring that summaries reach the appropriate agencies.

Follow-up

Supervised by the assistant director. The parents sort the DBI, are interviewed by a senior ward person and are observed in their interaction with the child. The child is interviewed by a psychiatrist or psychologist, who completes a standardized assessment and dictates a narrative summary. If possible, the child is engaged in free play with the other children and is observed in interaction with the parents. A Draw a Person, WRAT, and Beery DVMI are also obtained.

The Goals of Residential Treatment

The goals of short-term hospitalization are to provide a comprehensive evaluation that can be meaningfully used by the child, parents, and involved professionals and sufficient therapeutic assistance to prepare the child for life outside a highly structured setting at the earliest feasible time (Petti, 1977a)—which might include intermediate care as a transition. Treatment goals should be geared to alleviating perceived distress, decreasing disturbing behavior, assisting with the overt and covert problems present on admission, providing a break in the vicious cycle of negatives captivating the child, his family and the community, and helping the child return to a state of mind and body that will permit more normal social, psychologic and cognitive maturation. Short-term care should have short-term results, and any long-term results are dependent on family, biological, social, and educational factors operating on the child (Barker, 1974; Herstein, 1975), and the task of treatment is integrating the intensive experience of the hospitalization into a comprehensive and long-term plan for the child. This can best be achieved by "carefully delineated treatments *specific* to the conditions involved, not simply general caretaking procedures—however well motivated and humane the caretakers. Careful, accurate, and detailed observations of the child's cognitive, social, self-care, and adaptive skills must be followed by precisely directed interventions which are documented and altered according to the results obtained in the individual case" (Conners and Delamater, 1976).

The inpatient unit offers hope to the child and his caregivers, and this can be therapeutically utilized when achieved gains, validated by the staff through objective standardized measures (CBI, SoSAD, direct observations, physiological data, improvement in cognitive skills, changed attitude toward school, and improved family interactions) are presented to the child and family prior to discharge. The follow-up evaluation should offer another form of assessment and feedback regarding the maintenance of goals.

The goals for intermediate residential care are generally less intensive but more extensive as they strive for longer-lasting, more global changes in the child and family. Their objective is to consolidate the therapeutic gains as the youth moves back into the community (Allerhand, Weber, and Haug, 1966; Garber, 1972). Both short- and long-term facilities have the responsibility to anticipate problems with a high probability of occurrence, to coordinate treatment and planning efforts, to minimize the difficulties and maximize the growth potential, and to facilitate a smooth transition into the community (Taylor and Alpert, 1973).

Comparison to Other Modalities

Short-term intensive evaluation and treatment is a very expensive proposition and its cost/benefit ratio compared to similar delivery of the service outlined above in conjunction with outpatient, day-hospital, foster or community group home, intermediate- or long-term residential treatment or any combination of the above has not been determined. Winsberg et al. (1976) described a comparison between intensive therapeutic community involvement versus short- to intermediate-term hospital care of children from the lowest socioeconomic levels who were described as "aggressive, hyperactive, impulse ridden, assaultive and destructive . . . [who] had been identified as unmanageable in the home and/or school." All children were admitted to a large county hospital's child psychiatry unit, spent one to two weeks having their medication stabilized, and were then randomly assigned to either group. The Winsberg group using standardized criteria found that such children may be as effectively treated in the community setting as in the hospital with a multifold difference in cost. The limitation of the study is the skewed population sample and the relative lack of resources a county hospital has at its disposal for the adequate treatment and evaluation of such children. The authors also raise the issue directed to the readiness of the community to implement such an innovative program.

Barker (1974) notes a major problem in comparing the effectiveness or desirability of inpatient care: aims of treatment vary according to the child; prognosis without residential care is difficult to assess; delineating contributors to change between the hospitalization itself and other forms of care prior to and after hospitalization; nature of hospital care varies from unit to unit and sometimes within the same unit. What he considers possibly the main aim, "relief for the community rather than radical care of the child's disorder" may be a unique feature of the hospital.

Weintrob (1975) suggests that acute hospitalization is the treatment of choice for some disturbed adolescents and bemoans the dearth of such facilities. Gralnick (1968) argues that the older adolescent 14 and up can be beneficially treated within an adult treatment program of a general hospital. Barish (1968) in response states that special programming devoted to the psychological and educational needs of the adolescent can only be accomplished within a special unit. He touches on the two crucial advantages that only a hospital environment can provide: (1) a 24-hour therapeutic environment, and (2) the ability to offer any variety of treatment modalities, singly or in combination with relatively high degrees of coordination and controlled conditions with the integrating influence of a "single frame of reference." Garber (1972) offers similar arguments for separate adolescent facilities.

Weiss and Pizer (1970) suggest that outpatient is preferable to inpatient treatment because the latter leaves the stigma of a label that can preclude the individual from later obtaining optimal education, employment, choice for marriage and military service. Weintrob (1975) echoes these sentiments comparing hospitalization and residential treatment. These arguments are spurious, since the assertions mainly apply to state hospitalization or juvenile detention. Morever, repeated frustrations from programs that elicit hope but fail to provide results are more destructive than all the potentially stigmatizing effects of inpatient or residential care.

Maluccio and Marlow (1972) review alternatives to residential treatment, most of which relate to facilities for intermediate type care: day treatment centers combining services with education; the innovative use of existing child guidance facilities with psychotic children and therapeutic nursery school programs. Many of these programs are not funded by third-party payers and depend on special grants for effective operation.

The short-term inpatient hospitalization is unique in that it offers the opportunity to closely observe the child totally apart from the noxious environment which he/she may have helped create, and to carefully and scientifically assess the degree of health, pathology and responses to specific interventions. The intermediate facilities offer the prolonged 24-hour-a-day care that allows growth which might otherwise be hampered by a toxic home environment (Whittaker and Trieschman, 1972). The child who needs regulated separation from his family but cannot tolerate the closeness of a foster home, or whose parents would resent and possibly undermine a foster placement as well as the child who needs more structure than a group foster home can provide should benefit from the structure and function of a residential treatment center (Reid and Hagan, 1952, p. 23). Both are costly. Neither has been documented to be other than subjectively better than other treatment modalities.

Summary and Conclusion

The recommendation for short- or intermediate-term residential placement for children is an important and difficult judgment for professionals to make (Berman, 1976). We are all aware that the outcome might be deleterious to the youngster in some instances. The professional must make the decision based on the needs of the child and family within the social context of the community. The outcome of residential placement depends on the reliability and extensiveness of data that are available at the time of admission and the motivation of the involved family and professionals to work conjointly in providing optimal services to the child and family both during and after the term of placement (Taylor and Alpert, 1973). When the system is working optimally, hospitalization or residential placement can be dramatically constructive. When the residential facility is shortchanged by unconscionable lack of funds, custodial rather than therapeutic outlook and aspirations, and the implied assumption by all involved that it is a "dumping ground," then the results are often disastrous.

Residential placement offers intensive treatment for the child and family, a training ground for professionals who will be servicing many such children in other settings, and the opportunity to define more clearly the more severe psychiatric disorders of children. It provides the conditions to develop rigorous methods for measuring and assessing the value and appropriateness of treatment modalities ranging from individual, group, biologic, psychologic to psychophysiologic and psychoeducational approaches. In many instances this can be accomplished only in a day hospital or residential setting. A special plea must be made for funding these endeavors so that motivated and competent staff can be recruited and the necessary therapeutic modalities based on the individual needs of the child can be provided. Only when we accept the needs of children as special and hospitalization for a very brief period of intense evaluation and treatment as beneficial can we remove the so-called stigma and provide the child with a fair chance at a reasonable crack at life. History comes full circle in that the lofty goals of residential treatment in the 1850's can be made a reality in the 1970's.

References

Abroms, G.M., C.H. Fellner, and C.A. Whitaker. (1971)The family enters the hospital. *Am. J. Psychiat.* 127:10, 1363–1370.

Adler, J. (1976) *The Child Care Worker: Concepts, Tasks and Relationships.* New York: Brunner/Mazel.

Ahnsjo, S. (1969) Residential care of children. In J.G. Howells, ed., *Modern Perspectives in International Child Psychiatry.* Edinburgh: Oliver & Boyd Publishers, pp. 764–784.

Aichhorn, A. (1925) *Wayward Youth.* New York: Viking Press, 1965.

Allerhand, M.E., R.E. Weber, and M. Haug. (1966) *Adaptation and Adaptability.* New York: Child Welfare League of America.

Alt, H. (1960) *Residential Treatment for the Disturbed Child.* New York: International Universities Press.

American Association for Children's Residential Centers. (1972) *From Chaos to Order: A Collective View of the Residential Treatment of Children.* New York: Child Welfare League of America.

Barish, J.I. (1968) The adolescent within an adolescent treatment program. In S. Nichtern, ed., *Mental Health Services for Adolescents,* pp. 131–142.

Barker, P. (1974) *The Residential Psychiatric Treatment of Children.* London: Crosby Lockwood Staples.

Barker, P. (1974) The aims and nature of the inpatient psychiatric treatment of children. In P. Barker, ed., *The Residential Psychiatric Treatment of Children.* London: Crosby Lockwood Staples, pp. 27–47.

Barker, P. (1976) *Basic Child Psychiatry.* 2nd ed. London: Crosby Lockwood Staples.

Bartley vs. Kremens. Civil Action No. 72-2272 (U.S.D.C., E.D., Pa., July 24, 1975).

Berman, S. (1976) Hospitalization of children and adolescents: The role of the referring child psychiatrist. *J. Philadelphia Assn. Psychoanal.* 3:3, 5–15.

Beyer, H.A., and J.P. Wilson. (1976) The reluctant volunteer: A child's right to resist commitment. In G.P. Koocher, ed., *Children's Rights and the Mental Health Professions.* New York: Wiley, pp. 133–148.

Bornstein, M.R. (1976) Social skills training for unsocialized aggressive children. Pittsburgh, unpublished manuscript.

Bornstein, M.R., A.S. Bellack, and M. Hersen. (1977) Social skills training for unassertive children: A multiple baseline analysis. *J. Appl. Behav. Anal.,* In press.

Brown, S., I. Kolvin, D. McI. Scott, and E.G. Tweedle. (1974) The child psychiatric nurse: Training for residential care. In P. Barker, ed., *The Residential Psychiatric Treatment of Children.* London: Crosby Lockwood Staples, pp. 273–293.

Burdock, E.L., and A.S. Hardesty. (1964) A children's behavior diagnostic inventory. *Ann. N.Y. Acad. Sci.* 105: 890–896.

Calpin, J., and L.F. Hertweck. (1977) Use of social skills training for the deviant child. Presentation given at the conference on acute hospitalization for the disturbed and disturbing child. Pittsburgh: Western Psychiatric Institute and Clinic.

Conners, C.K., and A. Delamater. (1976) Behavioral pharmacologic model for inpatient treatment—Research and teaching with disturbed children. Panel discussion, American Association of Psychiatric Services for Children, San Francisco.

Conners, C.K. (1977) Psychotropic drug research with children and public policy: A scientist's point of view. Paper read at the Annual Meeting of the American Association for the Advancement of Science, Denver.

Copeland, A.D. (1974) An interim educational program for adolescents. In S.C. Feinstein and P.L. Giovacchini, eds., *Adolescent Psychiatry, Volume III—Developmental and Clinical Studies.* New York: Basic Books, pp. 422–431.

Curran F.J. (1939) Organization of a ward for adolescents in Bellevue Psychiatric Hospital. *Am. J. Psychiat.* 95: 1365–1388.

D'Amato, G. (1969) *Residential Treatment for Child Mental Health.* Springfield, Ill.: Charles C Thomas.

Davis, J.K. (1976) Systematic Use of Data in Human Service Settings. *Prof. Psychol.* 147–152.

Delamater, A., N. Rosenblum, C.K. Conners, and L. Hertweck. (1977) The behavioral treatment of hysterical paralysis: A case study. Submitted for publication.

Easson, W.M. (1969) *The Severely Disturbed Adolescent: Inpatient, Residential, and Hospital Treatment.* Toledo: International Universities Press.

Evangelakis, M.G. (1974) *A Manual for Residential and Day Treatment of Children.* Springfield, Ill.: Charles C. Thomas.

Forehand, R., and H.E. King. (1977) Noncompliant children: Effects of parent training on behavior and attitude change. *Behav. Mod.* 1:1.

Forness, S.R., and F.H. Langdon. (1974) School in a psychiatric hospital. *J. Am. Acad. Child Psychiat.* 13:3, 562–575.

Foster, G.W., K.D. Vanderven, E.R. Kroner, N.T. Carbonara, and G.M. Cohen. (1972) *Child Care Work With Emotionally Disturbed Children.* Pittsburgh: University of Pittsburgh Press.

Garber, B. (1972) *Follow-up Study of Hospitalized Adolescents.* New York: Brunner/Mazel.

Grace, H.K. (1974) *The Development of a Child Psychiatric Treatment Program.* Cambridge: Schenkman.

Gralnick, A. (1968) The adolescent within an adult treatment program. In S. Nichtern, ed., *Mental Health Services for Adolescents,* pp. 117–130.

Hanf, C. (1970) Shaping mothers to shape their children's behavior. University of Oregon Medical School, unpublished manuscript.

Herstein, N. (1975) The challenge of evaluation in residential treatment. *Child Welfare* 54:3, 141–151.

Hobbs, N. (1975) *The Futures of Children.* San Francisco: Jossey-Bass.

Johnson, H.L., C. Nutter, L. Callan, and R. Ramsey. (1976) Program evaluation in residential treatment: some practical issues. *Child Welfare* 55:4, 279–287.

Joint Commission on Accreditation of Hospitals. (1974) *Psychiatric Facilities Serving Children and Adolescents.* Chicago: Joint Commission on Accreditation of Hosptials.

Kahn, A.J. (1963) *Planning Community Services for Children in Trouble.* New York: Columbia University Press.

Kanner, L. (1964) *A History of the Care and Study of the Mentally Retarded.* Springfield, Ill.: Charles C. Thomas.

Kester, B.C. (1966) Indications for residential treatment of children. *Child Welfare* 45: 338–340.

King, J.W. (1974) Teaching goals and techniques in hospital schools. In S.C. Feinstein and P.L. Giovacchini, eds., *Adolescent Psychiatry, Volume III—Developmental and Clinical Studies.* New York: Basic Books, pp. 419–421.

Koocher, G.P. (1976) A bill of rights for children in psychotherapy. In G.P. Koocher, ed., *Children's Rights and the Mental Health Professions.* New York: Wiley, pp. 23–32.

Koocher, G.P. (1976) *Children's Rights and the Mental Health Professions.* New York: Wiley.

Krueger, M.A. (1977) The program day as school day in residential treatment. *Child Welfare* 56: 271–278.

Langner, T.S., J.C. Gersten, E.D. McCarthy, E.L. Greene, J.H. Herson, and J.D. Jameson. (1976) A screening inventory for assessing psychiatric impairment in children 6 to 18. *J. Consult. Clin. Psychol.* 44:286–296.

Lewis, M., and A.J. Solnit. (1975) Residential treatment. In A.M. Freedman, H.I. Kaplan, and B.J. Sadock, eds., *Comprehensive Textbook of Psychiatry—Volume 2,* 2nd ed., pp. 2246–2250.

Maluccio, A.N., and W.D. Marlow. (1972) Residential treatment of emotionally disturbed children: A review of the literature. *Social Service Rev.* 46: 230–250.

Mandelbaum, A. (1962) Parent-child separation: Its significance to parents. *Social Work* 7:4, 26–35.

Marks, R.B. (1973) Institutions for dependent and delinquent children: Histories, nineteenth-century statistics, and recurrent goals. In D.M. Pappenfort, D.M. Kilpatrick, and R.W. Roberts, eds., *Child Care.* Chicago: Aldine, pp. 9–67.

Mayer, M.F. (1958) *A Guide for Child-Care Workers.* New York: The Child Welfare League of America.

Millman, H.L. and Schaefer, C.E. (1975) Behavioral change: Program evaluation and staff feedback. *Child Welfare* 54:10, 692–702.

Monkman, M.M. (1972) *A Milieu Therapy Program for Behaviorally Disturbed Children.* Springfield, Ill.: Charles C Thomas.

Ney, P.G., and W.A. Mills. (1976) A time-limited treatment program for children and their families. *Hosp. Comm. Psychiat.* 27:12, 878–879.

Nichtern, S. (1974) The therapeutic educational environment. In S.C. Feinstein and P.L. Giovacchini, eds., *Adolescent Psychiatry, Volume III—Developmental and Clinical Studies.* New York: Basic Books, pp. 432–434.

Novick, J., E. Rosenfeld, D.A. Bloch, and D. Dawson. (1966) Ascertaining deviant behavior in children. *J. Consult. Psychiat.* 30:3, 230–238.

O'Leary, K.D., and G.T. Wilson. (1975) *Behavior Therapy.* Englewood Cliffs: Prentice-Hall.

Orvin, G. H. (1974) Intensive treatment of the adolescent and his family. *Arch. Gen. Psychiat.* 31:6, 801–806.

Pancost, R.O., and H.L. Millman. (1975) Program evaluation in a residential treatment center. A paper presented at the 52nd Annual Meeting of the American Orthopsychiatric Association, Washington, D.C.

Petti, T.A. (1977a) Who should be hospitalized and why? Presentation given at the conference on Acute Hospitalization for the Disturbed and Disturbing Child. Pittsburgh: Western Psychiatric Institute and Clinic.

Petti, T.A. (1977b) Depression in hospitalized child psychiatry patients: Approaches to measuring depression. *J. Am. Acad. Child Psychiat.* 17:49–59.

Petti, T.A., M. Bornstein, A. Delamater, and C.K. Conners. (1977c) Evaluation and Multi-Modality Treatment of a Depressed Pre-Pubertal Girl. In press.

Rees, H.M.N. (1974) Assessment and treatment of language-disordered children. In P. Barker, ed., *The Residential Psychiatric Treatment of Children.* London: Crosby Lockwood Staples, pp. 205–234.

Reid, J.H., and H.R. Hagan. (1952) *Residential Treatment of Emotionally Disturbed Children.* New York: Child Welfare League of America.

Rinsley, D.B. (1980) Principles of therapeutic milieu with children. In G.P. Sholevar, R.M. Benson, and B.J. Blinder, eds., *The Treatment of Emotional Disorders in Children and Adolescents.* New York: Spectrum Publications, Chap. 12.

Rinsley, D.B. (1974) Special education for adolescents in residential psychiatric treatment. In S.C. Feinstein and P.L. Giovacchini, eds., *Adolescent Psychiatry, Volume III—Developmental and Clinical Studies.* New York: Basic Books, pp. 394–418.

Robins, L.N. (1966) *Deviant Children Grown Up.* Baltimore: Williams & Wilkins.

Robinson, J.F. (1957) *Psychiatric Inpatient Treatment of Children.* Report of the Conference in Inpatient Psychiatric Treatment for Children held at Washington, D.C., October 17-21, 1956, under the auspices of the American Psychiatric Association and the American Academy of Child Psychiatry. Published by the American Psychiatric Association, Washington, D.C.

Rogers, W.J.B. (1965) Children's in-patient psychiatric units. In J.G. Howells, ed., *Modern Perspectives in Child Psychiatry.* London: Oliver & Boyd, pp. 534–561.

Sackin, H., and A.D. Meyer. (1976) In-patient care for disturbed children: Criteria for admission. Paper presented at the 23rd Annual Meeting of the American Academy of Child Psychiatry, Toronto.

Shaw, C.R., and A.R. Lucas. (1970) *The Psychiatric Disorders of Childhood*, 2nd ed. New York: Meredith Corporation.

Silver, L.B. (1976) *Professional Standards Review Organization: A Handbook for Child Psychiatrists.* American Academy of Child Psychiatry.

Solow, R.A. (1974) Planning for educational needs. In S.C. Feinstein and P.L. Giovacchini, eds., *Adolescent Psychiatry, Volume III—Developmental and Clinical Studies.* New York: Basic Books. pp. 391–393.

Sonis, M. (1967) Residential treatment. In A.M. Freedman and H.I. Kaplan, eds., *Comprehensive Textbook of Psychiatry.* Baltimore: Williams & Wilkins, pp. 1472–1478.

Taylor, D.A., and S.W. Alpert. (1973) *Continuity and Support Following Residential Treatment.* New York: Child Welfare League of America.

Thies, A.P. (1976) The facts of life: Child advocacy and children's rights in residential treatment. In G.P. Koocher, ed., *Children's Rights and the Mental Health Professions.* New York: Wiley, pp. 85–96.

Trapasso, K. (1977) The role of a hospital based psychoeducational approach for disturbed and disturbing children. Presented at the conference on acute hospitalization for the disturbed and disturbing child. Pittsburgh: Western Psychiatric Institute and Clinic.

Tucker, G.J., and J.S. Maxmen. (1973) The practice of hospital psychiatry: A formulation. *Am. J. Psychiat.* 130:8, 887–891.

Wardle, C.J. (1974) Residential care of children with conduct disorders. In P. Barker, ed., *The Residential Psychiatric Treatment of Children.* London: Crosby Lockwood Staples, pp. 48–104.

Weintrob, A. (1975) Long-term treatment of the severely disturbed adolescent: Residential treatment vs hospitalization. *J. Am. Acad. Child Psychiat.* 14:436–450.

Weiss, H.H., and E.F. Pizer. (1970) Hospitalizing the young: Is it for their own good? *Ment. Hyg.* 54: 498–502.

Whittaker, J.K., and A.E. Trieschman. (1974) Current issues and problems in residential treatment for emotionally disturbed children. In J.K. Whittaker and A.E. Trieschman, eds., *Children Away From Home: A Sourcebook of Residential Treatment.* Chicago: Aldine Atherton, pp. 4–35.

Winsberg, B.G. (1976) Home vs. hospital care of behavior-disordered chidlren. Unpublished report.

Wolfensberger, W. (1974) *The Origin and Nature of Our Institutional Models.* Published by Human Policy Press.

Treatment of Emotional Disorders in Children and Adolescents

Commentary: Short-Term Child Psychiatric Inpatient Unit

G. Pirooz Sholevar

The short-term psychiatric inpatient unit for children and adolescents is one of psychiatry's most misunderstood offspring. This type of unit has an autonomous existence from other psychiatric facilities (i.e., intermediate or long-term facilities) that is unique and essential to the health and welfare of children. Lack of understanding of the special mission of this service can result in its poor utilization and in the demoralization of the staff. This commentary's purpose is to highlight these special characteristics and underline further the differences in settings documented in Dr. Theodore A. Petti's excellent chapter (Chapter 13).

The short-term psychiatric inpatient unit for children and adolescents is a new type of psychiatric facility. There are probably twenty to forty such units existing in this country, with their numbers growing rapidly. The length of stay in this unit is generally from four to twelve weeks as compared to six months to four years in long-term units.

Its purpose is to provide a full-time setting where a child exhibiting behavioral disorders can be evaluated comprehensively within his familial and ecological context resulting in an appropriate and well-thought-out treatment plan. If this type of evaluation is attempted for the child while the child is an outpatient, important resources and liabilities are often missed due to the lack of systematic, around-the-clock observation of his behavior. As a result, a multi-problem child may end up with an inappropriate diagnosis and treatment plan requiring later multiple reevaluations. Thus, the high cost of the short-term unit is offset by the prevention of multiple-treatment failures, which are costly financially and in human suffering.

Location, Space, and Facilities

Short-term inpatient units are located usually within community general hospitals, which provide two main benefits. First, the unit is easily accessible to the community residents, allowing for increased contact between the child and his family and between the staff and the child's family. The family may also be familiar with the hospital's medical or emergency services. Second, the proximity of other medical services allows for concurrent and thorough evaluation and treatment of surgical, medical, neurological, and psychiatric difficulties.

The main limitations of the general hospital

setting are insufficient and expensive space. Other community recreational and educational facilities must be used to compensate for the limited open space within the unit. Staff office facilities are limited also.

Population Characteristics

The population in a short-term unit is more heterogeneous than the population in any other psychiatric setting. This is related to several factors operative in short-term inpatient units including (a) lack of intensive preadmission assessment and (b) multiple and diverse referral sources, ranging from mental health centers, social agencies, and courts to schools and families. Therefore, a short-term unit may concurrently serve children who are quite different behaviorally, such as delinquent, emotionally disturbed, brain-damaged, mentally retarded children, and children reacting to inadequate living arrangements.

The absence of strict admission criteria is desirable for such a unit in order to make its services available to the largest possible segment of the population.

The diverse clinical picture and wide age range result in several distinguishing features. The different behavioral manifestations of the children cause anxiety and confusion. Aggressive children may bring about severe degrees of agitation in psychotic or highly disturbed children, while mentally retarded children often mobilize the hidden fantasies of emotionally unstable children who may feel defective. Exposure to physically and sexually abused children can be particularly troublesome to more protected and intimidated children, while sexual overtures toward these same youngsters by more aggressive street-wise children may precipitate panic, which may cause premature discharge from the hospital.

The wide range in age and behavioral manifestations in the patient population make the programming for everyday activities next to impossible. For example, a severely retarded or brain-damaged child may not be able to participate in any unit activities, and this child would therefore require individual programming.

Due to the emergency and crisis nature of admission to a short-term unit, there is usually a high level of turmoil. Agitated and angry children introduced into the unit tend to provoke or get irritated by the others, which can result in great distress.

The rapid turnover of the children heightens the level of turmoil in the unit. In a short-term unit, there are generally two to four children who are discharged or admitted in a particular week. The departure of the children, particularly at the point when they are more stable and a source of support to more disturbed children, mobilizes a strong loss reaction in patients by reminding them of the many losses in their short lives. The collective loss reaction often results in great distress in the unit.

These difficult situations intrinsic to a heterogeneous psychiatric unit should be countered by a high staff-patient ratio, by frequent staff meetings to promote teamwork and share observations concerning the children, and by community meetings.

Staffing

There are some important considerations in the staffing of a short-term inpatient unit. A heavier level of professional and para-professional staffing is often required due to the characteristics of the unit. An 18-to-24-bed unit is the optimum size from the staffing point of view. For such a unit, two full-time child psychiatrists and a child psychiatric resident can provide an acceptable level of psychiatric coverage. The level and the quality of staffing in other clinical and administrative categories can change the level of needed child psychiatric input. A pediatrician should be available to such a unit on a part-time basis for provision of pediatric care and prevention of the inappropriate use of a child psychiatrist as a pediatrician.

A heavy level of child psychiatric coverage is needed for daily contacts with the patients, for frequent testimony in court, for daily communication with milieu and social work staff, for daily participation in community meetings and in family therapy, and for administrative and teaching activities on the unit. The child psychiatrist should rely heavily on the input from other unit staff, but he should remain as the final coordinator of treatment planning if serious accidents, treatment failures, or embarrassing clinical situations are to be avoided.

Clinical social workers provide a central role in the unit's functioning by evaluating and treating the family unit and by working closely with other agencies. Recreational therapists must coordinate programming for all age and skill levels, using the in building space along with other community resources (YMCAs, libraries, free concerts and sports events, etc.) to help determine the child's social and motoric skills.

A child inpatient unit will require an adequate

number of nurses for its functioning. Having two or three nurses on at all times, including evenings and weekends, prevents staff feelings of isolation and demoralization. Although the nurses in such units are generally new and have limited knowledge of psychiatric disorders in children and adolescents, their knowledge of the hospital setting and procedures, their punctuality, and their ability to relate to other medical components make them a vital part of the unit operation.

A higher child-care worker-patient ratio is needed in a short-term inpatient unit. This is related to a number of factors, including a high level of turmoil in the milieu due to the rapid turnover of the children, the wide range in age and diagnoses, and the need for systematic around-the-clock observation of the children and the reporting of the observation for the establishment of a clear diagnosis and treatment plan. The combined number of nurses and child-care workers in the unit at any particular time will provide the bulk of the staff covering the milieu.

In a short-term unit, the families of hospitalized children play an extremely active and significant role in the maintenance of the pathology, and they are therefore required to be actively involved in the treatment program. All staff members need information about family functioning, since family members can actively and overtly undermine the treatment process or disrupt the program in the unit. For example, the family members may come into the unit drunk and threaten or beat up their child in front of other children. The incidence of such undesirable events is high in the short-term unit, as the admission to the unit is the result of severe familial crisis.

Special Functions

Although the function of evaluation, treatment planning, short-term focused psychiatric treatment and disposition are attended to in a short-term unit, the special emphasis is on the treatment planning, and the other three functions become subordinate to this particular one.

Evaluation

The type of evaluation done in the unit is an extensive assessment of the areas of strength and pathology in the child, the family, and the total ecological system surrounding them. As a result of such a thorough evaluation, the continuum of dynamic forces operating within the child and his family (which is covertly or overtly extended into the social system around them) can be accurately and confidently recognized. The cognizance of such dynamic continuity enables the therapist to intervene at all appropriate levels to correct dysfunctional forces and produce the best therapeutic results in the shortest possible time. For example, family crisis can cause highly disruptive behavior in the school resulting in dysfunctional responses from the school personnel. Due to the confusing nature of an emergency situation and the high level of projection on the part of the child and the people around him, the problem-solving capability of everyone involved is significantly decreased and all feel misunderstood, accused, exploited, and mistreated. It is the task of the evaluative team in the initial diagnostic contact to map out the course of the development of the disturbance, the contribution of different people to the crisis situation, and the separation of acute disorganizing factors from longstanding deficiencies in all the systems surrounding the child. The initial diagnostic impression should result in a tentative treatment plan that will support or refute the first picture of the child: this is based on the data obtained by intensive diagnostic observations by *everyone* in the unit.

This systematic observation by the unit staff is reported at the beginning of the day and at the time of the change of shift. The milieu staff and other clinical and teaching staff members should meet as frequently as necessary and in weekly scheduled meetings to reformulate the diagnostic and therapeutic plans as well as to make arrangements for final disposition. The community meeting is also an invaluable source of diagnostic information. In summary, one of the values of the short-term psychiatric unit is that observation of the child's everyday behavior is more thoroughly and frequently documented and reported to other personnel for immediate clinical utilization.

Treatment Planning

After an in-depth analysis of the child and his living situation is made by the multidisciplinary team, the results are synthesized into an appropriate treatment plan. The acute and chronic disorders in the child, family, and ecological system are delineated and multilevel intervention plans for correction of the deficiencies are developed.

In a traditional type of mental health or residential treatment center, there is a tendency toward utilizing a more restrictive facility for supervision and treatment of the child and reducing the responsibility of the family and other social agencies. A short-term inpatient unit relies heavily on the input from familial and social resources in developing a child's treatment plan. Efforts are made to keep these important resources involved during and after the period of hospitalization. Critics charge that the most restrictive environment is sought following discharge; in fact the staff may actually recommend that the child should not be placed in a long-term hospital setting if the active undercutting of such a facility by the family would make the placement pointless. The short-term unit staff can sometimes work with the family to decrease this possibility by helping the family to understand and accept the rationale behind the treatment plan. Home visits and family therapy sessions can be used effectively to point out the inadequacies of an alternative plan.

Short-Term Treatment

Although the total functioning and personality structure of the child as well as his familial resources and deficits are taken into account, only the presenting symptom or the chief complaint is a focus of immediate treatment. The longer-term deficiencies are addressed in long-term treatment planning rather than immediately.

The treatment aspect of the short-term inpatient unit is *focused* and limited in duration and scope. Emphasis is on the treatment of the target symptom that has brought about the hospitalization. It should be noted here that the target symptom is usually the culmination of interlocking pathologies of the child, the family, and others in his social setting. The target symptom might be chronic running away, aggressive and destructive behaviors, drug abuse, or uncontrolled sexual behavior.

The practical aspect of dealing with the target symptom is to enable the child to return home by reducing the stress-producing behavior. Then the family can continue in long-term outpatient treatment with the hope of further therapeutic gains. The modification of the target symptom also makes it possible to place the child in a less restrictive residential facility rather than pushing him toward the most intensive hospital or correctional settings. The unique capability of a short-term inpatient unit is delineating and changing individual, family, and institutional dynamics, which can result in a rapid reduction in the intensity of the presenting symptom.

One important function of a short-term inpatient unit is the simultaneous undertaking of psychiatric, medical, and surgical procedures with the patient. Many of the emotional disorders experienced in this population are chronic and have resulted in the medical and surgical neglect of these children, as they were considered unmanageable in a hospital setting prior to this placement. Due to close proximity of such facilities, surgical and medical procedures can be carried out when the child's behavior is under control. The child can be prepared psychologically for the procedure by the staff and be reassured and supported emotionally before and after surgery.

Some of the combined medical and surgical procedures are diagnostic in nature. About 5% of the patients admitted to such units will suffer from complicated or rare medical conditions including neurological or systemic disturbances in addition to behavior disorder. These units are ideal places for diagnostic workups of children with these disorders.

Disposition

The dispositional aspects of a short-term inpatient unit are more significant than those of its longer-term counterparts. In essence, a short-term inpatient unit has no investment in or easier access to any particular type of facility or intervention. Thus the short-term unit is in the position to assign objectively the treatment of the patient to the most appropriate, least restrictive, and least expensive facility.

Due to the heterogeneity of the population, the children are usually discharged to a variety of places. In addition to returning the children to their homes and the same living conditions they had prior to admission, the children may be sent to foster or group homes with or without outpatient therapy recommended, institutions for mentally retarded or brain-damaged children, while long-term hospitals or residential treatment may be appropriate for more disturbed children. Facilities for delinquents are sometimes recommended when children are primarily in need of intensive supervision rather than psychiatric treatment.

The placement of the child in different residential facilities requires overcoming the institutional barriers to admission. Many institutionalized children have voluminous, inaccurate, and exaggerated histories highlighting their deficiencies and leaving out their assets which result in their inappropriate exclusion from many agencies. Equipped with a total and up-to-date picture of the child and his family, equally emphasizing their assets and deficiencies, the inpatient staff can act as the child's advocate in encountering and overcoming institutional admission barriers.

The disposition of the child by the short-term inpatient unit marks a new beginning. All records are wiped clean and the child walks into the community to actualize his potential.

The Community Meeting: A Dynamic Approach to Diagnosis and Treatment

The daily community meeting is an integral part of the short-term inpatient unit. It is at the community meeting that the child can receive support for difficulties that may arise because of the heterogeneous population and learn to be part of a cohesive and supportive group created by the staff and the children. It is also a stage where the children can act out their interpersonal difficulties and exhibit their severe behavioral disorders. Often the children are the products of families who blame and project their motivations onto their children and other adults while denying their own contributions to the conflicts; not surprisingly, the children adopt their families' patterns and project the difficulties they have to their peers and staff on the unit, while denying their own contributions to the problems. The community meeting can be used to highlight everyone's contributions to the problems, reduce the amount of projection and increase the self-observation ability of the children. In other words, "collective group ego," created with the help of the staff, provides the children with their missing ego functions so the children can recognize their part in the problems and choose the most promising solution.

The reduction in projection must be complemented by a similar development in the family therapy sessions if the treatment is to be successful.

Another use of the community meeting is for diagnostic purposes. The different strengths and deficiencies of the child are often exhibited as a result of group interaction. Here the staff can make an accurate diagnostic assessment of the level of reality testing, impulsiveness, provocativeness, irritability, agitation, destructiveness, and threat to others in each child. The capacity of the children to deal with loss and separation is manifested following the frequent discharge of patients. A staff meeting is held afterward to discuss all of the data from the community meeting and how it can be used.

The ideal frequency of community meetings is one in the morning and one in the evening on a 7-day-a-week basis. The needs of the children rather than the schedule of the professional staff should be kept in mind when determining the adequate number of community meetings. A community meeting in the morning can start the children and the staff off positively by dealing with the anxieties and frictions aroused among children during the night. An evening meeting is a helpful way to discuss the interactions and conflicts that occurred during the day.

Community meetings on the weekends are important, as most of the children in a short-term unit are in the hospital during that time and do not leave for more than six hours on a therapeutic pass. It is unacceptable to deny the children the necessary supports of a unit on a weekend because it coincides with the weekly break for the staff. The staff unwittingly may deprive the children of group support on the weekend due to the competition between milieu and other clinical staff, and the lack of confidence in milieu staff by themselves and by other clinical staff. This is one strong argument to have the milieu staff participate regularly in a leadership role in all the community meetings.

The bare minimum number of community meetings on weekends is one on Sunday nights, when some of the children are returning from their short home visits. They are aroused generally by their family and externalize their familial conflict on the unit staff or on other children. The children who are not allowed to go home often take their bitterness out on other children, resulting in great chaos. The institution of a community meeting on Sunday night can decrease significantly the Monday-morning chaos on the unit and enhance the implementation of the treatment programs.

Summary

This commentary underlines the differences between short-term child inpatient psychiatric units and intermediate or long-term units. The special characteristics of the short-term inpatient units are clarified, while the importance of these units in the establishment of comprehensive evaluative and treatment planning services is presented.

Acknowledgement

The valuable editorial assistance of Ms. Marilyn Luber is acknolwedged.

References

Blinder, B.J., Wm. Young, K.R. Fineman, and S.J. Miller. (1978) The children's psychiatric hospital unit in the community. *Am. J. Psychiat.* 135(7):848–851.

Schowalter, J.E. (1971) The utilization of child psychiatry on a pediatric adolescent ward. *J. Am. Acad. Child Psychiat.* 10:684–699.

Treatment of Emotional Disorders in Children and Adolescents

CHAPTER 15

Day Treatment

M. Evangelakis

Introduction

According to the National Institute of Mental Health, "A psychiatric day-night Service is one having an organized staff whose primary purpose is to provide a planned program of milieu therapy and other treatment modalities. The service is designed for patients with mental or emotional disorders who spend only part of the 24-hour day in the program. A psychiatrist is present on a regularly scheduled basis, and assumes medical responsibility for all patients, or the psychiatrist may act as consultant to the staff on a regular basis. Under the latter arrangement, at least one of the following then assumes professional responsibility for the program: a physician, a psychologist, a psychiatric nurse, or a social worker" (*Partial Hospitalization*).

The setting where the treatment is provided for the emotionally disturbed and/or mentally ill children or adolescents has been variously named "day hospital," "day care clinic," "day care center," "youth day treatment center." "children's day treatment service," and "threshold center." Our definition for the day treatment center for children and adolescents is: a clinical setting where full hospital treatment is given under medical supervision and the patients return to their homes each night. Such an arrangement offers an alternative to inpatient treatment for those patients for whom outpatient treatment is not helpful, yet suitable for those of the mentally ill who are well enough and do not need inpatient hospital setting. The day treatment does not isolate them from home, family and community (Evangelakis, 1974).

The critical issue about a day treatment center is not where the child spends his days, but where he spends his nights. A day treatment center is really a night-at-home hospital; since the nights are different, the days are qualitatively different. Almost by definition, a day treatment center expends intensive efforts working with the families of these children. The contact with the family makes each case a major case; the stated maximum stay for patients quickly becomes the expected length of hospitalization. Treating a child while he resides in the community places great demands on staff, which, however, may be well worthwhile. Proponents of the day hospital report that all types of mental illness are treatable in the day hospital. As with so many previous innovations in psychiatry, a great deal has been promised and is still expected from day psychiatric treatment of children and adolescents. These expectations for day treatment for young psychiatric patients were expanded to include day treatment clinics, programs, and settings for children and adolescents.

While this section restricts itself to the description and current status of day treatment programs for children and adolescents, much of what is to be presented is relevant to other treatment programs as well. What follows is an attempt to present the early expectations from day treatment of emotionally disturbed and mentally ill children and adolescents, the types of their psychopathology and developmental stages, the criteria for admissions, the reasons for referral, contraindications and indications for day treatment. Also brief descriptions on the structural arrangements, materials, staffing patterns, and staff-patient ratio, treatment and education programs, duties and responsibilities of staff, methods of management and control, and necessary support facilities. Finally, a comparison will be attempted between day care, outpatient and inpatient treatment and education.

History

Although other countries should claim pioneering work (1932–1946) with the concept of day treatment of mentally ill patients—"medical office for the ambulatory ill" (Austria); "off-hospital ill" (Greece); "non-bed patient" (Spain); "day-hospital" (Russia)—the day hospital movement was founded through the evangelism of the British and the Canadians (Cameron, 1947; Bierer, 1951) with units independently established in Montreal and London. In the past thirty years there has been reported a rapid growth in the numbers and types of day treatment programs for adult patients. Recently, the question has arisen whether the growth is more apparent than real. Although the number of units has increased, partial hospitalization is an essential requirement for community mental health center funding. In spite of this, the total census of active day hospital patients is not appreciably greater than it was a few years ago.

Day treatment in the form of organized day hospital for young patients began in the United States only in 1958. For children and adolescents, the emergence of the day psychiatric treatment might best be viewed as a technique designed to fill the need created by gaps in the historical development of the treatment of children and adolescents with behavioral, emotional, and mental disorders. Lowrey (1944) informs us that prior to 1909 psychiatric efforts in treating mentally ill children were primarily concerned with the care and training of the defective or mentally retarded children. Only in 1919 did child guidance clinics start getting concerned with the mildly disturbed and mentally ill children. These two methods of management of children with psychiatric difficulties were the most common methods used up to 1958. Up to that time the children were taken care of either in an outpatient clinical setting (physician's private office, clinical social agency, clinic of a general hospital, child guidance institute) or in a residential treatment center.

Both outpatient and inpatient treatments often prevented the rational therapy of the mentally ill child, which was based upon techniques which stimulate the harmonious maturation in all areas of functioning. Donald Bloch, in his 1958 paper "A Study on Children Referred for Residential Treatment in New York State" (Annual meeting of the American Orthopsychiatric Association), observed that there was no overall plan for emotionally disturbed children and pointed out that the treatment facilities come in isolated and discreet packages. He therefore advocated a flexible network of facilities available to the seriously disturbed child. It was felt these intermediate facilities would hopefully bridge the gap between the outpatient clinics and the residential treatment centers.

Also, Friedman and his associates, in the annual meeting of the American Psychiatric Association in San Francisco, described the emergence of the day hospital as an alternative to an outpatient facility or residential center. Also that the lack of differential local treatment centers results in the inappropriate placement of a large number of mentally ill children in residential treatment centers. They recommended the "day hospital" as an ideal intermediate facility that would not only serve the mentally ill children but also help the parents and by its presence the community and serve as a center for alerting the community to its mental health needs and gain its support for the expansion of appropriate programs. Tobin and Turner indicated that day-hospital care for mentally ill children is controversial because the autistic children, those with severe brain damage, the mentally retarded, and those with behavior disorders have rather special needs. They thought that special effective units should be organized to meet the needs of a particular group of children. They also agreed that residential care with available educative and training facilities appeared to be the choice, if the child's family setting was remarkably unfavorable.

In 1959, Freedman mentioned the possibilities and effectiveness of a day hospital for schizophrenic children and referred the reader to the history and current status of the League School in Brooklyn, which was founded in 1953 by the parents of schizophrenic children who had been barred from public and private schools. Although the parents were eager to keep their children at home, they were overwhelmed by the daily necessities of taking care of a disturbed child without relief. The school was founded on the hypothesis that many schizophrenic children can be adequately managed at home if there is available a day hospital setting that provided academic opportunity. As such, the school fulfills the need for an intermediate facility for the care of schizophrenic children and takes its place as an important installation in the community mental health program.

Thus the emergence of the day treatment concept as a treatment modality was the result of several developments in contemporary child psychiatry. First, a growing awareness of the unintended but antitherapeutic effects of traditional "training schools"—i.e., mental hospitals for the psychotic child—and increased interest in more democratic concepts of care with fewer restraints and restrictions. Second, the fact that children and family could seek treatment earlier and more readily in a less disruptive, part-time facility closer to their homes. Third, the economic advantage of a five-day-a-week facility over a residential treatment center requiring seven-day-a-week, twenty-four-hour staffing and complete isolation of the child from the family. Fourth, from the vantage point of family psychodynamics, there appear to be advantages in bringing into the treatment situation the family forces tending toward both illness and recovery by having the patient reside at home. Fifth, the major advances in psychopharmacology, permitting earlier and greater control of psychotic symptomatology.

Objectives of Day Treatment

The objectives of the day treatment program can be stated in a variety of ways that reflect differences in conception, theoretical framework, and value systems. The functions of the day treatment program are several.

To provide an alternative to hospitalization for children and adolescents facing emotional crisis, who may not need twenty-four-hour inpatient care and treatment.

As is well known, many severely emotionally disturbed and mentally ill children cannot be adequately treated while they remain in their homes or in the community. Direct psychotherapy is not sufficient to meet their needs, and a new gratifying living experience in a therapeutic milieu is required. Some neurotic children cannot be helped without intensive direct individual psychiatric treatment and a benign and positive living experience in a controlled situation. Also, some children with educational deficits and specific school problems require a controlled therapeutic school situation. Such a treatment setting provides a milieu that the child knows will tolerate deviation and help him in his attempts to deal with his problems.

To provide a period of intensive treatment that might noticeably alter the pattern of dependence upon various medical inpatient and outpatient psychiatric facilities.

Underlying the basic functions of the day treatment program is the idea of reversing the traditional "patient role," a role perpetuated through long-term residential or outpatient treatment where staff members are seen as caretakers, not as therapists. The traditional approach is all too often embraced by parents who seek a sanctuary for their child from the world of reality. The parental feelings of self-castigation, emotional inaptitude, and helplessness, characteristic of parents in despair who seek refuge in state hospitals or outpatient clinics are legion. Given this low self-image, the effects of institutionalization or the so-called permanent outpatient treatment can cause irreparable damage to the child's and adolescent's self-concept. These effects are often less treatable than the symptoms that precipitated admission.

Thus, in order to reverse the traditional "patient role" at the time of admission, instead of agreeing with the parents to allow the child or adolescent to participate in the day treatment program until the patient has "solved" his problems, and/or the members of the family "feel better," the staff agrees to accept the patient only for a period of "extensive diagnostic evaluation of the patient and his family." This approach seems to have several advantages: it puts the emphasis on a mutual endeavor between patient, parent, and staff to determine why there is a difficulty; and it avoids deceiving the child or adolescent or the parents into thinking that the association with the day treatment program would be a long-term supportive relationship. Many children become identified as "mental patients," implying that the single most important thing about them is their illness label. This usually encourages the child to develop a sick way of life that is accepted by his family and the community. This position does not ascribe to the philosophy of behavior analysis, which challenges this role by implying that the patient can understand his own behavior and modify it. Rather, it emphasizes that with the resolution of innate conflictual forces with those of the environment it may be possible to return to mental health and social acceptance, a more satisfying way of life.

To provide day psychiatric treatment and education for the emotionally disturbed children and adolescents under the supervision of the child psychiatrist who operates on an interdisciplinary team basis.

The general orientation of the day treatment program is based mainly on psychodynamic concepts that are utilized diagnostically and therapeutically. The treatment consists of individual and group psychotherapy, social group work, activity therapies, family therapy, and chemotherapy. For adolescent patients emphasis is on chemotherapy and group therapy as well as adolescent counseling, prevocational and vocational instruction and orientation. In general, the treatment program aims at developing social skills and interpersonal relationships, which in turn seem to influence intrapsychic processes rather than the reverse. This program is unique in that professionally trained nonmedical staff members form a vital team involved with the evaluation and active treatment of patients utilizing the psychiatrist as consultant and supervisor.

The individual treatment program is organized in accordance with the staff's understanding of the patient's needs. The staff members evaluate the patient with respect to his surroundings. The symptoms and behavior are seen in terms of intra- or interpersonal conflicts the patient is experiencing at the time. Symptoms, even those that may be ego-syntonic for the patient, alienate him from his family and from the community. Removal of the symptoms is therefore essential in the initial phase of the treatment. The next step is to understand the patient as a person and to try to see what is making him act or think in the way he does. The staff believes that the opposite of love is indifference, not hate. It combines the focused attention with psychological safety—i.e., listening to what the child is saying and entering into his experience.

Even though the staff is antiauthoritarian in large measure, it insists upon structure, on visibility and openness, and on teamwork. The program's philosophy does not subscribe to the stereotypes of "total approach therapy," "therapeutic educational experience," or "program specifically tailored to the child's individual strengths and weaknesses" as parts of a whole. The prescription of chemotherapy for children is not encouraged, nor are the theories of practice of the time-out or seclusion or quiet rooms and other isolation therapies in the name of "recompensation of defenses"! Computerized behavior modification is not prescribed, and there is no review of the literature or statistical analysis of the "cures" obtained in other programs. Nor is there any belief in the self-interest serving and grandeur research results reported by various "investigators of behavioral sciences" whose projects are supported by grants from the public health service and/or pharmaceutical companies.

To provide a treatment modality in the form of a milieu as effective therapeutic tool in the modification of symptomatic or abnormal behavior.

Since the program follows the clinical model, the individuals that come are viewed as patients. Therefore, children who are in need of help are treated through specialized means. Theoretically, they are understood in accordance with the school of ego psychology—i.e., when a patient is severely disturbed, his ego is impaired to the point that it prevents him from using whatever resources are available to him. Therefore, the first phase of treatment consists in taking over the decision-making aspects of the patient's life while he is in a treatment program, and also—through the social worker—working with the patient's family. Usually, this first phase is very demanding and requires a great deal of involvement on the part of the staff, who receive training and supervision so that they will not become enmeshed in the patient's pathology and so that professional potentials may be developed. Once the acute stage is over and the patient begins to show increased signs of ego strength, the second phase begins. There is a change in the staff's attitude and the patient becomes very active in terms of his participation in the treatment.

In this milieu, avoidance of physical punishment is assured, and in its place provision is made for the direct relation of consequences to causes. The emotionally disturbed children are treated in this environment, which calls attention to the slightest successes that they achieve. Through this consistent kind and firm environment the children are enabled to identify with accepting adults, become part of a group of peers, and give free expression of their hostile and pent-up feelings. Since the children admitted represent various levels of emotional development and behavior, the treatment programs are flexible; however, realistically, they are not planned to meet the individual needs of each. The children are gradually forced into a scheduled program of activities. Encouragement toward conformity is not avoided. It is believed that emotionally disturbed children cannot be treated in a permissive environment. Intense supervision and restrictions are prescribed for infractions to help the children regain some stability from vicarious retribution.

The children are provided with planned and supervised activities on a group basis that teaches them to react in a socially acceptable way within firmly set controls. The use of closely supervised groups with scheduled activities permits a greater degree of permissiveness than would be possible without the limitations set up by such a structured situation. Experience indicates that children need more than a benign or kind and stable environment that provides custody, healthful care, training, and education. The program requires that the child's physical and intellectual development be taken into consideration, and that opportunities for creativity be provided. All these are coordinated through continuous diagnostic and appraisal staff conferences.

The staff's orientation concerning the etiology of emotional disturbances and all mental illnesses in children and adolescents places emphasis in their phylogeny and ontogeny, both pivotal factors in the development of their personality and the etiology of their emotional and behavior disorders. In other words, the staff believes the majority of these disordered children are the products of biological and environmental disharmonies and contradictions and of harassed idealistic or pragmatic parents whose crisis of identity is a part of the history of our times.

The work of the staff of the day treatment program is responsible for a unique system in which dual controls and supervision of the staff by the immediate supervisor and the director of the discipline are the rule rather than the exception. The staff is trained to observe behavior and functioning. It evaluates the patients by using various activity programs as bases for observations. Patients are usually admitted and observed in activities for at least two weeks. The information is then organized, and an assessment of the patient's present condition is made. The psychiatrist takes part in the assessment, and the diagnosis and goals of treatment are defined. This becomes successful only by the implementation of the concept of interdisciplinary teamwork. This closely knit group continuously analyzes and works through intragroup tensions and conflicts. This gives the group members the cohesiveness and sense of identity which permits them to utilize all their individual energies in their constructive task, which is to treat the patient. This close emotional and intellectual contact among the members of the group allow the staff to conceptualize and implement a treatment program for the patient.

The daily living experiences of the children—their relationships with adults and with each other—are significant for their emotional growth, as the staff of the day treatment program bases its work on a team organization considered to be consistent with principles of child psychiatric treatment in which each participant has authority and freedom to select and use his own therapeutic tools within the general framework of treatment prescribed by the medical director of the program and his advisory council. The program's staff insists on a certain degree of firmness because not only do the children need a fixed, uneventful, predictable schedule, but they also need the comfort and security afforded by strict rules of behavior. A mild degree of reasonable permissiveness common to everyday living characterizes the therapeutic milieu. Certain behavioral manifestations are frowned upon and others are discouraged. Thus a quality of firmness that expresses itself without excessive disciplinary action by friendly but sound attitude, is always present. No child is ever reprimanded in anger: firmness is compatible with love and interest.

To provide a well-rounded special elementary and junior high school program and curriculum for the patients.

The staff believes that education is the business of the educator; that it is based on the reality principle, and that it is the imposition of the process of learning of discipline and purpose. The staff also believes that the pleasures experienced by children with some indulgent teachers who are desirous to touch, and in certain instances to fondle affectionately a child's face, head, or shoulders as a means of establishing relationship, cater only to the pleasure principle. Psychiatrists know that the sublimation of aggressive and sexual needs is not accomplished exclusively by the ego. Superego activity is very much a requirement in the process of sublimation and in motivating a change from pleasure to the reality principle.

The school, as part of the day treatment program in general, follows the public school curriculum, which is modified and supplemented by courses to meet the changing individual interest of children. The special education programs, employing skilled educational staff, are generally individualized with curricula geared to the emotional limitations and therapeutic needs of the children.

The curriculum of the education programs for children under psychiatric care provides for their social and emotional as well as for intellectual development. Every child is helped to develop optimally his capacities for communication, self-help and management, social skills, the acquisition and adaptive utilization of knowledge, and other functions and skills necessary for independent living. Adequate organization and firm expectations in the classroom appear to be effective stimulation to the child's cognitive and social development. We are aware, for example, that black teachers appear to be inhibited in disciplining the white children in the integrated classroom and are not aware of their reluctance. Their personalities in general tend toward being overly permissive with the children. However, black teachers may fail in their teaching goals with the white children if they avoid the necessary firmness which they use with black children. The white teachers seem to maintain better discipline in the class, using incentive techniques for performance and showing no favoritism, and their class shows good motivational responses to learning. However, white teachers may fail in their teaching goals with black children if they avoid the necessary firmness which they use with white children. The same issue applies to any teacher-child relationship, but where new arrangements occur, the teacher must be alert to the unconscious inhibitions (Berman and Eisenberg, 1971; Marcus, 1971).

We believe that as there can be no democratic voting in the interpretation of a disease, the same is true in interpretation matters of education. Many teachers feel that application of mental hygiene principles to the classroom is associated with the emphasis upon what is being called "tolerance" and "democracy in education." These overdemocratized teachers feel that the spirit of democracy encourages careful vigilance to make certain that the emotionally disturbed child receives full share of any improvement in the field of education. They often choose to change from a frontal attack on behavioral problems to an indirect approach (searching for causal factors, defining misbehavior as simple calls for help, an attempt to satisfy some pressing emotional inner needs, the search for security, or desire for attention)—i.e., to cultivate democratic relationships and tolerant attitudes in the class, a feeling of friendliness, of good will. These overdemocratized teachers perceive the classroom as a workshop in democratic living—i.e., the child is tolerated, is not forced to control himself, is allowed to feel that he has a choice in the management of affairs (in the name of "relief from tension"), is allowed excessive verbalism (in the name of "free speech" or "individualistic competition").

Efforts for management and control of the emotionally disturbed children force us to reexamine the usual broad diagnostic categories in order to achieve the educational philosophy that every child should have an opportunity to learn to the best of his ability. In working with these children we found many whose symptomatology is not simple learning or reading disability but suggests the presence of true emotional disorder or mental illness which fails to fall into neat categories but presents itself in the form of transient mood disturbances, periods of decreased efficiency, times of irritability, disinterest in the world around, and feelings of inadequacy and incompetency. If such children are indulged with overpermissiveness or in various ways babied at home, as well as in school by overpermissive "progressive" teachers, the classroom experience becomes a repetition of the situation encountered in their own family and deprives the children of stimulation towards self-discipline necessary in the learning process.

Schoolteachers need to be assured that too much permissiveness is perceived by children as a lack of interest. The child may withdraw from the relationship and become passive, with low self-esteem because he feels he cannot win love or approval and begins to daydream and become variously inattentive. On the other hand, he may become angry and act out his hostility through varying means. Many teachers have low self-esteen themselves, fostered in no small way by our culture. They feel their work is not appreciated, that others "intrude" with their recommended various methods of teaching and management. The teachers find it very helpful from the beginning to make the atmosphere in the classroom as comfortable as possible by providing structure. Children cannot sit where they wish. Formality is the keynote of the teacher's attitude. Initially some children may appear quite apathetic, yet when their interest can be aroused and their attention obtained, they become very active. Drills and repitition are very helpful for those children who cannot concentrate. Gaity and earnestness are not at all exclusive, and both may be necessary to draw out an inhibited child. A firm and understanding teacher seems to be the most important single factor in stimulating and motivating a child to learn, especially in the earliest grades. It helps even those children with obviously limited skills or less than average intelligence, or internal pressures that push them into hyperactivity. This educational process seems to lead from learning for love (reward, punishment) to a love of learning (insight, identification). These can be accomplished only through planned ego development.

To provide ongoing casework, parental counseling, and family therapy for the parents of the child and adolescent.

One of the preconditions for the child's admittance to the day treatment program is that the parents would be helped to take a stand. When the parents take a firm position, the child perceives this as an overt show of interest, an answer to his various signals for more guidelines, with the result of a tremendous relief for the child, and better relationship with his parents. Some of the children are taught to be ashamed of their parents and their traditions. Some of them demand to be treated with a pill for whatever ails them. Casework with parents reveals that for years they had been watching many problems with their child go on and had been standing on the sidelines feeling impotent, not being able to take a stand. Others felt that their parental authority had been weakened by the overunderstanding fostered by newspapers and magazine pseudo-counselors and pseudo-experts. The parents felt forced to become a party to the child's problems by not paying attention, by letting the child lie to them, by bailing him out of trouble, by showering the child with "rewards" for good behavior and "aversion therapy" for misbehavior—prescribed by behavior modificators and other "instant therapists"—by tossing the child out of the home or by providing him with financial support or by using the police and juvenile courts.

The day treatment program's philosophies are based on the idea that there must be active participation by children and adolescents as well as their parents or guardians in all areas of their treatment. Endemic to the program is the belief that the additional gulf separating children and adolescents from staff must be bridged through their conjoint planning of an involvement in almost all phases of the program. Confrontations over inappropriate behavior and high expectations regarding general demeanor and appropriate dress are also exerted by patients and staff. Within the milieu, behavioral changes are facilitated through the power of ongoing relationships and the sanctions of the community. It is essential that an atmosphere prevail whereby patients can feel the power to effect change in their own lives and influence others in a positive way in the process. The parents who are responsible legal guardians are requested to maintain an active association with the child during his treatment so that the meaningful tie with therapists does not easily take on the aspects of parent-child relationship. This allows the treatment staff to be completely free, warm and accepting of the children without placing themselves in the position of becoming the providing parents who will care for the child indefinitely.

Also, an important objective of the day treatment is community linkage—i.e. (1) to serve as a bridge for children and adolescents in transition from the residential treatment to the community outpatient clinics for treatment or complete discharge; (2) to maintain the children's ties with the family and community so the day treatment program can counter the regressive pattern that is usually associated with becoming a psychiatric inpatient; (3) to develop liaison services with the community agencies for the provision of the best possible psychiatric, psychological, and psychoeducational help for the child who requires the service of a day treatment program; and (4) to develop channels of public relations to acquaint the community with the day treatment modality as a concept and not as a place.

The day treatment setting is an excellent resource for the education and training of resident psychiatrists, students of social work, psychologists, and nurses, as well as activity therapists and mental health technicians. Also, as a research resource it can contribute in the further knowledge of the best techniques of day treatment for children and adolescents. It can also develop better admission criteria for the types of children and adolescents needing the day treatment services.

Applicability

Questionable Criteria for Day Treatment

A wide variety of reasons is offered for referral to day treatment. Some of these do not always seem valid to the day treatment staff, and this adds to the number of rejections. So far, most of the reasons that follow have proven to be inadequate justification for day treatment in the majority of cases.

The subject of contraindications for day treatment is timely not only in view of plans for opening new day treatment programs but also for existing programs. It is particularly important in view of the number of referrals made for day treatment in contrast with the number of available vacancies and the consequent ill-will that is generated when a referral has to be refused.

1. *Inadequate or pathological home environment.* It is frequently stated that the child cannot improve if he has to continue to live with a problematic

family or a disturbed home setting. This is often the reason for referral irrespective of the child's diagnosis or degree of disturbed behavior. An inadequate home environment does not constitute a bona fide reason for day treatment. Instead, the family should be worked with, or if this is not possible, the child should be placed in another type of "treatment" facility, such as a foster home or group living home in one of the many sectarian or nonsectarian agencies. If individual treatment is required in addition to such a placement, this may be obtained in a community clinic or by means of psychiatric consultation to an agency. Simply to remove the child from a difficult home situation is never a justification for such an expensive and potentially traumatic situation as placement in a day treatment program often integrated with residential treatment.

2. *Required more "intensive treatment" than is available in the community.* This occurs with various diagnostic pictures from milder disorders to more seriously disturbed delinquent and psychotic children. The need for intensive treatment is not sufficient justification for day treatment. Often we are confronted with the complaint that there are not enough outpatient psychiatric facilities in the community to afford the child adequate intensive treatment. Most child guidance clinics offer treatment once or at most twice a week. This, again, is not a problem for the day treatment programs, but rather a problem in community clinic organization. The fact that the average community clinic is not equipped to offer the kind of treatment a certain child requires is certainly not a reason for referral to day treatment.

3. *Insufficient response to clinic treatment in a prescribed period of time.* For some clinics, this is based on calendar considerations rather than on the needs of the child. If a child in truth needs intensive treatment once a week, outpatient treatment will not likely alter the patterns sufficiently to effect a cure. In time, the clinic will tire of such cases, often after a succession of therapists have failed to help the child, and day treatment becomes a way out for the outpatient clinic to "unload" the case. What is needed, instead, is more careful clinical diagnosis and treatment planning in the beginning, which would help to avoid the phenomenon of disposing of so many burnt-out or partially treated outpatient clinic cases.

4. *Uncooperative or untreatable parents or child requiring "enforced" treatment.* Such referrals are not usually justification for day treatment. Most progressive day treatment units insist on the cooperation and participation of the parents in the treatment program so that the child does not become dependent on the day treatment agency, but instead he may be returned to the community, hopefully to a better integrated home environment. Parents who are uncooperative in a clinic are likely to be even more so with a day treatment program and will tend to "dump" the children and forget about them.

5. *Inadequate diagnosis requiring more prolonged observation for establishing a better diagnosis.* Impressive diagnosis is not a justifiable reason for commitment to day treatment. One cannot in clear conscience commit a child to such a difficult experience as day treatment without being perfectly certain that this drastic step is absolutely indicated. Diagnosis is much better made by a community clinic with the child living at home. There are very few cases, indeed, in which it is necessary to remove a child from home to make a diagnosis. Often the reason given for wanting day treatment for diagnosis is that "more prolonged observation is required to establish the diagnosis." Longer observation may well be required, but a day treatment unit is not necessarily the place for such observations.

6. *Court Orders.* Unfortunately children on court orders are all too frequently inappropriately committed irrespective of their diagnosis or the scope of a particular agency's intake policy and treatment program. A child should seldom, if ever, be admitted to day treatment program by court order. Many of the present-day problems besetting day treatment programs are based on the fact that children have been committed by court order and cannot be removed, when indicated, without a further order. Some of the large state-operated day treatment programs have become greatly overcrowded with children of all diagnostic categories, many of whom could be managed elsewhere if other provisions could be made. If a child is dependent and neglected, the court might well instead commit the child to the custody of a social agency, which can assume the responsibility for the child's care and can arrange with the administration of the appropriate day treatment program for admission if this is indicated. Then, upon completion of treatment, the child can be released to the supporting agency without a court order.

7. Often less severely disturbed children with neurotic or behavior disorders are referred. School phobias, psychosomatic cases, and school problems are usually better treated at home and do not often require day treatment.

8. Many children are referred specifically for consideration for the residential treatment program. Evaluation takes place after some period of outpatient treatment and considerations around retardation, brain damage, and academic performance.

Indications for Day Treatment

The decision for day treatment is usually made on the basis of not only the severity of the child's or adolescent's symptomatic behavior but also how successfully this behavior can be contained within the context of human relationships. For day treatment it is more difficult to define exact criteria than it is to list the contraindications. Following are some of the reasons why children and adolescents are treated in a day treatment program.

1. The child who is diagnosed as being potentially dangerous to himself or to others is usually placed in day treatment. However, this does not mean that the first time a child says that he has suicidal thoughts or indicates hostile intentions, one should immediately refer him to a day treatment program. Many such children can be maintained at home and treatment is offered on an outpatient basis. This is always preferable if at all possible, since the child has a better chance of recovery if treated as normal and with as little disruption of his life as is consistent with good judgment.

For more destructive problems—suicidal, homicidal, or seriously antisocial conduct that cannot be contained within the context of an interpersonal relationhsip—more secure, residential placement is appropriate. Such placement makes individual court hearings appropriate, but the basis for predicting such conduct by the patient should be made explicit. Placement in facilities with a capacity for effective security is mandatory for patients who would act in ways that are seriously dangerous to themselves or others if they were free in the community.

2. The child who continually causes a disturbance in the community and who has been treated with no success while at home may need day treatment as a means of protection for society. The negative effect of his behavior on the community may have so much "feedback" that the child may have a better chance of improvement if he can be placed in a therapeutic environment even on a part-time basis where the grownups do not react so negatively to his behavior. The adolescent who is drug-dependent, who runs away from school, or who seeks nurture in sexual promiscuity cannot be helped by outpatient intervention unless he makes a very rapid attachment to the therapist. Usually no individual can offer the adolescent the gratification obtained from these regressive activities. If his ability to make positive one-to-one relationships is inhibited, day psychiatric treatment is appropriate, as it can be used partially to remove him from a psychonoxious environment and permit the inittiation of problem solving.

3. The child whose acting out may be either sexual or aggressive and may require placement in a day treatment to avoid the serious consequences to the child which too much freedom might permit. Miller and Burt (1977) have described adolescent groups that would seem to benefit from day treatment programs: e.g., the protesting adolescents who protest their admission to the residential treatment setting (RTC, children's psychiatric hospital, children's-adolescent unit of state hospital); the acting-out adolescents who obtain impulsive relief of internal tension or externalize their internal conflict by the conscious or unconscious manipulation of external reality; the acting-up adolescents with socially unacceptable behavior designed to test the adult's capacity for care and control (e.g., delinquent behavior); the play-acting adolescents whose experimental behavior is designed to gain personal experience of the environment and to test oneself (e.g., sexual activity); the adolescents whose nonsupportive parents are reluctant to engage in therapeutic endeavors; the adolescents whose parents are overanxious to abdicate their responsibility and dump them on the mental health system; the struggling-for-autonomy adolescents who deny any need for adult assistance and act out their independent wishes, act up to test the strength of the external world, and play-act the experience of defiance; the adolescent who benefits from the introduction of formal adversarial techniques into parent-child relationships that reinforce the disintegration of the family unit (e.g., treatment of venereal disease or drug abuse without the knowledge or consent of the parents).

4. The severely regressed, chronically psychotic child who is not the very young psychotic child who may still benefit from outpatient treatment, but rather the older child of perhaps 12 to 15 years of age where everything else has been tried. If adequate outpatient treatment has been offered and if the child is unmanageable at home and unable to be contained in any community program or special class of any kind, he may well require day

treatment program. It is unfortunate that the psychotic child with severe symptoms of a chronic nature often does not respond to treatment by any of our presently known methods. The child may well require prolonged residential care and treatment and may become a chronic adult psychotic.

A common tendency on the part of many clinics and practitioners is to refer immediately every case of childhood psychosis for day treatment as soon as the diagnosis is established. In my experience, a great deal can be done to help many psychotic children on an outpatient basis. Often these children require prolong ego support by a competent child psychiatrist who will help them adjust to the community. This is a very worthwhile endeavor if one can maintain such a child outside of a costly day treatment or inpatient residential psychiatric setting.

Also, it is particularly important not to attempt to separate psychotic children in the symbiotic face of their development from their symbiotic objects. Severe regression occurs if this is done. As pointed out by Mahler, it is logical to support the mother-child relationship, which is a step toward progression and development, rather than forcing an interruption in this stage of development. Needless to say, it is essential to make a very thorough and careful diagnosis of each case of childhood psychosis in order to determine the individual child's particular reactions in this rather heterogenous syndrome.

5. The brain-damaged—such as post-encephalitic child with hyperactivity, distractibility, and acting out—who cannot be managed in the community, frequently requires day treatment and considerable supervision at home at night. Such cases may be accommodated in a special group in the day treatment program.

6. The child with severe psychosomatic disorders may be studied and treated in adequate day treatment programs.

7. A special case may of course be admitted to a day treatment program to provide case material for research and training in a particular setting. Here, the needs of the program are taken into consideration, along with the child's needs.

Diagnostic Evaluations

Every child, with few exceptions, deserves an adequate attempt at outpatient treatment first before resorting to day treatment or inpatient treatment. The determining factor for admission is the child's diagnosis, his ability to be integrated into existing treatment groups, and his ability to function within the day treatment program on at least a minimal basis. Children to be committed are assumed to have the capacity to use the psychiatric modalities, educational programs, and the group experiences offered. Thus in order to determine the need for day treatment, one must study each case completely from every point of view, including the child and his symptoms; the family and the family constellation, psychopathology, and the patient's position and role; the sociological setting and the child's relationship to the community, the school, and the neighborhood. In addition, one must see the problem of treatment in a broad context, considering all possible forms of treatment before deciding on day treatment.

Making a recommendation that a child be admitted to the day treatment program comes after a very difficult decision, a decision that on the one hand admits that other treatment methods have failed and/or that the child must be removed from his usual living situation during the day in order to be helped. On the other hand, the decision suggests that day treatment can and will do better. The broad consideration of recommendation for day treatment might be broken down into four areas, which lend themselves as criteria for arriving at the decision to recommend day treatment.

1. *Severity of the child's emotional disorder*. How sick is the child? How much danger does he constitute to himself? Can he respond to a possible treatment program short of day treatment? How has he responded to treatment in the past? How does he respond to parental figures and figures of authority? Are his relationships with adults so intense and so mutually destructive that they indicate removal during the day from his present situation? Do his relationships with adults indicate that the controls and positive influences of a peer group within a well-structured day treatment program may be the only treatment avenue open, at least for the moment? Has outpatient treatment failed because of acting out stimulated secondarily by the outpatient treatment itself? Does the behavior of the child require the limited demands of interpersonal response imposed by a day treatment setting, and does he need the consistent structure, limits, controls, and decreased provocation that can be maintained there? Is the child's emotional and mental stability so precarious that he needs a special living situation that can tolerate at the same time the marked intermittent regression as well as the extensive experimentation necessary for gaining

greater inner controls and less acting-out expression?

Children who to a large extent have failed in the effort to live continuously with their families may create such problems of tension and anxiety within the family group that unless they are removed, even temporarily, the family will suffer breakdown and disintegration. It is not enough to say that day treatment is required where all else has failed, for while this is in some measure true, previous treatment failure may also have served to clarify the diagnostic picture and made it more possible to understand the fragile strengths and profound weaknesses that have made it impossible for the child and his family to strive any longer together in an outpatient treatment effort. Indeed, as we are learning more about which children need day treatment, and what kinds of exacerbations flow between a child and his family, such children are being admitted more swiftly and directly into day treatment.

2. *Severity of the child's disorder in terms of the family.* Suitability of children for treatment is determined also by the parents' potential for becoming involved in the child's treatment program and for working through their own problems to the extent that the child could sustain treatment again after returning home.

Can a child be maintained at home? Can the family further tolerate the child and his illness? Can the family provide an atmosphere of consistent acceptance and permissiveness—and at the same time maintain indicated understandable and appropriate limits and controls? Can the parents allow support and sustain the indicated treatment program with the child remaining in the home? What part do disturbed child-rearing practices and parental expectations contribute to the problem? How emotionally disturbed in themselves are either or both parents? Does immaturity, hostility, projection, and unconscious stimulation by the parents add to the child's difficulty? Is there a disturbing symbiotic relationship between the child and mother? Does the mother or father gain unconscious release of pathological impulses by transplanting them onto the child? Would such parents have the capacity to accept help for themselves? If the child were accepted for day treatment would the parents disrupt or interrupt treatment?

The parents of a seriously disturbed child may seek to give all of the child's upbringing to others at a point of threatened family breakdown. Sometimes it is the result of a crescendo of tension and anxiety that threatens the mental breakdown of the mother or father or even threatens the dissolution of the family itself. The clinician who is assisting the parents must be sensitive to the ways in which pathogenic parental patterns contribute to the child's disturbance, and he must raise the question as to whether the child's illness is modifiable while he remains in the home situation. The parents themselves can be helped to give a careful assessment of their own available strengths and of the motivations driving them to seek day placement. Very often the parents will reveal how keenly they feel in imminent danger of being destroyed, either because of the child's destructive impulses or their own inner anger and tenuous control over their rage.

Frequently parents contribute to the child's "problems" and "difficulties," necessitating his admission to the day treatment program, because of their abdication of traditional responsibilities and their insistence that public institutions assume some of the burden. The day treatment program and particularly its school are asked to compensate for the parents' failures. The parents usually display evidences of disorganization in their home and lack of sensitivity to the child as an individual. Many of these children are indulged with permissiveness, or they are ignored at home, which is characterized by its lack of self-discipline. The parental claim of "tough treatment" is not apparent in our interviews with them, contradicting the idea that a punitive approach is the style of control to which they are accustomed and understand. Day treatment seems a necessity where the following patterns of severe family disturbances are seen. The child and his parents have repeatedly gone through extreme and hostile and traumatic experiences to the extent that few positive values seem to remain in their relationship experiences. The child is placed in situations where the threat of abandonment and loss felt by the mother in her own early life with her own mother are now also placed onto the child. The child is early a subject to repeated scenes of quarrels and violence, with only brief and fleeting positive relationship experiences. The parent or parents use the child openly and manipulatively to give equilibrium and balance to their own precarious existence. The aggressive acting out in the child is unconsciously encouraged by the parents.

3. *Severity of the child's disorder in terms of the school.* Often a child with severe learning disabilities accompanied by detachment, withdrawal, or stormy behavior requires day treatment. The child may seem bland and unconcerned by his failure to learn, but underlying this is an enormous hyper-

alertness to the relationships flowing between the teacher and other students, and a tendency to interpret suggestions or requests from the teacher as unjustified demands and pressures. The child may conceal under blandness and unconcern his poor concept of himself and his enormous fear of inadequacy. He has a deep sense of panic as he compares the increasing knowledge and gain of the other children with his own poor fund of information, which he feels can never increase. In addition, for the child, learning is dangerous, for it means new orientations, flexibility, and growth, and perhaps further challenge and demands to give as well as to receive. The child scoffs at the future and dismisses concern for it in favor of the present avoidance of reality considerations, which for the moment keep away frustration and anxiety. His relationships with the other children consist of encouraging them to resist and defy authority and secluding them away from the classroom. His behavior frightens and repels some children, and is wildly overstimulating to others. Soon the good and sincere intentions of the teachers may be transformed into anger and frustration, with subsequent guilt for those forbidden feelings.

4. *Severity of the child's disorder in terms of the community*. To what extent has acting out involved the community? To what extent is the child's behavior destructive and dangerous outside the family? What has been the response and degree of success of the help-oriented individuals and agencies in the community? What further help might they contribute? Are there other help-oriented forces in the community to call upon? It is in the community that the child may show the greatest loss of impulse control. If the child should be profoundly distrustful of adults—angry toward those who show too much interest lest they touch the deep hidden core of vast unmet and intense dependency needs and hurts him badly—then he may project himself into a repetitive situation where retaliative and punitive measures are brought against him. By doing this, he can maintain his hostile concept of the world but can bring upon himself destructive consequences. If the child should be in outpatient treatment, such aggressive acting out places this treatment in constant hazard, making it still more difficult for the therapist to deal with the countertransference feelings which such children are capable of arousing and capable of sensing. Further, the form of the action and the aggressive act may be a communication to the parent, to the therapist, or to the authorities that the child feels within himself too much anarchy, too much chaos for him to master while being in the community, and his need, therefore, for a more firm and stable structure.

Inclusion into the day treatment program should not be made solely on the ground that the community must be protected; such a placement can be equally, if not more, against the personal interests of the patient. The inadequacies of juvenile court placements in this country militate against such favorable results. Although the task of designing effective day treatment programs for disturbed juvenile offenders is formidable, we do not think that wholesale jettisoning of the rehabilitative ideal serves any useful purpose. The arguments of those who would radically change the law seem to mirror adolescent delinquent reasoning. Magic answers are sought for complex problems; magic fails to work then punitive reactions take place.

Methods

Form of organization

Physical Plant

It goes without saying that in order for a day treatment program to function as a partial alternative to a residential or outpatient program, produce the best results, and be of the greatest service to the community and to the state, it needs adequate facilities, adequate staff, and financial support from its incipiency.

Ideally the day treatment program is conducted on the grounds of the parental institute or center and should use all the facilities and equipment of the institute or center. It is provided with operating space for its daily treatment program, educational and adjunctive therapy supplies, and janitorial service.

Cost

Regarding comparative cost, much depends on the size of the professional staff. Day treatment programs generally cost less to operate than psychiatric units in residential centers.

Types of Day Treatment

Day treatment centers for children and adolescents have a wide variety of treatment programs ranging from informally organized small facilities with a small number of staff members to highly structured programs with intensive treatment goals. Their particular approach seems to depend to a large extent upon local demands for psychiatric services, existence of other resources, community interests, availability of professional staff, and the state of psychiatric know-how in the locality.

In recent years, the following day treatment programs have been established:

a. *Preschool therapeutic nursery and kindergarten.* This program offers to children with a variety of disorders, where group interaction and contact with their peers seem indicated, help with their poor social adjustment. Thus the program is able to accept earlier referrals and initiate treatment before the child's patterns have become so fixed and long-standing that prognosis is poor. The type of children accepted for the preschool day treatment program ranges from borderline psychotic through behavior disorders and socialization problems. Many of these children have been nursery or kindergarten dropouts who were not able to adjust to their school environment. The therapeutic groups are necessarily small and vary in size from 3 to 6 children, depending on the severity of their disturbances. After the children in the nursery therapeutic groups progress to a point of being prepared for reading readiness and participation in a more highly structured school program, but not yet sufficiently fitted for public school, they are offered a wide variety of kindergarten activities including education, work, reading readiness, field trips, and exposure to appropriate educational stimulation. Programs of art, music, and socialization with refreshments and recess (much the same as a regular kindergarten group uses) are also employed.

b. *The special day treatment program for severe learning disabilities.* This program is usually conducted five days a week during the regular school hours of 8:30 to 3:15 and is established to provide for the needs of a number of children with a number of severe learning difficulties. These children are nonpsychotic but have learning disabilities that make them operate at two or three years below their normal grade placement. All of the children have average or above-average intelligence yet are suffering from neurotic interferences with their learning process to such an extent that the public school programs cannot adequately cope with their needs. These children live at home and commute by themselves much as they would to any special school setting. Casework for the families and therapeutic programs for the children are provided in addition to the school classes. A complete school program with music, art, recreation, and physical education is supplied, in addition to the specialized educational program designed to meet the needs of children with severe learning difficulties.

c. *The preadmission (residential) day treatment program.* One of the most difficult periods in the child's life is during the time that he is first hospitalized. A day treatment program may therefore be utilized as a preliminary to admission. Each child who would come into the residential treatment is allowed to participate in the day treatment program integrated in the residential unit. He can bring his belongings and establish some relationship to the surroundings, the other children, and the workers before coming to sleep in the residential treatment unit. This arrangement is established for variable lengths of time, depending how long it takes the child to adjust to the unit. It has proved to be a highly successful and beneficial step, making hospitalization much easier for the child to accept. When the family lives at some distance from the unit, it is often asked to stay near the hospital to facilitate such a program.

d. *The transitional day treatment program (from residential to outpatient treatment).* This type is integrated in the residential unit setting and helps children to accept leaving the hospital. It usually begins gradually, with the child first making overnight and longer weekend visits at home. If it is indicated, the child may continue on a day treatment status in the residential unit for a period of time before being referred to outpatient treatment. Thus there are available flexible facilities to meet the needs of the disturbed child if he moves in and out of residential treatment.

e. *The day treatment program for adolescents.* This program serves disturbed adolescents, many of whom have formerly been patients in the residential setting or other inpatient programs and have progressed to the point of being able to live at home but are not yet well enough to attend public school and be in the community all day. Many of these teenagers are able to commute from home by themselves and participate in a full day program five days a week. This program is highly structured with group psychotherapy, school activities, adolescent counseling, music, art, recreational, and other therapeutic services designed to meet the needs of adolescents.

With all the above types of day treatment programs, transportation difficulties are usually worked out in most cases by the use of the regular school bus or car pools or volunteer drivers.

Staff: Administrative, Clinical

The staff in the day treatment program consists of two types: the budgeted staff professional and nonprofessional and volunteer staff. For a capacity of 30 preadolescent and adolescent patients, the day treatment program should have a well-trained staff of at least 24 members under the leadership of a child psychiatrist. These members should be two clinical psychologists, two social workers, five teachers, five adjunctive therapists (recreational, music, arts and crafts), one nurse, six child care workers, one secretary, and one clerk-typist-receptionist. Also, supportive staff from the residential treatment program (dietary, maintenance, etc.) should contribute in the implementation of the day treatment program. This would depend on the realities of staff allocation, space, and transportation.

In a day treatment program, for administrative and clinical reasons, the social work staff is viewed as the axis around which all other staff members revolve in their efforts to enable the child to use the various facilities and services for the purpose of ego-building and the development of self-confidence; also, to help the child through insight in recognizing his behavior patterns, the genesis of his disturbances, and the part which he himself can play in order to overcome them. In contrast, the residential treatment program revolves around the nursing staff, which is considered the axis of the program.

Even though maintenance, dietary, and office personnel are not encouraged to have contacts with the children on an individual basis, such staff are involved to some extent with the children, the usual pattern being for the professional staff to keep them informed in a general way regarding the problems of the children and of the importance of their attitudes toward them. These staff members are often the source of emotional satisfaction and support in their passive relationships for those children who at first are not able to relate to others. To provide this, such staff members are exposed to in-service training and are integrated into the total therapeutic milieu.

The structure under which the staff operates and the relatively small size of the staff group in the program permits adequate communications. Feelings, criticisms, and commendations are freely expressed, and observations and ideas about the patients are continually exchanged informally. There is a minimum need for formal meetings. There are, however, problems in a group with this close-knit quality. The group members may resist suggestions or criticisms regarding the program by staff from other areas of the parental institution. The group process also presents a problem in absorbing new workers into the system. These issues are usually resolved, and they do not overshadow the optimism of the staff in the continuation of the existing program format. In agreement with Redl, we too avoid calling the staff's attitudes and feelings all "transference" (1959).

Supervision

Each staff member is closely supervised in two main areas. One focuses on the patient's behavior in his activities, and the other on the staff's individual discussions with him. One of the areas stressed in supervision is the staff member's feelings regarding working with a particular child, so that each staff member helps to reach maximum effectiveness in working with or in treating patients.

In-Service Training

The extent to which the staff becomes involved with the patients depends very much on its ability to deal with the problems that come up with the patients as well as on the feelings that arise within themselves in relation to the patients. Therefore, a very viable part of the program consists of in-service training carried out on an interdisciplinary level. Team members in each discipline are able to share the knowledge of their special training with other staff members. This seems to eliminate or at least diminish feelings of dissension on the part of the staff in regard to specific professions—a situation that often exists in psychiatric settings. All areas of knowledge are pooled in order to implement a more effective treatment program. All staff members participate in organized reading groups and individual and group discussions based on psychodynamic concepts. Regardless of the kind of formal training a person may have, he learns first to work in a one-to-one patient relationship as well as in a one-to-one supervisory relationship. Emphasis is, therefore, placed upon experience in dealing with "others." Staff members record their observations in regular progress notes that are useful in furthering their capability to observe and describe patient behavior.

Functions and Duties

For any description of a treatment program it is not enough to state only the number of professionals involved and their job titles. It is also important to know what actual functions and duties these individuals perform and even more important to know something about them as individuals. We feel the staff members should be valued for their person and their competence rather than their academic degrees. They should be able to function within a team which does not play the decision-making game by vote. They should know that the leadership of the team rests with the child's psychiatrist, who has the responsibility as a supervisor of the whole host of assistants who may or may not have less training but do expect their service to be used and their opinion to be heard.

Psychiatric Service—Child Psychiatrist; Director

The child psychiatrist is the official head of the day treatment program and supervises all staff assigned to it. He is charged with the administration of all aspects of the day treatment of children and adolescents and is directly responsible to the clinical director of the parental institute or center (usually residential psychiatric) for carrying out administrative, clinical, and staff educational duties. He also treats patients with chemotherapy and individual and group psychotherapies.

Psychology Service—Clinical Psychologist

The psychologist provides psychological evaluations to aid in admission decisions, in initial and progress diagnostic and treatment formulations and in discharge planning. He conducts psychotherapy in various settings (individual, group, and family therapy), as well as individual and group parental counseling.

Social Work Service—Social Worker

The role of the social worker in the day treatment program differs from the traditional role of the social worker in the adult or child inpatient or outpatient services. In the day treatment program the social work service is the axis around which all other services revolve. The social worker is constantly asked to make judicious use of her authority role affording a medium in which the child can find a place according to his own interests and tendencies. The social worker represents authority insofar as the center takes over responsibility for control in the life of a child from 8:30 A.M. to 4:00 P.M. The social worker, who is not actually a substitute parent but is seen as such by the whole group, spends a great deal of time working directly with children as well as with all the members of the team in general and with the nursing and school staff in particular in terms of being able to understand the purpose of the day treatment program and how it affects children and adolescents. This work is interpreted to the patient's family, who are actively involved in the day treatment program. The social worker helps the family to provide for the child much of the same type of structure at home in the evening as is found in his day treatment program during the day. This is not to be construed as an attempt to make therapists of the family members. Rather, it is to help the family extend the milieu program throughout the time the patient is away from the day treatment center. This helps the family members change some of their own behavior and the psychopathology underlying their behavior. Such family psychopathology may either contribute to the child's difficulties or may interfere with the staff's ability to help the child with the problems which he is attempting to solve in the treatment program.

The social worker provides evaluation of the family's strengths and weaknesses and treatment needs, during the child's evaluation period, during the day treatment and during the discharge planning. The social worker shares the responsibility with the psychiatrist for an interpretation conference with the family. She also provides individual and group as well as family therapy using casework and psychotherapy or any combination that is appropriate.

Adjunctive Therapies Service—Adjunctive Therapist (Recreational, Industrial, Music, Occupational)

The adjunctive therapist aids the child in developing the proper attitude toward self and others and helps him develop skills that allow him to pursue activities of interest to him upon return to his home. The adjunctive therapist assists with personality evaluation and treatment recommendations through observation of the child while he is participating in activities.

School Service—Schoolteacher

The schoolteacher provides the educational testing and evaluation services for admission, placement and discharge purposes. He also integrates day treatment children into school programs together with residential treatment children and recommends special services for them (speech evaluations, audiometry, etc.). The program aspires that during the child's months of enrollment in the day treatment program he experiences physical, mental, and social growth ranging from nearly total dependence to nearly total independence. The policy of the program, in relation to the disciplinary problems that may arise, is to support the schoolteacher in the need for obeying rules and regulations. No corporal punishment of any kind is permitted, no isolation rooms are used, no aides or crisis intervention personnel are assigned, no comprehensive behavior modification schemes are used, nor are staff allowed to give individual children gifts, candy, or toys.

A child with self-destructive tendencies might require a companion to hold him constantly in an attempt to prevent him from injuring himself or others. Teachers try to familiarize themselves with some of the dynamics underlying each child's behavior in order to anticipate and tolerate aberrant and destructive conduct. In order to accomplish this, the schoolteachers try to achieve a balance between undue repression and the absence of restraints—that is, avoiding the extremes of instinct gratification or restriction. Thus they set up minimal educational and behavioral goals for each child and use symbolic objects of acknowledgement of progress in the form of certificates and stars—never candy, chips, or tokens, never permitting these "reinforcers" to accumulate toward a longer-range goal. Also the children are helped to realize that they are working for the schoolteacher's approval and love or for the sake of achievement itself. The veteran schoolteachers have found the expression of approval and love more useful than their inexperienced—and oversold in the concept of mechanical devices—colleagues.

Children in the day treatment program are not permitted to bring toys, radios, athletic equipment, or other distracting items to school. Such articles are held by the schoolteacher or turned in to the school office, to be returned to the child's parents at the end of the child's school day. Chewing gum is also prohibited. Harmful or potentially dangerous items (such as knives, matches, cigarettes, lights, etc.) are confiscated by the schoolteacher, labeled with the date, child's name, and name of the staff member who confiscated the item. The item is returned to the school office and transmitted to the child's psychiatrist and eventually to the child's parents or guardians. Schoolteachers are expected to maintain professional objectivity at all times in their contacts with the children and to refrain from use of inappropriate gestures or language. The children are expected to be adequately dressed upon arrival at school. By "adequate" is meant shoes and reasonably clean outer garments in good condition. Shirttails will be tucked in. Students deemed improperly dressed are reported to the principal, who coordinates the problem with the appropriate service. Schoolteachers make every effort to anticipate and counteract disturbed behavior within the classroom. In the event assistance is needed for student control, the schoolteacher may use the emergency key to signal the school secretary, who immediately ascertains what help is needed. If it becomes necessary to remove a child from the classroom, he may be sent to the schools's hallway for a cooling-off period or a conference with the principal if available. If the child is completely out of control, the school secretary may notify the appropriate on-duty social worker for assistance. In the event of an injury to a child that requires more than cleansing with cold water, the school secretary is requested to notify the appropriate nurse.

Nursing Service

The nursing staff are chosen on the basis of their firmness and ability to identify themselves with the children. Both male and female nursing staff wear white uniforms and white shoes while on duty, with the exception of field trips. The program does not subscribe to the philosophy that nursing staff are fitted to be substitute parents for emotionally disturbed children and adolescents. The real parent retains his parental role in the child's life, even though the child spends the major part of the day with the day treatment program. We believe that if the child were to relate to the staff as parental figures, there might be further conflict in his familial relationships. The chief job of the nursing staff is seen to be the physical care, supervision of the child, reeducation of poor habit patterns by establishing routines that are tolerable to the child and yet have reeducational value. The nursing staff's function is also conceived as involving ego training within an affectional relationship. The development of this relationship is geared to the child's readiness for it, since his capacity to accept such a relationship is often one of the most serious areas of his disturbance.

Psychiatric Nurse

By the very nature of her training, the nurse is alerted to crises and how to handle them. She is especially trained in a one-to-one relationship with patients, to be an extension of the physician and therefore can readily and effectively interpret his treatment philosophy to other staff members or to supervisors. She is trained to make responsible decisions under pressure and to carry out these decisions in an emergency. Her diagnostic acumen for physical symptoms and her knowledge of pharmacology are available to other staff members. This quality is extremely important in this type of setting, since the physician is not always readily available. A nurse serves as clinical assistant to the child psychiatrist, as liaison with residential treatment nursing service, and functions as co-therapist under the direction of the psychotherapist. She supervises the child care personnel, delegating authority and responsibilities to them according to their capacity, and obtains, supervises, and administers medication. She also supervises the charting of related materials on children and the 24-hour clinical report.

Child Care Worker

The child care worker supervises children's schedules and activities, and in liaison with adjunctive therapies and school services he conducts small group meetings daily, at the beginning and end of the program day, with the purpose of improving group and peer relations and allowing the expression of thoughts, feelings, and self-evaluation within a supportive, reality-oriented environment.

Program

One distinctive aspect of the day treatment program is the utilization of group processes for treatment by group workers (mostly utilized in preadolescent children) and the program of adolescent counseling (mostly utilized with adolescents) by mental health technicians functioning as counselors. Each children's group has a group worker who is involved with them throughout the day. A brief meeting of the group at the beginning and the end of each program day helps in the development of group relatedness. The staff is oriented to the philosophy that it is trying to adjust the child in treatment and education at the day treatment program and to the traditional American family and community life and not to an ideal fantasy world in which it might like to have him live.

General Policies and Procedures

The day treatment program runs on a five-day-per-week basis from 8:30 A.M. to 4:00 P.M. It operates twelve months each year, as with residential treatment programs and is closed on state-designated legal holidays and other days specified in the day treatment calendar. A copy of this calendar as well as an information-for-parents form is given to the parents, and any changes are promptly acknowledged. Extended holiday periods, such as during Christmas season and the summer, may be granted to individual children at the discretion of the treatment team members.

Integrative Methods

A variety of formal and informal meetings take place within the day treatment program. Day treatment meetings are held twice a week for one hour each, as well as weekly progress and diagnostic and appraisal conferences (D and As). Staff members of the day treatment program participate in meetings of other discipline departments as well as in administrative meetings of the parent institute.

Assignment to Treatment Modalities

The child is assigned to special treatment modalities for specific purposes: to become adjusted to his situation, to help build effective defenses, to help better organize his life, to raise his self-esteem, to alleviate depression, etc. These psychiatric goals are accomplished through various therapeutic activities in the setting. Often the "traditional" type of treatment for certain types of patients, particularly for depressed patients, is to put them on a strict antidepressive regimen, which means more or less menial tasks with no gratification. We rarely utilize this model in treating children. Another specific feature in the program is along with, and in conjunction with, the activities, a group worker (nursing staff) or adolescent counselor (mental health technician or other mental health paraprofessional), who talks with the child each day, discussing problems centered around what is going on in the program and occurrences at home and in the community.

Treatment modalities offered in the day treatment include individual and group psychotherapies, family therapy, counseling, chemotherapy, educational experiences, adjunctive therapies (recreational, music, industrial, and occupational), as well as prevocational and vocational orientation for adolescents. If the child becomes physically ill, the necessary examination and treatment is given locally on an emergency basis; otherwise the child is referred to the family physician.

Psychotherapy Service—Structural Arrangements

The child receives a pass from his day treatment nurse for his psychotherapy interview. While in school, adjunctive therapies, or other activities, he shows his pass for permission to go to his psychotherapy appointment. Some children are expected to keep track of the appointment without reminder, while for others the psychotherapist may ask other staff to take this responsibility and the children are reminded of their special passes and when it is time for their appointments. Children are expected to keep appointments with their psychotherapists even if they do not wish to do so. If a child strongly resists going for his appointment, his psychotherapist tries to work through with him his reasons for not wanting the appointment.

Psychotherapists are instructed to limit the unnecessary changes in psychotherapy sessions which create inconsistency in the staff's and in the children's functions; not to schedule sessions during the times that are inconsistent with school class and adjunctive therapy hours; to supervise the departure of their patients after psychotherapy sessions; to make as few changes as possible in psychotherapy hours; to be on time for their appointments, and to accompany the child to the reception room and see to it that he returns to his school class or other activity. At times they may have to accompany the child to the school or other activitiy.

Methods of Management and Control

For the proper management and control of children, a degree of reasonable permissiveness within the limitations of a group structure common to everyday living is found to be satisfactory. Experience has shown that staff members develop effective limit-setting measures only within an administratively determined framework. The most effective controls are believed to be those which derive from good relationships between adult and child. However, there are times when the staff's understanding attitudes toward the children's problems, acceptance of them, and willingness to give endless attention and affection are not enough. Often tensions build up among the children to such a degree that some of them become almost completely out of control.

The value of limit-setting has been proven by the children's positive response to it. As the children recognize that the staff are in control of the situation and that limits are meant to be enforced, there seems to be less need for disciplinary measures. The limits also permit some children to become less overanxious about their own behavior, and they realize that the use of external controls is present for their benefit. When the staff can accept the fact that limit-setting is as necessary to a child's development as love and security, they are ready to make every effort to assume the responsibility for implementing controls without defensiveness, apology or irritability. The goals of discipline are the anticipation of problems and their prevention by distraction, by the use of guidance, and by the removal of certain privileges rather than punishment.

For more efficient management and control of the disturbed children, the program implements general and specific policies and guidelines, which include privileges and restrictions, limits and deprivations, prohibition of physical punishment, stability and maintenance of the authority of the staff, provision of the "psychiatric first aid," verbal control and temporary removal from activity, "holding" control (physical and verbal), complete removal from an activity, partial restitution on the part of the child in case of careless loss of property, the child's help in the cleanup and order and repair of property, help in his refusal to be in a certain place, to attend treatments, school, and adjunctive therapies, and help during his threats or attempts of truancy and running away.

Prohibition of Isolation Rooms

The theories that "isolation of a child can be used as a protective device in controlling his disturbed behavior" and that "isolation therapy contributes to the recompensation of defenses" seem to be psychiatric fantasies. The seclusion, isolation, quiet, blue or aversion rooms must be prohibited in all treatment programs, including the day treatment programs. In recent years doubts have developed as to the faith in the sanctity of the prescribed "isolation." We believe that instead of isolation rooms, normal living areas can be provided where the child and staff member can sit and talk. Thus the whole concept of isolation and a room designated for such purpose becomes unnecessary. We believe also that the existence of such rooms in reality limits operational flexibility and creates an environment in which the staff is prone to treat "behavior" rather than treating people. Where there is a standard procedure for isolation, there is also expected standardized behavior quickly learned by children that provokes isolation. Thus children who might desire to be alone learn to exhibit and utilize purposely the very behavior we consider pathological and which may actually be initiated or molded by the practice of isolation.

Holding the patient responsible

By policy, some day treatment programs charge the patient—in an accounting separate from the center's bill—for destruction of property. It is felt there is a relationship between an aggressive act and the patient's need to make reparation and that if this need is not met by holding the patient responsible, the loss not only of therapeutic effect but also of the patient to therapy may result. The child should be encouraged to put his feelings into words instead of breaking things. This seems to be critical in the management of property destruction in general as a symptom—to make the act one for which the patient is responsible. The therapeutic rationale is that the patient should not be automatically branded as irresponsible; rather, the patient should be offered the chance to prove that he is responsible for (directly or through parents) by paying for damage to property. In addition, charging permits the staff to present a unified and consistent front to the child as regards accountability. Such unification prevents a commonly encountered potential split between the staff (who have to deal at first hand with this disruptive behavior) and the therapists (who might otherwise be viewed as the patient's advocate, tending to excuse the child's actions instead of holding him accountable).

Most day treatment programs for children, for some unknown reason, have an unusual number of windows. Window-breaking by emotionally disturbed children is a problem handled by a motto, strongly believed and implemented by the staff, that "no windows are to be broken." Some-window breaking is rare because of shatterproof glass, screened-in windows, threat of instant transfer of a patient to a more restrictive facility, perhaps even a form of "program pride" to the effect this is not done. The billing of the patient is not a simple method of management (state-supported day treatment center that pays the bill, milieu countertransference and channeling of staff's anger, etc.).

Window breakage seems to occur from the actions of four types of children: severely psychotic children in panic or rage; children with organic brain syndrome associated with convulsive disorder and psychosis; children with behavior disorders of the unsocialized-aggressive reaction type; and children in the borderline categories, who break windows with the purpose of wrist-scratching or superficial slashing as an attempt of attracting attention and/or of releasing certain degree of accumulated tension. In some children this is a deeply ingrained habit pattern providing discharge of unverbalized frustration of specific or nonspecific, acute or chronic nature.

Problems in the Operation of the Day Treatment Program

Two types of problems are usually present in a day treatment program. First, problems inherent in the operation of the day treatment program, and second, problems generated by the changing objectives of a day treatment program embedded in a residential treatment center. An intensive day treatment program is usually planned at three levels: individual, group, and family. Ideally, staff psychotherapists treat their patients individually a minimum of twice each week. Also they treat them together with their families at least once a week. The social worker usually makes an evening home visit at least during the first two weeks of day treatment and at the time of the approaching discharge of the child from the day treatment program. Perhaps the most distinctive aspect of the program is the utilization of group process for treatment, especially for treating adolescents. Children are assigned upon admission to psychotherapy groups of six to eight patients each. Each group has a psychiatrist, social worker, or psychologist as a therapist and a co-therapist who usually comes from the ranks of nursing. Small-group cohesiveness is fostered by one or more in-group discussions and a moderately structured group activity program.

The handling of adolescents in a day treatment setting has its unique problems and techniques. It is known that adolescents differ in their communication techniques from adults and young children. Depending on their maturational age, adolescents may be highly concrete in their thinking and may have little or no effective awareness that their present actions influence the future. The important communication techniques of adolescents are behavioral—i.e., acting out (impulsive relief of internal tension or externalization of internal conflict by the conscious or unconscious manipulation of external reality), acting up (socially unacceptable behavior apparently designed to test the adult capacity for care and control; some types of delinquent behavior may fall into this group), and play-acting (experimental behavior designed to gain personal experience in the environment and to test oneself; initially, sexual activity may involve play-acting). Adolescents struggling for autonomy may deny any need for adult assistance. Thus they act out independent wishes, act up to test the strength of the external world, and play-act the experience of defiance. These communication techniques may become developmental stumbling blocks if they are inappropriately gratifying (Miller and Burt, 1977).

Some day treatment programs are experiencing complications of day treatment offered to adolescents. Legislators and courts have not substantially attempted to improve the inadequacies of facilities for disturbed and disturbing adolescents. However, these bodies have chosen to intervene most dramatically in parent-child relationships in the provision of psychiatric treatment. Recent rules from courts and legislatures disregard central issues of adolescent psychology. In adolescents there is inevitably a covert and often an overt conflict between parents and child if only because the child is struggling for autonomy. Laws that automatically give unexamined authority to parents to make a wide range of decisions on behalf of their children support family units, which are historically part of a stable network of human relationships. Thus to some extent the law reinforces a preexisting sense of value that adolescents accord to parents even though conflicts might exist.

By introducing formal adversarial techniques into parent-child relationships, recent changes in the law reinforce the likelihood of the disintegration of the nuclear family. The problem in the psychiatric treatment of disturbed adolescents often appears to be the reluctance of parents to support therapeutic endeavors, not their overanxiety to dump their youngsters into the mental health system. There are many psychiatric day treatment programs that refuse to consider admitting young people who are likely to become involved with the courts. The settings reason that the treatment of disturbed adolescents is sufficiently difficult without the complications of attorneys, who are easily seduced by adolescents and who appear competitive with physicians (often because of the automatic application of an adversary relationship). Psychiatrists also recognize their own defensiveness with attorneys and prefer not to be involved with them.

Information for Parents

The staff's communication with the parents is of extreme importance for the children's treatment. This is accomplished by regular casework sessions by the social work service with the parents or guardians who inform the day treatment staff of unusual or significant occurrencces in the family situation during nights, weekends, and holidays, while the child is at home. Staff is also available to the family in times of crisis by phone or by special interview during working hours.

The treatment team members usually experience considerable difficulty in obtaining accurate behavioral observations by the parents about the child during his staying at home at nights, holidays, and weekends. Another difficulty experienced is that the parents do not notify the day treatment staff promptly if the child, for various reasons, cannot attend for the day. Also, for several reasons, the parents are neglectful in removing the child promptly from the day treatment campus at 4:00 P.M. As "guesting" is not allowed, the child cannot be kept as an inpatient in the residential center.

Although threatened or attempted suicide is infrequent in day treatment programs, when such do occur it is of sufficient concern to call an emergency meeting of the treatment team. The child is immediately reevaluated and may be considered for residential treatment or any other plan that provides adequate supervision. At times the day treatment program is seen by the child as a way of getting away from the family, the teacher, or as a means of obtaining recreational activity. For the family, the day treatment may be seen as a type of "hospitalization" that creates little guilt or shame because it is less of a stigma than "inpatient commitment" and does not exile a child from the home. At other times both parents and child lose sight of the goals for day treatment, and the staff is obliged to confer with them, either to confirm the original goals or establish new ones.

Criteria for Discharge

A reasonable six-month length of stay is considered as an adequate period of day treatment. The child and the parents are reevaluated and a decision whether the child should continue in the program or be transferred to another program or terminate his treatment at the center and be referred to an outpatient program is made.

The child is considered ready for discharge whenever he is functioning in a socially acceptable manner and can function in a regular or special school setting, and the family is ready to keep him at home without undue anxiety. If the child is in need of further treatment that can be provided on an outpatient basis, he is referred to such a program. However, if the child is in need of a longer or more structured program than provided either in the outpatient clinic or day treatment setting, he is referred for admission to the residential setting.

Comparison

Day Treatment versus Day Care

The concept of day treatment differs from that of day care. Day care usually is considered as a service for children 2½ to 5 years of age that substitutes for home care or provides various enrichment programs. Often that purpose is to make jobs possible for mothers who without day care arrangements might have to stay home with their children and subsist at a poverty level.

The day treatment concept, on the other hand, is active and treatment-oriented, geared to the needs of emotionally disturbed and/or mentally ill children and adolescents, and is far removed from the custodial or babysitting approach. The day treatment center is a concept of a treatment modality. It is not a place. The primary distinction between "treatment" and "care" involves the concept of change. Treatment implies potential for change and optimism about resources, whereas care at best means maintaining a certain level of functioning, and at worst, a condition of hopeless stagnation. It is not surprising that our society, which puts a high value on change and demands technological breakthroughs, produces few professionals willing to identify themselves with purely custodial institutions or status quo operations. Day treatment settings must reckon with this value system.

Also, the day treatment program is unique and rests in its own network of agencies and service demands. More than most psychiatric settings, it is intimately tied in the social system from which it receives participants each morning and to which it returns them each evening. Its philosophy is shaped by such things as local mores, availability of staff, professional know-how, and administrative lines. More striking are some unique adaptations of the day treatment program. These seem to be intrinsic to the day treatment model itself, which demands strong convictions that human beings, "sick" or not, have the capacity to learn and change. Nightly, the staff is forced to place sufficient trust in the children to send them home, and daily they hear about decisions made in their absence.

In the context of the child's here-and-now family and community relationships, he emerges as a person who possesses strengths as well as weaknesses, health as well as pathology. His individual initiative is necessary to the day treatment system, in contrast to other approaches where the child is expected to be "patient and passive." Artificial distinctions between staff and patient roles are minimized and the social hierarchy altered to improve communications and emphasize responsibility. Also, activities of the day treatment program tend to be more reality-oriented because the outside world clings to day treatment patients.

Day Treatment versus Outpatient Treatment

The outpatient treatment, particularly for the moderately or severely disturbed child, it is felt is not enough (1 to 5 hours per week). Also, there are difficulties for the school to tolerate the manifest symptomatology of the child who is treated on an outpatient basis. The "outpatient" disturbed child is often forced to remain at home and unnecessarily drain and exhaust all parental energies. Often younger siblings are neglected because of the demands of the disturbed child. Most often such a child is placed to the other extreme—the residential treatment center which also has its limitations.

Day Treatment versus Inpatient Treatment

Rising costs, the shortage of highly trained personnel, demands for treatment and for cures, and criticism of delivery of services have combined to put the hospital system in this country under close scrutiny. The psychiatric hospital for children is no exception. Often, at the nub of the dissatisfaction has been the large state psychiatric institution, where under the guise of psychiatric hospitalization many injustices and inadequacies have been perpetrated. Other limitations of the inpatient treatment are: location a considerable distance from the child's home, thus parental visits are problematic and staff-parents' contact and close casework difficult; child loses positive aspects of family life when removed from the family and becomes accustomed to an institutional environment; the family becomes reorganized and its members regroup and can no longer accept the mentally ill child back into the household.

It is not surprising to find community and mental health advocates as well as many private practitioners who consider psychiatric hospitalization to be of low priority and are prepared to use this resource only with considerable misgivings. Adding to the negative view concerning psychiatric hospitalization is the proliferation of alternative resources that have developed during the last ten years. These include mental health centers, day treatment programs and the growing number of "nonprofessionals," self-styled therapists in the community who are prepared to treat emotionally ill persons.

Michaux and his associates (1972) reported full-time hospitalization is more effective than day treatment in reducing certain symptomatology, particularly in the differential treatment effects in a schizophrenic subsample when full-time hospitalization was compared with day treatment. Other studies, however, have indicated that for some diagnostic categories, full-time hospitalization seems to be no more effective than day treatment. We are among those who believe that the integration of a day treatment program into a residential treatment program with positive treatment results is possible.

It is our strong impression that many day treatment children see themselves as less sick than their residential counterparts and that their continued residence in the community permits them to return there with less difficulty in making the transition from residential treatment life. Among its many expectations was the hope of circumventing inpatient hospitalization, thus avoiding the undesirable aspects of inpatient confinement. This of course implied that the patients coming for treatment were at best representative of inpatient admissions and at least hospitalizable.

In general, patients suitable for day treatment are those who are able to function in this setting without the need for a more structured kind of care and treatment. By definition this group is different from those who cannot be maintained in such a setting. It is not valid to compare diagnostic categories in patients who are able to function in a day treatment setting to patient groups with the same diagnostic label who are unable to function in such a setting. All other things being equal, the day treatment group represents a less sick population.

One other source of error that should be commented on is the intensity of treatment. In the minds of many people, day treatment is a less intensive form of treatment, since it goes on for less than 24 hours in the day. This view of treatment would then see a state hospital as offering a more intensive mode of treatment because the patient is physically there during the entire 24 hours. Clinical experience is such that we all know in practice a patient may have much more staff contact in a day hospital setting than the same patient would receive in a state hospital. It follows, then, that any comparison that is made between treatment modalities must take into account the actual level of treatment intensity and not the assumed level.

With day treatment the drawbacks of residential programs that occur when there are so many workers on several shifts can be avoided, since it is possible for the children to relate to one group of workers rather than to several groups on changing shifts. Other advantages are found in that the bedtime and night patterns of the children do not need to be interrupted, and the children can maintain their roots at home, which in many cases proves quite therapeutic.

Looking back over our experience in residential placement, it seems to us that there are many cases where complete separation from the parents and the home has not proven therapeutic, but in fact the reverse is true, since many psychotic children have regressed severely when separated from home. This should move us toward more day treatment with the view aimed at maintaining the child's contacts with his family and community at night and on the weekends and holidays while he is participating in the full treatment program by day. The point here is not whether day treatment is better than inpatient treatment or vice versa. Each is one point on a continuum of services. Each may be appropriate for a particular patient, from a particular family and community, at a particular phase of the child's illness.

Summary and Conclusions

In the United States, the concept of day treatment of children and adolescents was variously implemented from the late fifties. As with other attractive innovations, the idea of day treatment has been attended by the enthusiastic reports of its pioneers. A major defect in traditional patterns of psychiatric care and treatment of children and adolescents had been the lack of options available. The professional worker was often forced to impose more or offer less treatment than the patient required. The alternatives for dispositions for children were usually limited to a locked ward in a psychiatric hospital versus an outpatient waiting list—two extremes on a possible continuum graded treatment alternatives. The opening of psychiatric wards has spawned night, weekend, and day treatment programs. The concept of an outpatient psychotherapy visit expanded to include walk-in clinics and clinic activity programs. Now the child may be exposed to increased or decreased gradations of stress, and he may enter the continuum at any point and exit at any point. As with hospitalization and outpatient services the continuum of day treatment programs is required to meet the individual needs of patients.

For adult patients, an evaluation of almost four decades of experience with the day hospital concept and its implementation has led to serious questions concerning the basic tenets of the day treatment philosophy. Early suggestions that this type of comprehensive day treatment will put mental hospitals largely out of business is seriously challenged today. Others doubt whether day treatment programs actually have reduced inpatient beds and even question the validity of comparing inpatients to day hospital patients. This author believes that the public—erroneously considered as being sophisticated in matters of mental health—realizes that day treatment is not useful for the majority of the emotionally disturbed and mentally ill children in general and adolescents in particular. The citizens and lawmakers who viewed the day treatment as a less expensive and more productive way of doing the job of the treatment of the emotionally and mentally ill children and adolescents found out that day treatment programs do not offer any opportunity for savings by providing day places rather than inpatient beds.

Many administrative and therapeutic problems still need to be solved. There are no available blueprints. The legal status and responsibilities of day treatment programs need to be further discussed and clarified. However, we doubt that these problems will impede the development of day treatment programs. Our own experience points up the number of children who can benefit by day treatment and whose relapses are often better controlled than by readmission to the residential program. Also, we believe that day treatment is much less expensive than keeping the patient in the hospital for a long time. Moreover, it frees beds for children who need them, and that long-term hospitalization often is a retreat from normal living. The day treatment challenges patient, family, and staff to close community ties and thus may be considered as performing a preventive function.

Two major trends are evident in day treatment. First, the past policies of inpatient services have become so flexible, day status is not uncommon. Second, outpatient services are beginning to offer morning, afternoon, and evening supportive and rehabilitative group programs. As of two years ago, many outpatient programs have expanded their services to cover weekend and holiday 24-hour continuous service. We believe that the day treatment programs have had a major influence in the expansion of treatment roles of these services. In time it will be difficult to tell where inpatient, day treatment, or outpatient programs begin and end.

Thus in keeping with current trends in child psychiatric treatment, we recommend the expansion of the day treatment programs. The cost for day treatment is lessened by the fact that day programs can be managed on one shift of personnel as compared with three shifts for residential 24-hour treatment services. All of the therapeutic aspects of the residential treatment program can be offered in the day time including psychotherapeutic casework with parents, educational, recreational, occupational, and other activity programs. In addition, many of the drawbacks of residential programs, which occur when there are so many workers on several shifts is possible to be avoided. The residential treatment programs have suffered the fate of overselling and then disappointing. Their critical evaluation and modification must begin immediately. We believe that two-thirds of inpatients in both adult and children-adolescents residential psychiatric settings can be responsibly treated in well-structured and directed day treatment programs.

References

Berman, G., and M. Eisenberg. (1971) Psychsocial aspects of academic achievement. *Am. J. Orthopsychiat.* 41(3):406–414.

Bierer, J. (1951) *The Day Hospital.* London: H. K. Lewis and Company.

Cameron, D.E. (1947) The day hospital. *Med. Hosp.* 69:3.

Evangelakis, M.G. (1974) *A Manual for Residential and Day Treatment of Children.* Springfield, Ill.: Charles C Thomas.

Freedman, A.M. (1959) Day hospitals for severely disturbed schizophrenic children. *Am. J. Psychiat.* 115:893–898.

Lowrey, L.G. (1944) *Am. J. Psychiat.* 101:375.

Marcus, I.M. (1971) The influence of teacher-child interaction on the learning process. *J. Child Psychiat.* 10:481–500.

Michaux, M.H., et al. (1972) Day and full-time psychiatric treatment: A controlled comparison. *Cur. Ther. Res.* 14:272–279.

Miller, D., and R. Burt. (1977) Children's rights on entering therapeutic institutions. *Am. J. Psychiat.* 134:153–156.

Partial Hospitalization: A Service of the Community Mental Health Center. U.S. Public Health Service Publication No. 1449.

Redl, F. (1959) The concept of a "therapeutic milieu." *Am. J. Orthopsychiat.* 29:721–736.

Treatment of Emotional Disorders in Children and Adolescents

CHAPTER 16

Community-Based Group Homes

Joseph L. Taylor

The community-based group home is the youngest among the several forms of full-time care of children away from their own homes. The concept was developed to meet a gap between foster family care and institutional life, primarily for adolescents who require a stable, small group living experience that provides structure and controls within a caring, therapeutic environment. This environment is intended to avoid on the one hand the emotional intimacy and demands of foster family living, and on the other, the greater isolation, impersonality, or depersonalization of institutions. Children below the age of adolescence who require separation from their families can generally be contained and treated adequately in foster family homes.

The origins of the group home movement are obscure, but they first appeared as a systematic orientation to child care in the early 1940's. Their growth was slow, for by 1961 a Child Welfare League of America survey could report only 13 agencies operating 30 group homes. The 1977 directory of CWLA member and associate agencies listed 141 organizations operating an unspecified number of these facilities. In New York State alone, a 1977 survey found 253 group homes, a 400% increase since 1967. In the late 1960's the group home movement received impetus as an alternative to the institutionalization of juvenile delinquents and patients in mental hospitals. In recent years the availability of government funding has encouraged group homes on a proprietary basis. Generally, however, group homes are sponsored by an authorized, often state-licensed public or voluntary social agency that offers the service as its only function or as one of multiple services for children. Although these various stages in the movement can be documented, no statistics are available on the number of children in group homes.

As noted by Shulman (1975), the group home represents a concept more than a consistent or standardized form of care, being defined more specifically by size and by setting than by program. Even the concept is loose, encompassing a variety of uses—short-term, long-term, emergency—and a variety of social and clinical states—neglected and dependent, emotionally and mentally ill, mentally retarded, sibling groups, delinquents. Some group homes serve only boys, some only girls; a growing number are co-ed. Whatever the conceptual or program differences, a group home is a small living unit, generally a house, sometimes an apartment, for 6 to 12 children, located in a neighborhood, owned or rented and operated by the agency (or institution) and staffed 24 hours a day by employees known traditionally as houseparents and more recently as child care workers. Some group homes operate as adjuncts to a hospital or residential treatment center, drawing their population from the parent organization. Agency or institutional ownership of the home is considered desirable to assure its stability (staff may leave but the home remains) and to assure control of the treatment program (in a foster home the family determines the style of living). To this basic setting can be added caseworkers, psychiatrists, psychologists, recreation specialists, tutors, and other professionals, depending upon the purpose and treatment objectives of the program.

Gula (1964) notes three types of group homes: (1) for adolescents who need a minimum of casework services but do need a constructive group living experience with helpful adults in a community setting; (2) for adolescents who need full casework services, occasional psychiatric consultation, professionally supervised group living, with child care staff collaborating closely with casework staff in a community setting; (3) for children and adolescents who need a maximum of casework service, regular psychiatric help, coordinated with therapeutic community living. The variables in these definitions are the amount and level of professional and child care service. The consistent factor is the group living experience in a community setting. This presentation of the subject will focus on the third of Gula's categories, since it subsumes the other types. The presentation will suggest an optimal model, based upon current theoretical views and accounts of experience.

The Population

Adolescents may come to a group home at different stages of problem and for different purposes. Some enter directly from their own homes as their first separation experience because a group home is considered the treatment of choice. Others enter after a prior stay in an institution, residential treatment center, mental hospital, or juvenile correctional facility has modified aggressive, impulsive, or destructive behavior sufficiently so that the adolescent no longer requires such stern structures and controls. Here the group home is a transitional step to consolidate gains before returning to one's own home or before moving on to independent living. Still others come after failures in foster homes had demonstrated an inability to tolerate the emotional closeness of family-style living or that suitable foster homes were unavailable.

The population also may differ diagnostically. Group homes that treat highly disturbed individuals accept those who demonstrate schizophrenia, borderline psychosis, ego-defective and other severe behavior problems. Some of these adolescents may be scarcely distinguishable from those in sophisticated residential treatment centers. The distinction generally is in the degree of impairment in reality perception and degree of impulse control. Behavior problems that cannot be tolerated in the open community and contained sufficiently to treat it, or suicidal behavior that requires more isolation and control than is possible in a community setting, is inappropriate for a group home. The adolescent who enters a group home following treatment in a hospital, residential treatment center, or correctional facility presumably has acquired a degree of insight and control over his behavior that is lacking in the adolescent who enters from his own home at the height of a turmoiled state.

Treatment Considerations

The clinical orientation of the group home movement is derived from the residential treatment center field. In fact many centers operate through small living units comparable in size to group homes. The concept of the milieu, the key notion in residential centers, is directly transferable to a group home. Thus the treatment effects of a group home are achieved through the operation and mix of its component parts. The community setting, the quality of the home itself, the child care staff, the professional services, the peer group, the daily living experiences within the home and social experiences outside the home combine to form a total experience for the adolescent that both rears and treats him. This is an expanded conception of treatment, in distinction to specialized therapies, such as casework counseling or psychotherapy, that utilize a professional therapist to address segments of an individual's experience through verbal transactions at stated intervals. The group home undertakes a more ambitious task. It presumes to supply a social system, a complete experience in constructive living that (1) encompasses all of the ingredients that go into an adolescent's normal rearing (physical care, food, clothing, medical care, education, recreation, religious training, etc.); (2) administers these ingredients through social structures and staff-resident interactions that form a therapeutic milieu; (3) adds specialized therapies (counseling, psychotherapy) to assist the adolescent in using the daily living experiences, the milieu, and the professional interventions constructively; and (4) integrates the social, educational, and psychotherapeutic activities so that all daily experiences can contribute to growth and development. (See later in this chapter for further discussion of therapeutic milieu.)

Limitations of space do not permit full discussion of the many components that constitute the group home orientation to treatment, but several of the unique features that distinguish such programs from other types of therapeutic interventions must be noted.

The Quality of Daily Living

Some of the treatment considerations may seem ordinary or self-evident, but the simplicity is deceptive. At the core a group home program attempts to influence personality and behavior through planned daily living experiences. The dominant treatment is improved daily living, the quality of life itself. Daily living involves raising children—that is, meeting their developmental needs from day to day, week to week, month to month, year to year. The group home thus has a parenting responsibility. Although raising children is an ordinary task, it is far from simple. The task is accomplished by attention to the multitude of self-evident details that constitute everyday life. The details are unspectacular, undramatic. But that is precisely what one must work with in real life, and that is what one must write about on the subject of group homes.

All details of daily living should support treatment. Thus authorities (Burmeister, 1960; Goldstein, 1966) attest to the therapeutic importance of an inviting, well-maintained, smoothly functioning home that through its very quality conveys caring and respect for its inhabitants. Sturdy but attractive furniture, books, magazines, flowers, plants, radio, television, indoor recreation space, a place for personal possessions, adequate sleeping quarters—all contribute to this objective. The very regularity of arising on time in the morning, getting off to school, household chores, homework hour, play time, meals served on schedule, all done today as it was yesterday and will be done tomorrow, help to create a sense of order and security in persons whose prior living had often been scattered, even chaotic. These considerations address the gaps in early nurturing that are universal among group home residents and can sometimes effect a connection to the nurturing environment that "holds" the adolescent until the clinical treatment program can engage him.

The parenting role also obligates the program to provide the growth experiences that adolescents need, whether or not they are in placement. The growth experiences include education, social relationships, religious education, and the opportunity to discover or express interests and to develop mastery of skills in the variety of activities that may attract adolescents.

Values and Standards

The objectives of a group home program, espousing real-life adjustments, achieved through rearing as much as through formal interventions by a clinician designed to alter intra-psychic states, virtually impose ego-directed maneuvers on the helping persons. Parenting requires that adults have a point of view about appropriate and inappropriate, right and wrong behavior. If children are to grow up with a sense of purpose, organization, and efficiency in dealing with life, they need adults who have a point of view. Character and personality, like muscles, need exercise to develop. That is the function of values and standards. In this view it is implicit that a group home program will take positions, that it will uphold expectations, standards, and values, Attention is given to how adolescents dress, their manners, habits of cleanliness, foul and abusive language, who their friends are, where they go, how much time they spend on homework. One is held responsible for his behavior. He does not escape responsibility on grounds of being emotionally disturbed.

Taking positions, however, is a posture that opposes what is ordinarily taught in the education of the professionals who work in group home programs. Traditional teaching encourages a therapist to take a neutral stance toward a patient's behavior, allowing for self-determination. Professionals who enter a group home program de novo must inevitably grapple with this issue. The resolution must observe the fine line between the use of authority and coercion that infantilizes or degrades, and permissiveness that both inflames the internal disorder of deeply troubled adolescents and exacerbates conflicts within the group.

The Community Setting

The typical group home is a large house or apartment in a residential neighborhood, indistinguishable from other dwellings. This location reflects the primary objective of the program—e.g., to help adolescents develop competence socially, educationally, and ultimately vocationally by living in the general community, using its services (schools, libraries, medical services, work opportunities, places of worship, etc.), and learning to make the personal accommodations necessary to become responsible members of society. Such a setting is more congruent with an emphasis on social competence than a setting in the country or on a separate campus within a city. The opportunity to gain experience in living as normal people do is diminished to the extent that one lives in a specially structured and protected living environment. It is one thing for an adolescent to have a temper tantrum or for a group of adolescents to be boisterous on a secluded campus; it is another for such outbursts to occur on a hot summer night within hearing of the neighbors when windows and doors are open. It is one thing to use a campus library, attend campus recreational functions, and attend a campus religious service; it is another to use a neighborhood library, belong to a community recreational center, and attend a neighborhood church. Through living as others typically do, the adolescent must conform to city curfew laws and learn neighborhood standards of dress and deportment, and he can participate in neighborhood cleanup or fundraising campaigns. Making friends is facilitated by walking to school with a neighbor, by having a classmate to the home for dinner, being invited to stay overnight with a friend, playing games in the yard, or getting together to hear records. Children learn that a house has to be painted, lawns cut, snow shoveled, the garbage put out. They must learn to have good relationships with neighbors to promote acceptance of the home. In short, the setting furnishes practice for living in the community. "Practice" is said advisedly, because the failure to learn or resistance to learning constitutes an arena, here in the community as it does around the daily living experiences within the home, wherein the adolescent is required to examine his behavior.

However, the resources to be found in a community, such as schools and recreation centers, do not come ready-made for use by a group home program. Because adolescents may not want to go to school or use a recreational center, or because they do not know how or are afraid to try, or will behave in ways that alienate people, considerable initiative and effort must often go into explaining the program and in building the relationships that obtain and sustain the desired service. As in planting and tending a garden, the community must be prepared and cultivated if it is to flower on behalf of the children.

A survey of 16 agencies and 28 group homes in New York City (Group Homes for the New York City Children, 1976) found that the location of the "community" within which a group home should operate is a matter of debate. One view holds that it should be located in a neighborhood of mixed ethnic and socioeconomic population, to promote interactions with diverse cultures, values, and lifestyles. The other view maintains that the residents should live in their own communities to strengthen identification with their own culture and ethnic group. Ironically, whatever the setting the initial step of obtaining a desirable location may be difficult because a zoning permit, often opposed by families in the neighborhood, is usually required. The same survey found that every agency in the sample had encountered community opposition in one form or another, from either public authorities or neighbors or both. A strategy for combating community resistance based upon experience in several communities has been published by Coates and Miller (1973).

The Child Care Worker

If the most important element in a group home program is the quality of the day-to-day living experience, then the child care worker is the key person in the program. It is possible to provide a day-to-day living experience without a caseworker or a psychiatrist, but it is impossible to furnish such an experience without caretakers who supervise the adolescents. The centrality of the child care worker is recognized by all authorities in the field, but for all of its importance the field has yet to reach agreement about the specifics of the role, including what persons make the best child care workers, how they should be educated or trained, what kinds of interactions they should have with children—and even what they should be called. The confusion about the role is evident in the titles attached to the work: houseparents, counselors, supervisors, child care workers, life skills educators.

In a perceptive observation, Mayer (1976) notes that the basic outlines of the role were established in the early 1930's when, to save themselves from obsolescence, the institutions of that day brought in caseworkers and other professionals. This introduced a middle level of professionals standing between child care workers and the top administrators. By their very existence (and the prestige of their professionalism), Mayer argues, this middle level keeps the child care workers in a lower classification. What might have happened had institutions professionalized child care workers instead, along the lines of the Educateur Model (Linton, 1971) developed in many European countries, makes for interesting speculation.

The subsequent evolution of the child care worker role has been in the direction of (1) making caretaking—e.g., the sum of the adult's activities in guiding, or supervising, the life of the adolescent—

therapeutic, and (2) giving the child care worker a more responsible role as a member of the group home team in planning and evaluating treatment of the individual child. The major objective has been to demarcate the role from other roles as a unique agent of help. The tasks expected of a child care worker are formidable. Simply to live with six or more emotionally and behaviorally disturbed adolescents is taxing and draining. But to survive is only the beginning. Beyond that, the child care worker must promote the physical well-being of the adolescent, hold him to standards of personal and social conduct, educate him to control his own impulses, protect him from the aggression of others in the group, and guide peer relationships. There is always the on-the-spot handling of deviant or disturbed behavior, the inescapable necessity to do something about it—intelligently, constructively, so as to make the multitude of incidents and episodes in daily living growth-producing. The worker must be able to accept the slow rate at which gains are made with highly disturbed adolescents and must be able to discipline his personal reactions to provocative children. He must be mindful of the individual and at the same time aware of the group. These responsibilities and functions require the talent and training of a counselor, a group leader, a recreation worker, a teacher, and a good parent. Polsky and Claster (1968) have grouped the above tasks of the child care worker into four major functions: monitoring (attention to dress, language, doing homework); guidance (encouraging innovations, such as in recreation); support (meeting emotional needs of individual residents; and integration (harmonizing relations among the residents and between residents and the staff.)

Since few persons come to a child care job already equipped for these functions, in-service training has been the principal vehicle for developing the worker's skills, along with short-term seminars and workshops at universities, national, regional, state, and local conferences. In recent years some community colleges and universities have established two-year associate-degree courses, designed to attract young people who wish to enter a helping profession.

The basic issue in arriving at a consensus about the purpose of the child care worker and the education to equip him is the distinction—or the blend—between the parenting function and the therapy function. Berwald (1970) supports the notion of parenting when he notes that the superintensive, around-the-clock treatment approach does not allow for the nurturant needs of the children, which he believes are met more adequately in a less intense atmosphere, and by persons who can better establish a more nearly homelike setting. The nurturance contributes to these other important needs (the development of ego and superego) in an environment where the accent is on controls, discipline, standards, and protection in an atmosphere of empathic understanding and affection.

The therapy model has been advanced by the field of residential treatment and extrapolated to the group home setting.

Advocates of both positions and positions in the middle agree unanimously that the status of the child care worker must be raised and that there should be training on a professional level.

The Director

Whatever the objectives or treatment sophistication of a group home, it needs a manager, or director. On several levels there must be an authority in charge. In the area of housekeeping the home must be kept in good repair and attractive; regulations concerning fire, health, and safety must be met; a network of suppliers and vendors for daily necessities organized. On the program level, child care staff must be selected, trained, supervised, and supported in the draining work. In planning admissions, someone must consider and prepare for how a new child will affect the child care staff, the group, and the neighbors. So that staff will know how to respond to a newly admitted child, someone must make sure that the psychodynamic formulations of the intake study are translated into hard techniques and methods for dealing with the daily life of the adolescent. Someone has to be called in an emergency or crisis, whatever the time of day or night, when a child runs away, comes home spaced out from drugs, or breaks down emotionally. There is the linkage role of conveying important information from one member of the group home team to another. These roles are normally carried by the director.

Some of the duties are more subtle. The use of authority can be a major problem in group care, both for the residents and the child care staff. Staff may use authority feebly for fear of being disliked by the children, or delay using it, making unnecessarily prolonged efforts to "reach" a child. The combined hostile pressures of an adolescent group may erode a staff member's ability to use authority. The failure to use authority has negative consequences for adolescents, because their own distortions are then reinforced by the adult's distortion of his own role. As Aarons noted (1945), for the superego to wage a successful struggle against regressive drive forces, parents and surrogates must remain constant and firm in maintaining ego ideals, both by espousal and example. Thus the director must be the ultimate authority to distinguish between right and wrong, between the permissible and the impermissible. The power to punish, to withhold, or to reward, and the recognition that he faces an unshakeable authority, is one of the things that the adolescent can relate to, and so the intelligent use of power is crucial.

In other areas, too, authority is needed. Although a team approach is useful and a consensus desirable, there are inevitable differences in a group of professionals and child care staff that stem from personal experience, personality and training. Yet at many points a clear decision must be made, despite the persistence of differences, whether certain behavior can be tolerated, whether an adolescent should change schools, have visits with parents, be restricted to the house, etc. The caseworker or psychiatrist may have an opinion, but they do not have to live out the consequences of their opinions in interaction with the group. Child care staff may know what is right but avoid the recognition because they fear living out the decision. Someone has to decide—based, to be sure, on available opinions and judgments—and then risk and live out the consequences in support of the child care staff and personally, no matter what becomes entailed in the way of worry, personal inconvenience, or hardship. The director is the logical person to assume the authority role in its various manifestations.

The Group

The professional literature is replete with testimony to the importance of the group. A recent follow-up study of a group home program for adolescent girls (Taylor et al., 1976) found that in their evaluation, the peer group was the most meaningful and helpful component of the program. Almost 75% of the girls' spontaneous memories involved pleasant, comradely, and highly supportive relationships with other girls. If the salience of memories is an indicator of important influences, then the relations among the girls emerge as the most significant factor in this group home experience. Polsky and Claster (1968) maintain that "the organization of the peer group to plan and execute the goals stemming from their own interests and needs is a crucial aspect of the treatment process in residential treatment." Many other authorities could be quoted to establish that the very bringing together of six to twelve adolescents who have common needs and experiences creates influences that go beyond the impact of individual children; that the processes by which groups are formed need to be understood so that their growth will be for the good of the program; and that the various uses to which groups can be put should be exploited.

The study of the group can be approached in terms of (1) the selection of the individuals who enter the program to form the group; (2) the spontaneous coming together of the individuals to support each other in their common situation; and (3) planned interventions by staff to organize groups for communal tasks that promote the home, participation in the management of the home, recreation within and outside the home, and for therapy.

The very selection and balance of the individuals that form the group is crucial. The group cannot have too many impulse-ridden, acting-out individuals. Some members of the group must have enough judgment and self-control to even out the disruptive behavior of others. Just as a symphony orchestra composed only of trombone players will give off a lopsided sound, so will a group home composed only of remote schizophrenics or violence-prone adolescents or runaways skew the character of daily life and interactions among everyone in the home to devastate the program.

The management function of the group can be achieved through regularly scheduled meetings that discuss chore assignments, study hour, use of telephone, visitors, rewards and punishments, etc. Here the residents are encouraged to appreciate the advantages that accrue to each from sacrifices that, by limiting self-indulgence (telephone, chores), assure an adequate level of gratification for all; and thereby develop a group morality for setting rules and regulations. The use of group techniques in therapy is self-evident, although there can be differences in goals and approach.

Communication Among Staff Members

The team approach in a group home program carries special opportunities and special dangers. It is an advantage that no single treatment component has to carry the sole or major responsibility for delivering help. The danger is that the team members may not be united on goals and objectives for the individuals in the program, or may not even be adequately informed on those day-to-day developments or happenings with the residents that form the base for staff responses to them. When team members are not adequately informed or united, children can exploit the differences to their own advantage, as children do in families when parents differ in their understanding, expectations, or discipline of the child. But when united, the members of the team have a unique opportunity to exercise the total impact of a therapeutic community. In overall planning, the individual roles of staff members can be integrated into a common purpose so that the components contribute to and support each other. In specific situations, the team can reinforce expectation, block evasion and denial, and create helpful influences toward the objectives in raising and treating children—e.g., learning to be clean and orderly about one's person, belongings, and room, going to school, doing homework, keeping therapy appointments, controlling destructive or impulsive behavior, dating habits, smoking, overeating, accepting and living within the reality of the natural parents' plans or capabilities for the child, etc.

Whatever the mechanics, there must be a daily exchange of relevant information in writing or verbally in emergencies (e.g., the therapist phones the home to advise that a boy left the treatment hour in an upset or destructive mood that may be acted out on his return to the home); and periodic summary reports by professional and child care staff, supplemented by periodic conferences among the team members to exchange perceptions and to review treatment plans and progress.

The necessity for free communication raises challenges to traditional notions about the confidentiality of case material. In this limited chapter it is possible only to recognize the issue and note that it is invariably resolved in favor of open sharing to facilitate a coordinated response to complex, often uncontrollable behavior that is at times dangerous to the child, to the other children, or to the community.

The Mix

While the separate components of the program contribute to growth and development, the elements also combine to create an influence toward treatment in which the whole is something more than its parts. Intended or not, the style of daily living, the activity of child care and professional staff, the peer group, and the dynamics of the community affect each other and interact to form a total influence. These effects are captured in the concepts "therapeutic milieu" and "milieu therapy." Therapeutic milieu, as defined by Polsky and Claster (1968) "is characterized by three orientations: democratic social structure, kind and understanding staff interaction and relations with patients, and efforts aimed at helping patients to achieve insight into their illness and develop more satisfying interpersonal relations." Milieu therapy is the fusion of all helping agents within the program into a coordinated, integrated helping thrust that encompasses the totality of living. The reciprocal influences among the separate elements in a therapeutic milieu and in milieu therapy generally make it impossible to separate out the impact of any single factor, but it can be assumed that the elements have an interlocking and reinforcing effect. Thus a mix of some kind takes place—as with light, make up of different rays that fuse into one visible beam unlike any in its spectrum, or like water that combines into something different from its ingredients. The mix generally includes:

1. A constellation of efforts and services that offers a caring environment. The style of living, the clinical treatment services, and the social services are all directed to creating a better life, but caring is what translates the abstractions of program into a meaningful experience among people.

2. A thrust within daily living that provides nourishment for growth and development. The nourishment can take the form of caring, encouragement, expectation, direction, pressure, and practical assistance toward self-improvement. The atmosphere is affirmative and forward-looking. Doing something about the present is more important than examining the traumas of the past. The knowledge base and the techniques of the helping professions are not yet precise enough to select and arrange the components of experience that will assure growth, but there is agreement that these aids create the climate and thrust for growth.

3. A total environment that contains a variety of potentially beneficial influences. If casework does not make a therapeutic impact, the peer group might, or the child care staff or psychotherapy. No one treatment has to carry the sole or major responsibility for delivering help. It is inevitable that adolescents will differ in their stage of problem, their needs, their readiness, and their ability to use the various therapeutic interventions available.

Despite the observations that can be made about a therapeutic milieu, there is no comprehensive theory at present to explain precisely how it operates to achieve constructive change. The principal action is thought to be on basic ego development. Andessa et al. (1972) have elaborated this conception. Noting first the common finding that some children improve remarkably in a good placement even when psychotherapy is not available, he goes on to say that humanistic factors within the environment itself can be assumed to exert beneficial influences upon the individual.

Milieu therapy assumes that a molding influence upon the psyche of the growing child is accompanied by action as well as by verbal intercession—by the act as well as by the word. For the child, residential treatment is life itself; it amounts to working through in the action of life what the neurotic classically does verbally in psychotherapy.

Thus changes in externalized behavior can be achieved through the improved quality of daily living experiences that relieve stress, provide protection, diminish anxiety, promote competent function, and thereby alter outlook.

However, change from within, or internalization, is predicated on affective investment. Affective relationship is grounded, in turn, upon need satisfactions, limit setting, basic protection, care and concern, personal safety and processes of identification with individuals and with the treatment center itself as existential fact. . . . Although milieu therapy is not psychotherapy, clearly it is of immense import in encouraging intrapsychic change. It could be said that psychotherapy is but a special case of milieu therapy, the therapist in the one-to-one relationship being the major environmental force working mainly through verbal-symbolic means. Milieu therapy operates not to make the unconscious conscious, but to build ego in place of id.

The frequency with which the terms "therapeutic milieu" and "milieu therapy" are found in professional literature would suggest that their attainment is commonplace. Polsky and Claster (1968) quote a number of research studies in mental hospitals and their own research and observations in residential treatment centers to suggest that they are not so easily attained. Andessa et al. note the forces, bred of inevitable variations among staff members in regard to attitudes, values, ego responses, and cultural background, that tend to disorganize a therapeutic milieu. The residents live with adults who are all too human and thereby complicated, subject to jealousies, rivalries, fears, and desires, as well as to motives of altruism and help. The conflicts this humanness create in the milieu interpose obstacles to the adolescent's developmental growth. It thus becomes a function of administration to recognize and temper the relationships among the adults in the program.

Under the concept of milieu belongs a point of view about treatment that has been advanced articulately by the correctional field, where community-based group homes are utilized extensively as an alternative to the institutionalization of delinquents. This orientation to treatment is a function of milieu because it invokes ethos more than method or technique. As presented by Goldenberg (1973), the view ascribes delinquent behavior to a malfunctioning social system, not to psychopathology of the individual. Democratization of daily life within the group home through joint planning and decision-making by the residents and the staff, and institutional change in the outer world subsystems that affect the growing adolescent, is the "treatment."

Group Homes for Mentally Retarded

The recognition that many mentally retarded persons do not require institutional constraints have sparked efforts to create other forms of living for persons previously institutionalized. This recognition, reinforced by the known horrors of shut-away care and the observations that institutions often reinforce retardation, has resulted in a variety of community-based programs, including group home living. The concept of normalization developed in Scandinavia by Nirje (1976), Bank-Mikkelsen (1976), and Gruenwald (1976) has revolutionized programs for retardates and increasingly determines the location of residential services. The emphasis is on socialization, including peer associations, leisure-time activities, dancing, trips, etc., and sheltered or other work, in an atmosphere of high expectancy for normal living. The literature in this field is mainly about the deinstitutionalization of young and older adults, but with appropriate extrapolations in objectives and programming, selection, and training of child care staff and tie-ins with community resources, the concept can be adapted to adolescents.

Research

The only major research published on group homes (Taylor et al., 1976), a follow-up study of adolescent girls in residence between 1959 and 1969, reported moderate but overall significant improvement in the lives of the girls due to the influence of the group home experience. Particular gains were made in adjustment to living situation, peer relationships, female and attitudes toward self. This research introduced the concept of a predicted rating scale with treatment and without treatment, against which baseline evaluations made at the time of admission to the program, and evaluations made at the time of follow-up, were compared. This study stands as one of the most comprehensive research evaluations that has been made in the field of residential living and treatment. Another section in this volume presents the most complete model of professional practice in a group home that has been published to date.

Concluding Remarks

The group home developed in order to fill a gap for children who could not adapt to or benefit from the then-existing two major forms of placement, foster family care and institutional care. Function preceded form, as it were, for proceeding from that generalized mission, the field has sought throughout the years to determine more precisely what children can be served best in group homes and through what methods. Given the many kinds of children and clinical conditions that group homes can theoretically serve, it would seem that the pertinent question should be—What disturbed adolescents does a particular group home want to serve? The basic advice given by writers is that a good story can tell only one tale. If it tries to tell too much, the story suffers. Analogously it would seem that a group home should have clarity about the purpose it wants to serve, the kinds of adolescents it wants to treat, a goal of treatment (basic personality change or social adaptation), and a firm ideological orientation to treatment. But at this point the reality of the community intrudes. The community that supports a group home usually expects it to serve a humanitarian purpose as well as a clinical function, the humanitarian purpose being to accept children who need a home, regardless of their clinical condition (assuming of course that the children are community-containable). This obligation conflicts with a selective admissions policy governed by whom the program can serve best.

Ultimately, however, the humanitarian values may be the crucial values. The research study noted above (Taylor et al., 1976) is instructive on this point. The comprehensive description of professional practice that accompanies the research report reveals that the impressive clinical equipment in the program was the servant of an enormous humanitarian effort. True, the program was rooted in a thorough philosophy of child care; it had a clear orientation to treatment; it had carefully rationalized the role and functions of the director, child care staff, caseworker, child psychiatrist, clinical psychologist, and volunteers who conducted the program. But such an effort, 24 hours a day, every day in the week, every week in the month, every month in the year, for years with some adolescents is a gigantic task, accomplished as often by patience and sheer will as by acts of program. Differences in degree create substantive differences. There are degrees of caring, tenacity, commitment, and intensity of involvement that are crucial to the outcomes that a group home program can achieve. That the humanism of the work is central is reflected in the major findings of the AJC study, for the peer group, the person of the director, and the stable, orderly, attractive home itself were identified by the study subjects as the major positive influences in the program. Moreover, there was remarkable job stability among the director, child care staff, caseworker, and child psychiatrist throughout the ten-year period studied. The unusual commitment of the staff in this program is evident in the many years they stayed with the exhausting work; in the amount of time they gave to it beyond the normal work week; in the way they worked together, abolishing traditional differences in their roles and subordinating or abolishing traditional differences in their role when necessary for the good of the adolescent and channeling the ultimate authority for the program in one person—the director—who established her right to this responsibility by the extent and quality of her involvement whatever the season or the time.

The operation of a group home for highly disturbed adolescents is thus much more than an exercise in clinical interventions. This does not mean that the clinical case can rest. The future of the group home movement is linked profoundly to the further understanding and the roles that will be assigned the child care worker and the psychotherapist. Allerhand, Waber, and Haug (1966) found in their landmark study of residential treatment that psychotherapy failed to prepare adolescents adequately for living successfully in the community when an internally oriented approach to the child dominated the treatment.

References

Aarons, A.Z. (1945) Normality and abnormality in adolescents. In *The Psychoanalytic Study of the Child,* Vol. 25. New York: International Universities Press, pp. 309–339.

Allerhand, M.E., R.E. Weber, and M. Haug. (1966) *Adaptation and Adaptability: The Bellefaire Follow-up Study.* New York: Child Welfare League of America.

Andessa, S. (1972) The elements and structure of therapeutic milieu. In *From Chaos to Disorder.* New York: Child Welfare League of America.

Bank-Mikkelsen. (1976) Kugel and Wolfensberger, eds., *Changing Patterns in Residential Services for the Mentally Retarded.* Washington, D.C.: U.S. Government Printing Office, pp. 227–254.

Berwald, J.F. (1970) Cottage parents in a treatment institution. *Child Welfare,* December 1970.

Burmeister, E. (1960) Living in a group home: From the professional houseparent. *Child Welfare,* March 1960.

Coates, R.B., and A.O. Miller. (1973) Neutralization of community resistance to group homes. In Y. Bakal, ed., *Closing Correctional Institutions.* Lexington, Mass.: D.C. Heath, pp. 67–84.

Goldenberg, I. (1973) Alternative models for the rehabilitation of the youthful offender. In Y. Bakal, ed., *Closing Correctional Institutions.* Lexington, Mass.: D.C. Heath, p. 50.

Goldstein, H. (1966) The role of the director in a group home. *Child Welfare,* November 1966, p. 504.

Group Homes for the New York City Children. (1976) A report of the Citizens Committee for Children of New York, XIV.

Gruenwald, K. (1976) Wolfensberger, eds., *Changing Patterns in Residential Services for the Mentally Retarded.* Washington, D.C.: U.S. Government Printing Office.

Gula, M. (1964) Group homes—New and differentiated tools in child welfare, delinquency and mental health. *Child Welfare,* September 1964, pp. 393–397.

Linton, T.E. (1971) The educateur model: A theoretical monograph. *J. Spec. Ed.* 5:155–190.

Mayer, F. Residential group care for dependent, neglected, and emotionally disturbed children in the United States and Canada. An unpublished monograph considered by the National Conference on Group Care in North American, New Orleans, January 1976.

Nirje, B. (1976) Wolfensberger, eds. *Changing Patterns in Residential Services for the Mentally Retarded.* Washington, D.C.: U.S. Government Printing Office, pp. 51–57.

Polsky, H.W. and D.S. Claster. (1968) *The Dynamics of Residential Treatment: A Social System Analysis.* Chapel Hill, N.C.: University of North Carolina Press.

Shulman, R. (1975) Examples of adolescent group homes in alliance with larger institutions. *Child Welfare,* May 1975.

Part III

Treatment of of Special Age Groups

Treatment of Emotional Disorders in Children and Adolescents

CHAPTER 17

Preschool-Age Children

John A. Sours

Childhood is a chrysalis from which each must extricate himself.
—D. H. Lawrence
Fantasies of the Unconscious

The aim of this chapter is to present a spectrum of treatments used for the preschool child. The age of the preschool child is customarily restricted to the span of brief years from toddlerhood (post-rapprochement) until entry into first grade—not nursery school, since children now start nursery school at 2 to 4 years old. But the term "preschool" is also used to refer to prelatency development—children, regardless of chronological age, between the separation-individuation phase and oedipal resolution who have not started the work of latency. The latter designation is not used in this chapter. Such children will be discussed in detail in the chapter on the treatment of the latency child. We shall restrict ourselves to the discussion of preschool children, ages 3 through 5 years or when the child starts first grade. For our purposes, this age span is appropriate, since children are seldom brought to a psychiatrist for treatment before the age of three (Geleerd, 1967). Younger children are usually referred to infant centers for developmental assessment and counseling of the parents.

In an area where child psychotherapy has been largely ignored, the treatment of the preschool child is a topic that has received little attention in both the child psychotherapeutic and psychoanalytic literature. This is largely due to the fact that children, particularly preschool children, are mainly the extraparental responsibility of nursery school and kindergarten teachers and tend not to be referred to therapists until latency years. The early Viennese teachers who later became psychoanalytic educators and practitioners were mainly interested in the primary and secondary school children. Except for Montessori, who came to early education by way of psychiatry, there was little interest in treatment of the preschool child between the world wars. Then the emphasis was on casework intervention aimed at the expression, clarification, and redirection of parental attitude that might help the preschool child to return to the expected normal path of development. This approach to child treatment, however, proved to be disappointing, but it later became one of the energies for the development of family therapy, with techniques questionably applicable to the direct treatment of the young child.

In the last several decades, analytic techniques have become increasingly applied to specific problems of the preschool child for both therapy and analysis. Increasing awareness of developmental issues has allowed a more precise diagnostic assessment of preoedipal psychopathology and de-

Appreciation is expressed to Dr. John B. McDevitt for his helpful comments.

velopmental deviation and given us an additional frame of reference for the understanding of treatment and the theory of technique (C.O.P.E.R., 1974).

The Developmental Approach to the Treatment of the Preschool Child

The developmental approach, in its emphasis on external-internal influences on ongoing development, phasic transitions, child observations, parental information about the child, and child-parent interaction, is complementary to the genetic reconstructive approach, which depends on the recovery of screen memories and fantasies, as well as the enactments of early affective experiences and patterns and somatic reaction. The genetic approach is predicated on the individual's perception of his traumas and developmental strains, along with the distortions of later developmental conflicts. Since the genetic approach depends largely on evocative memory, secondary process dominance, and an introspective stance, it is less useful in the treatment of the preadolescent child and markedly so for the preschooler.

The developmental approach to the treatment of preschoolers is ideally suited for treatment with children of this age group. It provides a broadened frame of reference that has grown from clinical and observational studies of psychic development and the widening scope of psychoanalysis as a clinical and theoretic instrument for understanding and treating the more severe forms of child psychopathologies. Traumatogenic experiences—separation, loss, deprivations, overstimulation, seduction, primal scene, etc.—are frequent experiences of young children and are potent forces in the formation of defensive pathology and character structure. Only by knowing human development of the first three years of life—namely, preverbal and preoedipal development, normal and abnormal structural development, neurophysiological and cognitive limits—can the therapist have a working concept of the therapeutic alliance and treatment process: the treatment of the fixated, aytpical and deviational development of self and object relations, as well as faulty and deviant ego functions (Shane, 1977). This expanded therapeutic thrust is directed at freeing up and facilitating the unfolding of impaired object relations and ego functions. In this regard the therapeutic alliance is pivotal to the therapeutic process and permits the emergence of transference manifestations and the transference neurosis in some oedipal and latency children. For example, dyadic-preoedipal transference is not the substance for interpretation of structural conflict but rather an instrument for facilitating development, warped by trauma and strain during the preoedipal period, by liberating innate developmental energies which thereby allow the progression of development.

The child therapist must understand the nature of development and its various lines, which are longitudinal and epigenetic, conflict-free and conflict-laden, conscious and unconscious, interpersonal and intrapsychic and somatic and psychologic. The developmental approach demonstrates that in the life-cycle psychic development originates from the tendency toward neurotic repetition, the tendency toward recapitulation of earlier developmental issues in later stages of development, and the progressive tendency of normal developmental forces. The concept of normative recapitulation is illustrated by the separation-individuation theory of Mahler (1968), which complements the theory of psychosexual phases and emphasizes the development of the capacity for object relationships and adaptations in their evolution along the lines of progressive ego development and self-object differentiation. And in the assessment and diagnosis of the young child, the developmental approach enables the therapist to detect ego arrests and deviations as well as structural malformations and imbalances before the child leaves the normal track of development.

Child Treatment and the Preschool Child

It is my purpose to review the contributions of child analysis and child psychotherapy, play therapy, family therapy, and behavioral therapy to the theory and technique of treatment of the preschool child. An attempt will be made to discuss the treatment process and the principles and procedures that are uniquely useful to this age range of children. I want to emphasize the richness of the treatment for this age child and especially the fascinating and effective child analytic work that is possible with many preschool children. The analytic material in preschool child analysis is strikingly clear and vivid, much less derivative than what is experienced in adult work. Externalizations, early transference manifestations, fantasies, play elaborations, thematic sequences, and verbalizations are part of the analysis of the preschool child. The rich and dynamic material results from the pressure of the child's instinctual drives, the immaturity of his ego and superego structures, as well as his intense desire for a new object—most apparent when he has attained some level of object constancy. All these factors make the preschool child an exciting and dynamic experience for the child psychotherapist and analyst.

The preschool child is a delightful patient in treatment even though he lacks an observing and critical ego. He tends to be enthusiastic, if not driven for contact with the therapist, imaginative, and frank. Since the preschooler has not begun resolving the Oedipus complex, the superego is not yet rigid, defenses are less rigid, and drives less neutralized. The force of the preschooler's drives impels him to verbal and play expression and communication. The preschool child's closeness to the unconscious and primary process makes him open to many levels of psychoanalytic communication (Bornstein, 1949, 1954; Fraiberg, 1952; Korhman et al., 1971; Malher, 1968; Pearson, 1968; Neubauer, 1972; Wolman, 1972). He can nakedly expose his fantasies and dreams with little self-consciousness. Treatment before latency, therefore, is easier and usually the results are superior.

The treatment of the preschooler is a remarkable demonstration of a number of developmental themes and issues seen during the separation-individuation subphases through phallic development and early stages of the oedipal period before the work of the latency phase begins. Most apparent in the treatment of the preschool child is the fact that the treatment material lies undisguised and readily open to developmental and analytic formulations. In addition, it offers stimulation and clinical data helpful to the therapist in areas outside of treatment where he can pursue various research issues in child development.

Treatment of the preschool child also gives the therapist a very intense experience with the interface between both child and parental dynamics and pathology. By working regularly with the parents, the latter become helpful suppliers of everyday information about the child's life and experiences. The complicated and intimate relation between the child's real and transference relationship with the therapist and his internal and external worlds becomes strikingly clear.

Contrary to what has happened in adult psychiatry, where many new psychological treatments have arisen in the last few years, there is a comparative paucity of parallel treatments for the preschool child. Obviously, therapeutic approaches, like Gestalt therapy, primal therapy, encounter groups, existential analysis, rational therapy, and biofunctional techniques, are not readily applicable to the preschool child. In some ways, the preschool child has been saved from this contemporary wave of new therapies; but on the other hand, except for some specific and notable therapists in this area, not enough has been done to make treatment for this age group better understood and formulated. In addition, much of the energy for helping young children has been directed to early childhood, where the emphasis is placed mainly on cognitive development and an adequate physical environment sufficient to enable mothers to take jobs outside the home.

Psychotherapy for Preschool Children

Indirect Treatments

There are a number of indirect treatments which have been used for children of all ages. These include attitude therapy (Levy, 1937), family therapy (Szurek, 1942), casework techniques (Coleman, 1949; Hamilton, 1947), as well as recently developed parent effectiveness therapies and crisis intervention over the last fifteen years. The preschool child may also be treated indirectly through the mother for conflicts and developmental disturbances not yet internalized (Furman, 1957). There has been increasing interest in family therapy, which draws its energy from psychoanalytic concepts and experiences as well as the psychology and sociology of small groups. Few family therapists have attempted to bring preschool children directly into family sessions. There are some reports of young children present during family sessions, but little systematic work has been done on this particular aspect of family treatment (Fieldsteel, 1974).

Direct Treatments

Outside of child analysis, which strongly uses interpretive activity, child therapies in general, whether they are supportive or expressive psychotherapies, tend to rely on abreaction, clarification, suggestion, manipulation, and the corrective emotional experience of the new object. In the treatment of the preschool child, the child's desire for the new object, if sufficient object constancy has been attained and narcissism decreased, draws him closely to the therapist, a new object, and provides him with an experience outside of his relationship with his mother and father. The therapeutic (working) alliance with the preschool child is based on the intrinsic need for a new object—the opportunity to displace current feelings toward his parents onto the therapist, with whom he can identify. He experiences sensations, perceptions, and feelings that occur at home with the parents and uses in the treatment situation his typical defensive configuration. The alliance is also driven by positive transference, special displacements to the therapist of feelings vis-à-vis the parents from an earlier period of development. The preschooler revels in the narcissistic pleasure of undivided attention from a new person (the therapist), who encourages guiltless unrestricted play and facilitates the shift from passive to active identification with the parents. In addition, the perception of the therapist as a helping person who wants to remove the child's psychic pain heightens the alliance once the child understands, by way of transference manifestations and displacements, current blurring of the past with the present and how he creates painful situations in the treatment. Then he identified with the therapist to the limit of his developmental capacity.

Child psychotherapies attempt to elicit both interactional and developmental-transferential material that can be utilized by the therapist in his work with the child, as well as in his attempts toward helping the parents understand the child and provide a new adaptive solution so the child can proceed smoothly ahead along healthier developmental lines.

Since World War II, play therapy has been less popular as a specific therapy. In 1948, for instance, *The Journal of the Nervous Child* devoted its entire issue to play therapy, and in 1955 a roundtable on play therapy appeared in the *American Journal of Orthopsychiatry.* Many of these approaches were quite specific in their aims and expressive of their originators' theoretical and tactical approach to child treatment (Schaeffer, 1976). The book Haworth edited (1964) reveals the nature of early play therapy, and James' monograph on theories of play therapy adumbrates the various techniques (1977). For instance, Solomon's active play therapy largely consists of the therapist selecting a doll that to his mind is symbolic of the patient's major conflict. From that point, the child is allowed to pick another doll in response to the therapist's and then play out what is considered pertinent to the material. This treatment claims to foster abreaction, increase verbal communication, heighten the child's level of consciousness about conflict, and permit more spontaneous and less stereotypic play. Active play therapy is considered particularly helpful for a specific situation or sympton, such as car sickness, a discrete phobia, and any circumscribed symptom in general. Implicit in this treatment is the therapist's deep awareness of not only the child's basic conflicts but also the parental home situation, so that the therapist is able to manipulate the play along these appropriate lines. Yet often the child therapist does not have sufficient comprehensive understanding of the child and the parents, especially early in treatment, to allow him to set up working treatment hypotheses and play them out therapeutically. Encouraging the child to throw himself into play for cathartic release only fosters repression and deludes the child in that there is a transient decrease in symptoms because of the discharge of instinctual tension. Consequently, the conflict between ego and id remains unchanged (Winnicott, 1971).

In 1939 David Levy recommended another form of active play that he called release therapy for the specific treatment of traumatic situations and experiences. These include separation and divorce, parental death, and birth of a sibling. The effectiveness of his approach, Levy thought, derived from release of drives and affects connected with the trauma. Release therapy retains some of its popularity today. It is, however, limited in its usefulness to traumatic situations such as elective surgery, post-traumatic reactions, and major disruptive events in a child's life. This therapeutic intervention is singularly helpful with children who face extensive dental or surgical procedures, or who have experienced the death of a parent. This approach is most useful in hospitals and rehabilitation institutions when a child is facing surgery and needs the opportunity of meeting with a child therapist for a few sessions. This treatment is also useful in the assessment and treatment of young children who have been attacked, molested, or raped; the play dramatizations allow the clinician to get some understanding of the extent of psychic trauma and the consequences of earlier conflicts and fixations reactivated by the recent trauma.

Another form of structured play therapy was described in 1955 by Hambridge. He advocated active play therapy. Play activity in this form is also said to foster creative free play, allow abreaction, permit mastery of anxiety, and facilitate separation and individuation. Treatment consists of structuring the play along the lines of sibling rivalry, separation, anxiety, awareness of genital differences, primal scene experiences, the birth of a sibling, difficult peer relations, and frightening dreams. This type of structured play therapy, much like release therapy, also requires that a therapist have a solid understanding of the child.

One other form of brief child therapy, also applicable to the preschool child, is Bender's puppet play (1936). In this treatment the child selects the puppets of his choice and uses them to play out fantasies, dreams, and actions. This treatment is most effective in a circumscribed situation for those children who have a natural leaning toward puppet play and are willing to remain with this play activity.

It was Axline in 1947 who strongly opposed both forms of structured play. She attempted to show that if the child has the opportunity to play freely without physical and emotional confines and the intervention of the therapist, he changes his attitudes toward both himself and the external world. She believed that every child has a growth potential that permits him to solve his own problems if he is encouraged in that direction. The child is given complete acceptance and permitted to play out his feelings at random, without clarification and interpretation. Unfortunately, cathartic release does not eliminate conflict between ego and id, and because of the discharge of tension, fleeting decreases in symptomatology may give the child a false sense of safety.

In the last ten years short-term therapies have returned to the structured approach. Gardner's use of the mutual storytelling technique is an example (1971). In this approach, the therapist makes up the child's story based on his assessment of the child's pathology and family's pathology and tells it to the child, who then responds to the symbolic content. With the therapist's help he elaborates the story and interprets it to the patient. This technique also presupposes the therapist's familiarity with the child's core conflict. Devaluing the conflict can transiently reassure the child, but at the same time it scotomizes the conflict. Likewise, connecting behavior at a later phase of development to an unresolved conflict from a previous phase is an exmaple of the fallacy of reductionism.

Whatever form of child therapy is used, there is always some degree of spontaneous play. The level of play can vary markedly from day to day for the child and is also quite different in terms of a patient's pathology and age. For the preschool child, it is essential that some level of free play be used in a spontaneous and unstructured way (Ekstein and Friedman, 1957). It must be kept in mind, aside from a very definite structured play situation for a traumatic situation, that whatever the analyst contributes, the play must be allowed to unfold smoothly. The therapist must not play beyond the child's level or interpret directly the play. Oftentimes, the play will involve aggressive and counteraggressive activities, attempts at object recovery and removal, masochistic defeats and maneuvers that foster identification. Free-flowing spontaneous play augurs well for therapeutic success, since it aims at restoring the child to normal involvement. Frequently, however, especially in latency children, play acceptance can lead to repetitive play, either reflecting a repressed masturbatory fantasy or a traumatic experience the child is not able to work out on his own. (These attempts include the desire to overcome passivity, the wish to be beaten, and affectionate yearning.)

In both child therapy and analysis dramatization, play often occurs and is another variety of free play. This involves the creative use of play materials that form the family constellation and express the emotional patterns among the family. This kind of play is ego-dominated and is striking in the structure that it presents and the control that the child is able to bring to it. It must be distinguished from acting out (A. Freud, 1965), and it carries with it the danger to the therapist that he may be swept into the play and respond with needless interpretation.

Whatever the therapeutic play situation is and the degree of structure and activity required, interpretation cannot be made directly through the play. One finds that this stops the play, contaminates the material and works against the child using the play situation as a sublimatory activity. The play should only be interpreted in those situations where the play is dangerous to the child or the therapist is apt inadvertently to allow sexual gratification.

Psychoanalytic Child Psychotherapy

Child therapy is basically a relationship between the child and the therapist. It is aimed primarily at symptom resolution and attaining adaptive stability. The objectives of child psychotherapy are basically symptom removal and modification of behavior. This is achieved through games and play activity—techniques that are not particularly useful in the treatment of latency and adolescent patients.

For the preschool child, interpretation, which must work in conjunction with verbalization and clarification, requires great care in application and the selection of language. The support and reassurances of the new trusted object (the therapist) are extremely helpful to the preschool child as well as abreaction and clarification of feeling. The preschool child, more so than any other patient in child therapy, requires trust in his development so he can move from action to games to play to fantasies, words and to symbolic functions. In addition, the therapist can help the child find more appropriate defense mechanisms. Child therapy, even for the preschool child, helps the child in effectively using defense against drives and allowing the child to discourage drive derivatives, decrease drive pressures and express affect.

It is also important that the parents be regularly seen, usually weekly, in the treatment of the preschool child. Their understanding of the child's behavior and pathology can only be attained through sharing information about the child's development with them. Using parental information directly within treatment—i.e., telling the child the parents have informed the therapist of events or his actions at home—can at times clarify a point in the treatment process, but it also can heighten the child's mistrust and make him less inclined to speak about events external to the treatment. The parents are helped to change their own attitudes toward the child. Parents must be on the side of the child's development, if treatment is to succeed, and be an auxiliary observing ego for the child in the informational relationship with the therapist. Direct advice to the parents is seldom effective, most markedly so if the parents' attitude toward the child is not empathic and their understanding not sufficient to enable them to speak properly to the child and play out some of the child's feelings. Except for traumatic situations external to the home, direct advice to the parents is not helpful. Explicit prohibition of parental seductiveness to the child is particularly not useful, at least in the early phases of treatment; and in general, attempting to change the parents' behavior will often confuse the child and muddy the therapeutic situation.

Indications for Psychotherapy

There are some specific situations calling for child psychotherapy. Neurotic conflicts that are not interfering with libidinal and ego development can often be worked out in psychotherapy. When internalization of conflict in the preschool child is minimal, there is a preponderance of external conflict and the balance between wishes and repression is not greatly out of kilter, psychotherapy can be most helpful. If, on the other hand, there is a preponderance of internalized conflict in the preschool child—sometimes found in those children with premature ego development—then child psychotherapy is not sufficient. Those preschool children with structural ego defects and deviation (preverbal disturbances and failures in separation-individuation) often require a very structured treatment that is provided best by child therapy.

These are preschool children who are autistic in the separation-individuation phase of development (Kernberg, 1972). To varying degrees they show distress in separating from the mother. Most seriously arrested are the symbiotic children who have not been able to differentiate self from object. A second group of arrested children appears symbiotic but yet shows a variable degree of object constancy and early signs of phallic-oedipal concerns. A third group is the phallic-oedipal children, who, although they have reached libidinal object constancy, slip back easily into preoedipal regressions.

After sphincter control is achieved and libidinal object constancy is consolidated, the preschool child displays clear-cut phallic behavior and the beginnings of oedipal preoccupations and ego autonomy. As he moves on to a higher level of phallic-oedipal development, there is differentiation and consolidation of the ego and superego. Some children at this level are able to maintain a high degree of ego autonomy without serious ego regression. But others lose ego autonomy and struggle with separation-individuation because of severe regression.

This latter group of phallic-oedipal children may be difficult to differentiate from preschoolers who have not fully passed through the separation-individuation phase, and although manifesting some phallic drive expression, are still dyadic in their object relations. Careful evaluation is necessary for this differentiation. At times diagnosis and developmental assessment can only be made by an extended period of consultation or an interval of therapy.

The frequency of sessions is related to the degree of defensive, structural, and adaptive change required. Twice-weekly psychotherapy does not provide the intensity necessary for such changes. The intensity of a four-to-five-session-per-week child analysis allows working toward a new balance of defenses, increasing the focus on a more progressive libidinal phase in the direction of neutralization of aggression and sublimation of libido, a wider range of affective responsiveness, modulation of primitive parts of the superego, and heightened self-esteem. Problems of passivity and strong negative yearnings, as well as those of intense aggression and masochism, are difficult to work through in a low-frequency treatment which cannot provide sufficient time for working through and termination.

For young children who develop mono-symptomatic neurotic problems (a specific fear, phobias, simple enuresis, sleep disturbances, etc.) without pathological personality structure and without being thrown off their developmental track, psychoanalytic psychotherapy may be sufficient to work out an isolated developmental conflict. But severe inner conflict or development arrest that looks as though resolution over time will not be possible suggests a full analytic therapy if it can be suppported by the parents. Having the mother present during therapy sessions may further help the preschooler (Furman, 1957) to express his feelings toward the mother, clarify feelings and use the therapist to verbalize confusing feelings. Advising the mother, separate from the child, on how to relate to the child and offering support is frequently helpful in establishing an equilibrium between parent and the child's ego (Bonnard, 1950; Bornstein, 1949; Fraiberg, 1952). The therapist, however, must be alert to the possibility that such young children may be found to have serious internalized conflicts or disturbances in early separation-individuation, requiring a therapy of higher frequency and longer duration. Likewise, preschool children with habit disturbances (sleeping, eating, toilet training, etc.) stemming from parental lack of environmental structuring and preschoolers who act out parental wishes can benefit from psychotherapy, in conjuction with parental counseling. Oftentimes, early treatment will avoid the development of later impulsive behavior disorders in latency and adolescence.

Therapy is indicated for those preschool children whose development is jeopardized by recent and severe traumas, often loss of a parent through divorce or death (Buxbaum, 1956). Giving the child a chance for abreaction and clarification of his experience may short-circuit transient symptoms and preserve future development. If not treated, often the child's character is molded around the traumas with a tendency toward repetition-compulsion.

The preschooler with difficulties related to developmental interference (harsh feedings, separations, losses, etc.) may not need therapy (Nagera, 1966). Counseling of parents or family therapy may be sufficient. Phase-specific interruptions in the unfolding of development do not necessarily warrant therapy of the child. Developmental conflicts can be brought about by phase-appropriate environmental demands. But if a developmental interference leads to a disruptive developmental conflict because of a traumatic event or environmental strain, and the parents are unable to help the child directly, then individual treatment, rather than family therapy, is needed. An example is a parent who responds traumatically to a preschool child's masturbation and sets up a developmental interference, which then is transformed into a developmental conflict by early phallic-oedipal wishes.

Without parental interference and traumatization, developmental conflicts expressed as behavior problems and symptoms may be fleeting. The child may find his own solution through reaction formation, early character traits, and sublimations. But if drive and age development are out of phase, external factors unresolvable, or the conflict simply too intense, the child may go on to have a monosymptomatic neurosis, which, if persisting into the oedipal years, can be internalized as an intersystemic neurotic conflict (A. Freud, 1965). In that case treatment of the child is not absolutely necessary. Educating and treating the parents are usually not enough to help for the child.

There are some preschool children with developmental arrests and deviations who do not benefit from psychotherapy. Interpretation of strong affects overwhelms their ego with secondary process thinking. These borderline schizophrenic or organic chldren first require strengthening of the ego through reassurance and educative intervention; the interpretation of defenses, transference manifestations, and resistances is possible. The same approach is necessary for those children who because of early deprivational experiences in object relations need an emotional experience to allow them to reach a level of object-relatedness sufficient for verbalization and interpretation. Weil (1973) suggests a similiar approach to borderline children with multiple imbalances between ego and drive endowment, between libido and aggression, and between hostile and nonhostile aggression. She believes preschool children with lack of object constancy, fear of object loss, maladaptive defensive structures against diffuse presignal anxiety require ego-strengthening psychotherapy, often with special tutorial help once the child goes off to school. Furman (1957) takes a similar position, using the therapeutic nursery school for ego-strengthening, which is then combined with psychotherapy and, if possible, analysis later.

Indications for Child Analysis

For children in general, analysis is the preferred treatment if there is permanent neurotic symptomatology that augers badly for future emotional development. If there is neurotic interference with libidinal development or neurotic interference with ego development, analysis should be considered. But the choice is more complicated for the preschool child. If object constancy has not been achieved, if he is vulnerable to anxiety, unable to tolerate frustration, and prone to outbursts of pathological aggression and omnipotence, then analysis of the preschool child is generally not indicated; at least, psychotherapy to strengthen the ego might well be used first until the child is less fearful of losing impulse control. Then child analysis can be used to turn id into ego content.

Child analysis is somewhat different from adult analysis, and this is even more the case in doing analysis with preschool cldren. They are not able to maintain verbal free association, but like the adult starting analysis, the child is told that he is in a special situation without the usual restrictions but is encouraged to limit direct drive gratification and communicate through play, toys, and actions on a semiotic-symbolic level. Parents usually encourage the child to play with the therapist, who in turn encourages the communication by helping the child with words for affect and connections, drawings for inchoate fantasies and toys for symbolic play. Because of the relative lack of inner restraints, the preschool child in terms of the semiotic function of sensory-motor representations, is inclined to free association.

Transference is limited to manifestations, displacements of the past mostly aggressive in nature. Transference neurosis is encountered more often in the analysis of latency chldren. The child analyst is a real object to the child and a source of support to the child, who is still living with the parents whom he needs for love and safety. Resistances in the child analytic patients are usually stronger; the child usually lacks conscious motivation. Preschool chldren, however, are often enthusiastic patients, eager to find a new object in the analyst. If the preschooler has achieved object constancy, this enthusiasm carries him into treatment and strenghtens the therapeutic alliance of the opening phase. In addition, the preschooler usually is active in sessions, bringing into treatment during the middle phase, play fantasies, dreams, drawings and dramatizations. And since structures are not yet well formed in the preschooler, the terminal phase moves quickly toward bringing the child back to his track of development.

Treatment Principles for Both Psychotherapy and Analysis of the Preschool Child

Both psychotherapy, to some degree, and analysis for the preschooler is a "defense analysis" whereby affect, resistance, and transferential material are analyzed. The thrust of both treatments is at symptoms and other defenses against painful effect. Ego resistances are analyzed before id content. Interpretation is of resistance before content and from surface to depth; it should be in the child's phase-appropriate idiosyncratic play, fantasy, and language. Phase-specific and phase-appropriate defenses, in keeping with the developmental model, are interpreted less than primitive and maladaptive defenses so as not to derail normal progressive development. The child is encouraged to use the therapist as a new object; and treatment moves from surface to depth, from motor activity to fantasy and eventually to verbal articulation and new object representations. Instinctual wishes are not interpreted until analysis of defense has proceeded well along. The interpretation of play is similar to that of fantasy—the interpretation of the defensive maneuver against dysphoric affect and then drive derivatives.

The opening phase of treatment is occasionally the first separation experience for the preschool child and can be a tense period for both mother and child. Yet there are many preschoolers who rush into the consultation room for a quick inspection of the playroom and display marked curiosity for the therapist, the new object in his life. Nevertheless, it is best that the therapist warn the parents in their initial interview that the child may be reluctant to separate from her. This is often the case of the child has not completed the rapprochement crisis—anal libidinal conflicts with the mother—combined with phallic or early oedipal apprehension. If this turns out to be the situation, then the therapist should try to distract the child from the mother and not linger in the waiting room. If the child refuses, then he can be promised that the office door will be left open. If this conciliation fails and the child panics, then the mother must come in with the child but remain detached from the work of the therapist and the child. The mother's presence is usually not a serious impediment. The child is not inhibited in play or direct communication and does not object to the mother overhearing the therapist's interpretations and general coments. The preschool child may in fact play out roles with the mother, giving the therapist another view of their interaction.

Parents of the preschool child in treatment must remain in touch with the therapist, not only in weekly meetings, but also through telephone conversations about interval occurences that bear on the treatment process. Because of his proclivity to fantasize his everyday life, the preschooler does not report his reality.

In the first sessions, little should be asked of the preschooler. Only comments that encourage play are useful in these early hours. Every effort should be made to help the child dramatize his fantasies about his family and family happenings, and intrapsychically, about good and bad representations of objects and self. A doll house and family are most helpful, as well as drawing, artistic, and instructional materials. These activities are necessary at this level of development and are not "acting out" in the sense of adult analysis. Games only work against spontaneity and creative effort. Drawing is particularly popular with the preschooler, although he may have to ask the therapist for help with details. Discharge of emotion through play, dramatization, and speech can lend to loss of control through fear of aggression and frightening libidinal gratification. Unable to contain his impulses through play—and too young to sublimate impulses through pretending, playing, or talking—the preschool child's play can erupt into action and acting out even if the analyst has told him that "no harm must come to himself, the doctor or the office." This disruptive activity often mobilizes countertransference, especially if the therapist must intervene by way of interpretation or physical restraint.

The choice for language for communication—notably interpretations with the preschooler—must be carefully made to ensure comprehension, maintain a balance between drive and defense and guard against narcissistic injury. Distancing devices ("I know another child who . . .") are helpful in reducing the pain of direct interpretative confrontation with the preschool ego. A full range of interpretations (those of defense, drive, transference, displacement, conflict, reconstruction, setting, attention, reductive and situational [Lewis, 1974] can be made to the preschool child, provided understandable language is used and not to close to his vulnerability. Sometimes, role-playing—the child telling an appropriate story—dampens for the child the strong affect a direct interpretation would evoke.

Transference reactions are the strongest and most plentiful during the middle phase of treatment. This is the time in therapy or analysis when the child's feelings increase in primitivity and strength, depending on the quality of defenses, the degree of frustration of drive, the intensity of the conflict, and the anonymous quality of the therapist as both a primary and real object.

Defenses in the opening phase are dealt with to clear the way for the working-through process of the middle phase, which is not as clearly demarcated as the opening and termination phases.

The middle phase is where the therapist usually sees development accelerating through the treatment. And when the child has been put back on his natural track of development, when conflicts, arrests, and deviations have been worked through and have led to considerable structural change, the decision must be made to end the treatment. The remaining transference meanings of termination are further worked through with the strengthening of ego and superego identification. Decision to terminate is made with both the child and parents, allowing them sufficient time to experience and work through the loss.

Because of unforeseen events in the preschool child's latency and adolescent years, termination should ideally be on a positive note for both child and parents. Additional treatment may be necessary. The child and his parents should feel that the therapist's door is always open.

Acknowledgments

Appreciation is expressed to Dr. John B. McDevitt for his helpful comments.

References

Adams, P.L. (1974) *A Primer of Child Psychotherapy.* Boston: Little, Brown.

Amster, F. (1943) Different uses of play in treatment of young children. *Am. J. Orthopsychiat.* 13:62–68.

Arthur, S.A. (1952) A comparison of the techniques employed in psychotherapy and psychoanalysis of children. *Am. J. Orthopsychiat.* 22:484–498.

Axline, V.M. (1947) *Play therapy: THe inner dynamics of childhood.* New York: Houghton-Mifflin.

Bender, E. (1952) Clay modeling as a projective technique. In *Child Psychiatric Techniques.* Springfield, Ill.: Charles C Thomas, pp. 221–237.

Bender, L., and A.A. Woltmann. (1936) The use of puppet shows as a psychotherapeutic method of behavior problems in children. *Am. J. Orthopsychiat.* 6:341–354.

Bernstein, I. (1958) The importance of characteristics of the parents in deciding on child analysis. *Am. J. Psychoanal. Assn.* 6:71–78.

Bernstein, I. (1975) On the technique of child and adolescent analysis, *J. Am. Psychoanal. Assn.* 23:190–232.

Bonnard, A. (1950) The mother as therapist in a case of obsessional neurosis. *Psychoanal. Study Child* 5:391–408.

Bornstein, B. (1945) Clinical notes on child analysis. *Psychoanal. Study Child* 1:151–166.

Bornstein, B. (1945) Emotional barriers in the understanding and treatment of children. *Am. J. Orthopsychiat.* 18:691–697.

Bornstein, B. (1949) The analysis of a phobic child. Some problems of theory and technique in child analysis. *Psychoanal. Study Child* 3/4:181–226.

Bornstein, B. (1954) Phobia in a two-and-a-half-year-old child. *Psychoanal. Quart.* 4:181–226.

Burlingame, D.T. (1951) Present trends in handling the mother-child relationship during the therapeutic process. *Psychoanal. Study Child* 6:31–37.

Buxbaum, E. (1951) Psychotherapy and psychoanalysis in the treatment of children. *The Nervous Child* 5:115–126.

Buxbaum, E. (1954) Technique of child therapy: a critical evaluation. *Psychoanal. Study Child* 9:297–333.

C.O.P.E.R. (1974) Conference on Psychoanalytic Education and Research. The American Psychoanalytic Association. Position Papers, Commission I and IX.

Coleman, J. (1949) Distinguishing between psychotherapy and casework. *J. Social Casework* 30:219–224.

Ekstein, R., and S. Friedman. (1957) The function of acting out, play action, and play acting in the psychotherapeutic process. *Am. J. Psychoanal. Assn.* 5:581–629.

Fieldsteel, N.D. (1974) Family therapy-individual therapy: A false dichotomy. In L. Wolberg and J. Aronson, eds., *Group Therapy.* New York: Grune & Stratton, pp. 44–45.

Fraiberg, S. (1952) A critical neurosis in a two-and-a-half-year-old girl. *Psychoanal. Study Child* 7:173–215.

Framo, J.L. ed., (1972) *Family Interaction.* New York: Springer.

Freud, A. (1974) Indications for child analysis. *Psychoanal. Study Child* 1:127–150.

Freud, A. (1946) *The Psychoanalytical Treatment of Children.* New York: Schocken.

Freud, A. (1965) *Normality and Pathology in Childhood.* New York: International Universities Press.

Freud, A. (1971) The Writing of Anna Freud. Vol. VII, 1966–1970. ***Problems of Psychoanalytic Training, Diagnosis and the Technique of Therapy.*** New York: International Universities Press.

Furman, E. (1957) Treatment of under-fives by way of parents. *Psychoanal. Study Child* 12:250–262.

Gardner, R.A. (1971) *Therapeutic Communication with Children.* New York: Science House.

Geleerd, E.R., Ed. (1967) *The Child Analyst at Work.* New York: International Universities Press.

Goodman, J.D., and J.A. Sours. (1967) *The Child Mental Status Examination.* New York: Basic Books.

Haley, J., and L. Hoffman, eds. (1967) *Techniques of Family Therapy.* New York: Basic Books.

Hambridge, F. (1955) Structured play therapy. *Am. J. Orthopsychiat.* 25:601–617.

Hamilton, G. (1947) *Psychotherapy in Child Guidance.* New York: Columbia University Press.

Harley, M. (1961) Panel report: Resistances in child analysis. *J. Am. Psychoanal. Assn.* 9:548-551.

Harter, S. (1968) Piaget's theory of intellectual development: The changing world of the child. *Conn. Med.* 332:444–456.

Haworth, M.R., ed. (1964) *Child Psychotherapy.* New York: Basic Books.

Heinickle, C.M., et al. (1965) Frequency of psychotherapeutic sessions as a factor affecting the child's developmental status. *Psychoanal. Study Child* 20:42–98.

James, D.O. (1977) *Play Therapy.* Oceanside, N.Y.: Dabor Science Publications.

Karasu, T.B. (1977) Psychotherapies: An overview. *Am. J. Psychiat.* 134:851–863.

Kennedy, H. (1972) Problems in reconstruction in child analysis. *Psychoanal. Study Child* 26:386–402.

Kernberg, O.F. (1972) Early ego integration and direct relations. *Ann. N.Y. Acad. Sci.* 193:233–247.

Kestenberg, J. (1969) Problems of child analysis in relation to the various developmental stages: Prelatency. *Psychoanal. Study Child* 24:358–383.

Klein, M. (1954) *The Psychoanalysis of Children* London: Hogarth Press.

Klein, M. (1955) The psychoanalytic play technique. *Am. J. Orthopsychiat.* 25:223–237.

Kohrman, R., H.H. Fineberg, R.C. Gelman, and S. Weiss (1971) Technique of child analysis. *Int. J. Psychoanal.* 52: 487–497.

Kramer, C.H. (1968) *The Relationship between Child and Family Psychopathology: A Suggested Extension of Psychoanalytic Theory and Technique.* Chicago: Family Institute of Chicago.

Lawrence, D.H. (1921) *Psychoanalysis and the Unconscious and Fantasia of the Unconscious.* New York: Viking Press, p. 150.

Levy, D. (1937) Attitude therapy. *Am. J. Orthopsychiat.* 7:103–113.

Levy, D. (1939) Release therapy. *Am. J. Orthopsychiat.* 9:713–736.

Lewis, M. (1974) Interpretation in Child Analysis. *J. Am. Acad. Child Psychiat.* 13:32–53.

Maenchen, A. (1970) On the technique of child analysis in relation to stages of development. *Psychoanal. Study Child* 25:175–208.

Machover, K. (1951) *Personality Projection in the Drawing of the Human Figure.* Springfield, Ill.: Charles C Thomas.

Mahler, M. (1968) *On Human Symbiosis and the Vicissitudes of Individuation.* New York: International Universities Press.

Nagera, H. (1963) The developmental profile. Notes on some practical considerations regarding its use. *Psychoanal. Study Child* 18:511–540.

Nagera, H. (1966) *Early Childhood Disturbances, The Infantile Neurosis, and the Adulthood Disturbances.* Monograph No. 2, Psychoanalytic Studies of the Child. New York: International Universities Press.

Neubauer, P.M. (1972) Psychoanalysis of the pre-school child. In B.B. Wolman, ed., *The Handbook of Child Psychoanalysis.* New York: Van Nostrand Reinhold, pp. 221–252.

Olch, G. (1971) Panel Report: Technical problems in the analyses of the preoedipal and preschool child. *J. Am. Psychoan. Assn.* 19:543–551.

Pearson, G.H.J. (1968) *A Handbook of Child Psychoanalysis.* New York: Basic Books.

Pearson, G.H.J. (1974–75) What is psychotherapy? Proceedings of the 9th International Congress of Psychotherapy, Oslo, 1973. *Psychother. & Psychosom.* 24, Nos. 4–6, 1974, and 25, Nos. 1–6 (1975).

Peller, L. (1954) Libidinal phases, ego development and play. *Psychoanal. Study Child* 9:178–198.

Schaefer, C.E., ed. (1976) *Therapeutic Use of Child's Play.* New York: Jason Aronson.

Shane, M. (1977) A rationale for teaching analytic technique based on a developmental orientation and approach. *Int. J. Psychoanal.* 58:95–108.

Smirnoff, V. (1968) *The Scope of Child Analysis.* New York, International Universities Press.

Sterba, E. (1959) Child analysis. In M. Levitt, ed., *Readings in Psychoanalytic Psychology.* New York: Appleton-Century-Crofts, pp. 287–310.

Szurek, S., et al. (1942) Collaborative psychiatric therapy of parent-child problems. *Am. J. Orthopsychiat.* 12: 511–520.

Weil, A.D. (1973) Ego strengthening prior to analysis. *Psychoanalytic Study of the Child.* 28:487–301.

Winnicott, D.W. (1971) *Playing and Reality.* New York: Basic Books.

Wolman, B.B., ed. (1972) *Handbook of Child Psychoanalysis.* New York: Van Nostrand.

Treatment of Emotional Disorders in Children and Adolescents

CHAPTER 18

Latency-Age Children

Charles A. Sarnoff

Introduction

The term "latency" refers to a specific potential found in children age six to twelve in the area of personality adjustment. Specifically, this is the ability to achieve a state of calm, educability, and pliability, using an age-appropriate organization of defenses. This state of "latency" is not always attained in children in this age group. Social and cultural influences determine the degree to which the available mechanisms are put to work producing states of latency.

The therapy to be described in this chapter will be concerned with the treatment of those aspects of childhood psychopathology that interfere with the development and organization of the ability to produce and maintain a state of latency. As such, the information contained herein will relate primarily to the neurotic and characterological aspects of children age six to twelve. Learning disabilities, symbiotic states, childhood psychoses, and organic brain disease are not the targets of the treatment modality to be described, although to some extent they may be useful in youngsters with these conditions in dealing with their social adjustment, especially where states of calm are striven for but poorly mastered by the child.

It is essential to the maturation of the child as a social being that these states of calm be achieved. It is during such states that most social learning is acquired. The ego skills exercised in the development of the mental functions (e.g., fantasy formation) that are used in maintaining the states of calm form the groundwork for the development of reality-oriented future planning as the child enters adolescence. Therefore, not only is therapeutic attention required for the states of disordered mood and behavior that mark failures in the attainment of the latency state, but attention should also be directed to the deficiencies that result when the development of latency fails.

History

Childhood has an history all its own. It is the history of a minority too weak to defend itself and in constant need of advocates. As strikingly portrayed by De Mauss (1975), the history of childhood is only just beginning to touch the cultural horizon at which children are perceived as individuals with needs and personalities independent of parental goals, and as creatures to be understood rather than to be herded and manipulated.

Within the history of childhood, the discovery that there is a specific organization of the personality, which imparts characteristics to the years six to twelve, which are independent of ordinary growth, subject to pathological alterations and influences, and able to be enhanced or modified by psychotherapeutic interventions, is a late and relatively tangential element. It has touched relatively few children. Usually these children are from highly child-oriented, educated groups in the upper middle-class suburban communities of Western society.

Prior to 1900, awareness that children's behavior

is motivated and that children have an emotional inner life appears in the writings of the occasional intuitive observer. *Lazarillo of Tormes*, the classical Spanish mock epic of the late Middle Ages, depicts a boy who is capable of self-reflection and remorse. In the mid-nineteenth century Felix Descuret (see De Saussaure, 1946) approached troubled children with an understanding of their needs and wrote of the resolution of jealousy and emotional discomfort, with insight into the psychological workings of the inner world of the child. A number of other sources could also be quoted to prove that awareness of the emotional life of the child has ever been available for use by gifted people in an occasional manner independent of organizations and educational disciplines.

It was not until 1896 that Freud (1950) first detected that there were distinguishing characteristics to the latency period that set it apart. At first all that was perceived was a relative paucity of recollections from this period during the psychoanalysis of adults. This was apparently sufficient to call attention to the period for further study. During the first quarter of the twentieth century, knowledge of the period grew till the point was reached that the latency period came to be viewed as a period of calm between the early infantile sexual life and the burgeoning sexuality of adolescence. The calm attained was explained on the basis of the growth of mechanisms of defense which were capable of transforming the moral demands of society into patterns of internal control that kept the drives in check and which shaped the drives when the efflorescence of bodily growth and instinctual energies that mark adolescence began. This view of latency held sway until 1926, when Freud declared that in latency "the sexual urges diminish in strength" (p. 210). From that point on, this became the most widely accepted general principle for understanding the quiet behavior of latency-age children. This theory obviated the development of concepts related to cognitive and ego growth that could be used as the basis for developing a psychotherapeutic strategy for dealing with troubled latency-aged youngsters. Fortunately, some workers continued to advance Freud's earlier ideas. Recently the concept of an "ego structure of latency" has been introduced to represent this point of view. In this way a theoretical orientation upon which to base a psychotherapy for latency-age children has been championed. The point of view that latency calm is the product of the utilization of maturing ego functions rather than of diminished drives is forced upon us by the observations that calm behavior is inconsistent in children, and that some children experience no latency at all.

Failure to enter latency and episodes of marked breakdowns in latency calm become important target syndromes in the psychotherapy of latency-age children. The appearance of such behavior, though not necessarily discomforting to child or parent, has predictive value in relation to social adjustment in adolescence and adulthood. The adjustments in fantasy that help the latency-age child master situations that are humiliating are the forerunners of the future planning skills that are vital to individual adjustment in the older person "on his own." The skills in abstraction and delay required for adolescent and adult functioning are developed and practiced in the production of states of latency. Failure to develop or maintain appropriate states of latency may be indicators that these vital cognitive skills are unavailable or are being bypassed and given short shrift in the development of the child.

Amongst those clinicians who were aware of the discovery of "latency," a growing body of knowledge about the psychology of childhood was organized. At first this had to do with reconstructions of the psychic life of children based on the analysis of adults (Freud, 1905). However, as early as 1909 (Freud, 1909), papers began to appear which described interviews with children as well as therapeutic interpretations based on psychoanalytic principles which had been directed towards children by meaningful adults. It is of interest that in one such case (Ferenczi, 1913) a child was thought to have lost interest in pursuing his wish to be a rooster when he ceased to talk in conversation and instead wanted to play with a toy rooster. Further investigation of the case described the observations of an involved adult.

Blocks to the direct role of a trained therapist in the work with children were removed when psychoanalytically trained people who worked with children were able to perceive that children of latency age symbolize their problems in their play much in the way that adults symbolize their problems in their dreams. Two prominent workers in this endeavor were Melanie Klein (1932) and Anna Freud (1946), whose books *The Psychoanalysis of Children* (Klein) and *The Psychonalytic Treatment of Children* (A. Freud) describe in great clinical detail the techniques they found to be effective in reaching children of latency age who have adjustment problems. This individual psychotherapeutic technique was practiced and developed in Europe. It was studied there by American psychiatrists. In

1935, Maxwell Gitelson brought the technique to Chicago, where it was integrated into the individualized approach to troubled children that William Healy had introduced through his child guidance demonstration programs some decades before. Thus was born in the United States dynamically oriented psychotherapy for children.

There have been few texts devoted to child therapy. There are case histories published, usually in paperback for mass consumption. Periodicals have been outstanding in chronicling the development of the field. A large body of data has been published in periodicals for use by the therapist in search of information about approaches to specific conditions. Useful periodicals are *The Nervous Child, American Journal of Orthopsychiatry, The Journal of the American Academy of Child Psychiatry, The Psychoanalytic Study of the Child,* and *Child Psychiatry and Human Development*. Recently the author of this chapter (Sarnoff, 1976) has published a book with an extended discussion of the psychotherapeutic approach to the latency-age child. Kramer and Byerly (1978) have described the psychoanalytic approach.

Theoretical Contributions

The psychotherapeutic approach to the latency-age child is predicated on the theory that the appearance of emotional symptoms and signs is determined in large measure by psychological influences. The concept does not in any way exclude biochemical or genetic factors. It merely places in a context which provides for psychotherapeutic leverage, such factors as social influences, cognitive development, maturation of the organization of ego defenses, and the vicissitudes of the instinctual drives.

As opposed to the theory of adults, which deals with internalized conflict and social maladjustments within a context of a stable cognition, psychotherapy with children must be shaped to fit the fact that one is dealing with a growing child. That which is acceptable and normal behavior changes with age. Symbolizing function and abstract cognition in the areas of comprehension and memory undergo marked changes during the latency age period. This necessitates framing and phrasing of interpretations in the context of an approach which takes into account the child's age appropriate capacity for comprehension and memory. Mechanisms of defense, such as projection, repression, and denial, serve a different function in latency than they ordinarily do in adolescence and adulthood. In addition, there is an organization of defenses, the structure of latency, which is unique to latency in that it channels drive discharge into fantasy during the latency years, while in itself serving as the groundwork for the ego capacity of future planning, which in turn becomes the bulwark of successful outcome in adolescence. In the psychotherapy of the latency-age child, the structure of latency must be encouraged at the same time that its products must be analyzed if one is to understand the drives and conflicts that the products represent.

Acceptable and Normal Behavior

During the latency age period, acceptable and normal behavior is defined differently at different ages. The young child in latency is expected to be close to his mother, with little in the way of interests outside the home. The late latency child is expected to show evidences of independence with plans of his own which are often derived from the influence of his peers. The early latency child opposes his parents' wishes with contentless negativism ("No, I won't"), while the older latency child opposes his parents by championing positive suggestions showing that he wants to do something on his own. Throughout latency, normal and acceptable behavior is defined in terms of obedience to parents and teachers, ability to achieve states of calm, quiet and pliability, coupled with an ability to let go and vent energy in appropriate times and places, such as gym, recess, and parties. A child younger than the latency age cannot be relied upon to have such well-differentiated responses to differing situations, for he has not yet developed skill in identifying and responding to the cues in a given situation that indicate which behavior is appropriate. The capacity to achieve behavioral constancy, the ability to behave consistently in given social settings, is not fully developed until the latency years begin. As the child enters late latency, ages nine to twelve, behavior is governed to a greater extent by peer pressures. In essence, this phenomenon, commonly attributed to adolescence, has roots that stretch back into latency. It is appropriate for children in late latency to show evidences of a process of individuation from the parent on the ethical level. This ethical individuation phase of late latency is a reflection of the cognitive maturation that places more emphasis on outside influences, reality, and the environment than internal, past, and family influences. The superego demands which are derived from internal past and family influences are usually linked with guilt and indeed actuated into influencing personal behavior through guilt. The acquisition of newer contents is contested by these affects of doubt and guilt. There is conflict and guilt when new influences challenge the child to seek new ways of doing things. Guilt is stirred when old ways of doing things are challenged and forbidden activities are encouraged by new influences. In marked cases of conflict involving ethical individuation, paranoid states, tics, urticaria, and obsessional symptoms of severe but transient character appear. They point to the presence of ethical individuation conflict, which should be explored in these instances.

Coupled with the problems of ethical individuation is the problem of passivity. This may also be marked in late latency. This is a conflict between the wish of the child to be cared for and to remain a child, and resentment of the loss of independence which fulfillment of this desire brings. Moods, temper fits, withdrawal to rooms, and challenges of authority take center stage clinically when these conflictual areas are most intense. Ethical individuation, with its emphasis on seeking new ways of doing things and new things to do, intensifies the passivity problems of late latency.

Symbolizing Function

The symbolizing function undergoes changes during the latency time period. Most striking are the changes in the symbols used for the production of fantasy. The prelatency child has very direct fantasies. ("When you die, Mommy, I'll marry Daddy"). The early latency age child shapes his fantasies with amorphous figures, especially of persecutors, who make him frightened, especially when it is dark. At about eight and a half there is a shift from amorphous figures to real figures who populate fantasies which are mainly lived out in the imagination or played out in fantasy play. In adolesence real people populate fantasies which are forced upon reality and are lived out in reality in what comes to be seen as neurotic behavior.

The symbols which play a primary role in the formation of latency states are a special symbolic form, called a psychoanalytic symbol. An ordinary symbol is an object, idea, or thing which in the process of memory represents in the awareness and communications of the person, another object or thing. It is a kind of convenient shorthand through which a great deal of information can be represented by a signal or sign which requires little effort. In the formation of a psychoanalytic symbol, the message to be conveyed is usually tied in with anxiety or another uncomfortable affect. To enable the expression of the message while maintaining comfort for the individual, repression of the connection between the symbol and the original information is effected. In this way fantasies can be created which express and discharge the urges implied in the original (latency fantasy) information package without revealing its content to the child or the casual observer. This sort of symbol becomes a highly useful tool in the process of mastery of uncomfortable experiences and in the discharge of drive energies for which the immature physiology of the child provides no other outlets for discharge. The latency play fantasy formed from psychoanalytic symbols becomes a means of reducing emotional tensions much in the way that masturbation, some categories of dreams, sexual relations, athletics, and adult sublimations are used toward the same end.

In keeping with the preponderance of inward-turning mental events in the latency-age child, the psychoanalytic symbols of the child have the characteristic that they do not take into account communicative potentials in relation to possible listeners and observers. The symbols serve primarily the role of a medium through which past experiences and memories can be evoked for the discharge of drive independent of objects in reality. Their nature and function is related most closely to the dream symbols of adults. Indeed, the play fantasies of children, which are constructed from these symbols, closely resemble the distortion-filled dreams seen in the treatment of adults. The play fantasies of children therefore serve in child therapy a role similar to the role of the dream in adult therapy. Because of the similarity of function, dreams are less frequently reported spontaneously in the psychotherapy of the latency-age child than they are by adults. The latency-age child (with the exception of bed-wetters) evidences rare dream reporting during therapy, though not rare dreaming. A special point can be made of encouraging dream reporting if this is desired.

Cognitive Growth

The predominant behavioral characteristics of the latency-age child which has the greatest impact on the moment-to-moment functioning of the child therapist is the level of cognitive maturation of the child. Symbols, fantasies, and the structure of latency contribute to the content of the therapy and the interpretations of the therapist. However, in a therapy in which the comprehension, appreciation, and memory for events and the interpretations of them by the therapist is the key to success, content is not the whole story. The therapist's approach, the patient's productions, and the very form of the therapist's interventions are determined by the level of cognitive maturation which the child has reached. Typically, a major portion of the child's spontaneous recall of events is channeled through the masked and highly symbolized medium of fantasy play. Therefore, the therapist must encourage this type of activity and pay close attention to it. When the time for interpretation and reconstruction arrives, the therapist is called upon to keep a point of reference in the concrete experiences of the child in the therapy session. The poor capacity for the recall of abstraction by the child in early latency militates against too abstract phrasing in these interpretations. Though the therapist may understand and theorize on an adult level of comprehension, cognition, and memory organization to his own satisfaction, molding of these insights into interpretations following adult patterns of phrasing and abstraction will fall upon the child's awareness as upon deaf ears.

In phrasing such interpretations, two areas of cognition are primary. They are the organization of the understanding of events, and the organization of the memory function. As Piaget has pointed out, children in the early latency years tend to understand the happenings about them in a magical, symbolic, and intuitive manner. It is only at about seven and a half years of age that the child can bring to bear abstractions in the interpretation of concretely experienced and observed events. In a child younger than seven and a half, interpretations should be concrete and aimed at reconstructing true experiences that the child has distorted into fear fantasies that are distressing, and at times, disorganizing. In the child older than seven and a half, interpretations can be more general and abstract, and relate seemingly disparate concrete elements. It is not until the child is at the very end of latency (12½) that one can expect to find abstract reductions of abstractions, universally. These can be understood at this age, and logical conversations can be conducted without breaks of attention and distractions into play by the child. In essence, it is at this age that the interpretation typical of adult therapy comes consistently into use. Such interpretations of content are used when the aim of the therapist is to help the child understand current behavior.

No matter what it is that the child can understand of his current behavior as a result of the level of cognitive comprehension that he has reached, it is only that which the child can carry with him and remember in the future that will have an impact. Where the therapist feels that insight and the ability to recognize repeated patterns of behavior is indicated in the therapy, the nature of the ontogenesis of memory function must be kept in mind.

The area of ontogenesis of the memory function is extraordinarily complex when related to the psychotherapy of the latency-age child. Every element brought into the session by the child is in whole or part a product of memory. Since at least three different memory organizations are at work creating the spontaneous recall that produces the contents of the therapy session, the therapist has to be tuned in on at least three levels of communication.

The earliest formed and most primitive memory organization used by the child is the affectomotor memory organization, which dominates until three years of age and bears the burden of the memory function until well past six years of age. The components of this memory organization are sight, sensations, and feelings which re-create the total life experience of the child, including associated affects. In the absence of verbal components, early life experiences can be recalled in terms of somatic sensations which are signifiers of the broader affectomotor imagery seeking representation in memory. Motor tone and posture, the selection of a broken toy that represents a recall of an old injury, angers, and sudden needs for toileting are all clinical manifestations that must be observed for and interpreted if the totality of the child's experience is to be brought into the psychotherapeutic field of view.

Fortunately for the therapist working with the latency-age child, the second form of memory organization, which is introduced at the end of the first year of life, begins to dominate the memory functions of the child at about the age of six. This is the verbal conceptual memory organization. At this age, the child is able to reduce memory elements from holistic, nonlinear affectomotor total memory elements to efficient and logically organized concepts locked into verbal representations. To some extent, their scope is limiting. The limitations are traded off against the expanding usefulness of elements based on memory in the sphere of communication. Thus, the child can talk about or represent in symbols that which he has experienced and must master. It is incumbent on the therapist to help the child to improve his verbal conceptual memory skills, and to help translate experience carried forward through affectomotor memory function into verbal concepts that can be shared, discussed, and mastered. While the child is in this phase (six to eight), there is little value in converting observations into abstractions, for there is less likelihood that children will be able to carry forward abstractions in memory than that they will be able to carry forward rote memory and verbally organized concepts.

The third level of the memory organization involved in spontaneous recall becomes available at about eight years of age. It develops as the result of social and parental encouragement, and may be absent, depending on the home environment from which the child comes. Called the "abstract conceptual memory organization," the third memory organization permits the child to recall spontaneously the intrinsic nature of things, rather than words.* As such, at this age, interpretations can be formed to take into account intrinsic relationships between related concrete experiences. (The application of abstractions to abstractions must await very late latency.) It is possible for the therapist to encourage the child to achieve skills in abstract conceptual memory at eight, and even for the child to show spontaneous evidences of this function at eight. However, it is the common experience of therapist and parents that it is not until age ten that there is a meaningful increase in the child's interest in current events, abstractions, and short, clearly thought out conversations.

Where the child has not reached a given level of memory organization, it is useless for the therapist to use its formal characteristics in the formation of his formulations and interpretations to the child.

Mechanisms of Defense

During latency, a number of mechanisms of defense undergo developmental vicissitudes. The pathology implied by their presence differs from that implied in a similar clinical manifestation in the adult. For instance, projection to transient persecutory fantasies serves an adaptive function in latency. There are defenses which are less strong in latency than they are in adulthood. For instance, direct questions can often bring out repressed material in the latency-age child.

Repression is less strong during the late latency years. Often in dealing with an obsessional symptom or a paranoid episode, all that one need do is ask some direct questions to bring forgotten events into consciousness. As the return to consciousness occurs, the symptoms clear. One child, a twelve-year-old girl who refused to go to school out of fear that she would be kidnapped by a group of men in a car that was following her, had a complete remission of symptoms when she was able to reconstruct the situation in which the symptoms had begun. The therapist, aware of the problems in ethical individuation that occur at this age (see above), asked the child if her friends had wanted her to do something that her parents would disapprove of. "Steal," said the girl, without hesitation. She then described stealing some gum at a candy store at the prompting of her friends. Though she had returned the gum, she was haunted by guilt, which had been dissociated from the theft and then expressed through the persecutory delusion. When the episode of stealing was restored to the center of her consciousness, the fear symptom cleared.

Projection is a symptom with strong pathological implications when it appears in adults. It is one of the mechanisms of the normal "fear fantasy" neuroses of latency. With the passage into adolescence, projection pursues a number of vicissitudes which include participation in sublimations, use as a bridge in object finding, and the projective-introjective process that contributes to modifications of the superego. If the projections of latency continue unaltered into adolescence, a pathological import may be inferred (see Sarnoff, 1976).

In early latency, the tendency to respond intuitively and to interpret the world and its events in terms of the child's self-oriented view of things permits the child to assume that what he wishes to see or not to see should be accepted by others as a true view of the world. Therefore any attempts to shatter denials are fraught with frustration, if not danger (Sarnoff, 1976). The children stare right through the therapist if challenged. In circumstances in which the therapist brings too much pressure to bear, aggressions and even destructive behavior aimed at the therapist or playroom can be expected. This is in marked contrast to the adult, in whom interpretations of denial usually produce new data.

* This should be differentiated from recognition, recall of similarities, and intrinsic characteristics, which are present in the second year of life. This is demonstrated by the child who can tell dogs from cats in a picture book.

The Structure of Latency

The organizations of ego structures that characterize latency and differentiate it from any other developmental period accompanied by age appropriate maturational steps are two.

These are the "mechanisms of restraint" and the "structure of latency." Both are important because they are organizations of defenses constantly found in a given individual and generally to be seen in any youngster who is able to achieve states of calm. Both have dual functions. They help to produce and maintain states of latency and continue on in the post-latency period as personality structures which are part of character. The mechanisms of restraint give shape to the superego and the control of instincts. The structure of latency becomes the core of the ego skill of future planning. Since these personality structures serve to produce and maintain one developmental stage and participate as character elements in subsequent stages, the child therapist is well advised to regard them with respect. These structures are not only useful to study in understanding the psychopathology and clinical psychodynamics of the child. Strengthening them is sometimes a necessary goal in the psychotherapy of latency-age children. This is especially so in those youngsters who show poor study skills, a short attention span, and impulsivity and explosiveness in chronic situations of psychological overstimulation.

These organized structures of the ego are best described within the context of the psychodynamic theory of latency. This is the theory that explains the fluctuations between excited states and calm, quiet malleable states in the latency-age child. The theory deals with the means of drive control during the latency age. The latency-age child has sexual and aggressive drives equal to that of the child in prelatency, though not as strong as that seen in adolescence. The drives are manifested in aggressive behavior, sexual excitement, and masturbatory equivalents. Such inner forces as powerful drives create a problem for the child in a society that considers acceptable behavior to be indicated by suppression of these activities. The situation is compounded by the fact that biologically, the child is no match for his elders physically, and has not yet been equipped by development and maturation with a mature genital organ capable of expressing the sexual drives in a realistic, object-oriented context. In essence, the child must seek the resolution of his need to discharge his drives, utilizing predominantly his inner ego resources.

If one adds to this situation the fact that the child is often seductively stimulated by adults, one sees that the inner life of the calm latency-age child has a greater analogous relationship to a steam engine sometimes pushed toward exploding, than it has to calm bays that invite one to meditation.

When confronted with distracting drive derivatives (e.g., sexual fantasies), states of goal-directedness and calm could be threatened. In early latency, the most common fantasy that threatens goal-directed, reality-oriented behavior is the oedipal fantasy. (This fantasy is characterized by sexual impulses in regard to parents associated with guilt and fear of retribution.)

These fantasies are uncomfortable for children. Any situation that stirs them up creates affects and excitements in the child which threaten the external appearance of calm and the availability of quiet moments which can be harnessed by educators as times for the transmission of culture.

Disruptions of calm need not take place. As Freud was the first to note, children who have reached the phallic-oedipal level resolve the threats involved in oedipal fantasy, whether spontaneous or induced, by retiring from the advanced lines of battle to reinvolve themselves in the conflicts of earlier ages. Usually this means that the child regresses to the anal-sadistic level. Oedipal sexual longings are replaced by more easily expressed urges to tease, to defy, to mess, and to smear. This is the level returned to by most children. Such behavior is seen in angry, excited youngsters. Rooms in which parties are given are often left in shreds by such youngsters. Mothers who drive car pools know well the back-seat society to which all children belong. It is a land which has as its main activity and shibboleth scatology and anal references piled high one upon the other. Although such behavior and sadistic teasing leak out from time to time, the majority of children express their anal regressions in a manner that is masked. This masked outcome is the product of maturity. The child has a stronger and more complex armamentarium of ego defenses for dealing with anal-sadistic urges than he had when first he encountered them around the age of two. Reaction formation, symbol and fantasy formation, repression, obessional defenses (e.g., collecting) all express the primitive drives and channel them into socially accepted patterns. The aggression and messing urges are turned into calm and neatness as a result of reaction formation. Aggressive fantasies replace actions, and collecting takes up energies in collecting and valuing stones that might otherwise be thrown.

These mechanisms are grouped under the rubric "the mechanisms of restraint." The patterns into which they shape the drives are guided by the expectations of parents and the demands of teachers and society. These patterns carry over into adolescence, where they influence strongly the attitudes of the child toward the burgeoning drives that threaten to overwhelm. This is the patterned shape of the prior experience that guides the child when pitted against the seductive demands of the adolescent peer group.

There are children who are unable to handle their drives on the anal-sadistic level. Excitements and humiliation call for comfort rather than responses of aggression. These youngsters regress further to the oral phase where they can be seen to comfort themselves with dreamy television watching, thumb-sucking, cuddling pets, and eating till they become obese. Maternal prohibitions that block phallic and anal assertiveness, leave the establishment of a pattern of defenses with an oral caste as the only outlet.

The child who is successful in using the mechanisms of restraint to transmute the potential tumult of his anal-sadistic urges into a period of calm, pliability, and quiet is a child who is capable of producing states of latency. This product of the mechanisms of the ego opens the door to education and the absorption of culture.

The process of producing states of latency is a dynamic one. Overstimulation and seductive behavior, beatings, and parental sarcasm can cause a flooding of the mechanism and a breakdown in the latency date. Aggressive behavior and regressed symbols are clinical expressions of failure in the latency. On the other hand, in situations involving parties, recess, free play, and athletics, such behavior is encouraged. It is a natural safety valve well recognized by the caretakers of children as a needed way of letting off steam. Another common means used by the child in decreasing the pressures of humiliation, stimulation and seduction is the use of talking, complaining, and seeking allies on a verbal level. This adjustment is important for the child therapist. Through it he establishes a rapport with the child, and if he can keep his phrasing simple, helps the child to reach verbal comprehension of his problems. In such situations, the slightest deflection of the therapist's attention from the child, as may occur when the therapist answers the phone, returns the child to motor syntaxes and other symbolic ways for the expression of conflicts.

The dynamic process of latency has yet another form of safety valve which is useful in maintaining the state of latency. This is "the structure of latency." This has been succinctly paraphrased by Donellan (1977) as a "configuration of defenses in the latency child which allows the expression of impulses through fantasy" (p. 141). The oedipal drives are turned into fantasy, and their energies discharged through fantasy, instead of being responded to by regression and adding to the burden of the mechanisms of restraint. This is accomplished in the following way. The oedipal fantasy either in part or as a whole undergoes repression. The repressed fantasy is fragmented, and the fragments are in turn represented by elements which, as the result of displacement, are divorced from the original, and not recognizable as related to them. This is the defensive role of psychoanalytic symbolization. The symbols are then drawn together into a coherent series of symbols, which make up the manifest fantasy of the structure of latency (i.e., the child who wants to kill his father, kills a king in fantasy instead). The coherency of the series is due to the fact that it is patterned by the influence of familiar tales and myths belonging to the child's culture. The appearance of this ability to adapt personal memories and fantasies (i.e., oedipal) to stories that have a social and cultural source becomes yet another conduit through which the potential for producing a state of latency can be used to enhance the socialization and acculturation of the child.

In children with impaired capacity for delay, displacement, abstraction, symbolization, or fantasy formation, the state of latency is unstable. Therapeutic goals take this into account. To bring a child into "latency" so as to produce states of calm and prepare for future planning in adolescence is an important goal in the therapy of a child with an impaired ability to produce states of latency. In all children who have a structure of latency which is at all operative, the fantasies produced and played out in the therapy sessions become an endless source of data. Like the dreams of adults, they provide the key to the complexes, sensitivities, and the instigators of regression in the individual child.

Applicability

As described above, analytically derived psychotherapy with latency-age children can be applied in situations in which there are problems of social adjustment, acceptance of self, and hypersensitive reactions to situations that induce feelings of humiliation. The child who has entered latency and manifests internalized conflicts such that they have the same patterns of behavior in disparate situations (i.e., sibling rivalry, jealousy of peers, being picked on and teased) can be helped to direct his energies away from his fantasies and toward the resolution of his reality problems. The overstimulated child can be helped to place his relationship with adults into perspective after the parents have been induced to stop the overstimulation. Children of parents who overemphasize needs for control and limit the rate of maturation of the child can be helped to bring their conflicts to the surface. This replaces battling within themselves to the accompaniment of guilt and doubt. This in turn alleviates the somatizations, paranoid symptoms, and tics, which defend against the guilt and doubt. The technique which will be outlined below entails the unraveling of the meanings of fantasies when direct verbal communication fails as a channel for bringing memories to the arena of consciousness and communication.

Children who fail to enter latency can be helped by the therapist who understands the mechanisms involved in the psychodynamics of the establishment of states of latency. The therapist can construct a therapeutic strategy that will diminish the pressure on the child at the same time that weak mechanisms are strengthened.

In children with delayed cognitive growth, child therapy can be applied with the aim of encouraging the establishment of more mature means of comprehending and remembering the abstractions necessary for school survival. Concurrently, improved cognition aids in the therapeutic process. There is established a means by which interpretations can be enhanced to achieve lasting impact.

Methods

An explanation of the therapeutic method through the use of extended case histories is beyond the space limitations and scope of this chapter. The interested reader is referred to the author's book *Latency* (Sarnoff, 1976) for such material. Here we will devote ourselves to specific procedures, activities, and interventions which are of therapeutic value in working with latency-age children. In essence the process of cure will be explored through an investigation of the nature of its effective components.

All therapies occur within a setting. For the therapist who wishes to work with the latency-age child with the great emphasis on play and fantasy that occurs, the nature of the setting and the things about are crucial. Therapists who work with latency-age children offer them settings of varying degrees of complexity and elaborateness. All have one thing in common. There is at least some material to which the child can turn at times when words fail to convey the concepts that the child means to communicate or when the use of words conveys threatening concepts so directly that uncomfortable affects are activated. In these circumstances, ego mechanisms are activated which shift the concept into fantasies, graphic representations, three-dimensional figures, doll play, movement patterns, and somatic responses. The structure of latency is related to the mechanisms involved in this phenomenon. The equipment of the child therapist's office is selected with an eye to its use in the service of techniques available to the latency-age child for using alternative media for the expression of concepts and conflicts, when words fail.

With this in mind, a therapist sets aside a drawer of his desk, a cabinet, a closet, a corner, or often a full room, for the purpose of fantasy play, and equips it with the necessary devices. There is some difference of opinion over whether one should undertake the expense of having a playroom, separate and distinct from the consultation room, with its decorations more in keeping with the mature style required for treating adult patients. One even hears of therapists who claim that they do not need a separate playroom or play equipment in the light of the fact that in their experience, they have never worked with or seen a child who made messes, was sadistic, tore things, or became openly destructive in their offices. Putting aside the implication that these therapists convey—that their skills surpass those of the ordinarily endowed therapist who feels a need for a playroom—the therapist without an independent playroom works under a limitation. He cannot encourage regression, follow fantasy undeterred, encourage the playing out of fantasy, or explore neurotic patterns expressed through motor syntaxes. So it has always been my custom to have a playroom available connected to my consultation room so that the child can move freely between each. In this way, the child who is given the choice of rooms from the start can wander between the "talking room" and the "playing and talking room." His movements are propelled by regressions, and the requirements of his need for ego distance from the latent content with which he is trying to cope.

The setting may be only a corner, or as much as

a room without outside views or noises, which is small enough and so simple of shape that the child cannot use distance or alcoves as means to hide.

Whether the setting be a corner or a room, the material required to furnish and equip it share certain characteristics. They call upon the child's resources and personality in a context of spontaneity. Patterned and organized play material, such as games with rules and games of chance, are less helpful than dolls, clay, and drawing material. The latter three, at every manipulation, are reflections of the inner life of the child. The basic principle is to place at the child's disposal, material that can be used to express what cannot be expressed in words. Fantasy play can reveal much while masking. Games with fixed rules mask more than they reveal, if only by dint of the fact that the time that is taken up with their formal aspects could be used for the spinning of fantasy. The child's personality is the subject, not the personality of the designer of the game or the personality of the therapist. When the therapist enters the fantasy of the patient as a character, he may not intrude his own fantasy but must seek the direction of the child as to his role. This is done, lest the adult intrusion be seen as leadership and the child be led from his thoughts and drives to follow a path that gratifies the therapist and reinforces the therapist's theories about the patient at the expense of true insight for both. When mutual storytelling is done, the therapist is best advised to avoid introducing his own fantasies and characters and instead seeking elaborations of the ideas of the child.

Sometimes it is necessary to use structured toys and board games when investigative therapy is to be avoided and the therapist's goal is to provide companionship or support for coping skills that are heavily loaded with obsessional mechanisms. I have a preference for keeping such games in a special place so that they are not available to be used by youngsters as a defensive maneuver, when such a maneuver is inappropriate to the therapy.

The nonstructured therapy materials consist of elements which reflect the two major regressive pathways observed in children. These are regression along the lines of cognitive skills involving media for the expression of recall of memory elements, and regression along the line of psychosexual development. The former, media for the recall of memory elements, relates to the formal nature of the material selected for play. The latter, regression of psychosexual development, relates to the symbolic content reflected in the way the material is used in play.

Memory elements are first expressed in the form of affects and body parts in motion. The memory function expands its horizon in the area of media used when music and rhythm and bodily motion, and form as expressed in pounding and shaping clay are added. Rhythm, motion, and shapes come to be recognized and can be used to express and master prior experience (end of the first year of life). Later, active shaping and clay play will reflect regression to this stage. The next step is the addition of the expression of memory (spontaneous recall) in the use of two-dimensional lines (three to four years of age) when the child begins to draw pictures. Often, hundreds of drawings will be made over a period of years, to the amazement of parents. These parents are equally amazed when this productivity ceases, and what had been seen as a potential artistic prodigy reveals himself to be "only going through a stage." Indeed, this is merely an age appropriate way of using media for mastering experiences, which is deemphasized when pictures give way to words. By the time of middle latency, the telling of tales, experienced both actively (by telling) and passively (by listening), becomes the means of mastering events. Now, symbols find expression in words, rather than plastic forms. The transition to the use of words is incompletely reached throughout latency. Clay forms and drawings persist. Repeatedly, the child is seen to require the participation of his whole body (body movements expressing his excitement), so that symbolized fantasy becomes fantasy play. Obviously, this is the time when play materials are of great value. Without them, the child is limited to words. Only part of the story that the child has to tell will be told. Only words as symbols will be available for translation into words as direct communications to the therapist. Affects and motor patterns expressible only in play will be deleted from the translating process, and no one will be the wiser.

Forward movement developmentally, in the area of media for memory, and spontaneous recall in the service of mastery, has been described. In reverse order, regressions along this developmental line traverse the following schema. What the child can say, he will say. What the child cannot say, he will put into action and fantasy. What cannot be put into play fantasy, can be drawn. What cannot be drawn, can be molded in clay, or more primitively, acted out directly in aggressive acts and discharges of affect. Thus, if a child cannot tell a dream, he may be able to draw elements from it. If he cannot draw, then let him try to work in clay. If the child cannot tell about himself, then introduce ego distance by having the child tell the story through the use of dolls with assumed names.

The regressive pull in child therapy is in the direction of direct physical expression and organ language. Therefore, the substitutions I have described have a danger in addition to their capacity to improve communication through placing the media with which the child is comfortable at his disposal. The substitutions can encourage too rapid regression in the borderline child. For this reason, for some children, the play material is used to encourage the child to use substitutions in the direction of less regressed activity. For example, there are times when the child has regressed to the point that he no longer expresses his latent contents through symbols and substitutes, but is actively involved in the expression of aggression through affective displays and discharge through motor syntaxes with the therapist as object. This is a technical way of saying that sometimes the kid gets temper tantrums and starts punching the therapist. At these times, substitutions should be upward, with the suggestion made that the child show the therapist what he has in mind using dolls or a punching balloon as a substitute object. Similarly, in children who have failed to develop verbal symbols of the psychoanalytic sort, it is necessary as a technique to encourage substitution upward through the creation of plastic elements, doll play, clay play, and drawings as a means of expanding the child's media for expressing and mastering events, displacing and binding affects, and delaying responses.

From the description of the material described above, a list of helpful play materials for the playroom can be derived. Clay, paper, pencil, water colors, scissors, glue, a punching doll, plastic toy soldiers, a doll house with a doll family, and toy cars are useful. There should be a bathroom available. Often the regression to body and physical sensations takes the form of masturbatory activity or the need to use the bathroom. Water should be available. I prefer a pump action sink with a self-contained cool water supply to a standard sink with hot and cold water and a head of pressure. Hot water can burn a child's hands. A head of pressure can be most unfortunate if the child places his finger under the faucet, then places himself between the faucet handle and the therapist and directs a spray of water at the therapist.

The levels of regression that have to do with psychosexual development pursue a developmental course consisting of an oral phase in which bottles, caretaking of dolls, stories of dependency using dolls, is pertinent. For this reason, dolls with bottles are useful items. Some therapists keep food around, recommending only small amounts. I find that the less children eat, the more they talk about their need to eat. The next phase is the anal phase. This finds reflection in latency in regressions to needs to smear and mess as well as sadistic and warlike fantasies. There are also fantasies of bombing, direct anal references, and projection. Clay and finger paints are most useful for expressing and letting off steam in this area. Toy soldiers are helpful in carrying out large-scale fantasies of omnipotent power. The child needs discharge in this area as well as analysis of content to help master prior experienced stresses. In addition, especially in dealing with the anal regression of the latency-age child, the mechanisms of restraint are in need of strengthening. The most useful and possible strengthening maneuvers during child therapy sessions in this regard are techniques that encourage the collecting and obsessional patterning mechanisms that are used naturally by most children. For this reason, games like dots (where lines connect dots to make boxes; each box completed belongs to the person who completed the box) are useful. Children can be encouraged to bring in pennies, baseball cards, etc., and organize them.

Doll play can be used to good advantage with the expression of anal phase material. It is important in this regard that each doll house be equipped with bathroom furniture. Clay should be around so that the child can use it to represent feces. A plastic clay that hardens can be useful for more general reasons. It holds its form. Therefore, figures made from such clay can be used session after session as the basis for the further elaboration of the fantasy or dream in which the figure appeared.

Next on the level of expression of psychosexual development are materials that can symbolize the elements of the phallic phase. Important among these elements is the Oedipus complex and sibling rivalry. Dolls of different ages and sexes, and a doll house, are invaluable in helping the child to portray the conflicts relating to this period. Guns are useful in helping children to express assertiveness, phallic penetrative urges, and oedipal aggression toward parents. Many family dolls which represent children invite the child to express feelings in this area.

The important thing to keep in mind about the cognitive and psychosexual determinants of the material used in the playroom is the difference in goal inherent in the selection of material for the expression and study of each of these developmental lines. The materials used in the cognitive area are chosen with an eye to the form of the media available for the expression on a symbolic level of latent memory elements. Motor syntaxes are learned at each phase for dealing with the media (clay, paper and pencil, symbolic motor patterns, words). Such phase-related motor experiences are retained in memory, either as the basis of building up a body of learning on which to base functioning and development, or as a mechanism for the continued processing of trauma with an eye toward mastery. Regressions can activate them inappropriately. The materials used in the area of psychosexual development are chosen with an eye toward their usefulness as symbols for the expression of latent, phase-appropriate content. The choice of material is based upon prior experience with the play of children and the dreams of adults. Certain symbols have been found to be consistently used to express certain latent contents. Thus a doll with a bottle has oral connotations. Clay and feces or finger paints and feces have come to be equated symbolically. This is a convention which is constantly reinforced by the spontaneous productions and associations of players and dreamers. A gun repeatedly appears in play and dreams as a phallic symbol. There are some who challenge these symbolic equations and their use. Indeed, even the relationship of fantasy and latent thoughts to symptoms and behavior is challenged. If child therapists who take such a stand, analytically derived child therapy becomes a therapy divested of much of its effectiveness. I recall from my college years, a young man who openly challenged the theory that dream symbols could have an unconscious meaning. He challenged the class to analyze a dream he had had the night before. He started off at first to tell the dream in words. "I was hunting. I had a rifle. I went into this cave after a mountain lion. I raised my gun to shoot. Just as I was about to shoot, my gun. . . ." At this point, he ceased using a verbal mode for relating his dream and shifted to a symbolic motor pattern. ". . . my gun went like this. . . ." He pointed his finger straight out as if aiming into the cave. Then, with the phrase "like this," the finger became flaccid and hung limp from the metacarpophalangeal joint. The class, who had maintained its demeanor up to this point, dissolved into uproarious laughter. The dreamer looked bewildered. A class of unsophisticated eighteen-year-olds knew something of the secret of dreams and put it to use that day. Experiences like this contribute to the advice that guns be present in playrooms so that phallic symbolism can be expressed.

The furnishing of a playroom has specific value. There should be low shelves in which play material can be placed in a haphazard manner, though easily available to the child. A table should be provided as a work surface. A formica top is preferable to a wooden one. Near enough to the table so that it can be reached, should be a low chest containing tools and equipment which can be brought out by the therapist as needed. A holder for paper and watercolor pens and pencils should be readily at hand for the child. Many people have a couch in the room so that the child can rest. A bin for each child is an excellent idea. Files can be useful for this. In these bins, whatever the child works on consistently or has produced and wants to keep for the next session can be kept out of harm's way and out of the hands of other children with sibling rivalry problems. There should be an open hard floor area in which the child can play by himself. The treatment of walls is important. Children often want to write on walls. This cannot be permitted, if only because one child can fill one wall in one day. Yet something is lost if the child is blocked in this. I've solved this problem by turning one wall into a chalkboard. Another wall, if covered with cork, can become a place where the child can exhibit with pride, his achievements in the area of drawing and design. In addition, the corkboard can be used to keep exposed and at hand pictorial symbolic elements that otherwise would be thrown away and which the therapist wants to keep in sight and available for future working through.

Of all the elements in the playroom, among the most important is the nature of the therapist, his personality, knowledge, and experience. Certain personal resources are required for the successful therapist. There must be a genuine liking for children. This does not refer to descriptions of the therapist made by others. This applies to the feelings of the therapist over prolonged periods of contact with individual children. If the impulse of the future therapist is to give the child something to do while he reads or if the potential therapist seeks to play games of chance, or if the potential therapist finds himself dozing when assigned the care of a child, the likelihood is that he should seek another profession. Gifted child caretakers and child observers may be insufficiently comfortable with children to be able to interact with them on a level that permits psychotherapeutic insight and communication. This may well explain why so many well-trained child therapists give up direct work with children to take on supervisory and administrative roles. The important positive personal attributes for the potential child therapist are warmth, a quiet and relaxed manner, a voice capable of modulation, and a capacity to remain cool and think in the face of sometimes destructive surprises. When these attributes are present, the child's needs in a therapist are satisfied, for a child can be comfortable in the presence of such a person. Of no less importance is the ability of the potential therapist to accept regressions that occur during the therapy sessions. He must be able to regress with the child and accept the stirring up of his own drives that this entails without the mobilization of defenses that would block communication or insight. He must be able to accept the child's behavior, think on the level that the child thinks, and still not regress himself to the level of playing and interacting with the child on a regressed level. Playing with the child and interacting in a way that expresses one's own infantile needs will intensify the child's regressions and problems. The troubled child needs an adult as a therapist, not a best friend. A child of his own age would serve the latter purpose better. In essence, the potential therapist should be comfortable with a child's regressed behavior, capable of regressing cognitively to be able to appreciate the communications and communicate in turn, but not to lose the sense of distance that permits reflection, free-floating attention, and awareness of the influence and the needs of society in guiding behavior.

It is very helpful if the therapist can draw or mold clay to the point that a recognizable representation can be made. This is in support of the use of figures as interpretations and in the passive introduction of symbols to children with poor symbolizing function.

Child therapy is an activity which does not require the use of medication or the "laying on of hands." As such, it is a field open to physicians as well as child-oriented people of many professional backgrounds. The experience of the physician equips him to deal with childhood psychopathology from the standpoint of differential diagnosis and physical or organic modalities of treatment. This does not bear a direct relationship to the therapy of the latency-age child as such. The experience of the physician in the treatment of physical disorders of mankind creates in the therapist what may be called a "feel for tissue." By this is implied that to administer any therapy one must be aware that the strongest forces for health lie in the natural recuperative and restorative processes of the body and personality. One must be able to put aside one's omnipotent fantasies and the search for hermetic magic in favor of choosing modalities of intervention that will not interfere with the natural developmental and curative processes. One must accept limitations on rescue fantasies and feelings of omnipotence so that interventions can be tuned to the pace and needs of the patient, not the therapist. There is a great deal to be learned from any physicianly ministrations governed by the rule "first of all not to harm" that can immediately be applied in the child therapy situation. Working with tissue as physicians do on an intensive level brings such skills into focus early in the career of the therapist. As seemingly distant an activity as learning to diagnose pathology slides has a bearing. There is an abdication of narcissism (as manifested in jumping to conclusions) in favor of the verifiable and consistent visual facts on the slide that is brought immediately to bear in child therapy. Here it is that the theories of the therapist take second place to the observable facts of the child's behavior.

In time all people who work in child therapy successfully can acquire the "feel for tissue." Knowing of it, in the hands of therapists without experiential background in this area, can hurry the process.

Those who come to child therapy from backgrounds related to child caring have had access to an invaluable knowledge base. Child therapy requires that the troubles of the child at a given age be familiar ground to the therapist. Knowledge of the typical fantasies and reality problems of each age helps the therapist to know where to look for trouble and what to talk about and encourage in the therapeutic situation. The parent of a verbal child, the student of child development, the worker in a child care institution have had invaluable experience in this regard. Those who do not have direct access to these childhood experiences can augment their knowledge through reading. The books mentioned above can be used in this regard. The author's book *Latency* (Sarnoff, 1976), other works (*Psa. Study of the Child*, Sarnoff, 1978), and the *Psychoanalytic Study of the Child* can be of use in this regard. The interested reader should search out works that are based on observations of direct communications with children rather than reconstructions based on the recollections of adults.

The implied message of this section of this chapter is that the child therapist needs to know about the experiences of childhood that lie behind the signs and symptoms of childhood psychopathology as well as the nature of the sensitivity of human tissue to therapeutic interventions and the strength of natural developmental and curative processes. Little is to be gained by lessening the value of the contributions of each of the backgrounds from which child therapists are derived. A study of each contributes to a comprehension of the breadth of experience required. It is incumbent on the child therapist to fill in those areas in which background is insufficient as soon as possible. Training programs often serve in the role of doing just this. It is of importance in seeking out a training program that one assures oneself that it is designed to fill these needs rather than the needs of the institution on the level of research or earnings. A personal analysis is an invaluable source of knowledge into the unconscious of Everyman. In addition, it helps the therapist deal with personal reactions, which would interfere with his capacity to participate in the therapeutic situation.

In child therapy, two areas, at least, are the forums of therapeutic attention. First, we focus on current stresses and humiliations that unsettle the child. Insulting and disappointing experiences trigger regressive behavior. Memory of the actual experiences may undergo repression. Defensive and regressive symptoms, as well as anxiety, appear in their stead. Personal insults are not the only current stresses that confront a child. Overwhelming of the ego by the drives, and developmental demands, also confound. Social pressures and the task of integrating newly acquired skills into peer accepted behavior can also unsettle a child. Psychotherapeutic activities must be aimed at helping the child deal with these difficult inputs and tasks, as well as resolving the use of defenses, when they are counterproductive or when their function produces symptoms. The second group of problems consist of unresolved humiliations and traumas from the past that were not mastered when they first occurred. These are manifested in self-defeating patterns of defense mechanisms, and internalized fantasy structures which dominate the child's behavior (e.g., sadomasochistic persecutory fantasies). They sensitize the child to turn current situations into insults.

Which of the usual activities that occur during child psychotherapeutic sessions is most effective in resolving these problems, both current and chronic? Of the many activities that take place during child therapy sessions, only a small percentage are effective in helping a child to resolve repressions, master trauma, deal with humiliation, give up symptoms, and progress from regressive behavior.

The understanding of the effective techniques helps the therapist to identify and to use them. To know them alerts the therapist to encourage their use and to enhance their effect. The portal to obtaining mastery of the facts of progress in child therapy lies in the area of understanding the functioning of the ego structures of the latency-age child. When the child's defenses do not permit him to talk of adjustment problems directly, the alerted therapist is aware that the ego structures of the child still may permit communication through fantasy play. In addition, the alerted therapist encourages fantasy play because fantasy play can also serve as a means of discharge and vicarious coping with the precipitating stresses.

The encouragement of fantasy and fantasy play is a therapeutic maneuver with multiple potentials. Coping, discharge, working through, and communication of information are all possible through fantasy play. Therefore, fantasy play becomes a means of helping the child to discharge and resolve in conflict areas, at the same time that it becomes a source of information for the working through of chronic problems of early origin. Strengthening the capacity to fantasize also strengthens the capacity of the child to enter states of latency, with the attendant calm cooperativeness and pliability that permits the child to be taught and to learn. This is done by encouraging the use of symbols and requiring delayed responses. If a child speaks of events haltingly, and with little spontaneity, one may ask if there are any "make believes" that the child has in regard to it. Play objects in the playroom encourage this. Just letting the child play in fantasy, and develop the fantasy, helps a child to work through problems. One can tell if this technique is working if the fantasies as told, gradually change. For instance, the child who starts off with fantasies that deal with fear of injury and loss of body parts, who goes on to fantasies of penetration and heroism, and the child who moves through fantasies of sadism towards siblings, to fantasies of the acquisition of objects to be used in adult occupations, is heading in the right direction. Often, little in the way of intervention is necessary on the part of the therapist. However, an occasional interpretation or discussion of a fear, coupled with reassurance, can hurry the child on his way to health. All that appears to be necessary is that the child be given place enough and time to pursue his fantasies undisturbed, and some progress is possible. The effectiveness of this technique can be checked by viewing the behavior of the child outside the sessions. Maturation of fantasy content (defined in terms of less regressed symbols, situations, and reactions) and improved behavior at home, coupled with appropriate "states of latency," are indicators that the therapy is effective.

Often, discharge through fantasy leads to improved behavior quickly. Parents tend to remove children from treatment at this point. It is well to forewarn the parents of this course of events in advance. In this way, one is permitted to work through the child's problems more fully. In addition, one is saved the problem of patients who drop out and then return to find no place in a busy practice.

Direct discussion of problems, and indirect confrontation of problems through fantasy play, are the most important of the effective technical activities in latency-age psychotherapy. Progress clinically through discharge with fantasy is often sufficient to produce improved states of functioning. It cannot be depended upon to produce lasting results. The child who improves on play therapy alone cannot be depended upon to hold his gains. Remissions are common. For this reason, interpretive interventions, improved communication, and sympathetic discussion are important factors in securing gains. The next section deals with selected activities that occur in child therapy sessions that are therapeutically effective. We deal here, not with the technique of cure, but with the activities which are the building blocks from which cure is constructed. Among these are the activities on the part of a therapist which the beginner needs to know in order to bring some order into his therapeutic activities and provide his teaching supervisor with material upon which to base advice.

Coping Skills

Coping skills are here defined as those aspects of the personality which may be used in confronting and dealing with day to day issues on a moment to moment basis. They are practical steps and manipulations used to handle pressures brought to bear by others, and to deal with tendencies within the child's own group of disorganizing defensive reactions. The child psychotherapist's role in regard to coping skills is, in essence, what one does while waiting for insight to arrive. The emphasis on coping skills early on, is one of the characteristics of child therapy which differentiates it from child analysis itself. In child analysis, manipulation through discussing coping skills is deemphasized.

Impaired coping skills are much in evidence in youngsters whose parents or teachers guide them to child therapists. To a large extent, this is due to the fact that these children come from homes in which the parental examples reflect less than adequate coping skills. Either as the result of chronic pressure from the disordered behavior of the child, as the result of preexisting disorders of adjustment, the parents themselves display poor coping skills. Thus, the children have poor models from which to derive their own techniques. For this reason, there are times when the management of coping skills entails direct work with the parent as well as with the child. The parent who responds to stress by running and panic, introduces the child to these techniques. If the parent is not worked with along with the child, the parent may undermine gains made in the treatment as a result of his continuing inappropriate behavior.

Years ago, I saw a sign in the office of a successful personnel manager, which said, "When in danger, fear and doubt, run in circles, scream and shout." This epitomizes the behavior of a person with poor coping mechanisms. Avoidance as reflected in withdrawal from sports or contact with aggressive peers is another. In instances where avoidance is used, one must especially beware the parent who quiets his own inner anxiety by limiting the activities of the child. The parent who drives the child to school when the child could walk or ride the bus, limits the child's future capacity to cope with situations requiring independent judgment, and the ability to evaluate and respond to danger potentials in new situations.

Working with coping skills usually requires direct intervention. It makes up a good deal of the pedagogical aspect of child therapy. For example, the child who has trouble doing his homework may be invited to do his homework in the therapy session. Direct tutoring help is obviously not the object of the therapist. Rather, an appraisal is made of the child's formal approach to the work. For instance, a child who repeatedly "forget all I know," when taking tests for which he had "studied hard," was found to have studied only to the point that he could recognize the material required. He had no ability to recall the material spontaneously. No amount of interpretation of motivation could have helped him to utilize his memory skills in a manner that was, until then, beyond his ken. Helping a child to set up schedules and to organize his approach to homework is useful in youngsters who tend to panic when they bunch all their work up to be done at one time. The youngster who is constantly teased and picked on will eventually cease to seek out the group of children whose level of sadomasochistic aggressive energies propel them into constant situations in which they are teased, or being teased. He will leave this group when the conflicts (i.e., castration anxiety) that have initiated his regressions are worked through. Early in the process, it is helpful to help the child to identify those aspects of his own behavior that exaggerate or call forth repetition and intensification of teasing. Provocations ("What did I do, I only stuck him with a pencil by accident." "All I did was curse at him, why did he hit me?" "The teacher punished me for kicking him when he started it by moving my paper!"), hypersensitivity ("I can't help crying when they tease me." "They sometimes bring friends along to see how upset I get. It's like I'm a show"), are explained to the child as activities which intensify the amount of teasing received. Two things happen when this is done. The child implements his knowledge so that the teasing decreases. The child is able to gain some distance from the situation, see his active role in the process and becomes more available for exploration into his unconscious motivation.

Direct intervention makes a large part of the work which involves coping skills in child therapy sessions. A not inconsiderable contribution, though often inadvertent, is the stance and behavior of the therapist. A ten-year-old boy, known for his temper tantrums as well as his tendency to respond to his teacher's questions in the classroom situation using expertly imitated French, German, or Spanish accents, came into a session in a furor. He railed against his soccer coach, who had criticized him that day. I sat quietly and listened. At one point, he seized a towel rack and pulled it from the wall. I interpreted his displaced anger. He responded with, "How can you sit there calmly?" "If I yelled back, there would only be a fight, and we would have learned nothing of what happened, and then we wouldn't be able to understand anything," said I. He seemed impressed with the use of calm to deal with an angry person. This impression was confirmed by his mother, who reported that within the week, he had used calm to deal with her. Upon returning home one afternoon, she found that he had left some dirty socks on the floor of his room. She called him from watching television, and began to scream her displeasure at him. Instead of his usual raised voice response, he calmly waited out the storm and commented to her on the value of discussion rather than yelling. She was doubly taken aback, once because of his new approach, and once because, in spite of his new approach, he still had not picked up his socks.

Obsessional Defenses

One of the mainstays of the mechanisms of restraint that produce the calm of latency states in the face of anal sadistic drive regressions is obsessional defenses. In states of latency, the clinical manifestations of these defenses consist of controlled patterns of behavior which bind such energy. These include collecting stones, coins, baseball cards, and toy cars, as well as playing board games built around complex rules, drawing pictures based on patterns of geometric forms, and setting up dominoes with great and meticulous care so that they can all fall in a row. These activities help to maintain for the child the state of calm which is part of an age-appropriate adjustment pattern. When this behavior appears in the session, it should not be directly discouraged, nor interpreted sui generis. Rather, discussion should proceed parallel to its appearance, with the therapist's awareness, at least in part, directed to the fact that the child is actively struggling to control regressive sadistic urges. The underlying problems can be dealt with without discouraging behavior within the therapy that has the therapeutic effect of strengthening the child's capacity to deal with intrusive regressive trends. In children who have failed to enter latency, and who show hyperactive, excited, at times destructive behavior in the sessions, or difficulty in achieving states of calm at home or in the school, the introduction of games with structure (such as checkers or board games) or counting, or watching the clock tick away minutes, or penny collecting, can introduce defenses that can help the child achieve a component of the ego organization that is necessary for achieving latency calm. This in turn permits the child to make progress in the works of maturing that must be done during the latency age period. This must be accomplished if the child is to be ready to negotiate the difficulties of adolescence and adulthood.

Repeating in Action

This refers to the fact that actions directed toward the therapist, such as silence, teasing, or striking, usually reflect or repeat an event of the day in which the child was the victim. In effect, the behavior of the child reflects an identification with a person who has behaved in an aggressive manner toward the child. The actions in the sessions serve to help the child to master the recent humiliation. The gain, though of importance, does not have much of an effect beyond the immediate session or relieving the immediate momentary distress. The child is only minimally aware that something is being mastered through the aggressions being brought to bear on the therapist. Through interpretation that causes a verbalization of the process, consciousness, consisting of verbal concepts, is widened to include an awareness of the defensive process that is going on.

The two therapeutic activities described just above consisted of strengthening ego function by changing defenses through encouragement or identification. As such, they are prime representations of nonverbal activities which are psychotherapeutically effective. In this section, we are turning to the role of verbalization and insight in the psychotherapeutic process. The emphasis turns from "what to do" to "what to say."

Often, if the therapist responds to the attack with questions such as "Who did this to you today?" or "Who teased you like this today?" The child stops, thinks, looks surprised, and then explores the half-forgotten humiliation which had returned with such force in masked form just moments before. As the child begins to talk of the experience, there is no longer need to relive it in action. Once the complex of events has been made expressible in verbal form, a kind of world picture painted in words begins to appear on the canvas, provided by the therapeutic situation. Unlike the descriptive process embodied in the process of action within the session or fantasies therein played out, the descriptive process that uses words can be directed and expanded so that it can explore with few limits. It can even open doors through the use of verbal deductive reasoning that could only be reached through arduous work, using actions and fantasies brought to the therapy through associations on the nonverbal sphere. The moment that the child's experience is transported from the world of affect and action to the world of words, there is a change in the quality of the therapy. Reflection, deduction, expanded detail, and manageable abstracts of extended events enrich the potential of the psychotherapeutic situation. Verbal insight becomes possible. Verbal memory becomes a therapeutic tool. Patterns of behavior can be recognized. Conflicting, often self-defeating activities can be considered simultaneously and recognized for what they are. Sources of anxiety in the child's own behavior, and potentially under his control, can be brought into focus. As a result, motivation for change can be introduced. The child who can see the origins of inappropriate behavior in the sessions in the misfortunes that befell him in the day just past, has learned to look for causes in unexpected places and can be induced to use such thinking in other situations. Therefore, working through (recognizing complexes and reactions and correcting them in all the places that they occur) may be introduced into child therapy, as it can in adult therapy. One is not always confronted with a child who takes out his humiliating experiences on the therapist. The therapeutic activity of getting a child to move his recollection of his experiences into the realm of words, does not always fall so easily into one's lap. (There are exceptions to this in the form of quite verbal children.) It therefore becomes necessary at times to encourage verbalization in other ways. The most common procedure is to question the child in such a way about his experiences, feelings, and fantasies, that he must put them into words, thus invoking a verbal mode of communication. Questions that can be answered with "fine," "good," "all right," and "no" are counterproductive. A very useful technique is to pick up the part of a child's sentences or activities that contain new elements, and ask for elaboration. One should be especially on the alert for sudden changes of topics or a switch from verbalization to fantasy play. This may indicate that material has been reached with which the child cannot deal. These "switch moments" are often the hinges around which therapeutic progress turns. Two possibilities are the most common causes of "switch moments." The child may have hit material that is too affect-laden to face. Possibly, the child's cognition has not matured to the point where he has reached the level of abstraction required to understand the therapist's recent adult-oriented interpretations and to remember them. In the latter case, the level of thought process needed to master the material on a verbal level is beyond the cognitive powers of the child. There are two technical psychotherapeutic procedures to be followed in this situation. If possible, the cognitive growth (see above) of the child should be encouraged toward a level at which comprehension, memory, and insight can be maintained at a sufficient level of efficiency for sustained behavior changes to occur. Cognitive potential often runs ahead of cognitive realization and actuated cognitive skills. Where this is not possible, greater emphasis must be placed on working through in fantasy. A brief description of these two psychotherapeutic processes follows.

Helping to Achieve Cognitive Maturation

At this point, the reader is referred to the section on "Cognitive Growth" (see above), and Chapter 4, "Cognitive Development," in the author's book, *Latency*. The mere act of verbalizing in a situation in which the child is a center of attention for a sustained period of time has a strong influence in making a child become more verbal. Pointing out connections is an important part of this activity. Showing the child the assembly of whole pictures out of smaller units such as lines, circles, and dots, with accompanying verbalization is useful. For example, draw a few lines which vaguely indicate an animal. Convey to the child the explanation that with each new line, the child will be able to recognize the image slowly being revealed. Add lines till the child links words to the concept of the animal conveyed in the simplest abstract reduction of its form. When a child speaks of a dream, or plays out a story, bring the nonverbal components into the realm of shared memory by having the child mold or draw the image. Then ask about details, seek verbalization. Hold the plastic form of the concept, and return to it again and again. Introduce it when concepts it represents are apparent in the associations of the patient. Concurrently, it behooves the therapist to ignore the implications of these communications as definitive interpretations. They do not serve as therapeutic tools over and above their role in encouraging cognitive maturation. Therefore, when the job of cognitive maturation has been achieved, they must be repeated.

Fantasy Play as a Therapeutic Activity

Playing out fantasies, even in the absence of communicative verbalizations that involve the therapist, and insight, can be of benefit in helping the child to abreact traumas and to work through fixations in psychosexual development. This was brought home to me strikingly by an eleven-year-old girl who had come to analysis some years before, dominated by the wish to be a boy. She refused to wear girls' clothes, was very athletic, and avoided dolls and such. Toward the end of her treatment, she insisted on extended periods of doll play. When I asked her what she thought was the reason for this, she said that it expressed and fulfilled her need to play out being a mother. This was something she had denied herself before.

At times a child has an absence of the ability to symbolize defensively. This interferes with fantasy play. Such children tend to have latency calm interspersed with episodes of marked anxiety, rather than excited behavior. Usually, it is active symbolization that is missing. They can passively use the symbols of others in the form of stories and TV dramas for hours on end. They cannot produce symbols on their own. Typically, these children fall into silence when they come upon material that is difficult to verbalize. This is in contradistinction to the shift into fantasy play that one usually sees in latency-age children. It is therapeutically useful to try to help these children create symbols of their own so that they can develop fantasy play to use in therapy and in life for the mastery of conflicts, humiliations, and fixations. How is this done? One technique is to introduce clay figures, doll figures, or drawings to represent the situation being described by the child at the moment he became silent. The next step is to ask the child what happens next, or even to suggest what may happen, using doll figures to illustrate the suggestion. As with most work which deals with cognitive growth in children, the symbolic potential of these children exceeds their functional capacity. This can be harnessed for therapeutic gain.

Fantasy play, like dreams, can serve as a source for information insights. More so even than in the therapy of adults, fantasies reflect the stressful events that have confronted the child prior to his coming to the session. The child who beats a punching "bop" bag for refusing to eat, may be telling the therapist of his own experience at the table with his parents. Repeated themes of punishment for refusal to obey brings into focus the character trait of stubbornness in a child. The theme, oft repeated, of protecting oneself from having a leg cut off, reflects castration fears. Stories of thefts, captures, and imprisonments have been signals to me, like the buoys in bays, that something lies just beneath the surface. In this case, most likely guilt. Not only recent events, but chronic stresses, fixations, and unresolved conflicts, form the precipitants of which the fantasy of the child consists. The current stress that is responded to by a fantasy defense in latency is usually an incident related in content and form to the pre-existing fantasy that it activates. New fantasy themes are rare. New fantasy elements are not. The repeated patterns of fantasies that are evoked in a child are usually related to unresolved antecedents and parental attitudes. Thus, the child who fantasies that he is an hero in the face of being called a name, is usually chronically sensitive to being called a name because of preoccupation with defects and inadequacies which had been part of his early life, and which he has been ever on the alert to conceal. The analysis of fantasy during psychotherapy is a topic that could fill an endless volume. These references are merely indications of the rich potential of the process.

Determining Outcome

There is little in the way of formal psychological testing for progress in therapy in the latency-age child, that differs from the standard available psychological tests. In situations in which the behavioral problems of the child are manifestations of a poor symbolizing function, and the usually associated inadequate latency, the progress of the child's improved symbolizing function with therapy can be followed with a test recently devised by Dr. G.J. Donnelly (1977), which detects the quality of a latency-age child's symbolizing function.

Clinical indicators are reliable and easily detected. Improvement in function is the primary goal of therapy in the latency-age child. Such improvement is defined in terms of the following key elements. The child should be able to maintain states of sustained calm, quiet, pliability, and educability in appropriate social settings. The child should be capable of symbolization, and resolution of situations of stress, through fantasy play discharge. This should be strongly differentiated from fantasy activity that is tinged with escape from reality. The eventual outcome of latency fantasy as defense, is the transition of its elements of trial action as compensation into the reality-oriented future planning of adolescence. The symbols and situations of late latency play fantasies should be strongly colored by appropriate tendencies toward realistic elements rather than improbable creatures. The child should be free of the symptoms which brought him to therapy. There should be good relations with peers, including acceptance of the child by other well-functioning children. Often, the progress of a child in latency-age therapy can be traced by following the changing nature and number of his friends. The march toward health is accompanied by an increase in the number of friends, with troubled and provocative children diminishing as companions, the further down the road to health the child goes.

Summary and Conclusions

The psychotherapy of the latency-age child requires special training because of the unique nature of the functioning apparatus of the ego in this age group. Because this ego function can often, when functioning well, mask problems that should be solved lest they menace adolescence, it is important to approach latency children as individuals, rather than to succumb to the use of modalities that put all children into one category, and create a buffer between the patient's needs and the therapist's response. In my opinion, such a situation can be produced by the use of such disparate modalities as drug therapy, and dynamically oriented therapy, that finds the source of interpretations in theories rather than in the associations and fantasy play elements of the child. Each child is an individual. Individuals should not be forced into molds of preconceived notion, constructed from the latest therapeutic fad. Such ephemera pass from positions of exaggerated importance into their rightful lesser place in the scheme of things, when their charismatic champions pass from power. Children, who have little capacity to discriminate between the effective therapist and the technician who diagnoses patients with the aid of cookie cutters in the shape of a personality pattern, deserve to be defended against emphases which are more of a fact of current trends in the literature of psychotherapy than reflections of the inner life of the child. In child therapy, the associations of the child should be the measure of all things. This is not meant to criticize the content of current theories. (In 1977, these were separation-individuation and object relations theory, with ego psychology beginning to fade and the symbol theory, cognitive development and the developmental approach used in this presentation just beginning to achieve popularity.) What comes under my criticism are therapists who would use any single theory to explain the processes within many different children. Advances in theory should expand, not limit, the number of psychotherapeutic possibilities and strategies. As I have noted, latency-age children should be protected from such limitations. They cannot detect such techniques, and cannot defend themselves. Therapists with the least amount of training, who are most apt to fall back on ready-made interpretations, are assigned to work with children. This is a product of the myth that children are little adults, and that there is little ego psychological development where calm is derived from diminished drives. This is not so. Therapists should, therefore, be selected from those specially trained to understand latency ego development.

References

De Mauss, L. (1975) *The History of Childhood.* New York: Atcom.

De Saussaure, R. (1946) J.B. Felix Descuret. In *The*

Psychoanalytic Study of the Child. New York: International Universities Press, pp. 417–424.

Donnelly, G.J. (1977) *Symbolization, Fantasy and Adaptive Regression as Developmental Tasks of the Latency Period.* Unpublished doctoral dissertation for the California School of Professional Psychology, San Francisco.

Ferenczi, S. (1913) A little chanticleer. In *Sex in Psychoanalysis.* New York: Basic Books (1950).

Freud, A. (1946) *The Psychoanalytic Treatment of Children.* New York: International Universities Press.

Freud, S. (1905) Three contributions . . . *Standard Edition* London: Hogarth Press.

Freud, S. (1909) Analysis of a phobia in a five-year-old boy. *Standard Edition* London: Hogarth Press.

Freud, S. (1926) The question of lay analysis. *Standard Edition* 20:179–258. London: Hogarth Press.

Freud, S. (1950) *The Origins of Psychoanalysis.* New York: Basic Books (1959).

Klein, M. (1932) *The Psychoanalysis of Children.* London: Hogarth Press.

Kramer, S., and L.J. Byerly. (1978) Technique of psychoanalysis of the latency child. In J. Glenn, ed., *Child Analysis: Technique, Theory, Applications.* New York: Jason Aronson.

Sarnoff, C.A. (1976) *Latency.* New York: Jason Aronson.

Sarnoff, C.A. (1978) Normal and pathological development in latency age children. In J. Bemporad, ed., *Normal and Pathological Child Development.* New York: Brunner/Mazel.

Treatment of Emotional Disorders in Children and Adolescents

CHAPTER 19

Psychotherapy with Adolescents

*Charles Jaffe**
Daniel Offer

Introduction

The years of adolescence, roughly those between twelve (the onset of puberty) and the early twenties (when the adolescent's developmental tasks have been mostly completed), have been romanticized and maligned. There have been theorists and therapists who have devoted a great deal of time to this period of life and who have warned of its difficulties. Holmes (1964) said that the intensity of an adult's interest in adolescence varies directly with his distance from adolescents. Josselyn (1957) described the psychotherapy of adolescents as "the most baffling, the most anxiety-arousing, and the most narcissistically gratifying experience a psychiatrist can have."

Adolescence is a phase in the life cycle, and along with childhood, young adulthood, adulthood, and old age, it has its developmental tasks, difficulties, pleasures, and opportunities.

It is the purpose of this chapter to discuss the outpatient, dynamically oriented, individual psychotherapy of adolescents (when using the term "psychotherapy," we intend to refer to this approach to treatment of adolescents unless otherwise indicated). We will examine some of the factors influencing the referral of adolescents to therapy and the suitability of this type of psychotherapy for certain patients. We will discuss the roles and qualities of the therapist, some of the elements in the development and process of psychotherapy with adolescents, and some goals and future potential of psychotherapy with adolescents. We emphasize the special problems in treating adolescents as opposed to other age groups.

Overview

There are many changes that occur in a person's life when he enters his teenage years. Adolescence can be conceived of as presenting four major developmental tasks to the person: separation from the family, development of a sense of identity, development of adult sexuality, and attainment of social and vocational competence. These tasks are interdependent and are met in parallel fashion (Hamburg, 1974). Puberty begins, and this means new discoveries and understanding of the body and its sensations. Sexual feelings are aroused, and the teenager learns to master these feelings as they affect relationships both inside and outside the family. The opportunity for adult sexual expression presents a significant challenge to the teenager. The adolescent learns the ways of skillful social interaction and to see himself as a member of a group in school, at a job, or in society as a whole. He begins the search for a vocation. Amid these tasks of finding a place in the larger context, the teenager

* This work was done while Dr. Jaffe was a Clinical Research Fellow in Adolescence at the Institute for Psychosomatic Research and Training, Michael Reese Hospital and Medical Center (Grant #T32 MH14668-01 of the NIMH, USPHS).

needs to develop a sense of his uniqueness within the community. He develops a sense of his special capabilities and limitations.

An overriding task seems to be the development of a sense of autonomy (Blos, 1967; Erikson, 1968), of self-reliance, with the ability to function as a separate individual, attached to others in a meaningful way, but not reliant upon others for the maintenance of abilities or sense of worth. This involves a separation from the infantile ties that have served as the groundwork upon which the developmental tasks until adolescence have rested.

The tasks of separation, development of adult sexuality, identity formation, and social and vocatinal competence involve a transition. Childhood is left behind and an adult life is in preparation. However, the joy of discovery, mastery, and the sense of personal uniqueness that can accompany the adolescent's expanding social and sexual opportunities and exploration cannot be overlooked in an examination of the developmental tasks and their liabilities.

Psychotherapy: Review of the Literature

The psychotherapy of the adolescent, with an emphasis on the relationship between the psychotherapist and the patient has been addressed by Aichhorn (1925), Gitelson (1948), Josselyn (1957), Holmes (1964), Meeks (1971), and others. Many of the thoughts on psychotherapy in the present chapter are drawn from these writings. Goldberg (1978) and Gradolph (1976) have presented an application of the work of Heinz Kohut (1971, 1972) to the psychotherapy of adolescents from the perspective of the development of the self.

Lorand and Schneer (1961) present works by sixteen authors on the psychoanalytic approach to adolescent problems. Their work includes, among others, chapters on homosexuality, masturbation, suicide, and psychosomatic disorders. Masterson (1958) has contrasted the psychotherapy of adolescents with the psychotherapy of adults.

Other works present papers on a variety of issues concerning the normal and pathological development, psychotherapy, and socially related problems of adolescents. Examples of these are Schoolar (1973), Howells (1971), Esman (1975), and the annual edited by Feinstein and Giovacchini (1970–1977).

Easson (1969), Holmes (1964), Masterson (1972), and Noshpitz (1959) are examples of work dealing with the inpatient psychotherapy of the adolescent.

Individual Psychotherapy of the Adolescent

In this section, we examine the individual, dynamically oriented, outpatient psychotherapy of the adolescent patient.

Understanding the theories of adolescent development with its vicissitudes of separation, narcissistic vulnerability, identity crises, and sexual impulses does not suffice when face to face in an interview with a patient. The adolescent's behavior can be understood by seeing it in terms of a theoretical model, and this may be helpful to the therapist. However, observing behavior and understanding it through theory does not help patients. What does help is applying this understanding in a way that the patient can use to help him negotiate his troubles.

In this section, we convey an approach to this endeavor. We look at how an adolescent is referred for psychotherapy and compare some aspects of inpatient and outpatient psychotherapy to illustrate the types of patients that may be best suited for individual, dynamically oriented outpatient psychotherapy. We discuss the roles and qualities of the therapist and some difficulties the therapist may have in treating some adolescent patients. We consider the role of the family in the treatment of the adolescent. We also address the process of psychotherapy with an emphasis on the relationship between the psychotherapist and the patient. Finally, we discuss what can be expected to be achieved with this approach to the psychotherapy of adolescents.

The population of patients who may benefit from individual, dynamically oriented outpatient psychotherapy does not necessarily lend itself to division into age, sex, socioeconomic, or diagnostic groupings. Generally, we are discussing the psychotherapy of adolescents who have the capacity to form a meaningful relationship with an adult they can use to help them make psychological changes. They display behavior that is not so self-destructive or destructive to others that it requires more complete supervision of their everyday lives. This may exclude some patients such as borderlines who act out in a variety of destructive ways and patients with active psychosis.

In our discussion of psychotherapy we make general statements that apply to many adolescent patients. Some of the areas addressed may be more applicable to either younger or older adolescent patients, although elements of the particular behavior or issue can be seen in adolescent patients in any phase of their development. Some patients may act out and have little ability to view their own behavior while others may be quite self-observant when they begin therapy. There may be some adolescent patients who will not approach therapy with significant misgivings about the ability of an adult to understand their problems and to help them. The degree to which any of the issues we discuss is applicable is dependent upon the characteristics of the patient. Just as with older patients, the psychotherapist treating adolescents needs to assess each patient individually.

When an adolescent is seen in a clinical setting, this represents a course of action initiated by people, in varying combinations, from important areas of his life, or by the adolescent himself. To understand how an adolescent comes to the attention of a therapist, we need to understand something about his behavior, the areas of his life that are affected by this behavior, and the reactions of people in his life to his behavior. We also need to understand something about the meaning of the adolescent's behavior in terms of its normality or pathology.

The adolescent is engaged in a reciprocal process of change and mastery between his growing external world and his developing internal capacity to negotiate successfully this larger world. This process involves action. For example, there is a need to test, to inquire, to try and fail and try again in many situations. The adolescent cannot accomplish the developmental tasks before him without this activity. The task of separation involves reworking of early relationships with family members, and attachment to people outside the family, and to do this the adolescent again and again tests his capacity to be autonomous. The development of adult sexuality means internal change regarding body image and sexual identity. This is accomplished through seeking actively new and different relationships and experimenting with sex, dating, and physical skills. Social competence and a sense of identity are acquired by the adolescent through repeated experimentation in social interaction by action or fantasy.

If adolescent behavior is viewed in the context of this activity it becomes apparent that an adolescent reaches a therapist's office when something about his best efforts to negotiate his world has attracted the attention of one or many people with whom he has contact. This may be school if the adolescent is truant, parents if there is excessive strife in the home, or the police if the adolescent's behavior involves illegal or destructive activity. There are times when an adolescent may seek a therapist on his own because he is aware that his feeling or behavior may not be adaptive. This usually occurs with older adolescents, particularly at the time they are beginning jobs or college education or have left home for the first time. Most of the time, however, the adolescent comes to the therapist at the behest of an adult in his life.

When the situation arises that the adolescent is referred by a parent, school authority, or some other adult in his life, some attention should be paid to the impact of the adolescent's behavior on the people with whom he interacts. When an adolescent is having a problem and is not seeking help for himself, he is dependent upon the adults in his life to realize that his efforts are failing. They may have difficulty with this for two reasons. Due to their own needs, significantly maladaptive behavior may be overlooked for some time, or some minor or transient deviation may be severely questioned. This issue is discussed below. A more general reason that adults have difficulty in responding to an adolescent's behavior is that there has grown a confusion about what is normal or abnormal behavior for an adolescent.

For many years, it was felt that it was expected that an adolescent would behave in an erratic, moody, fickle, even hypochondriacal fashion and that this was due to the intrapsychic changes occurring within the adolescent. Symptoms that in any other period of life would be considered evidence of psychiatric illness were viewed, in the adolescent, as the normal, even necessary, vicissitudes of development. Anna Freud (1958) states: "Adolescence is by its nature an interruption of peaceful growth, and . . . the upholding of a steady equilibrium during the adolescent process is in itself abnormal. It is normal for an adolescent to behave for a considerable length of time in an inconsistent and unpredictable manner." This approach led clinicians to treat symptoms in an adolescent as a consequence of normal development—adolescent turmoil—and to adopt an attitude that "They'll grow out of it."

More recently, however, this view has been questioned. Offer and Masterson, especially, have studied the issue of adolescent turmoil.

Offer and Offer (1975) studied 61 white, middle-class, normal adolescent males over an 8-year period. They found that they followed three general routes of development, which they called the continuous, surgent, and tumultuous growth groups. Only in the tumultuous growth group did the adolescents display the behavior usually referred to as adolescent turmoil. "These adolescents have been observed to have recurrent self-doubts and braggadocio, escalating conflicts with their parents, and often respond inconsistently to their social and academic environments." The continuous growth group showed no overt clinical symptoms. They had stable relationships with their parents, grew smoothly into extrafamilial relationships, particularly sexual relationships. They had no superego problems. The balance between their increased drives and ego capacity to handle them was without fluctuation that showed distress. They were goal-directed. The surgent growth group had some greater trouble with ego capacity to handle increased drives, and there was evidence of discord in the family, but overall they were as well adjusted as the continuous growth group.

Masterson (1967) studied 72 outpatients over a five-year period. He found that turmoil was "at most an incidental factor subordinate to that of psychiatric illness in the onset, course, and outcome of the various conditions in our patients. [Turmoil] exerted its effect primarily by exacerbating and giving its own coloring to preexistent pathology. It . . . is not so pronounced as to blur the substantial differences between healthy and sick."

It is our view that if an adolescent has been referred by any of a variety of sources for behavior that has been persistent and that has shown the adolescent to be unsuccessfully coping in some area of his life, this behavior must not be dismissed as "normal" adolescent turmoil. It must be explored in the context of some breakdown in his adaptive capacity.

Part of the evaluation for psychiatric treatment of an adolescent involves a decision about what form of intervention would be most beneficial to him. The major differentiation involves the inpatient versus outpatient care of the patient. It is our intent to present points of distinction in selecting inpatient versus outpatient care. The forms of outpatient therapy also include group and family therapy. These modalities are addressed elsewhere in this volume.

In order for an adolescent to be able to use outpatient therapy, he ought to think he has a problem, be able to attend sessions regularly, form a meaningful relationship with his therapist, and use the relationship, and possibly psychological insight into himself, for making psychological changes and growth. He should be able to handle his behavior in socially acceptable ways, and have family that can either grow with him or tolerate the changes he might make in treatment. Easson (1969) has stressed the idea that in order to use outpatient psychotherapy, the patient needs to have the ability to use relationships to help him with self-control and self-direction, and the ego strength to deal with controlling his impulses. Masterson (1972) and Meeks (1971) have also commented on the criteria for selection of inpatient or outpatient care for adolescents.

These criteria are consistent with the view that the adolescent is engaged in mastery of his feelings and his environment. If he can use the accomplishments he has made on his own to support his efforts to learn to resolve areas of conflict, he should be encouraged to do so. Major decisions regarding everyday life are made for a person in a psychiatric hospital. Admission to a psychiatric hospital should be reserved for those adolescents who have not developed the underlying personality structure that allows them to be their own major source of psychic structure and impulse control. For these adolescents, the external control, consistent and predictable environment, and ready availability of helping staff can provide a place to grow. Since major decisions regarding everyday life are made for a person in a psychiatric hospital, hospitalization can undermine the independence and self-esteem of an adolescent with greater inner structure.

When an adolescent can be treated on an outpatient basis in individual psychotherapy, some determination of the choice of long- or short-term psychotherapy is useful. The choice may depend on the desires of the patient and the family and on the preferred mode of intervention of the therapist as opposed to any theoretical justification. Generally, however, long-term psychotherapy is the treatment of choice when it can be demonstrated that the adolescent's problems are the result of prior failure to accomplish necessary developmental tasks. These problems may vary in their behavioral characteristics, but often are not of acute onset with a clear precipitant and do not involve a few focal symptoms. They are of a more general nature that involves the patient's perceptions of himself, and of his world and they may be traced over a significant part of the patient's development. Short-term psychotherapy is more appropriate when the adolescent's problems seem to be of acute onset with a clear precipitating factor, of short duration, situationally induced, a clearly felt problem to the patient, and available for change by suggestions and manipulation. Of course, these terms are themselves somewhat arbitrary. Even in long-term psychotherapy, crises may emerge that require active suggestion and manipulation by the therapist, and patients can develop lasting change and insight in even the shortest and most circumscribed interventions.

The Psychotherapist: Role and Qualities

The relationship between the therapist and patient is of primary importance in the psychotherapy of any patient, and particularly in that of the adolescent. The adolescent's struggles involve developing adaptive ways to live in society, as well as the resolution of unconscious conflict. The adolescent learns by exploration. He uses his actions in his environment to learn more about reality and about himself. The adolescent will use his psychotherapist in a similar fashion. The therapist becomes the embodiment of qualities that the adolescent may strive for or rebel against in the adult world. If the adolescent is mistrustful of adults because of past experience or because he is actively engaged in separation struggles, he may be rebellious, negativistic, and devaluing of his therapist. The adolescent may use the therapist as a standard for thought and behavior. The sexually developing boy or girl may use an opposite-sex therapist to test the effects of his or her sexuality. In all cases, the therapist working with adolescents should be prepared to be cast in, and to take, a variety of roles.

Some therapists may have qualities that allow them to treat most adolescents more easily than others. A therapist who is comfortable being verbally active and can engage in conversation or debate will be able to relate to his patient in a way that is familiar to him. The therapist who can engage in discussions or even arguments with his questioning patient may be using a valuable way to relate. Since sometimes information may be all that is necessary to help the patient, the therapist who can feel comfortable in the role of information giver may find this quite helpful to his patients. There are some adolescent patients, particularly the older ones, who may not need the same sort of activity and verbal involvement from a therapist. These adolescents may be treated by therapists who are usually more comfortable and effective with adult patients.

Adolescents can ask some penetrating questions. At one moment the patient can attack and devalue or be provocative with the therapist and at the next moment strive to be like him. His unconscious purpose in all this is to get some better idea about his own identity as a separate person. The adolescent often uses the therapist as someone to "bounce off of" in order to gain a more accurate sense of himself. Josselyn (1957) refers to this as the patient's use of the therapist as a "sounding board." The therapist who can respond to questions with candor, revealing things about himself where appropriate and useful to the therapy, can present a real picture of himself that the adolescent can use in his own efforts to develop a clearer self-image. This requires that the therapist be comfortable with his own fallibilities and limitations, as well as confident about his strengths and areas of particular knowledge.

Adolescents can be as sensitive to their therapist's vulnerabilities as they are to their own, and will often try to prove that their assumptions about the therapist are correct or to use the therapist's vulnerabilities to make him feel like the patient. If the therapist is himself conflicted in his areas of strengths and weaknesses, the adolescent will surely know it.

The therapist may be called upon to assert control of his patient's behavior. He may need to set limits or confront a particular behavior. If he is not secure in what he knows and does not know, he will not be able to confront the adolescent or handle the angry response he is likely to encounter in return. The therapist's confidence about himself is necessary if he is to be able to allow his patient to enter into the process of idealization, by which he can use the therapist as a model to help him find more adaptive ways to solve his conflicts.

The therapist needs to be flexible in his view of his patient's capacity to behave responsibly. It is most helpful if the therapist does not have stereotypical attitudes about adolescents, such as the idea that they are really only children in rapidly maturing bodies, or that they are adults who take advantage of their youth to avoid adult responsibilities. The adolescent may at times behave as a responsible adult, quite capable of taking care of himself, achieving in his world, and behaving with sensitivity towards others. At other times, he may act irresponsibly, and cope with his feelings in a manner befitting a much younger child.

Obviously, the therapist lacking the qualities of flexibility, candor, comfort with an active stance, and security with his own limitations and strengths will not have an easy time treating many adolescents. Another problem exists if the therapist has not developed his own sense of identity. If, for example, the therapist has not developed a perspective regarding the productive as well as the destructive aspects of society, he may have trouble with the concept that the adolescent's rebelliousness and negativism are representative of his own struggle to see himself as separate as well as to use newly found moral and intellectual skills. He may, instead, unconsciously encourage the adolescent to continue his rebellion. If the therapist is struggling with his own sexual urges, he may find it difficult to confront the provocativeness of the sexually acting out patient. If the therapist cannot see himself clearly in regard to his own developmental stage but really wishes to be like he thinks his adolescence should have been, he may have trouble in remembering which person in the therapy session is the adolescent and which is the mature adult.

In short, the therapist who has not himself established a knowledgeable, firm sense of professional identity and a realistic sense of comfort with himself, is subject to being stimulated by those areas of conflict in his patients that correspond to his own. In this case, he may respond with anger, rejection, or passivity, or he may enter into a collusion with his patient. He may enter into his patient's conflicts and not view them from the vantage point of the consistency, predictability, and reality-orientation that are needed to allow the patient to develop. The therapist then becomes a reflection of rather than a regulator of the patient's emotional climate.

The Working Alliance

There is an adage in medicine that goes: "If you talk with a patient long enough he'll tell you what's wrong, and if you talk with him a little longer, he'll tell you what to do about it." This adage illustrates some important aspects of the beginning, and the foundation, of psychotherapy with the adolescent. It touches on the respect accorded to the patient that allows him the chance to define and to solve his own problems, and it recognizes his ability to do this. For the adolescent, this is tied to his search for an increased sense of autonomy and self-direction. The adage also speaks to the humility of the therapist in realizing that the discovery of his patient's problems is something that results from, not results in, psychotherapy. There is an equal participation by the growth-directed, reality-oriented parts of two people. The patient is neither a child, for whom all things must be done, nor a completely autonomous being who can survive without assistance.

In the beginning of psychotherapy with an adolescent, the therapist concerns himself with these fundamental aspects of his relationship with his patient. This conscious, rational relationship that forms between a psychotherapist and his patient who are working toward the common goal of helping the patient to understand himself better has been most aptly described by Greenson (1967) as the working alliance.

There are, certainly, common factors about the working alliance that apply to work with patients of all ages. However, for the adolescent, who is in the process of developing capacities to view himself and his world in a realistic fashion, development of this working alliance takes on special importance and emphasis in his psychotherapy. The development of a good working alliance is in itself therapeutic. It helps the adolescent patient develop an ability to view himself; to learn to see himself, his thoughts, his behavior. It is this ability to view oneself, to develop an observing ego, that allows one to examine and to understand feelings and reactions in greater depth (see, for example, Meeks, 1971).

Much of the beginning of psychotherapy with adolescents can be seen as helping the patient stay around long enough to tell you what's wrong. With adolescents, unlike adults, the therapist cannot rely upon an already established capacity in his patient to realize, at least on a conscious level, that the therapist is a helpful person. That is, the adolescent patient may not be able to separate and identify certain concerns about coming to therapy that could be considered resistance rather than reality based. Therefore he has trouble putting aside the concerns at least long enough to come to psychotherapy sessions and work with these feelings. The adolescent's desire for self-direction places him in a position of going to the very same type of person he sees himself trying to break away from, an authority-bearing adult. Otherwise stated, the adolescent must seek help from a person whom he links with those internal parental representations from which he is trying to emancipate himself. Although he has suffered some inadequacy in his development that has made this process particularly difficult, he still sees coming to a therapist as a threat to whatever gains he has been able to make on his own.

The psychotherapist must help his patient solve this paradox. Gitelson (1948) refers to the "narcissistic contact" that the therapist must establish with his patient to help keep the patient engaged on a level that will transcend the emotional shifts of adolescence that make many relationships fleeting. Gitelson states that since the adult psychotherapist does not share with the adolescent the similarity of adulthood, nor the emotional position of the benign understanding parent, he must rely on "comparable experience, comparable anxiety, and comparable emotional direction and tendencies which are mutually sensed but the therapist has mastered." Masterson (1958) also remarks on the burden of the therapist to establish a relationship with his patient. He emphasizes the point that the adolescent may have been traumatized by his parents or coerced into therapy. He notes that the first efforts of the therapist should be to dissociate himself from the parents' behavior.

Those areas of therapy that have to do with testing the therapist, setting limits to behavior, active intervention on the patient's behalf or to protect him, can be seen as ways in which the therapist and his patient work actively to develop a good working alliance. These situations are action-oriented and have the exploring, experimenting flavor to them that is consistent with the ways that adolescents learn about themselves in the world. Through these maneuvers and interactions with the therapist, the adolescent can gain a sense that the therapist is interested in helping him establish a more realistic, adaptive view of himself and of his world. He learns that his therapist is not interested in infantilizing him by removing his attempts at self-direction and self-control, yet his therapist is also not interested in allowing him to become overwhelmed by embarking on a course of action that obviously reflects his inability to handle adequately the situation at that moment. The adolescent learns that, unlike many adults he may know, his therapist does not have a particular self-serving investment in his patient's behavior or feelings.

This method of interacting is different from therapy of adults. As Masterson (1958) notes, the emphasis here is on increased reality testing by interacting with the therapist rather than a controlled regression with increased insight into unconscious processes. The activity of the therapist to set limits and to interpret the adolescent patient's testing and acting out behavior is intended to create a dependable, rather than a dependent, relationship (Gitelson, 1948). As Gitelson points out, it is this difference between dependability and dependence that allows the patient to work productively in therapy rather than becoming helpless and more vulnerable. This distinction separates the influence of guiding authority from suppressive authoritarianism.

The therapist sometimes sees that his patient is acting in a way that is dangerous to future relationships or of immediate danger to himself. The patient, on the other hand, may see this action as quite reasonable and defend it on the grounds that it supports his right to make his own decisions. Attempts to disagree with the patient are met with complaints that the therapist is just like all the other adults, who are trying to keep his freedom from him.

The therapist has to draw some line of reasonable action. To allow his patient free reign is doing him no favors. In fact, it probably denies him the chance to explore the limits of reasonable behavior. The process in which the adolescent and his therapist discuss the limit and its meaning for both therapist and patient helps the adolescent view his behavior in a more realistic way. He uses his therapist as a guide to help him establish more effective ways to achieve his goal. He sees also that he may not be as free as he thinks he is just by asserting his right to make choices at all costs. He can gain a greater freedom by being able more fully to sense and understand his feelings. He can then see more clearly his need to behave a certain way, and he can more effectively control the response of his environment to him. In order for the process to occur, there has to be some working alliance already established, but the process also serves to enhance the alliance.

When an adolescent tests his therapist, it provides a similar opportunity for building a working alliance and increasing the patient's realistic view of himself. An adolescent can test his therapist in many ways. He may call him at home at night or not show up for a session. He may demand special attention or be silent, attacking, or demeaning. The adolescent patient has no reason to believe that his therapist will be any different from any other adult. He has also developed a view of himself that he expects to be confirmed in his interactions with adults. Why should he venture into yet another relationship that may simply re-create the painful feelings from which he has acted to protect himself? Through the process of testing, the adolescent can learn whether his therapist will accept him as a person with strengths and weaknesses, or will reject him for his failings. He learns whether his therapist can tolerate strong feelings of rage, disappointment, and dependence. He also learns whether his therapist can tolerate his increasing autonomy and growth. As the therapist negotiates these tests by identifying them and understanding them with his patient, the adolescent can allow himself to enter more freely into the relationship, and to allow his therapist to become the guide he needs.

Here again, we see that for the adolescent patient, the very process of establishing a working alliance with a therapist is an integral part of his therapy. By active examination of the patient's behavior by both the patient and his therapist, a more realistic, mutually interactive relationship is built that allows the patient to see himself in a more productive way.

The Role of the Family

The work to establish an alliance with an adolescent does not occur in a vaccuum. Unless the patient is older and has already achieved a significant degree of emotional and economic independence from the family, the adolescent patient is likely to be in an environment at home that continues to exert a strong effect. As we mentioned above, one of the criteria for the suitability of outpatient psychotherapy for an adolescent is the ability of the family to tolerate, if not support and encourage, the patient's progress in therapy.

Parents may find it difficult to have their child in treatment. They may experience guilt or anxiety over their child's problems. Parents may not know the right thing to do for their child. They may not be able to support their child toward appropriate growth due to their own conflicts over such issues as independence or sexual development. Parents may need their adolescent to act out their unresolved conflicts or they may subtly encourage their child to remain symptomatic as a way of preserving a family equilibrium that protects marital or other family problems from emerging.

Such conflicts within families may result in parents becoming intrusive in their child's psychotherapy, or in their becoming almost totally uninvolved in their child's attempts at growth. Parents may demand that their child and the therapist tell them everything that occurs in treatment. They may fail to recognize that the adolescent's therapy is for the adolescent to work on those areas that disturb him, not those areas that the parents find disturbing to them. Parents may also avoid any involvement with their child's therapy out of fear that they may open themselves to criticism from the therapist, or because they are truly not concerned with their child's development. The therapy, in this case, becomes a way for the parents to let someone else raise their child in a way that the parents can at least say they've done all they could for their child.

Therefore, an assessment of the whole family constellation is a necessary part of the initial phase of the psychotherapy of the adolescent. The actual type of involvement of a family in an adolescent's psychotherapy is variable. It may be appropriate for parents to keep in touch with the therapist occasionally, to have family sessions, or to help the parents seek therapy for themselves as individuals or as a couple. The initial evaluation of the family provides an opportunity for the therapist to view the patient in the context of his whole family and to establish a relationship with the parents that serves as a foundation for future contact.

Williams (1973) describes a family diagnostic method to assess the intrapsychic aspects of the patient and the family interactions that may be factors in the treatment of the adolescent and in planning for future family involvement. He states that seeing the family can shed light on whether the patient's intrapsychic distortions are internalized and fixed or if they are currently subject to parental influence. Family sessions can also illustrate how parents may present resistance to change in their child through double-bind communications or by use of the patient to protect against the emergence of marital conflict. Williams suggests flexible use of family sessions throughout the adolescent's therapy to deal with resistance to progress in the patient from his family, in overcoming resistances in the adolescent that are not available to interpretation, and in demonstrating how the adolescent creates resistance by restimulating anxiety over his behavior in the parents.

Offer and Vanderstoep (1974) suggest a somewhat broader view in their article on indications and contraindications for family therapy with adolescent patients. They feel that, in general, "for the relatively healthy adolescent, most psychotherapeutic methods used by an expert will prove helpful. For the very disturbed, most psychotherapeutic technique is inadequate. A firmly developed therapeutic alliance is often more important than the type of intervention used." They do, however, feel that family therapy may be particularly useful for the acting-out adolescent, because family sessions can illustrate that the patient's behavior may be a response to cues from other family members.

It is generally agreed that parents should be involved in treatment when their behavior seems to encourage inappropriate development in their child. Josselyn (1957) suggests that the degree of involvement of the parents in the adolescent's ongoing psychotherapy depends on the emotional maturity of the adolescent, the degree to which the adolescent's problem is internalized, the parents' response to the problem, and the parents' role in creating or fostering the problem. She recommends a thorough understanding by the therapist of the parents' behavior and their attitude toward treatment as a way of fostering a relationship with the parents that will be beneficial to them and to their adolescent in treatment.

The Middle Phase of Psychotherapy

The maintenance of the working alliance is an integral part of the ongoing psychotherapy with the adolescent patient. Attention must be paid to its status throughout. At any time, this alliance may be called forward for reexamination and reappraisal. As Meeks notes (1971), since no other, more self-observing or introspective work can occur without the firm foundation of this mutual, dependable relationship, whenever a break in the relationship occurs, the other work also stops. When the patient begins to test his therapist, by not attending sessions, not talking, demeaning himself or his therapist, or returning to previously discarded acting-out behavior, this can be seen as a break in the working alliance. At these times, the focus of the therapy needs to turn to the state of the relationship between the patient and his therapist to examine what has occurred. For some adolescent patients, the development and exploration of the working alliance may comprise the entire course of therapy.

When the working alliance is solid, the adolescent can use his therapist for more insightful work. The formation of a relationship with an adult who has presumably successfully negotiated some of the life tasks the patient presently confronts, and who can help the patient negotiate these tasks, is of real therapeutic value.

Masterson (1958) refers to the patient's use of his therapist as an idealized figure. The adolescent uses the idealized therapist as a kind of bridge between the demand of his archaic superego and the more flexible, reality-based superego that fits the demands of his larger world. Gradolph (1976) further refines this aspect of therapy by addressing the narcissistic aspects of the adolescent superego. He states that the patient uses the therapist as an idealized self-object to help maintain a cohesive sense of self during the period when the adolescent de-idealizes, modifies, and reinternalizes the internal parental standards. One way this use of the therapist is illustrated is when the therapist acts as an educator to his patient. An adolescent may be uninformed about the adult demands concerning sexual behavior, vocational choice and achievement, and changing patterns and roles in relationship to family. He may not know the details of sexual relationships or the ways in which adults handle their changing relationships with parents. The lack of information can place the patient in a situation where he feels guilty, isolated, or ashamed. When he feels comfortable enough to express concern in a particular area and is given information, he can often make positive use of this on his own. The therapist is seen as someone who knows more and can supply helpful information. Since the adolescent does not have to be concerned with the therapist being judgmental or offended by his concerns, the patient is free to make use of the information given him rather than having to worry about the fact that he needs the information in the first place.

The patient may also use his therapist as a person on whom he can try out new ideas. As the patient discovers his growing intellectual capacities, he may develop all kinds of fantasies or schemes that explore the limits of his intellectual power. This is more than the use of intellectualization as defense as described by Anna Freud (1946), it is more like the child's use of play to master new situations. By playing with ideas and tossing them around with his therapist, the patient can learn a great deal about his ability to use abstract thought.

The development of the ability to use abstract thought has significance for the therapeutic process itself. In order to develop an observing ego, it is necessary to be able to think abstractly. Therefore, as the patient discovers and enlarges his ability to think abstractly about the world, he also increases his ability to think about himself, and to help himself in therapy.

As therapy progresses, the patient can begin to evaluate his own behavior. Action without self-observation begins to be replaced by thinking over impulses before one acts. The adolescent increases his ability to sense his feelings and his reactions to them. Choice becomes a more meaningful part of his repertoire. The difference between real emancipation based on self-awareness and self-control as opposed to a struggle for freedom based on opposition and a need to defend against ambivalent feelings begins to be appreciated by the adolescent.

An important issue in the psychotherapy of an adolescent involves the patient's and therapist's stance toward the issue of attainment of autonomy from the parental family. The prevalent American cultural value that achievement of autonomy though self-reliance is a virtue may lead the patient to feel that autonomy and self-direction are synonymous with an absence of a need for close intergenerational family ties. The reality of family life is that interdependence between the generations is more the norm than complete autonomy. Historical studies of the family in Western Europe since the Reformation suggest that the family was never more of an extended kinship unit than it is at the present time (Laslett and Wall, 1972). Sociological studies have suggested that the majority of adults live in close physical proximity to their own parents and maintain frequent contact with them, even while achieving occupational mobility (Adams, 1968; Litwak, 1960, 1965).

Such findings from the social science literature suggest that we should question the emphasis prevalent in the mental health literature on the desirability of complete psychological autonomy from the parental family as the ideal outcome of successful development to adulthood or successful psychotherapy (Goldfarb, 1965). From this perspective, it is important that we should help the adolescent to accept not only his desire for autonomy and independence but, of equal importance, his desire to remain within the family as an interdependent family member, neither totally dependent nor totally isolated and autonomous. Autonomy and self-direction relate to the ability to choose whatever is most comfortable and fulfilling, regardless of its current popularity.

As the patient develops his ability to look at himself, not only does he learn what he feels and needs and who he is but he also learns an approach to new problems. New experiences occurring in the patient's life situation, such as starting a first job, moving out of the home, beginning college, or an involvement in a serious emotional and sexual relationship, may be stressful for the adolescent. Through therapy the patient learns to approach new situations and relationships with a sense of being able to gauge himself in response to his environment and to master new problems on his own. This increases the adolescent's self-esteem and sense of self-direction.

One aspect of growing up and becoming part of a larger society is that there are a number of transition points that mark the occasion. Adolescents may be involved in graduations, confirmations, bar mitzvahs, weddings, or ceremonies in various community organizations. The therapist who is treating a patient involved in these activities may be asked to attend. There may be many reasons why a patient may request this. He may wish to have an important, respected adult share in his achievement, or he may be relying on the therapist's presence for support or to act out a specific aspect of his problems. He may also feel the therapist's presence represents a competition for parents. When such a request is made of a therapist, the meaning of the request to both patient and therapist needs exploration. The therapist is a real, vital person in the patient's life, and it is consistent with the needs of an adolescent for him to wish his therapist to participate in a real way in his life at certain times. Therefore, there is no rule of thumb. The more standard analytic position of nonintervention in a patient's life does not offer guidance here. It is up to the patient and the therapist to decide if the therapist's participation in this direct way in the patient's life contributes to the patient's increasing growth and autonomy or if it is motivated by regressive or defensive needs.

Termination

In some cases, termination of psychotherapy with an adolescent occurs as part of the natural progression in the relationship. The patient came to therapy for a reason. The reason was identified and explored and the patient made use of his relationship with his therapist to learn more about himself. As the adolescent meets and masters new challenges and becomes increasingly comfortable with himself in relation to his world, he may feel his need for therapy lessens. He is able to turn his attention to the events in his life and to handle them without the help of his therapist. A progression toward autonomy that first involved the use of the therapist to help with separation from the family now becomes involved with the added independence from the therapist. Termination, then, presents an opportunity for the patient and his therapist to work through the feelings generated by this separation. The therapist can act as a model, much like an accepting parent who sees his child grow and leave home. Although saddened to see him go, he can help him to leave and take pride in his ability to enjoy life on his own. The therapist can express his sense of loss while showing his patient that he is not dependent upon him for gratification. The patient can see that despite the pain of separation, it does not mean that he must remain in therapy for the therapist's sake. He also learns that he cannot allow his own feelings of loss to keep him from continuing to progress and grow.

In most instances, termination is not smooth. It is sometimes difficult to know if a patient is leaving therapy because of the natural progression discussed above or if he is leaving for some defensive reason because of some break in the working alliance, or because of a reality interference. Some adolescents may deal with the anxiety of termination with a flight response and invoke changes in their life situation such as getting a job, leaving home, or moving to college to rationalize their behavior. It is up to the therapist to make this differentiation and to help the patient understand his behavior. If the therapy has been successful in establishing a good working alliance, the patient will be able to remain in therapy long enough to make the separation process more understandable and part of his growth experience.

There are also adolescents who deal with separation by an increased dependence on the therapist. Here, too, the therapist must distinguish a real need for continued therapy from a transient regression that necessitates helping the patient leave therapy.

Although the course of psychotherapy has been described as having beginning, middle, and termination phases that are identifiable and grow from a process of interaction of patient and therapist, this is often not the way that therapy actually occurs. Adolescents tend to come to therapy at a time when they cannot master a particular aspect of their development by themselves. When they have learned enough to meet the task at hand, they leave and face the next challenges on their own. This means that many psychotherapies of adolescents stop precipitously.

Psychotherapy with adolescents is often accomplished on an intermittent basis. The patient may come and work for a while, then need to consolidate his gains and continue on his own, then return to treatment at some later date. The therapist has to have a feel for his patient's ability to make progress on his own as opposed to his need to flee from therapy. Josselyn (1957) refers to this as being in touch with the state of the patient's ego and intervening only to help an overtaxed ego gain control. It is not useful therapy to let a patient's behavior go unquestioned when it indicates that he cannot handle his feelings adequately. It is also not useful therapy to keep an adolescent from managing as much of his life as possible on his own. This can often be a difficult determination to make.

Therapists treating adolescents have to deal with the idea that they may have a limited usefulness and that they may not get the gratification of seeing their patients develop over a long period of time.

Goals of Psychotherapy

The adolescent is usually seen for a slice of time during a phase of his life that is full of change and is in itself a slice of a larger process of change and growth. The patient enters therapy in a stage of transition and usually leaves it before he has fully developed his personality structure or his life direction.

Some reasonable goals for psychotherapy with an adolescent are helping the patient to strengthen his ego capacities and supporting his efforts to find successful ways to meet the challenges of his currently developing internal and external world, as well as preparing him to meet the new challenges ahead by understanding and having some control over his behavior. This increases the adolescent's ability to make choices for himself about his present and future behavior.

The adolescent is developing his personality and a goal of psychotherapy is to help the patient develop a positive and realistic view of himself and of his capabilities and limitations. If he has encountered difficulties in an earlier developmental stage that now interfere with his ability to meet the demands currently facing him, therapy can work toward the goal of removing these interferences. The analysis of unconscious conflict, genetic reconstruction, and reorganization of personality structure are too ambitious for most patients. This is usually reserved for older adolescents who have the emotional and cognitive ability to tolerate this more intensive kind of work.

For the therapist whose personal goals involve delving as deeply as possible into the roots of his patient's problems, therapy of adolescents may be quite ungratifying and appear incomplete. But the adolescent's development is incomplete, and to the patient, therapy is more a stop along the way than a time to stop and review his personality growth in depth. The goal is to help the patient learn to meet the challenges of life and to enjoy the process along the way. The goal is to provide the adolescent with the tools to develop and grow successfully on his own in his future.

Epilogue

When everything is said and done, the theories have been understood, and the psychotherapist's techniques worked through, what remains is the cultural and societal place of the psychotherapist. How does he see himself vis-à-vis the family, the school, the communities, the patient's peers, and finally, the teenager himself. There is no question but that in some social groupings within the American scene, the psychotherapist is an accepted commodity. He is someone to whom one turns if things do not go well. After all, so many other families do so. In other social settings (for example, in inner-city minority groups), the psychotherapist is viewed with much more suspicion and mistrust. He is often seen as the "tool" of the established middle class, and hence not to be trusted. This may mean for similar symptoms (e.g., severe reactive depression) teenagers are treated differentially, and not always because the psychotherapist is biased. True, the lower-class adolescent is much more likely to receive antidepressive drugs, without a psychotherapeutic trial period, than his middle-class peer. However, some of the reason behind this differential therapeutic approach lies in the patient population as well as in the mental health profession.

It is important to comment that we believe that a well-trained psychotherapist is more than our understanding distant uncle or a parent surrogate. The use of transference for psychotherapeutic reasons is essential. The psychotherapist might decide to spend most of his session discussing baseball with his patient, but he does it based on his knowledge about the psychodynamics of his patient. He does not do it at random, or because he is scared to discuss deeper issues with the patient. The psychotherapist, then, contributes something special to our understanding of, and helping, the youth. It is a perspective different from that of parents, teachers, peers, community leaders or other interested adults.

In this chapter we have attempted to demonstrate what that "something special" is and how it is utilized. We might add that, at times, the personal style of the psychotherapist has great significance as to whether a particular psychotherapeutic relationship would work. The clothing, accent, age, sex, and background of the psychotherapist is obviously a factor in influencing his particular style. Particularly in the beginning of psychotherapy it determines whether treatment will ever get off the ground. It is important for all psychotherapists, and particularly the young ones, to remember that skill aside, not every kind of patient can be treated by him. As a psychotherapist grows older, he knows that by instinct. Therefore, all the above is really applicable only after psychotherapy has been launched, even if we are talking about the first five minutes in the interaction of two human beings.

In conclusion, it is important to state that evaluative research on outcome of psychotherapy is sorely needed. The few research projects on outcome are retrospective in nature (e.g. Hartmann et al., 1968; Garber, 1972). There are no prospective research reports on outcome in psychotherapeutic work with adolescents. It seems to us that one of the priority areas in clinical research over the next decade is evaluative research. It will help us understand the process, the psychodynamics, the theories, as well as simply the outcome of psychotherapy.

References

Adams, B. (1968) *Kinship in an Urban Society.* Chicago: Markham.

Aichhorn, A. (1925) *Wayward Youth.* New York: Viking Press.

Blos, P. (1962) *On Adolescence.* New York: Free Press.

Blos, P. (1967) The second individuation process of adolescence. *Psychoanal. Study Child* 22:162–186.

Easson, W. (1969) *The Severely Disturbed Adolescent.* New York: International Universities Press.

Erikson, E. (1968) *Identity: Youth and Crisis.* New York: Norton.

Esman, A., ed. (1975) *The Psychology of Adolescence: Essential Readings.* New York: International Universities Press.

Feinstein, S., and P. Giovacchini, eds. (1970-1977) *Adolescent Psychiatry: Developmental and Clinical Studies,* Vols. I-V. New York: Basic Books.

Freud, A. (1946) *The Ego and the Mechanisms of Defence.* New York: International Universities Press.

Freud, A. (1958) Adolescence. *Psychoanal. Study Child* 13:255–278.

Garber, B. (1972) *Follow-up of Hospitalized Adolescents.* New York: Brunner/Mazel.

Gitelson, M. (1948) Character synthesis: The psychotherapeutic problem of adolescence. *Am. J. Orthopsychiat.* 18:422–431.

Goldberg, A. (1978) A shift in emphasis: Adolescent psychotherapy and the psychology of the self. *J. Youth Adoles.* 7(2):119–134.

Goldfarb, A. (1965) Psychodynamics and the three-generation family. In E. Shanas and G. Streib, eds., *Social Structure and the Family: Generational Relations.* Englewood Cliffs, N.J.: Prentice-Hall.

Gradolph, P. (1976) Developmental vicissitudes of the self and the ego-ideal during adolescence. Paper presented at the Central States Conference of the American Society for Adolescent Psychiatry, Chicago.

Greenson, R. (1967) The working alliance. In *The Tech-*

nique and Practice of Psychoanalysis, Vol. 1. New York: International Universities Press.

Hamburg, B. (1974) Early adolescence: A specific and stressful stage of the life cycle. In A. Coelho, D. Hamburg, and J. Adams, eds., *Coping and Adaptation*. New York: Basic Books.

Hartman, E., B. Glasser, M. Greenblatt, M. Solomon, and D. Levison. (1968) *Adolescents in a Mental Hospital*. New York: Grune & Stratton.

Holmes, D. (1964) *The Adolescent in Psychotherapy*. New York: Little, Brown.

Howells, J., ed. (1971) *Modern Perspectives in Adolescent Psychiatry*. Edinburgh: Oliver & Boyd.

Josselyn, I. (1957) Psychotherapy of adolescents at the level of private practice. In B. Balser, ed., *Psychotherapy of the Adolescent*. New York: International Universities Press.

Kohut, H. (1971) *The Analysis of the Self.* New York: International Universities Press.

Kohut, H. (1972) Thoughts on narcissism and narcissistic rage. *Psychoanal. Study Child* 27:360–400.

Laslett, P., and R. Wall. (1972) *Household and Family in Past Time*. New York: Cambridge University Press.

Litwak, E. (1960) Occupational mobility and extended family cohesion. *Am. Sociol. Rev.* 25:9–21.

Litwak, E. (1965) Extended kin relations in an industrial democratic society. In E. Shanas and G. Streib, eds., *Social Structure and the Family: Generational Relations*. Englewood Cliffs, N.J.: Prentice-Hall.

Lorand, S., and H.I. Schneer, eds. (1961) *Adolescents: Psychoanalytic Approach to Problems and Therapy*. New York: Pane B. Hoeber.

Masterson, J. (1972) *Treatment of the Borderline Adolescent: A Developmental Approach*. New York: Wiley-Interscience.

Masterson, J. (1958) Psychotherapy of the adolescent: A comparison with psychotherapy of the adult. *J. Nerv. Ment. Dis.* 127:511–517.

Masterson, J. (1967) *The Psychiatric Dilemma of Adolescence*. Boston: Little, Brown.

Meeks, J. (1971) *The Fragile Alliance*. Baltimore: Williams & Wilkins.

Noshpitz, J. (1957) Opening phase of psychotherapy of adolescents with character disorders. *Bull. Menninger Clin.* 21:153–164.

Offer, D., and J. Offer. (1975) *From Teenage to Young Manhood*. New York: Basic Books.

Offer, D., and E. Vanderstoep. (1974) Indications and contraindications for family therapy. In S. Feinstein and P. Giovacchini, eds., *Adolescent Psychiatry: Developmental and Clinical Studies*, Vol. III. New York: Basic Books.

Schoolar, J., ed. (1973) *Current Issues in Adolescent Psychiatry*. New York: Brunner/Mazel.

Williams, F. (1973) Family therapy: Its role in adolescent psychiatry. In S. Feinstein and P. Giovacchini, eds., *Adolescent Psychiatry: Developmental and Clinical Studies*, Vol. II. New York: Basic Books.

Part IV
Treatment of Psychosomatic Disorders

Treatment of Emotional Disorders in Children and Adolescents

CHAPTER 20

Treatment of Psychophysiological Disorders

Stuart M. Finch
Ronald C. Hansen

Introduction

For many years the term "psychosomatic" was utilized only to be replaced by the term "psychophysiologic," which has not really caught on. According to the American Psychiatric Association's *Diagnostic and Statistical Manual of Mental Disorders*, 2nd ed. (DSM II), "This group of disorders is characterized by physical symptoms that are caused by emotional factors and involve a single organ system, usually under autonomic nervous system innervation. The physiological changes involved are those that normally accompany certain emotional states, but in these disorders the changes are more intense and sustained. The individual may not be consciously aware of his emotional state. If there is an additional psychiatric disorder, it should be diagnosed separately, whether or not it is presumed to contribute to the physical disorder."

The Group for the Advancement of Psychiatry in its report on theoretical considerations and a proposed classification of emotional problems in youths (1966) has said:

Following the Standard Nomenclature, this term is used in preference to the term, psychosomatic disorders, since the latter refers to an approach to the field of medicine as a whole rather than to certain specified conditions. It is preferred to the term, somatization reactions, which implies that these disorders are simply other forms of psychoneurotic disorder.

The term, psychophysiologic (or vegetative) disorder, refers to those disorders in which there is a significant interaction between somatic and psychological components, with varying degrees of weighting of each component. Psychophysiologic disorders may be precipitated and perpetuated by psychological or social stimuli of stressful nature. Such disorders ordinarily involve those organ systems that are innervated by the autonomic or involuntary portion of the central nervous system. The symptoms of disturbed functioning at the vegetative level are regarded as having physiological rather than psychological symbolic significance, in contrast to conversion disorders, which usually involve voluntary innervated structures. Structural change may occur in psychophysiologic disorders, continuing to a point that may be irreversible and that may threaten life in some cases. Such disorders thus do not seem to represent simple physiologic concomitants of emotions, as may occur in psychoneurotic disorders of anxiety type, reactive disorders, or other pictures, including healthy responses. Biologic predisposing factors of genic or inborn nature, developmental psychological determinants with a limited kind of specificity, and current precipitating events of individually stressful significance appear to be among the multiple etiologic contributions to these disorders.

Although conflict situations of particular types may be consistently involved in the predisposition toward and precipitation of these disorders, no type-specific personality profile, parent-child relationship, or family pattern has as yet been associated with individual psychophysiologic disorders. Many similar psychological or psychosocial characteristics may be found in children having other disorders without psychophysiologic disturbances. Psychophysiologic disorders may also involve more than one organ system in sequence, with the occasional occurrence of more than one disorder simultaneously. Psychological factors may be implicated minimally in some disorders, while in others such influences may play a major role, together with somatic factors. Certain psychophysiologic disorders are associated with chronic and/or severe personality disorders of varying types, some even bordering on psychosis, while others may occur in conjunction with milder personality disorders or reactive disorders. Developmental considerations are involved, as in the more global, undifferentiated responses of young infants.

A secondary diagnosis of the type of personality picture seen with the psychophysiologic disorder should be specified. If conversion mechanisms in structures with full or partial voluntary innervation overlap with psychophysiologic mechanisms—as in the vomiting which may occur in adolescents with anorexia nervosa—this should be added as a separate diagnosis and the particular symptomatic manifestations should be drawn from the Symptom List. As indicated earlier, responses to predominantly somatic illness of acute or chronic nature should be classified as a secondary diagnosis; reactive disorders are frequently though not exclusively seen in reactions to acute illness, and a variety of personality disorders, from overly dependent to overly independent, or other pictures are associated with chronic illness.

As one can easily see, both of these primary references concern themselves with physiological systems and the amount and importance of the emotional component involved in whatever disease is being considered. When one looks at these two sources, one quickly realizes this is an attempt to categorize a wide variety of syndromes, some of which have a high emotional input and others relatively less. Apley (1973) has recently developed a model that emphasizes the multifactorial nature of psychophysiological symptoms and illnesses (see Figure 1). Central to this schema are the factors of vulnerability and conditioning. Understanding this complicated interaction allows one to intervene at various levels, both medically and psychologically, in the management of these disorders.

The fact that a pediatrician and a child psychiatrist are co-authoring this chapter means that we will choose those syndromes that are known to both specialties and recognized as having, at least at times, a strong emotional component. We are both aware that children come into the world with different constitutional variables. The work of Birch and Chess (1968) as well as Solnit and Provence (1963) have given strong evidence in this direction. Why one child develops asthma and another colitis and another eczema remains a mystery, but presumably there is a constitutional or heredity background to this type of differentiation.

We propose to discuss the following disorders, some of which are more clearly recognized as psychophysiologic and others less so: colic, rumination syndrome, enuresis, colitis, recurrent abdominal pain, asthma, obesity, diabetes, skin disorders, and dysmenorrhea. The authors have decided to make teamwork in the treatment of psychophysiologic disorders the main thrust of this chapter, and we have each written a view of our own specialty on each disorder. It is our impression that pediatricians see large numbers of cases that are rarely referred to the child psychiatrist, especially for a symptom such as colic or rumination, but such conditions often come to light during therapy of a parent and the child psychiatrist should be aware of the pediatric aspects.

There are many children who have physical ailments in which varying degrees of emotional input are present. Some of these are primary in nature, thus leading or contributing to the beginning of the disorder, while in others the emotional factors are secondary but increase the physical disability. These children can present a variety of somatic complaints including headaches, stomach pains, leg pains, etc., and might be labeled psychophysiologic, while others might be conversion reactions.

There is widespread misunderstanding, both among pediatricians and child psychiatrists, as to the difference between conversion reactions and psychophysiologic disorders. Part of this stems from the fact that there can be an overlap. Conversion reactions are a form of neurosis and the symptom has a symbolic meaning. This is in contrast to psychophysiologic disorders, which usually involve the autonomic system rather than the voluntary. There are certain disorders which would appear to be psychophysiologic, but are rarely referred to a child psychiatrist. Infantile colic would be an example of this, as would alopecia areata.

The question arises as to how many of these children should be labeled psychophysiologic. The pediatrician, often in frustration, comes to the conclusion that the youngster is malingering, but this is uncommon in both children and adults. More often than not, they represent some type of unconscious avoidance mechanism, perhaps for school and possibly for other activities. For example, the father who pushes his son toward baseball or football may find the youngster suffering from an increasing number of physical complaints for which no organic reason can be found. The child who does not wish to participate is often fearful of voicing his reluctance and his symptoms are real, although unconsciously derived.

Basically, it is important to attempt to determine whether the child with a physical disability has, in fact, a conversion reaction, which implies a different kind of personality than the one who has a psychophysiologic disorder. The treatment is usually easier in the former and much more difficult in the latter. The conversion reaction youngster is more suggestible and a symbolic meaning for his symptom can often be uncovered and thus eradicated. While it is true that some authors have proposed symbolic meanings for psychophysiologic disorders, these are usually quite vague and difficult to replicate. It has also been suggested that some mothers, and even fathers, need a "sick" child. There is some, but not much, evidence of this in conversion reactions as well as psychophysiologic disorders.

The youngster suffering from a psychophysiologic disorder has both psychological and somatic problems. Depending upon the particular disorder, the youngster may need two or more professionals collaborating in his treatment. For example, in treating obesity, a pediatrician, a child psychiatrist, and possibly an endocrinologist or nutritionist may be necessary. If we look at ulcerative colitis, one has to add a pediatric gastroenterologist or surgeon, and if we consider asthma, an allergist is usually required.

The main point is that the treatment of these

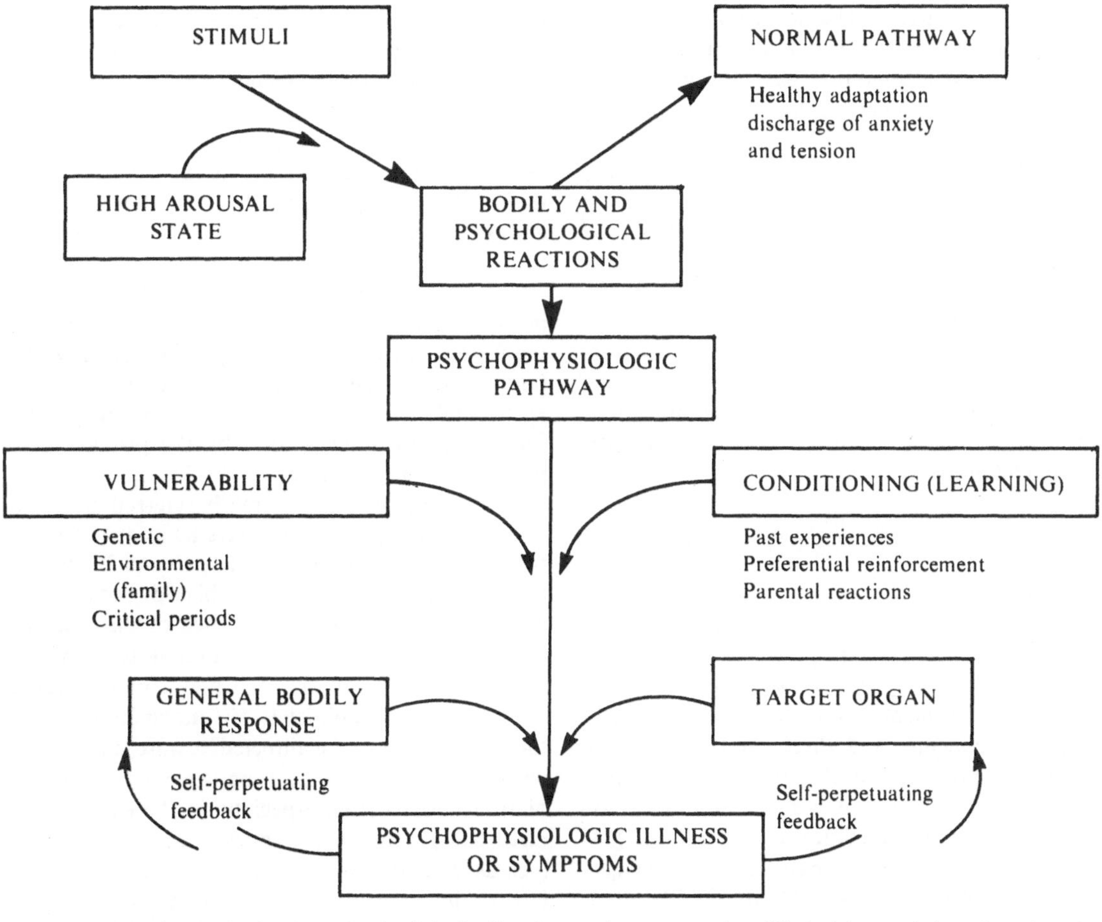

Fig. 1. Schema for the basis of psychophysiologic disorders and symptoms (modified with permission, from J. Apley, [1973] *Brit. Med. J.* 2:756-761.

youngsters requires that several specialists must work together and understand each other and their individual contributions. One usually thinks of the "primary physician" asking for consultations from other specialists and then designing a treatment program, but for many physicians such an approach does not come easily. There are psychiatrists who feel that a disease such as ulcerative colitis can be managed by psychotherapy, while other physicians may feel that colectomy is the only answer. Each has learned and practiced in his own field and cooperation in treatment is sometimes difficult. A further complication in the mental health field is that there are those who prefer family therapy, some prefer behavior modification, some prefer psychoanalysis, and others a type of crisis intervention. When one adds up the multiplicity of possible approaches, one can only assume that we do not have the one right answer. One also has to consider the so-called symptom choice question. Psychophysiologic disorders are generally divided into physiological systems, and their malfunction is enhanced by psychological tension.

For the most part, psychophysiologic disorders recognize no particular age nor ethnic group nor sociocultural status. It is probably fair to say that the earlier such a condition develops in life, the more severe the problem. Emotional and physiological factors operate together, and the earlier in the life span the disorder develops, the probability is greater that the disease will be more serious. If one is to accept the concept of early childhood autism and symbiotic psychosis of childhood as early schizophrenia, this makes a good analogy to the above. There are certain children who come into the world predisposed toward ego development problems, and others whose ego development is poor and who then develop a symbiotic psychosis. Still others become borderline psychotic later in childhood.

Infantile Colic

Early infantile colic, or paroxysmal nocturnal fussiness, is a poorly understood and ultimately self-resolving problem. Etiological studies are generally unconvincing, and there are a number of therapeutic approaches to this problem. One might perhaps view infantile colic as a tension release phenomenon, with the clinical appearance of gastrointestinal spasm predominating. Hence, the gastrointestinal tract has received considerable attention, although it may not be the target organ in each baby. One working definition of colic is that of a baby who, despite proper and adequate feeding and being otherwise healthy, has violent and paroxysmal periods of irritability, fussing, or crying. These periods last more than three hours a day, occur more than three of seven days per week, and are seen over longer than a one-week period (Carey, 1968).

Infantile colic usually begins about the third to fourth week of life, peaks in intensity (manifested by nocturnal crying) at about six to seven weeks of age, and declines thereafter, usually stopping by eight to twelve weeks of age (Brazelton, 1962). Colic is extremely common, with one study indicating an incidence of nearly 50 percent in normal infants (Wessel et al., 1954). Because it is so common, it will create an extreme life stress in certain families who deal poorly with stressful situations. Consequently, both pediatricians and psychiatrists must be sensitive to its occurrence in a family who may be unable to cope.

There is some indication from the pediatric literature that maternal anxiety is a major contributor to the colicky picture (Carey, 1968; Paradise, 1966). Whether or not maternal anxiety or mental status produces the colic, it seems clear that a vicious cycle is set up in many cases, wherein parental anxiety is picked up by the baby, making it nearly impossible for such infants to be comforted by their well-meaning parents. Such a situation causes an escalation of the baby's fussiness, and may cause gaps in the formation in the parental bonding and acceptance of the child. Beyond that, there are instances where child battering have occurred in the framework of infantile colic. Consequently, the family who is raising a colicky baby must be viewed as a family at risk, and represents fertile ground for therapeutic intervention by the primary care physician or psychiatrist.

The child psychiatrist is rarely referred an infant with colic. He usually discovers its existence while treating one or another of the parents. It may be that his sample of colic is biased because his patients are emotionally disturbed parents, but he has come to believe that maternal tension will increase and prolong colic, while a more relaxed atmosphere will diminish it. His therapeutic efforts, therefore, tend to be directed toward the parent while leaving the physical management to the pediatrician. It is true, especially in the emotionally disturbed parent, that a colicky baby can produce increased anxiety and tension in the parents, which, in turn, increases the baby's tension and colic. One task of the child psychiatrist is to break the cycle, with the help of the pediatrician.

Infantile Colic: Case History

A 6-week-old male infant is admitted to the pediatric ward because of a fractured femur. The mother's initial story is that he got caught in crib rails, during a colicky episode. Child abuse, of course, is foremost in everyone's mind.

Extensive interviews with the mother and father clarify the situation. This is the first baby born to a 17-year-old mother and 18-year-old father. Both parents grew up in abusive homes. The mother had seen marriage as an escape, and hoped that a baby would love her. The family had moved to the area just six months previously because of a job opportunity for the father in a copper mine. He was laid off ten days before the admission to the hospital.

The infant by history had become increasingly fussy, gassy, and disruptive each evening, starting at age three weeks. The mother had been especially pressured to keep him quiet after the father returned home from work at 6:00 P.M., but had been totally unable to accomplish this. She had at first felt her husband might hurt the baby and kept him away from it. Later, as it became clear she could not comfort the infant, she began to resent the problem as much as he did.

Shortly after the father was laid off from his job, the problem became unbearable. He left for twenty-four hours, on a drinking spree. The mother, at the end of her rope, wrenched the baby by the leg during one of his "colic" spells. Later that evening the father returned; both parents noted the swollen, immobile leg, and decided to come to the emergency room.

This case is a classical study in child abuse, where contributions are present from parental background, environmental stresses, and a "special" child. In this case, the infant did seem to have colic, a minor problem for most families, but in this instance, intolerable. There seems little doubt that infantile colic is worsened where parental anxiety mounts, causing a vicious circle of events.

As in most cases of child abuse inflicted by parents, it makes little difference which parent did the abusing, as the other is either passively participating, or at least acquiescing. In this instance, there was a coordinated follow-up through the pediatrician, social worker, and child psychiatrist. The psychiatric approach was basically one of family therapy. As some productive avenues of tension release were explored, and as they gained some positive feelings about themselves as parents, the mother and father began to accept the infant and his behavior. After six months of follow-up, the family structure had stabilized to the extent that no further involvement of the social agencies was deemed necessary, although intermittent contact with the pediatrician and psychotherapist was maintained.

Rumination Syndrome

Infantile rumination is a bizarre problem of early infancy, whose origin remains controversial. Fortunately, it has become increasingly rare during this century, and again, the reasons for its decreasing frequency are obscure. It is characterized by the apparently voluntary regurgitation of large amounts of food after feeding. In the past, this problem was attended by very significant mortality and morbidity, due to supervening malnutrition and cachexia.

Frequently, the regurgitation is preceded by semi-purposeful movements of the tongue, mandible, or by the placing of fingers or entire hand into the mouth. As infants acquire experience in rumination, they seem to reduce consciously the visible preliminary components to a minimum, and will not regurgitate while they are being observed.

Controversy exists as to the etiology of this disorder. One recent study (Herbst, Friedland, and Zboralske, 1971) has shown that there are hiatal hernias associated with the rumination syndrome in some of these infants. Gastroesophageal reflux in these infants may at times be difficult to detect even by the best pediatric radiologists. Consequently, there appears to have developed a physiologic explanation for the ability of some of these infants to regurgitate. However, the disturbed maternal-infant interaction has been noted for decades. Richmond (1966–67) had indicated that the rumination act in some of these infants provided a type of stimulation and gratification that was otherwise lacking. Additional evidence of the psychogenic contributions come from follow-up studies into adulthood, which indicate that childhood ruminators usually present a variety of personal adjustment problems (Kanner, 1948).

Although a rare problem today, infantile rumination represents a psychophysiologic disorder, frequently with clear-cut contributions from both disturbed maternal-child interaction and an apparent physiologic tendency toward gastroesophageal reflux. The child psychiatrist and pediatrician should be aware of both elements in approaching this problem.

Rumination Syndrome: Case History

A 3 month-old black male infant was admitted to a children's hospital because of the rumination syndrome. He had suffered persistent and progressive vomiting since age one month. It was noted to occur after each feeding and intermittently between feedings. Although frequent and voluminous, the vomiting was seldom observed, and seemed to occur the instant the nurse or mother turned her back on the child.

When the vomiting or regurgitation was observed, it was usually noted to be preceded by unusual movements of the tongue, mandible, or the infant's putting his fingers or his entire hand into his mouth. Other than signs of malnourishment, the child's physical examination was otherwise normal. Noteworthy was the very intense and searching eye contact of this baby. Radiographic studies of the esophagus, stomach, and small bowel were normal.

This was the first baby for this 20-year-old mother. There were no significant problems with pregnancy, delivery, or the nursery course. Through the first three weeks of breastfeeding this infant, the mother had experienced problems with the nursing process. Specifically, the baby did not gain weight well, the mother did not seem to empty her breasts well, and the efficacy of breastfeeding was questioned. Her family physician advised that she stop nursing at about one month of age, and this advice was taken. Subsequently, the regurgitation and vomiting ensued on formula feedings. The mother was admittedly disappointed because she had to stop nursing, and felt that this did interfere with her bonding with the infant. The emesis continued unabated through multiple formula switches and changes in feeding technique. Consequently, the admission to the hospital was precipitated.

The treatment in this case involved the standard approach to the ruminating infant. Thickened formula was given in reduced volume plus an increase in solid food. A nurse was constantly assigned to be with the baby during the first hour after feeding. At the first sign of a preliminary mouth, tongue, or hand movement, which might signal the onset of rumination, the child was immediately distracted, picked up, and, if necessary, the child elevated to prevent rumination. Initially the mother was not given the responsibility for such treatment herself, but was gradually worked into this schedule. Concurrently, because of admitted bonding problems with her infant, she was involved in weekly psychotherapy sessions.

Over a six-week hospitalization course, the infant's rumination gradually decreased to a negligible amount. At the same time, the mother became fully involved in the techniques by which his rumination was discouraged, including the intense stimulation and attention shortly after feeding. Follow-up visits indicated that there was subsequently no problem with food retention, and the maternal-child interaction was improved.

Enuresis

Enuresis: Medical Aspects

Enuresis is the involuntary noctural discharge of urine during sleep. Although there has been recent excellent reviews of this subject and considerable research devoted to various aspects of etiology and treatment, enuresis remains a confusing and frustrating problem for patients, parents and physicians. Each individual professional discipline has taken a different approach to the problem, causing the literature to be so divergent in views that no unifying approach has received widespread acceptance.

For practical purposes, enuresis is defined as nighttime wetting beyond the age of five in girls and in boys beyond the age of six. Additionally, it may be useful to distinguish between those children who have primary enuresis (never having been dry), and those with secondary enuresis (having experienced dryness for up to three to six months). This becomes particularly significant with the older children, since the secondary enuretics form a larger percentage of the total group with increasing age. (Oppel et al., 1968).

As with the acquisition of other skills, development of urinary control in children varies from child to child. Accordingly, only 81% of children will have achieved cumulative nighttime dryness by age 5 (Oppel et al., 1968), and of that population only 64% will have no relapse to wetness. Cumulative nighttime dryness will not be achieved by 95% of the population until age 10. Other studies have given essentially the same data relative to percentages of children still wet, varying with age (Blomfield et al., 1956).

As previously noted, there is a sexual difference

in the prevalence of enuresis. For example, at age 6, 12% of males and 8% of females will be enuretic. The familial incidence of enuresis is noteworthy, with the occurrence of the symptom in multiple members of 70% of the families. Additionally, if a parent of an enuretic child had a history of enuresis, 40% of male siblings and 25% of female siblings would be similarly affected (Hallgren, 1958).

The etiology of enuresis has received extensive attention from various health professions. Depending on the speciality and bias of the particular investigator, enuresis has been attributed to largely urological, psychological, allergic, or maturational causes. In view of widely discrepant opinions, it is unlikely that any single theory will be universally accepted. However, the theory that enuresis typically represents an hereditary delay in neuromuscular maturation, is perhaps most popular today among pediatricians. Some of the following is offered to support this theory:

1. Enuretic children frequently have small bladder capacities.
2. Possibly related to the small bladder capacity is the increased frequency in voiding and increased urgency to enuretic children.
3. The familial aspect of enuresis.
4. The high spontaneous cure rate noted with increasing chronological age (Cohen, 1975). At some point when neuromuscular maturation is likely to have occurred, persistence of enuresis may then be attributed to other causes, including psychological.

Enuresis occurs during arousal from deep, non-REM sleep, as has been recently demonstrated by Esmon et al. (1977). Imipramine possibly works by lessening the depth of sleep during the first part of the night's sleep, although other autonomic nervous system (bladder) effects may also be operative. Accordingly, other REM-related phenomena are probably not inherently associated with enuresis. When large populations of enuretic children are examined, the paucity of significant psychiatric problems is evident. Even in psychiatric circles, an opinion is evolving that enuresis itself, even when persistent, should not generate psychiatric treatment unless other symptoms suggest a significant emotional problem (Simonds, 1977).

Thoroughness and reassurance by the pediatrician in the initial encounter may be a major therapeutic intervention in the management of enuresis. A complete history and physical examination is essential before the parent can be confident in the pediatrician's assessment.

The history of the enuresis itself is a crucial area to explore. Aggravating and alleviating factors must be identified. It must be determined whether the problem is improving or worsening, and how both the child and the other family members react to the symptom. Whether any life compromise is present, such as avoidance of overnight activities, camp, etc., should be determined. Primary enuresis should be distinguished from secondary enuresis, in as much as urinary-tract infections are much more frequent in the secondary form. Daytime wetting may be associated with more significant psychological factors or may be related to an organic etiology. Although its precise importance remains somewhat unclear, most clinicians would view the so-called diurinal-enuretic as being in a higher-risk group for organic or psychological problems. The review of symptoms in most enuretic children will be largely noncontributory. However, it is especially important to review in detail any possible symptoms referable to the genital urinary tract, especially those which might reflect a urinary tract infection. Any neurological dysfunction, especially suggesting lower spinal cord dysfunction, would be most important and might indicate a neurogenic bladder as the basis for the incontinence. However, since a true organic basis is generally lacking, the review of symptoms is more apt to disclose problems in the area of adjustment and adaptive difficulties. A fairly commonly associated symptom is encopresis, and may reflect a common problem in early approaches to toilet training. Physical examination rarely discloses an organic etiology, but some of the possibilities will be mentioned. Presence of hypertension may reflect an underlying renal disease. Suboptimal physical growth might also reflect chronic renal disease, including recurrent urinary tract infections. Malformations of the external genitalia, meatal anomalies, or inflammation again may be of significance. A neurological examination, especially with regard to the lower extremities and rectal sphincter tone, might suggest a neurogenic bladder.

In general, laboratory investigations should be minimized, except in those cases where history and physical conditions draw attention to specific diseases as possibilities. For most children, a complete urinalysis and a screening urine culture suffice for the basic laboratory testing.

Reassurance and support, as previously noted, during the initial encounter may itself be therapeutic. Both patient and parent may be comforted by the relatively optimistic view of enuresis as a maturational problem.

There is no good evidence that restriction of fluids in the evening, elimination of specific fluids or routine voiding at bedtime or awakening to void during the hours of sleep have beneficial effects of hastening acquisition of bladder control. In actuality, such attempts are often a focus for struggles between the parent and child and may unduly complicate the psychological picture.

Some pharmacologic agents have been found to be superior to placebo in the treatment of enuresis, and the most currently popular of these is Imipramine. In general, Imipramine is given one-half hour to one hour before bedtime in a dosage of 25 ml. in children under age 12, 50 ml to those over age 12. In general, 75 mg. is not exceeded in terms of a single daily dosage. On such a regimen, approximately 40% of enuretics may respond with improvement or cure, but relapses occur in 40% to 60% after discontinuation of the drug (Kardish et al., 1968; Meadow, 1970). The side effects of Imipramine are generally well known to psychiatrists, but include nervousness, sleep disorders, and mild gastrointestinal disturbances.

Conditioning devices or "bed buzzers" are probably as effective as medication, such as Imipramine, and may cause success rates about 75% in those series which have been studied (Werry, 1965). This therapy is based on accepted learning theory, but the success is highly dependent on the quality of the instrument and the degree of cooperation achieved with the child and parents in this mechanical approach to the problem. Relapse rates are probably in the same range as with medication.

Investigators have reported cure rates of 30% using a program of "bladder stretching," wherein the child holds his urine as long as he can once a day (Starfield, 1972). Others (Marshall et al., 1973) have similarly advocated this method. One criticism of this approach is that it utilizes a negative sensation (bladder discomfort) as a reinforcing experience.

Although enthusiasm for urological manipulation still exists (Arnold et al., 1973; Mahoney, 1971), its position seems to be diminishing in the overall approach to enuresis, and it probably should be utilized only for those children who have documented distal obstructive lesions.

Enuresis, from the pediatricians' standpoint, should be viewed as a maturational phenomenon with an optimistic outlook in most cases. Primary and secondary psychological features are operative in a number of these children with persistent enuresis, and psychological help does need to be solicited in those cases. The reader is referred elsewhere (Cohen, 1975) for a recent comprehensive review of the subject from a pediatric standpoint.

Enuresis: Psychological Aspects

Enuresis is still poorly understood from the psychological standpoint. Although its frequency diminishes markedly by puberty, a few refractory cases persist into early adult life. In general, it can be assumed that the older enuretic will be less amenable to either medical or psychological therapy.

Most children with enuresis are not referred for psychological evaluation. Hence, it is usually assumed, and generally true, that only the more refractory difficult cases reach the psychiatrist's office. However, it appears that some well-adjusted children, from supportive and adequate families, can have persistent enuresis of the maturational-delay variety. These children may need no psychiatric therapy at all, other than to assure that the symptom does not compromise their life outside the home. This point is made to emphasize that not every child with enuresis, even refractory to medical therapy, is appropriate for psychiatric intervention.

Most commonly, however, the symptom is an extremely problematic one for the child and family by the time referral is made. Perhaps even more frequently, the enuresis is not mentioned as a primary problem, but emerges as an issue in a child referred for other problems. The pattern of enuresis may be primary, secondary, nocturnal, or *diurnal*. It may be associated with other symptoms such as hyperactivity and *encopresis*. Some children become dry following an initial evaluation, or even psychological testing, whereas others may undergo months of apparently successful psychotherapy, but continue to wet the bed.

Before initiating therapy, the child psychiatrist must be comfortable that a competent clinician has ruled out organic pathology. As previously noted, this usually consists of a complete medical history, physical examination, urinalysis, and urine culture. Urine infections, renal disease with hypertension, nocturnal epilepsy, and diabetes are potential causes. The actual form of psychotherapy will vary considerably depending on the individual case and the preference of the therapist. Simple counseling frequently suffices for the less refactory cases, but behavior modification and dynamic psychotherapy with or without medication may be indicated in other instances.

Certain pathogenic parental attitudes must be considered, since the therapy will be directed toward the correction of that attitude. Examples of these include: punitiveness, neglect, oversubmissiveness, and perfectionism.

Although uncommon, certain children may consciously or unconsciously wet in order to provoke their parents, typically the mother, in response to hostility engendered by parental punitiveness. Such a family will probably live with the enuresis until the cycle of punitiveness-hostility-retaliation is broken.

Neglect may play a role in persistent enuresis, especially in larger families where several children sleep together, and a harassed mother has little time or inclination to provide the patient supportive incentive to achieve dryness. In this regard, one could contrast a deprived, emotionally tumultuous family from Appalachia, with a tendency toward neglecting the symptom, with a suburban, achievement-oriented middle-class family, who might encourage the symptom through perfectionistic attitudes.

Perfectionistic parents unwillingly perpetrate the symptom in their child, even though they are quite disappointed that this infantile habit persists. Repeated episodes of belittlement induce shame and inadequacy feelings in a child who wishes to please. He may scold or criticize himself prior to sleep, making promises to awaken and avoid wetting. The enuresis may represent a wish-fulfilling dream, or merely neuromuscular delay, but in either case the perfectionism is a destructive and self-perpetuating attitude. These children need to understand that wetting is not bad, and the parents need to depressurize the process described. Any therapy with Imipramine may be quite useful, as these children gradually learn to be kinder to themselves and simultaneously achieve more selfconfidence when their enuresis improves.

Conversely, certain oversubmissive parents may impair the development of impulse control in their children. These may be the classically "spoiled," uncontrolled children, where few limits or expectations are set by the parents. Such children may need to develop areas of responsibility (chores, expectations with respect to behavior), and consequently gain impulse control relative to enuresis. Medication with *Imipramine* or the use of conditioning devices may be helpful *adjuncts*.

Cohen (1975) has summarized certain elements that are necessary goals in the counseling process:

1. Understanding by parents of the multifactorial nature of enuresis. This of course implies the willingness of the physician to individualize each case.

2. Acceptance of the child, with his symptom, by the parent, and willingness to support change through positive involvement. Since the enuresis question often becomes a major family battleground, parents must be willing to reduce negative feedback.

3. Achieving a sense of optimism by the child and family. Since virtually all enuretics eventually become dry, it is crucial, and often therapeutic, that the whole family realize the end of the symptom will come, and that they can meanwhile survive and cope.

4. Understanding of his symptom by the child, especially with the realization that each child *develops* different skills at different ages. Many parents and children feel as if their problem is especially unique and are surprised to know that as many as one in seven children the same age may share that symptom.

5. Appreciation by the child that he, and not his parents, will eventually acquire the body control to stay dry.

In most cases, the child will benefit by being primarily responsible for his symptom and making some active choices in his therapy. Marshall (1973) has suggested one such approach, utilizing "responsibility plus positive reinforcements."

That small group of youngsters who continue to be enuretic into adolescence and even into adult life is no better understood than young children with this problem. They are seen infrequently by child psychiatrists, at least primarily for this symptom. Perhaps the time it comes to the surface most obviously is during periods of military service. The symptom is either picked up at induction or shortly afterwards. Although not much has been written about the symptom in inductees, many professionals feel that the enuretics often came from deprived and hostile home atmospheres. In some such homes, the wetting had been accepted and special "corn" beds made to absorb the urine. Since various ways were found to discharge those young people, there is little reliable data on the frequency and associated problems.

We do know that enuresis is more prevalent in delinquent youngsters and those from emotionally troubled or broken homes. Some parents of adolescent as well as preadolescent youngsters often either did not make clear efforts to train their children or even at times unconsciously supported and approved the symptom. As with younger children, contributions by punitiveness, neglect, perfectionism, and oversubmissiveness may have been important.

Whatever the reason for enuresis during adolescence, efforts should be made to rule out organic pathology. This is especially important is those cases that began the symptom at or after puberty. Some teenagers have had the symptom since childhood and have had various types of therapy without success. Many others have not had any treatment of the enuresis and it has been ignored until time for summer camp, joining the military, or spending time away from home. This is a relatively small group, since most children stop bedwetting by puberty.

It is frequently unclear whether some of the emotional problems seen in such adolescents are primary and the enuresis is caused by the psychological problems, or the latter are mostly due to the wetting. It seems apparent that cultural differences may play a part. Consequently, with these teenagers, as well as their younger counterparts, full exploration of the family attitudes toward the problem is essential. Many of these young people already have or subsequently develop various psychiatric syndromes with a mixture of characterological and neurotic elements. They may have *fantasies* that there is some organic problem in spite of repeated physical examinations. Others drift toward passive-aggressive, passive, or aggressive character patterns.

Therapy, as with all adolescents, requires the development of a good relationship with the physician. Even more than their young counterparts, they need to feel optimistic about the treatment and play an active role in planning it. Fantasies need to be explored and corrected. Since teenagers are strongly invested in their bodies and preoccupied with potential damage or deficiency, these areas require delicate but reasonable exploration and education. Once the adolescent becomes convinced his body is sound, he can then take an active role in treatment plans. These may include a combination of approaches as long as the youngster has an optimistic attitude. Dynamic psychotherapy, behavior modification, and medication are examples.

These are refractory cases and it requires time, skill, and effort on the part of the therapist (Pierce, 1975; Umphress et al., 1970).

Enuresis: Case History

George was a 5½-year-old boy when first seen by the child psychiatrist after having been referred by the pediatrician. He was an only child and his mother was highly overprotective. The main complaints were that he was destructive in the home, often doing things he had been told not to do. A symbolic example was that they were trying to teach him to pour milk on his cereal which he promptly spilled all over the table. He had difficulty going out in public places, particularly with his mother, because he would wander off and be generally disobedient. He had entered kindergarten but was found to be quite immature and unable to get along with his peers. The parents were also quite concerned that he soiled in addition to the enuresis.

The father's work took him away from the home a great deal of the time, leaving the mother and child alone. The father had told the psychiatrist that he felt the "big battle" was between the mother and son. The parents had tried a variety of means—bribing, cajoling, threatening to reduce or eradicate the encopresis and enuresis—but to no avail.

In this case, the mother was quite insecure; she compensated by overprotecting the youngster and at the same time yelling and screaming at him for a number of things. The boy was rapidly learning how to push his mother's "red button" and upset her. He was much less successful in doing this with his father. A school conference was held and the child psychiatrist explained to the school personnel that George should be treated as a normal youngster and things of age appropriatness should be expected of him. His school behavior rapidly improved but continued much as before at home.

When George was first seen by the psychiatrist, he proved to be initially a clinging type of child but finally joined the doctor in his office, where he proceeded to be disruptive, but eventually calmed down and his behavior became more age-appropriate. Slowly over a period of a few weeks, he began to socialize at school and even improved his behavior at home. The enuresis did not disappear completely as did the encopresis but he has continued to show improvement. Incidentally, he had been thoroughly tested and found to be of normal intelligence and physically healthy.

Ulcerative Colitis

Ulcerative Colitis: Medical Aspects

Ulcerative colitis is the most common chronic inflammatory bowel disease in young adults and children. As with Crohn's disease (regional enteritis), the other closely related bowel inflammatory disorder, it is apt to begin in the second decade of life. Consequently, when seen, bowel inflammatory disease is prone to be superimposed on the problems of adolescence.

With ulcerative colitis the mucosa of the colon is friable, often frankly ulcerated, and inflamed. The patient usually complains of abdominal pain, bloody diarrhea, mucus, and pain on defecation. Frequently, the entire colon is involved.

The cause of ulcerative colitis is unknown. Because of the wide range of systemic and extra-intestinal complaints (skin lesions, arthritis, iritis, hepatic involvement, etc.), an immunologic basis is frequently postulated. Psychophysiologic determinants in the pathogensis of ulcerative colitis have been suggested for some time.

Engle, for example, noted in a large review of ulcerative colitis patients, that these people tended to be obsessive-compulsive and somewhat immature (Engle, 1955). Recently, more controlled studies have tended to cast doubt on the relationship of psychogenic factors to the causation of ulcerative colitis (Feldman et al., 1967; Mendeloff et al., 1970; Monk et al., 1970). The debate about causation relating to psychogenic factors is perhaps a moot point. There are clearly individuals with ulcerative colitis who have significant psychogenic components. That is to say, their disease is worsened by certain stresses, and their perception of pain and diarrhea is altered by their frame of mind. Perhaps the psychological features are no more prominent in bowel inflammatory disease than they are in any other severe, incapacitating illness, but they are clearly present in some colitis patients. Consequently, the child psychiatrist will see some patients with ulcerative colitis or Crohn's disease. Both forms of inflammatory bowel disease are apt to cause severe life impairment, with bloody diarrhea the prominent symptom in ulcerative colitis and pain predominating in Crohn's disease.

Optimal medical and in some cases surgical management is of course imperative. Many patients with colitis can be symptomatically improved with medication such as Azulfidine, corticosteroids, and antidiarrheal compounds. Fortunately, the most severe patients can be managed by protocolectomy, but again this is attended by psychological adjustment problems in many cases. In the future, because of the large risk of carcinoma of the colon, more and more children will be subjected to protocolectomy for this chronic disease. As with the other psychophysiologic disorders discussed in this chapter, close cooperation between the psychotherapist and the physician primarily treating the colitis must be achieved. In this regard, the surgeon, pediatrician, gastroenterologist, and child psychiatrist must have their plans for the patient clearly coordinated.

Ulcerative Colitis: Psychological Aspects

To the child psychiatrist, ulcerative colitis is an enigma. There are many views on not only the cause but also on the treatment of this chronic disorder. It may begin as early as infancy or in adult life, and we do not know how many individuals may have brief periods of ulcerative colitis that are not recognized. From the psychiatric studies done thus far, it would appear that emotions do effect the exacerbations and remissions in this disease. Few would argue that emotions are primary, but certainly most would agree that they are markedly influential in the course of the disorder. Secondary emotional input to the family is obvious. Any child who is having multiple bloody stools each day, losing weight, and not eating well will be a source of concern to any parent. In addition, the constant threat of potential surgery and body mutilation brings anxiety not only to the youngster but to the parents as well. Studies done on the personalities of these youngsters show two distinct types. One is the serious, compulsively oriented child and the other the more passive-aggressive child. The former would seem to outnumber the latter considerably.

The treatment of ulcerative colitis is a good example of the necessity of teamwork. To some physicians, the initial diagnosis should lead to immediate colectomy and ileostomy. Others prefer medical management and psychiatric input. The surgeon quite naturally prefers not to have a moribund child delivered for surgery because he is a poor surgical risk. The pediatrician is concerned with anemia, growth levels, and such things, while the psychiatrist is concerned about the emotional atmosphere in the family as well as the emotional status of the child (Finch and Hess, 1962).

Once such a team becomes organized, it is essential that they remain with the family and youngster throughout the illness and agree on the treatment program. If exsanguination, bowel perforation, or other such serious complications arise, decisions must be made promptly. If the child is getting along reasonably well even though symptoms are still present, it is worth while to continue to work on the emotional problems to lessen whatever tension may exist.

Ulcerative Colitis: Case History

Jimmy was a 7-year-old boy when first referred by the pediatrician to the child psychiatrist. He was an extremely immature, small boy who clung to his mother in an obviously dependent manner. The father was distant and relatively uninvolved. Jimmy's growth was far behind schedule, and because of his illness he had missed a great deal of school. He was put into dynamic long-term psychotherapy, but unfortunately, every new situation caused exacerbations in his colitis. These included such things as a move of the family to a new home, starting school, and so forth.

After a number of admissions to the pediatric ward, Jimmy was finally transferred to the psychiatric ward, where progress was made, but on a limited basis. A medical team was formed and the youngster was seen by each member who then met to discuss the various possibilities of how the child and his family could be managed. Jimmy's mother remained highly overprotective in spite of all efforts to change this, and the father's attitude remained much the same. Finally, a team decision was made that the child would need a colectomy and this was performed.

Following surgery, Jimmy was able to make a limited adjustment as an outpatient. He had few friends, participated little in the activities of his peer group, and continued to be very dependent on his mother. While many children improve after colectomy and psychotherapy, Jimmy's improvement was minimal, largely due to the refusal of his family to mitigate his dependency.

Recurrent Abdominal Pain

The syndrome of recurrent abdominal pain may be defined in a child who has had three attacks of pain, severe enough to affect activity, occurring over an interval longer than three months. Surprisingly, 10% of school children between the ages of 10 and 12 are affected (Apley, 1964). The etiology of this extremely common syndrome is not understood, but it is presumed that there are major genetic, psychogenic, and in some cases, organic contributions. It most commonly begins before age 10 years, but may be seen in children in ages 4 through 15.

Although the yield of treatable organic problems is notoriously small, of the order of 5%, in the workup of these patients, a meticulous history and physical examination by the primary care physician is mandatory. This is necessary both to rule out those few plausible organic causes, but also to make the presumption of psychophysiologic abdominal pain on a firm, rather than statistical, basis. Sometimes this may take several visits on the part of the primary care physician.

Of particular concern are such issues as: Why did the child or parent decide they needed help at this point? Whose idea was it to come? What do both the parent and the child think the problem is? How long has the problem been going on? How has it affected the child's normal activities and family relationships? Since school phobia (avoidance) may be present with abdominal pain, school attendance must be assessed. In addition to such specific interview questions, the primary care physician must obtain an extremely complete past medical history relative to the characteristics of the pain, associated symptoms (headache, pallor, dizziness, etc.), medical history (relative to colic, eating habits, and constipation), review of systems, family history (50% of these children will have a parent with functional gastrointestinal problems), and a survey of personality and emotional makeup (Roy, Silverman, and Cozetto, 1975).

From this process will often evolve a picture of a child who is perfectionistic, achievement-oriented, and as in the case history presented, under significant stress. These factors are extremely important when identified as they add great support to the diagnosis. This is not to deny that a psychophysiologic abdominal pain picture can be present without them. The number of organic causes of recurrent abdominal pain are legion, but few of them are seen with any frequency. As noted, the large preponderance of these children have their symptoms due seemingly to only genetic and psychophysiologic factors. Leading organic causes for this syndrome include: urinary tract infection, peptic ulcer disease, and chronic constipation. Consequently, the medical workup, after the complete history and physical, should usually be limited to studying these possibilities. In many instances, a urine culture is the only screening test necessary. The pediatrician or family practitioner must then be as understanding, reassuring, and supportive as possible for the child and his family, once the diagnosis is made. A contract for follow-up and availability for support must be made. Some of these children require referral to the child psychiatrist. Considering the huge number of such children with symptoms, it is apparent that only a tiny fraction reach the child psychiatrist. Those that do will often require the utmost in cooperation between the referring pediatrician and the psychotherapist.

Recurrent Abdominal Pain: Case History

A 15-year-old prominent attorney's son presents with recurrent abdominal pain of three months' duration. The pain is episodic, brief in duration, with periods of well-being interspersed. It occasionally follows meals, and typically in that regard the evening meal . There is no associated nausea, vomiting, decreased appetite, or stool change. He occasionally feels relieved after a bowel movement, but this is not a consistent report. The a pain seldom awakens him at night, and seldom lasts more than one hour in duration. Certain conscious stresses, such as an upcoming athletic event in which he is participating (e.g., wrestling), or certain school-related stresses seem to precipitate the pain. However, most episodes of pain, which occur two to three times per week, have no relationship to any conscious stress.

Family history reveals that the father is a prominent defense attorney and his mother is a housewife, but also holds a master's degree in library science. There are five siblings. The mother relates that three of the siblings have suffered from migraine, and two from recurrent abdominal pain. Physical examination is completely negative, except for a very minimal epigastric and periumbilical tenderness, from which the patient can be distracted by conversational diversion. Rectal examination is negative, and there is no occult blood in the stool. Because of the persistence of the symptoms, and the occasional awakening at night, an upper GI series is done. It is reported as negative for peptic ulcer disease.

Interviews alone with this young man reveal that he is under an inordinate external and internal pressure to achieve. He is concerned that he is about to receive his first academic B in high school, whereas his two older brothers never got a grade below A. Although it is fully two months before his first competitive wrestling meet of the season, he is already anxious as to what the outcome will be. He admits that concerns about athletic competition and school achievement cause him gastrointestinal distress, but that they are not responsible for all of his pains.

The pediatrician elects to follow this young man on a regular basis.

Asthma

Asthma: Medical Aspects

Asthma in children is characterized by recurrent, paroxysmal episodes of wheezing, cough, and breathlessness. There is usually some extrinsic, precipitating factor in childhood asthma, although the nature of that factor or agent may at times be elusive. Agents or factors that precipitate or worsen asthmatic wheezing include all allergens (a wide range), dust, climatologic changes, air pollution, infections (especially viral respiratory infections), exercises of various types, and psychogenic factors.

Pure psychogenic asthma is rare in children, if it exists at all. A significant psychogenic component is undoubtedly present in certain children, and a panic reaction at any time might worsen even the child whose previous course had no obvious psychophysiologic component. The impression of some allergists is that emitional factors play an increasing role in the older asthmatics; hence, they are a greater problem in adolescents and young adults (Hugh Thompson, personal communication, 1976).

The asthmatic child frequently finds himself in a family where one parent had asthma or severe allergies as a child, and consequently a framework of overprotection, hovering, or in some cases, denial of the illness develops. Each family is affected significantly by the illness of the severe asthmatic child. Frequent trips to the emergency room, and occasional hospitalizations to interrupt severe wheezing, leave the child and his family fearful relative to both ease of breathing and survival. In general, the child psychiatrist will be referred only the most disturbed patients.

Unfortunately, the worst bronchospasm may coexist with the most emotionally labile child. Consequently, a vicious circle of dyspnea wheezing-panic-increased wheezing is set up, and the interruption of that cycle is difficult. Emotional distress alone may trigger bronchospasm in such a patient. Inadequate treatment may lead to feelings of insecurity, further aggravating the emotional disturbance, which will, in turn, cause worsening of the asthma. The parent and child must express confidence in their physician, or his impact will be lessened and any emotional component intensified.

Asthma management is much improved today,

compared with previous decades. Injectable adrenalin, oral and nebulized bronchodilators and steroids, hyposensitization therapy ("allergy shots"), and the newer asthma preventative, cromolyn sodium, are all within the armamentarium of the physician who treats childhood asthma. Most of these drugs are aimed at modifying or treating wheezing once it has developed, but some (e.g. cromolyn) are purely prophylactic. Prophylactic treatment with cromolyn sodium (an agent which prevents exercise-induced and allergen induced asthma) has made it possible to keep many of the most difficult asthmatics relatively symptom-free while reducing or eliminating steroid dosage. Since oral steroids can have such disastrous cosmetic, medical and psychological side effects, it is important for the child psychiatrist to know something of therapeutic alternatives for the severely affected children referred to him.

Where hospitalization is needed, advances in respiratory therapy have made possible better intensive-care treatment, and have decreased deaths from asthma. Since fear of breathlessness is such a reality-based problem, proper medical control of the asthma itself must be assured. These medical aspects should be treated by a pediatrician or pediatric allergist who is comfortable with asthma and the emotional needs of the asthmatic.

Ultimate prognosis is good from the medical standpoint. One review (Rachemann and Edwards, 1952) noted that 39% of childhood asthmatics were cured completely; 20% developed other allergic symptoms, but their asthma remitted; 20% had occasional wheezing; 28% still had severe recurrent wheezing; and 2% died. Thus, a 70% favorable result can be anticipated.

Asthma: Psychological Aspects

To the child psychiatrist, bronchial asthma represents a graded series of emotional problems which may be primary, secondary, or both. In some children, the emotional factors are large and the allergic factors smaller, while in other youngsters, it is reversed. There are, of course, many children in between the two extremes.

By primary, we mean that an emotional factor contributed to the onset of a disorder. Secondary refers to those emotional problems arising as a result of the asthma itself. For example, it is almost impossible for a child and his family not to react to repeated asthmatic attacks in the youngster. The severity and unpredictability of the attacks may frighten everyone involved. Emotions of various kinds are stimulated and will need to be taken into account in any therapeutic approach. It is also to be expected that the various restrictions imposed will create emotional reverberations within the youngster and his family. For example, house pets may be banned and siblings will resent this. Rugs and other household furnishings may have to be changed, and everyone, particularly the parents, may inwardly resent this.

Psychiatric treatment modalities vary for asthma. Perhaps one of the better known is often referred to as "parentectomy," namely, separation of the child from his family by sending him to special units at a distant place such as the National Asthma Center at Denver, Colorado. While the climate may have something to offer in ameliorating the symptoms, it remains that the separation from the family is an important aspect.

This leads naturally to the question of whether the asthmatic child needs inpatient care or can be managed on an outpatient basis. The answer depends primarily on severity of the asthma and the emotional problems. It is a dictum of child psychiatry that a youngster should always be treated as an outpatient whenever this is feasible and only be hospitalized when it is essential. There is a small number of youngsters whose emotional problems, along with those of their families, are so severe that they cannot be managed on an outpatient basis. Others are so physically debilitated that they must be hospitalized on a pediatric ward. The former usually require longer hospitalization and therefore are better off in a good children's psychiatric unit. The latter may only need temporary hospitalization and would be better cared for on a pediatric ward. Various psychiatric approaches have been proposed for these youngsters.

A number of modes of therapy have been utilized in the treatment of this as well as other psychophysiologic disorders. Behavior modification is a popular method of treatment, but probably used less in this type of disorder than other forms of therapy. As a treatment philosophy, it is based on the Skinnerian philosophy of positive and negative reinforcment. In bronchial asthma, which has a large emotional component, especially of the secondary type, it may be quite useful.

Family therapy has grown in popularity in the last few years and is applicable in certain cases of asthma. It is, of course, almost the antithesis of "parentectomy." The family with an asthmatic child must feel some impact from the youngster's disorder. This would include both parents as well as siblings. As alluded to previously, the asthmatic child is often overprotected by parents, and the siblings may suffer. Once such a child becomes used to this type of "special attention," he may increase his demands and thus begin a vicious cycle. At times, it is wise to see the entire family as a unit and clarify what the various emotional factors are.

Individual dynamic psychotherapy for many asthmatic patients is often beneficial. It is useful to uncover the emotional factors whether they be primary, secondary, or both. Imagine for a moment a 14-year-old who is not allowed to participate in the ordinary activities of his peer group, whose household arrangements must be changed and toward whom parents are unconsciously hostile and yet outwardly overprotective. There are occasions when separation of the child from his family members would be the wisest course, but whenever possible all the family members would be taken into account (Schneer, 1963).

Another form of therapy which has seen a good deal of research of late (Davis et al., 1973; Khan, 1974; Philipp et al., 1972) is that of a counter-conditioning or biofeedback approach to the asthmatic child. In essence, various relaxation and self-hypnosis techniques are utilized. The aim is to decondition the aggregate of emotional factors that may contribute to wheezing, and to acquire some control over the bronchial musculature through biofeedback. The patient actually acquires a real sense of awareness of the state of his bronchial tree, and, contrary to the older thoughts of a purely involuntary control in the autonomic processes, can actively achieve bronchial dilatation. Although some of the work done has involved the use of sophisticated feedback devices outside the range of most psychiatrists' and allergists' offices (e.g., pulmonary function machines with rewarding red light to signal when a desired expiratory flow rate has been achieved) (Khan et al., 1973), the principles of relaxation and systematic desensitization are well known in behavioral and learning theory (Wolpe and Lazarus, 1966). This therapy form is becoming more popular and may evolve into a major approach to asthma and other psychophysiologic diseases. However, its precise usefulness in children awaits further study.

Bronchial Asthma: Case History

John was 11 years old when first seen by a child psychiatrist. He was suffering from moderate bronchial asthma which was never severe, but unpredictable in onset. Allergy tests and histories suggested allergies to a number of things, including certain animals, house dust, and some types of grasses. Various medications had been prescribed, some of which were effective for a brief time, and he had come to rely heavily upon them.

He was the third of three children, having two older sisters. He had been a much-wanted child, since the parents wanted a son. He was a normal full-term baby but suffered bouts of colic, did not eat well, and was slow in physical development. His intellectual capacity seemed normal. When the asthma became an obvious symptom at about kindergarden, the parents were alarmed and began a frantic search for an answer to the problem.

The pediatrician eventually recognized the emotional problems contributing to the disorder and made a referral to a child psychiatrist. On initial interview, the mother proved to be the dominant parent and the father relatively passive. There was obviously a close tie between mother and son and a rather distant relationship between father and son. The mother had taken what she wanted to hear from various physicians and had put rather severe limitations on the boy's physical activities, which only further widened the distance from his father. The latter resented not being able to participate in activities with his son. There had also been the trauma of removing all household pets and changing some of the household furnishings.

When seen for the first time by the child psychiatrist, John proved to be a rather frail youngster, small for his age, but otherwise physically normal including his pulmonary vital capacity. Initially, he was reluctant to relate to the psychiatrist because, in spite of parental reassurance, he expected more "needles." When his asthma was discussed, he agreed that it was quite a problem for him and he wished he did not have it. When asked what he thought caused the attacks, he said, "Sometimes I don't know, and sometimes I make it happen when I get upset." When the doctor expressed surprise at the statement, the patient said, "Watch, I'll show you," and he proceeded to hyperventilate to the point of producing a typical mild asthmatic attack.

Therapy consisted of casework for the parents and individual psychotherapy for John. This was done in cooperation with the pediatrician and the allergist, and gradually the situation improved. John was allowed more liberties in terms of physical activities, and the mother became less protective. Although the youngster continued to have occasional asthmatic attacks, he became more integrated with his peers and involved in their activities.

This short history illustrates that while there may have been some initial allergic input in the asthma attacks, there certainly were secondary emotional problems that developed. It required the efforts of several specialists to intervene in the parents' medical shopping and unite in the effort to cope with John's problems.

Obesity

Obesity: Medical Aspects

Obesity in childhood and infancy is being recognized increasingly as a major medical problem, and its roots are being traced clearly back to early infant feeding. Therefore, from the pediatrician's standpoint, the major task is to prevent early overfeeding, and to intervene as early as possible where children have become obese. Data on children who are markedly obese prior to the age of 15 (weight that is 20% more than allowed for that person's height and build) stand a greater than 90% chance of never staying thin as an adult.

The best predictor of juvenile obesity is excessive weight gain in the first year of life (Eid, 1970). Consequently, the obese infant tends to become the obese child, the obese child tends to become the obese adolescent, and by then the trend may be irreversible. That is to say, it is reversible only with the greatest difficulty. Consequently, numerous medical, nutritional, and psychological approaches to obesity will have unpredictable and generally discouraging results.

There is significant theoretical basis for suggesting a psychophysiologic cycle in obesity, One mechanism (Mayer, 1966), the glucostatic mechanism, suggests a feedback to the satiety center in the hypothalamus which indicates increased glucose utilization (dependent on the large body mass) which, in turn, stimulates the hunger mechanism. A similar "lipostatic" theory postulates a direct feedback between adipose mass and the hypothalamus, although direct evidence is lacking. Further evidence of a vicious cycle setup, which perpetuates the physiologic need for food and the hunger mechanism, is provided by the marked reduction in appetite shown is some intestinal bypass patients, once their body mass has been markedly reduced due to the bypass surgery. Although one would expect such a person, who is given an iatrogenic malabsorption setup, to continue merely to eat the same huge volume of calories, and lose weight only because of malabsorption, in fact, they tend to have, in many cases, a large reduction in caloric intake once the oversized body is reduced.

Hence, there is reason to suspect that the obesity, at least to some extent, may take on a life of its own, which can only be managed in some cases once the weight reduction has already taken place. This may account for some of the intractability of obesity treatment. In the context of a person's emotions "speaking through his body," the drive to eat can well be considered a psychophysiologic syndrome.

An approach to adolescent or childhood obesity must recognize both the physiologic and psychologic contributions. It is said that those with early-onset obesity will have less clearly identifiable psychologic factors than those who had a late-onset obesity. Whereas a sensible program of weight reduction is advisable in adults, for a teenager who is in a rapid growth phase, stabilization of weight and waiting for growth in linear height to catch up with weight might be more reasonable. Unrealistic goals must be avoided.

Obesity: Psychological Aspects

As with most other psychophysiologic disorders, obese children are usually referred to the child psychiatrist only when all other methods have failed. The child psychiatrist is fully aware that there are constitutional and genetic factors operating in many cases. Some families remain slim, while others constantly fight problems of weight. Most pre-pubescent youngsters are not particularly concerned about their own weight unless they are teased by their own peers. It is also recognized that the eating habits of American youngsters have changed from "three square meals a day." Today, eating habits in a busy family are often erratic, and the youngster frequently snacks and does not have a well-balanced diet. Most obese youngsters who have been said to have eaten a reasonable diet will, if put in a hospital where the diet can be rigidly controlled, lose weight. However, in most cases, the weight is regained when the child returns home.

Hilde Bruch has written extensively on this topic and has made some excellent observations, beginning in early life and continuing into the teenage years and later. The normal mother recognizes the different cries of her infant, such as being cold, wet, or hungry, and reacts accordingly. The immature, unintuitive mother may respond to all crying by feeding. This temporarily quiets the infant, and there is implanted a kind of automatic reaction that unhappiness can be relieved by food. In other words, the emotional intake that would be present is replaced by food intake.

During preschool and grade school years, obesity, unless it reaches remarkable proportions, does not come to the attention of the child psychiatrist. It is often handled by pediatricians of family physicians, and in many instances with some success. One problem lies, however, in the family battles that may take place over how much the child should eat, what he should eat, and the child's own decision about what he will eat.

Obesity really becomes a problem to the child in early adolescence when he or she wishes to be attractive, but finds himself singled out as physically unattractive or athletically incapable. They are often overtly jovial youngsters and yet basically depressed. The treatment of obesity by the psychiatrist usually begins during this period when the youngster has a strong motivation to correct the problem. Until that time, treatment can be difficult and unrewarding. In the adolescent age range, considerable success has been found in group therapy where the teenagers can share their feelings.

It should be mentioned that there are many parents who feel that they are doing a good job of parenting only by providing great quantities of food to the child. If the youngster is to be on a diet and siblings and parents consume large amounts of food, this makes it more difficult for the obese child, and parents often need counseling in managing the situation.

Obesity: Case History

This 11-year-old black girl was admitted to the Children's Psychiatric Hospital weighing approximately 190 pounds. She was thoroughly checked by pediatricians and endocrinologists and no physical problems were found. She was the oldest of six children and said she wished her parents had never had any children other than herself. She wanted all their attention and resented sharing it with others. Initially, during her three-month stay in the hospital, she was allowed to eat family-style with the rest of the children and staff and to eat whatever she wanted. Eventually, she asked to have a diet prescribed to which she promised to adhere. She did lose approximately twenty pounds, but still remained preoccupied with food and made few friends with the other children or the staff. At this point and against medical advice, the parents removed the girl from the hospital. Unfortunately, given the same family situation and lack of further help, the girl will probably remain obese for the rest of her life.

Diabetes Mellitus

Diabetes mellitus is one of the classical chronic diseases in medicine. The juvenile, or strictly insulin dependent form, usually has its onset in the pediatric age group, and certainly in most cases before age thirty. The etiology of diabetes remains unknown. Insulin replacement corrects the major metabolic derangements, but the degenerative vascular complications seem unaffected.

Consequently, unlike asthma, this is a disease whose ultimate outlook is either unpredictable or poor. The major psychological complications are usually of a secondary nature, and are those associated with any chronic disease. Especially important to recognize is the interaction of adolescents with diabetes. The adolescent diabetic attempts to normalize his life, throw off restrictions, rebel against those who are restraining him, and picture himself as much less vulnerable to his illness than parents and physician may accept. Accordingly, failure to take insulin, total inattention to dietary consideration, and using the diabetic control issue as a weapon in the dependence-independence struggle, are common problems in this age group.

However, there is some evidence that emotions may cause a primary aggravation of diabetes, and not just be a separate, adjustment-related issue. At least three groups (Baker et al., 1969; Hinkle, Evans, and Wolf, 1951; Nabarro, 1965) have now suggested that acutely stressful situations can exacerbate the diabetes in selected patients.

Therefore, the child psychiatrist may occasionally see a diabetic youth whose emotional problems affect his illness at more than one level. Baker's limited experience suggested that psychotherapy (as well as beta-adrenergic blockade to inhibit catecholamine secretion) could be very helpful in selected cases in establishing diabetic control. Until more data are available, it seems prudent to consider diabetes mellitus as a disorder with a potential psychophysiologic component, as well as the ever-present psychological ramifications of chronic disease.

Diabetes Mellitus: Case History

Jane was 15 years old when the pediatric and psychiatric services converged to coordinate her care. By then she had had diabetes mellitus for 10 years, and had been admitted to the Children's Hospital approximately twenty times. Over the previous two years, she had missed half of her classes at school, and had spent approximately 10% of the time in the hospital. Her medical management was becoming increasingly confused, increasingly difficult, with a "brittle aspect" of her diabetes evidence. That is to say, she varied from being in insulin shock to "out of control" over very short periods of time.

When first seen by the child psychiatrist, in consultation with the pediatric endocrinologist, several points came to light. First of all, there were numerous psychiatric factors that had previously not been explored. Jane was extremely stressed by the marital friction that had gradually evolved between her father and mother. It was learned that they were close to divorce, and that her periods of lack of control frequently coincided with worsening of this relationship. Whether inattention to management of her diabetes or emotional factors worsening the diabetes were the major operative agents is not clear. Probably, there were contributions from both. Additionally, Jane was having extreme difficulty adjusting to the vulnerability of her body. As with other teenagers, she wished to view herself as a healthy, invulnerable person, and the fact of her dependency on insulin and special diet was very distressing to her. She was also acutely aware of the eventual complications of diabetes, and at times was overtly depressed with the outlook for her disease.

In retrospect, it became clear that in many ways, Jane's diabetes followed her emotions. Although she was not overtly noncompliant, it was clear that when she was depressed, her interest in managing her disease diminished.

Both the pediatrician and the child psychiatrist adopted a positive outlook, and compared notes frequently in Jane's follow-up. The marital discord became a point of open communication, and was eventually resolved through family counseling. It then became an issue that Jane could deal with directly, and soon vanished as an issue. Jane began to communicate her feelings about the outlook for her disease, and soon began to appreciate that her life could be relatively normal and unrestricted, if she wished it that way. However, six months of biweekly visits to both the pediatricain and child psychiatrist were needed before these improvements were evident. Within one year, Jane's diabetes was much easier to control, and her school attendance was markedly improved. In times of stress, however, she continued to need the support of both the peditrician and child psychiatrist. Perhaps most importantly for Jane, was the emergence of a single pair of physicians to follow her, rather than the mixture of attending and house staff physicians who had dealt with her in the past. Only by careful communication between this pair of physicians was Jane able to maintain the gains that she made over the first year of involvement.

Skin Diseases

Skin Diseases: Medical Aspects

The following are some of the problems in adult medicine which have been noted to have important emotional factors (Obermayer, 1955): pruritis, atopic dermatitis (neurodermatitis or eczema), neuronychia, dyshidrosis, urticaria, lichen urticatis, rosacea, acne vulgaris, alopecia areata, sudden graying of the hair, psoriasis.

Among these, only atopic dermatitis, urticaria, and perhaps acne and dyshidrosis find any significance in pediatric practice. Although none of these is likely to be primarily referred to the psychiatrist, except perhaps after prolonged and unsuccessful handling on the part of a primary care dermatologic physician, some children may present to the psychiatrist with these dermatoses as a part of their problem. The psychophysiologic aspect of the skin disease must, at that time, be dealt with.

The most common of these entities would be atopic dermatitis. The atopic diathesis probably affects 20% to 30% of the population to some extent. Atopic eczema is characterized by an abnormal and heightened skin reactivity, and is accompanied by severe, spasmodic itching and its consequences. It affects all age groups, commonly begins in infancy, and is often associated with other aspects of the atopic diathesis, including hay fever, asthma, and other allergic symptoms. Precipitating factors may include specific allergens, cold, heat, certain foods, clothing, soaps, friction, and of course, psychogenic factors. Basic to the production of the eczema is the itch-scratch cycle which is self-perpetuating. Consequently, once set up, the original inciting event may be less important and the eczema in many ways develops a life of its own.

Since itching is to a large extent a subjective phenomenon (Jordan and Whitlock, 1972), emotional factors may well play into the itch-scratch cycle (Robin, 1973). Medical therapy is aimed at altering the cycle by appropriate measures. These include softening of the skin with a lubricationg cream or ointment. Since dryness or xerosis is a basic part of the atopic skin problem, this lubrication, by itself, may be sufficient for milder cases. Topical corticosteroids have now become a mainstay of treatment, and are useful because of their anti-inflammatory action, which in turn affords major relief from pruritis. Specific oral antipruritics are often useful, because of their sedating or tranquilizing effects. Where identified, of course, removal of the specific antigen or inciting agent is of major use. Specific immunotherapy, or "allergy shots," may be useful in selected cases. The most severe cases of eczema often require the coordination of both a dermatologist and an allergist. Atopes, of course, may have a tendency to have more than one severe problem, for example, both eczema and asthma.

Little is known of the psychogenic basis of the other diseases of the skin in childhood. Alopecia areata is so rare as to be almost never encountered. Urticaria in childhood is unlikely to have a psychogenic component. Acne vulgaris is apt to have more hormonal than psychologic contributions, but may well be seen in an emotionally disturbed teenager, and hence is worthy of the child psychiatrist's full understanding.

Acne is the most common significant dermatosis is the teen-aged youth, and may well be seen in a poorly adjusted individual with a poor body image. The medical treatment today is so successful in as many as 90% of the cases that most teenagers should be spared the spectre of a scarred, pitted, and inflamed face. The dermatologist or pediatrician attempts to:

1. By topical means, degrease and peel the skin in order to prevent comedone formation.
2. Suppress bacterial flora with oral tetracyclines, thereby reducing the free fatty acids of sebum, and controlling skin inflammation.
3. Remove formed comedones by mechanical means, and open (acne surgery) cystic acne lesions where indicated.

Skin Diseases: Psychological Aspects

The skin is well known as a reflector of the emotions. We blush when we are embarrassed, turn pale when we are frightened, redden in anger, and anxiety may produce excessive perspiration. Most of us have experienced any or all of these transient symptoms.

There is a large group of disorders of the skin, not always well defined, which can become chronic in nature, and some have more emotional input than others. For example, eczema can be mild to moderate to severe and reveal different types of skin problems. The word eczema has come to be used in a broad sense, and the same could be said of neurodermatitis. Another common skin problem, seen particularly during adolescence, is acne. This also varies in degree and even varies with the degree of emotional tension. This is not to say that acne is primarily caused by psychological problems, but certainly can be affected by them.

There is not too much scientific information on the psychological aspects of skin disorders, but most pediatricians and dermatologists are aware that the psyche does play a primary or secondary role and would agree that depression and stress can play a strong part. Articles written in this area usually recommend "supportive psychotherapy," and much of this type of therapy is done by the pediatrician or dermatologist, as it is uncommon for a youngster to be referred to a psychiatrist for skin problems alone.

Skin Diseases: Case History

John, a 10-year-old boy, was transferred from the pediatric ward to the child psychiatry ward suffering from generalized severe eczema. It had been present since his preschool years, but had gradually gotten worse in spite of all forms of therapy.

He was the second of four children from a disturbed family. His siblings had emotional problems of various kinds, the parents were incompatible, and the emotional atmosphere in the home was poor, to say the least. John was an intelligent youngster, but difficult to manage on the ward. He was constantly in trouble and often the brunt of attacks by the other children in which the staff frequently had to intervene.

It was the custom of the unit to send children home for short periods as soon as this seemed feasible, and this was attempted with John, with the pediatrician's approval, about two months after his admission. He had agreed to spend a weekend at home, but when the time came, he refused to leave the hospital with his parents. The decision was made for him to go home in spite of his refusal to see what the results would be, and it was contrary to the behavior of most of the children who welcomed the opportunity to return home for a visit.

In therapy, he proved to be an intractable youngster. Medication for the skin disorder was continued, but psychotherapy proceeded very slowly. He gradually improved over a period of months and was finally discharged to outpatient treatment with only remanents of the eczema. John was basically an angry boy who related poorly to others, but eventual results were reasonsably good, and the family situation improved with casework help.

Dysmenorrhea

Dysmenorrhea: Medical Aspects

By dysmenorrhea is meant the "painful period," or dysfunctional menses, which constitutes the most frequent cause of pelvic pain in the young female. It is also the leading cause of absenteeism from work or school in the female who is in the reproductive age group.

Painful periods are, in fact, so common as to-make dysmenorrhea an entity that cannot always be separated from the norm. Fully two-thirds of schoolgirls studied complained of painful menses (Sloan, 1972), although the degree of discomfort was minimal in half of those with symptoms. The other symptomatic schoolgirls required relief from their daily activities and hence would be among those who would miss school and require rest and analgesia. In its broadest application, these young women and schoolgirls would be said to have primary dysmenorrhea, that is, painful menstruation without any pelvic pathology. Secondary dysmenorrhea, where a pelvic lesion is present, does occur, although infrequently. Consequently, a gynecologist, or primary care physician competent in gynecologic diagnosis must thoroughly evaluate the young girl with painful periods.

Numerous theories have been advanced concerning the etiology of primary dysmenorrhea, but none explain convincingly why some girls suffer and some do not. Consequently, the psychogenic aspects have been widely emphasized as responsible for the incapacitation experienced in the more severe cases. Most gynecologists would endorse this psychogenic basis for primary dysmenorrhea. However, one should be aware of an opposite view, paralleling the women's movement, which deplores the tendency to label as psychosomatic an affliction occurring in this large percentage of women exposed to the same physical stress (Lenane and Lenane, 1973). This group would point out that other persons with visceral colic are afforded rest and relief of pain, withour accusation of oversomaticizing, whereas the psychosomatic label is automatically applied in dysmenorrhea. Supporting the "visceral colic," organic theory is the evidence that dysmenorrhea is usually not present in the early, anovulatory cycles, immediately after menarche, plus the quite significant success rate of ovulation suppression via the oral contraceptive agents in relieving dysmenorrhea.

Additional therapeutic approaches that have met with success include physical excercise (Golub et al., 1968), and in the most refractory cases, surgery. Each modality, including psychotherapy, has its enthusiasts, and the success rates, even of surgical approaches, vary with the enthusiasms of the physicians involved. It would appear, therefore, that each case must be individualized, followed closely by both medical and psychiatric practitioners, and the approach tailored to the need of the patient, rather than a preconceived plan.

Psychological Aspects: Dysmenorrhea

Dysmenorrhea is a common complaint in females from puberty onward. It is relatively rare that a teenager is referred to a child psychiatrist for this complaint alone, but it often arises as a concern during the course of treatment for other problems. There are, of course, many reasons why a girl or woman may have painful menstruation, and some of them have nothing to do with the psyche. The average child psychiatrist who sees dysmenorrhea among his patients would have a biased sample, since they also have emotional problems. He would not necessarily see those young girls whose painful menstruation is a result of physical causes.

It is important for the psychiatrist to keep in mind the significance of the beginning of the menses. Some adolescents look forward to the whole process of growing up, including menstruation, while others have been taught, directly or indirectly, that it is a "curse" which must be suffered. And here we are in the gray zone where dysmenorrhea could be psychosomatic, conversion reaction, or organic in nature.

If, for example, a young girl has been almost programmed by her mother to expect suffering, this would probably be in the category of conversion reaction. If a young girl has a fear of growing up, and menstruation exemplifies a portion of this, she might be called psychosomatic rather than conversion. The important point to be stressed is that some youngsters have been taught and shown that the whole maturation process can be enjoyable, while others have been led to believe that it is difficult and painful. Menstruation is an obvious, overt sign of the process and therefore may be focused on by the youngster in a general way. An example of the degree of emotional input into menstruation is found in anorexia nervosa, which often leads to amenorrhea.

Something should be mentioned here about the usefulness of sex education classes in schools. The grade level at which these begin varies from one school to another, and the skill with which they are taught also varies. It remains, however, that the knowledge a child receives is intellectual and does not necessarily change or improve sexual attitudes. In general, sex education classes are beneficial but not the panacea many parents and teachers anticipated. A young girl may learn a great deal about the anatomy and physiology of menstruation, but if she has emotional problems and fears of growing up, these classes will not prevent dysmenorrhea of a psychosomatic type.

The treatment of psychosomatic dysmenorrhea is not focused on the symptom itself, but rather on the overall emotional growth process of the girl. Once she has decided both consciously and unconsciously that it is desirable to become a woman, the dysmenorrhea will usually abate. During treatment, distorted ideas about menstruation are often presented along with family attitudes that contribute to the problem.

Dysmenorrhea: Case History

Mary, a 14-year-old girl, was first seen by the child psychiatrist at the request of the pediatrician because of a multitude of vague physical complaints. During the initial phases of treatment, it became evident that menstruation had begun and was quite painful and incapacitating.

Mary was the youngest of three children, having two older brothers. She had been overprotected by both her mother and father. Her family was extremely rigid emotionally, and there had been no discussion of sexuality. Mary suffered most from this rigidity. She had been given little, if any, preparation for menstruation, although she had heard vaguely and in a distorted way from other girls about it. Her mother literally went to bed for about three days each month and Mary never understood why.

At the onset of her first menstrual period, she was quite upset assuming that something was physically wrong with her. Only after finding her stained underpants did her mother give her a brief description of menstruation and did it in such a way that Mary assumed it would always be painful and it was something through which she would have to suffer.

The dysmenorrhea was not the primary reason for which she was referred. She was a youngster who had never been given much imformation about growing up and the pleasures of femininity. She had developed a number of emotional complaints, including minor phobias. She was upset about breast development and axillary and pubic hair growth, but these also were never discussed. During the course of therapy, she was helped to understand the normality of the changes in her body. At the same time, a social worker talked with the parents about becoming more flexible in these areas and discussing things with Mary. She gradually became a more normal adolescent who accepted the concept of maturation and eventual adult femininity, and as a result, suffered less dysmenorrhea. The child psychiatrist and the pediatrician shared discussing these things with her, and many of her previous distorted ideas were removed.

Summary

The child psychiatrist, although trained in medicine, spends the majority of his time with emotionally and mentally disturbed children and frequently loses sight of those whose emotions disturb physiologic function. In this chapter, we have attempted to present a view of psychophysiological disorders by both a pediatrician and a child psychiatrist. It is important that the child psychiatrist retain an interest in pediatric medicine, keep abreast of developments in that specialty, and establish a good working relationship with pediatricians in order to combine efforts when needed in the treatment of these disorders.

References

American Psychiatric Association. (1968) *Diagnostic and Statistical Manual of Mental Disorders,* 2nd ed. Washington, D.C.: American Psychiatric Association.

Apley, J. (1964) *The Childhood Abdominal Pain.* Oxford: Blackwell.

Apley, J. (1973) Which of you by taking thought can add one cubit to his stature? Psychosomatic illness in children: A modern synthesis. *Brit. Med.* J. 2:756.

Arnold, S.J., et al. (1973) Enuresis: Incidence and pertience of genitourinary disease in healthy enuretic children. *Urology* 2:437–442.

Baker, L., et al. (1969) Beta adrenergic blockage and juvenile diabetes. Acute studies and long-term therapeutic trials. Evidence for the role of catecholamines in mediating diabetic decompensation following emotional arousal. *J. Pediat.* 75:19–29.

Blomfield, J.M., et al (1956) Bedwetting prevalence among children aged 4–7 years. *Lancet* 1:850.

Brazelton, T. (1962) Crying in infancy. *Pediatrics 29:579.*

Carey, W.B. (1968) Maternal anxiety and infantile colic. Clin. Pediat. 7:590.

Cohen, M. (1975) Enuresis. *Pediat. Clin. N. Amer.* 22:545–560.

Committee on Child Psychiatry, Group for the Advancement of Psychiatry. (1966) *Psychopathological Disorders in Childhood: Theoretical Considerations and a Proposed Classification.*

Davis, M.H., et al. (1973) Relaxation training facilitated by biofeedback apparatus or a supplemental treatment on bronchial asthma. *J. Psychosom. Res.* 17:121–128.

Eid, E.E. (1970) Follow-up study of physical growth of children who had excessive weight gain in the first six months of life. *Brit. Med. J.* 2:74.

Engle, G.L. (1955) Studies of ulcerative colitis, III. The nature of the psychological processes. *Am. J. Med.* 19:231.

Esman, A. (1977) Nocturnal enuresis: some current concepts. *J. Am. Acad. Child Psychiat.* 16:150–158.

Feldman, F., et al. (1967) Psychiatric study of a consecutive series of thirty-four patients with ulcerative colitis. *Brit. Med. J.* 2:14.

Finch, S., and J. Hess. (1962) Ulcerative colitis in children. *Am. J. Psychiat.* 118:9.

Golub, L.J., et al. (1968) Exercise and dysmenorrhea in young teenagers: A three-year study. *Obstet. Gynec.* 32:508–511.

Hallgren, B. (1958) Nocturnal enuresis: Etiological aspects. *Acta Pediat.* (Suppl.) 118:66.

Herbst, J., G. Friedland, and F. Zboralske. (1971) Hiatal hernia and rumination in infants and children. *J. Pediat.* 78:261.

Hinkle, L.E., Jr., F. Evans, and S. Wolf. (1951) Studies in diabetes mellitus. III. Life history of three persons with labile diabetes and relation of significant experiences in their lives to onset and course of disease. *Psychosom. Med.* 13:160.

Jordan, J., and F. Whitlock. (1972) Emotions and the skin: The conditioning of scratch responses in cases of atopic dermatitis. *Brit. J. Derm.* 86:574.

Kanner, L. (1948) *Child Psychiatry,* 2nd ed. Springfield, Ill.: Charles C Thomas.

Kardish, S., et al. (1968) Efficacy of Imipramine in childhood enuresis: A double-blind control study with placebo. *Can. Med. Assn. J.* 99:203.

Khan, A. (1974) Mechanism of psychogenic asthmatic attack in children. *Psychother. Psychosom.* 24:137–140.

Khan, A., et al. (1973) Role of counter conditioning in the treatment of asthma. *J. Asthma Res.* 11:57.

Lennane, K.J., and M.B. Lennane. (1973) Alleged psychogenic disorders in women—A possible manifestation of sexual prejudice. *New Eng. J. Med.* 288:288.

Mahoney, D. (1971) Studies of enuresis I. Incidence of obstructive lesions and pathophysiology of enuresis. *J. Urol.* 106:951–958.

Marshall, S., et al. (1973) Enuresis: An analysis of various therapeutic approaches. *Pediatrics* 52:813–817.

Mayer, J. (1966) Some aspects of the problem of regulation of food intake and obesity. *New Eng. J. Med.* 274:610, 662, 772.

Meadow, R. (1970) Childhood enuresis. *Brit. Med. J.* 4:787.

Mendeloff, A., et al. (1970) Illness experience in life stresses in patients with irritable colon and with ulcerative colitis. *New England. J. Med.* 282:14.

Monk, M. et al. (1970) Epidemiological study of ulcerative colitis in regional enteritis among adults in Baltimore—III. Psychological and possible stress-precipitating factors. *J. Chron. Dis.* 22:565.

Nabarro, J. (1965) Diabetic acidosis: Clinical aspects. In B.S. Leibel and G. Wrenshall, eds., *On the Nature and Treatment of Diabetes.* The Netherlands: Excerpta Medica Foundation, pp. 545–557.

Obermayer, M. (1955) *Psychocutaneous Medicine.* Springfield, Ill.: Charles C Thomas.

Oppel, W., et al. (1968) The age of attaining bladder control. *Pediatrics* 42:614.

Paradise, J.L. (1966) Maternal and other factors in the etiology of infantile colic. *J.A.M.A.* 197:191.

Philipp, R., et al. (1972) Suggestion and relaxation in asthmatics. *J. Psychosom. Res.* 16:193–204.

Pierce, C.M. (1975) Enuresis and encopresis. In Freedman et al., eds., *Comprehensive Textbook of Psychiatry.* Pubtown & publisher, pp. 2116–2124.

Rachemenn, F., and M. Edwards. (1952) Asthma in children. *New Eng. J. Med.* 246:815.

Richmond, J. (1966–67) Rumination. In S.S. Gellis and B.M. Kagan, eds., *Current Pediatric therapy.* Philadelphia: W.B. Saunders. Robin, M. (1973) How emotions affect skin problems in school children. *J. School Health* 43:370.

Roy, C., A. Silverman, and F. Cozetto. (1975) *Pediatric Clinical Gastroenterology,* 2nd ed. St. Louis: C.V. Marky.

Schneer, H.I., ed. (1963) *The Asthmatic Child.* New York: Harper & Row.

Simonds, J.F. (1977) *Clin. Pediat.* 16:79–82.

Sloan, D. (1972) Pelvic pain and dysmenorrhea. *Pediat. Clin. N. Amer.* 19:669–680.

Solnit, A.J., and S.A. Provence. (1963) *Modern Perspectives in Child Development.* New York: International Universities Press.

Starfield, B. (1972) Enuresis: Its pathogenesis and management. *Clin. Pediat.* 11:343–350.

Thomas, A. et al. (1968) *Temperament and Behavior Disorders in Children.* New York: New York University Press.

Umphress, A., et al. (1970) Adolescent enuresis. *Arch. Gen. Psychiat.* 22:237–244.

Werry, J.A. (1965) Enuresis—An etiologic and therapeutic study. *J. Pediat.* 67:423–443.

Wessel, M.J., et al. (1954) Paroxysmal fussing in infancy, sometimes called colic. *Pediatrics* 14:421.

Wolpe, J., and A. Lazurus. (1966) *Behavior Therapy Techniques: A Guide to the Treatment of Neuroses.* New York: Pergamon.

Treatment of Emotional Disorders in Children and Adolescents

CHAPTER 21

Psychosomatic Disorders and Family Therapy

G. Pirooz Sholevar

Psychophysiological disorders are defined as a group of disorders "characterized by physical symptoms that are caused by emotional factors and involve a single organ system, usually under autonomic nervous system innervaton. The physiological changes involved are those that normally accompany certain emotional states, but in these disorders the changes are more intense and sustained. The individual may not be consciously aware of his emotional state." (DSM II, 1968).

The term "psychophysiological disorder" refers to certain specified illnesses and should therefore be differentiated from the expression "psychosomatic medicine." Psychosomatic medicine refers to a complete approach to the patient and the problem of his illness, including the social and psychological as well as genetic, physiological, and biochemical factors that may play a role in the predisposition, inception, and maintenance of many diseases. Those propounding this approach are concerned with the adaptation of human beings to stressful personal and interpersonal conditions and the psychological reasons for the failure of this adaptation to occur. Also, they are more concerned with the predisposition to the disease and its inception than with pathophysiology (Weiner, 1977).

Recently, the interest in the pathology of human illness has been expanded into a concern about the ecology of human conditions. Understanding of the different aspects of the patient's ecology is deemed necessary for the comprehension of human illness. "The patient's emotional involvement in the family system constitutes a major aspect of that ecology which we can no longer afford to ignore" (Meissner, 1977). Therefore, attempts at understanding and treating the illness in its natural context—as a dysfunction of the family system—has gained particular significance.

Recent observations strongly suggest that emotional and social interactions can markedly effect such bodily functions as blood circulation. Emotional phenomena can lead to physical phenomena and psychological reactions can greatly influence the course of a disease. In more recent studies it has been noted that family interactions can be significant in the generation of psychophysiological phenomena. In fact certain types of continuous family interaction may provoke certain illnesses. Other forms of family interactions may constitute a necessary—but not sufficient—condition for the onset of a certain illness; certain precise patterns of family interaction may therefore be necessary for particular agents to be effective. This is consistent with the observation that pathogenic agents are omnipresent but only produce illness in certain individuals (Weiner, 1977).

A brief exposition of the basic premises of family therapy may be helpful in the examination of possible relationships between family relational patterns and psychosomatic disorders. Family systems theorists' views differ from those using linear models (such as practitioners of individual psychology), since the former group looks at the individual in his natural setting—the family. Family therapists view the whole family system—rather than the individual—as the locus of dysfunction and treatment. They are concerned with family homeostasis and circular causality involving multiple feedback loops that act as important reinforcers to maintain the behavior of family members. The dysfunctional processes within the psychosomatically or psychologically disturbed family are seen as influenced by and influencing each family member according to numerous feedback mechanisms. The vulnerable child is viewed as a manifestation of the family response to intrafamilial or extrafamilial stresses.

An instructive example of the interrelationship between the family interaction and physiological changes in family members has been provided by Minuchin and his co-workers (1978). In an experimental family interview, conflict and stress were stimulated between the parents while their child watched behind a one-way mirror. The child was asked to enter the room when parental stress was at its greatest intensity. This format enabled study of the way parents in a psychosomatic family utilize the child during parental conflict. A valuable physiological coincidence, blood-free fatty acids (FFAs), was also used during the family interview; FFAs have been shown to be indicators of emotional arousal and precursors of the ketone bodies that give rise to diabetic ketoacidosis. The periodic measurement of FFA levels in family members during the family interview allowed a comparison of FFA levels in the child with the level and the patterns of his parents. The concomitant FFA levels during the family interview exhibited the physiological correlation to the observable behavioral events. Entry of the psychosomatic diabetic child into the room at the time of greatest parental stress caused the child's FFAs to rise and remain high while the parents' FFA levels dropped as they involved the child in their conflict. The physiological changes correlated with the behavioral change in the family members. The alterations in the FFA levels provided physiological evidence of the harmful effect of dysfunctional family patterns and faulty conflict management in the psychosomatic diabetic families. The crossover phenomenon, in which the parent's FFA levels decreased as the child's FFA level rose following his entry into the room and involvement in parental conflicts, corresponded with the dysfunctional patterns of family interaction (Hodas, In press).

In this chapter, we review family relational data described in the individual and family psychotherapy literature, followed by a discussion integrating seemingly divergent points of view. The therapeutic implications of family relational findings are then discussed.

Family Data Obtained from Individual Psychotherapy

The interpersonal and familial aspects of psychosomatic disorders have been described frequently in the literature on psychophysiological disorders in children and adult patients. In spite of the knowledge of the interpersonal dimension of psychosomatic disorders in many cases, therapists have often utilized inadequate measures for correcting the underlying relational disturbances correlating with psychosomatic disorders. Some of the commonly described deficiencies in family relationships are described below.

Stressful family situations. Many psychosomatic reactions are a response to familial stress. The familial response can be to a stressful situation outside of the family such as loss of a job, moving to a new location, precipitating separation from the familial and social support systems, or internal family stress, such as the birth of a baby. The relationship between familial stress and psychosomatic disorders has been particularly well documented in infantile colic, recurrent abdominal pain, and many other psychosomatic disorders (Finch and Hansen, Chapter 20, this volume).

Poor response to stress. The psychosomatically disturbed families do not deal effectively with extra- and intra-familial stresses. One of the reasons given for poor response to stress is the poor alignment between husbands and wives, who do not support each other emotionally to solve problems. This often results in the husband's making himself less available and the wife's attempting to assume much of the responsibility for handling the family. This pattern has been frequently described in families with infantile colic, recurrent abdominal pain, asthma, and other disorders. The families with infantile colic were particularly prone to further unadaptive responses to stress such as child abuse, especially if there had been a multigenerational history of abuse or neglect in the family (Finch and Hansen, Chapter 20, this volume).

Parental and maternal rejection have been described in asthma and rheumatoid arthritis. Parental rejection may take the form of overt rejection, overprotectiveness, and love that is conditional on certain behavior. *Maternal rejection* has been particularly well documented in children with infantile rumination syndrome. The rumination has been viewed as a self-stimulating activity on the part of an infant reared by neglectful parents.

Disturbances in parental functioning have also been described in many psychosomatic families, particularly in those with asthmatic children. The poor parental functioning has been correlated with poor social adjustment and significant impairment of pulmonary function in asthmatic children (Weiner, 1977).

Marital disturbances have been frequently described in psychosomatically disturbed families, particularly in female patients with rheumatoid arthritis (Moos and Solomon, 1965, Shocket et al., 1969) and in some asthmatic families. The dysfunction often takes the form of a stormy marriage where marital partners are constantly fighting. At times the marriages are characterized by profound hidden dissatisfaction between the marital partners, but the marriages appear stable on the surface, as is seen in the marriages of male arthritic patients (Cobbs and Kasl, 1968).

Dysfunction of sexual roles is described in female arthritic patients and patients with dysmenorrhea where the feminine role is conflicted or rejected. The disturbance in the male role is described in enuretic families where men are seen as little boys who are infantile and incapable of responsible functioning.

Personality structure of parents. The mothers of some psychosomatically disturbed children (such as asthmatics) are described as domineering and rejecting. The fathers in all psychosomatically disturbed families are characterized as passive and uninvolved with the family's life. Compulsive personality structure with isolation of affect, perfectionism, and emotional coldness among family members is described in the parents of many psychosomatically disordered children, especially in children with ulcerative colitis; these children are particularly dependent on their parents.

Control and suppression of affect is commonly described in psychosomatically disturbed families. The expression of emotions is undervalued; parents make little attempt to express their own feelings and discourage self-expression in their children. Asthmatic families suppress or are overly concerned with the crying of their children.

Collusive relationships between a child and one of his parents are well descirbed in enuretic families. Here, the parents—who are reluctant to fight each other directly and openly—develop an emotional pact conspiracy in which the child fights one parent on behalf of the other. There is a tendency for the development of such collusive relationships when one of the parents has a positive history for the same disorder; enuresis, bronchial asthma, and recurrent abdominal pain are examples of such disorders.

Familial or genetic factors. A positive parental history for a particular psychosomatic disorder is common. The emergence of the similar illness in the child frequently revives the old unresolved feelings and memories in the afflicted parent. The parent may respond to the revival of the past painful experiences by becoming overpunitive or overpermissive toward the child exhibiting the symptom. Although the occurence of the symptom in the child can be genetically determined, it becomes part of the intra-familial pattern of coalition formations and alliances. Then it gains a homeostatic function within the family and can be utilized by different family members to further their own wishes.

Family Therapy and Psychosomatic Disorders

Family systems theory began in the late forties and early fifties with the notion of conceptualizing and treating the individual as part of a larger family system. Behavior, motivations, and reaction of the individual were considered to be regulated by the whole family unit; thus symptomatic behavior of an individual was viewed as an expression of family dysfunction and the unmet needs of the members of his family unit. The family unit has an homeostatic property; any action of a family member results in reactions by other members who attempt to reestablish family balance. Psychological or physiological symptoms often develop in a family member as a byproduct of system imbalance and loss of homeostasis.

Early family therapists such as Ackerman, Jackson, Bowen, Lidz and Haley showed considerable interest in psychosomatic symptoms in families. They noted the concept of *reciprocal pathology*—improvement in a patient associated with the deterioration in the condition of another family member—on psychological and psychosomatic levels. It was observed that the improvement of schizophrenia in a family member could be followed by the development of ulcerative colitis in another family member—i.e., *transfer of illness* (Haley, 1963, 1964; Jackson, 1964, 1966).

Bowen described situations where the *soma* of one family member reciprocated with the *psyche* of another. He gave an example where a mother was constantly concerned with the inadequacy of her own internal organs. However, her worries focused on her son's bowels, skin, and sinuses. The son had multiple physical complaints.

Kanner (1948) described a child serving as an "organ of parental hypochondriasis." In his example, the mother lost her constipation after the birth of her daughter but proceeded to complain about her child's constipation. Once the daughter's constipation improved, the mother's constipation recurred.

Jackson (1964; 1966) noted rigid homeostatic patterns in the psychosomatic families and described them as being "restrictive" types who denied their members free expression, especially disagreement with other family members.

Contemporary Family Therapy Views on Psychosomatic Disorders

Important recent contributions to the understanding of psychosomatically disordered families have been made by family theorists with psychodynamic or structural approaches to treatment. In *psychodynamic* and *psychoanalytic* family theory, the continuation of the past dynamic forces in the family and their impingement on the current relationships are given particular weight. The therapist attends to the conflicts, persisting from previous developmental stages, that distort the current object relationships. The conscious and unconscious representation of early objects are seen as limiting the choice and the accurate perception of contemporary objects (Bahnson, in press).

The psychodynamic family therapist describes the psychosomatic disorders as occurring in centifugal family types. The centrifugal family type is characterized by isolation and early individuation of family members, poor communication of emotions, and early departure of family members from the family unit. The emphasis in such families is on individuation, mobility, and the individual's thrust for success coinciding with a similar emphasis in industrial societies. Youngsters in centrifugal families separate early from their parents in terms of physical closeness, emotional expression, and personal goal setting. There is only minimal sharing of affect and motivation, forcing the individual to turn to his own resources for handling of emotions and conflicts; this encourages somatization rather than sharing of the experience with other family members. Later in life, these families generally enter a somatic path of regression when encountering object loss or frustration by the object. Within centrifugal families, two different types have been described—one with special emphasis on independence and a second type emphasizing social success, achievement, and adaptability (Bahnson, In press).

Murray Bowen is a significant contributor in this area. Many of his concepts such as "family projective system," "differentiation and undifferentiation," "overfunctioning and underfunctioning" family members are applicable to the field of psychosomatic medicine (Bowen, 1978). According to Bowen's theory, psychosomatic dysfunction is one of the mechanisms by which people at the lower end of his maturity scale "control the emotion of too much closeness." This refers to a failure to resolve the mother–child symbiosis after adolescence and the resulting functional helplessness, which may find expression in somatic illness. Bowen has developed the notion of physiological reciprocity of the overfunctioning person in a family system. Here, in families with a seriously ill member, another member must remain healthy while laboring under heavy strain in order to maintain the "ill" one in his/her role as the sick member. Bowen has also described the phenomenon of the mother's functioning as "family diagnostician," deciding who is sick and what is to be done, and denying the possibility of being mistaken.

The *structural* approach to family therapy emphasizes the significance of contemporary relational patterns within the family system and the dysfunctional or functional family patterns that inhibit or promote successful adaptation. There is particular interest in the relative weakness or strength of boundaries between the family subsystems and individuals within the larger family context, as well as a special focus on the family's reaction to external and internal (family) stresses. Inappropriate responses to stress can result in dysfunctional unadaptive family patterns such as designation of one of the family members as a sick person. The structural family therapist emphasizes attention to data that can be observed, recorded, and directly altered.

The structural psychosomatic model was developed by Minuchin and his co-workers (1978) through the investigation of families with young children who had unstable diabetes, intractable asthma, or anorexia nervosa. Their attempts at inducing family crisis—rather than shielding the patients from stress—have been quite successful in the control of these conditions. They found the following functional characteristics present in the psychosomatic family: enmeshment, overprotectiveness, rigidity, lack of conflict resolution, and involvement of the child in parental conflict (Hodas, In press).

Enmeshment is "an extreme form of proximity and intensity in family interaction." Enmeshed family members are overinvolved with one another, rendering subsystem boundaries weak and interpersonal differentiation poor: "In enmeshed families the individual gets lost in the system."

Overprotectiveness in the psychosomatic family involves "the high degree of concern of family members for each other's welfare." In overprotective families one family member does for another what that person can and should do himself. The overprotection inhibits the development of competence and autonomy in children.

Rigid families "insist on retaining the accustomed methods of interaction" even when these methods are no longer applicable. As a result, these families have great difficulty "when change and growth are necessary," and they are "highly vulnerable to external events."

The psychosomatic family either denies or diffuses conflict; in either case, there is an inability to disagree within the family and a lack of effective conflict resolution. The result is that "problems are left unresolved, to threaten again and again . . ."

A major characteristic of the psychosomatic family is the involvement of the child in parental conflict. The child's involvement helps regulate "the internal stability of the family," but at the cost of reinforcing the psychosomatic symptom and the dysfunctional family organization. The child may be triangulated (caught) between his two parents, he may be in coalition with one parent against the other, or he may be a detour circuit through which the parents unite to express either concern or anger toward their sick child (Hodas, In press).

Critique of Psychosomatic Family Models

Minuchin and his co-workers' treatment of psychosomatic illness has been some of the most recent and exciting work to date in the field. This group has demonstrated convincingly (1978) the effect of family interactions on the physiological processes of the family members, and through active restructuring of the family's patterns, they have been successful in ameliorating psychophysiological disorders. They have made strong attempts to measure the effectiveness of their family intervention by submitting their technique to evaluative study using reasonably objective physiological symptoms as criteria (rather than the more subjective psychological symptoms). They also included a followup at a later date.

In spite of Minuchin and his co-workers' contributions, there are a number of drawbacks to their studies. First, they have implied that their approach is effective with all psychosomatically disordered families—a claim unsubstantiated by their data. Their studies have primarily involved families of very young patients (Bruch, Chapter 22, this volume), with illness of recent onset—usually in the preceding six months. In the anorexic group, for example, the median age of the patients was 14½ years old and the oldest child was no more than 21 years old; 25% of the designated patients were under 12 years old. More data on structural therapy's effectiveness with older and more chronically and severely disturbed patients is needed. It is quite possible that the latter group and their families are more resistant to an active restructuring of their family unit and could not be helped by the exclusive use of this particular method.

The group included in this study may have been pulled from a very selected sample, as most of the therapists involved in the study were identified with one group and one situation. It is also feasible that only the families who could relate well to this treatment chose to participate in the study—or were subtly chosen by the therapists—while those with different characteristics were excluded. These points need further investigation.

Although the approach by Minuchin and his co-workers has been effective, their attempts to predetermine what is the significant family interaction in relation to the illness may be premature. As Weakland has stated, (1977) "any attempt to predetermine just what must be viewed and the means of its viewing is apt to be not only useless but self defeating. In such an enterprise, fixed targets and instruments can only focus attention on things that are prominent or that one assumes *must* be important . . . Meanwhile, wide ranging but careful scanning of the terrain is obstructed."

The data gathered by Minuchin and his co-workers are concerned primarily with the contemporary patterns and structures of the families and the effectiveness of restructuring them in line with his treatment methods. He omits any data about the long-standing interactional patterns of the family and its families of origin; in fact, Minuchin makes a deliberate distinction between his working in the "here and now," as opposed to the "there and then" focus of psychodynamic therapists, who deal with interactions from the past that are "inactive" at the present moment. This is a major misinterpretation of the views of the psychodynamic therapist and an underestimation of the depth of the family's pathology. No dynamic therapist treats what is not active and alive at the present time; only the issues that have remained active for a long time and interfere with the family's adaptation in the present are the focus of treatment. Psychosomatic disorders, like other severe family pathologies, are probably the result of multigenerational family dysfunction. The family members require resolution of the family's longstanding conflicts if they are to forge forward and meet their full potential.

The psychodynamic model of psychosomatic disorders addressed itself well to the longstanding and multigenerational conflicts and deficiencies in the families. It allows for wide-range research in psychosomatic disorders and prevention of similar disorders in the next generations. It can easily be combined with other therapeutic systems for psychosomatic disorders. It lends itself also to a more extensive attempt at enhancement of adaptation than the correction of the illness in family members.

The drawback of the psychodynamic model is in its lack of sufficient emphasis on the current dysfunctional family patterns leading to psychosomatic crisis. This can limit the effectiveness of therapeutic interventions in reducing the risk to the patient and encouraging the family to participate in treatment.

In our view, the structural model of psychosomatic disorders is an important discovery consistent with the findings of psychodynamic and multigenerational family therapists and individual psychotherapists. The structural approach is helpful in the initial stage of treatment of families with psychosomatic disorders, and clinicians should be well grounded in its use. Also, attention to contemporary dysfunctional sets often can lead to the uncovering of the dynamic underpinnings of the family pattern. However, the model does require supplementation from psychodynamic models of the family and individual treatment in order to be effective with severely and chronically disturbed psychosomatic families.

Discussion

The description of deficiencies and relational patterns in psychosomatic families by individual psychotherapists and psychodynamic and structural family therapists may appear contradictory. In our view, there are no significant inconsistencies in the observations and conceptualizations of the above three systems. In fact, recognition of the related and complementary natures of the above systems can assist us in arriving at a comprehensive model allowing for scientific research and effective intervention into these disorders.

One basic deficiency in the psychosomatic families is the emotional unavailability of the marital partners to each other. As a result of their particular rearing and position in their families of origin, they have not developed the ability to recognize their needs or satisfy those needs through another person. This leaves the couple in a state of frustration and tension with little vision or hope for satisfaction and fulfillment. Unaware that they can achieve satisfaction and fulfillment through each other, the couple drifts away from attending to each other's needs by failing to communicate and by not seeking out and correcting areas of interpersonal conflict. As a result, they attempt other means to reduce the marital tension; this often results in inappropriate overinvolvement between a parent and one child or other mechanisms such as work compulsion.

It is within this familial context that a psychosomatically vulnerable child is raised. Since a child does not recognize his needs—such as hunger—innately, he requires the appropriate response on the part of the parents to recognize his needs and seek satisfaction. The parent who is unprepared and incapable of this level of functioning because of his/her own childhood and current marital and personal life responds to the child in a way that is motivated by his/her own frustrations and tensions and inappropriate to the needs of the child. The functional absence of the other parent reduces the possibility of corrective feedback in this dysfunctional system and allows the vicious cycle to perpetuate itself. As a result, the dysfunction of the family system increases and allows the utilization of the child as a detour for marital dissatisfaction and conflicts. The child develops as a person unaware of his needs, incapable of self-expression, unable to utilize others as a source of relief and satisfaction, and limited in his coping capacity. He may seek to reduce tension by dependent behavior, social withdrawal, or compulsive adherence to school work. Furthermore, having experienced inappropriate and insensitive responses to his actions in early childhood and being covertly exploited by the parents for the reduction of their tension, he grows vulnerable and fearful of criticism by others, misinterpreting many interpersonal events as insulting. He lacks self-awareness and the capacity to discriminate stimulating and responsive behavior from provocative and frustrating actions. The height of family dysfunction is reached at the outbreak of psychosomatic crisis.

We suggest that the basic psychological deficiency in psychosomatically disordered families is one of weakness or deficiency in the *integrative-expressive function* in more than two generations of the family. The "integrative-expressive function" (Parsons and Bales, 1965) pertains to how families regulate tension and how they supply oral and affectional needs. The disturbance of this function is present in the families of origin of parents and is evident on the marital and parental level in the psychosomatic families. The *adaptive-instrumental* function pertaining to the establishment of prestige and social position of the family is unaffected or defensively used to an exaggerated degree in psychosomatic families.

The multigenerational deficiencies in the intergrative-expressive function weakens the marital relationship and distorts the parent-child relationship. The couple do not support each other by searching for problems and resolving them together; thus they encourage dysfunctional patterns in lieu of functional family interactions.

Chronic psychosomatic disorders usually are found in families where family dysfunction on a psychological or physiological level have been manifest in three or more generations. Restriction in expressing affect and negative feelings, and rigidity of relationships are prominent characteristics in these families. Acute psychosomatic disorders particularly affecting young children are seen in less rigid families whose dysfunction has been manifest in only two or more generations.

Treatment of Psychosomatic Disorders

A number of principles and methods should be kept in mind while treating psychosomatically vulnerable families. Furthermore, mastery of a variety of methods is necessary for optimal treatment of families with psychosomatic disorders and will be described below.

In gathering family diagnostic data, the guideline suggested by Weakland (1977) can be very helpful. First, demographic data about the family should be collected. Then the views of the family concerning the nature and the history of the disease—with particular attention to the existence of similar or related illness in the nuclear or extended family members—is needed. Probing the way the disease creates—or resolves—a problem for the family members at the present time illuminates the psychosomatic syndrome further. The ways family members cope with the problems created by the illness and the alternative ways open to the family for dealing with the disease increase the therapist's grasp of the situation.

The emerging of psychosomatic symptoms in the course of psychotherapy has been described by a number of contributors. Many of these symptoms are not severe and do not create major problems in therapeutic management. However, critical psychosomatic breakdowns can occur in families during the course of treatment when the family abandons its practice of avoiding conflict. Rapid confrontation in a family that has avoided disagreement for years or has pretended confrontation but never actually taken a stand can result in serious complications, such as rapid increase in blood pressure, cardiovascular accidents, or myocardial infarction. Jackson (1964, 1966) and Ackerman (1950, 1955) have alerted us to such therapeutic mismanagements; in fact, Ackerman considered serious vulnerability to psychosomatic breakdown as a contraindication to family therapy (although he did prescribe family therapy for psychosomatic crisis).

Concurrent medical and psychiatric evaluation and treatment are necessary, particularly in the acute and initial phases of evaluation. Medical personnel such as pediatricians or internists should take charge in acute phases of disorders such as in the cachetic phase of anorexia or in the ketoacidosis of diabetes. Once the urgent medical aspect of the condition is under control, the therapist can take over primary responsibility for treatment. Medical support, however, should remain available throughout the treatment.

Delineating the functional and dysfunctional family patterns in psychosomatic disorders is helpful in designing highly effective strategies during the acute phase of disorders—particularly with young children suffering from anorexia nervosa, unstable diabetes, and asthma. Minuchin and his fellow structural therapists initially treat families with an anorectic child by family lunch sessions.

By underfocusing or overfocusing on the issue of food during the lunch session, the therapists are able to have the family reenact their dysfunctional patterns. These interventions help change the parents' perspective so that they begin to focus more on helping their child become competent and autonomous and less on forcing the child to eat.

Structural family therapists adopt clear strategies for dealing with enmeshment, lack of boundaries, overprotection, rigidity, and conflict avoidance in the family. They counter enmeshment by supporting individuation and autonomy, challenging intrusion of other family members and increasing the life space for each family member. They support the establishment of functional boundaries between family members and family subsystems and protect the family hierarchy. Overprotection is frustrated by supporting coping behavior in different family members. The myth of helplessness and incompetence underlying the rigidiy of the family system is confronted by helping the family explore alternative ways of coping rather than nontherapeutic symptom-reinforcing behavior (Hodas, In press). A major goal in structural family therapy is to disrupt the conflict-avoidance and conflict-detouring mechanisms of the family; dyadic disagreements are prevented from diffusion by blocking entrance of third parties. Periodically the family therapist joins with strategic family members to bring out the hidden conflicts in the family (Hodas, In press).

The goal of psychodynamic family therapy is to enhance functional relationships among family members by improving communication, expression of needs, and responsiveness to each other's expectations. The recognition and expression of affect are necessary for the establishment of the communication of needs within the family. With the establishment of effective communication, family members feel less isolated, helpless, and prone to somatization.

Often the disturbed relationships in psychosomatic families are a continuation of similar dysfunctional relationships in the parents' families of origin. By assisting the family in recognizing the parellels between current family relationships and those of the parents' families of origin, old conflicts are opened up, providing the opportunity for resolution. The working through of multigenerational conflicts enhances the differentiation and individuation of family members so that members are free to satisfy their needs through their current relationships.

In psychosomatic families where members are significantly attached to their families of origin, multigenerational deficiencies often are present (Bowen, 1978; Boszormenyi-Nagy, and Spark, 1973). Family therapy may be fruitful in enhancing differentiation of the family members from their families of origin. However, even when differentiation is not possible—due to the rigidity of the family system—an attempt for better integration at the same level of functioning should be attempted. This goal can be accomplished by helping family members express their needs and feelings and seek comfort and support from each other.

The structural and psychodynamic models of family treatment do not contradict each other, nor do they preclude individual psychotherapy for psychosomatically disordered family members. The best results are accomplished by combining the methods according to the needs of the specific families and the stage of treatment. Judicious utilization of structural models is helpful and frequently necessary in the initial stage of treatment—particularly with more acute problems. However, structural therapy should not be applied in a way that would prevent longer-term dynamic psychothererapies. The recognition and delineation of contemporary family patterns often lead to the uncovering of the dynamic underpinnings of family relationships; often this is helpful in dealing with the strong defenses of the more severely and chronically disturbed families. At times the reorganization of the family allows one of the family members to enter family-oriented individual psychotherapy with the hope of further differentiation and individuation.

The psychodynamic model of family therapy can be of great assistance in helping the psychosomatically disordered family achieve differentiation. However, this process may be too slow-moving in the acute stage of the disorder, where quick action and results are needed to protect the lives of some family members as well as to keep the family in treatment. The combination of the psychodynamic model with structural therapy and other treatment modalities such as individual psychotherapy or behavior modification may prove to be the essential elements of success in treating psychosomatic disorders.

Acknowledgment

The valuable editorial assistance of Ms. Marilyn Luber is acknowledged.

References

Ackerman, N. (1950) Character structure in hypersensitive persons, in life stress and bodily disease. *Proc. Assn. Res. Nerv. Ment. Dis.* 29:903.

Ackerman, N. (1955) Family psychiatry: Some areas of controversy. *Comp. Psychiat.* 7:375.

Bahnson, C. (in press) A historical family systems approach to coronary heart disease and cancer. In K.E. Schaefer, ed., *A New Image of Man in Medicine*. Mount Kisco, N.Y.: Futura Publishing Co.

Boszormenyi-Nagy, I., and G.M. Spark. (1973) *Invisible Loyalties*. New York: Harper & Row.

Bowen, M. (1973) *Clinical Family Therapy*. New York: Jason Aronson.

Cobbs, S., and S.V. Kasl. (1968) Epidemiologic contributions to the etiology of rheumatoid arthritis with special attention to psychological and social variables. In P.H. Bennet and P.H.N. Woods, eds., *Population Studies of the Rheumatic Diseases*. Amsterdam: Excerpta Medica.

Diagnostic and Statistical Manual of Mental Disorders, 2nd ed. (1968) American Psychiatric Association.

Haley, J. (1963) Marriage therapy. *Arch. Gen. Psychiat.* 8:213.

Haley, J. (1964) Research on family patterns: An instrument measurement. *Fam. Proc.* 3:41–65.

Hodas, G. (In press) Psychosomatic families. In G. P. Sholevar, ed., *Continuing Education in Family and Marital Therapy*. New York: Medical Examination Publishing Co.

Jackson, D. (1964) *Family Illness and the Principles of Homeostasis*. Unpublished manuscript.

Jackson, D., and I. Yalom. (1966) Family research on the problem of ulcerative colitis. *Arch. Gen. Psychiat.* 15:410.

Kanner, L. (1948) *Child Psychiatry*, 2nd ed. Springfield, Illinois: Charles C. Thomas.

Meissner, W.W. (1977) *Psychobiology and Human Disease*. New York: Elsevier North Holland.

Minuchin, S., B. Rosman, and L. Baker. (1978) *Psychosomatic Families: Anorexia Nervosa in Context*. Cambridge, Mass.: Harvard University Press.

Moos, R.H., and G.F. Solomon. (1965) Psychologic comparison between women with rheumatoid arthritis and their non-arthritic sisters. II. Content analysis of interviews. *Psychosom. Med.* 27:150.

Parsons, T., and R. Bales. (1965) *Family Socialization and Interaction Process*. Glencoe, Ill.: Free Press.

Shocket, B.R., E.T. Lisansky, A.F. Shubart, V. Fiocco, S. Kurland, and M. Pope. (1969) A medical psychiatric study of patients with rheumatoid arthritis. *Psychosomatics* 10:271.

Weakland, J. (1977) "Family somatics": A neglected edge. *Fam. Proc.* 16:263–272.

Weiner, H. (1977) *Psychobiology and Human Disease*. New York: Elsevier North Holland.

CHAPTER 22

Obesity and Eating Disorders

Hilde Bruch

This chapter will concern itself with children and adolescents who misuse the eating function in their efforts to solve or camouflage problems of living that to them appear otherwise insolvable. They are characterized by the abnormal amounts they eat and they show this by becoming conspicuous in their appearance. They may eat excessively and grow fat, or they restrict their intake to the point of becoming dangerously emaciated. Clinically these conditions are known as *obesity* and *anorexia nervosa*. Though they look like extreme opposites they are closely related through common underlying problems. Their treatment requires integration of various factors. There is need for psychotherapeutic help for the severe underlying emotional and personality problems of these young patients; at the same time the interactional conflicts within the family demand resolution, and the abnormal nutritional state must be corrected.

Neither obesity nor severe undernutrition represent uniform clinical and psychiatric pictures. There are many overweight youngsters who are just that, without being emotionally disturbed. In a large group of obese children who were followed into adulthood, about a third did fairly well, outgrew the excess weight or remained moderately overweight, but were generally well adjusted (Bruch, 1973, Chapter 8). However, two-thirds grew progressively fatter, and exhibited various degrees of maladaption, some with severe personality problems or manifest psychiatric illness (Bruch, 1973, Chapters 9 and 10). These emotionally disturbed fat youngsters suffered excessively from the hostile social attitude, and their abnormal eating and activity patterns were recognized as intrinsically related to other disturbances of growth and maturation. In the sufferers of developmental obesity, concern with size and weight and inability to delay gratification or to tolerate frustration appear as central issues throughout their development.

In anorexia nervosa a distinct syndrome needs to be differentiated from various unspecific forms of psychogenic malnutrition (Bruch, 1973, Chapter 14). In the typical, primary picture *relentless pursuit of thinness* is the main issue. This preoccupation with size can be recognized as a final step in a desperate struggle for a sense of control and the achievement of personal identity and effectiveness. This struggle usually has gone on in various disguises for some time. Perfectionistic academic performance and excellence in athletics are common early manifestations. In these patients the term *anorexia* is a misnomer; they do not suffer from true loss of appetite. On the contrary, they experience tormenting hunger pains, though they may deny it during the illness and confess it only much later; like other starving people they are frantically preoccupied with food and eating. The self-starvation is strenuously maintained with the goal of obtaining the ultimate in thinness. In the atypical forms, the eating function itself is disturbed and food is endowed with various threatening meanings (Bruch, 1973, Chapter 13). The weight loss is incidental to this avoidance of food and often complained of, or valued only for its coercive effect, in contrast to the pride with which the true anorectic defends her skeleton-like appearance as beautiful or delusionally denies the emaciation. These atypical cases vary considerably in the severity of the illness and accessibility to treatment. I shall limit my discussion here to the psychotherapeutic problems encountered in developmental obesity and primary anorexia nervosa, which appears to be on the increase.

Psychodynamic Diagnosis

It is common practice to rate the severity of obesity and anorexia nervosa in terms of the weight deviation, in absolute figures or as percentage deviation from the norm. In anorexia nervosa this figure is supplemented by references to amenorrhea, constipation, dry skin, etc. These measurements describe the visible aspects of the clinical picture, but contribute little to the understanding of the underlying psychologic problems. Though anorexia nervosa and developmental obesity look like extreme opposites, they have many features in common. In both conditions severe disturbances in body image and self-concept are dominant; food intake and body size are manipulated in a misguided effort to solve or camouflage inner stress or adjustment difficulties.

These youngsters do not feel identified with their bodies, but look upon it as an external object over which they must exercise rigid control (anorexia nervosa) or in relation to which they feel helpless (obesity, with its lack of will power). Though stubbornness and negativism are conspicuous in the clinical picture, these youngsters suffer, behind this facade, from a devastating sense of ineffectiveness; they feel powerless to control their bodies and also to direct their lives in general. They experience themselves as empty and lacking in the sense of ownership of their bodies and as controlled by others. They are helpless and ineffective in all their functioning, not self-directed or truly separated from others. They act and behave as if they were the misshapen and wrong product of somebody else's actions, as if their center of gravity was not within themselves. They lack discriminating awareness of bodily needs; specifically they are unable to recognize hunger and satiation. They also fail to identify other states of bodily discomfort such as cold or fatigue, or to discriminate bodily tensions from anxiety, depression, or other psychological stresses.

These deficits in the sense of ownership and control of the body color the way obese and anorectic youngsters face their problems of living, the relationships to others, and in particular the problems of the approaching adolescence. Like other youngsters they must prepare themselves for self-sufficiency and independence, and emancipate themselves from the dependency on their mothers and families, but are poorly equipped for these tasks. Not infrequently they have been overprotected, overcontrolled, and overvalued, with few experiences outside the home, so that adolescence with the need to grow beyond the family attitudes and values becomes a threatening demand. The parents, in their dissatisfaction with themselves and each other, have invested great expectations in them to compensate for their own frustrations. Frequently these youngsters feel deprived of the support and recognition from their peers that helps normal adolescents in this process of liberation. Recognition of these deficits is not always easy because these problems are overshadowed by the visible symptoms and the struggle over food which is conducted with mutual blame and increasing rage. The obese, when unable to adhere to a diet, is condemned as greedy and weak-willed, and the anorectic's refusal to eat is experienced and responded to as a hostile attack on or rejection of the parents.

Conceptual Model of Early Development

Inability to eat normally sets fat and anorectic youngsters apart. Traditional psychoanalysis explains this as resulting from the attachment of sexual and aggressive impulses to the hunger drive. My own observations led to the conclusion that hunger awareness is not innate knowledge, but that it requires for its proper organization early learning experiences that may be correct or incorrect, depending upon whether the responses of the food giver fit the child's needs (Bruch, 1973, p. 396). Detailed reconstruction of the essential early experiences of these patients suggests that expression of their needs and discomforts as infants has been disregarded or inadequately responded to. Characteristically, they had been given adequate, even excellent physical care, but it had been superimposed according to the mother's concepts instead of being geared to the clues given by the child.

A simplified model of early interactional patterns was constructed, with the assumption that from birth on, two basic forms of behavior need to be differentiated—namely, behavior that is *initiated* in the infant and behavior in *response* to stimuli; this distinction applies to both the biological and the social psychological field. Behavior in relation to the child can be described as *responsive* or *stimulating*, and the interaction can be rated as *appropriate* or *inappropriate* depending on whether it fits the need expressed by the child.

Appropriate responses to clues coming from the infant are essential for the organization of his initially diffuse urges into differentiated patterns of self-awareness, competence, and effectiveness. If confirmation and reinforcement of expression of his needs and impulses are absent, contradictory, or inaccurate, then the child will grow up perplexed when trying to identify disturbances in his biological fields or to differentiate them from emotional and interpersonal disturbances. He will be apt to misinterpret deformities in his self-body concept as externally induced, and he will be deficient in his sense of separateness and experience his body image in a distorted way. He will be passive and helpless under the influence of internal urges or external forces. These features are also characteristic of schizophrenia. This developmental scheme offers a clue to the close association of severe eating disorders and schizophrenic development.

The reconstructed early feeding histories are often conspicuous by their blandness, particularly in anorexia nervosa. The parents stress that the patient has been unusually good as a child, never giving any trouble or fussing about food, eating exactly what was put before him. If the mother's concepts are not out of line with a child's physiological needs, everything may look normal on the surface. Obesity in a child may be a measure of a mother's overestimation of his needs or of her using food indiscriminately as a universal pacifier. The gross deficits in initiative and active self-awareness, the lack of inner controls, including the inability to regulate food intake, become manifest only when the child is confronted with new situations and demands, for which the misleading routine of his early life has left him unprepared. Not having developed an integrated body concept, he will feel helpless when confronted with the biological, social, and psychological demands of adolescence. If every tension is experienced as "need to eat," instead of arousing anxiety, anger, or other appropriate emotions, he will become progressively obese. The anorexic tries to compensate for this deficit in inner controls in an exaggerated way by denying the need for sufficient food. The manifest clinical picture may develop under the stress of puberty itself; in others only at times of additional new demands, such as entering a new school, separation from home, or when a reducing regimen is rigidly enforced.

Weight Change

For effective and lasting correction of the abnormal body weight, the dietary program must be coordinated with psychotherapy and resolution of the family conflicts. All too often the abnormal weight is approached as an isolated symptom and weight loss or gain are enforced from the outside (Bruch, 1973). An unending stream of publications report successful dietary treatment, but rarely with information on the long-term results. The psychiatrist is apt to see the failures of this simple approach.

In obesity it will depend upon the severity of the condition whether and when to recommend a reducing program. Viewed as a manipulation of the energy balance, treatment of obesity is simple; reduction of food intake and increase in exercise accomplishes a predictable loss in weight or stabilization at a desirable level. Commonly mothers are instructed about such dietary restrictions. The more important task would be to teach them how to recognize a child's real needs and how to encourage him to find satisfaction other than through food. Characteristically, fat children are passive, immature, and helpless, and a dietary regimen should help them develop the capacity for inner controls and not be something superimposed by others. This is of particular importance for adolescents, who will diet only when it is a challenge to their initiative and responsibility.

In anorexia nervosa correcting the abnormal weight is often a matter of great urgency; the very survival of a youngster may be at stake. There have been continuous debates on how to accomplish the seemingly impossible task of getting food into patients who are stubbornly determined to starve themselves. As in obesity the physiological principles are simple: increase the intake and restrict the activities of these starving but hyperactive youngsters. The question is how to persuade, trick, bribe, cajole, or force a negativistic patient into doing what he is determined not to do.

Recently, behavior modification has been described with great enthusiasm as a method that guarantees rapid increase in weight (Agras et al.,

1974). The first report by Stunkard and his co-workers recommended freely chosen activities as a reward for gaining weight (Blinder, Freeman, and Stunkard, 1970). One of their four patients with satisfactory weight gain committed suicide after discharge. The method has since been refined by depriving patients of all desirable activities and permitting access to them only as "reinforcement" for weight gain. It appears that with this approach faster gain in weight is achieved than with any other method. However, the long-term results dramatically illustrate that weight gain in itself is not a cure for anorexia nervosa. I have observed catastrophic long-range effects in a series of patients previously treated with behavior modification (Bruch, 1974b). Serious depression, psychotic disorganization, and suicide attempts follow this method of weight gain so often that it must be considered dangerous. Without psychologic support and help toward better self-understanding, this method undermines the last vestiges of self-esteem and destroys the crucial hope of ever achieving autonomy and self-determination.

The enthusiasm about behavior modification is not quite so great as a few years ago. Follow-up observations have shown that the weight gain is often short-lived. Services who use this method have become selective and will accept only patients who come "voluntarily" and who make a "contract" to gain weight. Others will make arrangements for work with the families and for psychotherapy for patients. The somewhat startling aspect of such reports is the minute detail with which the behavior technique is described, whereas family therapy and psychotherapy are only briefly mentioned as something to be carried out by auxiliary personnel. The more drastic approaches, such as tube-feeding as punishment for not gaining weight, seem to be on the way out.

It is equally dangerous not to correct the weight and to permit a patient to exist at a marginal level of safety. This error is not uncommonly committed by psychotherapists in the unrealistic hope that once the underlying unconscious conflicts are recognized, the whole picture will correct itself. Sometimes years are spent in such a futile effort and precious time is lost and patients stay excluded from the necessary experiences of the adolescent years. The starvation itself has such a distorting effect on all psychic functioning that no true picture of the psychological problems can be formulated until the worst malnutrition is corrected. Only then will important underlying problems become accessible to therapy. The same applies to the handling of binge eating and vomiting, which may have become habitual by the time a psychiatrist is consulted. Without interrupting this behavior, for which hospitalization may become necessary, the basic problems, in particular the fear of emptiness, loneliness, and conviction of helplessness, cannot be clarified. A passive attitude on the part of the therapist implies that he condones the abnormal behavior camouflaging the underlying psychological issues and treatment may be unnecessarily prolonged.

Family Involvement

There are few conditions that arouse so much frustration, alarm, panic, anger, rage, and mutual blame as the spectacle of a starving child stubbornly refusing to eat or vomiting what has been taken in. One might say that paradoxically a "low weight" carries much weight in the family. Though less dramatic, but usually of longer duration, in obesity, too, all family concerns seem to focus on what the patient eats and weighs. Meaningful therapy is not possible unless the fighting forces are disengaged. A series of enthusiastic recent reports have dealt with crisis-oriented family intervention with immediate changes of the ongoing patterns of interaction (Barcai, 1971; Liebman, Minuchin, and Baker, 1974; Selvini, 1971). They usually deal with young patients, in the beginning of the illness, before the complicating secondary problems have become entrenched.

As an example of a relatively uncomplicated situation I wish to give the story of Betty, who grew up on a Western ranch and who had been considered happy and healthy until her fourteenth year; she was well-built and had menstruated early. After some teasing about being chubby, when her weight was one hundred and twenty pounds, she suddenly decided she was too large. She also felt that her schoolmates didn't like her anymore, that they felt her family was stuck-up and rich. The ranch was successful and was well known for its breeding stock. Betty began to stay away from teenage activities, with the explanation that she lived too far away from town, and she also went on a diet, ate less and less, and her weight fell from 120 to 85 pounds within four or five months. Her menses stopped soon after she began her reducing regime. She did not follow the instructions given by the local physician and a specialist in the larger town. She looked severely emaciated, her weight being down to 72 pounds, and she was listless and depressed when she was seen in consultation about ten months after the onset of her illness. She had kept very active in spite of her weakness.

During several family sessions the focus was on the question of "What makes it necessary for Betty to go to the extreme of self-starvation to get attention?" As a child she had been "father's helper," but now her place in the family had become undefined and she had regressed to being clinging in her relationship to her mother. The mother, too, had felt of diminished value, since an active grandmother had kept the reins on the ranch. It was possible to give some simple recommendations, such as the father reporting to his wife first, and also doing things with Betty, such as going somewhere together at least one evening every other week. Supplemental nutrition was prescribed in addition to regular meals. It was also mentioned that hospitalization would become necessary if there were no appreciable weight gain in the immediate future.

Five weeks later Betty had gained weight and spoke optimistically about wanting to weigh one hundred pounds at the next visit. The situation seemed generally improved, and she had enjoyed the evenings with her father and they felt much more comfortable with each other. But then Betty became alarmed about gaining too much and she had lost some weight at the time of the next visit. By that time, however, school had resumed and she claimed she felt again accepted by her classmates. When hospitalization was proposed, Betty pleaded not to miss school, that she would eat as much as was needed. This she did and at the next visit, four weeks later, her weight had risen to 99 pounds. She was in excellent spirits and had enjoyed a large party which her family had given for her classmates. Her father described Betty's new relationship with her peers with an interesting comment: "They are all so happy that she is back with them, and they have welcomed her back." By Christmas Betty seemed back to normal and she had since maintained her weight at a desirable level. She had maintained her open relationship with her father, is less dependent on her mother, and enjoys her school and has many friends. A letter two years later confirmed that improvement had persisted.

This family was open-minded and not defensive in its approach to the illness. Not all families are as ready to reexamine their position and some are outspokenly hostile to the idea.

Therapeutic involvement of a family needs to be conceived of as occurring in several phases. Resolving the acute conflicts over the eating is necessary, but it alone is not enough. To recognize and resolve the life-long patterns of interaction is of even greater importance, since they have resulted in this abnormal development of a youngster without a competent sense of identity. In anorexia nervosa the surface picture is often that of a smoothly functioning family; however, underlying the apparent marital harmony there is often a deep sense of disappointment with each other, with the patient feeling obligated to compensate for this. The overintense involvement with one or the other parent often expresses the parent's need for closeness. Clarifying this enmeshment requires that the parents acknowledge their own problems which they need to resolve in grownup terms, by finding comfort in each other. This is a prerequisite for patients becoming liberated from the bondage, free to pursue their own life as a basic right.

The need for family therapy has become widely accepted, but unfortunately it is often carried out without recognizable benefit. Though a family has met regularly, over a considerable period of time, with a therapist, a positive understanding of each other may not be achieved, especially when the focus is only on the family's shortcomings, or the sole recommendation is a hands-off policy. One patient described it as: "The therapist would just sit there and we would argue and fight and lash out in a kind of raw anger, but nothing would get accomplished. We never listened to each other and he did not help us to recognize what the others were saying." She contrasted this with a helpful experience during which the excessive mutual concern was pointed out as a problem, with each one taking over the feelings and goals of the others. The emphasis was on the loving aspects of the family interaction, which gave them a sense of confidence that there was something positive to work for.

No general outline can be given how best to conduct work with families, and how to combine it with individual psychotherapy; the focus, length, and intensity will vary considerably in different cases. Whether a patient can be treated effectively while living at home depends to a large extent on whether the family conflicts are handled successfully. Hospitalization may be necessary, not only to effect a weight gain but also to institute psychotherapy and to clarify the underlying family problems in the absence of the patient. Treating only the patient while hospitalized, without involving the family, will nearly unavoidably result in a relapse when the patient rejoins the family group.

Psychotherapeutic Intervention

The theoretical considerations that were previously discussed are the outcome of continuous reevaluation of the therapeutic results, in particular of the failure of the traditional psychoanalytic approach. The literature on the value of psychoanalysis for the treatment of eating disorders is hopelessly inconclusive, and clarification was not possible until distinct clinical pictures were described. Authors with extensive experience with true anorexia nervosa and also with developmental obesity have recognized early that conventional psychoanalytic explanations did not apply to these patients and that psychoanalytic treatment was ineffective (Eissler, 1943; Meyer and Weinroth, 1957).

My own investigations of the therapeutic situation as a transactional process led to the conclusion that the classic psychoanalytic setting, where the patient expresses his secret thoughts and feelings and the analyst interprets their unconscious meaning, contains for patients with eating disorders elements that represent the painful repetition of patterns that had characterized their whole development—namely, of being told by someone else what they feel and how to think, with the implication that they are incapable of doing it themselves (Bruch, 1973, 1974a; Selvini, 1971). The profound sense of ineffectiveness that has troubled them all their lives is thus confirmed and reinforced. The essential task of the therapeutic intervention must be correction of this deficit by offering patients assistance in developing awareness of their capabilities and potentials and thus helping them to become more competent to handle their problems of living in less painful and less ineffective ways. These modifications are in good agreement with modern concepts of psychotherapy that have been developed for the treatment of schizophrenia, borderline states, and narcissistic personalities. To meet the needs of such patients special consideration must be given to the deficits in their sense of autonomy, and the disturbed self-concept and self-awareness.

The approach to obesity and anorexia nervosa, even of experienced therapists, seems to have remained tied to ineffective and outmoded concepts, such as considering the psychological disorder as the outcome of oral dependency, incorporative cannibalism, rejection of pregnancy fantasies, or similar unconscious conflicts. With the new formulation, the therapeutic focus is on the patient's failure in self-experience, on his defective tools and concepts for organizing and expressing his needs, and on his bewilderment in dealing with others. Therapy represents an attempt to repair the conceptual defects and distortions, the deep-seated dissatisfaction and sense of isolation, and the underlying sense of incompetence.

The therapist's task is to be alert and consistent in recognizing any self-initiated behavior and expressions on the part of the patient; to do so he needs to pay minute attention to the discrepancies in the patient's recall of his past, and to the way he misperceives or misinterprets current events to which he will then respond inappropriately, and he must be honest in confirming or correcting what the patient produces. When held to a detailed examination of the when, where, who, and how, real or fantasied difficulties and emotional stresses will come into focus and the patient will discover the problems hidden behind the facade of his abnormal eating behavior.

Although inability to identify bodily sensations correctly is the specific disability in eating disorders, other feeling tones are inaccurately perceived or conceptualized. These patients suffer from an abiding sense of loneliness or from the feeling of not being respected by others, and this is related to the inability to recognize interpersonal implications. They often feel insulted and criticized, though the realistic situation may not contain these elements. The anticipation or recall of a real or imagined insult may lead to withdrawal from the actual situation and to flight into an eating binge—or to reinforcement of the self-starvation. Exploration of the realistic aspects of these experiences and examination of alternatives in such situations eventually help a patient to experience himself not as utterly helpless or as a victim of a compulsion that overpowers him, but as increasingly competent to deal realistically with problems. Having functioned as an active participant in the treatment process, and with increasing awareness of impulses, feelings, and needs originating within himself, he will learn to recognize appropriate feelings and reactions in areas of functioning where he had been deprived of adequate early learning. Gradually he becomes more competent to live his life as a self-directed, authentic individual who is capable of enjoying what life has to offer.

Under this approach even patients who had been in treatment unsuccessfully for several years, and who were filled to the brim with useless, though not necessarily incorrect, knowledge of their psychodynamics, will begin to change and then relinquish their self-punishing rituals. The important point is that patients learn to examine their own development in realistic terms, with emphasis on their own contributions, or on defining the areas where they had felt excluded from active participation. Examining their own development in this way becomes an important stimulus for acquiring thus far deficient mental tools and for a repair of their cognitive distortions; they learn to rely upon their own thinking and can become more realistic in their self-appraisal.

This approach implies a definite change in the therapist's concept of his role, and it is not always easy to make this change. It involves permitting a patient to express what he experiences without immediately explaining or labeling it; in other words, it requires suspending one's assumed knowledge and expertise. Some of the current models of psychiatric training emphasize early formulation of the underlying psychodynamic issues, and they may then stand in the way of learning the truly relevant facts. A therapist who assumes that he understands the patient's problem is not quite so alert and curious in unraveling the unclear and confused periods. He may be tempted to superimpose his prematurely conceived notions on the patient or become preoccupied with what he will find, whether it confirms his assumptions, instead of engaging the patient into becoming a collaborator in the search for unknown factors. It is important that a therapist recognize meaningful messages in seeming generalities that are often labeled as evasive; never having experienced confirmation for anything they expressed, these patients, though often unusually gifted, can verbalize their state of profound bewilderment only through such stereotyped complaints.

Part of the therapeutic role is to make it possible for patients to uncover their own abilities, resources, and inner capacities for thinking, judging, and feeling, and they will respond well when they recognize the therapist's fact-finding attitude, that he does not have some secret knowledge that he withholds from them. Once the capacity of self-recognition has been experienced, there is usually a change in the whole atmosphere of involvement in the treatment process.

In spite of the overt negativistic attitude these patients are unusually alert to what is going on, and indications of some change may become apparent in the first few sessions—namely, when they recognize that what they have to say is listened to as important. Instead of focusing on the motives underlying the overeating or noneating, I find it useful to inquire about their general development in the spirit of getting acquainted, about their feeling of self-confidence and satisfaction with themselves. Most will reply that they never had any confidence in themselves, that they had lived by doing only what was expected of them. Some will name a definite event which made them aware that something was wrong with their way of life.

To give just one example: Joyce was nearly eighteen years old when she and her parents came for consultation. She had been anorectic for two and a half years, and she, and also her parents, had been in treatment throughout this period, with two hospitalizations to enforce weight gain. However, her weight was only 32 kg. (height 165 cm.). In the expectation that she would again be exposed to a weight-gaining regimen she had lost 5 kg. during the month preceding the consultation. She was an only child born to middle-aged parents who were deeply devoted to her and had encouraged all her intellectual and artistic talents. As the consultation progressed it was recognized that this very giftedness and success in all undertakings had left Joyce with a distorted sense of value, that this was what she owed her parents who enjoyed and cherished her successes. Unless an activity required great effort and strain she rated it as "ordinary" and of no value to her; only the "eccentric," or extraordinary, gave her a feeling of worthwhileness in her own right.

During the first session in which the parents participated, Joyce mentioned that she felt the true onset of her illness had occurred much earlier, when she was about twelve years old; while having tea her mother told her not to take a third cookie. When this was taken up during the next session, the parents shrugged it off as one of her attempts to blame them for her illness. Joyce had mentioned this episode to her previous therapists, who had called it "intellectualizing" or who had paid no attention to it. She definitely felt this episode was important though she did not know why. To my question whether she might have become aware at that moment that mother had control over her body and told her what she needed because she did not trust Joyce to rely on her own sensations and judgment, she smiled for the first time and asked: "Is that why I get so angry when father tells me I am tired?"

From then on she appeared like a changed person who spoke freely about her long-standing anguish that nothing was her own, that she had felt obliged to live her whole life as her parents had planned it; in particular she had been horrified about having to lead the life of a teenager to satisfy them. This issue had not come up at all with her former therapists, whom she described as having been silent and expecting her to keep on talking, and who would then tell her what it meant. She never felt that they were right or that it mattered what they said. Within a few sessions she expressed openly that up to now she had resisted the idea of "getting well" because this had meant only having weight put on her and being told what to think and how to behave. For the first time she was confident that therapy might help her in becoming her own person and to be someone individual.

What a patient offers as a vital issue varies of course from case to case. The important point is that seemingly ordinary, even silly memories are taken seriously, and then used as a meaningful explanation of the illness which may be defined as a fight against the feeling of nothingness, or ruthless punishment for not living up to expectations. Having never trusted themselves to acknowledge their own needs, they need to experience in therapy that they have the right to express and pursue their own wants and wishes.

Once patients feel understood and respected in their deepest concerns and experience that the therapist follows their lead about important issues, they are more apt to listen to his explanations, that meaningful psychotherapy is not possible as long as they are in the state of acute starvaton, since that in itself makes their psychological reactions abnormal; that the cadaverous appearance arouses strong reactions in others that interfere with all human relationships, and that the therapist's anxious concern might interfere with the progress of treatment. Once rapport has been established, a patient is willing to accept that the problems that precipitated the whole illness will remain inaccessible to clarification as long as the nutrition is abnormally low. Thus they will come to the point of permitting the weight to rise gradually, without experiencing a loss of self-esteem and pride, and become capable to face the problems of increasing independence, autonomy, and maturity.

Conclusion

Anorexia nervosa and juvenile obesity have the reputation of offering unusual treatment difficulties, and relapses or outright failures are not uncommon. This appears to be related to erroneous or inconsistent treatment efforts. Results are closely linked to the pertinence of the psychodynamic understanding, and the pursuit of meaningful treatment goals. If the unrealistic expectations with which many obese youngsters approach dieting remain uncorrected, or worse, if the therapist shares them, the outcome may well be the repeated sad cycle of frantic reducing and even more rapid regaining. However, with realistic goals, focused on achieving a more competent, less painful way of handling problems of living, including the ability to establish weight control at a reasonable level, the long-range treatment results are surprisingly good. Progress needs to be evaluated not only as weight stability but also in terms of adequacy of living. Those fat youngsters who had gained insight into the underlying problems achieved a high level of functioning, were successful in their work, got married, and functioned adequately as marriage partners and parents. They raised their children with good control over their eating, so that they grew up slim, not plagued by excess weight as the parent.

In anorexia nervosa the relationship of treatment success to the pertinence of the approach is even more apparent. Though early institution of a meaningful comprehensive therapeutic program improves the chances of recovery, long-standing illness does not preclude good results, even after many years of futile effort, by making underlying lack of autonomy the focus of therapy. Evaluating the long-range outcome led to the conclusion that no one factor of the clinical picture is predictive of success or failure, but that they are directly related to the competence and adequacy of the therapeutic interventon, and its integration with nutritional restitution and correction of the faulty pattern of family interaction.

References

Agras, W.S., D.H. Barlow, H.N. Chapin, G.G. Abel, and H. Leitenberg. (1974) Behavior modification of anorexia nervosa. *Arch. Gen. Psychiat.* 30:279–286.

Barcai, A. (1971) Family therapy in the treatment of anorexia nervosa. *Am. J. Psychiat.* 128:286–290.

Blinder, B.J., D.M.A. Freeman, and A.J. Stunkard. (1970) Behavior therapy of anorexia nervosa: Effectiveness of activity as a reinforcer of weight gain. *Am. J. Psychiat.* 126:77–82.

Bruch, H. (1973) *Eating Disorders: Obesity, Anorexia Nervosa, and the Person Within.* New York: Basic Books.

Bruch, H. (1978) *The Golden Cage: The Enigma of Anorexia Nervosa.* Cambridge, Mass.: Harvard University Press.

Bruch, H. (1974a) *Learning Psychotherapy: Ratonale, and Ground Rules.* Cambridge, Mass.: Harvard University Press.

Bruch H. (1974b) Perils of behavior modification in

treatment of anorexia nervosa. *J.A.M.A.* 230:1419–1422.

Eissler, K.R. (1943) Some psychiatric aspects of anorexia nervosa, demonstrated by a case report. *Psychoanal. Rev.* 30:121–145.

Liebman, R., S. Minuchin, and L. Baker. (1974) The role of the family in the treatment of anorexia nervosa. *J. Child Psychiat.* 13:264–274.

Meyer, B.C., and L.A. Weinroth. (1957) Observations on psychological aspects of anorexia nervosa. *Psychosom. Med.* 19:389–398.

Minuchin, S., B.L. Rosman and L. Baker (1978) *Psychosomatic Families: Anorexia Nervosa in Context.* Cambridge, Mass.: Harvard University Press.

Selvini, M.P. (1963) *L'Anoressia Mentale.* Milan: Feltrinelli. (London: Chaucer Publishing Co., 1974)

Selvini, M.P. (1971) Anorexia nervosa. In S. Arieti, ed., *The World Biennial of Psychiatry and Psychotherapy,* Vol. 1. New York: Basic Books, pp. 197–218.

Selvini Palazzoli, M. (1978) *Self Starvation: From Individual to Family Therapy in the Treatment of Anorexia Nervosa.* New York: Jason Aronson.

Treatment of Emotional Disorders in Children and Adolescents

CHAPTER 23

Vomiting

Charles W. Davenport

Many children's diseases are initiated or accompanied by vomiting. The causes may be infectious, toxic, neurologic, or psychogenic. The vomiting may be the first indication of emotional disorder in an infant or child and the only objective symptom reported. Laybourne reported in 1953 that a review of the child psychiatric literature dealing with vomiting revealed very few papers devoted to this topic. A recent review of the psychiatric literature would indicate that there have been few subsequent reports. This chapter will consider three types of vomiting syndromes: (1) rumination; (2) neurotic or psychogenic vomiting; and (3) cyclic vomiting. These categories are somewhat artificial because ruminating and cyclic vomiting are generally proceeded by either physiologic or psychogenic vomiting. However, there are some unique distinctions between these forms of vomiting and their treatment.

Rumination

Rumination is a well-defined syndrome in which infants bring up food without nausea, and rechew and reswallow the food. At times, fluid is also ejected from the mouth or allowed to run out. The mouth is kept wide open, the head often held back, and sucking movements of the tongue are observed. It is noted that the activity is profoundly gratifying. This syndrome is not without risk, as considerable amounts of food and particularly fluid loss may cause threat to life if the process is not interrupted. It appears this syndrome was considerably more prevalent at the turn of the century than it is reported at this time.

An early report by Cameron in 1925 eloquently describes this syndrome: "All my cases have been in artificially fed infants. After taking a meal in the ordinary way, the baby, as a rule, lies quietly for a time, then begins certain purposive movements by which the abdominal muscles are thrown into a series of violent contractions, the head is held back, the mouth is opened, the tongue projects a little and is curved from side to side as to form a spoon-shaped concavity on its dorsal surface. After a varying time of persistent effort, sometimes punctuated by grunting or whimpering sounds, expressive of irritation at the failure to achieve expected results; with each contraction of the abdominal muscles, milk appears momentarily at the back of the mouth. Finally a successful contraction ejects a great quantity forward into the mouth. The infant lies with the expression of extreme satisfaction upon its face, sensing the regurgitated milk and subjecting it to enumeral sucking and chewing movements. It is evident that achievement of this produces a sense of beatitude. Failure produces nervous unrest and irritation. The power to regurgitate successfully is not suddenly acquired. In the early stages before rumination has been achieved the act differs relatively little from that of vomiting. In its earlier development, therefore, rumination is very apt to be mistaken for habitual vomiting due to other causes and may require careful observation to make the distinction evident. Nor are such babies easy to observe. This characteristic of the ruminating child is that it sins; sins only in secret. To watch it openly is to put a stop to the whole procedure. Only when a child is alone and in a drowsy vacant state, while nothing distracts its attention or excites its curiosity, does the act take place."

Rumination begins during the first year of life, between two and twelve months. There is a history of vomiting due to virus or other illness before the development of rumination. The infant learns that vomiting reduces tension and is pleasurable. The capacity to vomit and ruminate becomes established, and rumination is reinforced by the high degree of satisfaction these infants seem to derive from the process.

Rumination occurs in isolation and it is not seen when there is significant stimulation. It is symptomatic of the failure in early object relations (Flanagan, 1977) and is a reaction to parental inability to relate to the infant. In essence, the infant gives up on gratification from the outside and turns inward for pleasure. Rumination re-creates the early feeding process which was gratifying. However, neurotic behavior such as rocking and sucking of fingers also replaces relationships with the outside world.

The health of such infants is not impaired if they either bring up small amounts or reswallow most of it. However, loss of large parts of the food results in weight loss, and these children frequently present to the pediatrician with failure to thrive. Richmond's (1958) four infants were 25–44% underweight, and we recently saw a 9-month-old youngster in our hospital who weighed less than 8 pounds. So much food may be lost that the patients present with malnutrition, dehydration, and lowered resistance to infections. The mortality rate in the past was estimated at 20–50%.

The mothers of these children have been described as immature, dependent, and suffering from deprivation in early lives themselves. There is a history of marital conflict, often quite overt. There is no specific maternal psychopathology; these mothers have been diagnosed pscyhopathic personality and pre-psychotic disorders. Something in common is the inability to relate to and comfort their infants. It was noted by Richmond (1958) that the mothers reported death fears preceded the onset of rumination. He felt that unconscious death wishes were defended against by conscious efforts of the mothers to avoid their infants.

Ruminating infants have received a variety of treatments. This includes a number of mechanical devices such as ruminating caps to tie the jaw shut, plugging the nostrils with cotton, and inflatable ballons in the esophagus. Williams (1955) studied the rumination of a Banta infant with x-ray and suggested that the rumination was the result of unusual sensitivity of the sphincters of the upper GI tract. This infant was treated with antispasmodics 20 minutes before feeding, and the ruminating apparently ceased.

Lang and Melamed (1969) reported the successful treatment of a ruminating infant with the use of electric shock as an aversive counterconditioning stimulus. These were youngsters who were in desparate physical conditions.

Psychological treatment of rumination is highly successful. Unless it alters the mother-child relationship, the infant will suffer future developmental disorders. The treatment is to provide an emotionally adequate mother substitute to help the infant to form a trusting relationship with his outside environment. The pattern of ruminating is observed (generally shortly after feeding). The mother substitute holds, carries, and stimulates the infant during those times he would ordinarily ruminate. A final step in the treatment is to substitute other developmentally appropriate stimulations. Finally, the natural mother needs to learn to provide appropriate care for her infant as demonstrated by the substitute mother. Treatment of the natural mother for her underlying emotional problems is also indicated, although they are often not available for such treatment. Like the mothers of children who fail to thrive, these mothers can learn to feed their babies appropriately. However, many fail to stimulate their babies in a manner that optimally promotes development.

Neurotic Vomiting

Some children vomit easily when exposed to stressful situations such as forced feeding, excitement, and riding in cars, and in relationship to school phobia. Other children seem to respond to the emotional tension and/or rejection in the home.

Infants have few ways to express overwhelming emotional tension. Vomiting is one response to stressful tension, and an emotional disturbance of the mother-child relationship is frequently the source of such tension. Exactly how such adverse emotional tension is transmitted to the child is unclear, but in a very general way the mother's disturbance in the relationship produces tenseness in the interaction between mother and child. Ferholt and Province (1976) report such an instance in a 10-month-old boy with a history of vomiting and failure to thrive. There was an impairment in the child's object relations. The emotional tie to mother was weak, and a persistent mild psychological tension was noted. Initially, this infant demonstrated no interest in others and his own body care. Treatment in this case was aimed at providing a primary caretaker to give nurturance, comfort, and pleasure. This resulted in a decrease in tension and an increase in active assertiveness and curiousness in his approach to the outside world. Prolonged holding and feeding led to attachment to the primary caretaker. Eventually, he became more independent and was placed for adoption, as his parents decided they could not appropriately care for him.

The forced feeding of children is a frequent cause of vomiting. In infants and very young children, vomiting may be a physiologic response to overfeeding by the mother, who equates acceptance with how much her food is appreciated. It also represents the child's mode of rebellion against excessive parental demands.

> Amy, 2½ years, was referred because of vomiting, sleeping disturbance, temper tantrums, and enuresis. Amy's sleep disturbance had begun four months before referral when her father was hospitalized with a terminal illness. Vomiting began shortly after her father's death, and it was associated with her mother's coaxing to eat more. Therapy was directed toward the mother's attitude about feeding Amy and its relationship to the loss of her husband. Amy's love and attention was important to her mother as a substitute for her losses. Once the mother recognized the connection between her forcing Amy to eat and the vomiting, she took the pressure off eating and was rewarded by the cessation of vomiting.

Some children vomit in response to a stressful situation. School phobia is a classical example in which children express their anxiety about separation from parents by the psychosomatic route of nausea and vomiting. Such youngsters complain of illness in the morning prior to school, and they vomit either at home or in the school. The symptoms have their onset after a significant loss, change of school, return to school after illness, or a minor episode of failure. These children are generally quite dependent upon their mothers, and when their self-esteem is challenged, they become anxious and seek closer contact with mother. Separation issues predominate, and school phobia is often precipitated by loss due to hospitalization or death of a family member.

> Sandy is a 10-year-old girl who had regularly attended school without difficulty until the fall of her fifth year. She had attended school for one week when she became ill with the flu and missed school for approximately three days. Subsequently, she became anxious, nauseated, and finally vomited when she was required to go back to school. Her fearfulness and vomiting had prevented attempts by school personnel and parents from helping Sandy to return to class. Significant in the history was the accidental death of her brother the previous summer. Although she had showed no overt signs of mourning, Sandy had always been close to this brother. She intiated her first interview by asking, "Did you know my brother is dead?" Sandy's brother was a favorite child in the family, and the parental rejection of her prior to his death and subsequently was obvious. Sandy's reaction was to feel somehow responsible because she had not gone with him on the day of his death. Brief crisis intervention was instituted to help the family and Sandy deal with the loss of the brother. Parents were only partially able to do this, but Sandy was readily able to give up her vomiting and return to school.

Death and separation seem to be important factors in vomiting. Hill (1968), in an article on vomiting in adults, found that ten of twenty patients had a childhood history of vomiting. Four related the onset to a separation, and nine had lost a parent by death before age fifteen. For example, one woman remembered starting vomiting at age seven when her parents reclaimed her from her grandparents, who had raised her from early childhood. Another reported her vomiting started at age 7 years when her nanny died. Another began vomiting when separated from her twin at 14 years of age. Finally, one began vomiting when removed to an orphanage after her father's death. Pederson (1965) reported a case of an 8-year-old girl who developed persistent abdominal pain and vomiting that began shortly after she and her mother were struck by an automobile and her mother died in that accident. Gradually, over the period of two months, the girl developed persistent vomiting and abdominal pain. These vomiting episodes often prevented her from going to school, and there had been a deterioration in her ability to perform in school as well. The girl reported that certain foods—cokes and cupcakes, to be exact—caused her to become ill, and eventually it was discovered that in the accident she was involved in followed a trip to the grocery store in which her mother had bought her a coke and a cupcake. This had resulted in her feeling responsible for her mother's death. Brief psychotherapy seemed to have a cathartic effect as well as to help resolve feelings of responsibility for the death of her mother.

Vomiting is reported to be a fairly frequent hysterical symptom in adults. Such hysterical vomiting is also seen in children and it may be related to other symptoms such as conversion disorders. A case like this was reported by Rock (1971) in his article on conversion reactions in childhood. In this case, an 8-year-old youngster had begun to have vomiting episodes after a mild illness. The history in this family included the fact that it was an illegitimate child with an overanxious mother and an overcontrolling maternal grandmother. The child was subjected to early training and demands, and denial of anger was firmly reinforced. When he transferred schools, he was subject to some scapegoating and he developed vomiting, coma, and astasia-abasia. Therapy revealed themes of depression and dependence, and his psychopathology was seen as representing an attempt to control hostility and anger toward peers and siblings. In a sense, he could not openly express such feelings. He first had nightmares and then began developing the psychosomatic symptoms. The minor illness had resulted in more positive attention, as did the subsequent vomiting behavior.

This group of vomiting disorders represents a wide variety of neurotic reactions to stressful situations in the environment. The treatment of choice in such cases is a psychodynamically oriented psychotherapy. In the infants, some form of surrogate mothering which offers warmth, object relations, and reinforcement of positive development is the key to treatment. In such cases, psychotherapy is aimed at parental disturbances. In some cases, the mothers are seen by themselves for psychotherapy to deal with their anxieties and rejection of the children. More frequently, it is necessary to see both parents conjointly. Although one parent may appear to be the most assertive member of the pair, their pathologies are often found to be overlapping and reinforced by each other.

As the children reach latency and adolescent years, more direct psychotherapy with the youngster is indicated. In latency-age children, traditional play and verbal psychotherapy are found to be most useful. The parents of latency-age children must also be seen to support the psychotherapy of their children. The adolescent with vomiting responds to individual psychotherapy, since parental involvement may not be indicated when the adolescent is in treatment.

Cyclic Vomiting

The syndrome of cyclic vomiting has also been known as recurrent, periodic, and acetonemic vomiting. This syndrome includes recurrent vomiting, headaches, fever, and abdominal pain. The children have vomiting attacks that may occur as often as every month or may only happen two or three times per year. Each episode lasts a few hours to five days. During a vomiting episode, children are withdrawn and irritable and demonstrate aggressive behavior. The vomiting is most severe when they eat or drink, but these children seem compelled to eat and drink in the face of the vomiting. During the spells, there is an associated ketosis which is characterized by acetone on the breath, ketone in the urine, and acetonemia. This syndrome is generally reported in girls. They are described as intelligent, high-strung, and emotionally unstable. The age of onset is between two and five years of age. Although it has been suggested that the majority of cyclic vomiters grow out of the disorder at puberty, this does not seem to be the situation for many of the cases. Indeed, Hammond (1974) found that vomiting persisted in seven of twelve patients who were followed up as adults.

In 1882, Dr. Samuel Gee of London reported nine cases of what he called fitful or recurrent vomiting in children. He stated that "these cases seem to be all the same kind, their characteristics being fits of vomiting which occur after intervals of uncertain lengths. The intervals themselves are free from signs of disease. The vomiting continues for a few hours or a few days. When it has been severe, the patient is left much exhausted. Pain in the upper part of the belly or around the navel often accompanies the vomiting. The state of the bowels during the attack is uncertain, the feces are whiter than usual."

Although most observers agree about the description of the syndrome, there is no accepted etiology. Gee (1882), Gordon (1935), Brown (1954), and Nelson (1959) describe fatigue as an important precondition. Brown reported on a 4½-year-old girl who died as a result of her vomiting, and he listed overexertion and fatigue as exogenous factors that led to the onset of the vomiting.

A number of clinicians have postulated auto-intoxication as a factor in etiology. Rachford (1904) suggested that certain toxins were absorbed in the gastrointestinal tract and acted selectively on the vomiting center in the medulla. Langmead (1907) noted that at postmortem, the liver pathology of a child who suffered from this syndrome resembled that of chloroform poisoning.

The fact that the urine is high in ketones and that acetonemia is present during the vomiting attacks led some investigators to hypothesize that ketosis was the cause rather than the effect of the vomiting. However, children placed on a ketogenic diet showed no symptoms, and patients with starvation ketosis did not develop recurrent vomiting. These findings seemed to have laid to rest the ketosis theory.

Much interest has been focused on the possible relationship between the recurrent vomiting and migraine headaches. In 1904, Rachford observed four children who suffered recurrent vomiting attacks and subsequently developed migraine headaches. C.H. Smith (1937) reported on 65 cases of recurrent vomiting and noted a close relationship with migraine. In his cases, there was a higher than normal incidence of migraine headaches in the family histories. He also noted a progression at puberty from vomiting to headaches and finally, in adulthood, to migraine headaches. Alvaraz (1957) also observed that children with his syndrome came from migranous stock. In the review of 44 cases, Hoyt and Stickler (1960) reported that 36% had headaches associated with vomiting attacks.

More recent studies have noted an association between cyclic vomiting and abnormal EEGs. In 1954, Vahlquist and Nylander reported two cases of severe vomiting accompanied by mental changes which showed abnormal EEG patterns. Subsequently, Millichap (1955) found that during vomiting, there were abnormal EEGs that looked like seizure discharges in 76% of his 33 patients. Others, however, could find no correlation between abnormal EEG and the vomiting episodes.

There have been a variety of other etiologic factors suggested, including allergy (Brown, 1954; Smith, 1937; Smith, 1934), faulty body mechanisms (Talbot, 1923; Talbot and Brown, 1920), infection (Gordon, 1934; Paterson, 1935; Richmond, Eddy, and Green, 1958), and refractive errors (Glaser and Lerner, 1937).

Although pediatric investigators who have studied cyclic vomiting often speak of the presence of psychological problems, there were few cases reported in the psychiatric literature until recently. Chester (1959) described a seven-year-old boy and a thirteen-year-old girl with recurrent vomiting. She implied that the conflicts between mother and child interfered with the initial process of identification, namely incorporation. The mothers themselves are described as dependency provoking; the child patients as passive, masochistic, and showing obvious ambivalence. These children were felt to be still involved in pre-oedipal relationships and an analogy was drawn between their illness and psychotic depression.

Sperling (1968), in her case of an adolescent girl who began vomiting at age 13, concentrated on the dynamic factors underlying this girl's symptoms. The patient was described as being dependent upon her mother in reality and able to rebel against her mother only by means of somatic symptoms. Sperling viewed cyclic vomiting as a revival of infantile vomiting. In this particular case, she also saw it as a conversion symptom based on unconscious specific fantasies (pregnancy, fellatio), in expressing both id wishes and superego demands. Despite the patient's attempt to rid herself of mother through her vomiting, the symptom made the patient even more dependent on her mother.

Davenport, et al. (1972), reported on three cases of cyclic vomiting. Although there were many individual differences among these cases, there were also some striking similarities. All three were girls, the duration of the episode was about five days, and the onset occurred early in life. There was a marked weight loss during the vomiting episode which was quickly regained. The children were extremely thirsty and excessively demanding of fluids in the face of their vomiting. Indeed, the drinking made the vomiting worse. There were frank personality changes with the vomiting episodes. The children became withdrawn and depressed. They regressed to autoerotic behavior, which included open masturbation. The level of regressed behavior seemed to relate to the level of development of the children prior to the onset of this syndrome. Developmentally, the children seemed to be unplanned but wanted. Conception had been a problem for all three sets of parents, and the children were the first-born of the family. The mother's pregnancies had been complicated by hyperemesis gravidarum. Eating patterns had been noted as different from early in life. The children varied from having ravenous appetites to being "fussy eaters." In each case, toilet training was early and rigid. There were striking similarities in the family backgrounds of these patients, and the mothers have been described as dependent and showing overt hostility to their vomiting daughters.

The mothers themselves had histories of vomiting some time early in life. The fathers were described as immature and adolescent in their own development. They were seen as seductive in their relationships to their daughters. Sibling rivalry was striking in these families, and the competition for paternal attention was quite high. Psychotherapy demonstrates these girls to be conflicted about sexual feelings, particularly about accepting their own feminine identity. Although the children show varying levels of personality development, they had all failed to resolve oedipal conflicts. They were involved in seductive relationships with their fathers and hostile dependent interactions with their mothers. The parents also demonstrated varying degrees of discord and sexual dysfunction. Oral dependent and oral aggressive behavior was noted in many of the children. The mode of expression of orality varied with their level of development. They all demonstrated anal aggressive and sadistic fantasies. One patient was openly assaultive. The EEG patterns were remarkably different, ranging from continuously normal to mild abnormalities during the vomiting episodes to continuously abnormal EEGs. It seemed that the severity of the EEG disturbance was related inversely to the severity of the psychopathology. That is, for the better integrated child, the EEG tended to be more abnormal. For the child with the normal EEG, the psychopathology was that of a psychotic depression.

Hammond in 1974 reviewed 35 cases of cyclic vomiting and stressed the psychological aspect of the syndrome. Twelve of their patients were seen for follow-up when they were between ages 17 and 27. They were compared to a control group who had been admitted to the same hospital at the same time with minor complaints. In their follow-up study, seven of the group had persisted in having vomiting spells into adult life. Abdominal pains, which had been seen in nine of the patient group, continued into adult life for six of the cases. As children, six of the patient group suffered from headaches, five developed severe headaches in their early teen years, and eight of the twelve patients suffered from migraine headaches at follow-up. Insufficient data was available for assessment of psychological status of the patients in childhood. However, the psychological findings at follow-up suggested eight of the patient group had symptoms indicating a psychological disturbance. Four were depressed, three had anxiety, and one had a personality disorder. Seven of the patient group gave a history suggesting the importance of emotional stress as a precipitating factor for the gastrointestinal symptoms and migraine. Such precipitating factors in childhood included parental disharmony, disturbed parent-child relationships, or illness in a parent. As teenagers and young adults, anxiety was again a prominent factor and was related to examinations, work, and family problems.

Reinhart and Evans (1975) reported on a follow-up study of five patients who had been seen for psychiatric evaluation with a diagnosis of cyclic vomiting and eleven other patients diagnosed as having cyclic vomiting who were seen for follow-up only. Four of the sixteen patients had a laparotomy with no specific pathology found. In these four cases, there was a fair amount of resistance on either the family's or the physician's part to psychological factors being involved in the etiology of the illness. The authors felt the adjustment of three to be suspect, but one who was seen for psychiatric reasons seemed to be functioning well. Seven patients were not seen for psychiatric evaluation and had no surgical intervention. Two of these children were reported to have no problems, three continued to have vomiting episodes, although apparently not serious ones, five had psychological symptoms that were described as tense, sensitive, and a loner. There were no complaints of headaches or abdominal pain. However, two patients had family histories of vomiting, migraine headaches, or peptic ulcer. Eight of the sixteen cases had a psychiatric evaluation. Of these eight, the authors saw five and three were seen in other clinics. These patients who were seen for psychiatric consultation seemed to have fared quite well, both in regard to vomiting and also in regards to subsequent emotional problems. Reinhart focused on the parental anxiety about their abilities to keep their children alive. Their cases seem to find the child being labeled by the parents as weak or ill and generally vulnerable. The children seem to be inordinately anxious and regressed too easily and they suggest a predisposition physiologically. Their view was that of a psychological problem in which prolonged dependent relationships and failure of the child to separate and individuate predominated. That is, the parent was seen as too involved in controlling the child's behavior at a time when he should have been asserting independence. Treatment in their cases was directed to having the parent give responsibility to the child as indicated by age.

The treatment of this syndrome has varied widely according to the postulated etiologic factors. A plethora of theories suggests that the cause is in fact unknown, and probably cyclic vomiting can be considered a psychosomatic syndrome. That is, a somatic reaction to psychological stress with an underlying physiologic predisposition. In the acute stages, pediatric hospitalization with fluid and electrolyte support is often indicated. The hospital may also be seen at such time as a refuge for these children, a place where they can avoid the considerable psychosocial stress in their homes and parents.

A child who presents a clinical picture of cyclic vomiting should have psychiatric consultations to assess the psychological and psychosocial factors involved in this disorder.

Although adequate medical evaluation of such cases is indicated, there is a tendency for children with cyclic vomiting to be investigated not only extensively but repeatedly. There is, indeed, a danger that these children are overinvestigated, thus aggravating the anxiety of the children and their families and perhaps reinforcing the illness. Indeed, when there is psychiatric disturbance within the family, the parents may be reluctant to face their own problems as precipitating factors and thus pressure the doctors to continue traumatic investigations. Indeed, exploratory operations are a further hazard for such children.

The other danger of overzealous medical evaluation is a delay in considering the psychological factors contributing to this syndrome. It would appear the earlier we can intervene to decrease the parents' anxiety about their child's illness, the better our chances are for successful treatment. Thus it is important for the pediatrician and psychiatrist to be decisive in making the necessary functional diagnosis.

It would appear from Hammond's (1974) study and other reported cases that cyclic vomiting does not always terminate with puberty, that indeed as adults, they remain sensitive to psychological stress which may cause vomiting, headaches, or primary psychologic symptoms.

A number of medications appear to have been useful in the treatment of some children. Those patients who have an EEG compatible with a convulsive disorder may respond to anticonvulsive medication.

Joan is an 8-year-old girl who was referred with a history of recurrent vomiting which had begun at four years of age. She had infrequent episodes of vomiting the first year and then almost monthly vomiting episodes between ages five and six and a half years. At that point, she began taking Dilantin and was referred for psychiatric treatment which she received for approximately one year. She had no more episodes until two months prior to her second referral. Three months before her family doctor had taken Joan off her Dilantin at the family's request. It was also noted that her vomiting was preceded by an infection and that her parents were on vacation at the time. At the time of her second evaluation, she had been out of the hospital for one week and had returned to school, where she was functioning quite well, and in general, the interval history suggested that the interpersonal problems that had been dealt with in therapy remained greatly improved. She was placed back on Dilantin and there have been no further vomiting episodes for one year.

In one of the patients who had a psychotic depression during her cyclic vomiting episodes, Imipramine brought about a complete remission of her symptoms. Indeed, when the medication was discontinued four years later, she had a recurrence of her episodes, which again were managed by treatment with Imipramine.

Psychotherapy has been helpful for these youngsters in understanding their families and dealing with internal conflicts. Although psychotherapy is not always accepted, in those cases where psychotherapy has been successful in bringing about a change in family dynamics, such treatment has been effective in alleviating symptoms.

Pat was ten years of age at the time of her admission to the hospital with a history of recurrent vomiting. Her first episode had been approximately three years prior to admission, and she began having regular vomiting episodes the year and a half prior to admission. Extreme weight loss was associated with her vomiting episodes but regained shortly after vomiting stopped. Hospitalization on the pediatric service for intravenous fluids was always necessary to terminate such episodes. Psychologically, she became apathetic, depressed, and irritable during her vomiting episodes. She continued to be hungry and thirsty in spite of vomiting whatever she took in. Pat described a prodronal stage in which she felt weak, lethargic, often had upper respiratory symptoms and a "grouchy feelings in her stomach." Psychologically, she had become dependent and attention seeking. Then she would begin to vomit both day and night. There were headaches associated with the vomiting which were relieved by rest. Occasionally she complained of blurred vision. During her episodes, she became more withdrawn and irritable. Also, it was noticed that she became sexually immodest, unkempt, and irritable, which was unlike her behavior in between episodes. The family was described as close initially, but eventually it was discovered that the parents had severe problems and indeed considered separation. They described Pat as seeking affection from her father and also as breaking up parental embraces. The father had a seventh-grade education and was from a lower-class Southern family. There were numerous signs of sadistic and violent qualities in this man. He enjoyed a rather seductive relationship with the patient, and indeed, the patient said "Dad likes me better than mother." Mother was a housewife with a high school education. She reported recurrent vomiting before puberty, suffered from hyperemesis gravidarum with her pregnancies, and "had a weak stomach." She was a constricted and "too sensible woman." The patient was described as having no developmental problems, and although she disliked school, she went without difficulty and seemed to do quite well. Indeed, she was an overachiever who had an average IQ but performed at a higher level. The patient was described as a fearful and withdrawn girl who was particularly upset by violent stories in newspapers. She herself was quite compliant, showing very little aggression or negative feelings. She described fears of growing up and also of having regular menstrual periods. Pat presented as a cooperative youngster who demonstrated no thinking disorder and was constricted in her affect. She seemed unconcerned about her situation and enjoyed the attention she received in the hospital, not even complaining when she received intravenous feedings. She clearly described her father as perfect and her mother as mean, and she saw herself remaining in the family forever. EEGs during vomiting episodes were markedly abnormal in this youngster and improved between episodes but were still mildly abnormal. The tracings were marked by 14-cycle-per-second positive spikes during sleep in both posterior quadrants but with right-sided dominance. Psychological testing revealed a mixed neurosis with conversion and phobic features. There were oedipal conflicts and concerns about feminine identity. Her anxiety about relationships with boys seemed to be translated into somatic symptoms, which resulted in removing her from school, placing her with parents and thus reducing anxiety. Psychological testing concurred with the history of the father as a provocative sexual object, and the mother figure was seen as hostile and dependent. The mother was seen as a disciplinarian and ineffective as a comforter.

In the early part of treatment Pat talked about the hospital being better than home. However, when unable to go home her first weekend, she had her first vomiting episode, but there was no anger associated with it. She tried to avoid classes in the hospital at that time, claiming that she was too sick to go and that her doctor had okayed it. It was also noted that she was secretive around adults but talked freely with the other children. During her vomiting episodes, she was quite immodest. Her second episode seemed to be triggered by anger at staff for not doing what she had wanted. The third episode started when she was home on pass and did not wish to return to the hospital. She was angry at both parents and hospital at that time and quite openly belligerent.

Initially Pat was overconcerned about being perfect and correct and seemed unable to talk to any adults in the milieu except in a most polite way. The exceptions to this were during vomiting episodes, when she would be belligerent. In therapy, she began to discuss some of her fears of her father's sadistic tendencies and to explore the relationship she had with both parents. She clearly described her competitive relationship with her mother, including getting up before her mother to get breakfast for her father and in other ways competing with her mother. Indeed, it became clear that when this did not work, she did other things to provoke discipline, both within the milieu and also when she went home. Secondly, she began to take a look at her fears of growing up, menstruation, and thoughts about sexuality. At such times, she had fantasies of doing "cruel, wild, and crazy things." This alternated with needing to be perfect and at times needing to be punished for the unconscious fantasies that she had. When her mother became pregnant again, Pat became transiently angry and aggressive, indeed somewhat disorganized in her thinking. She then focused on realistic reasons for complaining about her mother in terms of age and only eventually was able to focus on the fact that she was afraid that she would once again be rejected by her mother. Following this, she seemed to accept her growing independence. Pat became spontaneous, happy, and outgoing in school.

The therapy of these children focuses on the dependent relationship and rejection in the family dynamics. The children cling to parents for support and deal with the rejection of mother by primitive defense mechanisms such as denial. Although triangular oedipal conflicts were seen in our cases, the children are also involved in preoedipal conflicts which became dominant during the psychological regression associated with vomiting. During their vomiting episodes, therapists gained insight into the underlying dynamics. However, patients needed a supportive therapeutic approach during these episodes because of the remarkable psychological regression they demonstrated. Once the children are able to recognize their role in the family dynamics, they can be supported in accepting their ability to become independent as is appropriate to their age and maturity.

Work with parents to support the growing independence of their children is essential. This frequently involves *conjoint therapy* of parents who are actively involved in the triangular struggle with their child. The parents have been seen as immature and dependent themselves. The marriages seem stable on the surface, but the alliance frequently is quite tenuous and conflicts have been suppressed. Such parents can be helped to support the growing independence of their children. They have been able to see their problems as stress factors for their children and to decrease the family pressure on them. However, the parents of the hospitalized children have been unable or unwilling to involve themselves in definitive treatment for themselves. In such cases it may be necessary to place the children out of the family home during adolescence.

The three cases reported by Davenport et al. (1972) were all hospitalized in a psychiatric hospital for the initial phase of their treatment. Subsequent children have not needed hospitalization, and the patients reported by Dr. Reinhart (1975) apparently responded to outpatient psychotherapy. The children treated as outpatients have been seen in the preschool or early latency years. In such cases one can intervene in the environmental stress and reinforcement of the symptom of recurrent vomiting, before the symptom becomes fixed.

References

Alvarez, W.C. (1957) Cyclic vomiting. *Gastroenter.* 33:1000.

Apley, J., and R. Mac Keith. (1962) *The Child and His Symptoms: A Psychosomatic Approach*, 2nd ed. Oxford: Blackwell Scientific Publications (1968), pp. 61–71.

Brown, R.J.K. (1954) A fatal attack of cyclic vomiting. *Brit. Med. J.* 2:1033.

Cameron, H.C. (1927) Ketonaemia, cyclical vomiting and some nervous disturbances in children. *Arch. Dis. Child.* 2:55–61.

Cameron, H.C. (1942) Fifty years of progress in paediatrics: Ketosis and recurrent vomiting. *Clin. J.* 71:6–12.

Chester, A. (1959) Psychodynamic mechanisms of children and adolescents with cyclic vomiting. Paper read at the American Psychiatric Association Divisional Meeting.

Davenport, C.W., J.P. Zrull, C.C. Kuhn, and S.I. Harrison. (1972) Cyclic vomiting. *J. Am. Acad. Child Psychiat.* 11(1):66–87.

Ferholt, J., and S. Province. (1976) Diagnosis and treatment of an infant with psychophysiological vomiting. *Psychoanal. Study Child* 31:439–460.

Flanagan, C.H. (1977) Rumination in infancy—past and present. With a case report. *J. Am. Acad. Child Psychiat.* 16(1):140–149.

Gee, S. (1882) On fitful or recurrent vomiting. *St. Bartholomew's Hosp. Rep.* 18:1–6.

Glaser, J., and M.L. Lerner. (1937) Cyclic vomiting of ocular origin. *Am. J. Med. Sci.* 120:553–567.

Gordon, T.B. (1935) Recurrent vomiting. *J. Mich. Med. Soc.* 34:537–541.

Hammond, J. (1974) The late sequelae of recurrent vomiting of childhood. *Develop. Med. Child Neurol.* 16:15–22.

Hill, O.W. (1968) Psychogenic vomiting. *Gut* 9:348–352.

Hoyt, C.S., and G.B. Stickler. (1960) A study of 44 children with the syndrome of recurrent (cyclic) vomiting. *Pediatrics* 25:775–780.

Lang, P.J., and B.G. Melamed. (1969) Case report: Avoidance conditioning therapy of an infant with chronic ruminative vomiting. *J. Abnorm. Psychol.* 74(1):1–8.

Langmead, F. (1907) The acetonaemic conditions of children. *Brit. Med. J.* 2:819–822.

Laybourne, P.C., Jr. (1953) Psychogenic vomiting in children. *Am. J. Dis. Child.* 86:726–732.

Millichap, J.G., C.T. Lombroso, and W.G. Lennox. (1955) Cyclic vomiting as a form of epilepsy in children. *Pediatrics* 15:705–714.

Nelson, W.E. (1959) *Textbook of Pediatrics*, 8th ed. Philadelphia: Saunders, pp. 695–696.

Paterson, D. (1935) So-called acidosis attacks: A plea for more accurate diagnosis. *Lancet* 1:917–919.

Pederson, W.M. (1965) A case study of neurosis secondary to trauma in an eight-year-old girl. *Clin. Pediat.* 14:859–861.

Rachford, B.K. (1904) Recurrent vomiting. *Arch. Pediat.* 21:881–891.

Reinhart, J.B., and S.L. Evans. (1975) Cyclic vomiting in children—through the psychiatrist's eye. Paper presented at the Robert B. Lawson Day at the Children's Memorial Hospital, Chicago, Illinois.

Richmond, J.B., E. Eddy, and M. Green. (1958) Rumination: A psychosomatic syndrome of infancy. *Pediatrics*, 22:49–54.

Rock, N.L. (1971) Conversion reactions in childhood: A clinical study of childhood neuroses. *J. Am. Acad. Child Psychiat.* 10(1):65–93.

Smith, C.H. (1937) Recurrent vomiting in children: Its etiology and treatment. *J. Pediat.* 10:719–742.

Smith, P.S. (1934) Cyclic vomiting and migraine in children. *Vir. Med. Mon.* 60:591–595.

Sperling, M. (1968) Trichotillomania, trichophagy, and cyclic vomiting. *Int. J. Psychoanal.* 49:682–690.

Talbot, F.B. (1923) Cyclic vomiting. *Med. Clin. No. Am.* 7(3):753–763.

Talbot, F.B., and L.T. Brown. (1920) Bodily mechanics: Its relation to cyclic vomiting and other obscure intestinal conditions. *Am. J. Dis. Child.* 20:168–187.

Vahlquist, B., and I. Nylander. (1954) Cyclic vomiting with recurring EEG changes and severe course: A report of two cases. *Acta Paediat.* 43(Suppl. 100):608–623.

Williams, C.G. (1955) Rumination in a Bantu baby. *So. African Med. J.* 29:692–695.

Treatment of Emotional Disorders in Children and Adolescents

CHAPTER 24

Treatment of Encopresis

Jules R. Bemporad
Richard A. Kresch
Russell S. Asnes

Introduction

Since the term "encopresis" was established by Weissenberg in 1926, numerous articles have appeared, sometimes offering conflicting views of etiology, diagnosis, and treatment. The major reason for this disagreement may be that all encopresis is not one single disease entity and that the symptom of fecal soiling may be observed in different types of children. Therefore, by way of introduction, it might be useful to differentiate the various types of fecal soiling and their respective causes.

The first consideration for the clinician should be to separate soiling due to organic gastrointestinal disease from soiling motivated by emotional or so-called functional causes. The primary medical or pediatric conditions that may cause either soiling or chronic constipation are a rectal fissure or stricture and Hirschsprung's disease. Rarer conditions which may manifest constipation as part of the symptom picture are hypothyroidism, hypercalcemia, and lead poisoning. Since this latter group of disorders present other striking pathognomic signs and symptoms, further discussion appears unnecessary. A rectal fissure, on the other hand, may present no other symptoms and may be confused with functional encopresis. A rectal fissure, which may result from a perianal infection or from straining during defecation, causes pain on elimination, and as a result, some children will withhold bowel movements. Chronic constipation unfortuately worsens the condition, so that the child may begin avoiding the toilet and display behavior similar to encopretics. A differential diagnostic sign is the child's obvious complaint of pain on defecation and the presence of discomfort from birth. There also appears to be a lack of voluminous stools. Rectal strictures essentially produce the same symptom picture. While these conditions can be easily resolved if diagnosed in time, a lack of proper management may lead to a power struggle between the parents and the child and predispose to later true encopresis. For example, Thomas, Chess, and Birch (1969) describe a 43-month old girl who was referred for psychiatric consultation because of withholding of bowel movements and refusal to use the toilet. This child had a rectal stricture that caused her to experience pain on elimination which although diagnosed shortly after birth was not properly appreciated by the mother, who mishandled the child. In this case, an initially easily remedial defect became in time a chronic, strongly entrenched emotional disorder.

Hirschsprung's disease is also not difficult to differentiate from encopresis on the basis of history and physical examination. In this disease, there is a marked reduction or absence of ganglion cells in the myenteric plexus of the muscle layer of a segment of the large intestine. As a consequence of this defect, the involved section of bowel does not conduct the normal peristaltic waves essential for the propulsion of fecal matter. The bowel proximal to the aganglionic segment becomes progressively dilated by retained and impacted feces. Although the major symptom is constipation, liquid feces may leak around the obstructed mass, giving rise to chronic soiling. Garrard and Richmond (1952) have outlined the clinical differences between this condition and encopresis. Hirschsprung's disease usually begins in the neonatal period with an initial history of obstipation. Children with Hirschsprung's willingly use the toilet and may produce characteristic pellet-like or ribbon-like stools. On clinical examination, these children show an absence of stool in the rectum, while encopretic children usually present with a feces-packed rectum. Finally, an intestinal mass may sometimes be palpated in children with Hirschsprung's disease. The diagnosis may be confirmed by radiological studies or a biopsy of the aganglionic segment.

After excluding gastrointestinal and metabolic conditions, a number of functional disorders that include chronic soiling and constipation must be considered. Often, encopresis is a minor manifestation of a different primary disorder. For example, in his pioneer paper on encopresis, published in 1938, Shirley found that of his sample of seventy children (using age 2 years as the training age), twenty had an IQ under 50, while fifteen more had an IQ under 80. In effect, half of his sample scored in the mentally retarded range, and in such children, fecal soiling appears to be part of the general delayed maturity of all functions. It is doubtful that in such children the soiling is a neurotic symptom which, as will be described below, becomes enmeshed in a long-lasting power struggle between child and parent.* In a related fashion, autistic children are sometimes encopretic as a result of their overall lack of socialization and their nonrelatedness to others, so that they do not become toilet trained in order to please their parents. The frequency of incontinence in both retarded and autistic children may have declined since the late thirties due to better institutional care and the widespread use of behavior therapy as a means of inducing continence (Neale, 1963; Doleys et al., 1975).

Another group of children whose fecal soiling appears to be the result of a primary underlying disorder is the varied types of children described by the "minimal brain dysfunction" (MBD) label. While some chronically encopretic children seem to have an innate organic defect and show evidence of mild neurologic difficulties such as "soft signs," they do not exhibit the characteristic hyperactivity, distractability, and emotional lability. On the other hand, an occasional child with MBD will present with fecal soiling. On evaluation, these children describe being so incessantly active that they do not take time to go to the bathroom when involved in some pleasant activity. These children do not present with the disturbed familial relationships or the particular unfriendly, passive-aggressive personality found in the chronic neurotic encopretic. The parents of these children do not appear obsessed with their soiling, which, again in contrast to the neurotic encopretic, seems sporadic and follows no particular pattern. With treatment of their primary disease, these children stop soiling and can sufficiently "slow down" to attend to body needs.

Another group of children who may sporadically exhibit fecal soiling are those (usually younger) children who involuntarily defecate under conditions of severe stress. One such four-year-child would pass feces when his father scolded him. When seen for evaluation, this child exhibited some minor neurologic signs of immaturity and stated that he became overwhelmed with terror when reprimanded. His inability to localize and contain his emotions appeared to result in his soiling. This child stopped soiling after the father, who was not aware of the extent of his effect on the child, no longer scolded him. Freud and Burlingham (1943) described soiling as a common regressive reaction in children who were separated from their parents in World War II. The association between involuntary evacuation and fear can also be seen in adults, as evidenced in the frequent soiling in advance troops entering combat. While this type of soiling in children responds rapidly and favorably to the removal of stress and to supportive psychotherapy, if the child is mishandled and the parents do not recognize the cause of the soiling, the child may begin to develop more frequent soiling and become truly encopretic. In most histories of en-

*Another difficulty in evaluating the literature is revealed by Shirley's study: the age at which a child may be considered encopretic. Most child psychiatrists today would not consider a two-year-old who is still soiling to be pathological. The cut-off age varies from study to study, so the samples may not be comparable.

copretic children, for example, it is noted that their soiling became frequent and chronic after some stressful life event that was ignored by the parent. The child may then learn that the soiling, and not his underlying emotions, is paid attention to by the parents, thus reinforcing the perpetuation of the symptom.

Finally, there is the group of encopretic children described by some authors (Anthony, 1957) as soiling as a result of never having been trained. Such children are reported as coming from lower socioeconomic families where soiling is tolerated and as requiring only retraining as therapy. Undoubtedly such children exist, especially in rural areas, but they are very rare in urban centers. A study by Carlson and Asnes (1974) showed the opposite trend: that in the inner city, hospital clinic mothers tended to train their children earlier than did mothers seen by suburban private pediatricians. The financially less advantaged appear to have less time and to be concerned with overwhelming everyday pressures to the point that they cannot afford leisurely and late toilet training. As a result, they train their children earlier and do not tolerate "accidents." A confirmation for the lack of relationship between poverty and continuous encopresis comes from a recent study by Levine (1975) on 102 encopretics seen at the Children's Hospital in Boston. In the primary continuous group, only 2 out of 40 primary wage earners were either unemployed or on welfare; while in the secondary (discontinuous) group, 21 out of 62 primary wage earners were not gainfully employed. Therefore, the families of the continuous encopretics appeared to be financially better off than the families of the discontinuous groups. The "never trained" children seen by the authors were incontinent because of family pathology rather than social or economic factors. The parental tolerance for a soiling child depended more on psychological than materialistic reasons. On the other hand, children who are never trained and whose soiling is no problem to the parent may not be brought for help and escape detection.

While the types of children noted above all exhibit fecal soiling, they do belong to the extensive category of chronic neurotic encopresis that is the prime subject of this chapter. Children with this disorder present with long histories of frequent soiling which continues despite extreme parental rewards or punishments. The soiling may be considered neurotic in the sense that it is ultimately self-defeating, that it is a substitute for and expresses emotions which would be unacceptable, and because it is intimately connected with pathological familial interrelationships. This type of encopresis may be considered a complex multi-factorial disorder, since it often involves an innate neurological defect, a developmental disturbance, a traumatic precipitant,a particular family constellation, and ultimately, a characteristic personality pattern. The authors have found that these are children that eventually are referred for psychiatric treatment, since their soiling becomes resistant to other forms of therapy.

In an initial study in 1971 (Bemporad et al.) on 14 such children, it was noted that they exhibited a surprising similarity in many aspects. In terms of family constellation, there was a high rate of divorce, but even in those families that were intact or where the mother had remarried, there was little communication between the parents. The fathers were characteristically withdrawn and uninvolved in family affairs. They often held two jobs and even when home did not interact with other family members. The mothers, on the other hand, were excessively domineering and intrusive. They demonstrated a strange mixture of infantilization and rejection toward their children. In addition to their inconsistency, the mothers showed peculiar areas of denial about essential everyday life activities. This last quality presented itself as a uniform and at times blatant lack of empathy for the children. The mothers often ignored serious pathology in their children (such as language disabilities, depression, psychopathy, and in a few cases quasi-schizophrenic symptoms, while obsessing over their soiling. This lack of empathy also took the form of openly revealing humiliating things about the child in his presence and in a shameless intrusion into the private affairs and property of other family members and then a public declaration of secrets that were discovered. It often appeared incomprehensible that intelligent, talented persons could be so insensitive to the feelings of others and blind to their needs.

A prominent reason for this maternal inappropriateness was their own self-preoccupation and depression. The mothers were dissatisfied with their lives and, indeed, often had valid reasons for complaint. Their husbands were emotionally unavailable, they were frequently in financial difficulties, and their own life histories revealed a pattern of rejection and disappointment. On the other hand, they seemed to perpetuate their own unhappiness by taking no pleasure in their children or in their career or family activities. Most mothers had few friends, rarely socialized, and expressed a suspicious attitude toward nonfamilial individuals. Yet they were unaware of their own participation in producing their unhappy situation.

The fourteen children who exhibited chronic neurotic encopresis were all latency-age males. Their personality characteristics could be briefly summarized as sullen, obstinate, and depressed. They were generally noncommunicative and kept their relationships at superficial levels, preferring to be alone most of the time. No particular diffferences were found between continuous and noncontinuous soilers. Psychological testing revealed a predominance of deprivation and hostile fantasies. Most showed evidence of some neurological defect, such as difficulties with fine or gross motor coordination, language disorders, or general immaturity. Half produced very immature figure drawings in spite of good to superior intelligence.

During the initial interviews and later therapy sessions, the encopretic children volunteered little, remained passive, and seemed either resentful or bored by the whole clinical procedure. This finding was fairly consistent despite a variety of therapists and settings. They did not like to talk about their soiling and often denied it. They all expressed a sense of hopelessness and emptiness regarding their relationships with their parents. When seen with their mothers, the boys seemed content to withdraw and to let their mothers dominate the interview, even though, as stated above, the mothers often embarrassed and criticized them. During these joint sessions, the mothers consistently focused on the soiling and ignored any other area of their children's unhappy lives, or else the mothers would take the opportunity to complain about their own problems, as if the child were not present. The most apparent type of transaction that emerged from these joint interviews was a lack of empathy for the child on the part of the mother and a total uninvolvement on the part of the fathers.

The histories of the encopretic children were significant in many respects. Eleven of the fourteen had been toilet trained prior to age eighteen months, and the training procedures were described as rushed, coercive, and generally unsuccessful. Eight children had actually achieved bowel continence, while the other six had repeated "accidents" prior to the onset of chronic, frequent soiling. The beginning of the daily soiling in the children was coincident with some sort of traumatic experience, usually involving separation. Five of the patients started frequent soiling when they enrolled in school, three others exhibited encopresis when their parents separated or divorced, two others after the birth of a sibling, and two others after abrupt changes in their environment. The mothers described the children as docile during infancy but as increasingly obstinate as they approached middle childhood; however, the accuracy of their reporting may be questionable in this area, since any opposition was perceived as spiteful by the mothers.

The patients' present behavior and histories indicated that they had never internalized control of soiling or acquired autonomous function free from emotional loading. In this regard, Anna Freud (1965) has carefully documented the child's progressive control over eliminatory functions in her description of developmental lines. Freud enumerates four stages in the process of achieving adult continence; (1) complete freedom to wet and soil; (2) a placing of value on excretory products, which are either given to the mother as a sign of love or expelled as a manifestation of anger; (3) the internalization of the mother's standards of cleanliness as part of a close, warm relationship; and (4) the autonomous control of soiling and wetting independent of object relations. Freud stresses that a positive relationship with the mother is a necessary condition for the normal progression along this developmental line. Furthermore, Freud believes that the internalization of maternal standards is not complete until latency, and that even then, any "child who is severely disappointed in his mother, or separated from her, or suffering from object loss in any form, may not only lose the internalized urge to be clean but also reactivate the agressive use of elimination."

This consequence appears to have been the case in the encopretic children described. As a result of the unsatisfactory nature of toilet training, these children continued or later reverted to using soiling as a means of expressing anger at others. Soiling does not progress to an autonomous stage but remains as a weapon in an emotional battle. The mother's extreme reaction to the soiling perpetuates the utilization of encopresis by the child in his relationship with her and further prevents elimination to advance to a conflict-free area of behavior.

Other authors have expressed similar views regarding the genesis of encopresis. Anthony (1957) has remarked on the difficulties of the mother-child relationship during toilet training (which he appropriately calls "the potting couple") as important in predisposing to encopresis. McTaggart and Scott (1959) comment on the family's attempt to encapsulate and deny the child's encopresis while exerting an intense interest in the child's bowel functioning. Bellman (1966) has noted that a disturbed mother-child relationship leads to errors in toilet training because of the child's inability to communicate his frustrations appropriately as well as the mother's insensitivity to his complaints. Baird (1974) conceives of the encopretic child as the symptom bearer for a disturbed family and the soiling as reflecting and concealing an underlying conflict between parent and child. The structure of the family is such, Baird observes, that it is able to displace hostility between family members onto the encopretic child, so that the maintenance of the symptom becomes essential for avoiding an awareness of other pathological transactions. In turn, the symptom serves the child to gain attention from the parents.

Hoag et al. (1971) has reported an intensive study of ten encopretic boys. Her group also found the fathers to be emotionally withdrawn and physically absent, while the mothers are described as unfeeling, hostile, rigid, and prone to intellectualization. The children were described as feeling unloved and generally unhappy, although they did not freely verbalize their frustrations. Similarly, Bellman (1966) gives a clinical picture of the encopretic child as prone to display anxiety reactions, lacking assertiveness, and being immature. According to Bellman, the encopretic child does not share in mutually enjoyable activities with his parents, has poor peer relationships, and is "fixated" to his mother. On psychological testing, Bellman found that the children revealed passive tendencies as well as evidence of inhibited agression. Other prominent themes were lack of maturity, feelings of failure and poor self-assertion, and, again, poor parent-child relationships.

These contributions are very relevant in that they indicate the extent of family disturbance in the life experience of the encopretic child and thus point the way to appropriate therapy. Without an amelioration of the family situaion that appears to evoke and maintain the soiling, it is doubtful that treatment can be successful. Instead of conceptualizing encopresis as symbolic of unconscious fecal fantasies or as a regression to the anal stage of libidinal organization, the chronic soiling becomes more comprehensible when seen as part of a total family problem, with the child's particular pathology being both an instigator and response to familial criticism.

As to why a particular child develops encopresis, other contributions have also found disturbances in toilet training and a preexisting neurological deficit which may predispose to both problems in achieving and later maintaining continence. Huschka (1942) and Lipshitz (1972) both found a high frequency of coexisting neurological immaturity and speech and learning problems. Bellman (1966) believes that encopretic children may be at the outside limits of normality in terms of neurological maturation which interferes with training.

Almost all contributors to the literature on encopresis have found difficulties in toilet training as a significant predisposing factor. There is a broad consensus among Sterba (1949), Shane (1967), Huschka (1942), Anthony (1957), McTaggart and Scott (1959), Silber (1969), and Bellman (1966) that toilet training that is unrealistic in terms of a child's capabilities is of prime importance in the etiology of encopresis.

Silber (1969) notes that cultural expectations of toilet training place undue stress on the toilet situation and that children who withhold stools tend to regard the consequent enemas as punishment. McTaggart and Scott (1959) found that premature and coercive training existed in the majority of encopretics and led to the development of psychogenic constipation as an expression of rebellion. Anthony (1957) notes a deficiency in the mother's understanding of "potting couple language," which results in mutual hostility characterized by a "battle of the bowels." Bemporad (1971) and Anthony emphasize that coercive toilet training is but one aspect in the genesis of encopresis, and that maturational vulnerability in the child and disturbed family interactional patterns are essential concomitants. Levine (1975) suspects that many encopretics are given an "anal stamp" when young, which he defines as the energetic use of enemas, suppositories, and digital disimpaction. However, Hoag (1971) observed that there was no uniformity in the method of toilet training, which led her to believe that the type of toilet training is not correlated with the symptoms. Baird (1974) also felt that toilet training is not of prime etiological importance due to lack of encopretic behavior in siblings from the same families. In the previously cited study (Bemporad et al. 1971.), the siblings of encopretic children were also found to have a high degree of psychopathology, especially of the acting-out variety. However, these nonsoiling siblings had not experienced the same type of toilet training, did not show equivalent neurological immaturity, and did not seem to have the same hostile dependent relationship with their mothers.

In summary, chronic neurotic encopresis appears

to be a fairly specific disorder that depends on a number of predisposing factors, organic, developmental, familial, and ultimately characterological, for its manifestation.

Approaches to Therapy

From the foregoing description of the encopretic child, it becomes evident that he is usually deviant in a number of significant areas. However, the one aspect of his life that appears most important in terms of the maintenance of the encopresis is his relationship with his parents. In the original sample of fourteen encopretic children, it was found that the soiling responded best to changes in family transactions. In some cases, greater involvement of the fathers in family life was sufficient to cause a cessation of the encopresis. In other instances, amelioration of the symptom was directly proportional to changes in the mother's attitude toward the child and his ability to communicate his needs with an assurance that he would be considered.

More encopretic children seen since then have confirmed the direct relationship between the course of the soiling and parental sensitivity to the child's needs and requests. It may be of significance that Baird (1974), on the basis of clinical experience with over forty encopretic children, reports successful results in cases where only the parents were seen. Without an alteration in familial transactions and attitudes, the soiling may stop temporarily, especially when the child is separated from his parents, only to recur when he rejoins the family unit.

The following two case histories are presented to illustrate in a detailed manner the factors responsible for soiling and the effect of differing therapeutic modalities. Care was given to choosing contrasting cases in terms of gender and chronicity, although basic similarities become clearly evident despite surface differences.

A patient who typifies the neurotic type of encopresis was Helen, a nine-year-old girl who was hospitalized for diagnostic studies because she had never achieved bowel continence. Helen's case is presented here not only because it is characteristic of the more severe cases of encopresis but in that it demonstrates the effect of the parent on the perpetuation of the symptom and the recurrence of soiling when the familial situation is not therapeutically ameliorated.

Helen's history is remarkable in many respects. Throughout her infancy she was hospitalized repeatedly for urinary tract infection and frequently seen by urologists as an outpatient for urethral dilatation. Despite these repeated medical contacts, it amazed Helen's pediatrician that Helen's mother had no knowledge of female genital anatomy. The mother believed that Helen's vagina had been stretched and did not know the difference between the urethra and the vagina. In addition, when Helen was hospitalized for her soiling, it was discovered that under her clean, neat outer clothing, she was physically dirty with filthy (not simply fecally stained) underwear. It appeared to the staff that the mother had totally denied the perineal area because of her own difficulties. This is a key example of the parent's apparent island of irrationality and inappropriateness, which is not infrequently found in the parents of the neurotic type of encopretics. It was also apparent that Helen's mother had never supplied the necessary structure to initiate and complete bowel training successfully. When asked about this, the mother answered that she felt Helen would learn to train herself. Helen was also incontinent of urine until age seven, when she did stop wetting on her own, although the fecal soiling continued. The manner in which the mother explained the frequent urethral instrumentation to Helen could not be determined. However, the mother was unaware of the possible psychological traumatic effect that the hospitalizations, the frequent medical visits, and the associated pain and fear would have on Helen. This, again, is a frank demonstration of the astounding lack of empathy on the part of the parent which we have so often found in the families of chronic encopretics. The mother did admit to keeping Helen in diapers until she was five years of age.

Other noteworthy aspects of Helen's past history are that her mother was forty years old when Helen was born and suffered from toxemia during the pregnancy. Although most developmental milestones were reported as within normal limits, the mother stated that Helen did not walk until eighteen months of age. Helen had a brother, ten years her senior, who lived away from home.

The parental relationship was similar to the type described previously in children with neurotic encopresis. The father was a limited, withdrawn, ineffectual man who worked two jobs and was rarely home. Even when home he took no interest in family affairs and isolated himself from his wife and daughter. During the family interviews, he let his wife do the talking for the family, and at times he would smile or quietly laugh as if he were not listening and was lost in a daydream. He showed little concern over his daughter's problems and was totally uninvolved, despite her extensive medical history. In contrast, the mother exerted a dominating influence on the family and controlled each interview by her complaints and criticisms. While presenting herself as a martyred, overburdened individual, she managed to downgrade her husband for his lack of economic success and to disparage her daughter for her soiling behavior. Beneath this façade of self-sacrificing concern, the staff soon learned that Helen's mother exerted complete control of her family unit and was morbidly resistant to changing her own behavior. She simply would not follow suggestions when they did not suit her, although she may have agreed to do so. She somehow managed to manipulate things so that she continued to have her own way.

Much of the controversy with the mother arose over the details of Helen's hospitalization. The mother wanted to stay with her, although "rooming in" did not appear indicated for a child of this age and with this type of problem. The mother insisted Helen would miss her family, although Helen gave no such indication. She kept inventing contingencies where she would be needed by Helen despite the admitting pediatrician's firm statement that she could not remain on the wards with her daughter. Throughout Helen's hospital stay, the mother kept insisting that Helen was miserable without her, despite blatant evidence to the contrary. The staff felt that "you cannot make a dent" in the mother's attitudes and beliefs. During this time, it was learned that the mother worked as a teacher's aide in Helen's school, managing to spend her time next door to Helen's classroom. She had done the same thing when her son was in elementary school, although she had to travel a considerable distance to be at his school.

During her stay on the pediatric ward Helen presented with numerous passive-aggressive maneuvers. She would take literally fifteen minutes to put on her slippers and robe if someone were waiting for her and would respond to coaxing with a silent smile. At other times she appeared not to hear requests or demands when they did not suit her convenience. On one occasion, she refused to change after spilling medicine on her clothing, and when she was not forced to, she changed clothes on her own initiative a short time later. In general, the staff tolerated her delaying tactics, avoided power struggles, and was responsive to her requests. At the same time, Helen joined in peer activities on the ward and in the playroom and occupational therapy unit.

Her pediatrician started Helen on a regime of mineral oil and having her stay on the toilet for fifteen minutes after each meal to "train" her bowel function to obtain some normal rhythmic function. Concurrently, she was seen daily by a psychiatric nurse and in family sessions once or twice a week. During the daily individual sessions, Helen was at first instructed in common sense hygiene in terms of caring for herself—bathing, combing her hair, etc. The stress was on accepting more responsibility for herself and for her own behavior, her soiling included. During these sessions, Helen was polite but not excessively warm or friendly. There was little indication of a sense of trust in the therapist, and she would purposely dawdle when asked to go to the sessions. Once with her therapist, however, she did follow suggestions and seemed interested in learning to care for herself. During this time, when Helen was given her bath, she remarked "it feels so good" and asked to stay in the tub longer. The request was granted, and it seemed that Helen was beginning to enjoy her body and to acknowledge a psychic relationship with her body.

In the family sessions, Helen usually remained silent and seemed content to let her mother dominate the sessions. At times, when her mother would complain about her soiling, Helen was noted to smile silently in the same manner as when she was being obstructionistic with the ward staff. During these sessions, and indeed throughout the hospital stay, Helen's mother refused to acknowledge any psychological causes for the encopresis or any psychological problems at all.

Psychological testing done at this time (which unfortunately was limited to psychometrics) revealed low average intelligence, which, however, was not felt to be a valid estimate because of Helen's erratic and oppositional behavior during testing. There was a large "scatter" on the WISC subtests, which seemed to reflect the amount of trying rather than any true measure of intelligence. The Bender-Gestalt showed evidence of minor organic problems. Her figure drawing was markedly immature, and in it she drew a "squiggle" in the lower abdomen which she described as a "stomach" but later described as intestines.. It appeared that she wanted to be sure to draw attention to this area of her anatomy. She had to be tested on two occasions because of her oppositionalism, and even under these conditions, the examiner was unsure of the accuracy of the test data. He described Helen as denying her mistakes, showing a surprising lack of self-evaluation, as obstinate and immature.

After one week of hospitalization, Helen was socializing well with other children and participating in ward routines. In this context, her soiling ceased and she regularly used the toilet. It would have appeared that the mineral oil regime had been successful and that Helen had needed only to be trained. This speculation was to be proved as overly hopeful after her discharge from hospital. The importance of psychiatric follow-up was repeatedly stressed to Helen's mother throughout Helen's hospital course. The mother initially agreed to have her child followed as an outpatient, but then protested that the hospital was too far from her home and that regular visits would cause too great an inconvenience. A suitable therapeutic clinic that was closer to home was found and contacted prior to Helen's discharge. Helen's mother never kept her appointment, and when contacted about this, it was learned that Helen had started soiling again. The mother said that Helen had begun soiling again because she refused to take the mineral oil regularly, but this excuse was of obviously questionably validity, as Helen had been continent in the hospital with sufficient regularity that the effect of the mineral oil at such a late date was doubtful. Of greater significance was the resumption of the hostile mother-daughter relationship that had been interrupted by hospitalization. Helen's mother stubbornly refused to seek further help, using one excuse after another. It may well be that her daughter's healthy individuation while on the ward had threatened the mother who needed to keep Helen dependent and immature.

Helen's case is important to the understanding of encopresis in that the role of parental participation in the perpetuation of the disorder is clearly apparent. Superficially it might appear that Helen had simply never been trained and that all that was required was to install the habitual use of the toilet. However, when studied more carefully, specific characteristics of other encopretic children come to light. The parental constellation fits the classic encopretic picture with a schizoid, impotent father and a domineering, critical mother who undermines the proper maturation of the child. Of greater significance is the peculiar lack of empathy and appropriate response of the mother. With regard to the patient herself, Helen demonstrated the mild neurological deficits and the immaturity commonly found in encopretics. Her history is significant in that there was no structure in terms of toilet training, and that furthermore, Helen was subjected to numerous medical procedures in the perineal area during the time when toilet training should take place. Helen displayed a strange ambivalence toward this area of her body in that she seemed to want to deny its existence, as did her mother, yet specifically drew a section of bowel in her figure drawings.

When Helen found her needs met by a responsive staff and by daily sessions with a supportive therapist, her anger and its mode of expression ceased. She not only stopped her soiling but became less obstinate and more relaxed and playful. Her symptoms rapidly returned as she was again faced with the frustrations of her life at home. Many encopretic children, in fact, may temporarily stop soiling when they are separated from the home situation only to begin again when they are with their parents. Most chronically encopretic children will only soil at home, and at first, Helen's soiling at school did not seem to fit this pattern. This situation may be explained by the fact that her mother was in the next room. The recurrence of Helen's encopresis underlines the need to work with the parents and to see encopresis as a family, and not simply an individual, problem. Successful therapy should involve the entire family in the attempt to alter pathological modes of interrelating that perpetuate the symptom. In successful treatment the soiling will usually disappear as the home situation improves and the child can relate in a healthier fashion. Even after cessation of the encopresis, treatment should continue, since the soiling is but a surface manifestation of an entrenched pathological family system, although the soiling will tend to obscure the other areas of difficulty.

The following case of an encopretic boy that was successfully treated may demonstrate the subtle power struggles and child-parent hostility that have to be resolved before treatment can be discontinued.

Tim, a nine-year-old while male, was first seen in the Pediatric Psychiatry Clinic at Babies Hospital of the Columbia Presbyterian Medical Center on September 16, 1975. He was referred from the Pediatric Clinic, where he was seen for evaluation of a two-year history of fecal soiling.

The patient was the 8 pound 7 ounce product of an uncomplicated full-term pregnancy and normal spontaneous vaginal delivery to an 18-year-old young woman. The labor, however, was somewhat precipitous, lasting only 3½ hrs. Postnatal course was unremarkable. In the first months of life he was described as a pleasant baby who ate well and slept well and presented no particular management difficulties. However, the mother stated that from approximately 3 months of age Tim was frequently "constipated" and required suppositories and enemas to produce bowel movements. She was unable to define what she meant by "constipated" in terms of frequency and character of bowel movements. Toilet training was begun at approximately age 2 to 2½ years, and bladder control was achieved before bowel control. The mother recalled that the toilet training period was difficult but was unable to specify the reasons why. After toilet training was completed, the patient had a bowel movement approximately every 2 to 4 days; however, the mother on occasion administered enemas. The enemas were given on an intermittent and unpredictable schedule which related more to the mother's whims than to the state of Tim's bowels. However, fecal soiling reportedly did not present at this point. The history obtained about Tim's infancy and toddlerhood is extremely vague, and few details are present. There was parental disagreement as to whether or not Tim ever actually had sustained periods of full bowel control. It also appeared that the parents were only superficially involved with Tim during this time, and that the vague history may result from a lack of knowledge about his actual development. At approximately age 7 years the mother noted for the first time soiling of his undergarments. This soiling increased in frequency and finally progressed to frank bowel movements, which were soft and formed in his pants. The mother reported that Tim "ignored the whole business" and would not change his clothes unless specifically instructed to do so. The frequency of the fecal soiling increased markedly in the eighteen months prior to the onset of treatment at the clinic. This period of time was associated with an intensification of serious marital discord between the parents.

The parents stated that the first evidence of behavioral difficulties with Tim occurred at about age 3 years, when he became somewhat fussy in his eating habits and a poor sleeper. Upon starting nursery school at age 4½, he objected to attendance but did not have tantrums. He showed a passive resistance, never displaying tantrums or active clinging behavior. In the nursery classroom he remained somewhat isolated and withdrawn and was a poor participant in group activities. In the first grade he was described by his teachers as being uncooperative and failing to do his homework. At home the mother noted the same type of oppositional behavior relating to household chores and general discipline. He was noted at about this time to be quite clumsy, frequently tripping and falling. He was also rather easily frustrated, excessively demanding of attention, and rarely satisfied when granted what he had asked for. He was lacking in individual initiative and would rarely do things on his own. At about the time of the first or second grade Tim began to lose all his friends, partly as a result of his foul smell and partly as a result of his unwillingness to share and participate equally in tasks. A review of school report cards in the first and second grades revealed teachers comments which centered around Tim's social immaturity, poor attention span, and lack of interest in classroom activities. He was described as either "wanting everything his way or not at all." From the very beginning Tim was quite reluctant to talk about his fecal soiling with his parents or teachers and would make somewhat half-hearted attempts to hide his soiled clothes. He would remove his clothing himself and place them in the hamper or hide them in various locations throughout the house. On occasion he threw them down the stairs and scattered them about the living room and his mother's bedroom in open defiance of maternal prohibitions against such behavior. Since the second grade Tim has had few friends and led a rather solitary existence. His only real playmates were his sister, three years his junior, with whom he gets along well, and a neighbor two years older than him who appeared to have an unusual ability to tolerate Tim's need to have his own way. His leisure activities were passive in nature, mostly involving listening to records, playing with a tape recorder, watching television, and spectator involvement in hockey and baseball. Until the onset of treatment Tim's soiling had increased in frequency, so that for the past 12 to 18 months he had rarely ever used the toilet bowl for elimination. The soiling was described by his parents as constant and bearing no relationship to time, place, or event. However, Tim disagreed and felt that he soiled himself mostly at home and less frequently at school or at play. It was noted by both Tim and his parents that he often awakened in the morning soiled.

Tim's family consists of his mother and father, both age 27, and a sister age 6. The parents began dating at age 13 and were married at age 17, when Mrs. S. was 4 months pregnant. Both parents dropped out of school and moved in with the maternal grandparents while the father held a full-time job and finished high school at night. This arrangement continued for approximately six months, at which time Tim's parents moved into their own home because of intolerable stresses in the maternal parents' house. A profound lack of parental involvement in Tim's care was evident from the time of his birth. During his infancy his maternal grandmother and great-grandmother provided most of the routine child care. Mrs. S. describes her activities at this time as "doing nothing." The father was rarely home, as he attended school during the days and worked at night. After leaving the maternal grandparents' home, Mrs. S. returned to work sporadically and Tim was left with a wide array of relatives and babysitters. Even while home, the mother described her behavior as unpredictable, with frequent temper outbursts and crying spells. She stated that she never felt close to Tim because of the adverse effect his birth had upon her life. Throughout most of his life Tim has spent a great deal of time staying at the home of either his maternal grandparents or his maternal great-grandparents. This was a child care arrangement similar to the way in which Tim's mother was raised. Frequent disagreements ensued between Tim's parents and caretakers over the methods of discipline and general child rearing. Tim's parents felt that he was "spoiled" by his great-grandparents, who were elderly and tended to grant his every wish while making no demands upon him for appropriate behavior. Toilet training was chaotic and inconsistent due to the large number of adults involved in the process. Mr. S. stated that Tim was sometimes unsure as to who his parents actually were, due to the multiple parent figures involved in his life. There was little organized planning involved in providing for Tim's care, and as a result he rarely knew where he would be staying from day to day and how long he would be there. The birth of a sibling when he was 3 years marked the onset of Tim's behavioral problems. At this point he became somewhat regressed and began having eating and sleeping disturbances suggestive of vegetative signs of depression. When asked if the second child was planned, the parents pleaded ignorance and seemed quite bewildered. Neither parent expressed any pleasure in the birth of the second child. The marital relationship was poor from the early stages, and both parents described a complete lack of communication. Very little overt fighting is described, although Mrs. S. stated that "I talked, he listened." Five years prior to the onset of treatment the parents were seen by a marriage counselor without change in the relationship. Three years later the parents were separated at the initiative of Mrs. S., who stated, "I just had it," there was "no communication." The primary issues in the marital discord appeared to be Mr. S's passivity and inability to tolerate a mutually sharing relationship and Mrs. S's seemingly constant hostility directed toward her husband. The marital separation coincides temporally with the onset of Tim's encopresis. At this time Tim's behavior became even more regressed, manifesting infantile play activities, and whiny, stubborn, and withdrawn behavior. After the separation toilet training was reinstituted in a harsh and punitive manner with frequent beatings and humiliation when Tim failed to perform to maternal expectations. His mother reported that she had no success in her attempts to train Tim and would frequently resort to physical punishment as a means of expressing her own fury at him. After the separation, the father was unreliable in terms of maintaining his financial and visitation obligations. This served to increase Tim's concern over separation and abandonment. Any hint of warmth or empathy was absent from Mrs. S's descriptions of their marriage. Both parents felt that Tim's birth represented an intolerable burden upon them, and they both expressed open resentment over the fact that Tim "ruined our lives." In February of 1975 the divorce was finalized and Mrs. S. remained in the family home with the two children while Mr. S. moved to an apartment nearby. After the divorce, the intense rage that both parents felt for each other surfaced. Bitter fighting ensued and was mostly centered about financial and child care issues. Mrs. S. displaced her anger at her former husband onto the children. She sought relief from the burdens of caring for the children by leaving them even more frequently with her parents and grandparents. She was rarely home, and there was a rapid succession of boyfriends. Mrs. S. had strong feelings that "she got the raw end of the deal" by retaining custody of the children, and in fact stated in the clinic waiting room in a voice loud enough for all to hear that "the men have it easy, they get divorced and go off and have a good time and the women get stuck taking care of the damn kids."

Mrs. S's lack of empathic response to Tim was exemplified by her description of him as a "rotten brat." Also because of his poor motor coordination, he became fearful of actitivies such as Little League baseball, but the mother would force him to attend such activities and then humiliate him publicly when the inevitable failure occurred. Mrs. S. also made it clear to Tim that her daughter was a "good girl," in contrast to his badness. She would continually compare them, with Tim always coming out on the short end. In addition, the issue of secondary gain in the maintenance of his encopresis arose at this point. Because of far-ranging family problems, Tim's relatives began attempting to avoid caring for him. His mother stated that she "couldn't get rid of him even for a weekend; nobody wanted a kid who stank." His fecal soiling thus enabled him to mintain at least increased physical proximity to his mother and gratification from the resultant hostile-dependent relationship was obtained.

On evaluation Mrs. S. presented as an attractive, stylishly dressed young woman who spoke in a voice always tinged with anger regardless of the topic of conversation. Her sense of humor was bitingly sarcastic. She described a life-long history of fighting with her own parents, resulting in her being cared for primarily by her grandparents, who lived next door. This pattern has repeated itself with Tim in that he spent more time with grandparents or great-grandparents than he did with his mother. At the time she became pregnant, Mrs. S. was an honor student at high school and had elaborate plans to attend college and embark on a career. At the time of Tim's treatment, she worked as a salesperson and was highly resentful of what she considered her "wasted life." During the course of the therapist's contact with Mrs. S., no evidence of warmth toward anyone was apparent. Her personality was characterized by an all-pervasive sense of self-pity, feelings of loneliness, her view of life as a vicious battle, and a startling lack of femininity and sexual interest in men despite her promiscuity. Her descriptions of her relationships with her numerous boyfriends revolved around her "using" them for their money and as babysitters. Her hostility toward the examiner was evident on the first visit as she began her discussion by giving a rather vituperative narrative of the failures of previous therapists who had attempted to work with Tim. Although she had read some of the psychiatric literature which discussed family problems relating to encopretic children, she remained adamant that such findings were not applicable to her and "it was all Tim's fault." The only descriptions which she offered of Tim were highly critical and deprecating. Works such as "selfish, nasty, and obnoxious" pervaded her descriptions. When asked if Tim had any admirable qualities she replied "None" without any hesitation.

Mr. S. was a flashily dressed, somewhat overweight man of limited intellectual potential who was rather withdrawn and excessively passive. He continually deferred to his ex-wife during the initial history taking. He seemed vaguely concerned about Tim's welfare, yet when asked about his day-to-day symptoms, Mr. S. replied, "You'd better ask my wife, you know I don't spend much time with him." Mr. S. saw his wife's family as a root of the problem, feeling that they spoiled Tim and that "they've never learned to mind their own business." He also stated that he had never directly confronted his in-laws concerning their activism in Tim's upbringing. His involvement with his children was minimal, having been detached when he was in the home and having been unpredictable as to when he would visit and rarely providing activities for them when they were in his care after the divorce. While superficially appearing to be a rather passive and gentle individual, Mr. S's attempts to toilet train Tim involved severe physical punishment and ridicule that increased in intensity as Tim grew older. Of note is that when Tim returned from a visit with his father, Mr. S. brought the soiled laundry with him rather than wash it himself. Mr. S. worked as a salesman and appeared overwhelmed and perplexed by the intricacies of his daily life. Superficially concealed by his outward passivity was intense rage toward his former in-laws, whom he felt were responsible for his marital discord as well as Tim's problems. He felt degraded by their constant reminders of his vocational failures. He attributed his inability to assume the role of the "man of the house" to the undermining of his position by his wife's family. He stated rather sadly that "my wife always listened to her mother even though they hated each other."

When seen in the clinic Tim was a thin, attractive, blond, fair-skinned boy of 9 years of age who was appropriately dressed in jeans and T-shirt. He was eager to start the session when greeted in the waiting room but then withdrew once in the consultation room. During the initial sessions he refused drawings and toys, preferring instead to talk. In fact, when asked if he wanted to play he replied, "I thought you were supposed to talk to a psychiatrist." In the early sessions he engaged in little spontaneous conversation but would answer questions fully and rather elaborately. He spoke with a slight lisp and had a repetitive mannerism of rubbing upwards the end of his nose with the palm of his hand. His mood was sad, and he showed little spontaneous smiling or response to jokes. He showed no evidence of thought disorder, depersonalization, derealization, delusional thinking, or suicidal ideation. His affect, although somewhat constricted, did possess a range of response appropriate to the stimulus. His reality testing was intact. His intelligence appeared to be about average. When asked what he would wish for if he could have three wishes he replied, "A baseball glove, lots of candy, and to be a lawyer." When asked his reasons for wanting to be a lawyer, he replied, "So I can divorce people when I grow up." Noteworthy is the fact that Tim's father had expressed a wish to return to school to study law. The father was seen as the person to turn to for help in times of stress or danger. A recurrent theme throughout Tim's therapy was persistent reunion fantasies with his father. When asked why he was coming to the clinic he replied, "You already know." Initially he avoided discussion of his encopresis, and when asked why he seemed so reluctant to discuss his symptoms, he replied: "I hate it" and "It embarrasses me and I want to stop." When the examiner responded that he would try and help Tim to stop it on his own by working together, he seemed physically relaxed and then began talking freely about numerous areas of his life. He discussed the absence of sensation during bowel movements and freely discussed the almost constant yelling and harsh discipline meted out to him by his parents for his failure to "keep my pants clean." When asked again to make a drawing he drew a boy with a terrified, angry look on his face. His associations to this drawing were "it's a boy, he's mad and frightened because his mother is coming to hit him because he was bad, broke a vase or something, his name is [B], that's my middle name and my father's first name." "After she hits him she'll send him to bed." When asked to draw, a female he responded with a rather infantile smiling figure somewhat larger than the male with the following associations. "This is a mother, his mother [referring to the previous drawing of the male], she's smiling because she likes to hit him." When asked why she liked to hit him, Tim responded: "Because she hates him."

Physical examination was within normal limits with the exception of an innocent cardiac murmur. Rectal examination was reported to show good sphincter tone with no tenderness and a rectum full of soft brown stool. Neurological examination revealed cranial nerves 2 through 12 intact, equal motor strength bilaterally, normal gait and mild difficulty wih tandem walking, poor backward walking, poor-finger-to-nose coordination, poor rapid alternating movements with mirroring, poor finger opposition wiih mirroring. There were no tremors noted, sensory perception and stereognosis were within normal limits; however, there was some decreased proprioceptive ability. The patient was also unable to distinguish right from left.

Psychometrics prior to the onset of therapy revealed a WISC Full Scale Score of 109 with a Verbal Score of 106 and a Performance Score of 112. Subtest scatter consisted of arithmetic and coding subtests, which were markedly lower than others. The Wide Range Achievement Test was administered and revealed that Tim's reading scored in the 93rd percentile, spelling scored in the 93rd percentile, and arithmetic scored in the 19th percentile.

An initial diagnosis of encopresis in a child with minimal cerebral dysfunction was made based upon the symptoms and the presence of "soft" neurological signs, subtest scatter on the WISC, poor attention span, and easy distractability. No attempt was made to distinguish between continuous or discontinuous encopresis, since it was not clear whether Tim had ever attained full bowel control, since the parents described frequent "accidents" prior to the onset of daily soiling.

When the results of the evaluation were discussed with the parents, the father remained silent and the mother said, "Okay, I'll give you three weeks." When she was informed that it would undoubtedly require a greater length of time than three weeks for successful treatment, she angrily replied, "We'll see." Plans for treatment were influenced by the mother's unwillingness to bring Tim to the clinic more than once weekly. Mr. S. quickly stated that he would be unavailable to attend the sessions. With these limitations it was decided that the family would be seen once weekly, and that Tim and his mother would be seen together except on occasion, when Tim or his mother would be seen separately. Often session time had to be split in order to accomplish this.

Psychotherapy with Tim consisted of 31 sessions spaced over a 9-month period. The therapy can, for the sake of understanding, be divided into three parts; the first was a period of opening of communications within the family, the second was the coming to awareness of repressed rage, and the third centered about insight into the dynamics of the symptom and consolidation of the clinical improvement.

Early in the treatment the focus of the therapists' attention was directed toward helping Tim verbalize anger and hostile feelings which were demonstrated in his drawings and play activities and seemed to overwhelm him. He would express such feelings in a passive-aggressive manner resulting in further punishment by his family, which then led to ever-increasing rage. Illustrative of this was Tim's reporting in a session of his pleasure in disrupting his grandfather's fiftieth birthday party with loud behavior and foul-smelling soiling. He explained that "it served him right because he forgot my birthday but didn't forget my sister's." Much effort was spent in pointing out the self-destructive nature of this type of behavior. It was explained to Tim early on that his encopresis was related to his inability to verbally express his anger. Within four to six sessions Tim began somewhat tentatively to assert himself at home. Initially this assertion centered about relatively minor issues such as choosing his own clothing for school, but it resulted in his getting his way and reinforcement for this more assertive behavior, such as explaining to his mother when he was angry at her rather than simply acting out his fury. Tim's increased assertion was accompanied by a slight decrease in his mother's domineering intrusiveness into minute aspects of his daily activities. During this period much support was lent to Mrs. S. in order to help her control her rage toward her son. The therapist encouraged Mrs. S. to discuss her feelings of rejection by her own parents, her exploitation by numerous men in her life, the economic hardship of single parenthood, the lost hopes for a good future and her wasted life, and her frustration brought about by Tim's symptoms. She spoke freely of her embarrassment in public places because of his odor and her reluctance to bring friends home because of the malodorous nature of her house. She sadly spoke of her isolation from friends, which was increased by her inability to visit with her children and particularly one friend to whom she had been very close and had been frequently invited with her children to spend time at a country retreat. Mrs. S. feared that Tim would never stop soiling and would become a social outcast during adulthood. Endless complaints about Tim's lack of cooperative behavior at home were empathically noted by the therapist. At approximately eight weeks into the therapy Mrs. S. reported a noticeable improvement in Tim's general behavior at home, as exemplified by cooperating with household chores, and obeying bedtime rules and at school with decreased oppositionalism, but no change in his encopresis. At this point, mother, father, and child were seen together for several sessions, as well as the father alone, and it became clear to the therapist that the father was unaware of the general problems at home. He expressed guilt over his lack of involvement with his children, and when this was brought to his attention, began to spend somewhat more time with them. The predominant issue with Tim during the early stage of treatment was fear of punishment by the parents and a longing to be closer to his father, by whom he felt utterly rejected. Efforts were made to bring to Tim's awareness the intensity of these feelings of abandonment and rejection and to help him gain some insight into the reasons for this situation. Tim was able to accept the notion that he bore some responsibility in driving away the father through his difficult behavior, and that a more successful way of achieving his goal of paternal affection was to make himself more desirable to his father. This insight resulted in Tim's attempts to gain attention by positive behavior rather than by a stubborn clingingness. As Mr. S. began seeing Tim more frequently, the second stage of treatment was initiated. However, Mr. S. encountered serious difficulty in being freely able to meet the needs of a child. This was exemplified by an incident in which Tim was brought on a hunting trip with his father and then left alone in a camouflage blind for over two hours. When Tim became frightened and began to cry, he was punished for chasing away the potential deer.

The second stage of therapy, that of heightened awareness of repressed rage, was ushered in by Tim's remaining symptom free for approximately ten days. The response of both parents to Tim's giving up of his encopresis was joyful, and the mother was able to give positive reinforcement such as rewarding Tim with money for specific tasks and freely dispensing compliments on his improved behavior at home as well as reinforcing his own pride in remaining clean. The mother then became somewhat more flexible and was able to set appropriate limits to which Tim could comply. At this point the mother made a decision, against the advice of the therapist, to embark on a rather extensive oral surgery treatment program for Tim. Despite detailed explanations of a child's propensity to react to painful medical procedures with regressive behavior and often to view the treatment as punishment, Mrs. S. persisted in her plan. She denied that the elective surgery might adversely affect Tim's recent symptomatic remission. She felt that no relationship existed between his encopresis and the proposed oral surgery, stating "Life is full of pain and he might as well learn how to handle it." It then became clear that Mrs. S. chose to institute the treatment on advice of her lawyer, whom she had engaged in order to force her ex-husband into increasing child support payments. Since he was faced with the imminent prospect of a job layoff, Mrs. S. was compelled to rush into the treatment for Tim in order to ensure that Mr. S., rather than she, would have to pay the bills. The procedure resulted in significant pain for Tim, and his mother was unwilling to or unable to provide support and comfort for him through this difficult period, instead punishing him for his complaints of continued pain. Stating he was unable to eat prompted his mother to force him, resulting in frequent dinner table fights. Tim's response to this lack of maternal sympathy was to resume his encopresis. Tim's rage was readily available for interpretation at this point. Also, the dynamics of his encopretic symptom were clear to him. During this time there emerged into consciousness intense rage and a feeling that he was unloved—in fact, hated and unwanted—by both parents. Building on his past therapeutic experience Tim directly expressed these feelings, which resulted in heightened maternal criticism. During this rather stormy period, sessions with Mrs. S. centered about discussions of her guilt and narcissism. Mrs. S. felt that she should love her child more than she did and had a dim awareness that she provided less than optimal mothering for him. However, she was unable to contain her rage over his demands. She felt that she had little to give when her need was to receive care and love herself. She felt deprived of love by her own parents and desperately sought to satisfy her dependency needs in her adult relationships. She resented Tim's pressing demands for the very same emotional support for which she was so desperately searching. Her anger toward Tim and her displacement of hostility toward males was directly interpreted to the mother, who found support within the sessions. Gradually his mother's anger turned to guilt, then to reconciliation. The culmination of the second period of therapy was his mother's offer to allow Tim to accompany her on a trip out West if he could remain "clean." Tim's response to this offer was mixed. On one hand, he was pleased at the possibility of such unknown closeness to his mother, yet on the other hand he felt totally defeated, and his firmly seated negative self-image stood in his way of overcoming his symptom. Conjoint sessions with mother and child facilitated the expression of their feelings. This openness of communication was followed by a period of improved general and school behavior much like that which had preceded Tim's prior clinical improvement. However, Tim's ambivalence was overwhelming, and he required an additional month to gain control over his bowel movements. During this time he was quite open in the expression of his intense need to retain the encopresis as his only way of gaining control over the family situation and attaining a degree of autonomy. It became clear that his bowel movements were the only area of his life which could remain uninfluenced by his mother. At this point Tim was begun on methylphenidate, 10 mg. daily, as treatment for his minimal cerebral dysfunction because he had begun to experience academic problems in school secondary to distractability. Although the reasons for the medication, which were primarily concerned with academic issues, were fully explained to Tim, he interpreted the medication as a gift from the therapist which would help him control his bowels. His intense need for emotional nurturance became tied to the pills, which became a substitute, within the transference, for maternal affection. The medication helped relieve his ambivalence, and he set a target date for overcoming his symptom. After the start of medication, school reports indicated that Tim's attention span and concentration had improved. During this period, Tim freely vented his anger over his feelings that he was not loved and that his sister got preferential treatment. He stated that "since I've been born no one loves me." Tim's rage was amorphous, directed toward his entire family, and he stated that he was willing to take the consequences of his continued encopresis for the sake of making his family angry in return. He believed that he deserved punishment because he was bad and that his family could not and would not help him. He felt an intense loneliness and became more depressed. During this time the mother was seen weekly, in addition to frequent telephone conversations, in an attempt to diminish her anger toward Tim, which was exacerbated by his openly rebellious behavior, in order to enable her to provide the support and caring that he so desperately needed. Despite these efforts, Tim's family expressed conflicting opinions as to whether or not he could eventually gain bowel control. Mother was finally able to muster a somewhat restrained enthusiasm, which appeared to be all that Tim required, as he then gained full control over bowel movements and was able to accompany his mother on a trip to California.

The third phase of treatment consisted of insight into the reasons for his encopresis and the consolidation of his symptomatic improvement. After approximately 7½ months of treatment Tim seemed to gain full control over his encopresis. Family sessions were then marked by a rather tentative communication and increased attention and support at home from his mother. At this point Tim showed a marked improvement in schoolwork and began to show increased interaction with peers and displayed a newfound sense of self-competency. During the next 1½ months Tim had somewhat frequent episodes of soiling clearly related to specific precipitants, such as mother leaving for an extended weekend without informing Tim, selling his toys in a garage sale, and scheduled visits from his father that never materialized. In fact, Tim was able to relate what caused him to soil, although he still felt that he had no control over the actual defecation. Tim became openly expressive of both hostile and loving feelings. For the first time since entering treatment he expressed feelings of love for his mother. He then went through another stage of feeling rejected, unloved, and unworthy but rather than experiencing a depressive episode as he had done earlier, he directed his rage toward the appropriate objects. The parental response was to "stop bugging him" and a type of détente was reached, with the result that Tim stopped soiling. After approximately 8½ months of therapy the mother reported that she was moving to California and promptly proceeded to sell her home. Tim spent much time in session discussing his ambivalence toward moving and his fear of living alone with his mother and sibling. When Tim was maintained symptom-free for approximately 3 weeks, the mother suddenly terminated Tim's treatment, saying that it was "too much of a hassle" to bring him any longer. Mrs. S. left for California one month prior to her children in order to find a place to live. Both children stayed with the father, who was seen by the therapist and given detailed instructions on caring for the children, which he proceeded to follow. While remaining with his father, Tim was given the responsibility of caring for himself until his father returned home from work in the evening. Household chores and cooking were mutually shared, and Tim successfully attended a day camp. The father found Tim to be less whiny, and stubborn and more assertive and cheerful. Mr. S. for the first time enjoyed the newfound closeness with his son. The change in Tim's personality at this juncture was dramatic. His feelings of inferiority had markedly decreased, and he no longer felt embarrassed about his odor. He reached out for friends and engaged eagerly in organized play activity. His mood was significantly elevated and he gave up his clinging behavior. His oppositionalism was attenuated. At last contact Tim had remained free of fecal soiling for approximately 16 weeks. The fantasies he had repeatedly expressed during his therapy of reunion with his father had finally come true. He has recently gone to live with his mother on the West Coast and is lost to follow-up.

In summary the foregoing case history is illustrative of the environmental, psychogenetic, and psychodynamic issues frequently observed in encopretic children and their families. Tim demonstrated an organic predisposition exemplified by his precipitous delivery and soft neurological signs. Added to this organic substrate, traumatic and unstructured toilet training tended to focus family conflict on bowel function. This then results in faulty internalization of sphincter control and poor body image. The absence of sensation of rectal fullness and passage of feces results from a denial of the perineum as a means of reducing conflict. Because of the repulsive nature of the symptom, the encopretic child readily presents himself for the role of family scapegoat. Feeling devalued, the child then experiences actual rejection and exaggerated fear of separation. The frequently observed family constellation of maternal depression and hostility and lack of emotional support from the father serves to intensify the symptom. In time, the symptom becomes self-perpetuating as the child's sole means of expression and control, which comes to rest in his bowel functions. The child's personality then further isolates him from key objects and fosters intensified dependency as a means of securing maternal attention. The treatment of such children must focus on breaking into this cycle. In Tim's case, this was done by permitting and encouraging the mother to ventilate her overwhelming rage, encouraging greater paternal involvement with the child, and encouraging the child to freely express his feelings directly in words rather than through his body.

Therapeutic Considerations

These cases demonstrate the difficulty as well as the need of a family approach to the therapy of chronic neurotic encopresis. Some general guidelines may be offered in the therapy of such children and their families which may be applicable despite specific differences presented by each particular case. As emphasized, this form of soiling should be seen as a family problem rather than a disorder restricted to the child himself. As such, both family and child require therapeutic intervention. While a straightforward family therapy approach with only family sessions might appear indicated, experience has shown that individual sessions with the child in addition to family sessions are helpful in allowing the child to freely express himself and to develop a trusting relationship with a significant adult. Therefore, therapy guidelines could be divided into goals with the family and goals with the individual patient.

In terms of family goals, therapy should initially stress a "defusing" of the situation. So often the patient is referred after a long series of unsuccessful trials with laxatives, enemas, diets, and other treatments that the mother is furious with her child and demands immediate results. The therapist should call for a moratorium on threats and promises regarding the soiling and explain that the encopresis is a symptom of other, more significant problems. Therapy should then shift the focus of attention and concern from the soiling to these other areas of pathology. The parents have to be made to appreciate their child's difficulties apart from the soiling. This is often a formidable task, since the family is more comfortable in continuing to view the child as the source of problems due to soiling rather than having to explore the various unmet needs of the child. In the sessions, it may be pointed out, at appropriate times, how the parents do not listen to the child or miss the meaning of what the child has to say for himself.

Concurrently, the relationship of the parents with each other may be examined, often without the child present. The major obstacle to this investigation is the chronic resistance of the father to participate in therapy. His absence is frequently reinforced by the mother, who finds it easier to deal with any problem without him and will help in his attempts at excluding himself. Despite these resistances, the participation of the father, or a father substitute, in the child's life has been found to be very significant in terms of successful treatment. While the old pattern of dominant wife and submissive husband cannot uniformly be changed, even some attempt at mutual activity and joint involvement can be most beneficial. Both parents should be given the opportunity to allow themselves to experience certain emotions that had been suppressed or repressed for many years. If this is possible, they will be better able to empathize with their child and to cease their insensitivity to his frustrations. One mother of an encopretic child who entered analytic therapy had presented a hard, businesslike exterior. In the course of analysis, however, dreams and later memories of romantic and tender yearnings were revealed. Due to a disappointment with her own father in childhood, compounded by a poor relationship with an overdemanding, critical mother, this woman had essentially stopped herself from feeling any emotion verging on tenderness or love since her early teens. She was typical of the massive restrictions that these parents put on their feelings and the threat that children pose to them, since the children reawaken painful memories and feelings. They prefer to deny behaviors and resist pleas for help than to face their own shortcomings and unhappiness. Yet an effort must be made for the parents to take the child's perspective and to attempt to view themselves from his eyes. With greater responsiveness to the child's needs, his reasons for anger, and its expression through soiling, gradually diminish. Verbal communication from the child is encouraged, and the parents should be made aware of the child's communications and to respond appropriately.

In terms of individual therapy, the first step is to create an atmosphere in which the child will feel comfortable enough to reveal his inner self. So often these children are accustomed to intrusive yet insensitive adults that they have developed a secretive, untrusting attitude toward others. They are usually passive in therapy, unwilling to volunteer information and reluctant to join in mutual activities. Extreme patience is needed, with the therapist taking a supportive but unquestionably active role. Discussions of the soiling are usually fruitless in the initial stages, and the child simply denies responsibility for his encopresis. The significant aspect of the beginning sessions is to attempt to build some sort of a trusting relationship through joint activities. A practical yet important aspect of the initial stages of therapy is to attempt to remedy the various other problems that encopretic children often present, such as learning disabilities, by indicating these to the parents in the family sessions in a noncritical manner. The point here is to show the child that his deficiencies are recognized but that he is not to be blamed for them and that rather there are ways of ameliorating them.

At the same time, the therapist should look for strengths in the child which can be used by the child to begin to build a sense of esteem and to allow him to individuate from the family unit. While most of these children are poorly coordinated so that they have come to view sports as a source of embarrassment rather than pleasure, they may display interests in other areas, from model-building to stamp collecting. These interests should be utilized as bridges to peer involvement, and the therapist may have to do some spade work in finding appropriate clubs or groups in which the child may participate.

Gradually the child must be encouraged to express his feelings verbally, first to the therapist and then in the family sessions. It is crucial at this time that the parents be ready to respond appropriately to the child's verbalizations so that he can feel that he can make his wishes known without recourse to soiling. Once proper lines of communication have been established with the parents listening to the child, the encopresis usually disappears without direct discussion of the symptom. By this time the child will have expressed his anger toward the mother in the individual sessions, and then the relationship of the soiling to suppressed anger can be explored in order to prevent future recurrences of the symptom.

A major danger at this stage of therapy is that the parents will wish to discontinue therapy once the soiling has stopped, even if the child has been continent for only a brief period. Here again the therapist must carefully explain that the soiling is only one manifestation of a whole complex of problems which ultimately may be more serious than the encopresis. Therapy is definitely to be continued until the child feels free to express himself without fear of retaliation, has established sources of self-esteem outside the home, has built some satisfying peer relationships, and realizes the connection between his anger and the soiling. Finally, the child should perceive the soiling as destructive to himself and not simply as a means of punishing the parents. The parents, on the other hand, should be aware of the child's frustrations and should be able to communicate with each other, and the father should play a greater role in family life.

These goals describe an ideal result which is not uniformly realized. As in Tim's case, resistance and regression continue to plague the progression of therapy and often try the patience of the therapist. Nothing can be left to common-sense judgment, and interpretations must be repeatedly spelled out in great detail. Since treatment of the encopretic child involves an alteration of the whole family equilibrium, it is a difficult and time-consuming task, and the therapist should be prepared for a lengthy, trying experience.

The scope of this chapter has been to present encopresis as a multifactorial disorder that occurs when a number of specific prerequisites are met. In the majority of chronic neurotic encopretics studied, it has been found that often there was an original organic defect which made toilet training difficult. Delayed milestones and continuing neurological deficits indicate that the child may not have been ready for toilet training when it was initiated or that a more supportive, structured type of training was indicated. Instead of this type of gentle training, most of the children were subjected to rushed, punitive training or essentially no training at all, with the mother expecting the child to train himself. In other children, traumatic life events occurred during the time of training, so that there was a disruption of the mother-child dyad during this developmental stage. Some mothers of encopretic children report that the child was stubborn, so that they had to "break his will" during toilet training; others report that the child seemed bewildered by the toilet training process, which was carried on nonetheless. In an initial study (Bemporad et al., 1971), it was found that many mothers of encopretic children became pregnant while the child was still a young infant and that toilet training was rushed because the mother could not conceive of having "two kids in diapers" at the same time.

Using Anna Freud's excellent theoretical model as a guide, the encopretic child appears not to have progressed along the developmental line of control over wetting and soiling. The encopretic child has not established autonomous control over his bowel functions but has continued to fuse these functions with his relationships with other people. The passage of fecal products or the failure to integrate the mother's standards of continence retain emotional value for these children and serve to express, in a grossly inappropriate manner, feelings and generalized tensions. In addition, the child does not appear to have truly consolidated the perineal area into his mental body schema and continues to deny responsibility for eliminatory functions. In keeping with this denial system, enuresis is often found to accompany encopresis, although for some unknown reason, the wetting usually stops while the soiling persists. It may be that the wetting is too uncomfortable to the child or that it does not sufficiently provoke the parent.

This lack of secure and autonomous control over eliminatory functions can also be seen in the frequent "accidents" seen in supposedly previously trained encopretic children. In periods of acute stress, such children appear to react with involuntary defecation. One striking example is of an eight-year-old boy who started soiling when a group of boys held him down and pelted him with water bombs. This child was truly terrified at the time and passed an involuntary stool during the harassment.

In reviewing the histories of encopretic children, it was found that very often recurrent soiling began after some type of psychological upset in the child's life. The most frequent precipitating event was the beginning of school, with parental separation and birth of a sibling as other common triggering events. While soiling often began after separation from the mother, it continued and became worse after reunion with the maternal figure. In retrospect, it would appear that the soiling may have been the last of a previous series of cries for help by the child which went unheeded.

Regardless of the initiation of the symptom, however, the perpetuation of the soiling seems dependent on a preexisting hostile-dependent relation with the mother who responds strongly to the encopresis.

The child learns that he has a powerful weapon against the mother in his persistent soiling. The soiling becomes an exceedingly important act for the child, since, as previously described, the mothers of these children are so lacking in empathy that they are impervious to appropriately expressed needs of the child. Encopretics may demonstrate other and much more serious psychopathology that is simply ignored by the mother. In a previous series, it was found that encopretic children displayed significant learning disabilities, marked character pathology in terms of obsessive and depressive traits, and even grossly quasi-psychotic symptoms which the parents simply did not recognize. In working with these children and their families, one begins to feel the child's sense of frustration and hopelessness over communicating needs and feeling to self-involved and withdrawn parents. Faced with a powerful, controlling mother who refuses to respond to usual signs of distress and unhappiness, and lacking the support of a father who is even more detached and usually absent, the encopretic child may well seize this opportunity to aggravate and to some extent control the mother.

The predominant feelings the child expressed toward the depriving mother are resentment and anger, which become the motive force behind the soiling. In evaluating the siblings of encopretic children, it was found that they were also angry and resentful but that they discharged these feelings in antisocial or in other forms of pathology. The siblings seemed to lack the predisposition of an organic defect and traumatic toilet training so that they did not soil. However, they did demonstrate a moderate degree of psychopathology.

In addition to serving as an outlet for feelings whose direct expression is forbidden, the soiling often brings the child a great deal of secondary gain. As in cases of psychosomatic illness or of anorexia nervosa, the encopretic child may be singled out among his siblings and become the center of attention within the family. The child may accept and enjoy the "bad" role rather than be ignored. The dramatic extent to which some mothers will go to curb the encopresis may serve to enhance the child's sense of power and control over the previously unresponsive mother and father. In this sense, most families perpetuate the symptom by focusing on it and by their extensive preoccupation with it. One of the initial steps in therapy, in fact, is to shift the concern of the family from the soiling to the habitual pathological patterns of interaction which are usually overshadowed by the encopresis.

As described above, the families of chronic neurotic encopretics are surprisingly similar, with fairly typical pathological modes of relating. The fathers are shadowy, uninvolved figures who are away from home and emerge only to exert a punitive effect on the child. The mothers are superficially domineering and critical. In therapy they gradually reveal their profound depression and dissatisfaction with their fate. From the child's point of view, however, their major flaw is their peculiar lack of empathy that results from their unhappy self-involvement and defensive need to deny feelings of tenderness and mutuality.

These are very often intelligent, capable women who resent their being trapped in what they feel is an inferior, degrading situation. They harbor grudges against their spouses' lack of financial or social success and take every opportunity to downgrade their husbands. Similarly, some mothers complain openly about being tied down by their children. There is a general sadness about these mothers, once one gets beneath their character armor, as if they had irrevocably lost their chance in life. As in Helen's case, the mother may cling to the child and become obsessed by the soiling while denying extremely important aspects of the child's life. For example, after Helen's extensive medical history, the mother was incredibly ignorant of female anatomy. Or, as in Tim's case, the mother may openly reject the child and use him as a scapegoat for her own unhappiness. In either event, the striking quality of the maternal relationship is its insensitivity to the child's requests and demands. It would appear that this lack of empathic understanding is the perpetuating agent in encopresis, since it constantly causes the child to react angrily from his frustrated attempts at open communication and allows him to seize on the one behavior that will upset, preoccupy, and bind the mother.

Given this familial constellation, therapy should

be directed at correcting the pathological transactions between family members so that the child's needs are more adequately met. From the parental side, this entails getting the father more involved in family affairs and to be more supportive of the mother's considerable burdens. Concurrently, the mother must be made aware of her child's needs and feelings, as well a her using the child and his symptoms as a cathartic vehicle for her own frustrations and resentments. These mothers also need to be made sufficiently comfortable in therapy so that they can allow themselves to experience feelings within themselves which they had suppressed years before. They require a sense of appreciation for their considerable abilities and often will perform their mothering functions better if they find some extra-familial activity that is enhancing in self-esteem.

In young children, changes in the family patterns will suffice to curb the soiling without the need for extensive therapy with the child himself. In older children, individual therapy in addition to parental therapy is necessary in that the soiling has become part of the child's emotional armamentarium and also because older encopretic children have developed other personality disturbances that require therapeutic intervention. With an amelioration of the home environment, these children require the therapist's encouragement for them to dare to communicate their feelings openly without fear of retaliation. Verbal communication should be encouraged as an appropriate substitute for the soiling as a message of anger and resentment. At this time it is crucial for the child and family sessions to be closely coordinated so that the parents will respond favorably to the child's attempts to openly express himself.

Individual therapy is equally important in order to let the child have one relationship that he feels is his own and in which he can feel free to divulge his suppressed anger and his sense of inadequacy. In the therapy sessions the relationship of the anger to the soiling should be made clear, but there should be no undue stress on the encopresis itself. Rather, therapy should be aimed at freeing the child's emotions, at helping him to open lines of communication, to find satisfying avenues of building esteem, and to form a close relationship with a responsive and understanding adult. If these goals are met, the soiling will usually stop on its own without any prolonged discussion. In the series of children seen, the soiling has never been found to be symbolic of some unconscious drive or to be understandable as a regression to an anal stage of libidinal organization. It has uniformly been most understandable as a pathological communication with the parents and has responded best to a family therapy approach.

The situation may well be different in those rare adolescents who are encopretic. In these patients, the soiling seems to have taken on new meanings, and it no longer responds to amelioration of family interactions. In those few patients seen with soiling well beyond puberty, the encopresis appears to serve a special intrapsychic function related to power and a thwarted sense of freedom. These adolescents were reminiscent of patients with sexual perversion who utilize bizarre rituals for a fantisied sense of grandiosity. Two encopretic adolescents seen were both socially withdrawn, and fearful while displaying a good deal of obstinacy and anger. Both were highly resistant to giving up their encopresis despite environmental changes.

Finally, a word of caution might be stated. As mentioned above, the cases described above are of chronic neurotic encopresis, which include a minority of children who will occasionally soil, usually in periods of stress. The findings of Freud and Burlingham (1943) on children who were separated from their parents during the London blitz should be kept in mind when considering encopresis. These perfectly normal children displayed a markedly high frequency of soiling when they were moved away from their parents in order to ensure their safety. Soiling can be a natural response to stress in children. Only when the soiling continues beyond the stress and is frequent, and there is clear evidence of its use in the service of feelings whose open expression is not allowed because of disturbed family relationships, can the diagnosis of "neurotic" encopresis be made with some certainty and the course of treatment outlined here be instituted.

References

Anthony, E.J. (1957) An experimental approach to the psychopathology of childhood. Encopresis. *Brit. J. Med. Psych.* 30:146.

Baird, M. (1974) Characteristic interaction patterns in families of encopretic children. *Bull. Menninger Clin.* 39(2):144–153.

Bellman, M. (1966) Studies on encopresis. *Acta Paediat. Scand.* 170(Suppl.):1.

Bemporad, J.R., C.M. Pfeifer, L. Gibbs, R.H. Cortner, and W.W. Blood. (1971) Characteristics of encopretic patients and their families. *J. Am. Acad. Child. Psychiat.* 10(2).

Carlson, S.S., and R.S. Asnes. (1974) Maternal expectations and attitudes toward toilet training. *Behav. Pediat.* 84:148.

Doleys, D.M., et al. (1975) Treatment of childhood encopresis: Full cleanliness training. *Ment. Retard.* 13(6):14–16.

Freud, A. (1965) *Normality and Pathology in Childhood.* New York: International Universities Press.

Freud, A., and D.T. Burlingham. (1943) *War and Children.* New York: Medical War Books.

Garrard, S.D., and J.B. Richmond. (1952) Psychogenic megacolon manifested by fecal soiling. *Pediatrics* 10:474–483.

Hoag, J.M., et al. (1971) The encopretic child and his family. *J. Am. Acad. Child Psychiat.* 10:242–256.

Huschka, M. (1942) The child's response to coercive toilet training. *Psychosom. Med.* 2:301.

Levine, M.D. (1975) Children with encopresis. A descriptive analysis. *Pediatrics* 56:412–416.

Lipshitz, M., et al. (1972) Encopresis among Israeli kibbutz children. *Isr. Ann. Psychiat.* 10(4):326–345.

McTaggart, A., and M. Scott. (1959) A review of twelve cases of encopresis. *J. Pediat.* 54:762.

Neale, D.H. (1963) Behavior therapy and encopresis in children. *Behav. Res. Ther.* 1:139–143.

Shane, M. (1967) Encopresis in a latency boy. *Psychoanal. Study Child.* 22:296.

Shirley, H. (1938) Encopresis in children. *J. Pediat.* 12:367–380.

Silber, D.L. (1969) Encopresis: A discussion by etiology and management. *Clin. Pediat.* 8:225.

Sterba. E. (1949) Analysis of psychogenic constipation in a two-year-old child. *Psychoanal. Study Child.* 3–4:227–253.

Thomas, A., S. Chess, and H.G. Birch. (1969) *Temperament and Behavior Disorders in Children.* New York: New York University Press.

Weissenberg, S. (1926) Uber Enkopresis. *Z. Kinderheild.* 40:674.

Treatment of Emotional Disorders in Children and Adolescents

Commentary: Persistent Encopresis in Preadolescence

G. Pirooz Sholevar

The majority of encopretic children suffer from developmental disorders, although many times in the literature they are referred to as neurotic. This is permissible—in its broad sense—as the symptom of encopresis, like many neurotic symptoms, expresses an underlying unconscious fantasy. However, that is where the similarity ends; the overwhelming number of encopretic children do not show the more advanced stage of ego development and the type of intrapsychic conflictual configuration typical of neurotic children. Encopretic children are better described as suffering from a developmental "arrest" or "disorder." The development of the ego and its many functions have been hindered—generally as a result of disturbed family relationships and poor parental functioning. The relationship between encopretic children and their families is frequently poor because of the parental deficiencies or pathology. It is the purpose of this commentary to examine the family's contribution to the genesis and maintenance of the encopretic symptom and to supplement Chapter 22, the excellent article by Bemporad, Kresch, and Asnes. In addition, this commentary takes a new look at the phenomenon of persistent encopresis where the symptom persists in spite of treatment.

Introduction

The symptom of encopresis ceases to exist around preadolescence or in the adolescent years except for a very small segment of the population who continue to suffer from encopresis in their adult years, and usually do not consult medical and mental health facilities.

The population described in this commentary consisted of a group of twelve encopretic children who remained persistently encopretic up to their preadolescent years. They were often difficult to treat and required from one to three years of treatment before achieving symptomatic improvement regardless of the treatment modality used, the skill of the therapist, or the frequency of the sessions. The slow response to treatment was due to many factors, particularly the longstanding and severe familial dysfunction that was the underlying factor for the symptom. In one case, the treatment failed and the encopretic symptom persisted, while in another case—even though the symptom was under reasonable control—the personality disturbances accompanying it continued.

The presence of pathology in parents and other family members was manifest usually in the initial phase of treatment. The disturbance included the personality and functioning of the parents, the relationship between the parents, and the parental relationships with their children. Sometimes, the disturbance in the parents' relationship with each other or their child was *covert* and it was only during the course of treatment that the relational disturbances and distortions in the parental self and object representation became evident. Then the interconnection between the behavior and the fantasies of different family members became manifest and suggested strongly that the encopretic symptom was the result of collective family pathology and expressed the "unconscious shared fantasy" of all members, including the encopretic child, who was an active and willing participant. More frequently, parental relational disturbance was *overt* and its influence on the child's behavior and development was manifested clearly. Therefore, the families were considered to be families suffering from chronic familial dysfunctions that failed to satisfy the needs of their members. They appeared stable on the surface (stable-unsatisfactory) or exhibited functional instability (unstable-satisfactory families) (Jackson, 1968).

The Characteristics of Encopretic Children and Their Families

The focus of this section is on the familial characteristics of our sample of severely disturbed children who suffered from persistent encopresis. Ten of the twelve children in the study were preadolescent boys, and of the remaining two, one was an adolescent girl and the other an eight-year-old boy. The encopretic children and their families were seen in individual therapy, in family therapy or a combination of the two for an average of two to four years. About half of the group received two to four years of treatment before the cessation of encopretic symptoms. The treatment was generally a family-oriented one taking into account all the disturbances in family relationships in addition to the behavior and functioning of the encopretic child.

The study suggests that the families of children with persistent encopresis demonstrate distinct personality characteristics and transactions that are related to soiling and will be explained below in greater detail.

The Mothers

The mothers of encopretic children showed all or some of the following characteristics. *Depression* was frequently present. At the onset of treatment, the mothers often did not recognize their "depression" and unhappiness. They could be referred to more appropriately as being in a state of covert or masked depression with generalized low ego activity, low ability to recognize their affective state, and inability to recognize and deal with losses (Cytryn and McKnew, 1972). The mothers became cognizant of their depression after their general condition and self-observation ability improved through treatment. One such mother described herself as having carried a cross for years without noticing it.

The mothers of encopretic children led lonely and *isolated* lives. They had tremendous feelings of mistrust toward others and saw people as a source of humiliation, pain, and danger. They felt cut off (Bowen, 1978) from friends, from family, and especially from men. One common way of distancing themselves from others was by failing to care for their physical appearance and allowing themselves to become obese. Significant *obesity* was a finding in about half of the members in the group studied.

One of the most striking features of the mothers of encopretic children was their *extremely low self-esteem*. They considered themselves failures in all areas of their lives; their parents were critical of them and they were not well regarded by their friends and neighbors. Educationally they had done poorly, which contributed to their negative self-images. As wives, they had failed, since their marriages were turbulent and unsatisfactory, or had broken up. They also felt inadequate sexually or unable to attract, enjoy, or gratify their sexual partners. And, if all that was not enough, they felt they had failed as mothers because their children could not even perform such a basic function as controlling their bowels. Their feeling of worthlessness and inadequacy predisposed them to assume a masochistic posture where they expected, sought and received poor treatment from others.

Their *masochistic posture* was similar to moral masochism but it was based on a predominant feeling of *worthlessness* rather than the unconscious feeling of guilt. However, their search for punishment was similar to patients with moral masochism. They sought out and accepted depreciating, sadomasochistic relationships with women and men and subsequently with their children. It was as if they felt unworthy or undeserving of good treatment by others because they themselves had never been treated well.

The narcissistic depletion and the inability of the mothers to value themselves was extended to their children as extensions of themselves. The children's needs were unattended, and they were seen as worthless or evil. They abandoned their children emotionally as they felt abandoned by everyone else, including their own parents, their spouses, and their children. The longstanding emotional starvation of the mothers and their unsatisfied narcissistic needs often resulted in the parentification of their child. Self-centeredness and immaturity were also present in encopretic children, who in turn exhibited the same behavior with their peers and teachers.

Mothers were generally dissatisfied with all aspects of their lives but resigned to their fate and therefore did not attempt to change the areas of their dissatisfaction. This lack of impetus to change could be attributed to chronic feelings of depression, resignation, worthlessness, and the conviction that they did not deserve much. These feelings were rooted acutally in the early experiences of the mothers as young children and their position in their families of origin.

Hostility and *anger* were prominent personality traits of the mothers of encopretic children. Their anger was so profound at times that some mothers avoided talking or even looking at other people, while others were constantly angry and sarcastic toward their children, husbands, therapists, and parents.

The mothers were easily angered by the therapist's expectation that they attend treatment sessions regularly, by any delay in their appointments, by persistence in the child's symptoms while in treatment, by falsely perceiving criticism during sessions, or even by the therapists's expressed hope in their success in any venture they undertook.

The mothers were *fearful of men* and harbored tremendous hostility toward them. This was rooted in their hostile, dependent relationship with their own mothers, where a third person was perceived as a threat to the tense mother-child dyad. Furthermore, it was related to their early unsatisfactory or nonexistent relationships with their own fathers, which were transferred later to their relationships with men. This resulted in brief, conflictual and unsatisfactory encounters with men. They chose men who were immature and infantile. If marriages occurred, they were unstable, conflictual, and usually ended in dissolution. This left the mothers with the viewpoint that men were irresponsible, selfish, and unavailable. Furthermore, men were seen as unappreciative of family life, since they exploited women sexually, made them pregnant, and then abandoned both mother and child. They viewed men as dangerous people who had temper tantrums and broke furniture or hit their wives. With the departure of the husbands, the wives' hositility was directed toward the male children. They reproduced the fathers' characteristics of irresponsibility, immaturity, and tantrums in their children in order to maintain their sadomasochistic relationship with the new object. It is therefore no surprise that encopresis was found to be much more common in boys than girls.

Together with a mistrust of men, there was a negative attitude toward sexual relationships. The mothers' *sexual problems* ranged from sexual abstinence and frigidity to frank homosexuality. Sexual conflicts were responsible for the breakup of many families in the sample. One mother left her husband due to his masturbation or "abnormal sexual practices," while another drove her husband to continual extramarital sexual relationships by refusing sexual intimacy.

To summarize, the characteristics of mothers of encopretic children were as follows: they were women who felt worthless and inadequate in coping with life and reacted to external demands with anger, hositility, depression, and withdrawal from society.

The Fathers

The absence of the fathers was a significant finding in this group of twelve encopretic children. This was generally the result of the marriages' disintegration following a prolonged period of conflict. Therefore, we were left with only a hazy picture of many of the fathers of encopretic children.

There was direct information from two fathers who had remained with their families and indirect information from wives about separated husbands. The indirect information about husbands was regarded with caution, as it was given by women who were hostile toward men and had severe personality problems. For example: Mrs. G. thought that the "abnormal sexual practices" of her ex-husband would ruin her son and that the father would teach her son to masturbate. She kept her son with her on dates to prevent him from visiting his father. The major reason for her attempts to compete with the father concerned her fear that the son would leave her just as other men had done in the past.

The presence of the father in the family was an unusual finding, both in our sample and for encopretic children at large. As Bemporad et al. (1971) have reported, there is a cessation of soiling once a man enters and stays in the family unit. An interesting finding in this sample was that in the two cases where the father was present at home, one of the encopretic children was a girl—an unusual finding—while the other child was adopted. In the former family, there was a significant degree of covert undermining among family members, with a strong coalition formation between the daughter and the mother against the father. In the latter family, the couple was emotionally divorced. The father was extremely passive and uninvolved with the care of his adopted son.

The fathers of encopretic children were described generally as immature, dependent, and infantile. Some of the fathers had a history of soiling to ages ten or eleven. Other fathers were very dependent on their own mothers even as grown men. Often they were totally passive and gave their wives free rein to rule the household while they themselves remained uninvolved in family life.

Three of the fathers included in the study were described as aggressive, impulsive, and violent, particularly when their wives rejected them sexually. This impulsiveness, when added to the sexual disinterest and rejection by their wives, gave rise to maladaptive or potentially destructive behavior such as incest, infidelity, or excessive masturbation, which made the husbands, at least on the surface, seem more responsible than their wives for the child's problems. The mothers used the action of their husbands as further rationalization to strengthen their original beliefs that men were perverted, selfish, and dangerous.

Some of the fathers remained interested in their children in spite of their wives' erecting all kinds of barriers—including legal ones—to make it impossible for fathers and sons to visit each other. The mothers frequently undercut the fathers by constant criticism, often finding fault with fathers for failing to plan activities for their children and only watching TV, a fault of which the mothers were also guilty. Some of the fathers actually planned more activities with the children than the mothers did.

Encopretic Children

The children with persistent encopresis in this study showed other behavioral disturbances in addition to the symptom of encopresis. Feelings of worthlessness and low self-esteem, as part of an underlying poorly organized and masked depressive syndrome—reminiscent of their mothers—were present in a number of children. When improvement occurred through treatment, the children began to recognize their feelings of rejection and depression. A clear example was a child who became depressed overtly and made several suicide attempts while in treatment in a psychiatric hospital. Another child had an accidental injury after he had expressed death wishes, while still another child complained constantly that his mother did not love him and was at the same time extremely jealous of his sibling.

More than half of the encopretic children showed significant limitations in their ability to relate to others and remained *isolated* and friendless and exhibited shallowness in their relationships. In one case, the child's behavior remained extremely withdrawn even after two years of outpatient treatment followed by two years of treatment at a residential center—he was probably the most withdrawn child in a large residential center. Isolation of affect was present to a lesser degree in half of the children. The children's relationships with their therapists deepened very slowly, this shallowness being a repetition of their distant, isolated, and disturbed family relationships in addition to the lack of basic trust, and the shame and embarrassment around the encopretic symptom. Other children used different modes of distancing in treatment, like constant provocation in sessions or frequently missed appointments that served as a barrier to closeness.

The encopretic children were often fearful of growing up and becoming men, which would have made them a clear target of their mothers' hostility toward men. This perception resulted in heightened castration anxiety, fear of bodily injury, feelings of bodily defectiveness, and lack of pride in their physical selves. Their strong fear of being bodily harmed resulted in their passivity and avoidance of competition and sports. The symptom of soiling here served as a manifestation of their anxiety about growing up and their wish to remain young. It also explained why encopresis occurred in eleven boys in comparison to only one girl in the sample.

Other associated behavioral disturbances in this group of children included: school truancy, learning disorders, fire-setting, poor impulse control, obesity, temper tantrums, and diurnal or nocturnal enuresis (present in less than half of the group).

In summary, the encopretic children manifested other symptoms in addition to encopresis, such as social withdrawal, isolation of affect, lack of self-esteem, depression, suicidal tendencies, and conflict over their masculinity. The combination of these symptoms caused their lives to be lonely and fearful.

Family Relationships

The families of children with persistent encopresis showed many signs of dysfunction in the nuclear family as well as in the relationship between the nuclear and extended families. The mothers were generally the "carriers" of the dysfunction between the extended and nuclear family systems. They felt rejected by their own parents, as they had often been severely exploited by one of their parents—usually the mother—against the father. Their mental representation of women was that of rejecting people and men as frightening ones. The mothers carried their feelings of rejection into their new families. Their attempts at forming their own families failed quickly due to severe distortions in their development and in their object relationships. Thus marital relationships were doomed from the onset. They found men who were equally incapable of relating, and then dealt with their fear of losing their newfound partners by denying relational conflicts. The inability to recognize and resolve conflicts was a contributor to the marital breakups. For example, one mother became furious with people who informed her of the infidelity of her husband. She preferred to "believe" flat tires or car breakdowns kept him away from home every night until early the next morning.

Embittered by the disappointments following their marriages, the mothers' self-esteem was lowered even further and they became even more disillusioned and isolated themselves not only from their families of origin but from acquaintances and friends. One of the children became the representative and recipient of all the bitterness toward the disappointing objects; boys, particularly, were chosen to be accountable for the action of the men (fathers and husbands). By keeping the child soiling and infantile, he would not grow up and become a frightening or rejecting man. At the same time, the encopretic child functioned as the covert "punisher" of the mother and satisfied her masochistic longings by acting as a substitute for her past "objects."

Encopretic children responded to their deeply felt rejection by withdrawal, isolation, and poor self-images. They felt unprotected, vulnerable, and fearful of being harmed; furthermore, they lacked the degree of self-observation, ego organization, and parental guidance to recognize their situation. As a result of this poor functioning, their relationships and academic work suffered and they remained infantile and constantly sought immediate gratification.

Denial of conflict and lack of conflict resolution were significant aspects of the dysfunctional family system and involved the marital and parental relationships in extended and nuclear families. An example of how far encopretic families went to avoid open conflict was a severely encopretic child who was excluded from basketball games by his peers because he "stank" (soiling). The parents did not "notice" an odor but kept the windows open in winter to have fresh air circulating in the room. This avoidance of conflict decreased the chance of conflict resolution and was motivated by the longstanding multigenerational relational difficulties in the family. They feared that any expressed conflict would unleash all the accumulated hostilities in past and present family relationships and result in a total breakup of the family unit. They therefore concluded that the only way of maintaining relationships was by denying differences and conflicts. This is similar to the "pseudomutual" pattern of relationship described in the literature (Wynne et al., 1958).

Treatment

Persistent encopresis in preadolescence is related to significant disturbances in familial relationships which effect many family members besides the encopretic child. The therapeutic approach should be family-oriented and should address the many unmet needs and deficiencies in the familial relationships.

A significant degree of dissatisfaction and depressive constellation is present in the mother, the child, and the father of encopretic families. The parents are usually unaware—at the initial phase of treatment—of their disappointments and miseries due to their low level of self-observation and poor ego functioning. A major therapeutic goal here is to make the family members aware of the pervasive and multiple familial sources of discontent beyond the symptom of soiling. Often this is accomplished by increasing the family's observational ability of themselves and other family members so that each has a better appreciation of his own needs and of the needs of other family members. This also helps them differentiate themselves from the fused family ego mass and begin the slow, painstaking process of individuation. As this process evolves, the family members begin to recognize how miserable they are and how little they do to alleviate it.

Social withdrawal is characteristic of the encopretic family. Again, all family members need help in recognizing how they mistrust and avoid each other. The therapist should attempt to develop an atmosphere of trust and recognition of mutual needs in the family and help the members satisfy their own needs as well as the needs of other family members. The unmet needs of *all* family members should be brought into the open. This phase of treatment should be followed by encouraging different family members to find active ways of satisfying their needs and building positive self-images. This will free the children to socialize, make friends, and act in such a way that would endear them to their peer group rather than drive their peers away.

The mothers of encopretic children will often prove to be resistant to the establishment of any relationship, so it is necessary to pursue a variety of possibilities to improve their social lives, such as reestablishing ties with their friends and families of origin or joining a church group. Obtaining a job helps to increase their feeling of self-esteem, improve their financial situation, and open up new vistas, since they have chances to meet new people. Taking care of their physical appearance enhances the possibility of developing new friendships and should be encouraged, but the building of relationships with men may prove to be extremely difficult for these women. This is related to their very low self-esteem as well as previous painful experiences with men, which have left them with tremendous hostility and feelings of anxiety. Therefore, the establishment of relationships with men cannot be one of the earliest steps in countering isolation and might prove unattainable even in the advanced stages of treatment.

The therapist himself is one of the most important tools used in the treatment of encopretic families. In his interactions with the family, the therapist should act as a model of openness, sensitivity, self-observation, self-expression, and responsiveness to the needs of the family. He establishes himself as an attentive, interested person who views each member of the family as a distinct and valuable person, treating him accordingly. He attempts to be insightful about himself, and avoids confusing his actions and motivations with those of family members. In addition to that, the therapist is not exploitative, intrusive, neglectful, or abusive, which are the characteristic modes of relating in families of encopretic children. Other important qualities the therapist brings to the treatment are feelings of positiveness, optimism, and adequacy. These feelings are contrary to the feelings pervading the families of encopretics that nothing good is going to happen.

The families of encopretic children also show a weakness in their *sense of reality*. As nothing is going to work out for them, they do not feel the urge to do anything. They act as if they do not have to do the necessary tasks. Translated into the language of everyday life, this means that the family rules do not require that a person go to the bathroom when the urge is present, nor does he have to go to school, to work, or to visit anyone. This weakness in the sense of reality and responsiblity is related to feelings of hopelessness, hostility, helplessness, resignation, and inadequacy. To counter these feelings, the therapist should present himself as someone who respects what has to be done, looks forward to challenges, does his best to succeed, and helps the family to do the same.

Successful solutions for persistent encopresis in outpatient psychotherapy is not always possible. At times the underlying strong negative feelings of rejection and hostility among family members persist in spite of prolonged or intensive therapeutic attempts. In such cases, the clarification of the motivations of different family members can actually unearth a persistent, deep-seated rejection of the child. For example, in one such instance, the perception of such negative attitudes by the child made him depressed and suicidal. These factors required additional intervention, and the child was admitted to a residential treatment center. Work with the family continued toward the exploration and elimination of the hostile and negative attitudes toward the child and mobilizing positive feelings for him. The mother was encouraged to take a more active part in fulfilling her life, and with her increased satisfaction in her own life, she reached a point eventually when she began to show more interest in her child.

When the encopretic child is admitted to a residential treatment center, the symptom of encopresis generally ceases immediately following admission for several reasons; these include peer and staff pressure, and reduction in covert family support for the symptom. However, sometimes the control of soiling in such circumstances is achieved through witholding of feces, severe constipation, and fecal impaction. This tendency is seen commonly when children are faced wit the prospect of loss (i.e., leaving home or a facility). Their inability to deal with loss results in their becoming possessive toward their feces. The absence of the encopretic symptom in residential centers brings the focus on other symptoms, such as poor peer relations, depression, suicidal thoughts, or impulsivity.

It is important for the residential staff to know if a child has a history of soiling, as it helps with the recognition of the child's personality structure. It also helps the staff recognize "the offender" when and if the symptom of encopresis reappears in the residence. For example, in a residential treatment center, some feces would periodically mysteriously appear in the swimming pool, and the staff was at a loss to determine where it had come from. The review of the record of the children in the residence showed that two out of sixty children had a history of encopresis. It was established very quickly that one of of the two previously encopretic children had been under stress and had temporarily resorted back to the symptom of encopresis. The knowledge of this historical fact was helpful to the staff in figuring out how to deal with the situation.

When encopresis persists into preadolescence and adolescence, in addition to the troublesome symptom itself, there is often damage to the personality, resulting in such maladaptive character traits as passivity, withdrawal, and isolation, or inability to respond appropriately in stressful situations without regressive soiling. An example of the latter situation was an encopretic child who became free of encopresis in the mid-phase of his treatment. Two years following the termination of treatment, when fearing a confrontation with his father about a stressful situation, the child became temporarily encopretic. Once the confrontation was over, the symptom of encopresis disappeared.

The suggested treatment of the persistent encopretic child and his family is family-oriented and entails many changes, including restructuring the family system and helping the family members to individuate and differentiate themselves from the undifferentiated family mass. In-depth focus on the relationship within the families of origin may be necessary for achievement of this goal; this may be a long and arduous process and take up to three to four years to achieve.

In summary, this commentary describes the family relationships and characteristics of the encopretic child and his parents and points out the difficulties in treating the persistent encopretic symptom that extends into preadolescence. Treatment goals and strategies for persistent encopresis are discussed.

Acknowledgement

The valuable editorial assistance of Ms. Marilyn Luber is acknowledged.

References

Bemporad, J.R., C.M. Pfeiffer, L. Gibbs, R.H. Cortner, and W. Blood. (1971) Characteristics of encopretic patients and their families. *J. Am. Acad. Child. Psychiat.* 10(2):272–292.

Bowen, M. (1978) *Family Therapy and Clinical Practice.* New York: Jason Aronson.

Cytryn, L., and D.H. McKnew. (1972) Proposed classification of childhood depression. *Am. J. Psychiat.* 129:2.

Jackson, D. (1968) *Communication, Family and Marriage.* New York: Science House.

Wynne, L.C., I. Ryckoff, J. Day, and S.I. Hirsch. (1958) Pseudomutuality in the family relations of schizophrenics. *Psychiatry* 21:205–220.

Part V

Treatment of Special Disorders

Treatment of Emotional Disorders in Children and Adolescents

CHAPTER 25

Borderline States and Ego Disturbances

Rudolf Ekstein

"All thinking is metaphoric."
—Robert Frost

"All our truth, or all but a few fragments, is won by metaphor."
"Literalness we cannot have."
—Clive Staples Lewis

Introduction to the Concept

In order to narrow down the task of defining the concept of *borderline conditions*, a concept now very much in vogue, used in many different ways, I have traveled back surveying my own labors in this field for some thirty years, and have found that the opening paragraph of a communication (Ekstein and Wallerstein, 1954, p. 344) prepared almost twenty-five years ago concerning *Observations on the Psychology of Borderline and Psychotic Children* fits today's task as well. We stated then:

He who ventures to accompany the borderline or psychotic child into the *terrain of his inner world* will find his journeys beset with many special hazards and bewildering phenomena. We refer not to *the fluid landscape* or to the archaic figures which emerge, coalesce and disappear, only to rise again in more monstrous display. For despite the dimness of the landscape, some maps have already been charted and reports of previous travelers are available for aid. However, even the most seasoned traveler will be puzzled by phenomena of *arrival and departure in this world of fantasy.* Once having communicated his readiness to embark upon these journeys in whatever guise the child requires, the traveler cannot but wonder at the exact moment and at the startling abruptness with which the voyages commence and terminate. Nor can he help but speculate that a knowledgeable grasp of *the time table* might provide him not only with more adequate preparation for the journey, but with the means for affecting the course and destination of his young guide as well.

We describe children whose adjustment was marginally located in their use of both neurotic and psychotic mechanisms, a clinical group described as borderline, as schizophrenic-like, as severely neurotic, as acting out, and the like. Certainly, these children did not fit the kind of ideal classification that Kraepelin strived for, that researcher dedicated to thoroughness and excellence, and whose classification for psychotic disorders, whose delineation of the symptomatology has dominated diagnostic classification systems for a long period of time. A marked and frequent, often abrupt fluctuation in ego states as they emerge during the treatment process characterizes the patient group of concern to us.

The map of the landscape we then described was certainly not drawn by Kraepelin, to whose enormous self-discipline we owe the classification of the psychoses, a system which had been generally accepted and still influences our diagnostic thinking. We cannot expect much help from his systematizing rigor as we attempt to define the nature of the borderline condition in childhood and adolescence. Since our earlier observations of borderline children and adolescents, and our psychotherapeutic experimentations, discussed and described in a variety of publications (such as Ekstein, 1966, 1971), many in the field have contributed to the challenging issue and have traveled in the terrain of the inner world of such patients, have described landmarks, discovered one or another path, but the *terrain* is still like the unknown jungle, *full of dangers and surprises*, and unsolved questions.

Historical Comments

Psychoanalytic contributions frequently describe these difficulties of the borderline conditions in terms of ego psychology (Geleerd, 1958) or in terms of object relations (Gilpin, 1976; Kernberg, 1975). It proves most useful to think of borderline conditions as a continuum from one extreme to the other, and to relate the nature of this continuum to the developmental scheme (Masterson, 1972).

We might choose to describe a continuum between the primary and secondary process, between autism, symbiosis, and object-self diffferentiation, or between a chaotic ego and a developed, mature ego structure.

Most authors usually refer to borderline conditions as lacking a clear point of diffferentiation, so that the child or adolescent may move quickly back and forth between regressed and progressing states of psychic functioning. No clear differentiation can be made, let us say, between a psychotic and/or neurotic state or between schizophrenic or psychopathic states of mind, between neurotic functioning and severe acting out, etc. The states of separation and individuation in each of these patients can never clearly be defined. They are as fluctuating as is the vulnerable, not yet consolidated ego, and that, of course, holds true for object and self representations.

Recently, in referring to the ever-growing literature on the borderline conditions in adults, in adolescence, and in childhood, I have attempted to use an analogy that will not allow for a concise definition of the borderline syndrome, but will point in the direction that clinical research must go. Previous writings of mine (Ekstein, 1966, 1971), of Kernberg (1975), of Mahler and Furer (1968), of Masterson (1972), and many others contain additional reviews of the major contributions and milestones, and I will not deal with them except whenever it will be necessary in developing my theme.

Theoretical Considerations

I will try now to develop some theoretical considerations I consider necessary in order to approach the issue of treatment techniques, limits of treatment, and further questions.

I spoke earlier about the confusing, bizarre, and often frightful inner landscape of the borderline child and/or adolescent. In a book review (Ekstein, 1973) concerning Masterson's work (Masterson, 1972) on borderline conditions, I wondered about the choice of the concept *borderline*. It makes one imagine a border existing between two countries. Usually, in many parts of the world this border is clear and well defined, recognized by both countries, respected, etc. We can cross these borders under certain conditions, such as showing a passport; we may need a visa to enter the other country, etc. It is usually quite clear to which country one belongs, and one knows the regulations permitting one's entry into the other country, or coming back to the country of origin, etc. We also know the rules permitting us to immigrate, to acquire another nationality, etc. But these conditions allowing movement back and forth do not always follow normal expectations.

By now it ought to be clear I refer to the difference between borderline and normal conditions of mental functioning. We may, in our fantasy, travel to the Land of Oz, but we can give up this fantasy quickly and return to normal thought, reality tasks, realistic considerations. We may fall asleep, have our ego regress to a hypnagogic or dream state, may even perhaps have a nightmare and for short moments be unable to differentiate between the waking state and sleeping state, but we usually recover soon, and know how to return to wakefulness, etc. We may for short intervals lose our temper and become slightly paranoid or over-anxious, and under stress we all have temporary breaking points, but we can usually return to the land of origin, the normal state of mind. To return to the geographic metaphor: not all borders are like the one between Canada and the United States, where citizens of both countries do not need visas and have comparatively easy requirements allowing movement across the borders. The condition is quite different on the Mexican border, where movement is not quite so easy. There are those who are allowed to move easily from one country to another, while others are illegal trespassers who will be returned if they are found; others who hide awaiting or avoiding legal complications, etc.

I am now speaking about trespassers, about border guards, and about the nature of the border itself. Between certain countries the borders are ill defined, and from time to time these countries are at war concerning the *clarification* of these border issues. There may be shooting at the border, and the terrain between two countries may be so ill defined that one may not know whether one is in China, let us say, in India, or in Tibet.

Usually we know our way in our own territory very well, but if we go into a foreign territory we may feel lost. We may not know the language spoken. We may not know the customs, the way to stay alive, the way to obtain a work permit, to work, and to understand the unknown reality.

If one were to speak about those who cross borders to work, one could think of all kinds of conditions that allow for normal crossings, as well as those crossing which are illegal, dangerous, and may end in a state of affairs where there is no return.

If we were to apply this simile to the inner world, the inner landscape of the individual child or adolescent, we will be able to come closer to certain considerations of importance to us. Suppose one could think of the human mind as a kind of geographical map with inner borders, lines of clear differentiation. Freud did this several times when he drew spatial models of the mind for us. First he did so more fully about 1900, introducing the topographic model which differentiates among three systems: the unconscious, the preconscious, and the conscious system of the mind. In 1923 he developed the structural model and drew a spatial picture of the mind in terms of ego, superego, and id, describing as he did the nature of the border between ego and reality; stressing that the id had a common border with the superego and the ego, but would have no common border with reality. He suggested to us that the borderlines between these different areas of inner territory are sometimes vague, and change from time to time. Each of these areas have different functions, and as suggested through his picture of the mind, the function of one area is often temporarily undermined and put out of action through invasions by the other, or as he suggested through the simile of the erection of dams creating the Zuider Zee, the Dutch people's struggle for the safety and creation and cultivation of farmland threatened by the flooding from the open ocean.

In hypnagogic states the ego functions would be invaded by border crossers of the id, or the superego, etc. Some of these invasions of welcome or unwelcome invaders are regular, well defined, and predictable. We could think of them in terms of the waking or sleep state, as predictable as the ocean tides. But some of these invasions are not predictable, and remind us of flood waters brought on by hurricanes or the destruction following a tornado.

Whether we use political analogies or those concerned with weather changes, we realize we describe travel uncertainties, and we need to stress that the difficulty may lie with the travelers or trespassers, their legal or forged documents, the border guards, or the nature of the border itself. If we are experienced travelers, we will try to predict possible diffficulties, and we may want to know the border conditions, the prospects of living in foreign territory, and about the possibility and ability to return.

Applicability

I can best characterize this uncertainty and its meaning by describing the opening few minutes, the first interview with a borderline adolescent. A few years earlier I had seen him at the end of puberty, and because of lack of time had referred him to a colleague. He did not maintain the treatment, had experimented with drugs for a couple of years, dropped out of school, associated with street people, lived away from home, etc. When he returned, he called me up at his own motivation, and told me that while the last time he had come under duress, he was now ready himself to start psychotherapy. He was quite candid about the happenings of the past two years, the frightful play with danger, and his increasing awareness of his inner turmoil. I was quite willing this time, having time available, to see him, and when he came to the moment of truth in establishing a schedule with me, he suddenly said he wondered whether it might not be a good idea for him, before starting formal psychotherapy, also expecting to be tied to a college schedule, if he made one more vacation trip to Afghanistan. I wondered jokingly if he would bring back one of those lovely coats that the young people were bringing home at that time, and he hinted he had much more in mind. I realized he spoke about smuggling drugs and bringing them back to the States for easy money. He had been dealing in a small way in drugs before. I wondered whether he knew what the prisons in Afghanistan were like. He said he knew about prisons from friends. I wondered whether he was more afraid of psychotherapy with me than he was of the Afghanistan prisons. I wish I could describe his face as he said to me: "I know what you mean. I am going to stay here and let's start."

He had confronted himself with the different borders he might have to cross. One was the *external border* that would lead to Afghanistan. Would he run away again from his inner conflicts, away from home, away from school, away from work in therapy here, and act out his deep anxiety, his problem of separation and individuation, the adolescent task; or should he risk it and cross the *inner border*, that hidden part of the preconscious mind, the memories of the past, the inner conflicts, the fear of trying to function in the territory of reality testing, or problem and task-solving? What would create more terror? Would it be the external danger that he must face and had faced in the past, the challenge of authority, of the adult world, or would it be the territory of inner chaos?

Would the holding action of psychotherapy, my holding him in the transference situation be strong enough to help him face his mind's jungle, the impulse-driven assocation with street people, the temptation to make an easy living through drug sales, the constant search for sexual partners who could not really satisfy nor maintain stable relationships? One might well say of this young man that he was afraid—were he to enter the inner territory, the forbidden chaos—that he could not return. He would rather chance traveling to Mexico or Afghanistan and deal with illicit drugs and with watchful border guards.

I would like to suggest that the psychotherapist is also a border guard, but a different kind of border guard, often a border guide. He guarantees that those who travel from reality to the Land of Oz, acquire a return ticket, have the inner capacity to travel both ways. He will have a psychological passport, so to speak, by means of which he can truly travel without fear and only with normal—that is, appropriate—restrictions which serve his and another's safety.

There was a time in Europe, following the First World War, when the empires were destroyed, making room for smaller republican states. Many people during that war and in its aftermath were dislocated, finding suddenly they had no country. They could not travel because they had no passports. They were acceptable in no country. Finally, the League of Nations, forerunner of today's United Nations, created the Nansen Passport for such people, and thus they would not need to stay in the middle of a bridge, not being allowed to move from one country to another, finally settling down to a life free from fear and hunger. Much of psychotherapy has to do with providing people with a Nansen Passport for travel in inner territory.

But what of the psychotherapist himself? In that paper written twenty-five years ago, it was suggested (Ekstein and Wallerstein, 1954, p. 368):

> The world of every child, his mode of thought and perception differs markedly from that of the adult therapist. And it is necessary in the therapy of all children to devise and create ways of living oneself into the world of childhood. This difference and attendant difficulties in understanding and communication increases seven-fold in work with the borderline and psychotic child. His psychological world is not only alien to the logical adult mind of the therapist, but is characterized by a fluidity of ego organization which can hardly be captured in the therapist's conscious recollection of his own childhood. This wide gulf separating patient from therapist has faced us with formidable problems of many kinds. At the same time it has provided the chief stimulus and challenge to the work we are attempting.

The therapist also needs a kind of Nansen Passport. He must learn how to travel into the child's inner territory which is frightful, strange, and beyond his understanding. Certainly it is often beyond any comparison to past personal experience still available to him. To what degree will he be capable of traveling with the young person into this strange inner territory? Whenever one travels into a foreign country and finds one is unable to speak the language, to communicate, one feels frequently misunderstood even when there are some who know his language. Certainly, the therapist, too, does not understand the language of the foreign country. But he tries. Frequently, he learns a bit of the new language, perhaps speaks it well enough to shop and try a few new foreign words. I certainly know how long it takes to be truly bilingual. Usually we need to get along with substitutes for full understanding. And that is the psychotherapist's problem who travels with a Nansen Passport into the Land of Oz, this Alice's Wonderland, and tries to understand the problems the borderline child poses.

I think I have made clear by now that the borderline syndrome refers to many a border crosser, to many a border trespasser, and to many different kinds of border guards, the inner watchdogs of the mind, some overstrict, some corrupt, some weak and unreliable. And this brings to mind, of course, that the children and adolescents of today, here in the States and also elsewhere, have gone through phases of growing up in the midst of borderline conditions of and in the world itself. It is not only they, the children and the adolescents, who have a borderline quality, but it is their parents, the educational systems, the conditions of the country that are unstable and fluctuating, and without directional signs. More than ever before, many feel that the value system is shaky, moral standards are shifting and drifting like the desert sands, and the opportunity reality offers, the nurture from civilization itself, are often impoverished, often seducing in the wrong direction and full of double cues. The psychotherapist who works with these borderline conditions cannot expect too much support today from parents, from the community, from the mental health movement, all being inconstant and unpredictable change. Therefore, he who intends to work with such children needs to have his compass as he ventures into borderline territory. I refer to his training, and we know the optimum training conditions for work with such children and adolescents are not always easily available.

I have found the best training for work with borderline conditions is one that is connected to research. We have no definite and certain answers to give to our students, but we may have them join us in search and research so we can find our way in uncertain inner and outer territory.

None of the examples of techniques used are meant to be final. They are meant to be experimental in nature. There is no clear map, no registry of streets, of starting points, of centers, but only vague characterizations of the psychic territory to be traveled and understood. Christopher Columbus had no clear map when he sailed for India and instead discovered America. The men and women who expanded the western frontier had no more than unreliable maps, but they went forward. The territory we are exploring as we help young people suffering from borderline conditions—a new frontier, so to speak—has no clear map either. But we have a general direction, and we have orientation points here and there for our travel, a cautious travel though it must be, always forward, but never without contact with those points we have left behind, without the reentry permit and reentry skill.

I have suggested earlier that this communication deals primarily with the psychotherapy of the borderline child and adolescent. Therefore, I stress in these observations the modes of psychotherapeutic communication. In the illustration of the adolescent who wonders whether it is more risky to travel to Afghanistan or to start psychotherapy, we have pointed, of course, to the use of the metaphor in order to bridge the world between the patient and the psychotherapist. The use of the metaphor in therapy is comparable to negotiating an unsafe, shaky suspension bridge. As we cross the bridge and look down into the waters' wild flow, we wonder if it might not be safer to have a bridge phobia that would prevent us from crossing. The young boy who speaks about the trip to Afghanistan may consciously think he is talking merely in concrete and realistic terms about a few weeks' vacation in a romantic, adventurous land. We know, indeed, that he tells us more as he talks about his compulsive need to act out, to get himself into a dangerous, precipitous situation, although we do not exactly know what is the meaning behind the compulsive drive. He touches on the problem, and we must hear it not merely in concrete terms, the way he hears it now, but we do well to hear it also as a metaphor, an attempt to relate to us his drivenness, his attempt to be successful with impossible means, his fantasy of omnipotence and his fear, perhaps his longing that he will be or should be destroyed. It is as if we are trying to discern behind the fog of his remark what he is really all about, what his personality makeup is. While we answer through another metaphor, and ask him whether he knows about the nature of prisons in Afghanistan, he understands but not completely. We try to point to his inner anxieties, not just to the fear of the police in Afghanistan, and we allude to his secret wish to defy all rules and law, his special problems with his parents, etc., but we merely hint at this. We allude and he alludes. But neither knows the full meaning of the allusion.

When we suggest he seems to be more afraid of psychotherapy than of Afghanistan prisons, we know, of course, that we speak about his fear of the transference, of the special relationships he yearns for and is also afraid of, his homosexual strivings and panic, and his defiance of the paternal love-hate object. But all this is not yet clear, only played with as a potential answer to the riddle, the unconscious dynamics. At the moment the psychotherapist responds to metaphor with metaphor, both the patient and doctor negotiating that unsafe, shaky, swinging suspension bridge. And I suppose the patient has as many questons about the therapist as does the therapist. Would he, the patient, be better off to run away to Afghanistan, to be counterphobic vis-à-vis the trip, and to be phobic vis-à-vis the trips to the therapist's consulting room? Would the psychotherapist not be better off being phobic about this kind of patient, remembering the patient broke off with another competent psychotherapist, and, therefore, again rather refer him to someone else than get stuck with him in a hopeless encounter? Or should he, the psychotherapist, be counterphobic, risk himself on that shaky suspension bridge and try to traverse it? We love to think of Coleridge's word about the *suspension of disbelief*. He will be the therapist of such youngsters successfully who suspends the disbelief in their stories, suspends also the disbelief in the impossibility to treat such people, and who himself takes the risk on that suspension bridge. The word "suspension," as we see, has many meanings. The acceptance of overdetermination of meaning must be the therapist's stock in trade, his trump card. Perhaps we can make our point concerning the treatment of borderline children clearer if we show the use of metaphoric language as applied in the treatment of a 13-year-old borderline boy who suffers from school phobia, and severe inability to learn. The diagnostic workup describes him as being in a symbiotic relationship with his mother. Self and object are not clearly differentiated. And his system of communication will therefore be more a search for communion than the kind of language that exists between people who are each fully separated individuals rather than still in part fusion.

Methods

The therapist tries to build a suspension bridge of communication, and we note the risk each takes as they traverse the bridge. The problem is how one can turn a conventional conversation into a therapeutic conversation. Before we turn to this interchange, a few additional remarks are in order regarding the use of metaphor, remarks based on a communication by Ekstein and Wallerstein (1957) on "The Choice of Interpretation in the Treatment of Borderline and Psychotic Children," and another by Caruth and Ekstein (1966), "Interpretation Within the Metaphor: Further Considerations."

We refer there to Ella Freeman Sharpe's classical paper (1950, p. 156) on metaphor where she suggests that:

> My theory is that metaphor can only evolve in language or in the arts when the bodily orifices become controlled. Then only can the angers, pleasures, desires of the infantile life find metaphorical expression and the immaterial express itself in terms of the material. A subterranean passage between mind and body underlies all analogy.

We understand her remark to mean that children who have not as yet truly acquired delay functions, have not established nor acquired the capacity for the secondary process and reality testing, cannot truly use metaphoric expressions, since, instead of their controlling language, language controls them. One might say that metaphor masters them just as they are often dominated by psychotic or psychotic-like language. Nevertheless, if we listen to them, we can see behind their language, experienced by them in a concrete way, deeper metaphoric meanings, since we, the therapist, control our own metaphoric language, and are not controlled by it. For the patient, the metaphor the therapist uses is often a path to regression, back to primary process, the language of the dream, the language of fantasy, uncontrolled by reality testing. Thus, the metaphor used by the therapist allows the child not only to be in touch with him, but also be in touch with his preconscious mind.

Caruth and Ekstein, quoting from John Middletown Murry (1922) as follows:

> The investigation of metaphor is curiously like the investigation of any of the primary data of consciousness; it cannot be pursued very far without or being led to *the borderline of sanity*. Metaphor is as ultimate as speech itself, and speech as ultimate as thought.

are able to pursue the meanings of metaphor as they allow themselves to go to and cross that borderline of sanity.

We thus learn to listen on several levels of

communication. Coming back to the treatment of the 13-year-old borderline boy, we seem to hear a merely conventional conversation in which he seems to try to talk within the area of secondary process language where reality testing rules. But we observe he is pulled away to primary process. We are now in the strange position wherein the choice is difficult, where we wonder whether we should accept his conversation as realistic or we are to understand his communication as a psychotic-like message. In one way, one may say the child tries to protect the therapist and himself by telling him he is talking his language; that the therapist will be able to understand him on his, the therapist's level. As the therapist listens to the young boy, he cannot be sure whether the youngster is talking his language or another language. Should he, the therapist, play naive? One might suggest they are meeting in the middle of that suspension bridge, the bridge between two countries where one is or perhaps both are forbidden to return to the old country but also forbidden to move forward. They now need to use a Nansen Passport confirming, so to speak, they are each without a country, without permanent commitment to one or the other language. The therapist is not a citizen in the country where the language of psychosis is utilized, nor is the 13-year-old boy a citizen in the reality-testing country of the therapist. We may hope the boy, now in treatment for a year or so, may someday become a *naturalized citizen* in the land of reality, even though he will continue to have an *accent* that indicates what his original language was, and we may see behind his naturalization papers for the country of his new choice, earlier loyalties to the Land of Oz, the psychotic process area of his inner landscape.

This child does not really have a true existence in his social environment. He behaves as if he indeed had one. He begins the therapy session by telling his therapist about actually nonexisting arrangements described as existing. He talks about meetings at school and community center, seeming reality situations in which he maintains a quasi-reality with considerable distance always remaining on the periphery of social events he describes. Wherever he goes, he tells us, he arrives late, and remains uninvolved. Soon, he leaves the presentation of quasi-reality and interrupts himself with a concrete but entirely inappropriate question which seems to require a direct answer from the therapist. He puzzles the therapist, who wonders how he is—when earlier he really was not permitted to enter the conversation—to react to all this. The patient wants to involve his doctor in an ordinary dialogue about ordinary events in everyday life, or so it seems. We know that contact-making is ordinarily beyond him. He is driven by his anxiety to leave his line of thought but he has learned to express the new thought which disrupts that line of thinking in a way as if it fits in with ordinary dialogue. He treats the material the way a dreamer does upon awakening, secondary elaboration as he remembers and reports his dream. In other words, he tries to maintain a sequence of thinking as though he were telling a meaningful story. These sequences almost give the impression that a story is told, a story that has a point, as if he actually were using the language of ordinary conversation. But at a given point, this does not work any longer. As he is flooded with anxiety, he is forced to disrupt the thought sequence in the very same way a child is overwhelmed by play disruption when the play material gets too near the hidden problem of conflict. In order to master his anxiety, he asks a quasi-question in the hope the outside authority will provide the matrix to glue his fragmented sentences together, and thus supply new, quasi-meaning.

He asks now in what branch of service did the therapist serve. The therapist, having to choose between the concrete meaning of the question and the potential metaphoric meaning, is presented with a dilemma. Can such a question be interpreted instead of being answered?

The boy is frightened at his loss of control as he recognizes that his thought pattern is disrupted, is falling apart, and one might well suggest that were he to know what goes on in him, he might think as follows: "As I see I am falling apart, I want to ask definite concrete questions, whether or not support will be forthcoming; and question I must in order to find out how reliable my psychotherapist is, whether he can put Humpty Dumpty together again who has just fallen off the wall of the secondary process, a mere thin veneer hiding the underlying turmoil."

Again, as he repeats the question as to where the therapist served in the war, in what kind of service he was, he is asking the question in such a way as to interrupt his flow of thought, as to stop the increasing loss of control, and to anchor his feet to the ground, the shifting ground of reality testing, of secondary process thinking, and he returns to the therapist in order to force support in his attempt to reconnect the feeble attachment to reality.

That particular therapist, overwhelmed for a moment by the sudden turn of events, the sudden change in the nature of the child's communication, now asks the boy what branch of service the boy thinks he was in; and thus he hopes to maintain the therapeutic process. What can the therapist accomplish with that question? What are his choices, his options in order to maintain himself and the patient on that suspension bridge? Is he to answer the question? Is he to give a concrete answer? Should he interpret the meaning of it, such as telling the boy why he, the therapist, thought the question was asked, and how it was to serve the purpose of dangerous flow of regressive thought fragments? Or should he say to himself that he does not as yet know what the material means; and that he would do better if he were to tread water? The therapist is in a predicament of finding himself now on the suspension bridge. On the surface it would appear that both therapist and boy are still carrying on a conversation, a system of communication that can be likened to secondary process. Is it really a realistic conversation concerning the question whether he, the therapist, was serving in the ground or air forces, or are we to allow ourselves to follow the boy's thinking on a different level? Should we say rather that at this moment he suspends reality testing and actually asks his therapist: "If I am up in the air, can you give me nurturance and support? Am I a *Luftmensch* lost in the air like a balloon having been torn from its mooring, and do I want to remain crazy, or can you give me the basis for returning to mother earth, back to the breast?" Suddenly, what started as an ordinary or perhaps at best a borderline conversation ends in the Land of Oz, the land of psychotic thinking. Although the therapist tries to stem the flood by asking the boy what he really meant, it becomes quite clear this boy will not have his feet on the ground as he proceeds to communicate. His next question is whether he, the patient, were to enter the air force, would he get attention. He tests the therapist, we now understand, whether he will provide him with nutriment even though he enters the land of craziness.

The therapist is placed in a dangerous predicament—that is, of facing the boy's direct questions, questions which if he answered either way only interrupt the psychotherapeutic dialogue. These questions are similar to the kinds of questions all patients ask when they want direct answers, when they want permission for something, direct advice one way or the other, challenges that always put the therapist in a position where he is wrong either way he answers, regardless whether he forbids or permits, whether he yields or does not yield, whether he answers directly or refuses to answer. One might very well say that these kinds of *questions are* foreplay, frequently merely the *overture to the psychotherapeutic dialogue*. One may well suggest this conversation is as yet an empty conversation, a dialogue for the purpose of not communicating, of avoiding the thoughts that really occur. They could be considered the obstacle to the royal road of saying freely what comes to mind. They are an expression of transference resistance in the service of controlling the dangerous, anxiety-arousing flow of thought, flowing as it does in the direction of the Land of Oz.

The boy does not respond to the therapist's question as to what he, the patient, thinks about the kind of service the therapist may have been in during war time, and of course he indicates he was not at all interested in an answer but rather used the question to block his own thoughts. He continued to talk about a meeting described in a brochure which he waves frantically in which there was to be discussed a high school program for the educationally handicapped. Rather than waiting for the therapist to answer, or asking him again, he is now wandering about aimlessly and again announces another projected outside meeting. What is his gambit? It is if he were to say to us, "I do not have my feet on the ground.I am up in the air. But here is the evidence—really the mere pretense—that I do have my feet on the ground." He tries to maintain the façade of secondary process with conversation about the proposed new high school program, proceeding with a quasi-dialogue. He pretends he goes to a normal high school, trying to maintain the façade in order to avoid the anxiety around the conflict that he is not capable of attending regular school, that actually he cannot even cope with quasi-dialogue.

The child at this point does not permit ordinary psychotherapeutic interventions, interpretations that speak for the underlying meaning, but rather he utilizes the therapist to maintain a facade of normalcy. He cannot permit the therapist to show him what he really is, a child unable to be maintained in a public school, a child unable to learn and meeting even the minimum requirements in a school for youngsters as severely handicapped as he. He must maintain that façade of normalcy. That, after all, is the external requirement of parents, of the world about him. But at the same time he also wants to convey to the therapist more about himself. Usually the psychotic denial then breaks down in his expression of desperation: "You cannot help me." He denies the reality of being unable to be maintained in a regular school setting by saying that he is allowed to go to a very special school. His "being up in the air" is described by him in such a way that his school success puts him into a situation that is "higher and better" and he says, "I am up in the air. I will prove I am better. I am not ill. I am better than normal."

What is the therapeutic problem at that moment? What can the therapist do in order to create insight for the patient so he will see his illness without bringing about an explosive destruction of the communication bridge? The constant denial is only maintained in order to break down in his plea of desperation.: "No one helps me." He describes his inner anxieties in terms of being dragged from doctor to doctor for medical treatment. He shows scratches on his arm and says they were received in a fight with his sister. The underlying theme that unites this material could be understood as follows: "I am better than anyone else; I am up in the air. I am higher and better. Mother expects me to be better than anyone else; therefore she sends me to doctors to fix me up, but instead they destroy me."

One could well think of this material as a borderline version of the oedipal conflict. It is as if he were to say to us that in order to get love from his mother he must be better than everyone else. But he is constantly afraid that he will be hacked to pieces, castrated, and destroyed, that he has no control. He wonders: Can the therapist help him if he is up in the air? He wants assurance from the therapist that if he never proves to be competent, he will still get the attention even if he were to remain crazy.

Is it possible now for the therapist to enter the problem in such a way that the patient will not feel completely exposed or trapped, and will be enabled to make use of the treatment?

If the therapist understands the material, he may well respond in such a way that the material is not directly translated into the kind of language we use when we have our feet on the ground, but is responded to in such a way that we take poetic license. Thus we make it possible for the patient to hear if he wishes to. Suppose the therapist would suggest that he indeed belonged to the air force, but the task of the air force was to be up in the air whenever necessary, and to land properly on firm ground when indicated. Nobody should be left in the air forever, but only for the time that it is necessary to see what is up in the air, what is up there. Airplanes can fly and can land. He, the therapist, if he flew with the young patient would want to help him learn the mechanics of taking off, of flying, of reaching the goal, of landing, etc.

He may wonder with the child whether the trip high in the air was really necessary, or whether after reaching one's destination, one could really go to that meeting, get together with the people, and get on with the task. As we suggested earlier, the therapist would need to suspend his disbelief that what the boy is saying about these meetings is true, is real. They are attempts at meetings, even if but fantasied meetings, fantasied tasks solved, and they are the child's attempt to maintain the veneer of normality. While it is clear this veneer must be considered a defense, it is actually also an adaptive maneuver. It is to acquire permission to enter the land of reality, to cross the suspension bridge, to go where the therapist, parents, and peers usually live. But the patient also wants to tell his story, which requires the therapist suspend his disbelief in some other way. He is to disbelieve that he cannot understand the child's underlying problems, the conflict that he expresses in that borderline language. Can one be sure that each partner will require the capacity to carry a Nansen Passport which permits exit and reentry? Suspense refers to the underlying anxiety in the process of the psychotherapeutic dialogue. We are referring to transference as well as countertransference anxiety; suspense, suspending refers to the necessary delay of process; the willingness to wait, to suspend sometimes one's own language and speak the language of the other, and to suspend also understanding when it is not yet fully available. The idea of the suspension bridge refers to a system of communication, a bridge suspended over two territories but firmly grounded. This bridge, however, is not only a borderline language. It is also the bridge between two human beings, an interpersonal bridge. It refers to the tenuous nature of object relations, the relations between object and self, and sometimes suspended in the other sense of the word, sometimes leading to fusion, to merging, but maintaining also the thin link between two human beings in the subtle process of interchange.

The example just discussed refers to a child, not yet an adolescent. With him as well as with younger children, the basic problem is one in which separation is opposed by the child's strong need to return to the mother matrix. This boy reminds one of the Greek myth which describes Hercules fighting with the giant Antheus. They are to wrestle each other to final defeat. No sooner does Hercules pin Antheus down to the ground, to mother earth, than does he, the giant, gain strength again and threatens to defeat Hercules. Hercules discovers that mother earth gives the giant strength. He uses a new technique now. He lifts Antheus up into the air and deprives him of mother earth's strength. He, the giant, grows weaker and weaker, and finally Hercules kills him. Antheus gained his strength by returning to mother earth. He must search for nutriment, and if deprived of that nutriment, he cannot sustain himself.

The young patient constantly tries, while experiencing himself up in the air, isolated, differentiated, prematurely individuated, to reconnect and restore the needed support; and he wonders whether the therapist will support him, even if he were crazy and up in the air.

The therapist must now be a different kind of Hercules. He does not wish to defeat his patient, but rather he wants to strengthen him so that he could be up in the air and nevertheless self-reliant, competent, truly individuated. Can he work in such a way that the patient establishes with him an enduring alliance in which the therapist for a time must be the auxiliary mother-matrix?

Can that suspension bridge of metaphoric communication be like an emotional umbilical cord which maintains them in a kind of understanding that is based on two languages, the primary and secondary process language? The glue that guarantees the effectiveness of that suspension bridge is metaphor.

Let us return to the original example concerning the adolescent who wants to wander off to Afghanistan before beginning psychotherapy. Here we observe the opposite constellation. The young boy creates a quasi-psychotic fantasy of eternal maternal support. The older adolescent does not try to return to the symbiotic matrix, but rather is on his way toward premature individuation. He wants to move away from family and country, and sees himself as the successful adventurer in Afghanistan. His language is the language of acting out, of unrealistic adventure, of substituting the home through drugs, and substituting lasting peer relationships through acting out of quasi-mature sexual fantasies. He moves toward psychotic-like individuation and separation. This patient's moves are premature experiments towards individuation while the child's experimentation is one of delayed holding on to earlier states of development.

It is not without interest that the parents of this adolescent were themselves people who played with schemes which included the idea of living in foreign countries, of being involved in dangerous economic adventures, their version of Afghanistan, while the mother of the younger boy participates in precarious symbiotic-like overattachment to the child.

Comparisons

In other communications, we described not only the use of metaphors of language, but also of action metaphors, a way of indirectly participating in plays in acting out in order to maintain a bridge of communication by means of which we bring about the psychotherapeutic process. It has been suggested that occasionally actions speak louder than words. Psychotherapists, of course, are committed to the idea that usually words speak louder than actions. But there are cases where the use of hospitalization, of day treatment centers, of special schools (Ekstein and Motto, 1966), of foster homes, special placements, living out of the home, group sessions, the use of special teachers, social workers, etc., in addition to individual psychotherapy are indicated, and all of them can be understood as action metaphors within the context of the psychotherapeutic dialogue.

Usually, the latter application of our theoretical considerations can best be carried out within a psychiatric team, best in a clinic or residential setting or hospital. Alone, a truth which must be learned by psychotherapists—we cannot always be successful. The problem then of collaboration both with parents or other carriers of modalities of treatment is an eternal one, never completely solved.

Actually, often we have found that professional discussions with other professionals, such as nurses, recreational therapists, occupational therapists, teachers, social workers also need the suspension bridge we have described. We must learn to have respect for the other's language, often a different technical language, frequently a different theoretical language, and accept it as such, perhaps as a metaphor that is a response to our own thinking, and we may well find our own language in relation to other professions is not more than that.

I am speaking of the respect necessary for the system of communication each of us uses whether he is a patient, or whether he is a colleague, a therapist, or one belonging to another profession. We cannot expect that each is to speak our own specific language. We must learn to be multilinguistic.

Summary and Concusions

Let us return then to the original issue of clarifying the notion of *borderline*. Is not this notion itself a borderline notion? Is it not merely a way of saying that we must individualize our treatment methods. The examples used are but exaggerations which can be applied to any psychotherapeutic treatment which is based on psychoanalytic principles, on the use of the patient's and therapist's inner world. That is true for metaphor in borderline situations, and it is also true within the context of treatment of more severely disturbed people, clearly psychotic, clearly autistic or schizophrenic, as well as for the use of metaphor in those conditions belonging to the neurotic range.

Perhaps the borderline condition is itself a kind of suspension bridge, helping us to see there is a wide spectrum, a wide arc from one condition to another, no clear-cut differentiation, but all of them united on a continuum which is to describe the functions of the mind, the functions as available during different stages of growth and development.

The borderine condition could be considered as a magnifying glass by means of which one can also see other conditions much better on that wide continuum of mental and emotional illness. The two cases discussed can also be used to describe the continuum. The younger boy longs for the past, the return to the maternal matrix, the breast, the paradise. The older boy yearns for the future, wants self-actualization. On the one end of the continuum is the wish to return to the secure world of yesterday in which self and object are united, fused, where one knows safety and warmth. Actualization and individuation are at the other end of the continuum. The price for the first condition is the lack of self; and the price for the latter condition seems to be desperate loneliness. But this just points to that continuum that describes the human life cycle moving from blind trust to individuation. One might well say as most authors today state that borderline problems can develop at any of the points of life crisis and life tasks. It is the task of the psychotherapist Hercules, to turn the crisis, the emergency into a task, into an emerging process. Such emerging process will permit the child, or the adolescent, to move toward a better-established identity, toward the solution of the identity crises—as they occur during the first and second individuation—in such a way so there will be established identity, a commitment to the psychic territory of one's choice. The achievement is to include the capacity to expand this territory and to be able to travel fearlessly into other territories having acquired the right of passage, the capacity to move forward without having lost the capacity also to go back, to return, to regress, to find one's psychological and one's social roots.

But then this was always the task of any psychoanalytic treatment. It aims at the restoration of the continuity between yesterday, today, and tomorrow. To what degree is this possible in psychoanalysis applied to children, adolescents, or adults? To what degree is this possible in modified treatment techniques such as suggested here, we do not fully know. We have seen immense improvement, but are still stunned by tasks beyond solution. Freud speaks about the necessity that each patient, after analysis, must learn to still bear some anxiety and a great deal of uncertainty. I suggest the same holds true for the psychotherapeutic profession itself. The study of borderline conditions may increase the uncertainty and that anxiety, and it will be our task to turn the anxiety and uncertainty of our search into further research into an area beyond our usual borders, an area that has no visible boundaries, and invites endless exploration, more like space travel than a trip across land and water, mountains and valleys.

References

Caruth, E., and R. Ekstein, (1966) Interpretation within the metaphor: Further considerations. *J. Am. Acad. Child Psychiat.* 5(1):35–45.

Ekstein, R. (1966) *Children of Time and Space, of Action and Impulse.* New York: Appleton-Century-Crofts.

Ekstein, R. (1971) *The Challenge, Despair and Hope in the Conquest of Inner Space.* New York: Brunner/Mazel.

Ekstein, R. (1973) The border: Its crossers and trespassers; its guards and guides. *Contemp. Psychol.*. 18(12):634–636.

Ekstein, R., and J. Wallerstein. (1954) Observations on the psychology of borderline and psychotic children. *Psychoanal. Study Child* 9:344–369.

Ekstein, R., and J. Wallerstein. (1957) Choice of interpretation in the treatment of borderline and psychotic children. *Bull. Menninger Clin.* 21:199–206.

Ekstein, R., and R. L. Motto. (1960) The borderline child in the school situation. In M. J. Gottsegen and G. B. Gottsegen, eds., *Professional School Psychology.* New York: Grune & Stratton.

Geleerd, E. R. (1958) Borderline states in childhood and adolescence. *Psychoanal. Study Child* 13:279.

Kernberg, O. (1975) *Borderline Conditions and Pathological Narcissism.* New York: Jason Aronson.

Mahler, M., and M. Furer. (1968) *On Human Symbiosis and the Vicissitudes of Individuation.* New York: International Universities Press.

Masterson, J. F. (1972) *Treatment of the Borderline Adolescent.* New York: Wiley-Interscience.

Murry, J. M. (1922) *Countries of the Mind.* London: Collins.

Sharpe, E. F. (1950) *Collected Papers on Psychoanalysis.* London: Hogarth Press.

Treatment of Emotional Disorders in Children and Adolescents

CHAPTER 26

Psychotic Disorders

Bertram A. Ruttenberg
Ashley J. Angert

Introduction

The treatment of psychotic children is one of the more controversial areas about which one could attempt an orderly set of principles. As most workers in the field would acknowledge, problems in the approach to therapy are often due to the confusion surrounding the definition of the various categories under the heading "psychoses of childhood" and exactly which disturbed children fit which category, as well as to lack of agreement on their etiologies. A survey of the literature reveals that the disorders included under the Psychoses of Childhood are heterogeneous, with different diagnostic labels given to similar or overlapping groups, and the same label given to different clinical descriptions. Nevertheless, all agree that precise diagnosis is essential for adequate therapy to be instituted. In the most general sense, the term "psychoses of childhood" is a broad generic designation for a group of clinical syndromes that present a picture of severe emotional disturbance which may appear any time from birth to the peri-pubertal period (Ruttenberg, 1977a).

Diagnoses generally subsumed under this heading include early infantile autism, atypical child, symbiotic psychosis, childhood schizophrenia, borderline psychoses, manic-depressive psychoses, and depressive equivalents in infancy—i.e., infantile rumination, hospitalism, marasmus, anaclitic depression, and primary agitated depression. Often conditions which may take a psychotic form are also included, such as elective mutism and folie à deux.

The confusion surrounding the use of these terms is easily seen. The American Psychiatric Association's *Diagnostic and Statistical Manual of Mental Disorders II* (1968) allows for only one inclusive category for childhood psychosis—i.e., "schizophrenia, childhood type"—and one category for "psychoses associated with organic brain syndromes." In recent years, early infantile autism has strayed far from the narrowly defined specific syndrome of Kanner and become to many a generic designation encompassing a wide variety of psychotic, organic, developmental, language, and learning disorders of early origin. For some, the presence of organicity means that a disorder should be excluded from the childhood psychoses (see the Group for the Advancement of Psychiatry [GAP] classification, 1966); for others, organicity is an integral part of the condition (Bender, 1960; Ritvo, 1977).

Many workers have addressed themselves to the problem of lack of clarity. Goldfarb (1970) noted how such semantic contradictions and confusion results in interference with treatment planning, clinical investigation, and reporting, and suggested careful definition of diagnostic criteria and description of the sample being reported. Wherry (1972) noted inadequate and biased sampling, sweeping inferences and generalization, and a dearth of well-designed studies of therapeutic efficacy. He suggested that for communication in the literature to be meaningful and results comparable, populations have to be descriptively and functionally compatible or comparable, and standardized methods of assessment and rating need to be developed. Ruttenberg et al. (1978) developed a Behavior Rating Instrument for Autistic and other Atypical Children (BRIAAC) which quantitates levels of function along eight scales of development, and provides numerical and graphic profiles for comparison between different psychotic populations and between psychotic and other low-functioning populations. Profiles define the nature of the population and may be used in assessing, reporting, and comparing therapeutic efficacy. DeMyer et al. (1971) compared five diagnostic systems for the childhood psychoses with goal of standardization, and recognized the difficulties presented by the terminology once the broad differentiation between psychotic and nonpsychotic had been made.

Diagnostic Classification

Many in the field have been struggling to set up a useful and universally acceptable system of diagnostic classification, without which it is difficult to develop individualized treatment plans, to transmit information about a child, or to provide accurate data for demographic, epidemologic, and other research purposes.

Among these have been Despert (1968), Anthony (1958), Bender (1960), Settlage (1964), Fish and Shapiro (1965), Eisenberg (1966), Bettelheim (1967), Wolman (1970), Menolascino (1971), and Ruttenberg (1971). Systems have been devised around age of appearance, acuteness of onset, degree of ego disorganization, specific clusters of symptoms, and etiologic factors. Some describe the disorders as separate and distinct entities, while others place them on a continuum.

Despite the varied approaches, the central core of each system remains the clinical description, and at this point it would be helpful to emphasize those clinically observed characteristics that are commonly found to a greater or lesser degree among the childhood psychoses.

A British Working Party (Creak et al., 1961) prepared a list of such characteristics, which, with a few additions, has become widely accepted. These are:

1. Gross and sustained impairment of a child's emotional relationships with people.
2. Apparent unawareness or distorted concept of the child's own personal identity to a degree inappropriate to its age.
3. A pathological preoccuptaion with particular objects or with certain characteristics of them.
4. Sustained resistance to change in the environment and a striving to maintain or restore sameness.
5. Abnormal perceptual experience, such as excessive or diminished response to sensory stimuli.
6. Acute and excessive anxiety, often in response to disordered thought or fantasy.
7. Loss or inadequate development of speech.
8. Distortion of motility patterns, such as immobility, hyperkinesis, bizarre postures, or stereotyped mannerisms.
9. A background of functional retardation in which islets of normal, near normal, or exceptional function or skill may appear.

A tenth point which might be added would include the thought disorder and peculiar often highly sophisticated symbolic language of the later-onset childhood schizophrenic.

In a review of 52 published reports featuring diagnostic symptomatology in childhood psychoses, Goldfarb (1970) felt that all behavioral symptoms described could be embodied within these points.

Probably the most significant development in recent years has been the recognition that the disorders known under the heading "psychoses of childhood" are frequently multifactorial, and that one reason for confusion has been that in fact a variety of etiologies can produce similar-looking syndromes, and any one syndrome often does have several etiologic factors. There is presently a tendency toward a multifactorial approach to both diagnosis and treatment.

A distillate of these current trends in the area of diagnosis and classification is reflected in two proposed systems of general psychiatric classification which are gaining wide acceptance. The first, formulated by the Group for the Advancement of Psychiatry (GAP) Committee on Child Psychiatry (1966), focuses on the functional psychoses and requires, in a developmental context, the absence of gross signs of brain damage and mental retardation for a primary diagnosis. The section on psychotic disorders is:

1. Psychoses of infancy and early childhood
   a. Early infantile autism (onset from first month to first year), which must be distin-

guished from autistic reactions secondary to brain damage or mental retardation.
   b. Interactional psychotic disorder (onset from 2nd to 5th year). Includes symbiotic psychosis and related disorders such as secondary autism.
   c. Other (children with atypical development).
2. Psychoses of later childhood
   a. Schizophreniform psychotic disorder (onset 6th to 13th year).
   b. Other psychoses of later childhood (affective, depressive).
3. Psychoses of adolescence
   a. Acute confusional state (pseudopsychotic reaction)
   b. Schizophrenic disorder, adult type (dementia praecox)
   c. Other psychoses of adolescence

The second system currently being developed is the World Health Organization (WHO) multiaxial classification (Rutter et al., 1969), which allows for three associated diagnostic dimensions:(1) the clinical psychiatric syndrome; (2) the level of intellectual function; and (3) etiologic considerations: biologic (organic), metabolic, and psychosocial factors. The new American Psychiatric Association *Diagnostic and Statistical Manual III*, unpublished at this writing, will have a similar multiaxial format, but will include a fourth axis citing the levels of pertinent developmental function.

In this multiaxial system the clinical syndrome and the time of onset remain predominant. The inclusion of the other axes provides a more complete diagnostic statement and invites a broader therapeutic approach.

The categories for the Psychoses of Childhood are delineated as:

1. Infantile psychoses (onset within first 2½ years): autistic, atypical, and symbiotic subtypes, characterized by disturbance in interpersonal relationships, delayed or disordered language development, ritualistic behavior, resistance to change, irregular intellectual development, and motor stereotypy. Those with accompanying signs of organic brain disorder or mental retardation are included.
2. Disintegrative psychosis (onset after 2½ years): normal development in the first 2½ to 3 years of life is followed by a severe disintegration of ego function involving emotion, behavior, relationship, and speech loss. This is frequently an organic process.
3. Schizophrenia (onset after the 3rd or 4th year of life): clinical picture is similar to that of adult schizophrenia.
4. Other psychoses (folie à deux, manic depressive)

This classification allows for the fact that etiology in many cases seems to be a biologic (genetic, congenital, or postnatal) substrate of vulnerability, even though environmental conditions seem to precipitate the onset of overt symptomatology, as contrasted with cases in which environmental factors predominate. The presence or absence of these factors may influence treatment modality.

History

Information on the historical development of the therapeutic management of the psychoses of childhood is more sparse than that of adult psychoses. This is consistent with the relatively minor position of the child in society until the most recent of times. Yet there have been those with an interest. Among these were the Holy Roman Emperor Frederick (1200 A.D.) and his ignoble experiment involving isolation and stimulus deprivation of an infant, resulting in what was apparently autism and developmental retardation. In the early 1800's Itard described, in what is now a classic work, his long-term therapeutic effort with Victor, the "Wild Boy of Aveyron." He was a feral child of about 10, descriptively autistic and retarded, whose condition Itard felt was due to environmental deprivation. His methods anticipated some of the relationship developing, stimulating, and conditioning methods used today. Kanner (1971) cited Maudsley's attempts in 1867 to implicate genetic predisposition and parental influence in producing insanity. The late nineteenth century was marked by attempts to classify mental disorders, and Kraeplin's introduction of the term "dementia praecox" emphasized description, organic etiology, and mental deterioration, thus discouraging attempts at treatment. In 1906, De Sanctis noted that some children who displayed psychotic behavior were neurologically intact and intellectually well endowed. He was the first to delineate childhood psychoses, which he termed dementia praecoxissma, as different from mental deficiency. Because they were not mentally defective, he felt they could profit from "medical-pedagogical treatment"—i.e., therapeutic education and training.

In 1911, Bleuler proposed a dynamic conceptualization of psychosis that stressed intrapsychic and adaptational processes. He coined the term "schizophrenia" to represent the split between feeling and thought. Freud's theories of infantile sexuality (1905) and constructs of id, ego, and superego and unconscious conflict, and Meyer's (1910) consideration of mental illness as a reaction of constitutional givens to environmental stress and parental influence, added to Bleuler's concepts, gave psychiatrists working with children some tools with which to attempt active treatment of the childhood psychoses.

In the 1930's and 1940's, clinicians turned their attention to the psychotic process and function. Potter (1933) described more clearly psychotic symptomatology and focused on developmental immaturity and parental pathology in treatment. Despert (1938) emphasized early traumatic experiences and lack of use of language for communication. She reported that individual psychotherapy was more effective than institutionalization, and worked on establishing contact and interpreting the child's symbolic language and disordered thinking. Bender (1947) emphasized the psycho-physiologic dysfunctions such as plasticity, pallor, flushing, incoordination, and others.

In more recent years therapeutic efforts have evolved in many directions, including behavioral, psychoanalytically oriented, family, and drug therapies, and the interest in developing an optimal combined approach is high.

Etiology

Theories of etiology can be categorized as those that emphasize (1) organic factors, (2) psycho-developmental failure, (3) psychosocial (parental) failure, and (4) multicausality. The time of onset of the illness is also an important consideration.

The psychoses of early onset tend to be categorized by withdrawal, overall developmental delay, and retardation, especially in the areas of communicative language, comprehension, and social behavior, and delays in the perceptual-cognitive and motor areas. Most but not all authors concede a biological basis for, or participation in, the etiology and process.

The psychoses of later onset, such as the schizophrenias, appearing after a period of normal or near normal development, show behavioral regression rather than developmental arrest, and there is a more evenly divided controversy over the "nature-nurture" or organic versus environmental theories of etiology.

Among the theories favoring the organic etiologies, the early-onset psychoses seem to be based more on "congenital vulnerabilities", while the later-onset psychoses present more research evidence for a genetic component. For example, Mosher and Finesilver (1971) reported a significant occurrence of schizophrenia in the adopted offspring of schizophrenics. Even here, the question was raised that a "predisposing vulnerability" was inherited.

Organic Theories

These imply a dysfunctioning central nervous system, with dysfunction genetically based or congenitally or perinatally acquired. Particularly in the psychoses of early onset there have been implications of dysfunction of the limbic and reticular activating systems (DesLauriers and Carlson, 1969), disturbances of arousal causing perceptual inconstancy (Ornitz, 1973), primary language and cognitive disorders (Rutter and Bartak, 1971), and multiple language, cognitive, perceptual motor, and autonomic impairments.

Biochemical studies, particularly of biogenic amine metabolism of the neurotransmitters, seek to implicate metabolic factors (Cohen, 1974). A review of the biochemical studies of schizophrenia (Guthrie and Wyatt, 1975) concluded that there is as yet no consistent evidence for a biochemical cause for or correlation with the etiology of the childhood psychoses. It must be noted that the majority of these studies have been done on autism and other psychoses of early onset. Recent studies (Coleman, 1976) raise the hope that precise analyses of metabolic products may someday differentiate even similar symptom clusters and determine in some cases the kind and amount of replacement or antagonistic medication required to restore normal mental function.

A growing number of prenatal influences on the developing fetus have been reported to cause damage to the function of the nervous system and its neurometabolic correlates (Chess, 1971). These include medications formerly taken with impunity during pregnancy, drugs and alcohol, viral infections, serious medical illnesses, trauma, and others. Ruttenberg (1971) reported that examination of perinatal hospital records of their child psychotic population, mostly of early onset, revealed a 50–80% occurrence of one or more of a list of these prenatal influences, including prenatal toxicity or distress. In 100 consecutive births at a university hospital this incidence was only 3–4%

Theories of Psycho-Developmental Failure and Regression

These theories emphasize disturbances in the normal psychological development of the young child as causative factors. Spitz's (1945, 1946a) well-known study of children in orphanages demonstrated that lack of mothering stimulation could produce anxiety, withdrawal from and rejection of subsequent human contact, profound regression, and developmental delays in the motor area, speech, and intellectual and social functioning. Anaclitic depression could occur in 6- to 11-month-old children when a mother figure was lost. Sally Provence and Selma Fraiberg have personally communicated data on normally developing 3- to 5-month-olds who developed fragmentation of ego function indistinguishable from signs of organic brain disorder after loss of the mother.

Mahler (1952, 1968; Mahler, Furer, and Settlage, 1959) applied her concepts of autistic, symbiotic, and separation-individuation phases of normal development to explain a continuum of syndromes of childhood psychoses. At each level there can be an interference in the system of reciprocal communication between mother and child which is necessary to stimulate continued development. This interference can be due to inconstant, skewed, inappropriate, or traumatic input from the mother, or can be due to a basic congenital vulnerability or incapacity of the infant to respond, or to both in combination.

Contributions of S. Freud (1924) and Melanie Klein (1932) in their attempts to understand the psychological aspects of psychosis are of course extensive and can only be noted here.

Beres (1956) applied concepts of ego psychology to the childhood psychoses and stated that because of developmental arrest or regression, the ego fails in the areas of reality testing, drive regulation, object relationship, and other adaptive functions. His therapeutic interventions were designed to correct the ego deviation and free ego development.

Applying the concepts of Beres and Mahler, Ruttenberg (1971) offered a unitary developmental theory of the childhood psychoses, explaining each clinical subcategory and diagnostic entity as the manifestation of a cluster of behaviors—i.e., a nodal point on a developmental continuum at which ego function breaks down. Because of a combination of intrinsic and extrinsic etiological factors, the ego can no longer sustain and shape further biologic development, modulate drive expression, elaborate character trait equivalents and a repertoire of defenses, develop and maintain age-appropriate object relationships, tolerate separation, and achieve subsequent individuation. He lists eight subcategories in order of increasing developmental sophistication. This holistic approach suggests therapeutic intervention designed to move the child along the developmental and maturational continua.

Theories of Psychosocial (Parental) Failure

These are theories that emphasize the quality of mothering and parenting in general as of greatest significance in causing psychosis in children. Kanner (1943), although he considers autism an inborn disturbance of affective contact, noted the rejecting "refrigerator" parent.

Rank (1949) stressed the role of the unresponsive parent. Ferster (1961) put this in operant conditioning terms and noted parents' failure to reinforce the infant's approach behavior, resulting in fixation, self-stimulation, aggression, or withdrawal. Reiser (1966) implicated prolonged subclinical maternal depression, often beginning postpartum, as a source of deprivation in production of childhood psychoses.

Bettelheim (1967) linked parental unresponsiveness to unconscious hostility, and stressed the psychotic child's resultant perception of the world as one in which he is intimidated and helpless, and against which his actions have no impact or meaning. Out of frustration he withdraws. Both he and Mahler (1968) note that overstimulating and overpossessive mothering also overwhelm the child's drive to explore and individuate, and the child withdraws. Wolman (1970) implicates an overdemanding parental attitude which expects the child to compensate for parental failures and frustrations. Szurek and Berlin (1973) emphasized the impact of continuous tension generated by parents in conflict which produces anxiety and early distortion of the child's emotional development.

Many authors, especially those involved in family approaches to evaluation and therapy, have noted the "double binding" or simultaneous communication of contrary messages, with an injunction to choose one, and with no escape permitted, which is often present in families of psychotic children (Bowen, 1960).

Theories of Multicausality

Increasingly, either by direct statement or by implication, teaching and clinical centers are adopting a multifactorial concept of etiology of psychoses in childhood. Goldfarb (1974) cited increasing empirical data pointing to an interaction of intrinsic and environmental factors. He proposed a theory of causality in which dysfunction of internal mechanisms and inadequacy of familial responses combine in different measures to produce psychosis.

Harper and Williams (1974) studied the pre-, peri-, and postnatal histories and clinical assessments of a large number of disturbed children and found a higher incidence of prenatal stress, perinatal complications, degree of environmental stress, and deprivation among autistic children than in those with any other form of emotional disturbance or with physical illness.

The Evaluation Process

The evaluation process for children who appear to be severely emotionally disturbed is at present used not merely to ascertain a diagnostic classification and subcategorization, but, given the important role accurate assessment plays in the development of a therapeutic plan, diagnosis is now a portion of the total goal of evaluation. The evaluation process should result in an accurate clinical picture of the child and a multiaxial diagnosis, with an assessment of the probable etiologic factors leading to that clinical picture. These should include presence of organicity, psychosocial, cultural, and environmental stresses, family dynamics, psychosexual development and conflicts, and neurologic and metabolic deficits.

The proposed American Psychiatric Association *Diagnostic and Statistical Manual* (DSM III) has recognized the need for a multidimensional approach to evaluation, and has included in its diagnostic breakdown: (1) the clinical psychiatric syndrome; (2) the disorder of personality; (3) the associated medical-organic factors; (4) the psychosocial impact; and (5) the capacity for ego-adaptive functioning. This approach was designed to encourage comprehensive treatment planning and to eliminate the either-or choices and simplistic categorization clinicians have been forced into in the past.

With this goal in mind, assessment of the childhood psychoses is best done from a maturational and developmental framework involving multiple disciplines. Maturation and developmental level is emphasized because the manifestations of a particular disorder will tend to vary and take on different forms depending on the child's level of development and function. Available specialists, in addition to the child psychiatrist, should ideally include a developmental pediatrician, pediatric neurologist, speech and hearing pathologist, psychologist, sensory integrative therapist (pediatric occupational therapist), and movement therapist. The process can be initiated by a private psychiatrist in an office setting, with referrals made to appropriate specialists, or it can be done at a clinic or hospital setting where services may be more centralized. In either case, it is of the utmost importance that those chosen to take part in the evaluation process have the patience and experience needed to work with these children.

Haslett (1977) presents an outline for a comprehensive child psychiatric evaluation.

One approach to the differential assessment of seriously disturbed infants and preschool children, outlined by Provence (1974), is that of the Yale Child Study Center. It requires 5 to 6 interview sessions with parents and 3 to 6 sessions with the child, and combines informal play, formal testing, and individually selected physical, neurological, and biological examinations. The formal "Revised Yale Developmental Schedules," derived from Gesell, Stanford Binet, Merrill Palmer and Viennese Scale items, with other supplemental tests, is used. This results in a developmental profile with four categories, including motor (gross and fine), adaptive (perceptive-integrative), speech, and personal-social. It covers communication, affective expression, perception, manipulation skills, sense of self, relationship to others, social skills, coping ability and major defenses, intelligence and levels of functioning, self-help, sensitivity and insensitivity to stimuli, impulse control, aggressive behavior, thought processes and content, body mastery and sphincter control, and autoerotic and auto-aggressive activities. When organized according to developmental assets and deficits and other parameters, this data contributes to formulation of the treatment plan, and provides a baseline for periodic reassessment.

Another approach to assessment of these children is practiced by the authors at the Developmental Center for Autistic Children in Philadephia, where a streamlined format has been designed in response to the length of time, often months, which it takes following usual procedures to formulate a diagnosis, recommend a treatment plan, and have that plan instituted. The major differences in the procedure of that center are that the major portion of the evaluation takes place in one 3-hour period, usually in the morning, and that the entire evaluation team is present for the evaluation. The team consists of a child psychiatrist, developmental pediatrician, perceptual-cognitive specialist, psychiatric social worker with background in family dynamics, speech pathologist, body movement therapist, pediatric occupational (sensory integrative) therapist, and early and special education specialist.

Following initial referral, all previous medical records of child and mother, including pregnancy and perinatal records, previous evaluations, and clinic, preschool, or school records are collected and reviewed by the team for appropriateness for evaluation. On the basis of this initial screening, some children are referred to more appropriate facilities for the evaluation. Further information and studies may be sought prior to evaluation day. A member of the team may make a home or school visit to observe and interview if this is indicated.

On the day of the evaluation the team, located behind a one-way mirror, observes the child in a playroom with various combinations of one or both parents and with several different therapists who conduct their own assessments, as well as adding specific tasks or interactions requested by other team members. The child may also be observed with other family members, familiar caretakers, or teachers. A snack is provided and a bathroom made available to add to the data observed. Opportunity is thus present to note many aspects of the child, his relationship to others, family interaction, gross and fine motor functioning, problem-solving ability, use of communicative speech—in short, most of the parameters required for the evaluation. In addition, a BRIAAC Rating (Behavioral Rating Instrument for Autistic and Atypical Children) assesses the child along the 10 levels of the eight scales of that rating system. This is used as a basis for comparison if the child is reevaluated at a later date. The observation period is also videotaped for further evaluation and for use as a baseline.

Following the observation period an hour-long team conference which includes the referring professionals takes place. All material is reviewed, a multiaxial diagnosis is proposed, etiologic factors are considered and given priority ordering, and a treatment plan is proposed. If further studies are warranted, these are arranged for. Immediately following the evaluation conference, the parents or guardians are met with and the findings and recommendations are discussed with them. Assistance is provided for the family until the appropriate placement has been achieved.

Basic Principles of Therapy

1. Multidisciplinary Approach. The basic goal of therapy with the psychotic child is to restart, redirect, or reshape the specific developmental processes found to be disturbed in the evaluative assessment. The nature of the treatment approach and emphasis has usually been a reflection of the therapist's training, conceptual orientation, and ideas about etiology and pathogenesis, as well as a need to "sell" his or her particular contribution. Those who have a psychoanalytic-developmental framework tend to focus on the establishment of relationship in individual or family therapy with the goal of effecting changes in personality and psychotic structure. Those grounded in learning theory apply these principles via behavior therapy and special eduation. Those with an organic orientation tend to use medication, physical treatment, body manipulation, and behavior training.

The growing trend toward a concept of multicausality has resulted in a broadening of the therapeutic spectrum in clinics that formerly emphasized one or another modality. Many prominent exponents of chemotherapy now warn that medication is an adjunct to total therapeutic management. Some psychoanalytically oriented milieu programs are integrating learning theory and more structured behavioral approaches as indicated. Special therapies such as speech, movement, music, art, and sensory-integration have also become significant and important. In short, while there may be the occasional superbly qualified and talented individual who can effectively single-handedly treat the young severely disturbed child, the trend is towards the multidisciplined team approach with integration of several different modalities as needed.

2. Approaching the Child at Its Level. Perhaps the simplest basic principle—and unfortunately, the least heeded—is that the child must be approached in each area of its development at the level at which he or she is functioning. Too often the nature and level of contact is geared to chronological age, to physical size or maturation, or to

the level of highest accomplishment or skill, no matter how narrow that area may be.

An example of the need to approach the child at his level is the initial contact with a 6-year-old autistic boy who could read and speak in full sentences but in a mechanical echolalic way. When approached frontally and greeted by name, he averted his gaze or "looked through" the therapist, and when pressured to make contact at the verbal and visual level, rolled his eyes up so only the sclerae showed. When touched on his shoulder he sank to the floor. When the therapist noted his infantile crib-like position on the floor, the therapist started to rock back and forth on his knees over him and hum. The child responded by babbling, looking at the therapist's face, and reaching up to grasp at the therapist's collar. Despite his age and apparent cognitive abilities, the child had to be engaged as if he were a crib-aged infant to initiate therapy.

With the younger, more pervasively delayed child, the approach can take the form of joining the child in his motor activity (rocking or spinning with him) or in his primitive vocalizations. At a higher level repeating his babbling may develop a communicative link. A music therapist might pick up the rocking or tapping rhythm or the tones and key of his crying. In each instance the goal is to have the child feel and give evidence that he has been contacted and accepted, and to respond with eye contact or expression.

3. The program should address itself to both intrinsic and extrinsic pathology. Not only the developmental psychological factors, behaviors, organic problems, and other "child-focused" problems as delineated in the evaluation must be programmed for, but also the child's environment, living situation, parental conflicts affecting the child, and general care must be attended to in a systematic way. A schizophrenic 5-year-old with separated parents who used her as a medium through which they communicated their hostilities, and from whom they could satisfy their needs for a captive provider of exclusive love, got progressively more psychotic despite intensive daily treatment in a day clinic setting until her mother and father were induced to receive individual therapy for their respective problems, as well as family sessions. This relieved the tension on the child, who then could progress.

4. The treatment plan must be repeatedly revised to reflect changes in each of the areas of disturbed development, including factors such as biological development, maturation, regression, and effectiveness of the treatment. The child who progresses from a state of autistic withdrawal through a symbiotic phase of clinging attachment to a more schizophrenic type of illness will need somewhat different therapeutic approaches at each stage, and emphasis may be switched from one therapist to another. A 6-year-old boy who followed just such a progression became so overwhelmed by the intensity and apparent reality of his psychotic fantasies about his male therapist, generated by the unaccustomed increase in relationship and closeness, that therapy was at a standstill. However, he was given the opportunity to develop a therapeutic relationship simultaneously with a female music therapist, could make an alliance with her and continue to progress, and was encouraged to become involved aggressively in sports and games. When he was more secure in his recognition of his fantasies as such, it was possible to shift the emphasis back to his male therapist again to work on these feelings. These changes were necessary because his ego was not strong enough to deal with the intensity of the relationship with a male therapist at a certain stage of his development, and this had to be reflected in his treatment plan. Later, overwhelming seductive fantasies concerning his female music therapist developed and had to be handled in a similar manner.

5. There should be an adequate therapeutic trial of at least three years with psychotic children before one can be sure that the level one has reached is a more or less permanent plateau beyond which there will be diminishing returns and limited therapeutic resources should be focused elsewhere. It often happens with the younger, more pervasively disturbed child that the first sustained signs of self-image and self-esteem and motivation do not appear until after two to three years of effort. Similarly, the first spontaneous vocalizations, practicing of lip and tongue movements, and simple words may not appear for a long period of time, yet eventually develop into some degree of communicability.

In assessing therapeutic effectiveness over time, it should be remembered that development in psychotic children of all varieties is irregular in both order and degree, with bursts of change and advancement occurring between long plateaus where there appears to be little change.

Schema for Therapeutic Management and Continuing Assessment

Of equal importance to the basic principles of therapy noted above is the attention given to the overall schema of therapy. It is essential that several key areas be consistently addressed and decisions made at the onset of treatment. Data for making these decisions will of course be derived from the initial evaluation and assessment. One approach is to review the four basic components of the therapeutic complex (adapted from Wenar, 1977) in setting up the treatment program.

1. The therapeutic setting: outpatient, home, day care, special class, therapeutic nursery, residential.
2. The therapeutic agent: professional therapist, child care specialist (para-professional) with professional supervision, parent.
3. The therapeutic approach: relationship, behavior therapy, drug therapy, education.
4. Target behavior: eye contact, relationship, rituals, self-stimulation, self-destructiveness, speech, imitation, cognitive function, and others.

All of these are highly dependent on the level of functioning of the child, and must be combined in individually indicated ways. In general, the younger the child and the earlier the onset, the more pervasive is the pathology, and the more comprehensive the approach.

From the outset, it is exptremely helpful to have a system of record-keeping for each child which simply and clearly delineates all of the problems in every area with opportunity for all those who may work with the child to add data. Some modification of a problem-oriented record system can be useful for this. In this type of a system, when a child enters a treatment program, the relevant team or the individual managing the case, be it in a private or clinic setting, opens a working record which begins with a data base consisting of no more than two paragraphs which describe briefly identifying data, age, family constellation, presenting problems, referring agency, previous treatment attempts, living situation, and educational status. Following this, several categories are set up to head lists of current problems. These are arranged according to the needs of the therapists, but can include categories such as social/family, psychological, educational, medical, abnormal behaviors, and so forth. Under each heading all problems as determined by evaluation are listed with a proposed plan of action, and the person responsible for following through on that plan. Target dates for review of progress are set. This record is then used each time the case is reviewed, with deletion of items no longer problems, and addition of new problem areas. Lengthy reports from various disciplines are placed in another part of the record for reference as needed. It should be emphasized that a big problem in treating very disturbed or multiply handicapped children is maintaining a constant awareness of all the problems the child faces, and maintaining communication between all those who may work with the child.

The Treatment Milieu

Milieu therapy evolved from the recognition of the therapeutic value of a planned environment in which the child's needs are provided, his anxieties alleviated, and his efforts to have an impact and communicate, however subtle or indirect, are sensitively discerned and responded to with consistency and availability. For the more pervasively disturbed younger child there are primary caretaking adults and a multidisciplinary team of therapists who attempt to reduce confusion, induce structure, and enhance the child's relational, cognitive, and adaptive activities. Such a setting may be offered on a residential or a day program basis.

Bettelheim (1974) feels that the child must be removed from what he views as the unconscious psychotogenic parental hostility. Parents are replaced by concerned caretakers in a 24-hour therapeutic environment where the psychotic process can be undone and relationship correctively reexperienced. The caretaker, under psychoanalytically oriented supervision, relates to the child on the level of his pathology and must be available on a 24-hour crisis intervention basis. Psychotic defenses are relinquished after trust is established, needs and desires are met, and the feeling of powerlessness from which the defenses arose is undone. The therapeutic milieu provides the experience in reality that one indeed has an impact on the environment and has a role in determining what happens to him without reprisal.

Goldfarb, Mintz, and Strook (1969) designed a residential therapeutic environment to provide "corrective socialization" through therapeutic and educative procedures which "focuses on every relational encounter." Goldfarb considers the essential therapeutic instrument to be the responses of the adult human environment, designed to clarify confusion, point out reality, and demonstrate coping and social adaptation. Self-awareness, time and space orientation, general awareness of the environment, and the development of a sense of identity and individuality are facilitated. This corrective social milieu is coordinated with individual psychoanalytically oriented psychotherapy. Weekend contact with the family is required, and relationship conflicts in this area addressed in preparation for eventual return to the family constellation.

Ruttenberg (1971) described a psychoanalytically and developmentally oriented relationship milieu therapy day program for autistic and other severely disturbed psychotic children. This has as its core the establishment of a positive emotional relationship with a warm, sensitive mothering person, who, as in the Bettelheim program, approaches the child at his level of functioning and attempts affective contact, which, if not overwhelming, will counter the child's tendency to withdraw and isolate. The relationship thus formed is used to develop self-concept and body image, and to enhance motivation to explore and master the environment. This first relationship becomes the child's prototype for a sense of trust, individuation, and ultimately object constancy. The child care worker, at the appropriate time, then provides a bridge to other therapists, as well as a means for presenting the child with developmental tasks as suggested by more specialized staff.

Initially the milieu encourages the 1:1 interaction, with a small cubicle to which each child and caretaker can retreat. This provides a degree of sameness as to surroundings, toys, and area to rest. Gradually group functions are entered into and intervention by other therapists occurs depending on the developmental stage. As sense of self and socialization skills increase, peer groups of two or three children are formed. Other types of therapeutic milieus emphasize learning theory and behavior modification, or group interaction (Goldfarb, Mintz, and Strook, 1969), and some combine behavior modification and psychodynamic developmental approaches (Helm, 1976; Davids and Berenson, 1977).

Individual Therapies Focused on the Child

Individual therapies involve a one-to-one interchange between the therapist and child which can be conceptualized in terms of specific theories of human behavior and according to special areas of stimulation needed by the child. Theoretical approaches include: (1) psychoanalytic concepts of ego function and development, object relationship, and drive development, conflict and defense, transference, psychic energy, and structure; (2) adaptational and interactional concepts; (3) learning theory; and (4) therapeutic approaches stemming from work with pathologic development in such special areas as speech and hearing, reflex development and body movement, as well as music and art therapy. No matter what the modality, all must recognize the importance of initial rapport, therapeutic alliance, and engagement of interest; in short, all those terms implying development of basic trust. It must also be stressed that individual approaches are most successful when correlated with the child's total environmental experience.

Psychoanalytic Approaches

Melanie Klein (1932) first gave detailed accounts of the psychoanalysis of psychotic children. McDougall and Lebovici (1969) report in detail the psychoanalysis of a 7-year-old schizophrenic boy who in earlier years had shown autistic symptoms. Use is made of transference phenomena. Through verbal questioning and discussion, and analysis of projective play and art productions, clarification, interpretation, and reconstruction are possible. This technique is usually reserved for the verbal schizophrenic or symbiotic child, although nonverbal and preverbal infantile behavior may provide clues for reconstructions and understanding in terms of transference.

Psychoanalytically oriented psychotherapies also use play and interview techniques and interpret symbolic meaning. The therapist makes freer use of information provided by outside sources and often will include the parents in the therapetuic situation. Less work with reconstruction of earlier traumas and transference is attempted. Rather analytic developmental concepts of relationship, development of sexual and aggressive drives, and defense are used to reactivate emotional progress along the developmental lines.

Initiation of the relationship, on which the subsequent therapy is based, should include (Holter and Ruttenberg, 1971): (1) total emotional availability and undivided attention; (2) sensitivity to the child's subtle cues; (3) ability to respond to those cues at the child's level; (4) comfortable selective participation in the child's discharge phenomena; (5) sharing of affect; and (6) sharing of experience. Once the initial intervention is successful and contact is made, a new approach reflecting the next developmental step is taken. Holter (in Ruttenberg, 1971) describes the technique of focal approach used to interrupt the repetitive plateau of sameness. Eye contact is pursued and focal involvement attempted in the mode of behavior the child is using as a defense.

Tinbergen and Tinbergen (1972) have proposed an ethologically based approach to the treatment of autistic and atypical children which fills the need for a nonverbal approach to nonverbal children. They note that with the possible exception of face aversion, all the other components of social reactions manifested by autistic children are to be found, albeit in an abbreviated manner, in the behavior of normal children. Every infant is seen to be in conflict between his bonding desires and fear, and that, normally, a positive reaction on the part of the environment allays these fears and encourages relationship. If genetic and/or traumatic early experiences produce a fearful, hypersensitive child, he withdraws into autism and has an aversion to the level of stimulation and the nature of the usual signals that encourage bonding. Therapy must take these sensitivities into account and employ a low-keyed approach. This view from an ethologist is interesting in that it independently arrives at initial therapeutic techniques similar to those of psychoanalytically oriented therapists.

Mahler (1968) sums up the psychotherapeutic goals as seeking establishment of body image integrity, restoration of ego functions and relationship, and neutralization of aggression with libidinal gratification. Interpretation of primary process behavior and fantasy leads to assimilation, integration, and synthesis. The therapist must provide auxiliary ego strength and support, and set limits to protect the child from destructive impulses which create panic, as well as help the child undo confusion and fragmentation and establish coherence through play therapy. Then relationship in time and space, bodily functions, and the realities of various social relationships can be taught.

Detailed accounts of psychoanlytically oriented psychotherapy of psychotic children are provided by Mahler (1968), her associates Bergman and Kupfermann (in McDevitt and Settlage, eds., 1971), Bettelheim (1967), Ekstein (1966, 1971), Szurek and Berlin, (1973), McDougall and Lebovici (1969), and others.

Behavior Modification

Systematic application of certain principles of learning theory, particularly learning through reinforcement, rather than those of learning by imitation, have effected relatively rapid acquisition of or change in specific behaviors (Ney, Palvesky, and Markely, 1971). Positive reinforcement (rewarding) tends to enhance learning of behavior, while negative reinforcement (punishing) or nonreinforcement (not responding) tends to diminish or extinguish behavior. Operant conditioning methods use contingent and immediate reinforcement. With psychotic children, positive reinforcement in the form of food, tokens, a desired activity, or a caretaker's hug or enthusiastic approval is used to motivate initiation or increase of specific desired behaviors such as attending, imitation, naming, eating or toileting behaviors, and accepting cognitive tasks. Negative reinforcements such as slapping, pinching, electrostimulating (shocking), isolating, or ignoring are used to reduce or eliminate bizarre mannerisms or speech, aggressive, destructive, and self-mutilating behavior, tantrums, uncooperativeness or inattention, and resistance to toilet training. (Lovaas, 1971; Churchill, 1969; Hingtgen, Coulter, and Churchill, 1967). Leff (1968) reviews the use of behavior modification techniques in the psychoses of childhood. Yates (1970) listed six uses of these techniques as (1) elimination of undesirable behavior; (2) manipulation of nonsocial behavior in a controlled environment; (3) teaching speech, (4) training capacity for imitation; (5) developing cognitive skills; and (6) social skills.

Behavior therapists are less concerned with etiology, especially in terms of conflict and defense. They view the psychotic child's behavior and low function as a consequence of an impoverished repertoire of behaviors with which to respond with adaptation, coping and relating. They (Ferster, 1961; Hamblin et al., 1971) postulate that this impoverishment came from a lack of parental reinforcement of the child's earliest attempts to explore and interact. Subsequently a wide range of behaviors that depend on social reinforcement for their unfolding failed to develop. The autistic and other psychotic behaviors tend to perpetuate this condition by warding off social reinforcement and shutting out experiential environmental stimuli via their self-stimulating repetitive and bizarre behaviors.

Though there are reports of machine-like application of reinforcement, including hundreds of persistently repetitive and methodical trials, behavior therapy is more often practiced within a total milieu of special education program with specific target behaviors in mind, rather than as an exclusive treatment approach. There are a number of behavior modification programs in the literature that can be referred to, which are designed to change any variety of undesired behaviors in emotionally disturbed and retarded children. These can be appplied by an individual therapist or an entire milieu can be programmed to focus on a particular behavior. Parents and teachers can be involved in the program. Again, this approach is most successful when used in a developmental and relationship context.

Lichstein and Schreibman (1976) report the use of electric shocks to extinguish a variety of behaviors such as self-destructiveness (head banging, skin tearing), antisocial behaviors (biting, smearing, screaming), autoeroticism, resistiveness, bizarre movements, and escape and avoidance behaviors. They review twelve studies, all of which found the aversive technique to be highly effective in removing the specific undesirable behaviors in autistic and schizophrenic children. Some response generalization, increase in social behaviors, and affective responses were reported. There was fear of the apparatus and some negative emotional responses (withdrawal, sullenness) occurred, but it was felt that positive responses outweighed negative ones.

Psychotic children do tend to respond to a consistent structured learning situation and environment. However, the ususal highly organized behavior modification program tends not to take into account the level and rate of emotional development, the defensive need, and the emotional significance of the behavior to be modified when targeting behavior goals.

Behavior therapy focuses on the achievement of specific tasks or modes of behavior. Limitations of this method include the lack of generalization from the specific learned behavior, the lack of general motivation toward learning and exploration, a lack of integration of these behaviors into an overall total alteration and breadth of personality change (humanization necessary to achieve clinical normality), and a lack of permanence of change.

A 10-year-old child who had been in a strictly controlled behavior modification program for autistic behaviors with an apparent organic substrate illustrated some of the problems that can occur. He had verbal responses, but they were mechanical, rote, without generalization, and without affect, and he would sit and wait for the next order. He reprimanded himself by slapping his own face or banging his head, had a general robot quality about him, and looked as if he were about to explode with intense rage. Recent experience has shown that children whose affect and behavior are contained and controlled by operant conditioning methods do not internalize these in the form of self-control, but require the outside reinforcer. They frequently "go wild" and lose all capacity for impulse control. The above-mentioned child was placed in a 1:1 millieu day program where he was helped to respond affectively. For an extended period there was a strong display of rage and disorganization, at times requiring that he be strapped in a chair to keep him from hurting others or himself. Gradually this was phased out and behavior became more cooperative. After 1 3/4 years of treatment he was able to initiate exploration and mastery, was pleased with his own image, and could express himself more spontaneously in full sentences. He could enjoy adults and was starting to interact with peers. Without the at-times chaotic process of rebuilding his ego functions, with increase in impulse control and affective response, his personality development would not have resumed despite the external behavioral approach.

Mahler's tripartite approach focuses on correction of the distortions which occurred during the symbiotic period of relationship development. The child reexperiences the traumatic symbiotic phase of development directly with his mother; then with the help of the therapist this is replaced with a higher-level less ambivalent relationship. Schopler and Reichler (1971) also report the use of parents as co-therapists.

Both DesLauriers (1962), for older childhood schizophrenics, and Schopler (1965) for early-onset psychotics, having implicated diminished ability to establish contact with reality by virtue of disorders of subcortical arousal mechanisms due to early sensory deprivation, advocate and describe intrusive approaches and bodily stimulation and contact. Piaget's (1951) concept that exploratory activity leads to relationship have contributed to this approach.

Later, DesLauriers and Carleson (1969) applied the principles of face-to-face contact and intrusive stimulation to the arousal system to the treatment of early infantile autism. The premise is that autistic children have not received adequate sensory stimulation, whether from environmental failure (stimulus deprivation) or from internal dysfunction due to an abnormally high threshold for sensory receptivity, or from failure to make the transition from proximal to distal sensory reception (Schopler, 1965). Lacking this, the child has been unable to delineate his body boundaries and his differentiation from the rest of the world. The therapeutic approach is to provide kinesthetic, tactile, and proprioceptive stimulation in a playful atmosphere. (These same stimuli are also provided by mothering, by the early levels of relationship therapy, and by body movement therapy.) Here the approach is an intrusive and insistent stimulating emotional reaction, albeit sometimes negative. The goal is to learn that human contact can be pleasurable and to afford affective experiences with which to identify.

Zaslow (1964) speculates that autism is due to maternal mishandling of the child's infantile rage by certain mothers who cannot tolerate rage and who withdraw or respond in kind, and he pushes the intrusion to the point of eliciting rage and panic, then proceeds to "take over" in the process of supplying physical control, with firm and nonanxious soothing, rocking, and love (see also Saposnik, 1967). All report positive affective response and ego function development.

Special Adjunctive Therapies

These modalities are avenues of initial contact and corrective psychotherapeutic experience as well as sources of stimulation of development in pathologic areas.

Sensorimotor integrative therapy (pediatric O.T.) assesses and corrects pathological and residual infantile reflexes that interfere with muscle tonus, posture, and motor skills; and compromise the development of mastery, gross and fine motor skills; and the attainment of adequate body image and self-esteem. The relief experienced by the child upon attaining proper muscle tone, stability, balance, and proprioception encourages relationship and general motivation (Ayres, 1973).

Language and communication therapy (Wolf and Ruttenberg, 1967) emphasizes the need to motivate the autistic and atypical language delayed child to become interested in listening to sounds and then in learning and practicing to produce sounds and to articulate words. Here, too, therapeutic rapport must be established, and the speech pathologist's knowledge of the developmental processes of hearing and speech formation and the hierarchical sequences of words, grammar, and language deployed. Verbal schizophrenic children are helped through the therapeutic relationship at the level of pronoun usage, communicative narration, symbolism, and concept formation. Schizophrenic thought disorder and clang associations are corrected through encouragement of an ordered thought process and expression through language.

Whereas language therapy employing operant conditioning methods may be more applicable to the disorders of early onset (Baltaxe and Simmons, 1975), with the schizophrenic child, the use of the therapeutic relationship and encouraging reality testing is the more effective vehicle for therapeutic change in language and communication (Hicks, 1972).

Body Movement Therapy uses the Laban notation concepts of effort-shape and the psychologic drive equivalents of muscle tension-flow patterns (Kestenberg, 1965). Kalish (1968) has developed techniques of assessment, approach, and movement interaction with young psychotic children in which the movement therapist mirrors and elaborates on the nonverbal activity of the child, establishing emotional contact through the mutual movement and eliciting in the child an awareness and use of his own body and its parts, adaptively and for expression, thus stimulating a body image. Verbal concepts such as up, down, in, out, fast, slow, on, under, etc., are introduced in the context of the interactivity. With more developmentally advanced symbiotic and schizophrenic children, correlation of body language cues and verbal language equivalents is attempted and an activity milieu is provided for acting out feelings and playing out infantile memories, fantasies, and aggressive impulses (Bernstein, 1972). This approaches Ekstein's (1971) therapeutic use of play-acting in the metaphor, and psychodrama with schizophrenics. Often long-term body movement therapy starting nonvocally can eventually develop into a predominately verbal-in-the-course-of-movement communication and psychotherapy.

Play and art therapy employ toys, hand puppets, dolls and doll furniture, clay and other molding, drawing, and painting materials, building blocks, and construction paper for cutting and pasting. These can be used as media for affective and drive tension discharge, and for projection of conflicts, reliving and reworking of traumatic experiences, and the expression of fantasy (Kramer, 1972). Elkish (1968) provides an illustrated case history.

In music therapy, Nordoff and Robbins (1965, 1976) have developed improvisational techniques that engage psychotic multihandicapped children at their level of musical function by picking up the basic beat and rhythms as found in their dancing, spinning, rocking, and finger movements, and joining in in the tone and key of their sounds, which include cries, humming, shrieking, and improvising music that gives the child the feeling that he has been sensitively "read" and picked up on. This provides a nonthreatening musical experience that expresses the child's unverbalized affects and moods and to which the child can respond or attend. Once engaged, the child can be influenced by changes in tempo, pitch, key, and rubato. Control can be induced by the child's following the beat, changes, rests, and stops. Question and answer, give and take, reciprocal musical games can stimulate interaction and vocalization. For example, a music therapist echoed a child screeching, whereupon the screeching settled down to a repetitive "ee-ah" that was exchanged alternately between the child and therapist with growing attention. Soon the child said it quickly and waited for the reply. Suddenly the child reversed the sequence to "ah-ee" and laughed. The therapist responded with the same reverse and also laughed, turning this into a game of change and surprise. The child obviously felt he had an impact, and contact was made between therapist and child. The child expanded his relationship and vocalizations, and in time words, concepts, and interpretations of feelings could be introduced through the medium of songs and lyrics improvised for the individual child. This, as in movement therapy, can gravitate to a more verbal psychotherapy. Nonimprovisational group music can introduce early education concepts of learning parts of the body, steps in dressing, taking turns, and other social interactions. Nursery school–type songs, either standard or written for the groups, can be used, and each child can use a simple musical instrument identified as his (whistle, tone block, horn, etc.). The music therapist chooses these special instruments and vocal activities to foster attention span, impulse control, and other basic skills needed for learning, socialization, and class interaction, and teaches self-help procedures. These unfold step by step to music and lyrics composed specifically for the purpose.

Some supposedly nonverbal children can sing words and express conflicts in song though they cannot talk them, and verbal psychotherapy can be conducted through this medium (B. Grinnell, personal communication). Interestingly, children who can sing but not talk are frequently the suspected victims of early child abuse, and are often the only left-handed child in a right-handed family, with specific language disabilities on an organic basis. We have postulated, based on the nature of their flinching, that they have sustained blows on the left side of the head dealt by right-handed abusers, with resultant brain damage and shift of dominance to the right side of the brain. Though an aphasic disorder results as far as the spoken word, it is known that the center for singing words is on the opposite (right) side of the brain and may account for the ability for verbal expression in song. Schizophrenic children often find it easier to express conflict through singing and dancing in individual and group sessions by reason of mobilization of their affect in motor expression (Heimlich, 1965).

Group therapies are designed to provide corrective socialization contact with peers, provide adult monitoring and role models, and the shaping of group expectation and reactions. Smolen and Lifton (1966) describe outpatient group therapy in a child guidance clinic setting. Each child was approached within the group at his level of function and appreciation of reality. Group interaction and response were encouraged. Expectations were conveyed and the underlying feelings of the children elicited or expressed for them. Parents were instructed to carry on the process at home rather than foster or accept infantile or regressive behaviors.

Group psychotherapy is usually conducted with verbal older schizophrenic children, often with a mix of lesser degrees of ego disturbance. Speers and Lansing (1965) undertook group psychotherapy with young psychotic children, associated with collateral group therapy with their parents. Coffey and Wiener (1967) report successful group treatment of autistic children.

At the Developmental Center for Autistic Children group experiences are a part of the total milieu and are therapeutic rather than therapy per se. They may involve (1) groups of two to stimulate peer interaction, including rivalry; (2) a daily group orientation on arrival, such as sitting forming a circle, with good-morning songs involving the name of each child, day of the week, and plans for the day; (3) a body movement group, where they learn social and game rules and taking turns, and experience both peer disapproval and support; (4) group singing of nursery school songs created or adapted for teaching body parts, concepts, self-help skills, etc.; (5) a transitional class group with a 1:2 or 1:3 teacher-pupil ratio easing the transition from the 1:1 relationship to the standard special class 1:4 ratio.

Educational and Remedial Therapy

The advent in 1975 of the U.S. Federal Right to Education for All Handicapped Act (P.L. 94–142) has defined the relationship between special education and its supportive therapeutic adjuncts and is responsible for a shift toward the provision of therapy for psychotic children of school age (4.7–21) within or in association with special school or classroom settings.

Pioneering examples are Highwick in England,

Southard School at the Menninger Foundation, Topeka, Kansas, Pendelton-Bradley in Providence, R.I., Fenichel's League School in Brooklyn, and Bettelheim's Orthogenic School in Chicago. At Highwick, the child's defenses are respected, but any signs of relationship-seeking are immediately gratified. Without demands and pressure, motivation for relationship and learning increase. Southard School provides psychoanalytic psychotherapy in a therapeutic educational milieu. Pendelton-Bradley evolved a balance between psychotherapy, operant conditioning, perceptual-motor training, and cognitive stimulation. The League School attempts to relieve anxiety and confusion, encourages social relationships, teaches skills, and facilitates success. It begins individually and introduces a group with limits and protection. Bettelheim's milieu has been described.

There is an increased interest in educational approaches that make use of teachers specially trained to stimulate cognitive and emotional development. Depending on the level of functioning of the psychotic child, the therapeutic process may involve infant stimulation, early education, and special education techniques. The latter is most useful when there is an accompanying substrate of organic brain dysfunction.

Psychotic children, particularly those with early onset, are woefully behind in their academic experience and achievement because of interference with the learning processes and autonomous ego functioning caused by the psychotic processes and the often underlying intrinsic disorders of language and perception.

Goals include increasing motivation for an interest in learning. Specific remedial targets include language and communication, reading, perceptual discrimination, motor skills, and sensory-motor coordination. Special modifications of infant stimulation techniques have been used, and with nursery school children Montessori methods have been developed and adapted. Frostig and Horne (1970) combine psychoanalytic principles with therapeutic education in three sequential stages of establishing initial rapport and relationship, building a body image, and then stimulating perceptual, motor, and cognitive-learning function.

The Dubnoff (1965) Center in Los Angeles, while recognizing these principles of ego and emotional support, has added a detailed series of structured sequential developmental learning programs involving behavior shaping techniques.

Whittaker (1975) lists seven problem clusters common to the wide group of disturbed children, including the childhood psychotics now served by mandate, in special classes: (1) poor impulse control; (2) low self-image; (3) poor modulation of emotions; (4) relationship defects; (5) upset family equilibria; (6) specific learning disabilities; (7) limited play skills. He proposes a devel-opmental/educational paradigm of the therapeutic milieu, wherein the daily living experience, routines, group interaction games, activities, classroom education, and adjunctive therapies become a medium for stimulation of expanded development and not just a program for behavioral management.

Drug and Other Somatic Therapies

Excellent reviews of this area have been done by Campbell (1973) and Campbell and Shapiro (1975). The increasing view of childhood psychoses as manifestations of organic, biological disorders or deficits has been reflected in widespread clinical trials of many drugs and other somatic agents. Unfortunately, reports of alleviation of symptomatology based on a few cases poorly classified as to subgroups and imprecisely described, rather than carefully controlled studies, are followed by too free use of the chemotherapy agents, especially by general practitioners, pediatricians, and psychiatrists under pressure to do something and looking for a "cure." They may be either incapable of conducting a psychotherapeutic program or supervising a broad-based therapeutic milieu, or unwilling or unable to commit the amount of time and money required. Ekstein, Bryant, and Friedman (1966) note that first reports of somatic therapies tend to come from centers that treat larger numbers of children and are under pressure for rapid admission and discharge.

Among the biophysical interventions reported, prefrontal lobotomy, insulin coma and metrazol shock therapies, and electroconvulsive therapies have been used with some general, limited, usually transient effect. Bender (1947) reported one hundred cases of childhood schizophrenia under 12 treated with electroconvulsive shock treatment and noted no change in the essential schizophrenic process, but did report improvement in the capacity to deal with anxiety and other secondary symptom formation (hallucinations and delusions). The children were reportedly better able to accept teaching and psychotherapy, but there was a flattening of affect. There was no deterioration in intellectual capacity, and prognosis improved when ECT was added to the total program. However, girls near puberty associated it with sexual submission and boys with punishment. Younger children submitted passively and with little overt anxiety. ECT is now in use only with adolescent manic-depressive and catatonic schizophrenics.

Biological therapies are directed to the central nervous system and influence its neurophysiologic and metabolic processes. Recent neuropsychopharmacological studies of transmethylation, neuro affector transfer metabolism, biogenic amine metabolism, and enzyme and protein metabolism envision the therapeutic correction of the specific metabolic defect by chemotherapeutic replacement, blocking, or neutralization. This would require specific metabolic assessment techniques not as yet available and might explain why drugs given to psychotic children with similar symptoms may have diametrically opposite effects.

Those who favor a biological basis for psychosis consider chemotherapy an essential part of the therapeutic program, and may report that medication is the only regimen that was effective, or the part of the regime that was most effective. Others with a multifaceted approach generally consider drugs as an adjunctive part of a broad based therapeutic regimen, inasmuch as the drug per se does not undo fixated patterns of learned responses or provide trust and relationship. Drugs have limited results and affect only specific portions of the clinical symptomatology, and they are not without serious side effects. They may be very helpful in reducing symptoms that interfere with the child's contact with his environment, and thus his learning, socialization, coping, and relating, by counteracting apathy and withdrawal, reducing hyperactivity, rage, self-mutilation, panic reactions, insomnia, and autoerotic preoccupation, and may help externalize internal rumination and enhance impulse control. Irritability and aggressivity, disorganization, confusion, and psychotic thought disorder may be reduced. Campbell (1973) has concluded that as yet, with the possible exception of lithium for the treatment of psychotic depressions or manic-depressive psychoses, there is no drug that in and of itself is a specific therapeutic agent for any diagnostic subcategory of the childhood psychoses. She also feels, however, that "drug treatment is an essential component of the total treatment of the psychotic child of preschool age," inasmuch as the psychoses of early onset are more pervasive and require broader, more intense treatment, and that such a child may be less responsive to drug treatment at a later age. The severity of the psychotic condition and the generally poor prognosis warrant the associated risks.

Campbell and Shapiro (1975) list general indications and guidelines for drug therapy, which include tables of classification and dosage. They stress the adjunctive nature of drug therapy, the purpose of which is to facilitate maturation and development through influencing not only immediate symptoms but also the long-term process of the illness. Should a drug interfere with maturation or learning (i.e., Dexedrine slowing physical growth, or chlorpromazine dulling affect, activity, and mental alertness), it should be discontinued. Thorough acquaintance with the "battery" of available drugs is essential in that side effects produced by one may be avoided by switching to another in the same subclassification with somewhat different properties. For instance, though in the same group as chlorpromazine, trifluoperazine tends to be less dulling. While still accomplishing a degree of control, it tends to counteract withdrawal into fantasy and to stimulate verbalization of the fantasy. At times one must balance the positive and negative effects and in a sense "orchestrate" the medication. For instance, a very angry, assaultive, or self-mutilative schizophrenic may need to be brought under control with the more sedating chlorpromazine to the point of depression of affect and activity and inaccessibility to teaching. Once the control is established, the child is not maintained in this state, but dosage is reduced, and a drug with more stimulating properties such as haloperidol or trifluoperazine is then substituted.

In the drug therapy of children the following special considerations should be kept in mind:

1. Before initiating chemotherapy with the major tranquilizers (neuroleptics), a complete pediatric examination should be performed, with a complete blood count including differential, a urinalysis, and liver function studies. Ideally the laboratory studies should be repeated weekly for the first month, and monthly thereafter.

2. A child is dependent on adult supervision for proper administration of medication. Thus the parent should be fully informed of the nature of the medication and anticipated therapeutic effects and side effects. Chemotherapy on an outpatient basis should be prescribed only if the responsible adult is deemed competent and reliable with regard to regular administration and keeping the drug in a safe place.

3. Parental attitudes toward medication may be positive or negative. It can be used as a way of imposing control over the child, or as a "magic cure" which will help keep the family from dealing

with its interactional problems. Some parents object to the use of medication because of a fear that this will lead to hard drug use or indiscriminate pill use at a later time. Usually, frank discussion about the real need and specific indications will allay these fears. For medication to be effective, interfering expectations and attitudes have to be dealt with.

4. These are powerful drugs with many side effects. These may be specific for the class of drug (dermatologic sensitivities, extrapyramidal system effects, etc.), nonspecific (irritability, loss of or increase of appetite, drowsiness), or true allergic reactions. A careful history should be taken of any allergic problems or drug sensitivities in the child and his family. A history of allergy mandates cautious administration, and in general, it is wise to administer only one drug at a time unless a special problem arises. Among the more common side effects of antipsychotic medications are loss of appetite, irritability, blurring of vision, muscle discomfort, and slowed reaction time. Extrapyramidal dystonias and dyskinesias are seen more frequently in the preadolescent and adolescent. These may be cause for reducing dose, changing drugs, or adding an anti-Parkinsonian agent. At times the reactions are severe enough that drugs must be discontinued.

Knowledge of long-term effects of these drugs is incomplete. Dextroamphetamine and methylphenidate depress the height and weight of children. Phenothiazines and lithium may affect the growth hormone. Because of lack of knowledge of long-term efffects of some drugs, and definite effects of others, long-term maintenance is open to question. Some problems of prolonged drug maintenance can be lessened by a one-day-a-week "drug holiday" and by gradual diminution and cessation of therapy for 10 days every 3 to 4 months, if possible.

5. Medication should be administered on an outpatient basis with provision for parental or teacher monitoring of the child's reactions between the physician's visits. Dosage should be built up from a low initial dose, to spot any serious reactions. Common errors are to continue the therapeutic trial on an insufficient dose, or to increase the dosage too fast, causing a worsening of behavior and lack of patient cooperation because of excessive side effects.

Classes of Drugs

1. Sedatives, hypnotics, anticonvulsant agents, and barbiturates have fallen into disuse for psychotic children because of the disorganization and confusion they frequently cause. Chloral hydrate (Noctec) is a safe and effective hypnotic to induce sleep. Diphenylhydramine (Benadryl) has been used effectively to curb anxiety and to reduce restlessness and some of the behavior disorder aspects of psychoses. It should be used in young children before trying a major tranquilizer because of its relative safety and lack of side effects, and its facilitation of sleep. It has a calming and organizing effect. Being an antihistimanic, it also reduces the upsetting upper respiratory congestion associated with chronic colds and allergies particularly upsetting to psychotic children. Diphenylhydantoin (Dilatin), phenobarbital, and other anticonvulsants have dropped from general use with psychotic children, but are still prescribed when there is electroencephalographic evidence of subclinical seizure patterns, associated with hyperkinesis and periodic psychomotor outbursts.

2. Stimulants: D-amphetamine (Dexedrine) and methylphenidate (Ritalin) have been used for their paradoxical effect in calming the organically driven hyperkinetic child by stimulating cerebral inhibitory areas. This has been effective in the younger child with psychosis of early onset when hyperkinesis is a part of the total clinical picture. However, if the child's hyperactivity is based on anxiety, as in the nonorganically based psychoses of early onset, or as in most childhood schizophrenics, where pervasive anxiety is one of the basic symptoms, the result may be increased withdrawal, anxiety, anorexia, and disorganization. Limited experience with L-amphetamine (Cydril) reports it effective in controlling hyperactivity and aggressive and self-mutilating behavior with less disorganization. The precise subgrouping of the psychotic children treated was not clear.

3. Tricyclic antidepressants: Nortriptyline was reported to be effective with most anergic psychotic children. Imipramine (Tofranil) has had little convincing therapeutic effect on psychotic children. It has been used to control enuresis in nonpsychotic children. The effect on this symptom in psychotic children is as yet unproven. Toxic side effects make their use in young children risky.

4. Neuroleptic Drugs (major tranquilizers and antipsychotic agents)

a. Phenothiazines: Among the major tranquilizers, longest used has been chlorpromazine (Thorazine), especially to control the acute psychotic disturbance of the school-aged child and adolescent. However, accompanying depression of psychomotor activity, lethargy, and extrapyramidal rigidity and dyskinesia limits the child's accessibility to psychotherapy, socialization, and education. Its use beyond the acute phase depends on the clinical need for increased sedative effect to control disintegrative anxiety. When possible, a switch should be made.

Trifluoperazine (Stelazine) and fluphenazine (Prolixin) are reported to have fewer side effects and seem to increase accessibility, counteracting withdrawal and internalization of fantasy, particularly in the prepubertal child. Reports of retinal changes and oculomotor spasm (oculogyric crises) with long-term use require opthalmologic consultation periodically.

Triflupromazine (Vesprin) and thioridazine (Mellaril) have also been reported as effective antipsychotic agents, with effects somewhere between those of Thorazine and Stelazine (less depressant than the former, less stimulating than the latter).

b. Butyrophenones and thioxanthenes: Haloperidol (Haldol) and thiothixene (Navane) have been introduced as effective antipsychotic agents in children with particularly chronic, apathetic, and resistive pathology. They are reported to facilitate socialization and thought content, reduce assaultiveness and self-mutilation, and stimulate accessibility without disorganization. The combination of activating and antipsychotic properties are desirable for young children. Though a safe therapeutic dosage margin is claimed, some clinicians have found that the margin between optimal and overdosage is not wide, and thus the progressive dosage steps when initiating therapy should be small with daily supervision required. Use in children under 12 requires careful monitoring. Haldol has been reported effective with Gilles de la Tourette's syndrome, which some consider a special psychotic-like disorder.

5. Minor tranquilizers: Meprobamate (Miltown), chlordiazepoxide (Librium), and diazepam (Valium) are ineffective in psychotic children and may cause worsening of anxiety and aggressiveness.

6. The use of hallucinogens is in the experimental stage. Groups headed by Bender et al. (1966), Simmons et al. (1966), and Fish et al. (1969) using LSD-25 and methysergide report increased motor activity, alertness, and affective responsiveness in the children with psychoses of early onset and autistic and atypical symptomotology. In the psychoses of later onset with schizophrenic symptomatology, there were mixed results or an increase of anxiety and disorganization.

7. Campbell (1973) noted in her review that the use of lithium reduced self-mutilating and explosive aggressive behaviors in psychotic and retarded children.

8. Campbell also reported her experiments with the use of L-dopa with severely disturbed preschool children, mostly psychotic, who gained in social initiation, affective responsiveness, verbal production, and motor activity and play, and decreased in withdrawal and psychotic speech. A decrease in brain serotonin is postulated to be the mode of action.

9. A consideration of psychoendocrine mechanisms has resulted in the trial use of a thyroid hormone (T3) by a number of investigators with preschool psychotic children. There was reported to be increased alertness, social and affective contact, and use of speech for communication. It is said to stimulate developmental lags by alleviating hormonal deficiency or metabolic defect.

10. Megavitamin therapy is based on the principles of orthomolecular psychiatry, which hold that certain mental disorders, including the childhood psychoses, may be the result of deficiency in certain metabolic nutritional substances including vitamins. Massive doses of water-soluble vitamins (B complex and C) have been used and significant improvement claimed, especially in the autistic and atypical child. Studies have suffered from lack of controls, and from lack of standard diagnostic criteria for subjects and for their improvement. An American Psychiatric Association task force (Lipton et al., 1973) concluded that the studies reported did not meet the tests of scientific validity and that megavitamin therapy had no demonstrated value in the treatment of the childhood psychoses. More recent reports (Autry, 1975) have reactivated the controversy.

11. Feingold (1975) has implicated food additives, dyes, and preservatives in the causation of hyperkinesis and associated severe behavior in autistic disorders. The therapeutic intervention would be in the form of a diagnostic elimination diet and the use of foods free of these additives. Bird, Russo, and Cataldo (1977), in a review of the subject, dispute the correctness of the implication.

Campbell (1973) concludes her comprehensive review by reemphasizing that drug therapy for psychotic children should be only one part of a comprehensive treatment approach, but one that is an essential component for treatment of the preschool psychotic child and for the psychoses of early onset. For the schizophrenic child with psychosis of later onset there is less consistent response to and thus less absolute indication for chemotherapy.

Treatment of Parents

Parents must be assessed as to their specific roles in relation to the child and his psychotic process. Therapeutic intervention must include steps taken to undo any attitudes, actions, and roles that contribute to the pathological development of the child and at times the parent may become the primary focus of the therapy.

With the very young child in whom the psychotic condition is just emerging and appears largely reactive, not yet pervasive, and fixated, it may be possible to treat the parents in lieu of the child. In other instances the parents, if problems are present, are best treated concurrently, paralleling that of the child. Occasionally at least part of the therapy time may be spent in integrative sessions together with the child.

The following factors and influences may require counseling or therapeutic intervention: (1) the genetic endowment; (2) the emotional and physical climate provided, including the state of the marital relationship (Wolman, 1970; Szurek and Berlin, 1973); (3) the amount, quality, and consistency of caretaking; (4) the models for identification; (5) the symbolic meaning of this child to the parent; (6) the use of the child as an extension of the self, as a scapegoat, or as the vehicle through whom to get at the other parent; (7) a need to have or expectation of having a damaged child; (8) anxious, symbiotic overconcern with separation or inappropriate overevaluation or underevaluation of the child and his capacities for autonomous functioning. Clinical illustration of each of these influences and corrective intervention with the parent are described below.

When marital discord undermines the treatment effort and puts the child in the middle, conjoint parental therapy is desirable. Often the hostile and even distress messages sent through the child, and getting at each other by getting at the child, can be alleviated by mobilizing the direct expression and confrontation of their feelings and disappointments in each other (often expressed in their blame of the other for the illness of the child) and working them through. Motivation to pursue this course may be elicited through demonstrating the destructive impact of their scapegoating and using the child as a foil.

Assessment of genetic endowment is especially important for counseling with regard to having further children. Evidence for genetic factors in etiology is great enough that the family with one psychotic child and several relatives who are schizophrenic should be advised of the higher risk factor. Such a family history may also lead one to advise the family that treatment may ameliorate the symptoms, but that the child may not be cured.

The emotional climate in the home between parents is extremely important. Marital discord can undermine the treatment effort and put the child in the middle. Hostile messages can be sent through the child in a very confusing way; parents can try to get at each other through the child, and often express their hostility by blaming each other for the child's illness. Paradoxically, a terrible relationship between parents may be improved if a child becomes psychotic, which then makes the child's illness the cause of their well-being, and makes it dangerous both for the child to give up his illness, and for the parents to allow him to improve. Conjoint parent therapy is often advisable in these cases, with mobilization of direct expression of feelings, and with open expression of their disappointments, blame, and so forth. Their conscious or unconscious use of the child to solve their problems must be pointed out, and alternatives found.

The amount, quality, and consistency of caretaking is important especially in assessing the degree to which deprivation may play a factor in an apparent psychosis. A mid-teenaged mother recently arrived from the South to a large city and found herself isolated in a small apartment with her 5-year-old child, with whom she rarely talked and did not know how to play. Because of the mother's fears, the child had no peers and was left to her own devices, albeit fed well and otherwise cared for. This child had developed behaviors that appeared schizophrenic, talking to herself or her fingers and withdrawing into fantasy. Focus on treatment was on the mother, with individual counseling, group therapy, and training sessions in how to cope with daily problems as well as how to relate to and play with her child, who was in a therapeutic nursery setting. After one year she was able to enter a public school, and six months later was doing well in first grade.

Pathologic parental models for incorporation can present serious problems for the therapist or case manager. One or both parents may be borderline schizophrenic or overtly psychotic but managing to function, albeit in a very brittle way. They may be severely obsessional, preoccupied with vague fears of a paranoid nature, and have a lot of magical thinking, and they may be very resistant to pressures to change. In fact, change may be disintegrating to them. Yet despite their abnormal effects on their child, these parents are often functioning satisfactorily in other areas, so there is no question of there being legal cause to have a child removed from the home to foster care. One solution frequently employed when the child's pathology is severe enough is to encourage placement in a residential treatment center, focusing on the child's need for total care rather than the parent's inability to change. Another possible solution is to provide, in a day program, a consistent caretaker of the same sex as the more disturbed parent in order to provide a corrective experience with a caring adult.

At times a child will take on a special symbolic meaning to a parent which will supersede the child's being an entity in its own right. Common examples of this are the child born out of wedlock who bears the burden of the mother's guilt feelings, the child who is seen as ugly, mean, or evil because he "looks just like" the father who had those qualities and from whom the mother is separated, and the child born just after the death of a same-sex close relative, especially the mother's mother or father, when the child can be seen in some way as a replacement and this is carried to a psychological extreme.

A child can be used as a pathologic extension of the self, especially by mothers who are schizophrenic. An autistic child of such a mother had little chance to develop a separate identity as long as her mother had the fantasy, openly expressed at times, that "she is me, I am her . . . she is the me I'd like to be . . . she is doing it for me . . . I will live through her." A great amount of therapy is required to get the mother to differentiate herself from the child, and to care for it as a separate entity, with appropriate affect.

There are cases in which there is an unconscious need or expectation, on the part of one parent, of having a damaged child. Examples are the mother with a withered right hand whose child was normal until just following eye muscle surgery, when she became incontinent, smeared feces, and stopped making eye contact. Despite all therapeutic efforts the child got worse because the mother would covertly sabotage treatment, and would not comply with suggestions for dealing with her child at home. It became clear that this mother needed to have a damaged child to compliment her own damaged state. She felt inferior and could disguise her own dependency needs in the help she could expect on behalf of her damaged child. The child (and the therapists) got the nonverbal message from the mother of the role expected of the child.

Anxious symbiotic overconcern can also be seen in some parents of disturbed children. A mother whose four-week-old child had a respiratory infection was told by her mother that "the baby sounds just like your little sister before she died of pneumonia when you were three years old" (and the sister was one year old). This evidently sparked old guilt feelings in the mother, who, although she had raised other children, panicked and began scrubbing the floors and walls, kept visitors away, and after mistakenly assuming a doctor to say her child had no gamma globulin, and thus no resistance to germs, kept the child isolated. From 3 to 15 months everyone who saw the child, except the doctor, had to wear a surgical mask at the mother's request. Human contact was limited. For six months, according to her older sister, the child reached out for contact, and then gradually gave up and became autistic.

Family Therapy

The general principles of family therapy are considered in another chapter. Observing and treating the patient together with the rest of the family, as a unit, brings the dimensions of family dynamics, interaction and roles into the total understanding of the factors enhancing and sustaining the psychotic process in the child and helps clarify the relationship between the nature of the family interaction and communication and the psychotic illness in the child. The objective in family therapy is not only to identify, clarify, and change family processes that might have led to psychosis, but also to identify and change patterns that tend to perpetuate psychosis no matter what the cause. Attempts are made to improve family communication and work out the conflicts and the double and ambiguous messages confusing and hindering the child's clinical progress.

The "family" may be defined as all members living under one roof (aunt, cousin, grandmother, etc.) having significant input into or responsibility for this child. It may be parents and the psychotic child, or in a one-parent family, mother, siblings, and child, mother, grandmother, and child, or mother, boyfriend, and child. In short, all the people who have significant impact on and input into the child's daily care are included. Family therapy may be a preparation for individual therapy, or may become an adjunctive part of the total therapeutic management. Indications for its use may become evident only through the resistances, undoing, and therapeutic stalemates that appear in the course of involvement with the family, and may follow home and parent/child observation.

With autistic and atypical children, supportive mobilization and integration of family resources, clarification of impact of the developmentally disordered child on siblings and parent (focus of attention on the sick child, greater expectations placed on the well one, placement of blame, etc.), and the correction of pathological adjustments are goals and indications for family therapy. Schopler and Reichler (1971) report that objective recognition of the autistic child's disabilities and their extent helps to increase family equilibrium, and encourages mobilization of the family's coping abilities. With symbiotic psychotic children, tripartite therapy (therapist, child, and mother) is often effective in uncovering the pathologic symbiotic pattern between mother and child.

Family therapy involving all members is also frequently employed as an adjunct to treatment of the child in a day therapeutic nursery setting. A frequently seen constellation is that one parent maintains a façade of overcompetence and dominance while the other, usually the mother, exhibits helplessness and passivity. Decisions can't be made. When the mother becomes pregnant, she takes on a feeling of strength relative to the fetus and worries about its intactness and helplessness. When the child arrives and starts developing, the mother infantilizes it, and gives the double-binding message that it should stay emotionally dependent and infantile to gain love, yet should achieve intellectually. There is at the same time an emotional distancing between parents. Often the father works odd shifts or travels at his work, or there is a formal controlled relationship with little sharing of feelings. This fosters an even more intense relationship between mother and child.

Bowen (1960) describes the changes in the mother/father/child triad as a result of family therapy:

1. Initial struggle between controlling mother and schizophrenic child as child begins to individuate and assert himself. Father remains peripheral.

2. As father begins to participate and challenge mother's dominance she becomes anxious and attacks him.

3. With therapist's support to assume an active, dominant position in the family, the emotional distancing between the parents disappears and emotional attachment builds.

4. As the relationship between the parents improves, the schizophrenic child becomes upset, feels left out, and tries to regain the lost symbiotic position.

5. If the parental relationship remains firm, and the child is no longer the focus of pathologic attention, the child improves and develops emotionally.

The child's pathology should be considered in terms of family interaction processes and dynamics, as well as in terms of developmental delay and disrupted ego apparatus. Whether perceptual and integrative dysfunctions are due to genetically or congenitally based deficiencies, to lack of organizing mothering stimulus in the early months of life, or to clearly delineated family pathology, there is no question that family assessment and therapy as indicated should be an essential part of the total conceptual approach.

Treatment Approaches to Specific Disorders

For the purpose of clarifying more specific treatment approaches, it is helpful to view the childhood psychoses differentially as those of early onset, prior to age 3, and those of later onset, age 3–4 on. The early-onset conditions include early infantile autism, children with atypical development, symbiotic psychosis of early childhood, and disintegrative psychosis of early onset. Those of later onset include schizophrenia in childhood, peripubertal, and postpubertal adolescent periods, borderline psychoses of later onset, manic-depressive and other depressive psychoses, severe psychosomatic equivalents of psychotic states, and conditions which can take on a psychotic form, such as elective mutism and folie à deux.

The division into early and late onset is helpful in that the earlier-onset conditions are more pervasive and debilitating and generally require intensive daily care in day treatment settings or residential settings with a variety of therapists available. Those of later onset may require hospitalization or residential treatment, but often can be treated with outpatient therapy and special but less intensive school placement.

Disorders of Early Onset

Early Infantile Autism

This syndrome was first described by Kanner (1943, 1944, 1949) as "an inborn disturbance of affective contact" with five main signs: (1) An inability or refusal to relate to people, with a withdrawal from contact from the beginnings of life. The child seems unhearing, gives no eye contact, smiles neither spontaneously nor responsively, and doesn't cuddle or assume an anticipatory posture. (2) An anxious, obsessive insistence on maintaining sameness of environment and routines. Changes cause negativism, withdrawal, or panic. Actions are perseverative and stereotyped. (3) A preoccupation with a few inaminate objects handled intensely in a repetitive, skillful, but bizarre, nonfunctional way, and a preoccupation with the sensory stimulation obtained. (4) Essential mutism or vocalization and echolalic speech not used for communication. (5) A clinical impression of intellectual and cognitive potential higher than the severe general level of retardation at which they function. Kanner implicated both inborn tendencies and a cold, rejecting environment.

To Kanner's basic criteria, Ruttenberg (1971), noting evidence for congenital vulnerabilities in the hospital birth records, and following Creak's nine diagnostic points (1961) for childhood schizophrenia, proposed additional diagnostic criteria. These included: (1) distorted or deficient body image; (2) abnormal or immature motility patterns; (3) distorted and inconsistent perceptual experience, with extremes of sensory sensitivity; (4) uneven body mastery and its use in a fragmented, disjointed way; (5) extremes of autonomic reaction (flushing, pallor); (6) a defensive alertness and hyperawareness of the environment, with overt anxiety present only when manipulative efforts at maintaining sameness or tuning out to maintain autistic aloofness are threatened; (7) preoccupation with kinesthetic, tactile-sensory, and proprioceptive modes of sensory input and autoerotic discharge (developmentally preoral), expressed by repetitive rocking, whirling, head banging, wall rubbing, hand mannerisms, and facial grimacing. With biologic maturation there develops polymorphous perverse discharge through oral, anal, and phallic areas; (8) auto-aggression.

Ornitz (1973) divides the functional disorder manifest as autism into five areas of dysfunction: (1) perception; (2) developmental rate; (3) relating; (4) speech and language; (5) motility. The presenting symptoms vary with the age of the child and influence the nature of the therapeutic intervention. Deviant behavior may be noted almost immediately postnatally as disinterest in sucking and stiffening when held. There may be extremes of reactivity, lethargy, and little crying, or hypersensitivity and irritability. Responsive cooing, smiling, and eye contact do not develop by the third month. The anticipatory and cooperative response to being picked up or dressed does not appear. The child does not cuddle, but becomes either rigid or limp. In the second 6 months of life solid food is often rejected and only the bottle or baby food are tolerated. This may persist for years. Initial babbling, used as a discharge phenomenon, fades or becomes echoing rather than progressing through jargon to communicative speech. By 12 to 18 months, rocking, head banging, and bizarre hand movements are noted and toys and other inanimate objects are fingered, mouthed, lined up, or otherwise used in a perseverative stereotyped way. By 24 months the child moves an adult's hand toward what he wants without giving eye contact.

In a secondary form of childhood autism, relatively normal behavior is reported until 15 to 24 months. The child has been no trouble, and often seems to have been too good. A few words have developed, then after some stressful situation, high fever, a new sibling, etc., these words (often basically babbling type—*ma ma, da da*, etc.) are lost and the other autistic criteria develop. This seems to be at a time when a degree of autonomy is beginning to be expected from the child, as well as verbal communications. The child regresses to a controlling autistic position. There is aloneness without the true individuation and age-appropriate independence of autonomy. Mahler (1968) sees this secondary autism as a defensive position taken because of an inability to go beyond the controlling symbiotic position, or to sustain it under pressure of environmental expectations. Others see the autistic position as a defense against sensed inner deficits and vulnerabilities. When the autistic defenses are given up under the influence of therapy, the underlying perceptual and mental disabilities when present will become apparent and available for special training. By the fourth year lack of communiative speech and relatedness predominate. "You" is substituted for "I," and the negative may be the expression of a positive wish. Where language is attained, its content is likely to be concrete. The child remains aloof with flattened affect and rigidity of behavior. Autistic children with no sign of organic predisposition or vulnerability are more likely to come from disturbed families, and unless the family or parental pathology is lessened, may progress from autism not to normality but to psychoses of higher and higher development and sophistication, using acquired cognitive and ego skills in their psychotic adjustments: symbioses, psychoses with oral and anal sadistic and phallic manifestations, schizophrenia or severe ego disorders of lesser degree.

In our experience autistic children with predisposing vulnerability are less likely to come from primarily disturbed families, though the families may be secondarily overwhelmed and upset by the stress of the dysfunctioning child.

Treatment: An adequate therapeutic approach to the autistic child almost always involves a multidisciplinary team. The major approaches include (1) psychoanalytically oriented relationship therapy; (2) behavior therapy; (3) body manipulation and movement therapies; (4) drug therapy; (5) early educational stimulation; (6) language therapy; (7) family therapy or simultaneous therapy and counseling for the parents.

Recent innovative approaches to the treatment of autism include the use of parents as co-therapists (Schopler and Reichler, 1971), use of the home environment as the primary therapeutic setting (Howlin et al., 1973), use of the stimulus of normal peers in a nursery setting (DesLauriers and Carlson, 1969), and application of ethological approaches and techniques (Tinbergen and Tinbergen, 1972). There has been expanded use, under professional supervision and guidance, of nonprofessional volunteers, mother's helpers at home, parents, and child care paraprofessionals.

The varied multidisciplinary approaches have developed primarily because of the pervasiveness of the pathology and the number of hours of daily input necessary to engage the child and reactivate development.

The age of the child influences choice of therapeutic setting. Children under 2 or 3 years of age would tend to have the focus of therapy in the home with, if available, a half-day infant stimulation nursery program. Specific therapies such as psychotherapy, speech, etc., are provided in the therapists' offices. Children aged 2½ to 6 or 7 are best treated in a special day care milieu. In the past such programs worked with children until age 10 or 11, when pending onset of puberty necessitated transfer. The recent passage of legislation mandating that departments of education provide special classes for all handicapped children, including those severely emotionally disturbed, has prompted the initiation of special class settings in some areas which can provide for some of the needs of these children, and allow for transfer from nursery-type settings at an earlier age. Psychiatrists and other adjunctive therapists will hopefully be working in cooperation with these new systems.

A typical autistic child entering a day nursery treatment program might be the 3½-year-old boy with symptoms of avoiding human contact, refusal to make eye contact, no interest in toys, refusal to eat solid foods, need for rigid routines, and no speech for communication, although he can sing songs and seems to like music. A brief review of this case will serve to illustrate several aspects of treatment. Careful evaluation revealed the possibility of an organic predisposing factor, as there was a complicated pregnancy and caesarean section delivery precipitated by placenta previa. There were developmental interferences and traumas in that the child had 3 reconstructive surgical operations on his penis for a hypospadias between the ages of 1½ and 2, and after each hospitalization of 48 hours he would not recognize or respond to his parents. At this time rocking and head banging started. Overall development was delayed, and there were serious problems in the parents' relationship which began prior to the child's birth. By 2 years of age he said a few words and learned to hum tunes, but by 26 months, he stopped saying any words, following a fall in which front teeth were knocked loose and removed, and by 3½ he was still untrained for bladder and bowel.

The initial treatment plan for this child focused on both child and parents. The child was assigned to a warm mothering child care worker on a 1:1 basis, and parents were worked with as a couple at first to support them and further delineate their problems, following which they sought individual treatment.

The child's target areas for therapeutic intervention were avoidance and withdrawal from relationships, tantrums, refusal of solid foods, repression of emotional expression, reaction to trauma to his penis, and the related lack of toilet training, and his resistance to cognitive functions. The child care worker initially developed a primary relationship by holding, rocking, caressing, and singing to him. Over a one-year period the child was walking around actively with her, and they were romping and playing together. The child was able to look at the world around him, and such cognitive tasks as naming objects, counting, and recognizing letters was casually begun.

It is a general principle with such a child that the relationship is restricted to only one person until contact is firmly established and there is some degree of trust. With this child, once the connection was made, a music therapist was added to the regime. She capitalized on his natural interest in music and developed musical games and ways of communicating emotionally through such things as speed and loudness of beating a drum, and "conversations" using basic instruments. In addition, such ego functions as waiting, pausing, control, fast, slow, etc., were stimulated through the music therapy. After two years he was in a music group and starting involvement in group activities. Throughout, after contact was firmly established with the child care worker, psychotherapy and therapist supervision of those working with the child was provided.

After 3 years of treatment, at age 6½, self-awareness as an individual became more and more evident; there was an ability for concept formation, and there were beginnings of reading and writing. Severe compulsivity and echolalia were reduced and there was an increase in self-control and frustration tolerance. At age 3½ a Vineland IQ was 59. At 6½ a WISC showed an IQ of 87, with a wide scatter from severe retardation in areas of visual-motor coordination and visual memory span to superior levels in conceptual ability and reality testing. He could analyze and synthesize complex perceptual material, but his ability to complete coding tasks was poor. There were many indications of mild but diffuse brain damage.

Speech therapy was added at age 6½, and vocal pitch, weak volume, articulatory substitutions, poor recall for words in sequence, and a tendency to repeat questions were worked on. In a 6-month period he could read and write 150 words and was developing great curiosity.

At age 7 there were intense behavior problems at home, and the child's parents were becoming overwhelmed. With his new verbal abilities and relatedness, he had become demanding and uncontrollable and still had eating difficulties. A temporary residential hospital placement with opportunity for frequent home visits and continuation of psychotherapy was decided upon. This allowed for a more controlled environment with attention to specific behaviors, continuation of analytically oriented therapy, and a respite for the parents, who continued in their therapy.

After 7 months he was discharged and enrolled in a small flexible private school near his home. Psychotherapy and speech therapy continued. After one year he was again in a residential setting. From age 8½ to 10½ he set rigid standards for himself and would have tantrums if he failed to meet them. Self-assertion and aggressiveness in looking after his own rights developed, and he responded poorly to criticism. In some areas he excelled (math and science), while in others he demanded a great deal of individual attention. He had many peculiar ideas of what was fair or unjust, and often lacked any feeling for the rights or needs of others. He was competitive in sports but grew angry when others did better. In his last year in residence these areas were worked on in therapy. By 11½ he entered a day school at a junior high level, and was then able to attend a regular high school. Electronics and mathematics became his whole life, but to the exclusion of peer relationships. He was able to carry a full academic program plus attend extra electronics and math courses in the afternoons. Currently he is in college, is an honor student, and serves as a research assistant. He is considered very good in math and the sciences, can solve complex mechanical and electronic problems and make circuit repairs, and can find work on his own. Peers phone him for help, which he gives, but he doesn't really relate to them in any other way. He appears to others to be the "absent-minded professor."

This case illustrates one of the more successful outcomes in a disorder of mixed congenital and environmental etiology, but a case which, despite anomalies and possible encephalopathy, seemed ultimately not affected in the areas of intelligence and language comprehension. The autism was primarily reactive to bodily deformities, and the traumata of injury and surgery which interfered at critical stages of the child's development. Although this family also had marital problems, this is different from the autism that appears to be primarily due to disorder in the parent-child relationship, or that is a defense against broad developmental and mental deficiency in which the child's autistic position is a defense against pressures for performance at levels at which he is incapable of complying. In either instance, when therapeutic management relieves the pressures and approaches the child at his level, symptoms begin to subside, relationships can develop, and depending on other damage which may be uncovered, development can proceed.

In this case, long and comprehensive therapeutic and educational management, including help for other family members, was provided. The child progressed from autism to aggression, and then to a rigid and schizoid adjustment. He is now happy in his own way, certainly heading for success in a career of his interest and choosing and perhaps making significant contributions in the field. Anna Freud has explained some kinds of narrow-based genius and idiot-savants as the focusing of that person's psychic energy on one subject. Widen the focus, normalize the person, and lose the expertise. One wonders if one should leave well enough alone, and not try, with our limited resources and knowledge, to make a conventional social being out of such a person, but just be satisfied to be available should there be decompensation or should he become aware of his differences from others enough to be unhappy about it and want help to change. At present this patient is happy with his adjustment. So be it!

Child with Atypical Development

The terms "atypical child" and "atypical development" were used by Rank (1949) and associates to refer to children "whose development has been arrested at a very primitive infantile level." Reiser (1963) states that the terms are now used to cover the range of psychoses of infancy and early childhood. Descriptively this designation would include infantile autism, but it also embraces a wider range of conditions whose age of onset is as early as that of the infantile autism but whose manifestations of ego disorder in the areas of relationship and affective contact may not be as severe and the levels of functioning not as low. There are more development irregularities, and substrate of organic brain dysfunction or ego fragmentation, which gives a similar picture, is more apparent. The American Psychiatric Association *Glossary of Psychiatric Terms* (1969) emphasizes the delay in emotional development and the disorder in personality development and associated ego functions. While primary brain deficiencies and disorders and mental subnormality are not included in "atypical development," their presence as predisposing factors creating vulnerability to stress and other etiological factors is acceptable.

Cohen and co-workers (1974) outlines his point-by-point clinical differentiation of infantile autism and atypicality. Differential diagnosis must be made between autism, atypicality, anaclitic depression, chronic stimulus deprivation syndrome, elective mutism, aphasia, perceptual impairment (auditory or visual), mental retardation, severe chronic brain syndrome, psychomotor seizure equivalents, and early childhood schizophrenia (beginning age 4 or 5).

Rank's original papers (1949, 1955) gave a rich description of these children, citing their outstanding symptoms as "withdrawal from people, retreat into a world of fantasy, mutism, or the use of language for autistic purposes, bizarre posturing, seemingly meaningless stereotyped gestures, impassivity or violent outbursts of anxiety and rage, identification with objects or animals, and excessively inhibited or excessively uninhibited expression of impulses." Other features common to all are lack of contact with reality, little or no communication with others and lack of uniformity (fragmentation) of ego development. She described extremes of activity and passivity and of abilities. She was convinced that hereditary and biological factors played a predisposing part; for treatment purposes she focused on the role of the "postnatal failure of the parent/child relation through disorders of fusion and attachment."

Treatment for the atypical child is similar to that for the autistic child, with perhaps a shorter, less intense initial focus on relationship and more emphasis on the ego defects in language and perceptual-motor coordination.

Rank and MacNaughton (1950) describe the use of a therapist as a mothering substitute in order to undo the developmental arrest and make restitution by accepting and responding to the child at levels at which the child presents himself. Ego development was activated in stages by: (1) stimulating the child's contact with the outside world through bodily contact and sensory stimulation; (2) taking over the child's executant functions and acting as a partial ego for incorporation and identification, and mirroring his behavior to stimulate self-concept and self-evaluative functions; (3) further differentiation of the child from the therapist through the use of toys and games (which also stimulate cognitive functioning) and through exploring reality in the person of the therapist. The child was protected from self-aggression, and externalization of aggression with its channeling into socially tolerated forms was facilitated. Play with toys, dolls, and animal figures was a major therapeutic vehicle.

Symbiotic Psychosis

Mahler (1952) first described this clinical subclassification as follows:

a. No conspicuous or grossly deviant behavior in the first year of life. However, low frustration tolerance and sleep disturbance are often reported and these children are described as having been "oversensitive" and "crybabies."

b. At the chronological period (age 1–2) when growing independence and separation from the mother is expected, anxiety appears and emotional development stops, or if it appears at a later date, there is regression to this level. The child resists separation and behaves as if his mental representation of the mother is fused with (not separated from) that of the self (the symbiotic position).

c. By age 2 to 3½ the child has separation anxiety and "affective panic reaction."

d. The child's body feels as if it is denying boundaries and melting into one's own when it is held.

e. The child focuses on parts of his own body excessively (hands, fingers, hair, etc.).

f. There is attempted restitution of oneness with the mother through delusions and hallucinations.

g. Attempts are made to maintain and control the presence of the person the child is attached to through the manipulation and maintaining of sameness of the environment, tantrums, and anxiety.

h. Symbiotic children are impulse-ridden. "Manifestations of love and aggression are utterly confused. They crave body contact and seem to want to crawl into you . . . yet, they shriek in panic if such bodily contact or overt demonstration . . . [is initiated by] the adult."

Mahler (1968) defined the underlying process in symbiotic psychosis as "a deficiency or a defect in the child's intrapsychic utilization of the mothering partner during the symbiotic phase, and his subsequent inability to internalize the representation of the mothering object." In a prior paper (1961), she stated that the major causal factor in infantile psychosis is the breakdown in communication between the mother-infant pair: "If the infant's signals do not reach the mother because he is unable to send them, or if the infant's signals are not heeded because the mother does not have the capacity to react to them, the mother-infant interaction pattern takes on a dangerously discordant rhythm."

Treatment is designed to facilitate the restart of developmental progression out of the symbiotic state and toward separation and individuation. Because of the symbiotic nature of the disorder, a therapeutic nursery group situation is contraindicated while the child is susceptible to symbiotic panic. The problem of the extreme anxiety and panic and tendency to retreat toward autism is crucial. In the symbiotic state the infant's mental image of self is fused with that of the mother. He may respond to any realization of separateness with panic and a need to manipulate and control the whereabouts of his mother and the environment. Approach must be cautious and not head on. A close informative alliance with the mothering figure is necessary. The therapist becomes a substitute mother, offering herself as a symbiotic partner with whom to relive earlier developmental steps more adequately—a "corrective symbiotic experience." In Mahler's tripartite therapeutic design, therapy involved the mother, child, and therapist. Mahler (1968) reported that the mothers were very helpful in being able to understand and interpret the child's nonverbal communications.

In the first stage, the therapist's presence is accepted as a part object, then is more and more involved as the symbiotic partner. The handling of aggression directed inwardly and outwardly in a way to minimize anxiety at threatened object loss is crucial. The therapist can act as a demonstrator of healthier interaction and then as a bridge between mother and child, with the goal of reestablishing the mother-child relationship at a post-symbiotic level.

Detailed case reports of therapy of symbiotic psychoses may be found in Mahler (1968) and by A. Bergman, P. Elkish, and K. Kupfermann, in *Separation-Individuation* (McDevitt and Settlage, 1971).

The developmental arrest at or regression to a symbiotic position and resultant symbiotic psychosis almost always requires as part of its etiology the complicity of the parenting figures. This may be the vicariously smothering, enveloping, infantilizing type of mother who clings or promotes fusion, or the passive masochistic or anxious-conflicted depressed type who invites or tolerates the manipulative efforts of the child to retain an orally focused omnipotent type of control and sameness. The parent, usually the mother, must be helped to give up her part in the symbiotic constellation, which often means an intensive therapeutic look at her own needs. The therapeutic approach must include demonstration and correction of the pathologic relationship in a supportive manner by way of tripartite conjoint therapy with parent and child, or family therapy.

There is often a great amount of unconscious resistance and intransigence in the parents of symbiotic children. This is not outright defiance, but more likely unwitting undoing and sabotage. Often a very structured and monitored plan is necessary to wean the parent, and at times forceful and direct orders are required to break the unhealthy bond. It is typical for the mother of a symbiotic psychotic child to attempt to remain in a treatment center with her child, initially refusing to leave out of fear that the child won't survive. Often she needs quite forceful persuasion to separate. At the same time the separation anxiety and guilt are dealt with in psychotherapeutic counseling. The therapist's support often substitutes for the gratification lost in the separation from the child.

In the therapeutic setting, the child is entered into a healthier, dynamic rather than static symbiotic relationship with limits, give and take, and an encouragement on the part of the mother substitute to explore, test out, experience, ask and do for one's self, and also control one's self. Along the lines of Mahler's corrective symbiotic experience technique, mother at scheduled times observes the therapist/child relationship and may partake in it, and gradually takes over in time for the psychological weaning within the therapeutic situation.

It is interesting to note that many autistic children go through a symbiotic psychotic phase after relinquishing the autistic state, and a mother may occasionally feel threatened rather than happy that her formerly autistic child is reaching out, wants to be picked up constantly, and won't leave her alone.

When symbiotic fixation has to be resolved if development is to proceed, it may be possible to make the change in stages. One child's mother was left by her husband with three children, of whom he was the youngest, at age 1½. She had to work and was at the mercy of a demeaning aunt and sister. He would refuse to go to bed until his mother came home from work late at night, then would insist on crawling into bed with her. Her life was rather empty, so this attention was not hard to take. With others, the child appeared autistic, and perhaps the need-seeking symbiosis with his mother was a way of including her within his autistic boundries. In treatment, the mother was getting an attentive outlet and support, and the child was responding to a very sparkling child care worker. Mother was advised that it was time to move her child out of her bed, which was upsetting to her and to him. The first stage was a cot at the foot of the bed, much as he had slept when father was there. Then, after parallel play peer involvement had developed with a cousin, it was arranged that he sleep in the room with this cousin. This was achieved after some struggle and the mother's realization that her weak no's were a sign of her own mixed feelings. The separation of the symbiotic bond was followed by therapeutic and developmental gains. Sometimes the promise of other desired developments in their own lives can be the inducement that will motivate parents to remain firm in the struggle to enforce the relinquishing of a symbiotic pattern.

Disintegrative Psychoses of Early Onset

Heller (1908) reported 6 cases of acute onset of "progressive infantile dementia" in the third or fourth year of life after relatively normal adjustment and development to that point. This begins with acute change in mood and the development of angry behavior, destructive rage and anxiety, hyperactivity, animal-like movements, postures, and grimacing. Incontinence develops. There is progressive dementia and regression, but intelligent facies. Destruction of ganglion cells has been reported. Laufer and Gair's review (1969) cites other reports of this rare condition, including Despert's (1938) report of cases of psychoses of acute onset and deep regression. Rutter (1972) reports also regressive loss of social skills and the development of mannerisms. A progressive encephalopathic process and temporal lobe and subcortical pathology have been suspected. Treatment is supportive and chemotherapeutically focused on the suspected encephalopathic process. Prognosis is usually poor, and the child remains mute and retarded.

Prognostic Expectations

For autism, atypicality, and symbiosis, prognosis varies according to the intensity and quality of therapeutic input (Wenar and Ruttenberg, 1976), as well as with the degree of disturbance and any uncovered underlying organic factors. Reports of marked and sustained improvement vary from 25-50% of the cases. Significant improvement is reported in an additional 25-50%, and no improvement in 25% (Brown, 1963, 1974; Bettelheim, 1967; Szurek and Berlin, 1973; Eisenberg, 1966). Often treatment succeeds in removing the psychotic symptoms only to reveal an underlying substrate of brain dysfunction or mental subnormality. Treatment and special educational training appropriate for these disorders is then employed. The psychotic reactions up to that point would have precluded the use of these procedures.

Often even with the best of results, certain residual stigmata remain. A post-autistic child may easily tune out or withdraw under certain situations, or retain the preference for sameness and routine, becoming "peculiar" and an "oddball" in his habits, character formation, and relationships.

An example of the residual symptomatology in a fairly successful case is the child first seen at age 4 for autistic symptomatology (withdrawal, little eye or peer contract, echolalic and noncommunicative speech, and rocking) which had not become apparent to his parents, both highly intellectual obsessive mathematics professors, until he was age 3. During therapy he became more and more schizophrenic in the quality of his symptoms, developing his own fantasy world which included an imaginary planet with its own rules and culture. By late latency he was able to sustain first special school, then regular high school. When he was in college, he was referred for therapy. The referral noted him to be eating food picked from garbage cans. He claimed in formal, stilted speech that he should eat no better than the starving people in India, and stared off into space as he talked rather than give eye contact. He walked 14 floors to the therapist's office because people in other parts of the world had no elevators to use, gave his ample allowance to charity, and conducted a Boy Scout troop. Under therapy he gave up some of the more flagrant peculiarities and recompensated sufficiently to finish college. He dated occasionally, after long and prolonged negotiations about time, place, what to do, etc. as if it were a formal contract. He obtained work as an actuary, lives alone on a very rigid routine, supports himself, and sustains relationships only with females in distant areas by letter. Should they move near him, the relationship cools or he ends it.

Other less successful cases may retain much of their original symptomatology and require permanent residential care. Unfortunately, these people at age 20 or 30 may seem much like autistic one- to five-year-olds in adult bodies.

Disorders of Later Onset (after age 3–4)

Childhood Schizophrenia (Schizophreniform Psychotic Disorder)

Childhood schizophrenia is the major subcategory of childhood psychoses of later onset. In contrast to the mute autistic or infantile, clinging, and manipulative children with early-onset psychosis, the schizophrenic child is usually capable of verbal communication, but exhibits disorders of thinking, bizarre ideation, delusions, active and unrealistic fantasy, volatile or flat but inappropriate affect, and distorted perception of and often withdrawal from reality.

Auditory hallucinations, ideas of reference, perplexity, disturbances of mood, posturing mannerisms, and grimacing are common, all of which require higher levels of function than in the austistic child.

Rimland (1964) noted the following additional characteristics associated with schizophrenia vis-à-vis autism: There is an initial period of normality in the first 2 to 3 years, with the child reported as a "best baby," or easy to care for. The full nature of the predisposing personality or prodromal signs and qualities is yet to be described. However, these children look sallow, and their bodies have a doughy, plastic feel (see also Bender, 1947). They may be immature, floppy, gravity-bound, and poorly coordinated in bodily movement. Whirling is often present. Capacity for perception of relationships between objects is impaired. The gestalt of the whole is lost in preoccupation with detail. Disorientation and confusion are present, but the child is accessible and may be engaged; however, these children relate in pathological and bizarre ways.

Ekstein, Bryant, and Friedman (1966), Laufer and Gair (1969) and others say that voice quality may be hollow and mechanical. Their language is characterized frequently by its seeming unrelatedness to the world about them. Word salad, neologisms, and clang associations and sequences are common, as are pronoun reversals. Even where vocabulary is precocious, syntactic usage is deficient. Language is symbolic but is concrete rather than abstract in conceptualization. Metaphorical expressions and punning are common. A fantasy world may be populated with imaginary companions, animals, and even a system of governing rules in an imaginary country or world that represent projections of the child's own libidinal and destructive impulses.

Anxiety and fear are intermittently pervasive and may be related to both the generally poor impulse control, and to the nature of the fantasies, which reflect confusion in sexual identity, body image, feelings of helplessness, fragmentation, defensive omnipotence, and oral, anal and phallic agression. Cognitive capacity and intellectual function are less likely to be impaired to the degree often found in the early-onset psychoses. Also, a substrate of organicity is less likely to be implicated. Focus on one subject, skill, or exceptional ability with precocity is common.

The Schizophrenic Process

Boatman and Szurek (1960) and Ekstein (1966) described the extreme and fluctuating variability and paradoxical nature of the symptomatic expressions of schizophrenic children and attribute this to their limited adaptive capacity, based on ego immaturities or deficiencies. The schizophrenic child responds to stressful environmental and interpersonal demands with anxiety when he feels they are beyond his coping capacity. His regressive behavior and fantasy are his defensive adjustment to avoid overwhelming anxiety. Bender (1956) would implicate an inherent defect in integrative capacity as the primary disorder. Smolen (1965) states "both prenatal and postnatal experience, if sufficiently noxious or non-supportive, may interfere with maturation and result in distortions of development, which can produce findings identical to . . . [actual] central nervous system damage." Goldfarb (1970), Ekstein (1966), and Beres (1956) all describe the ego adaptive vulnerability acquired from the impact of earlier psychosocial and familial tensions. McDougall and Lebovici (1969) describe how organic defects are nevertheless, through projection, experienced as if they were the consequences of environmental trauma and maternal frustration, and are attributed to the "bad mother." Fragmentation and splitting occur. An ambivalent relationship develops rather than a symbiotic attachment or an autistic aloofness.

These children do not withdraw, but express their ambivalent relationships through states of motor excitement, sadomasochistic attack, verbalization of fantasy and phobic anxiety. The nature of these relationships indicate that these children have achieved a degree of separation and individuation. The child's hallucinations are considered to be a primary process distortion of reality, time, space and perception, colored by the child's inner fantasy life. The quality of the fantasy ideation and symbolic language of the schizophrenic child usually indicates that a level of intellectual and developmental function had been reached commensurate with the capacity, however disturbed, for object relationship and internalization of its mental representations.

McDougall and Lebovici (1969) and others of the French school feel that the psychotic defensive system ultimately involves the hitherto conflict-free autonomous ego functions. Language may then distort or lose already established semantic and symbolic functions. Oedipal reactions are premature and preoedipal in mode of expression.

Mahler, Ross, and DeFries (1949) explained the schizophrenic symptomatology on the basis of primary disintegrative, secondary self-integrative and restitutive and tertiary neurotic-like defense mechanisms. Ekstein (1966) describes how schizophrenic children express their conflicts through peculiarities of their verbal and nonverbal language and acting out, playing out, and symbolic and metaphorical language. What was a pathological symptom can gradually become an avenue of communicative expression and restitution.

Clinically one is impressed by the relative intactness of perceptual-cognitive functions in contrast to autistic children. When organic symptomatology is present it tends to be manifest in terms of vasovegetative pallor, vestibular clumsiness, and floppiness. Bender's hypothesis of a schizophrenic core of defective integrative capacity is given support by the clinical course in many cases, in which despite improvement in relationship, impulse control, cognition and mastery skills, a residual core of "schizophrenic" thinking disorder, concreteness, and ritualistic bizarreness remains.

The treatment of childhood schizophrenia involves a different emphasis from the disorders of earlier onset. Overt symptoms of childhood schizophrenia do not appear until after the age of 3 to 5 and may not appear until the prepubertal period. Therefore even the youngest schizophrenics have achieved higher levels of psychosexual and emotional development and ego function. They can relate, make affective contact, and communicate verbally. Where there is plasticity and floppiness in motor tone and integration, it is in most cases the result of ego fragmentation and splitting, rather than actual organic brain dysfunction. In general, there is less likely to be the presence of congenital organic vulnerability as an etiological factor than in the disorders of early onset. There is more likely to be a familial history, suggesting either a genetic predisposition or the passing on of pathology from generation to generation by direct contact and opportunity for incorporation of and identification with the psychotic attitudes and behaviors. Also, the incidence of severely disturbed families predating the appearance of the clinical onset of the child's disorder is considerably higher. There is less developmental delay and less impairment of intelligence and cognitive capacities. The major disorder is one of thinking and fantasy. Accordingly, there is less need for a total multidisciplinary approach, less need for and emphasis on basic and general reactivation of development including relationship and learning milieu, therapeutic educative infant and cognitive stimulation, and less emphasis on learning theory-based behavior modification. Body image and language have been attained. Focus may be more on correction of distortion, and synthesis and integration. Relationship milieu therapy will involve a corrective relationship experience, providing models for incorporation of attitudes for identification rather than the establishment of a relationship per se. Play therapy, art therapy, verbal psychotherapy, and psychoanalytically based techniques are available to the child by virtue of his higher level of functioning. Parental involvement is not on the basis of their co-therapist role in or reinforcement of therapeutic input but more likely in active individual psychotherapy or in conjoint or family therapy in which their own pathology and its role in the development or enhancement of the child's disorder is studied and actively worked on. Chemotherapy is directed to specific goals of increasing contact with reality reduction of agitation and anxiety, reduction of hallucinations and delusions, externalization of ideation, and bringing fantasy in contact with reality. The therapeutic milieu attempts to provide both psychotherapeutic intervention and the protective and corrective social and relationship experiences. This may be provided as a total experience on a residential basis.

In general the nature of the treatment approach reflects the therapists' formulation of etiology and pathogenesis. Those who emphasize psychological factors favor individual and family therapy. Those who hypothesize organic factors tend to use physical or chemotherapeutic means coupled with behavior training and the special education techniques.

Again the trend in treatment planning is the integration of a combination of several types of therapy, as indicated by the evaluation, which with schizophrenic children can make more use of standard psychometric intelligence and projective tests for children. The full range of disciplines is seldom required as it is for optimum effect of the psychoses of early onset.

Of course, when one begins prompt treatment of a 3- or 4-year-old with schizophrenic symptoms, the tendency is to deploy a wider range of development stimuli than one would find necessary for an older child. Anna Freud has stated (personal communication—Hampstead Clinic, London, 1975) that a child who has been prematurely stimulated sexually often develops compensatory precocious verbal abilities that may at first mask the seriousness and depth of the disturbance.

Psychotherapeutic approaches combine the following goals:

1. Reversal of the intrinsic pathological process and restoration of ego function, body image, psychosexual development and reality testing, with a shift from primary process to secondary process thinking through a supportive, educative and corrective interpretive therapeutic relationship and milieu.

2. Correction or removal of the contributive factors in parental and family psychopathology.

Wolman (1970) outlines four principles of directive treatment:

1. Graded reversal of deterioration: A step-by-step building upon the levels of functioning found toward higher levels of function and defense. Care is taken lest direct confrontation or disruption of defenses be precipitous and overwhelming and provoke further withdrawal and regression.

2. The principle of constructive progress: New, more attractive and mature elements are introduced to the child's experience to replace the less mature ones expected to be relinquished.

3. Education toward reality: Reality testing takes top priority in the ego supportive therapy of the schizophrenic child, with the goal of shifting attention from his inner fantasy world to the real physical and social world.

4. Direct guidance: Encouragement toward the sociocultural goals. A geniunely interested friendly therapist is required who can withstand with rational equanimity hostile defensive attack by a patient. Wolman predicts poor prognosis unless there is simultaneous change in the intrafamilial patterns that engendered the schizophrenic reaction in the child. He requires parental participation.

Mahler (1968) and Mahler, Furer, and Settlage (1959) present a more psychoanalytically oriented interpretative approach with supportive parameters. The goals are establishment of body image integrity, restoration of ego function and relationship, and neutralization of destructive aggression and libidinal gratification. The pointing out and interpretation of primary process behavior and fantasy leads to incorporation, assimilation, integration, and synthesis. The therapist must provide auxiliary ego strength both for motivation and for the purpose of setting limits to protect the child from his own panic-creating, destructive fantasies and impulses. Emotional adjustment can be achieved only after a measure of impulse control can be established through first counteracting the child's fragmentation and attaining coherence in play and other functions. Basic concepts and social relationships in time and space, body functions, and the reality of social relationships may have to be painstakingly taught. Parents are often involved in a tripartite approach including therapist, parent, and child.

Ekstein (1966, 1971) also views these relationships as crucial and approaches them therapeutically through the messages contained in the symbolism of the child's behavior and speech, and by making use of the fluctuating availability of the various ego functions. Interpretation within, and at the level of, the child's metaphor or regressive acting behavior leads to joining the child therapeutically in his fantasy, play-acting, and play. At each stage, engagement in a working alliance with the child must be maintained in this manner. Work with the parents and the development of environmental support systems must go on simultaneously to provide the proper milieu to sustain positive change and to undo the tendency for the child's illness to organize and control family life.

Szurek and Berlin (1973), implicating the psychotogenicity of parental anxieties and family tension, describe both simultaneous treatment of the schizophrenic child and his parents, and milieu treatment programs, the latter providing learning, living, and socializing experiences.

Milieu therapy programs providing corrective relationship and socialization experience have been described by, among others, Bettelheim (1967, 1974), Goldbarb, Mintz, and Strook (1969) (residential), and Ruttenberg (1971) (day care).

Both Szurek and Ekstein have made careful studies of countertransference reactions on the part of the therapist toward parental authority figures which may evoke rescue fantasies, taking sides against the parents, and may compromise clinical judgment.

According to Despert (1968), breaking into the child's fantasy world and into his defensive neologisms is the core of the therapeutic process. She illustrates her techniques, which differentiate reality and unreality, reestablish ego boundaries, and reduce the pervasive anxiety making self-realization possible.

McDougall and Lebovici (1969) report the psychoanalysis of a 10-year-old verbal schizophrenic child and give a session-by-session record of the rich verbal fantasy, behavior, and drawings as well as the analysts' interpretation, management, and discussion for the reader. Distorted perception and reality were expressed through the transference relationship. The affectomotor lability, fantasies of incorporation, sadistic attack, and magical influence were well illustrated.

Other psychotherapeutic approaches include those of DesLauriers (1962), who advocated intrusive approaches and bodily contact, based on his belief that schizophrenia represents inability to establish contact with reality by virtue of disorders of subcortical arousal mechanisms rather than a withdrawal from or conflict with reality.

Bender (1967), based on her concept of an all-pervasive, immutable schizophrenic core of disordered function, focuses her therapeutic effort on facilitating and sustaining maturation of function through physical and psycho-educational care and providing remedial training and transitional socialization directing the child back toward the mainstream of school and community life.

Chemotherapy is an important adjunctive modality in the treatment of childhood schizophrenia, as noted in the section of general principles of treatment. The so-called major tranquilizers or antipsychotic agents are the drugs of choice, and are used for reduction of delusional thinking, hallucinations, extreme disintegrating anxiety, and ego disorganizations. There are secondary effects of some of these drugs which may also be useful, such as sedation during agitated periods and at night if sleeplessness is a problem.

Among the major tranquilizers used, chlorpromazine (Thorazine) is used specifically for the acute disturbance of the school-aged and adolescent child. Trifluoperazine (Stelazine), triflupromazine (Vesprin) and thioridazine (Mellaril) have less depressant effect, and increase accessibility and verbalization of fantasy, counteracting withdrawl. Haloperidol (Haldol) and thiothixene (Navane) are reported to be effective in cases where the chronicity, apathy, assaultiveness, self-mutilation, and resistiveness are important impediments to therapeutic intervention. Many cases become accessible only to psychotherapy, increased socialization, and continuation of education after medication has been used to diminish the acute phase of the illness.

Other organic therapies such as electroconvulsive therapy and insulin and metrazole shock treatments have given way to the major tranquilizers, although electroconvulsive therapy is still used by some in older adolescent schizophrenics in cases of persistent withdrawal, catatonia, self-destruction, and extreme agitation. It is claimed that when square wave type electrostimulation is used with the near threshold power level, there is no residual brain dysfunction, memory loss, or loss of cognitive function.

Group therapies make use of the childhood schizophrenic's capacity for verbal expression of fantasy and reality and for interaction with peers. Acting out of fantasies with the group and projection of delusional inner fantasy onto the group provide grist for the therapeutic mill, and enable introduction of corrective socialization. Jensen et al. (1965) developed a "total push" program for schizophrenic children in a therapeutic community.

Behavior modification is reported primarily for

its use with the psychoses of early onset. It is used with childhood schizophrenics for removal of specific targeted symptoms such as bizarre socially alienating behavior, or to motivate participation and cooperation in a group or class, using a special group technique such as a "token economy," where rewards for desired behavior, control of impulse, learning, or social achievement are earned in the form of tokens or script that may be cashed in for a movie, trip, dessert, or in the form of desired privileges or group activity, or otherwise serve as a reinforcer of social interaction.

Educational therapy or therapeutic education is a more recent concept. There has been a growing movement to base the schizophrenic child's therapeutic management within the context of a special school or classroom for the seriously emotionally disturbed. Ego supportive structuring and consistency of milieu and therapeutic educational program, with the goal of expanded socialization and development, along with individual psychotherapy and adjunctive therapies, is favored. Many of Ekstein's case reports originated in the Southard School associated with the Menninger foundation, Topeka, Kansas. Bettelheim's case reports (1955, 1967) derive from the Orthogenic School, Chicago. Also see Goldfarb, Mintz, and Strook (1969) and Ekstein (1966, 1971).

The recent Federal Right to Education of All Handicapped Act reemphasized the role of the school in providing therapeutic education supports for seriously disturbed children, virtually mandating the integration of the therapeutic and educational approaches to the schizophrenic child.

A low teacher-pupil ration (1:4) and opportunity for 1:1 interaction with the special teacher, with psychotherapy, adjunctive therapy, and parental or family therapy rounds out the multidisciplinary approach needed to support the therapeutic education effort. The daily living experience, the routines, peer group interaction, in-class games, adjustment to and acceptance of the adult authority in the classroom, education, therapies, and community exploration all have the goal of expanded physical, cognitive, and emotional development.

Adjunctive therapies as described earlier are modified to fit the developmental needs of the schizophrenic child. The level of biologic maturation and physical size must be considered. A 100-pound body-movement therapist might have difficulty with a 125-pound pubertal disorganized male child who emotionally enjoys being rocked while simultaneously wanting to bite and devour, and is at the same time responding biologically with an erection and open masturbation. Her closeness would be overstimulating and disorganizing to him, as well as an assault on her defenses. Thus the degree and nature of body contact and closeness needs to be adjusted according to such factors.

With the ability for verbal expression and expression through art, music, and play available to the therapist, the therapeutic focus with a schizophrenic child is on conflicts, fantasies, anxieties, and fears and distorted self and reality images of the past and present. The adjunctive therapist finds himself moving further away from a focus on basic early developmental stimulation and more to aspects of specific conflicts, many of which were hitherto unexpressable or unconscious.

Though the sensori-integrative (OT) therapist's work is largely with the younger children, he will work with any residual infantile or pathological organic reflexes. These would be found in the floppy, plastic "Bender type" of organically and genetically based schizophrenics, and with those who may have an associated learning disability. The speech therapist will help the schizophrenic child at the level of correct usage of pronouns, narration, and transition from concrete to more abstract use of symbolism and concept formation as expressed in the schizophrenic thought disorder.

Music therapy can be an effective medium through which a schizophrenic child can have an alternative to an obsessive-compulsive rigid defensive post-schizophrenic adjustment. Percussion instruments and singing can provide an acceptable outlet for unacceptable aggressive impulses that would otherwise be rigidly repressed. After initial expression of strong feelings through singing and dancing has been experienced without fantasied destruction of the self or others, trust toward the one who supported and allowed the expression and still showed acceptance develops, and fantasies and realities are confided by virtue of that trust, enabling evolution of a psychotherapeutic relationship.

A review of special considerations related to age of onset of acute schizophrenic symptoms may be helpful. Prelatency (age 3-5) symptomatology may present in a previously relatively normal child who is vulnerable and who is overwhelmed in some way by his environment, or may present in a child who has been developing from an autistic or symbiotic syndrome into a more sophisticated schizophrenic syndrome. At the developmental stage when earlier instinctual impulses are supposed to be controlled by the ego and superego controls which are forming, so that latency age priorities of cognitive functioning and formal learning in a classroom social group can be achieved, ego function breaks down and the transition fails. If at the beginning of the disintegrative process the ego can mobilize certain symptom compromises (phobic anxiety, obsessive-compulsive preoccupation, conversion or psychosomatic equivalents), then an infantile or childhood neurosis would develop and the child would be able to continue in some way through latency. The psychotic process, however, results in an arrest of development in the pregenital-prelatency phallic oedipal period, and usually with regression to earlier developmental levels (probably to points of traumatic fixation that will be uncovered only through careful history taking and/or psychotherapy or analysis).

Therapy at this early age retains the aspects of (1) developmental reactivation and training, (2) environmental support and therapy, direct working out of conflicts, and reworking and mastery of repressed traumatic experiences. The therapist or total therapeutic environment must represent a stable auxiliary ego, providing information, limits, guidance, and values and mirroring perspective and understanding.

The stresses of latency (age 6–10) involve the requirement for peer relationship and play, and conformity to authority requirements in the classroom. Individual desires must give way to group rules. Although the child may have made a marginal adjustment to age 7 or 8, when pressures for learning, productiveness, and achievement increase, the child breaks down. At this age there is generally less regression to overt infantile behaviors. Instead, the child tends to withdraw into a world of his own and develop a delusional system. The fantasy may be elaborate and represent the complex conflicts troubling the child. Whereas the key complaint about the younger schizophrenic is the severe regression, in the latency age the complaints are often of unexplained destructive outbursts of anger and rage, anxiety-driven hyperactivity, withdrawal and preoccupation, and failure to learn. Often there are exaggerated fears of specific people, animals, or the dark, and unusual or severe eating disorders may occur. A 10-year-old girl developed a preoccupation with brain tumors, injury, death, and delusions of being looked at and talked about, and became unable to leave her mother or go to school. A 9-year-old boy who was severely withdrawn and fearful received no treatment because, with his IQ of 140, he could get by in school. By puberty he developed anorexia nervosa and lost weight down to 60 pounds because of his fear of becoming fat and female.

Therapy at this level should include chemotherapy, psychotherapy to work through the delusions and fantasies, provide support, and help promote socialization, maintenance of a close liaison with a special school program, and work with any family pathology present.

The pubertal period (11–13) provides stresses of a different nature, with the biologic impact of growth and sex hormone induced changes. The ego is hard put even in a hitherto normal child to integrate the sudden and often uneven body changes, the resurgence into a predominant role of the sexual (first homosexual, then heterosexual) and associated aggressive sadomasochistic drives and fantasies, and a reappearance of the oedipal fantasies. Parental seductiveness, overstimulation, or actual incest may be a precipitating factor. The child is bombarded with conflicting double-binding messages. At the same time the child is encouraged to play grown up, yet directed to conform and abstain sexually; to be independent and a man, yet to submerge his identity and submit to authority at home. The precocious expectations attributed to the opposite sex and often laid on them by adults in the guise of liberality and freedom are overwhelming. Frequently the paralysis of parents who are afraid to set limits, their blindness to the actions of their children provoking and begging for these limits, and their reluctance to be less modern and progressive than their child's friends' parents, confuses the child. At the same time, by sixth to eighth grade, full class rotation begins, there are a number of teachers to adjust to, and there are variations in the composition of each class. There is strong peer pressure to conform and even to try daring things—pot, sex, etc. Rejection by cliques is rampant.

The psychotic defensive tendency is once again that of regression and also of delusional adjustment. Therapy at this level may require chemotherapy for an acute, agitated, or destructive period. Analytically oriented psychotherapy coupled with life support at home and school is the treatment of choice and may continue intermittently into or through the high school period. A special school or class for the emotionally disturbed may be necessary for a period of time.

Postpubertal schizophrenic breakdown, in adolescence proper, is identical with the dementia praecox of later adolescence and early adult life. Rather than being the response primarily to the impact of biologic hormonal and physical changes and associated impulses and fantasies as with the peripubertal reaction, this is usually precipitated by a specific real-life situation or traumatic incidient that a latently weak ego, or a momentarily overwhelmed ego, cannot cope with, and which produces a schizophrenic reaction that may clear up rapidly or fixate into a prolonged schizophrenic state.

These older children are treated much as adults, with use of short-term hospitalization and medication as indicated, and with psychotherapy both for resolution of conflicts and overcoming of severe distintegrative anxiety, and for the great deal of support as an "auxiliary ego" which these people need. In addition, special schooling may be required, but this is less often the case in the older child. Any of the adjunctive modalities mentioned may be employed as needed, but the approach is more like that for the adult, which won't be detailed here.

The "benign" deviational and borderline psychoses of later onset include the group of children who, despite a relatively better contact with reality and better general ego function than the schizophreniform psychosis, remain severely disturbed and are similar in many ways to Bender's descriptive category "pseudo-neurotic schizophrenia." Given the concept of nodal points of breakdown of ego function on a developmental continuum, these cases fall between the full psychoses of later childhood and the neuroses and personality disorders of latency. Mahler, Ross, and DeFries (1949) describe latency-aged children whose symptoms develop insidiously, manifesting low frustration tolerance, emotional immaturity, impulsivity, lack of control over aggressive and sexual impulses, mood swings, shallow, tenuous relationships, and poor reality testing. They also have neurotic defenses and symptoms (phobias, hysterical and hypochondriacal traits). When frustrated, they withdraw into fantasy or are very demanding and resort to tantrums. They are usually not delusional. Under stress they may break down into frank schizophrenic-like psychotic episodes in late latency or puberty. Geleerd (1946, 1958) described similar groups, and emphasized the inability to relinquish the fantasy of an omnipotent hold on the family, the anxiety, the diminished interest in human relationships (except anaclitically), and the reaction to frustration as a total loss, with the need for supportive-auxiliary ego and mothering to maintain their hold on reality.

Weil's cases (1953, 1956) are somewhat less severe and have not had frank psychotic breaks. There are signs of delayed and deviational development from infancy (poor integration, unevenness of general maturation and of the physiological and psychological apparatus). She describes decreased "ego stamina" to cope with the diffuse anxiety and overload of tension. Treatment requires the long-term ego support of an anaclitic relationship with a parent/mothering type substitute. Chronicity is usual. Prognosis is guarded. Therapeutic goals are to strengthen the child's ego function, increase frustration tolerance, and decrease the feeling of helplessness that drives the child to need and to cling to his fantasies of omnipotent control. Chemotherapy has been found to be useful in the reduction of anxiety and in the enhancement of impulse control.

Weil (1973) reports prelatency aged children (before age 6 or 7—but over age 3 or 4) whose disturbance falls midway between a psychotic basic pervasive disturbance of ego development and a clear-cut neurotic disturbance. These children are termed variously "ego deficient," "ego disturbed," "deviational," and "borderline." She feels that certain of these children can be prepared for psychoanalytic psychotherapy or a more classical child psychoanalysis, using parental guidance and participation and/or therapeutic education.

These children show disturbances in integrative functioning which often derive from initial regulatory instability between mother and infant (Sander, 1962), often due to predisposing vulnerabilities. These result in imbalances between ego and drive, within and among ego functions between libido and aggression (with aggression prevailing), and between hostile and non-hostile aggression. The ego deficiencies are preoedipally based, and apparent growth is really an "as-if" imitation. Especially before latency, deficient, distorted, or traumatic past experience can be made up (or corrected) by special therapeutic educational work with a skilled teacher or a sensitive, motivated supervised mother. This may be used as a preparation for psychotherapy or may be continued as the therapeutic agent of choice.

Manic Depressive Psychoses and Other Severe Depressive States of Childhood and Adolescence

Until recent years it has been uncommon to use "depression" as a diagnostic entity in children. It is not mentioned in the standard diagnostic schemata and official classifications like the APA DSM II. One is told that manic-depressive psychosis is nonexistent in prepuberty and rare in adolescence. However, the child psychiatric and psychoanalytic literature is replete with terms and symptoms descriptive of aspects of depression. Children are commonly seen to be very unhappy, apathetic, withdrawn, and guilty. Some question equating this with clinical depression. Depressed affect is associated with grief and mourning over loss (death or psychological separation from a love object). Bowlby (1960), for instance, proposes that grief and mourning occur when the infant experiences loss and frustration of attachment needs, caused by maternal unavailability.

Depression is considered to be associated with feelings of helplessness (derived from oral phase trauma) and hopelessness (phallic anxiety based), with consequent frustration and giving up. Rochlin (1961), as others before, implicated childhood deprivation, or actual loss leading to fear of subsequent loss, abandonment, and severe loneliness. From that follows a feeling of worthlessness leading to self-rejection (loss of self-esteem), self-abandonment, and self-destruction. The early object loss may predispose the person to psychotic depressive reactions in adolescence and adulthood.

Melanie Klein's (1932, 1952) formulation of the early (6 month to 1 year) and central depressive position is based on the concept of the capacity for very early superego formation, which can produce a sense of impending loss and anxiety created by the child's own ambivalent (and unconscious) oedipal fantasies, putting the ambivalently loved object in danger from the child's own destructive wishes.

Rene Spitz (1945, 1946a) studying children in orphanages in their first two years of life, reported withdrawal from, and anxious reaction to, human contact, profound regression, delays in motor and speech development and intellectual and social functioning, marasmus, and frequently death despite good physical care when there was a minimum of environmental stimulation and human contact. This condition, which he termed "hospitalism," did not occur in another nursery where mothering and environmental stimulation was present, despite a lower level of initial function and family background. These children in both nurseries had shown no sign of neurological impairment at the beginning of the study. In the same year, Spitz (1946b) reported "anaclitic depression" in children aged 6–11 months who, after having established a relationship with a primary mothering figure, lost the love object. Depression, withdrawal of interest in the outside world, retardation of function, marasmus, and even death resulted unless the love object or an adequate substitute was restored within three months. Spitz demonstrated the necessity of the continuity of mothering and environmental stimulation from the beginning of life for normal development, and described the serious disintegration of ego functions that resulted from its deprivation, producing clinical symptoms not unlike those described in the most serious psychoses and amentias.

Putnam, Rank, and Kaplan (1951) report a case of "primal agitated depression" in a 3-year-old following a two-week separation from his parents and the birth of the sibling. Frequent frustration had occurred even before the two-week separation. The child was in a state of agitated depression with depressed affect, constantly masturbating and biting himself, with low frustration tolerance. The mother participated in the sessions and the relationship between mother and child observed and reworked. Earlier experiences of loss had led to chronic mild depression which preceded the agitated state.

The literature refers to the rarity of the affective psychoses in childhood. However, Langdell (1973) noted the growing mention of marasmus, anaclitic depression, and other reactions to loss and deprivation in early childhood. He felt that many subtle forms of depression, in the forms of low self-esteem and self-punishment, go unrecognized. Other manifestations may be truancy, runaway, and accident proneness. Depression, self-destruction, and suicide in latency are reported with increasing frequency. The early psychic roots of depression are to be found in early loss or deprivation of mothering and the anxieties of frequent separation. Harsh superego pressures and oedipal guilt are responsible for the self-defeating and deprecating attitudes. The establishment of the familial nature of manic-depressive psychosis has led to its being looked for and found with greater frequency in the latency age. Feinstein and Wolpert (1973) describe the characteristic sensitivity to loss, and the affective instability in the manic-depressive child and suggest a treatment plan utilizing both psychotherapy and lithium. Anorexia nervosa, asthma, and obesity can be seen in part as psychosomatic depressive equivalents.

Treatment involves:

1. Chemotherapy: preliminary studies using lithium (Campbell, 1973) suggest that it may be a specific medication for periodic depressions, affecto-manic episodes, and the auto-aggressive and self-destructive phenomena of young schizophrenics.

Monoamine oxidase inhibitors are not recommended for children because of their toxicity. Except for the use of imipramine (Tofranil) in enuresis with children over age 6, the use of tricyclic antidepressants (imipramine, amitriptyline, and nortriptyline) is not recommended for prepubertal depressed children, though they can be used with adolescents to alleviate depression and anxiety.

2. Hospitalization may be required in children of any age if there is overt or covert suicidal behavior.

3. Psychotherapies for the infantile depressions (anaclitic, marasmic) evidenced by eating and sleep disturbances, head banging, withdrawal, and apathy involves the provision of emotionally warm and nurturing mothering in the form of a substitute mother. If the real mother has been only psychologically absent due to her own depressed state, appropriate support and therapy for her is indicated so that she may be returned to the active and effective care of her child.

Head banging and other self-destructive activities may require helmeting and physical or chemotherapeutic restraint and/or aversive and extinguishing behavior modification techniques until the underlying environmental situation and, with older children, the internal conflicts, may be affected psychotherapeutically.

Depression in an older child may be expressed by whining, tantruming, and a general unhappy affect. Truanting and runaway tendency are also manifestations of feeling unwanted. Feelings of unworthiness result in an unspoken invitation to be picked on and chased by peers, and failure in school. Accident proneness, self-destructiveness, and feeling bad and evil are the pubertal child's reactions to the reemerging oedipal fantasies and unacceptable sexual impulses, especially if a punishing superego has developed. Self-punishment and self-rejection can lead to a psychotic degree of depression or depressive equivalent behaviors.

Though the individual symptoms and behaviors must often be dealt with on an immediate and socially related basis, the underlying causes of these symptomatic behaviors must be identified and corrected. Both the home situation must be corrected and the child given support, insight, and help in expressing and directing his anger and frustration outward instead of on himself.

It must be determined whether the feelings of unworthiness and the associated anger at self are the result of earlier object loss, or are based on sensed deficits and on the hopelessness of not being able to learn in an MBD child, or not being able to speak in a true expressive aphasic.

Conditions That May Take a Psychotic Form

For the sake of completness, it should be noted that some severe psychosomatic disorders may be physical equivalents of psychotic depression. Examples would be severe exfoliative dermatitis, usually related to anger, severe asthma, often related to loss, and anorexia nervosa, often related to guilt. These can be life-threatening, and require well-managed combined medical and psychotherapeutic approaches.

Other conditions which may present in a psychotic form are elective mutism and folie à deux.

Elective mutism is commonly defined as a condition wherein the child is mute in most situations outside the home, where it is claimed he comunicates with speech. It is usually picked up in the school or preschool day care or nursery environment where verbal communication is an integral and expected part of the learning situation.

Though it is usually considered a nonpsychotic, neurotic defensive or phobic condition, as a reaction to family disturbance (Pustrom and Speers, 1964), or to developmental immaturities and a vulnerable self-image which includes timidity, hypersensitivity, inability to cope, minimal speech deficiencies, and a fear of loss of control over verbal impulse and power (words can destroy) (Halpern et al., 1971), cases associated with psychosis do appear.

Hayden (1977) at the October 1977 Meeting of the American Academy of Child Psychiatry presented her comprehensive studies, which noted four types of elective mutism. In a controlled study she found that the behavioral characteristics of these types conformed more closely to those of the neurotic control group rather than to either the speech-impaired or to the normal groups. She described her four types as: (1) symbiotic mutism with a strong dependent relationship to the caretaking/mothering source; (2) speech phobic mutism, the rarest type, in which the child seemed afraid to speak, afraid of his own voice and words, often associated with "warding off rituals"; (3) Reactive mutism, in which the mutism was precipitated by a single event or series of traumatic events, including trauma to face and mouth in the years when speech develops (this group seemed closest in description to the psychotic); (4) Passive aggressive mutism, in which the child was tenaciously resistive, withholding, uncooperative, and frequently a victim of neglect or child abuse at home.

Elective mutism is placed in with the consideration of the childhood psychoses because it appears frequently (referred by school or day care center) for evaluation as "autistic" or "psychotic" behavior, with incomplete home history. It must be differentiated from childhood aphasia, retardation (in which speech development is more vulnerable than motor development), childhood autism in which child has never developed speech, or secondary autism or schizophrenia in which speech was lost, or a retreat from the confusion of bilingualism in the home.

Folie à deux again is not in itself a psychotic disorder but may produce symptoms and whole clusters of behavior which are psychotic-like. This transference of psychotic behaviors and delusional ideas from one child or adult to another child who has been in close contact is rarely reported in the literature. Simonds and Glenn (1976) have reviewed the literature and presented a case history of a 10-year-old girl who had a close relationship with a paranoid incestuous stepfather. There is some question as to whether a child subjected to psychotic and incestuous parenting, stimulating sexual drives and fantasies, would not be driven into a psychosis per se. Certainly with only pathological models to incorporate and identify with, a pathological ego would develop.

Anthony (1970) reported folie à deux-like reactions in two 5-year-old children of psychotic mothers who perpetuated the symbiotic relationship and compromised the child's reality testing by perpetuating their delusions about the world and prolonged the separation-individuation phase. He felt that some degree of vulnerability existed in these children making them more susceptible to the conditions. Diagnostic criteria include:

1. An intimate association with the "infecting" person, who is in a dominant position.
2. The prepsychotic personality of the "infected" one being seclusive, dependent, and suggestible.
3. Delusional content and thinking of the parents is modeled after and communicated by the child,
4. Child's close relationship is maintained for reasons of secondary gain.
5. Remission occurs after separation, following initial heightening of anxiety.

Treatment requires separation from the "infecting" parent or environment and provision of a milieu in which anxiety is relived (chemotherapeutically where indicated) and the child's confusion and delusions are corrected through relationships with a therapist and staff who support correct reality testing.

Direction and monitoring of healthy peer relationships and community activities helps as a preparation for return to full community and school life. Social work counseling and therapy for the family, especially the "infecting" member, is necessary. Serious consideration should be given to finding other residential facilities or foster family placement.

To a lesser degree folie à deux-like reactions are to be found among peers. In the case of the young teenage boy who killed a 4-year-old girl, his best boyfriend developed severe anxiety and the fear that he too would kill a little girl, that he too was bad, a potential murderer, and he began hearing voices telling him to do so. He developed an acute hysterical state which quickly subsided under reassurance and a two-week vacation with his parents away from the newspaper and radio reports and neighborhood activity concerning the case.

It also occurs in treatment centers that better-functioning children can tend to copy the behaviors and speech of lower-functioning children. When this occurs, steps should be taken to separate them from their pathologic models as much as possible, and consideration given to transfer to a higher-functioning milieu.

References

American Psychiatric Association. (1968) *Diagnostic and Statistical Manual of Mental Disorders*, 2nd ed. (APA DSM II). Washington, D.C.: American Psychiatric Association.

American Psychiatric Association. (1969) *A Psychiatry Glossary*, 3rd ed. Washington, D.C.: American Psychiatric Association.

Anthony, E.J. (1958) An experimental approach to the psychopathology of childhood. *Brit. J. Med. Psychol.* 31:211–225.

Anthony, E.J. (1970) The influence of maternal psychoses on children. Folie à deux. In E.J. Anthony and T. Benedek, eds., *Parenthood: Its Psychology and Psychopathology*. Boston: Little, Brown.

Autry, J.H. (1975) Report of workshop on orthomolecular treatment of schizophrenia. *Schizo. Bull.* 12:94–103.

Ayres, A.J. (1973) *Sensory Integration and Learning Disorders*. Los Angeles: Western Psychological Services.

Baltaxe, C.A.M., and J.Q. Simmons. (1975) Language in childhood psychoses. *J. Speech Hearing Disord.* 40:439–458.

Bender, L. (1947) Childhood schizophrenia: Clinical study of one hundred schizophrenic children. *Am. J. Orthopsychiat.* 17:40–56.

Bender, L. (1956) Schizophrenia in childhood—Its recognition, description and treatment. *Am. J. Orthopsychiat.* 26:499–506.

Bender, L. (1960) Treatment in early schizophrenia. *Prog. Psychother.* 5:177–184.

Bender, L. (1967) Theory and treatment of childhood schizophrenia. *Acta Paedopsychiat.* 34:298–307.

Bender, L., L. Cobrinik, G. Faretra, and D. Sankar. (1966) The treatment of childhood schizophrenia with LSD and UML. In M. Rinkel, ed., *Biological Treatment of Mental Illness.* New York: L.C. Page.

Beres, D. (1956) Ego deviation and the concept of schizophrenia. In *Psychoanalytic Study of the Child,* Vol. II. New York: International Universities Press, pp. 164–235.

Bernstein, P.L. (1972) *Theory and Methods in Dance-Movement Therapy.* Dubuque, Iowa: Kendall-Hunt.

Bettelheim, B. (1955) *Truants from Life.* Glencoe, Ill.: Free Press.

Bettelheim, B. (1967) *The Empty Fortress: Infantile Autism and the Birth of the Self.* New York: Free Press.

Bettelheim, B. (1974) *A Home for the Heart.* New York: Knopf.

Bird, B.L., D.C. Russo, and M.F. Cataldo. (1977) Consideration in the analysis and treatment of dietary effects on behavior. *J. Autism Child. Schizo.* 7:373–382.

Bleuler, E. (1911) *Textbook of Psychiatry.* A.A. Brill, trans. New York: Macmillan.

Boatman, J.J., and S.A. Szurek. (1960) A clinical study of childhood schizophrenia. In D. Jackson, ed., *The Etiology of Schizophrenia.* New York: Basic Books.

Bowen, M. (1960) A family concept of schizophrenia. In D.D. Jackson, ed., *The Etiology of Schizophrenia.* New York: Basic Book.

Bowlby, J. (1960) *Grief and Mourning in Infancy and Early Childhood. Psychoanalytic Study of the Child,* Vol. 15. New York: International Universities Press.

Brown, J.L. (1963) Follow-up of children with atypical development (infantile psychoses). *Am. J. Orthopsychiat.* 51:855-861.

Brown, J.L. (1974) Further follow-up of children with atypical development at J.J. Putnam Center, Boston. Infantile autism reconsidered. Paper presented at American Orthopsychiatric Association Annual Meeting, April 1974, San Francisco.

Campbell, M. (1973) Biological interventions in the psychoses of childhood. *J. Autism Child. Schizo.* 3:347–373.

Campbell, M., and T. Shapiro. (1975) Therapy of psychiatric disorders of childhood. In R.I. Shader, ed., *Manual of Psychiatric Therapies.* Boston: Little, Brown.

Chess, S. (1971) Autism in children with congenital rubella. *J. Autism Child. Schizo.* 1:33–47.

Churchill, D.W. (1969) Psychotic children and behavior modification. *Am. J. Psychiat.* 125:1585–1590.

Coffrey, H.S., and L.W. Wiener. (1967) *Group Treatment of Autistic Children.* Englewood Cliffs, N.J.: Prentice-Hall.

Cohen, D.J., et al. (1974) Biogenic amines in autistic and atypical children. *Arch. Gen. Psychiat.* 31:845–853.

Coleman, M. (1976) *The Autistic Syndromes.* New York: North-Holland.

Creak, M., et al. (1961) Schizophrenic syndrome in children. Progress report of the British Working Party. *Brit. Med. J.* 2:889–890.

Davids, A., and J.K. Berenson. (1977) Integration of a behavior modification program into a traditionally oriented residential treatment center for children. *J. Autism Child. Schizo.* 7:269–286.

DeMyer, M.K., D.W. Churchill, W. Pontius, and K.M. Gilkey. (1971) A comparison of five diagnostic systems for autism and childhood schizophrenia. *J. Autism Child. Schizo.* 1:175–189.

DeSanctis, S. (1906) On some varieties of dementia praecox. *Rivista Sperimentale di Freniatria* 32:141–165. English translation in S.A. Szurek and I.N. Berlin, eds., *Clinical Studies in Childhood Psychoses.* New York: Brunner/Mazel (1973).

DesLauriers, A. (1962) *The Experience of Reality in Childhood Schizophrenia.* New York: International Universities Press.

DesLauriers, A.M., and C.F. Carlson. (1969) *Your Child Is Asleep—Early Infantile Autism.* Homewood, Ill.: Dorsey.

Despert, L. (1938) Schizophrenia in childhood. *Psychiat. Quart.* 12:366–371.

Despert, J.L. (1968) *Schizophrenia in Children.* New York: Robert Brunner.

Dubnoff, B, (1965) The habilitation and education of the autistic child in a therapeutic day school. *Am. J. Orthopsychiat.* 35:385–386.

Eisenberg, L. (1966) Psychotic disorders in childhood. In R.E. Cook, ed., *Biological Basis of Pediatric Practice.* New York: McGraw-Hill.

Ekstein, R. (1966) *Children of Time and Space, of Action and Impulse.* New York: Appleton.

Ekstein, R. (1971) *The Challenge.* New York: Brunner/Mazel.

Ekstein, R., K. Bryant, and S.W. Friedman. (1966) Childhood schizophrenia and allied conditions. In L. Bellak, ed., *Schizophrenia: A Review of the Syndrome,* 2nd ed. New York: Grune & Stratton.

Elkish, P. (1968) Nonverbal, extraverbal, and autistic verbal communication in the treatment of a child tiqueur. In *Psychoanalytic Study of the Child,* Vol. 23. New York: International Universities Press, pp. 423–437.

Feingold, B.F. (1975) *Why Your Child Is Hyperactive.* New York: Random House.

Feinstein, S.C., and E.A. Wolpert. (1973) Juvenile manic depressive illness: Clinical and therapeutic considerations. *J. Am. Acad. Child Psychiat.* 12:123–136.

Ferster, C.B. (1961) Positive reinforcement and behavioral deficits of autistic children. *Child Develop.* 32:437–456.

Fish, B., M. Campbell, T. Shapiro, and A. Lloyd. (1969) Schizophrenic children treated with methysergide. *Dis. Nerv. Syst.* 30:534–540.

Fish, B., and T. Shapiro. (1965) A typology of children's psychiatric disorders. *J. Am. Acad. Child Psychiat.* 4:32–52.

Frederick II. (1949) In J.B. Ross and M.M. McLaughlin, eds., *The Portable Medieval Reader*. New York: Viking Press, pp. 366–367.

Freud, S. (1905) Three essays on the theory of sexuality. In *Standard Edition*, Vol. 7, pp. 125–244. London: Hogarth Press (1953).

Freud, S. Neurosis and psychosis. In *Collected Papers*, Vol. II. London: Hogarth Press (1950).

Frostig, M., and D. Horne. (1970) *Charting and Evaluating the Therapeutic Process with Autistic Children*. Los Angeles, Calif.: Marianne Frostig Center of Educational Therapy.

Geleerd, E.R. (1946) Contributions to the problem of psychosis in childhood. In *Psychoanalytic Study of the Child*, Vol. 2. New York: International Universities Press, pp. 271–292.

Geleerd, E.R. (1958) Borderline state in childhood and adolescence. In *Psychoanalytic Study of the Child*, Vol. 13. New York: International Universities Press, pp. 279–295.

Goldfarb, W. (1970) Childhood psychosis. In P.H. Mussen, ed., *Carmichael's Manual of Child Psychology*, Vol. 2. New York: Wiley.

Goldfarb, W. (1974) *Early Childhood Psychosis: The Variety of Its Forms, the Vicissitudes of Change, the Complexity of Its Causes.* The 42nd Salmon Lecture, New York Academy of Medicine. New York: Psychosocial Process (1975).

Goldfarb, W., I. Mintz, and D. Strook. (1969) *A Time to Heal*. New York: International Universities Press.

Group for the Advancement of Psychiatry. (1966) *Psychopathological Disorders in Childhood: Theoretical Considerations and a Proposed Classification.* New York: Group for the Advancement of Psychiatry.

Guthrie, R., and R.J. Wyatt. (1975) Biochemistry and schizophrenia III—A review of childhood psychoses. *Schizo. Bull.* 12:19–30.

Halpern, W.L. (1971) A therapeutic approach to speech phobia—Elective mutism revisited. *J. Am. Acad. Child Psychiat.* 10:94–107.

Hamblin, R.A., et al. (1971) *Humanization Processes: A Social-Behavioral Analysis of Children's Problems.* New York: Wiley-Interscience.

Harper, J., and S. Williams. (1974) Early environmental stress and infantile autism. *Med. J. Austral.* 1:341–346.

Haslett, N.R. (1977) Treatment planning for children. *Psychiatry Dig.* 16:21–34.

Hayden, T.L. (1977) Elective mutism. Paper presented at the annual meeting of the American Academy of Child Psychiatry, October 1977.

Heimlich, E.P. (1965) The specialized use of music as a mode of communication in the treatment of disturbed children. *J. Am. Acad. Child Psychiat.* 4:86–122.

Heller, T. (1908) Infantile dementia. Reprinted in J.G. Howells, ed., *Modern Perspectives in International Child Psychiatry*. Edinburgh: Oliver & Boyd (1930).

Helm, D. (1976) Psychodynamic and behavior modification approaches to the treatment of infantile autism: Empirical similarities. *J. Autism Child. Schizo.* 6:27–42.

Hicks, J.S. (1972) Language disabilities of emotionally disturbed children. In J.V. Irwin and M. Marge, eds., *Principles of Childhood Language Disabilities*. New York: Appleton-Century-Crofts.

Hingtgen, J.N., S.K. Coulter, and D.W. Churchill. (1967) Intensive reinforcement of imitative behavior in mute autistic children. *Arch. Gen. Psychiat.* 17:36.

Holter, F.R., and B.A. Ruttenberg. (1971) Initial interventions in psychotherapeutic treatment of autistic children. *J. Autism Child. Schizo.* 1:206–214.

Howlin, P., et al. (1973) A home-based approach to the treatment of autistic children. *J. Autism Child. Schizo.* 4:308–336.

Jensen, S.E., et al. (1965) Treatment of severely emotionally disturbed children in a community. *J. Can. Psychiat. Assn.* 10:325–331.

Kalish, B. (1968) Body movement therapy for autistic children: A description and discussion of basic concepts. *Proc. Am. Dance Ther. Assn.* 3rd Annual Conference, Columbia, Md. A.D.T.A. pp. 49–59.

Kanner, L. (1943) Autistic disturbances of affective contact. *Nerv. Child* :217–250.

Reprinted in *Childhood Psychoses: Initial Studies and New Insights*. Washington/New York: V.H. Winston & Sons/Wiley (1973).

Kanner, L. (1944) Early infantile autism. *J. Pediat.* 25:211–217.

Kanner, L. (1949) Problems of nosology and psychodynamics of early infantile autism. *Am. J. Orthopsychiat.* 19:416–426.

Kanner, L. (1971) Childhood psychosis: A historical overview. *J. Autism Child. Schizo.* 1:14–19.

Kestenberg, J.S. (1965) The role of movement patterns in development 1. Rhythms of movement. *Psychoanal. Quart.* 34:1–36.

Klein, M. (1932) *The Psycho-Analysis of Children*. London: Hogarth Press.

Klein, M., et al. (1952) *Developments in Psychoanalysis*. London: Hogarth Press.

Kramer, E. (1972) *Art as Therapy with Children*. Springfield, Ill.: Charles C Thomas.

Langdell, J. (1973) Depressive reactions of childhood and adolescence. In S.A. Szurek and I.N. Berlin, eds., *Clinical Studies in Childhood Psychoses*. New York: Brunner/Mazel.

Laufer, M.W., and D.S. Gair. (1969) Childhood schizophrenia. In L. Bellak, ed., *The Schizophrenic Syndrome*. New York: Grune & Stratton.

Leff. R. (1968) Behavior modification and the psychosis of childhood: A review. *Psychol. Bull.* 69:396.

Lichstein, K.L., and L. Schreibman. (1976) Employing electric shock with autistic children: A review of the side effects. *J. Autism Child. Schizo.* 6:163–175.

Lipton, M.A., et al. (1973) *Megavitamin and Orthomolecular Therapy in Psychiatry*. Washington, D.C.: American Psychiatric Association.

Lovaas, O.I. (1971) Considerations in the development of a behavioral treatment program for psychotic children. In D. Churchill, G. Alpern, and M. DeMyer, eds., *Infantile Autism*. Springfield, Ill.: Charles C Thomas.

Mahler, M.S. (1952) On child psychoses and schizophrenia: Autistic and symbiotic infantile psychosis. In *Psychoanalytic Study of the Child*. Vol. 7. New York: International Universities Press, pp. 286–305.

Mahler, M.S. (1961) On sadness and grief in infancy and childhood. In *Psychoanalytic Study of the Child*. Vol. 16. New York: International Universities Press, pp. 332–351.

Mahler, M.S. (1968) *On Human Symbiosis and the Vicissitudes of Individuation. I—Infantile Psychosis*. New York: International Universities Press.

Mahler, M.S., M. Furer, and C. Settlage. (1959) Severe emotional disturbances in childhood: Psychosis. In S. Arieti, ed., *American Handbook of Psychiatry*. New York: Basic Books.

Mahler, M.S., J.R. Ross, and Z. DeFries. (1949) Clinical studies in benign and malignant cases of childhood psychosis (schizophrenic-like). *Am. J. Orthopsychiat.* 19:295.

McDevitt, J.B., and G.F. Settlage, eds. (1971) *Separation-Individuation: Essays in Honor of Margaret S. Mahler*. New York: International Universities Press.

McDougall, J., and S. Lebovici. (1969) *Dialogue with Sammy: A Psychoanalytic Contribution to the Understanding of Child Psychosis*. New York: International Universities Press.

Menolascino, F. (1971) The description and classification of infantile autism. In D. Churchill, G. Alpern, and M. DeMyer, eds., *Infantile Autism*. Springfield, Ill.: Charles C Thomas, pp. 71-97.

Meyer, A. (1910) The dynamic interpretation of dementia praecox. *Am. J. Psychol.* 21:385–403.

Mosher, L., and D. Feinsilver. (1971) *Special Report: Schizophrenia*. Rockville, Md.: National Institute of Mental Health, Center for Studies of Schizophrenia.

Ney, P.G., A.E. Palvesky, and J. Markely. (1971) Relative effectiveness of operant conditioning and play therapy in childhood schizophrenia. *J. Autism Child. Schizo.* 1:337-349.

Nordoff, P., and C. Robbins. (1965) *Music Therapy for Handicapped Children*. New York: Rudolf Steiner.

Nordoff, P., and C. Robbins. (1976) *Creative Music Therapy: Individual Treatment for the Handicapped Child*. New York: John Day.

Ornitz, E.M. (1973) Childhood autism: A review of clinical and experimental literature. *Calif. Med.* 118:21–47.

Piaget, J. (1951a) *The Child's Conception of the World*. London: Routledge & Kegan Paul.

Piaget, J. (1951b) *Play, Dreams and Imitation in Childhood*. New York: Norton.

Potter, H.W. (1933) Schizophrenia in children. *Am. J. Psychiat.* 89:1253–1270.

Provence, S. (1974) Developmental assessment and its implications for individualized treatment plans for atypical and autistic children. Paper presented at the American Orthopsychiatric Workshop, April 1974, San Francisco.

Pustrom, E., and R.W. Speers. (1964) Elective mutism in children. *J. Am. Acad. Child Psychiat.* 3:287–292.

Putnam, M.C., B. Rank, and S. Kaplan. (1951) A case of primal depression in an infant. *Psychoanalytic Study of the Child*. Vol. 6. New York: International Universities Press.

Rank, B. (1949) Adaptation of the psychoanalytic technique for the treatment of young children with atypical development. *Am. J. Orthopsychiat.* 19:130–139.

Rank, B. (1955) Intensive study and treatment of preschool children who showed marked personality deviations or "atypical development" and their parents. In G. Caplan, ed., *Emotional Problems of Early Childhood*. New York: Basic Books.

Rank, B., and D. MacNaughton. (1950) A clinical contribution to early ego development. In *Psychoanalytic Study of the Child*. Vol. 5. New York: International Universities Press, pp. 53–65.

Reiser, D.E. (1963) Psychoses of infancy and early childhood as manifested by children with atypical development. *New Eng. J. Med.* 209:790–798, 844–850.

Reiser, D.E. (1966) Infantile psychosis. *Ment. Hyg.* 50:588–589.

Rimland, B. (1964) *Infantile Autism*. New York: Appleton-Century-Crofts.

Ritvo, E. (1977) National Society for Autistic Children: Definition of the syndrome of autism. Los Angeles: Professional Advisory Board.

Rochlin, G. (1961) The dread of abandonment—A contribution to the etiology of the loss complex and to depression. *Psychoanalytic Study of the Child*. Vol. 16. New York: International Universities Press.

Ruttenberg, B. (1971) A psychoanalytic understanding of infantile autism and its treatment. In D. Churchill, G. Alpern, and M. DeMyer, eds., *Infantile Autism: Proceedings, Indiana University Colloquium*. Springfield, Ill.: Charles C Thomas.

Ruttenberg, B.A. (1977a) Childhood psychoses. In B. Wolman, ed., *International Encyclopedia of Psychiatry, Psychology, Psychoanalysis and Neurology*. New York: Human Sciences Press.

Ruttenberg, B.A. (1977b) Autism. In B. Wolman, ed., *International Encyclopedia of Psychiatry, Psychology, Psychoanalysis, and Neurology*. New York: Human Sciences Press.

Ruttenberg, B.A., M. Dratman, J. Fraknoi, and C. Wenar. (1966) An instrument for evaluating autistic children (BRIAAC). *J. Am. Acad. Child Psychiat.* 5:453-478.

Ruttenberg, B.A., B. Kalish, C. Wenar, and E.G. Wolf. (1978) *Behavior Rating Instrument for Autistic and Atypical Children (BRIAAC)*. Chicago: Stoelting Co.

Rutter, M. (1972) Childhood schizophrenia reconsidered. *J. Autism Child. Schizo.* 2:315–337.

Rutter, M., S. Lebovici, L. Eisenberg, et al. (1969) World Health Organization: A triaxial classification of mental disorders in childhood. *J. Child Psychol. Psychiat.* 10:41–61.

Rutter, M., and L. Bartak. (1971) Causes of infantile autism: Some considerations from recent research. *J. Autism Child. Schizo.* 1:20–32.

Saposnik, D.T. (1967) An experimental study of rage reduction treatment on autistic children. Master's thesis, San Jose State College, California.

Schopler, E. (1965) Early infantile autism and receptor processes. *Arch. Gen. Psychiat.* 13:327–335.

Schopler, E., and R.J. Reichler. (1971) Parents as cotherapists in the treatment of psychotic children. *J. Autism Child. Schizo.* 1:87–102.

Settlage, C. (1964) Psychoanalytic theory in relation to the nosology of childhood psychic disorders. *J. Am. Psychoanal. Assn.* 12:776–800.

Simmons, J.Q., O.I. Lovaas, B. Schaeffer, and B. Perloff. (1966) Modification of autistic behavior with LSD 25. *Am. J. Psychiat.* 122:1201–1211.

Simonds, J.F., and T. Glenn. (1976) Folie à deux in a child. *J. Autism Child. Schizo.* 6:61–73.

Smolen, E. (1965) Some thoughts on schizophrenia in childhood. *J. Am. Acad. Child Psychiat.* 4:443–472.

Smolen, E., and N. Lifton. (1966) A special treatment program for schizophrenic children in a child guidance clinic. *Am. J. Orthopsychiat.* 36:735–742.

Spitz, R. (1945) Hospitalism: An inquiry into the genesis of psychiatric conditions in early childhood. In *Psychoanalytic Study of the Child.* Vol. 1. New York: International Universities Press, pp. 53–74.

Spitz, R. (1946a) Hospitalism: A follow-up report. In *Psychoanalytic Study of the Child.* Vol. 2. New York: International Universities Press, pp. 113–117.

Spitz, R. (1946b) Anaclitic depression. In *Psychoanalytic Study of the Child.* Vol. 2. New York: International Universities Press, pp. 313–342.

Szurek, S.A., and I.N. Berlin, eds. (1973) *Clinical Studies in Childhood Psychoses.* New York: Brunner/Mazel.

Tinbergen, E.A., and N. Tinbergen. (1972) *Early Childhood Autism: An Ethological Approach.* Berlin and Hamburg: Verlag Paul Parey.

Weil, A. (1953) Certain severe disturbances of ego development in childhood. In *Psychoanalytic Study of the Child,* Vol. 8. New York: International Universities Press.

Weil, A. (1956) Some evidences of deviational development in infancy and early childhood. In *Psychoanalytic Study of the Child,* Vol. 11. New York: International Universities Press, pp. 292–299.

Weil, A. (1973) Ego strengthening prior to analyses. In *Psychoanalytic Study of the Child,* Vol. 28. New York: International Universities Press.

Wenar, C. (1977) Treatment of autism. In B. Wolman, ed., *International Encyclopedia of Psychiatry, Psychology, Psychoanalysis, and Neurology.* New York: Human Sciences Press.

Wenar, C., and B.A. Ruttenberg. (1969) Therapies for autistic children. In J. Masserman, ed., *Current Psychiatric Therapies.* New York: Grune & Stratton.

Wenar, C., and B.A. Ruttenberg. (1976) The use of BRIAAC for evaluating therapeutic effectiveness. *J. Autism Child. Schizo.* 6:175–191.

Wherry, J.S. (1972) Childhood psychosis. In Quay and Wherry, eds., *Psychopathological Disorders of Childhood.* New York: Wiley.

Whittaker, J.K. (1975) The ecology of child treatment: A developmental/educational approach to the therapeutic milieu. *J. Autism Child. Schizo.* 5:223–238.

Wolf, E.G., and B.A. Ruttenberg. (1967) Communication therapy for the autistic child. *J. Speech Hearing Disord.* 32:331–335.

Wolman, B. (1970) *Children without Childhood: A Study of Childhood Schizophrenia.* New York: Grune & Stratton.

Yates, A.J. (1970) The psychoses—Children. In *Behavior Therapy.* New York: Wiley.

Zaslow, R.W. (1967) A psychogenic theory of the etiology of infantile autism—Implications for treatment. Paper presented to the California Psychological Association, San Diego, California.

Zaslow, R.W., and L. Breger. (1967) Theory and treatment of autism. In L. Breger, ed., *Clinical-Cognitive Psychology Models and Integration.* New York: Prentice-Hall.

Treatment of Emotional Disorders in Children and Adolescents

CHAPTER 27

The Treatment of Minimal Brain Dysfunction

Dennis P. Cantwell

Introduction

The syndrome of minimal brain dysfunction in children is a rather controversial one. There are those who feel that it is the most common of all psychiatric disorders of childhood and that it is the most common cause of referrals to child psychiatric clinics in the United States. On the other hand, there are those who feel that minimal brain dysfunction is a "scientific myth." Part of the reason for the controversy of opinion is the wide variety of terms that have been used to describe children with ostensibly the same disorder. These terms include: minimal brain dysfunction, minimal cerebral dysfunction, brain damage syndrome, minimal brain damage, hyperactivity, hyperkinesis, hyperactive child syndrome, the hyperkinetic syndrome, and more recently the attentional deficit disorder syndrome with and without hyperactivity. This diversity of terminology has had both theoretical and practical implications. These terms have been used in widely different ways by different people. Thus children with the same disorder have been described by different terms, while children with different disorders have been described by the same terms. Thus research findings from different centers cannot readily be compared, and treatment studies of all types are difficult to compare if fundamentally different disorders are being treated but are being given the same name.

This difference in terminology also has theoretical underpinnings and implications. Terms such as brain damage syndrome, minimal brain damage, and minimal brain dysfunction imply an organic etiology. However, terms like the hyperactive child syndrome, hyperkinetic syndrome, and attentional deficit disorder are basically behaviorally descriptive terms with no implication for etiology. If brain damage is used in its literal sense, to mean structural abnormality of the brain, then brain damage syndrome is an inaccurate and misleading term. While some children who present with the clinical picture of hyperactivity, short attention span, distractibility, etc., may suffer from frank brain damage, it is clear that the majority do not. Most brain-damaged children do not present with the clinical picture of hyperactivity, short attention span, and distractibility (Cantwell, 1975b).

Brain dysfunction may be a more accurate term than brain damage to describe those children who present with less well-defined disorders manifested by more subtle neurological signs. These more subtle defects in coordination, perception, and language may occasionally be associated only with actual damage to the brain. However, many children considered to have this disorder on the basis of behavioral diagnosis do not demonstrate even these subtle neurological signs. Thus brain dysfunction syndrome would be an inappropriate term to describe the large percentage of children who present with primarily behavioral abnormalities. Finally, prefixing a word like minimal to a term like brain dysfunction implies that we can quantity something for which we do not have reliable and accurate techniques to detect in children.

Historically the terminology for this disorder has moved from those terms suggesting an organic etiology to those which are more behaviorally descriptive. Following the encephalitis epidemic of 1917–1918, there were a number of children who did present with a behavior disorder characterized by hyperactivity, short attention span, distractability, impulsivity, and aggressive behavior. The name given to this disorder was the "brain damage behavior syndrome" (Rutter, Graham, and Yule, 1970). And indeed, in these children the disorder was due to true brain damage produced by encephalitis. However, the corollary that developed from this was not true. This was that in every child who presented with a syndrome of hyperactivity, short attention span, distractibility, etc., there was brain damage even if one could not demonstrate it by standardized techniques. In fact, as late as 1966, Bakwin's (1949) textbook continued to carry the statement that brain damage in children of any etiology presented with a uniform behavioral picture of hyperactivity, short attention span, etc.

In the 1960's an NICHD (Clements, 1966) task force proposed the term minimal brain dysfunction. Since true brain damage could not be demonstrated in the majority of these children, this term, minimal brain dysfunction, became very popular. Perhaps the most comprehensive and clearest description of the term minimal brain dysfunction is that put forth by Wender (1971). Wender's view of the minimal brain dysfunction syndrome in children is a rather broad one. He feels that the behavior of these children is not qualitatively different from that of normal children, but rather it is the intensity of their behavior and it is the persistence and the particular clustering of symptoms that distinguishes the MBD child from the normal child. He lists as key core symptoms that are found in the "classical" type of MBD as

1. Motor behavior, which includes increased level of activity and impaired coordination.
2. Attentional difficulties.
3. A variety of perceptual and cognitive difficulties.
4. Learning difficulties.
5. Impairment of impulse control.
6. Impairment of interpersonal relationships.
7. Emotional abnormalities, which include increased lability, altered reactivity, increased aggressiveness and dysphoria.

He points out two salient problems in the clinical diagnosis of this disorder. First, *all* of these abnormalities are found only in the classic case, and second, that the manifestations of these abnormalities tend to vary with age; thus the clinical picture will vary in the same child, depending on the age at which it is seen. In his clinical experience he feels that MBD children run the gamut from those who possess all of the classical signs and symptoms listed above, to those who possess only a few. He likens the diagnosis of minimal brain dysfunction to that of rheumatic fever. With rheumatic fever there are clinical empirical rules which strongly suggest that if the child has at least two major, or one major and two minor, symptoms or signs of rheumatic fever, it is highly likely they will have the characteristic underlying tissue pathology of rheumatic fever. However, since we have no characteristic underlying pathology of MBD, it is not possible to establish major and minor criteria for the syndrome and thus the boundaries of the syndrome are difficult to define.

In contrast to this rather broad view, most recently the DSM III committee charged with the drafting of the new official diagnostic nomenclature for psychiatric disorders of childhood and adolescents has adopted a more narrow and phenomenologic view. They describe two disorders: attentional deficit disorder with hyperactivity (ADDH) and attentional deficit disorder without hyperactivity. It is the first of these two disorders that corresponds most closely to what has been traditionally subsumed under the minimal brain dysfunction or hyperkinetic syndrome rubric. In this chapter it is the diagnosis and treatment of the attentional deficit disorder with hyperactivity (ADDH syndrome) that will be discussed, since most of the published literature have used criteria similar to the DSM III criteria.

The Diagnostic Evaluation

The diagnostic evaluation of a child referred for minimal brain dysfunction is geared to answering several questions. First, what is the clinical picture that the chiid presents with. Second, what, if any, associated developmental disabilities does the child have. Third, what, if any, associated biological factors are important in the genesis or the management of the case. Fourth, what, if any, associated psychosocial or familial factors are important in the genesis or management of the case. Fifth, what is the level of impairment produced by the disorder? Sixth, what is the likely natural history of the disorder if left untreated? And finally, what are the proper therapeutic modalities, and what is the evidence for their efficacy?

The diagnosis of the ADDH syndrome is essentially a clinical diagnosis. It should be based on a comprehensive diagnostic evaluation. This evaluation should include a detailed interview with the parents, a detailed interview with the child, a parent behavior rating scale, a teacher's behavior rating scale, a physical examination, a neurological examination, and appropriate laboratory studies. A useful framework for integrating the information obtained from this diagnostic evaluation is the five-phase multiaxial framework proposed for DSM III. Axis I describes the clinical psychiatric syndrome, the clinical picture with which the child presents. Axis 2 describes any associated developmental disabilities. Axis 3 describes any associated biologic factors that may play a role in either the genesis or the management of the clinical psychiatric syndrome. Axis 4 describes the type and severity of any psychosocial factors and stresses that may play a role in the genesis or the management of the clinical psychiatric syndrome. Axis 5 describes the level of impairment produced by the clinical psychiatric syndrome and the highest level functioning reached by a patient during the previous year. This framework will be used to describe the clinical picture of the typical ADDH child as well as the typical diagnostic evaluation.

Axis 1. Clinical Psychiatric Syndrome

The *primary symptoms* of this syndrome include: attentional difficulties, excessive motor activity, and impulsivity. Children with this disorder are described in school as having a short attention span, as being impulsive and distractible, as failing to follow through on instructions and complete work, and as being disorganized and inattentive. In addition, the children are reported to be fidgety, restless, overactive, overdemanding of the teacher's attention, and disruptive of others at play and at work.

At home, attentional problems are characterized by a failure to follow through on parental requests and instructions, or by the inability to engage in most activities for periods of time appropriate for age.

In young children hyperactivity is manifested by excessive gross motor activity such as running or climbing. In older children and adolescents, hyperactivity may be indicated by extreme restlessness and fidgeting. Often the impression obtained is that the *quality* of the motor behavior is what distinguishes this disorder from ordinary overactivity. The activity tends to be haphazard, poorly organized, and lacking in clear goal orientation. However, in situations where a high level of motor activity is expected and appropriate, such as the playground, children with this disorder do not obviously display more activity than others.

The behavior of children with this disorder is extremely variable. Typically, symptoms fluctuate across as well as within situations, and inconsistent functioning is a very common characteristic. A child's behavior may be well organized and appropriate on a one-to-one basis, but become disorganized in a group situation or in the classroom. Home adjustment may be satisfactory, and difficulties may emerge only in school. In addition, the child's level of motor activity may vary considerably within any situation. The usual pattern is an inconsistent one. It is the rare child who displays uniform, constant symptoms of hyperactivity either within or across settings.

In addition, there are many *associated symptoms* that often change with age. These include obstinacy, stubborness, negativism, bossiness, or bullying; increased lability of mood, low frustration tolerance, or temper tantrums; low self-esteem; lack of response to discipline; and antisocial behavior, especially in adolescence. Specific developmental disorders such as reading and other learning disabilities are also common and will be described on Axis 2.

ADDH children are often not brought to professional attention until the advent of school, when the demands imposed by the classroom create symptomatology which leads to a referral. And many of the children are referred not for the primary symptoms of the disorder but rather for associated symptoms, such as learning disabilities or acting-out behavior. A careful developmental history will reveal the presence of a typical ADDH syndrome from an early age. The clinical picture of the ADDH syndrome is best delineated by: the interview with the parents, the parent and teacher behavior rating scales, and the interview with the child.

Interview with the Parents

The spontaneous complaints of the parents to the physician will generally be around several major areas such as activity level, attentional behavior, excitability, and impulsivity. If all of these areas are not covered spontaneously by the parents, specific questions should be asked. Some suggested questions in this area are listed below:

Activity Level: Is he more active than his siblings? Is he more active than his peers? Is he, for example, unable to sit through a meal, school period, TV program, movie, haircut? Is he unable to stay in a doctor's or dentist's office waiting for an exam? Does he wear out things like shoes, clothes, bike, etc.? Does he run over desks, furniture, bookshelves, etc.? Is he fidgety (wiggles his hands, rocks his legs, etc.)? Is he into things that don't concern him (breaking dishes, tools, appliances, etc.)? Is he overtalkative? Does he monopolize the conversation?

Attentional Behavior: Does he have trouble completing projects? Does he daydream? Is he unable to listen to a story or attend to a TV program for any length of time? Is he easily distracted from projects by stray outside stimuli? Is he unable to follow through a set of directions or instructions?

Excitability: Is he easily upset by rather trivial things? Does he have a low frustration tolerance? Is he irritable or quick-tempered? Does he get wound up and overexcited in stimulating new situations? Does he have trouble taking no for an answer? Does he have trouble taking corrections?

Impulsivity: Is his behavior unpredictable or variable (like Jekyll and Hyde)? Does he tend to do reckless or dangerous things like climb out onto the roof and out of upper windows? running out into the street? riding his bike in front of cars?

Parents should be asked for a more detailed description of the symptoms that they mention spontaneously as well as those that are elicited by more specific questions around the cardinal symptoms of the syndrome. *Recent examples* of behavior in question should always be obtained, as well as the *frequency* of the behavior, the *severity*, and the *context of its occurrence.* What is "hyperactive" behavior to a parent with one child may be considered quite normal by a parent who has three or four children who are equally as active. Also, "aggressive behavior" to one parent may mean he hits his sister once a week, while to another parent it may mean the child chases people with an axe. The importance of obtaining specific examples of behavior cannot be overemphasized. The circumstances that appear to precipitate certain aspects of behavior and those which ameliorate difficulty should always be noted. The physician should attempt to find out what methods have been used to deal with the problem by the parent.

After completion of a detailed description of the core symptoms, it is useful for the physician to proceed with more systematic questions on other recent behavior and other aspects of the emotional state of the child. Some of these, such as antisocial behavior and cognitive and learning disabilities, will be very common in ADDH children. Others will be less common, but they should be inquired into, nevertheless. Areas that should be covered in such an inquiry include: school adjustment, aggressive and antisocial behavior, affective state, neurotic symptoms, psychotic symptoms, sexual behavior, neurologic symptoms, peer relationships, relationships with adults, and general physical health.

An important aspect of the interview with the parents also includes a detailed family history. Several family studies have shown that the biologic parents of ADDH children have a high prevalence rate of hyperactivity themselves in childhood and also high prevalence rate for certain specific psychiatric syndromes in adulthood—alcoholism and sociopathy in fathers, and hysteria in mothers. Hyperactivity in childhood and these specific psychiatric syndromes in adulthood also are found to a high degree in the extended relatives of hyperactive children (Cantwell, 1975c).

When interviewing the parents it is important to keep the age of the child in mind. In the early preschool years mothers often report the baby seemed to be unusually active, hyperalert, and difficult to soothe. General irregularity of physiological functions manifested by colic and sleeping and eating disturbances are common but not characteristic of ADDH alone.

When the child begins to walk, other symptoms begin to emerge. It is at this point that the activity level and attentional difficulties become more noticeable. The typical child seems to have a distinct lack of a sense of danger, moves from one activity to another very quickly, and is relatively impervious to disciplinary measures that the parents found effective with their other children. It is when the hyperactive child reaches the school system that the diagnosis is often the most easily made. Behaviors that were disturbing but tolerable in the home setting are not so easily tolerated in the classroom setting. Academic problems increase with passage of time, and antisocial behaviors become more prevalent. In adolescence, educational retardation, antisocial behavior, depression, and low self-esteem are the most common presenting problems. Combined with a diminution in the classic symptoms of hyperactivity, inattention, impulsivity, and excitability, the primacy of the secondary problems during adolescence often obscures the diagnosis. A careful developmental history will usually reveal the earlier symptoms of the ADDH child syndrome.

Behavior Rating Scales

A number of rating scales of children's behavior for completion by parents and teachers are available. For a complete discussion of this area the reader is referred to a recent review by Conners (1973b), who is also the author of the three scales recommended for use in evaluating hyperactive children: a parent symptom questionnaire, a teacher's questionnaire, and an abbreviated symptom questionnaire.

Conners Parent Symptom Questionnaire (PSQ)

Conners has devised a rating scale for completion by one or both parents which consists of 93 items of behavior grouped under 25 major headings. Each item represents a symptom commonly seen in behavior disorders of childhood. The parents are asked to rate their child as he is currently functioning with regard to each symptom on a four-point scale: not at all, just a little, pretty much, or very much. They are also asked to indicate the items they are most concerned about or those they think are the most important problems their child has and to rate the overall severity of their child's problems. Space is also provided for the parents to describe in their own words any other problems they have with their child. Scoring is achieved by giving a numerical weighting (0,1,2,3) to the parents' rating of each item. The higher score indicates greater pathology. A total symptom score can be obtained by totaling the 93 weighted items. In addition, Conners has carried out a factor analysis of the questionnaire on a sample of normal children and a sample of clinic outpatients between the ages of six and fourteen. Eight factor scores can be obtained by totaling the weighted ratings for 42 of the PSQ items. The eight factors are labeled: conduct problems, anxiety, impulsive-hyperactive, learning problems, psychosomatic, perfectionism, antisocial, and muscular tension. Discriminant function analysis has shown that 70% of clinic outpatients, 83% of normal controls, 77% of neurotic children, and 74% of hyperactive children can be identified from factor scores. The factor scores have also been shown to be relatively stable across ages and a wide range of social class.

Conners Teacher Questionnaire (TQ)

The questionnaire for completion by teachers consists of 39 items of behavior grouped under three major headings: classroom behavior, group participation, and attitude toward authority. The teacher is asked to rate the child with regard to each item of behavior on a four-point scale: not at all, just a little, pretty much, or very much. In addition, the teacher is asked how long she has known the child, to describe briefly the child's main problem, and to rate globally the child's behavior compared to that of other children the same age on a five-point scale from much worse to much better. The teacher is also asked if any children in the same family attend the school and present any problems. Finally, she is requested to add any information concerning the child's family relationships that might have bearing on his attitudes and behavior. The first page of this questionnaire contains areas for filling in results of standardized intelligence tests and most recent achievement test, the child's actual level of classroom performance in school subjects, and any special placement or help the child has received. Thus the questionnaire gives a very complete picture of the child's functioning and achievement in school. Scoring is achieved by giving a numerical weighting (0,1,2,3) to the teacher's rating of each item of behavior, with a higher score indicating greater pathology. A total symptom score can be obtained by totaling the 39 weighted items. Factor analysis of this questionnaire has yielded five factors: aggressive conduct, daydreaming/inattentive, anxious, fearful, hyperactivity, and sociable/cooperative. These five factors seem to have high test-retest reliability and to be quite sensitive to changes due to medication. This questionnaire seems to be the most widely used teacher evaluation procedure for ADDH children. Normative data have been obtained for the questionnaire, and it has been shown to distinguish normal children from ADDH children.

Ten items on the PSQ and TQ are identical and have been combined to form an abbreviated symptom questionnaire (ASQ), which can be used to obtain frequent follow-up assessments of the child by both parents and teachers. This abbreviated scale has been found to have almost the same sensitivity in obtaining statistically significant differences in psychotropic drug studies of hyperactive children.

Interview with the Child

The interview with the child is the diagnostic tool for delineating the clinical picture. However, it is probably the least valuable in itself. In a one-to-one setting with a strange interviewer, the child is likely to look quite normal.

The interview can be considered as consisting of two parts: an unstructured part and a relatively structured part. The interview also provides two different types of data: behavior of the child observed during the interview and information offered by the child during the interview. A detailed description of aspects of the interview with the child has been provided elsewhere. However, certain points are worth emphasizing here. One is that in order to assess attention span, distractibility and persistence, the child must be given some tasks during the interview. These tasks need to be near the limit of his ability, but within them, since the intent is not to test his cognitive abilities. A child can be asked to get paper and pencil, to write his name, to draw a picture of anything he likes. He could be asked to draw a picture of a man and woman and then make up a story about each of them. He may be asked to copy some designs, such as the Bender-Gestalt figure. He can be asked to give the days of the week forward and backward, as well as the months of the year, and to do some simple arithmetic. Recognition of words and reading of paragraphs or other tasks might be employed. During this period of the interview the child's response to a task including the physical behavior, attention, persistence, fine coordination, and visual motor functioning should be carefully noted. Besides noting how much the child is distracted by incidental noises, movements of the examiner, people passing by the room, etc., the physician should make an effort to distract the child by coughing, jingling coins in his pocket, tapping a pencil and dropping a book on the floor. The author finds it useful to rate the child's behavior on the Rutter-Graham rating scale, which has been shown to have good inter-rater reliability and validity.

Axis 2. Specific Developmental Disorders

These are diagnosed when there is a *specific* delay in development, which is not simply an essential criteria for another disorder—for example, language delay in infantile autism. Likewise, a child who shows only a general delay as part of mental retardation would not be considered a *specific* developmental disorder.

Each aspect of development noted in the DSM III classification of specific developmental disorders is related to biological maturation. However, they are also affected by nonbiological factors. Specific development disorders occur very frequently in conjunction with all childhood psychiatric syndromes, but particularly in conjunction with the ADDH syndrome.

Those specific developmental disorders to be considered in children with the ADDH syndrome include: specific reading disorder, specific arithmetical disorder, developmental language disorder (expressive and receptive types), developmental articulation disorder, enuresis, and encopresis. The interview with the parent and the behavior rating scales are often the first indication that a specific developmental disorder is present. The interview with child is likely to reveal language and articulation disorders if they are present. However, it is also likely that specific psychological testing will be necessary to document the nature and severity of the specific developmental disorders present. A proper psycho-educational assessment should be part of the evaluation of every child with the ADDH syndrome. This should include an assessment of general academic achievement, general intelligence, language functions, motor functions, memory, and perception. Specific deficits in cognitive or perceptual motor functions may be uncovered in an individual ADDH child which need to be remediated. The presence of such specific developmental disorders as reading or language disorder necessitates the introduction into a therapeutic program of specific remedial therapeutic procedures, which will be described later. These would not be necessary in a "pure" case of ADDH without an associated specific developmental disability.

Axis 3. Biological Factors

The ADDH syndrome as a behavioral syndrome may occur in the absence of any known biological factors, and in fact generally does so. However, a physical examination and neurological examination and any appropriate laboratory studies should be done to reveal any possible remediable physical or neurological problems. Listed below are some of the findings that may be gleamed from a typical physical, neurological and laboratory workup of a child with the ADDH syndrome.

Physical Examination

If one excludes the rare ADDH children with demonstrable organic brain damage, the physical examination is usually completely normal. In a minority of children defects of vision or hearing may be picked up (Stewart et al., 1966), as well as abnormalities of speech (De Hirsch, 1973). One group of investigators (Waldrop and Halverson, 1971) has reported a high incidence of minor physical anomalies in ADDH children such as: epicanthus, widely spaced eyes, curved fifth finger, adherent earlobes, etc. Their findings were more consistent for boys than for girls with the syndrome. These authors have suggested that the same factors operating in the first week of pregnancy led to both the congenital anomalies and the hyperkinetic behavior.

In a study of 76 hyperkinetic boys Rapoport et al. (1974) confirmed this increased incidence of physical anomalies. If an index population of ADDH children are divided into those with minor physical anomalies and those without minor physical anomalies, do these two subgroups differ in other ways? The evidence suggests that those ADDH children with the minor physical anomalies are also characterized by differences in *clinical picture:* earlier onset of the disorder, greater severity of hyperactivity and more aggressive behavior; other *physical factors:* history of obstetrical difficulties in the mother; *laboratory studies:* higher level of plasma dopamine betahydroxylase activity; and *family studies:* history of hyperactivity in the family (Quinn and Rapoport, 1974).

Moreover, those fathers of the ADDH children with minor physical anomalies who were themselves hyperactive in childhood also had higher plasma dopamine betahydroxylase activity. Finally, it is notable that within the group with minor physical anomalies, there is littler overlap between those with a history of hyperactivity in the father and those with a history of obstetrical difficulties in the mother. This suggests that there may be two distinct subgroups of ADDH children with minor physical anomalies—a genetically determined one and one determined by adverse events occurring early in pregnancy. If so, comparing the "genetic" with the "obstetrical" group should result in finding differences between the two groups in clinical picture, laboratory findings, natural history, or response to treatment. The finding that the ex-hyperkinetic fathers also had a high plasma dopamine betahydroxylase levels would support the idea of a genetic subgroup.

Neurologic Examination

Again, if one excludes the rare ADDH child who has demonstrable organic brain diesease, "hard" neurological signs are likely to be absent. There is a general consensus that certain "soft" neurological signs are more frequent among behaviorally defined ADDH children (Werry, 1972); however, the results are not conclusive. Moreover, most studies have methodological deficiencies, such as absence of proper control groups and failure to use a reliable, standardized neurological examination (Schain, 1972; Werry, 1972). While there has been a tendency to infer brain pathology from these soft signs (Kennard, 1960; Laufer and Denhoff, 1957), the evidence for doing so is lacking (Rutter, Graham, and Yule, 1970; Werry, 1972). It appears that only one study has compared carefully matched ADDH neurotic, and normal control groups of children using a standardized neurological examination of demonstrated reliability (Werry, 1972). The ADDH children did have an excess of minor neurological abnormalities indicative of sensory motor incoordination. However, the ADDH group did not have an excess of major neurological abnormalities, of EEG abnormalities, or histories suggestive of trauma to the brain.

The relevant question then is *not:* Do ADDH children have an excess of soft neurological signs compared to normal children or compared to children with other deviant behavior? The more important question is: Do those ADDH children with soft neurological signs differ from those ADDH children without soft neurological signs?

Evidence on this is limited. However, there is some data indicating that those ADDH children with soft neurological signs are distinguished from those with no such neurological signs by a greater likelihood of response to stimulant drug treatment (Mendelson, Johnson, and Stewart, 1971; Satterfield, 1973), suggesting that they may form a meaningful subgroup.

Laboratory Studies

Laboratory findings are generally more reliable, more precise, and more reproducible than are clinical descriptions. If some laboratory measure could be found that was uniquely and consistently associated with the ADDH syndrome, it would make diagnosis easier, and would permit possible subgrouping of the syndrome. No such laboratory study exists at the present time. However, it is possible that there are some relevant laboratory findings which might be used to divide the children with the syndrome into meaningful subgroups whose condition differs in etiology, prognosis, or in response to treatment. Some relevant laboratory studies will be summarized below.

Electroencephalographic Studies

Electroencephalographic findings with ADDH children are quite variable. Studies have reported that 35-50% of ADDH children have abnormal EEGs (Satterfield, 1973; Werry, 1972), with an increase in slow wave activity being the most common finding. There are no EEG abnormalities specific to the syndrome. There is even some question whether ADDH children have a greater number of EEG abnormalities than carefully matched normal and non-ADDH emotionally disturbed children (Eeg-Olofsson, 1970; Petersen, Eeg-Olofsson, and Selden, 1968; Werry, 1972).

Do ADDH children with an abnormal EEG differ in other areas from those ADDH children with a normal EEG? The evidence suggests that those with an abnormal EEG have been found to differ from those with a normal EEG in *clinical picture*: greater anxiety at home and school, greater motor restlessness in the classroom (Quinn and Rapoport, 1974; Satterfield, Cantwell, and Satterfield, 1974) *laboratory studies*: significantly higher WISC full scale and performance IQ, significantly lower Bender perseveration scores; and *treatment*: greater likelihood of response to stimulant drug therapy. Thus the EEG also seems to select out a meaningful subgroup of the total population of ADDH children.

Neurophysiologic Studies

Neurophysiologic studies of ADDH children have been limited in scope and number and have reached somewhat different conclusions. Satterfield and his associates (1974) have suggested that ADDH children can be divided into two subgroups based on neurophysiological data: those with evidence of "low central nervous system arousal" and those with "normal or high central nervous system arousal." In a series of four studies they first identified a subgroup of ADDH children who had low central nervous system arousal levels as measured by skin conductance level. They also found that methylphenidate raised the central nervous system arousal levels in ADDH children to a normal or near-normal level. In their second study, these authors replicated both of these findings using two additional indicators of central nervous system arousal: the auditory-evoked cortical response, and the EEG with the child at rest. In this second study, excessive slow wave activity (as measured by power spectral analysis of the EEG) indicated low central nervous system arousal in the subgroup of ADDH children who obtained a positive response to methylphenidate. In a third study the authors found that a low central nervous system arousal level in a population of ADDH children was associated with a greater degree of behavioral disturbance in the classroom, as well as with a positive clinical response to central nervous system medication. In a fourth study it was shown then that those ADDH children with excessive EEG slowing (another indication of low central nervous system arousal) obtained the best response to the central nervous system stimulant medication.

In summary, Satterfield et al. (1972) found that ADDH children had lower skin conductance level, larger amplitude, and slower recovery of evoked cortical responses than normal children. These measures together with high amplitude EEG and high energy in the lower frequency (0–8 Hz) band of the resting EEG also distinguish ADDH children who responded best to stimulant drug treatment from those who obtained a poor response. In all, the Satterfield group found eight laboratory measures associated with a positive resonse to methylphenidate. All of these are consistent with the hypothesis that there is a subgroup of ADDH children who have lower levels of basal resting physiological activation than age-matched normals. This subgroup differs from other ADDH children in two other important areas: *clinical picture*: more restlessness, distractibiliity, impulsivity, and attentional problems in the classroom; and *treatment*: a greater likelihood of positive response to stimulants (Satterfield, Cantwell, and Satterfield, 1974; Satterfield et al., 1972).

However, not all neurophysiologic studies of children have produced such consistent results. Many of the differences may be due to different patient populations and diagnostic criteria and to differing experimental stimulus conditions.

Biochemical Studies

The positive response of many ADDH children to central nervous system medications such as the amphetamines and to the tricyclic antidepressants, both of which affect the biogenic amines, offer indirect evidence that a disorder of monoamine metabolism is an etiologic factor in some ADDH children. There are several other lines of evidence to support this hypothesis. Dextroamphetamine is thought to be ten times as potent as its isomer, levoamphetamine, in inhibiting catecholamine uptake by norepinephrine terminals in the brain. The two isomers are of approximately equal potency in inhibiting catecholamine uptake by dopaminergic terminals (Snyder et al., 1970). There is a suggestion that these two isomers have a differential affect on the aggressive behaviors and hyperactive behaviors of ADDH children. These data offer indirect evidence that some symptoms of ADDH children are mediated by dopaminergic systems and others by norepinephrinergic systems.

More direct studies of a possible metabolic abnormality have been limited. Wender, et al. (1971) failed to detect any differences in metabolites of serotonin, norepinephrine, or dopamine in the urine of ADDH children compared to a group of normal children. However, the study population was very heterogeneous. Wender (1969) did find very low concentrations of serotonin in the blood platelets of three children with the syndrome, all of whom were from the same family. In the rest of the study population, the platelet serotonin levels were normal or in the borderline range. Coleman (1971) demonstrated low platelet serotonin concentrations in 88% of 25 children with the syndrome. In a group of ADDH boys, Rapoport et al. (1970) found an inverse relationship between the degree of hyperactive behavior and urinary norepinephrine excretion. In addition, there was an inverse relationship in response of the hyperactivity to dextroamphetamine and urinary norepinephrine levels. Shekim has recently reported a relationship between urinary MHPG and response to dextroamphetamine.

All of these studies are suggestive of a possible disorder of monoamine metabolism in the ADDH syndrome. However, urinary and platelet data reflect only imperfectly brain monoamine metabolism. Since direct measurement of central nervous system monoamine metabolism is not a possibility, the measurement of monoamine levels and turnover in cerebrospinal fluid, as has been done in adults with affective disorders (Goodwin and Bunney, 1973) might offer a more fruitful approach. Shaywitz, Cohen, and Bowers (1975) have reported a study suggesting that HVA is reduced in cerebrospinal fluid of children with the ADDH syndrome following probenecid blockade.

Thus there does seem to be an emerging body of evidence that at least in some ADDH children there may be an abnormality of monoamine metabolism. Moreover, the limited studies that have been done suggest that laboratory studies in this area may pick out children with somewhat different clinical pictures with regard to hyperactivity and aggression and that urinary norepinephrine and MHPG excretion may be related both to the degree of hyperactivity and to response to stimulant medication (Shekim, Dekirmenjian, and Chapel, 1977).

Axis 4. Psychosocial Factors and Stressors

Children with ADDH syndrome are just as likely as other children to be affected by some psychosocial and familial stress. There are studies suggesting that certain types of psychiatric illness are common in immediate family members of children with the ADDH syndrome, and also that certain patterns of family interaction may be related to ultimate prognosis and to response to drug treatment. Two studies of biologic parents of ADDH children revealed increased prevalence rates for alcoholism, sociopathy and hysteria (Morrison and Stewart, 1971; Cantwell, 1972). One of these studies also reported a high prevalence rate for these same psychiatric disorders in the biologic second-degree relatives of ADDH children (Cantwell, 1972). In both studies it was noted that the ADDH syndrome also occurred more often in the biologic first- and second-degree relatives of ADDH children than in the relatives of control children. Two further studies of the nonbiologic relatives of adopted ADDH children revealed no increased prevalence rates of psychiatric illness or the ADDH syndrome (Cantwell, 1975; Morrison and Stewart, 1971). These data suggest that genetic factors may be important in the etiology of the syndrome. They also suggest that ADDH children may be at risk, for both genetic and environmental reasons, for the development of significant pathology in adulthood.

Several psychiatric studies of the siblings of ADDH children also show they have increased prevalence rates of certain types of problems. Welner et al. (1977) and Cantwell (1975) in separate studies have looked at the prevalence of the ADDH syndrome in the siblings of probands with the disorder. Welner found that 26% of the brothers and 9% of the sisters met the criteria for the hyperactive child syndrome; while Cantwell found that 22% of the brothers and 8% of the sisters met the same criteria. Cantwell used the DSM III criteria for attentional deficit disorder with hyperactivity to make a diagnosis.

Cantwell also looked at the prevalence of a new disorder that is described in DSM III, attention deficit disorder *without* hyperactivity. Two percent of the brothers of ADDH children met the criteria for attentional deficit disorder without hyperactivity, and 11% of the sisters met the same criteria. Thus 24% of the brothers of ADDH children and 19% of the sisters met the DSM III criteria for attentional disorders. Safer (1973) examined the full and half siblings of 17 index cases of "minimal brain dysfunction." Of the 19 full siblings, 10 were considered likely to manifest minimal brain dysfunction, while that diagnosis was given to only 2 of 22 half-siblings. Thus 55% of full sibs were considered likely to manifest the symptoms of hyperactivity, short attention span, and impulsive behavior, as opposed to only 9% of the half-sibs. The data for the Cantwell sibling study that found increased prevalence rates for the ADDH syndrome in the brothers and sisters of hyperactive children have not yet been completely analyzed. Eventually specific diagnoses will be made using the DSM III criteria of all the brothers and sisters of the index ADDH children. This will allow for tentative conclusions about other types of psychiatric disorders seen in brothers and sisters of children with this disorder. The Welner study did this to some degree, but did not make specific psychiatric diagnoses. They did find that in the nonhyperactive brothers of ADDH children there was an increased amount of depressive *symptoms*. However, the authors did not attempt to make a case for increased prevalence rates for a depressive *syndrome* or a depressive *disorder*. In the nonhyperactive brothers, there was also a lower full scale and verbal IQ as measured by the Weschler Intelligence Scale for children (WISC), as well as lower spelling and math achievement as measured by the Wide Range Achievement Test (WRAT)(Fish, 1975). In the nonhyperactive sisters of the ADDH probands, WRAT testing revealed lower reading and spelling achievement scores. This might suggest that the nonhyperactive siblings of hyperactive boys may also suffer from some degree of learning disability, but a much more systematic study is needed to answer this question.

It is not surprising that the sibs of ADDH children might demonstrate increased prevalence rates for psychiatric problems. First, the studies of the psychiatric problems of parents of ADDH children show that the parents have increased rates of certain specific psychiatric syndromes in the "antisocial spectrum." This in itself for both genetic and environmental reasons may lead to the development of psychiatric disorder in sibs (Cantwell, 1975a). Moreover, the problems of a child with any type of handicap or psychiatric disorder is likely to increase family disorganization, discord, and turmoil. This discord and disorganization may then lead to problems in sibs as well as to increased problems for the ADDH child.

Studies of family interaction have often assumed a unitary parent-to-child direction, when in actual fact, as pointed out by the seminal studies of Bell (1968), children themselves also play a role in the genesis of parent/child interaction. Three recent studies dramatically demonstrate this in children with the ADDH syndrome.

Campbell (1975) observed three groups of children: 13 hyperactive, 13 learning disabled, and 13 normal boys interacting with their mothers in a structured problem-solving situation. The data indicated that the mothers of the ADDH children made more nonspecific suggestions and more suggestions about impulse control, were both more encouraging and disapproving than were the mothers of the learning disabled and control children. Mothers of the learning disabled and control children did not differ significantly from each other on any of these measures.

Conversely, the ADDH boys made significantly more requests for feedback as well as more comments about the tasks and on their own performance than the learning disabled and control population, who did not differ from each other on any of these measures. The data suggests that the mothers of the ADDH group were responding in the interaction situation so as to structure the task and thereby optimize the performance of their children.

In the same vein, the ADDH boys elicited and maintained a high level of interaction by requesting more feedback and by making more comments throughout the interaction session.

Humphries, Kinsbourne, and Swanson (1978) reflected on the work of Campbell by asking the question: does reducing the impulsivity of the ADDH child by use of methylphenidate lead to an improvement in performance achieved by the child and by his mother on a task which requires them to work cooperatively to reach a common goal?

Moreover, they sought to ask whether or not an improved performance was also accompanied by a more favorable social interaction between the ADDH child and his mother. They used a commercially available toy, an Etch-a-Sketch, to present a two-dimensional "self-paced contour tracking task." The original task required the child to use both hands to control horizontal and vertical movement in navigating a maze. Humphries had previously found that the use of sttmulant medication improved the child's performance on this task when he worked alone compared to placebo.

In a modification of the task involving the parent, the mother controlled one dimension of the task while the child controlled the other. Twenty-six ADDH children and their mothers took part in the study, once while the child was given an acute dose of methylphenidate and once while given a placebo in a double-blind fashion. The results indicated that mothers and children performed significantly better when the child was on stimulant medication. While medicated, the child directed the mother more and in a more positive fashion. Conversely, the mother behaved in a less controlling way and reacted more positively to the child. Humphries and his colleagues concluded that the use of the medication produced a more favorable interaction between the ADDH child and the mother, which resulted in a less constrained learning experience on the part of the child. They concluded that it is unlikely that the controlling behavior supposedly demonstrated by mothers of ADDH children is anything more than a response to the way that the children act when in nonmedicated state.

Barkley and Cunningham (1978) expanded on the type of study conducted by Humphries. They observed 20 ADDH boys interacting with their mothers during 15 minutes of free play and a 15-minute task period in three separate situations: unmedicated, placebo, and medicated with methylphenidate. A triple-blind crossover design was used to study the effects of methylphenidate. The children demonstrated significant improvement in activity level and sustained attention. As a result, they became more compliant to the commands of their mothers and also more attentive to the mothers' commands. In response to this, the mothers displayed increases in attention to the child's compliance and reduced their directiveness and negative behavior toward the boys. The boys increased their level of independent play, and the mothers responded with an increased positive attention to and decreased control over such play.

All three of these studies suggest that the hyperactive child does in fact play a large role in initiating and maintaining certain aspects of mother/child interaction. Moreover, they suggest that not only do the mothers respond to these interactions initiated by their children, but that these interactions demonstrated by the mother and the child can be modified by the use of central nervous system stimulants.

There are a number of psychosocial and familial factors that may be related to type of long-term outcome in ADDH children. Each of these will be reviewed in turn.

Family Structure

An examination of the census data for 1970 focusing on living arrangements of children and adolescents in the United States reveals that a significant number of those under 18 years of age in the population are living in a stressful situation. That is they are living in families broken by marital disruption, in families at the lower socioeconomic levels, in nonfamily situations, and in institutions. These are all circumstances that create potentially high risks in the development of emotional and mental disturbances, delinquency, truancy, and other manifestations of maladjustment.

In a comprehensive review of this topic, Rutter concluded that children, especially boys, not brought up by their two natural parents have an increased risk for delinquency. This association does not apply to neurotic types of disturbance but may apply to depression as well.

More recently, Kellam, Ensminger, and Turner (1977) at the University of Chicago have examined family structure and its relationship to the mental health of children as part of their Woodlawn Mental Health Project. In their study, family type was found to be a strong predictor of the child's social adaptational status as well as behavior and psychological well-being. Children in "mother alone" families had a high incidence of psychiatric disturbance, indicating that the presence of certain other adults may have important protective functions. "Mother/grandmother" families were nearly as effective as "mother/father" families with regard to risk to the child. The data also indicated that the absence of the father was less important than the aloneness of the mother in relation to risk of psychiatric disturbance on the part of the child.

Shinn has recently reviewed the evidence for the relationship between father absence and children's cognitive development. She reviewed literature showing detrimental affects of father's absence on children's cognitive development as assessed by standard IQ and achievement tests as well as by school performance. The evidence suggested that in father-absent families or in families in which fathers have little supportive interaction with their children, there is often an associated poor performance on cognitive tests. Differential effects are obtained associated with: (a) certain characteristics of the father absence, such as cause, duration, age of onset; and (b) with certain characteristics of the child, such as age, sex, race, and socioeconomic status; and (c) with the skill tested (quantitative versus verbal). The evidence suggests that financial hardship, high levels of anxiety, and particularly low levels of parent/child interaction are important causes of poor performance among children in a single-parent family while sex role identification does not seem to play as an important role. The degree to which mothers are able to compensate for the loss of the father also is obviously an important factor.

In summary, the weight of the evidence suggests that children who are brought up in homes with one parent are more likely than other children to show academic problems, psychiatric problems, and become delinquent. To the author's knowledge, there has been no systematic study of the effect of family structure on the long-term outcome of ADDH children.

Family Discord

Closely related to family structure is the question of family discord. While there is an association between a "broken home" and an increased risk of delinquency and antisocial behavior, the risk of delinquency is greatly increased if the parents are divorced or separated. The risk is only slightly raised if one parent dies. This suggests that it may be the family discord and disharmony, rather than the break-up of the family per se that leads to antisocial behavior in the children.

It has been shown in several independent studies that boys from unbroken homes rated as quarrelsome and neglecting of the children were more likely to become delinquent than boys who came from cohesive unbroken homes or from broken homes (Rutter and Hersov, 1977).

In short, antisocial disorders and delinquency tend to be commoner in children with unhappy unbroken homes than in harmonious but broken homes. This suggests that it is the ongoing disturbance of family relationships rather than the family break-up per se which leads to most of the problems.

It seems that children may be harmed either by open hostility in the home or by a lack of warmth and positive affection. When there is *both* overt quarreling and discord *and* a lack of affection, this has the most deleterious effect. By itself, overt quarreling and discord seems to be most serious. The effect on the child is also worse if he becomes embroiled in parental disputes, and the child is more likely to develop a psychopathology if the discord is prolonged for many years.

The child is especially at risk if in additon to marital discord one or both parents have a psychiatric illness or personality disorder.

Finally, it seems that a good relationship with one parent can somehow mitigate against the effects of family discord. There is only scanty evidence, but family discord does seem to play a role in the outcome of ADDH children as noted below.

Psychiatric Illness in the Families

There is a good deal of evidence that children with parents who have a mental disorder are at risk themselves for mental disorder (Rutter, 1966). This may be for genetic reasons, environmental reasons, or both.

A large body of studies also suggest that parental criminality is associated with delinquency in the child. There are several family studies showing that parents of hyperactive children have increased rates of psychiatric disturbance in the "antisocial spectrum": namely, alcoholism, sociopathy, and hysteria (Cantwell, 1975). As noted below, there is also some suggestion that this type of family pathology is associated with an antisocial outcome for hyperactive children, although this needs replication in a systematic fashion (Cantwell, 1975a).

Family Size

Several studies have shown that individuals from large families tend to have lower levels of verbal intelligence than those from small families (Rutter and Herzov, 1977). There are probably several reasons why this is true. There is some evidence that children from a large family receive less adequate infant care and less encouragement in school than other children. Financial and material resources may be considerably less in large families. There is also a suggestion that the linguistic environment of young children with many older siblings is different from that of older children or children in two or three sibship families. There is probably less intensive interaction and less communication from the parents in large families; thus children from large families tend to have lower verbal skills. Chldren from large families with at least four or five children are twice as likely to develop antisocial problems and become delinquent. The question of family size and its relation to eventual outcome has not been studied systematically in ADDH children.

Social Class

The question of social class in ADDH children has not been addressed properly. There is good evidence that the syndrome occurs across a wide socioeconomic range (Loney, in press). There may be a disproportionate occurrence in disadvantaged populations. However, that has not definitely been proven. However, it does seem that being hyperactive in childhood is associated with the attainment of a lower social class in adulthood (Borland and Heckman, 1976).

Patternite, Loney, and Langhorne (1976) suggested that the primary symptoms of the syndrome are not related to social class, but the secondary symptoms (such as aggressive behavior and self-esteem problems) are more severe among lower SES children. They felt that this difference was related to differences in parenting styles related to social class. The intriguing question of whether low social class for whatever reason is associated with a poorer outcome for ADDH children has never been systematically investigated.

In summary, there are a number of factors relating to family structure, family size, ordinal position, family discord, and family illness which are related to the development of psychopathology in childlren, particularly to the development of antisocial and delinquent behavior. Only lately have a few of these factors been looked at in conjunction with the outcome in adolescence and young adult life of ADDH children. It can be hypothesized that they should be expected to be affected by essentially the same familial and psychosocial factors to which nonhyperactive children are sensitive. Moreover, because of their intrinsic problem, they may be more sensitive to familial and psychosocial factors that may impair their development.

What evidence is there that these family factors actually play a role in the outcome of children with the syndrome? Mendelson, Johnson, and Stewart (1971) and the Montreal group (Minde, Weiss, and Mendelson, 1972; Minde et al., 1971; Safer, 1973) found certain familial variables to be associated with an antisocial outcome. Those children with the most antisocial behavior at follow-up in the Mendelson study were more likely to have fathers who had learning or behavior problems as children and who had been arrested as adults. Weiss found that the families of the ultimately antisocial children had been rated as significantly more pathological in initial evaluation. Three specific items on the rating scale—poor mother-child relationship, poor mental health of the parents, and punitive child-rearing practices—distinguished the families of the ultimately antisocial children from the rest of the group. Minde, Weiss, and Mendelson (1972) found that one of the four factors associated with poor outcome of the ADDH children in their group included more unfavorable ratings of their family environment. Thus certain aspects of family interaction and family pattern of illness do seem to be related to a specific type of outcome in ADDH children.

Do these familial factors play any role in affecting response to stimulants among ADDH children? Few studies have attempted to look at family variables in any systematic way. Conrad and Insel (1967) found that children whose parents were rated as "grossly deviant" or "socially incompetent" were less likely to respond positively to stimulant medication even in the face of other factors which tended to predict a good outcome. Their criteria for "grossly deviant" and "socially incompetent" indicate that most of these parents were either alcoholic or sociopathic.

Studies of family interaction in relation to drug response have been limited and inconsistent. The Montreal group (Weiss et al., 1968; Werry et al., 1966) found that the mother-child relationship and the quality of the home were unrelated to drug therapy, but in a later study (Weiss et al., 1971a), there was a positive association between response to stimulants and the quality of the mother-child relationship. Other authors (Knobel, 1962; Kraft, 1968) have noted that the attitude of the family to the child taking medication is likely to affect treatment response. Undoubtedly there are other areas of psychosocial factors that are related to outcome in children with this syndrome and also to response to various types of therapeutic modalities. But this remains in the area of speculation at the moment, since no definitive studies are available other than those mentioned above.

Axis 5. Level of Impairment and Highest Level of Adaptive Functioning

Here the clinician should make some effort to rate the level of impairment produced by the clinical psychiatric syndrome of the attentional deficit disorder. It is also helpful to see how well the child has functioned during the past year. The child may be severely impaired by the syndrome at the time that he is seen but six months earlier may have been functioning fairly well. This is important in planning which therapeutic modalities are necessary and for how long. A chronically ill child who has been impaired in many areas for a long period of time is much more likely to need intensive and extensive therapeutic intervention than a child who has been functioning reasonably well but has taken a recent acute turn for the worse.

The diagnostic evaluation when conducted as outlined above—using an interview with the parents, an interview with the child, and behavioral rating scales to identify the clinical syndrome; and an interview with the parent along with physical examination, neurological examination and appropriate laboratory testing to identify any associated developmental disorders, biological factors, and psychosocial factors—will provide answers to a number of the questions outlined earlier in the paper.

The next important question to answer is what is the natural history of the ADDH syndrome? Or put more simply, with an individual child: If I do nothing in the way of therapeutic intervention with this child, what is likely to happen?

While the symptom of hyperactivity may diminish with age, it seems now that the initial optimism about the eventual outcome of ADDH children is unjustified. Retrospective and prospective studies paint the following picture of ADDH children in adolescence. Hyperactivity per se seems to diminish with age, but the children are still more restless, excitable, and distractible than their peers. Attention and concentration difficulties remain as major problems. Chronic, severe underachievement in almost all academic areas is a characteristic finding. Low self-esteem, poor self-image, depression, and a sense of failure are common. Marked antisocial behavior occurs in up to one-quarter of the children, and a significant number have police contact and court referrals.

The clinical picture of the ADDH child as an adult remains unclear, as there are no prospective studies following hyperactive children into adulthood. There are reports of young adults still requiring stimulant medication, and the follow-up study of Menkes (Menkes, Rowe, and Menkes, 1967) suggests that in some cases the syndrome may be a precursor to psychosis and other types of severe psychopathology in adulthood. Two family studies also support the notion that the hyperactive child syndrome is a precursor to the development of psychopathology in adulthood, and that alcoholism, sociopathy, and hysteria are the most likely psychiatric outcomes in adulthood.

Since antisocial behavior, alcoholism, and hysteria are disorders for which we have no specific treatment in adults and for which treatment of any type has not been shown conclusively to be effective, it would seem likely that early intervention with ADDH children to *prevent* these outcomes would be the most profitable type of therapeutic program.

The rest of this chapter will outline what is known about effective therapeutic modalities for ADDH children.

Therapeutic Interventions

After a comprehensive diagnostic evaluation has been completed, the next step is deciding which therapeutic modalities are useful for an individual child with the ADDH syndrome. For management purposes, a child with this syndrome is best considered a multihandicapped child requiring a multiple modality treatment approach. Any treatment should be individualized and based upon a comprehensive assessment of each child and his family. Any single individual treatment modality used *alone* is unlikely to be completely successful.

Involvement of the Family

Involvement of the family is probably the first step in all therapeutic interventions. The parents should be told about the nature and the phenomenology of the ADDH syndrome. The nature of the child's symptoms and how they can handle specific difficulties of the child should be explained thoroughly. Parents can be taught the principles of structuring their child's environment so that there are regular routines and proper limits are set on the child's behavior. Specific areas such as temper tantrums, fighting with siblings, etc., can be focused on in individual sessions with the parents. More intelligent and involved parents can be taught basic tenets of social learning theory. Two books by Patterson—*Families* and *Living with Children*—can be quite helpful in giving the parents techniques in how to deal with specific aspects of their child's behavior. Two other books that offer excellent advice to the parents of hyperactive children on day-to-day management of their children's problems are *The Hyperactive Child: A Guide for Parents* by Wender, and *Raising a Hyperactive Child* by Stewart and Olds.

The use of parent groups modeled after those described by Patterson has been found to be an effective treatment modality in the absence of psychopathology in the parent. In these groups the parents are taught the basics of social learning theory and behavior modification. The importance of avoiding stressful situations known to cause difficulty, overstimulation, and excessive fatigue are emphasized. Videotaping segments of parent-child interaction and playing back these behaviors with explicit instructions to the parents as to how to deal with them has also been found to be helpful. The use of two group leaders, each with different roles, has been found to be a useful therapeutic technique. One group leader concentrates on more dynamic and interpersonal issues for about half the group's session, and for the other half of the session the other group leader concentrates on the parent training. The group format allows the parents to give one another mutual support and provides for an exchange of information regarding community resources, school funding, parent organizations and other issues. An often-neglected aspect of management of the family is referring the family to groups of other parents whose children suffer with this disorder or other learning disabilities. Organizations such as the National Association for Children with Learning Disabilities, which has local branches in almost every major city, allow parents to give each other mutual support and provide for an exchange of information in regarding community resources, school funding, other parent organizations, and other issues. Of course, if the parents have their own psychopathology this must be dealt with separately by referral to the appropriate professional individuals or agencies. There are situations in which the hyperactive child has become enmeshed in a pathological and dysfunctional family system, often becoming the family scapegoat. In these cases, a more dynamically oriented family therapy approach may be a necessary therapeutic intervention.

Medication

The ADDH syndrome can be considered to be the condition "par excellence" for childhood psychopharmacology. The central nervous system stimulant drugs are currently the drugs of choice. The tricyclic antidepressant imipramine is a second choice should the child not respond to any stimulant medication. There exists now a number of well-controlled clinical studies of the amphetamines, methylphenidate, and magnesium pemoline, indicating that they are effective with this disorder. This literature has recently been reviewed by Barkley (1977). Fifteen studies of children treated with amphetamine involving 915 subjects revealed that 74% improved, while 26% were unchanged or worse. Fourteen studies with methylphenidate involving 866 subjects revealed an improvement rate of 77%, while 2 studies involving 105 subjects with magnesium pemoline produced an improvement of 73%. Clearly, then, the stimulants are the drugs of choice for this condition and are quite effective. There is little to choose between the three major groups of stimulants, the amphetamines, methylphenidate, and pemoline regarding the percentage of children with the ADDH syndrome who will show improvement. However, there are idiosyncratic children who respond well to one stimulant and not at all to another, or respond slightly to one but much better to another, or who respond equally well to both stimulants but have more side effects with one. Thus it is worthwhile in individual cases to switch medications to see which child will benefit most from which medication.

There were earlier favorable reports that deanol and caffeine were effective drugs with the ADDH syndrome. However, these earlier clinical studies have not been replicated by systematic controlled studies (Conners et al., 1972).

The stimulants, like all medications, affect many functions. All of these need to be kept in mind when stimulants are used to treat children with the ADDH syndrome. From the clinical standpoint, the most important effects are those on cognitive function, activity level, behavior, and academic achievement (Cantwell and Carlson, in press). While there is no good evidence that stimulants improve performance on general cognitive measures such as tested intelligence, reading achievement, language skills, and complex learning, there is solid evidence suggesting that stimulants do positively affect such cognitive functions as attention, perception, and memory. There's also evidence that they influence cognitive style and improve laboratory measures of learning. Stimulants have been found to produce a significant degree of reduction in errors of omission in laboratory situations where sustained performance is required. Likewise, stimulants produce an increase in accuracy in tasks requiring vigilance and in tasks requiring immediate or delayed perceptual judgment. Stimulants lead to a more deliberate response in reaction-time tests when the desired response is one of less impulsive responding. On the other hand, they have also been shown to reduce response latency and to increase reaction time in tasks where the required response is a rapid one. Taken together, the results of stimulants on cognitive function suggest that they improve performance in tasks requiring sustained attention. Inattentiveness has indeed been found to be the best *single* predictor of a positive response to stimulant medication in children with the ADDH syndrome.

Probably the most common symptom for which stimulant medications are prescribed is "hyperactivity." There are contradictions in the literature regarding the effects of stimulants on activity level. There are a variety of reasons for this contradiction. First, there is varied usage of the term "hyperactivity." Second, there are different measurement techniques used to quantify activity. Different *types* of motor activity are often measured and compared as being the same; and finally, the *situations* in which the activity is measured often differs from study to study.

During performance on laboratory tests measuring attention and cognitive style and concept attainment, there are consistent reports of activity level being decreased along with an accompanying decrease of task-irrelevant motor behavior when stimulants are used. However, there are also studies which show that children who are reported by parents and teachers behaviorly improved after treatment with stimulant medication actually have an inceased amount of activity level in a free field situation such as on the playground. Thus the likelihood is that the stimulants probably affect the *quality* of motor activity at least as much if not more so than the quantity.

There is a solid body of evidence from well-controlled methodologically sound studies which suggests that the most consistent positive effect of stimulant medication is on disruptive and socially inappropriate behavior, both as perceived by teachers and by parents. Although there is less consistent evidence of a positive effect on emotional symptoms such as fears, phobias and anxiety, there are those who feel that stimulants do have a positive effect on shy children who are stimulated to a more active outgoing behavior. Fish (1975) felt that the ADDH children who responded best to stimulants in her practice were those with predominantly anxiety and neurotic mechanisms. Thus it may be that stimulants produce changes in both types of children, overcontrolled and undercontrolled, depending on which set of symptoms are severe enough to show change.

Despite the well-documented effects of stimulants on cognitive functioning there is little or no evidence to support the view that stimulants positively affect problem-solving ability, classroom learning, or reasoning. However, it must be said that a proper study evaluating the effects of stimulants on academic achievement in the classroom has not yet been carried out. Such a study presents a difficult methodological problem. First, the time frame must be long enough for actual achievement in the classroom to have occurred. Second, the effect of stimulants must be singled out from a combination of other factors that may affect academic achievement. For example, Satterfield and the current author (Cantwell and Satterfield, in press) have recently reported changes in the reading comprehension and recognition, arithmetic, and general information subtests of the Peabody Individual Achievement Test in a group of children intensively and consistently treated with methylphenidate over a one-year period. However, these children also received a wide variety of other forms of treatment including individual psychotherapy, group therapy for children, and family therapy, and some were in individual educational therapy. The effects of these various treatment modalities cannot be reliably separated out from the effects produced by stimulant medication alone. Third, the actual measurement of such academic changes presents some difficulty. The question to be answered is whether or not an individual child makes as much or more progress in an academic subject over a year's time than we would predict for him. Prediction for an individual child probably needs to be done by using a multiple regression equation involving intelligence, chronological age, and academic achievement. This has rarely, if ever, been done in long-term studies of academic achievement and their effect by stimulant medication. Although there is no positive evidence that actual academic achievement in the classroom is facilitated by use of stimulant medication, there is as yet no study which definitely and conclusively proves that it is not.

The mechanism of action of the stimulants is not

definitely known. It is postulated (Snyder et al., 1970) that amphetamine and related drugs act by enhancing catecholamine effects, particularly neurotransmitter actions, both centrally and peripherally. This enhancement is achieved by blocking catecholamine reuptake into presynaptic nerve endings, thus preventing inactivation by monoamine oxidase. With regard to what particular catecholamines are involved, there is evidence to suggest that a variety of similar effects can be specifically explained by both dopamine and norepinephrine enhancement.

Wender (1975) has postulated further that children with the ADDH syndrome have a preexisting metabolic abnormality, involving the central nervous system neurotransmitters. Thus the so-called paradoxical effect that stimulants have in these children is not paradoxical at all. According to Wender, the medications have stimulant effect just like they do in normal children, but it is correcting a preexisting metabolic deficiency.

There are also neurophysiologic mechanisms used to explain the so-called paradoxical effect of the stimulant drugs for children with the ADDH syndrome. As reviewed above, Satterfield and his colleagues have postulated that there is a subgroup of ADDH children who have lower levels of basal resting physiological activation than age-matched controls. They further postulate that stimulants have a physiological stimulant effect on these children, increasing arousal and concomitantly increasing cortical inhibition and decreasing sensory and motor system activity. In these studies, those hyperactive children who did not have a positive response to central nervous system stimulants had normal or high levels of basal resting physiological arousal. They also have a physiological stimulant response to the stimulant medication, but because of the different pretreatment levels of arousal, they have a negative rather than a positive behavioral response to the medication.

Finally, Rapoport recently conducted a study of normal children treated with amphetamine on a one-shot basis, using a variety of tests that have been used to study drug response in ADDH children. She demonstrated that these children who had no attentional problems or hyperactivity had responses in the same direction on these tests and measures as ADDH children do. Thus it seems unlikely that stimulants exert any type of "paradoxical" effect on these children.

In addition to the positive effects produced by the stimulants there are some undesirable side effects that need to be monitored, although it is noteworthy that there are few published reports of significant side effects, offering at least indirect evidence that they are relatively uncommon. The common short-term side effects include: headaches, stomach aches, increased talkativeness, and moodiness. Stomach aches usually pass with time, although they may be associated with other GI symptoms such as nausea. An initial period of insomnia is common, particularly if more than one daily dose of stimulant tablets or long-acting forms are used. An initial period of anorexia is also common. Tearfulness and irritability may accompany moodiness. There may be a slight but perceptible change in the personality of the child which the parents find not to their liking even though the medication is producing positive effects in other areas. The short-term side effects of the stimulants are generally temporary and usually of minimal clinical significance; only rarely are short-term side effects enough of a problem to cause discontinuation of the medication (Cantwell and Carlson, in press).

Much less can be stated with certainty about long-term side effects of the stimulants. There is no evidence that children who are on chronic stimulant medication tend to become drug abusers in later life. There is now evidence that the retardation of growth rate that occurs with stimulants in a temporary phenomonon lasting for about a year or two, and there does not seem to be any permanent effect on adult height and weight (Roche and Jackson, in press).

For those children who do not respond to any of the stimulants, it is worthwhile trying a tricyclic antidepressant such as Imipramine.

Imipramine has been found to be effective with a large percentage of ADDH children (Rapoport and Mikkelsen, in press). It has been reported that the bedtime does is effective the next day. This is distinctly different from the antidepressant effect of these medications, which takes two to three weeks to occur. This nighttime dosage schedule offers a distinct advantage. However, there is some indication that the likelihood of toxicity is increased by a single dose at nighttime. The effects of tricyclics on activity level, behavior, cognitive functioning, academic achievement, and other functions are similar to those of the stimulants, although there is not as much evidence for their effect on cognitive functioning. However, there is also an indication that tricyclics are not tolerated as well as the stimulants. The main side effects include: anorexia, nausea, weight loss, insomnia, and dry mouth. Also, surprisingly they often produce negative effect on mood in ADDH children, in contrast to their antidepressant effect in adults. As of yet, Imipramine is not approved by the FDA for use in children under the age of 12 except for enuresis. Moreover, the recent reports of EKG abnormalities in children treated with Imipramine has led the FDA to improve investigational protocols for its use only within certain dosage ranges for children with regular EKG monitoring being recommended.

If a child does not respond to any of the stimulants or to tricyclic antidepressants, it is the author's opinion that none of the other psychoactive drugs will likely be effective (Cantwell, in press). There is general agreement that the major tranquilizers produce deleterious effects on learning and cognitive functioning even though they may produce a decrease in activity level, and although antihistamines such as diphrenhydramine have been advocated by some, their effectiveness with ADDH children has not as yet been proven in a comparative trial using objective measures of evaluation. Anticonvulsants are only useful for ADDH children if they have a seizure disorder. There is no evidence that in the absence of seizure activity, anticonvulsants are indicated for ADDH children even if they have abnormal EEGs. In the extremely rare case of mania which may present with hyperactivity in prepubertal child, lithium may be effective. But certainly it has not been shown to be effective in the usual child with the ADDH syndrome.

Regardless which drug is used, in treating the ADDH syndrome there are certain general principles to be followed.

An older and tested drug should be used in place of a new drug unless there is a great deal of experimental evidence for superiority of the newer medication (Eisenberg, 1968).

Baseline assessments of the child's behaviors that are expected to be affected by the medication must be obtained systematically. The same instruments should be used to record the same behaviors at regular intervals during the course of treatment. Response to treatment is probably best *singly* evaluated by the physician from reports of behavior at school. However, the more standardized ratings made by different observers in different settings, the greater the likelihood that the physician will obtain a true picture of the effect of the medication. The author recommends that the physician use the Conners Parent Symptom Questionnaire (PSQ), the Conners Teacher Questionnaire (TQ), the Conners Abbreviated Symptom Questionnaire (ASQ), and the Rutter-Graham Psychiatric Rating Scale for children (Gofman, 1973) as baseline and follow-up measures to judge the effectiveness of the medication (HEW, 1973).

Side effects should be assessed and monitored in the same systematic fashion as the expected behavioral effects of the medication. There are systematic rating sheets for side effects to be completed by parents and to be asked of the children that are quite useful for this purpose (Gofman, 1973).

The initial dosage of any drug should be the smallest available dose of the medication being used. A knowledge of the duration of action of the medication is necessary in order to know whether to prescribe the drug on a once-a-day basis or on a two-or-three-times-a-day basis, depending on how long the physician wishes the medication to be effective. Starting with the low dose, the physician should then titrate the medication and raise the dosage until either clinical improvement is noted or until side effects occur which necessitate discontinuation of the drug. At present there are no laboratory measures against which one can titrate the medication. The physician must use his clinical judgment based on the information he obtains from the parents, the school, and his own observation of the child.

While there are *rough* guidelines that one can use for optimal dosage of individual drugs on a milligram of drug per kilogram of body weight basis, this is a controversial area.

It is well to remember that an individual child may require a great deal more medication than would be expected, since there are large individual differences in blood levels of medication for comparable doses of the same drug in children of the same body weight. Moreover, one drug may have a therapeutic effect for a particular child only at a particular blood level. Children considered "non-responders" to medication often simply have not been given an effective dose (Conners et al., 1972; Wender, 1971).

If improvement occurs, then seems to disappear, the dosage should be increased, since tolerance to the effect of the medication often develops. Although the literature on drug treatment of hyperactive children generally seems to ignore the fact that tolerance does develop, clinical experience and scientific data support that it does (Arnold, 1973). Just as the amount of medication that an individual child might require is highly idiosyncratic, so is the development of tolerance. There are many children who can remain on the same dosage of medication for a year or more, and others become tolerant to the effect at a much earlier period of time.

All children on chronic medication should be given a drug-free trial at some time during the course of the year. This can be done by substituting placebo without letting the child or the schoolteacher know and obtaining a rating scale to see if there is deterioration of behavior. Each child should also start school in September without medication, and after several weeks a rating scale should be obtained to see how it compares with the teacher's rating obtained at the end of the school year when he was on medication. If it looks like the child no longer requires medication he should be followed more closely to see if his behavior deteriorates over time. Abstinence syndromes do not seem to develop during a drug-free trial.

At present there is no good way for determining when a child should be completely taken off medication. The popular idea that ADDH syndrome disappears and medication has a "reverse effect" at puberty has never been established scientifically. No medication should be stopped because a child reaches a certain age, but only when the clinical picture indicates the child no longer requires it.

A good deal of preparation must be done with both the child and the parents in conjunction with the use of medication. At the very least, the treating physician should help the child understand the nature of his difficulties and how the medication (and other therapeutic interventions) are intended to help the child help himself. The role and action of the medication in his life then can make more sense to the child and he will hopefully see the medication as one of *his* tools, not something forced on him by his parents, his teachers, or his doctor (Kehne, 1974; Wender et al., 1971).

The parents should also be prepared in a rational way for a trial of any medication. The physician should state that since ADDH children are likely to have different causes for their condition, there are medications which may help one child but not another. Moreover, there is no sure way of telling ahead of time which medication might work for which child. The parents should also be told that a dose of a particular medication that is effective for one child may not be effective for another child. For any particular drug that is used, the physician should explain in great detail to the parents what the expected benefits from the medication are and what the medication will *not do*. Expected side effects should also be gone over in great detail and the parents encouraged to observe their child carefully for any likely side effects. The time invested in this type of preparation of the child and his family will reap its benefits should medication have to be changed or should dosage have to be changed over a long period of time in order to find the optimal dose of the optimal drug for each child.

An important and often neglected part of the physician's work in treating children with medication is establishing contact with the school. The physician should make direct contact with the child's teacher either in person or over the phone. Without cooperation from the school in reporting both positive and negative effects of the medication, it is the author's opinion that it is impossible effectively to manage a child on any psychoactive medication. The teacher is likely to be the only person to see the child regularly in a group setting where he is required to do the same tasks as a large number of peers of the same age. Thus in a sense the teacher is in a position to compare the performance of the ADDH child with a "control group" on a daily basis. This is not meant to imply that the teacher has control of either the prescribing or the regulation of medication dosage, but that the physician needs to be in contact with the teacher in order for him to make the proper adjustments in the dosage of medication.

Using the general principles outlined above it can rather rapidly be determined whether or not the child will respond to any of the medications, and if so, what aspects of his disorder the medication positively affects. The next step will be selecting the therapeutic modalities that are necessary based on an individual child's presenting complaints.

Educational Intervention

Since about 75% of school-age ADDH children also present with educational problems, the necessity for educational intervention should be determined next. However, as is noted by Keogh (1971), there has been little research aimed at specifying the nature of the educational problems of ADDH children, or at documenting their natural history, or at delineating the variables leading to school failure in individual children with the ADDH syndrome. Clearly the educational problems of the ADDH children are not all due to the same cause. It is probably safe to say that if an individual child with the ADDH syndrome also presents with lowered academic achievement, that even if he responds positively to some medication that alone will not be enough to significantly influence his academic problems. Thus some type of educational intervention will be ncessary, although what *type* that should be and in what *type of setting* is an open question. For example, Conrad and Insel (1967) attempted to assess the effect of tutoring and medicatiion in a groupd of 68 children with the ADDH syndrome. All experimental groups were matched for intelligence and degree of hyperactivity. One of the groups received dextroamphetamine alone, one received tutoring and placebo, one received placebo alone, and one received both dextroamphetamine and tutoring. The results were disappointing in that only three of the 68 children progressed to a point that they no longer needed remedial educational help at the end of one year. However, more importantly there was no evidence that the improvement produced by the use of dextroamphetamine alone could be significantly enhanced by the addition of tutoring. However, in a well-designed study by Wolraich and his colleagues (in press) of ADDH children in a special class, behavior modification and stimulant medication were found to be effective in different situations (group versus individual) and on different behaviors (attentional versus motor and verbal overflow).

It has often been stated that different types of classroom structure may affect behavior and academic competencies in children with the ADDH syndrome, but *few* studies have addressed this question in a comprehensive fashion, and none has studied the problem of classroom structure and its affect on academic achievement over a long period of time. Despite the lack of hard evidence for generalized classroom special education intervention for children with the ADDH syndrome, there is a good deal of evidence that specific cognitive training procedures are indeed effective for individual children with the syndrome. Douglas (1972, 1974, 1975, 1976) has reviewed evidence strongly suggesting that ADDH children have a pattern of cognitive deficits suggesting a major problem with attention-impulsivity. She has described this problem as an inability to "stop, look and listen." She concludes further that the activity and distractability problems are most likely secondary to an attentional deficit. Following from this, it seems to be a logical assumption that training the ADDH child to overcome some of these functional deficits could lead to benefits in a number of areas. There are a number of studies that in fact suggest just that. Palkes (Palkes, Stewart, and Kahana, 1968) taught ADDH children to develop self-control over their voluntary behavior by teaching them to verbalize self-directed commands. Ten boys were taught to vocalize a set of self-directed commands before responding to any task or subset of a task. Cards bearing instructions such as "Before I start any of the tasks I am going to do, I am going to say 'Stop, listen, look and think before I answer' " were used as training aids. Pretest was done with the Porteus Maze and then the investigator presented a series of tasks to the boys to be performed. These included Kagan's Matching Familiar Figures Tests (MFF), the Embedded Figures Test (EFT), and the Trail Making Test (TMT). The experimental group verbalized the set of self-directed commands before responding to any of these tasks or any subset of the tasks. Another control group of boys were given the same tasks without being trained in the self-directed command procedures. The next day both groups were seen for about a period of one-half hour, and all procedures were repeated. Results indicated that there were no significant pretest differences on the Porteus Maze between the two groups of ADDH children. However, on post-test the group who received the verbal training had significantly higher PQ scores, suggesting that the use of the self-directed verbal commands training procedures was effective in increasing their overall performance on the Porteus Maze. The training group also received significantly higher Q scores at post-test, suggesting that the self-directed verbal commands also reduced the number of qualitative errors. ADDH children who received the verbal training cut fewer corners, crossed over fewer lines, lifted their pencils less and threaded the Porteus Maze with fewer irregular lines than did the control group. The conclusion was that the improvement in the performance on the Porteus Maze was due to a more prudent approach to the solution of the problem learned by the group who received the verbal training procedures.

Egeland (1974) compared a group of impulsive ADDH children who were trained to use more efficient strategies and scanning techniques with a group who were trained merely to delay their responses. The predictions were that the training procedures would lead to the following changes: (1) an increased amount of time prior to making a response; (2) a decrease in the number of errors on the MFF immediately after training; (3) a decrease in the number of errors on the MFF two months after training; (4) a generalization of the improved performance to measures of reading achievement.

The subjects were 24 boys randomly assigned to each of three groups. One group trained to improve search strategies and scanning techniques, a second group trained only to delay their responses at least 10-15 seconds and a control group of impulsive, hyperactive children who received no training at all. A variety of different materials and exercises were used to train children to process information more effectively and to solve match to sample visual discrimination problems. Another group was trained to delay responses by showing examples of the kind of work they would be doing during the training session and explained to them that one way of increasing the likelihood of getting the correct answer was to think about your answers and to take your time. Results indicated that both training methods were effective in the short term in reducing the number of errors on the MFF. However, it was noted that two months after training only the group who were trained to use more efficient search strategies maintained their new skills and continued to make fewer errors. The group who were trained only to delay their responses actually showed a significant increase in errors two months after follow-up. Some measure of generalization to actual academic achievement in these children was provided by results from a reading test that showed that the group trained to improve their search and scanning techniques was achieving at a higher level of reading comprehension at the end of the school year than either the control group or the group who was trained only to delay their strategies. Thus the training given to the group who learned new rules and new strategies for attacking problems produced a durable effect on the error scores on the MFF, both immediately after training and 2 months later. Moreover, this improved performance seemed to generalize to some extent to the child's performance in reading achievement.

More recently Douglas and her colleagues (1976) reported on an attempt to use modeling and self-instructional techniques to improve attention and to reduce impulsivity in ADDH children. Subjects consisted of 18 boys and a control groop of 11 boys. Both groups were well-matched. The training program included consultation sessions with both parents and teachers and training sessions with the children themselves. Modeling, self-verbalization, and strategy training techniques were based on the work of Meichenbaum and Goodman (1969, 1971). The assessment battery included the MFF, the Story Completion Test (Parry, 1973), the Porteus Maze (Porteus, 1969), the Bender Visual-Motor Gestalt (Bender, 1938), Memory tests from the Detroit Tests of Learning Aptitude (Baker and Leland, 1967), the Durell Analysis of Reading Difficulty (Durell, 1955), the Wide Range Achievement Test—Arithmetic Subtest (Jastak, 1946), the Conners Abbreviated Parent Rating Scale (ASQ) (Conners, 1973b). Results at the end of the three-month training period and also three months later after no training had taken place indicated that the group that had received the training showed significantly greater improvement on most of the measures.

All of these studies taken together, and others that are reviewed by Douglas et al. (1976), suggest that it is possible to teach ADDH children to change their impulsive approach to problems and possibly to improve academic achievement as a result of this training. Much more research is needed to determine which materials, which exercises, and which training methods are the most efficient for which hyperactive children. However, it is unfortunate that none of these studies involved a comparison between training methods alone, stimulant medication alone, and both together. As is shown by the Gittelman-Klein et al. (1976) comparative study of behavior modification and methylphenidate, it may well be that a training program might be effective for improving certain deficits in ADDH children. However, this does not mean that the training program will be better than or even equivalent to another form of therapy (such as medication). It might well be that similar changes in the measures used in these various studies might have been produced equally well by stimulant medication. In fact, performance on the Porteus Maze has been shown to be significantly affected by stimulant medication. Furthermore, the combination of stimulant medication plus a cognitive training program might be even more effective than either alone. Only the type of study conducted by Gittelman-Klein (1976) can provide the answer to this vital question. In the absence of specific research studies that allow us to state whether these cognitive training programs are effective over time and whether or not they are enhanced by medication, the physician must use his clinical judgment in the analysis of each child's learning strengths and disabilities and also on the analysis of available community resources to make a decision about what type of educational program might be best for an individual child. The availability of specialized individual training programs such as those outlined above in the ordinary public school is limted at best. One is often forced to accept an "educationally handicapped" program or a "learning disability" program which may not have any demonstrated effectiveness but may be the only thing available. However, it is clear that most ADDH children, at least when initially evaluated, are not doing well on the regular classroom setting. It is also clear that stimulant medication *alone* has not been shown to produce a demonstrable effect in academic achievement over time. Thus most of ADDH children who do present with poor academic achievement as well as with their behavioral symptoms will need some type of educational intervention. Since each year an individual child spends about 1,400 hours out of 8.716 waking hours in school, it is vitally important that as a minimum, the teachers be familiar with the syndrome and that there be a consistency of expectations between the home and school. Efforts should be made to ensure that methods of behavioral reinforcement between the home and the school are consistent.

From the practical standpoint most ADDH children will probably have to remain in a regular classroom setting. In these cases, individual tutoring for specific problem areas in combination with the use of stimulant medication in those children whom it benefits is likely to prove the most beneficial over the long haul.

Behavior Modification

There is a great deal of solid evidence to suggest the effectiveness of behavior modification techniques for changing a variety of the behaviors that characterize children with the ADDH syndrome. However, a great deal of the behavior modification literature suffers from methodological problems such as small sample size and lack of evidence for generalization of effects. Moreover, diagnostic criteria very often are not spelled out in the behavior modification literature so that one gets a picture of *what behaviors* are modified but not in *what type of children*. It may be that activity level, attentional problems, distractability, and other behaviors characteristic of children with the ADDH syndrome can be brought under significant control in certain types of children but not in others. In general, behavior modification studies do not spell out the clinically defined syndrome the children are manifesting; rather they concentrate on behaviors only. Finally, a serious lack in behavior modification literature is a lack of attention to measures of learning and academic achievement as measures of outcome.

Gittelman-Klein and her colleagues (1976) have conducted the best comparative study of behavior modification in children with the ADDH syndrome. They have reported results on 34 out of a planned 75 children. Prior to any intervention pre- and post-treatment data were obtained from several sources, including an interview with the child, observations by psychiatrist, parental evaluations, and teacher evaluations. Classroom observations were also carried out. Three groups of children were studied from the intervention standpoint. One group received behavior modification alone both at home and school. One group received behavior modification procedures plus methylphenidate. One group received methylphenidate alone. A consistent pattern of treatment effects was obtained in that all treatments produced significant clinical improvement. At the end of 8 weeks, the children who received the behavior modification alone were significantly improved as were children who received behavior modification plus methylphenidate and children who received behavior modification alone. However, the combination of methylphenidate and behavior therapy was not statistically significantly better than methylphenidate alone. Both of these treatments, the behavior modification plus methylphenidate and methylphenidate alone produce statistically better results than behavior modification combined with placebo. Thus the study would suggest that stimulant medication is the intervention of choice for ADDH children, and that if medication alone does not produce significant improvement in certain areas, behavior modification techniques could, and probably should, be added. However, the reverse strategy—that is, medication is to be used only *after* behavior modification techniques have been used first, which is advocated by some—does not receive support from the data in this study. Further research in this area of intervention is needed with larger numbers of children studied over longer periods of time with multiple measures of outcome being used, particularly measures of academic achievement. The evidence does suggest that behavior modification techniques are useful for many of the behaviors, such as overactivity, distractability, and attentional problems that characterize the children with the ADDH syndrome. As mentioned above, one of the aspects of involvement of the family can be the training of both parents and siblings in behavioral modification techniques to modify certain aspects of the ADDH child's behavior.

Psychotherapy

As with the other psychiatric disorders of childhood, outcome studies of the results of psychotherapy of children with the ADDH syndrome are few and far between. There is also very little written about the techniques of psychotherapy useful with these children. Probably the leading writer in this field is Gardner (1973), who divides the types of psychogenic difficulties of children with the ADDH syndrome into two types. One group of psychogenic difficulties arises in direct response to organic deficits which he sees as etiologic in this syndrome. The second group are those symptoms to which any child is susceptible. The second group of symptoms have their origins in difficulties between the child and his environment. Gardner views treatment modalities of hyperactive children as consisting of four basic interventions: medication, special education, parental guidance, and psychotherapy, in that order. His conceptualization of therapeutic intervention is similar to that of the present author but in a somewhat different order. Gardner has written extensively about the types of difficulties amenable to psychotherapy with these children and also about the types of techniques used. He feels that therapeutic sessions need to be well-structured because ADDH children need organization more than they need the opportunity for free expression. He sees predictability and reasonable limits as being vital to these children. He has developed a number of therapeutic techniques including: a mutual storytelling technique, a board of objects game, a bag of objects game, and others to deal with these psychogenic difficulties of the ADDH child. These difficulties include such things as ignorance of any distortions about reality, denial, fear, and withdrawal from involvement with others, immaturity and regression, impulsivity, perseveration, and low self-esteem. In this author's experience, low self-esteem is probably the most common symptom of children with the ADDH syndrome for which psychotherapy is indicated. Group therapy as well as individual therapy, has found to be useful.

Clearly there are symptoms that the ADDH child presents which are identical to those that any child with any psychiatric disorder presents. Some of these will be amenable to psychotherapy, others will not. It is unlikely that psychotherapy will have any effect on the basic core symptoms such as the attentional deficit. However, psychotherapy is probably the most overlooked therapeutic modality with these children.

Other Forms of Therapeutic Intervention

When one is presented with a disorder of unknown etiology, such as the ADDH syndrome, for which a variety of therapeutic modalities are available, there are always a number of "fringe" therapies which are advocated. Those advocated for this disorder include: neurophysiological retraining such as patterning, optometry, sensory-integrative therapy, megavitamin therapy, elimination diets, and hypoglycemic diets (Silver, 1975). At this time it is the elimination diet, which consists of the elimination of salicylates, food colorings, and food additives, which is currently undergoing the greatest popular vogue (Feingold, 1973). As with other types of "magic cures," promotion of this type of intervention far outstrips the scientific evidence on which it is based. A recent article by Esther Wender has critically reviewed the published available literature concerning the effectiveness of additive free diets on children with this syndrome. In her view there is little hard evidence to support the rather extravagant claims for the effectiveness of this therapeutic modality, just as there has been essentially no evidence for megavitamin therapy and others mentioned above. It is well for the clinician to remember that parents are quite likely to be familiar with the latest "fad" and the clinician can play a major role by discussing their assets and liabilities with the parents. It is best probably to take a nonjudgmental approach and to explain to the parents what scientific evidence exists, if any, for the effectiveness of the therapy that they are asking about. If none exists, the physician should say so, but should not attempt to prevent the parents from trying it if they so desire, as long as the physician does not feel that the intervention is actually harmful. It behooves the physician to be well aware of what the popular literature and media are saying about the treatment of children with this disorder.

Summary and Conclusions

Children with the ADDH syndrome should be considered to be at serious psychiatric risk. Published studies, both prospective and retrospective, indicate that this disorder is not simply one of childhood which disappears with time. Rather, they indicate that this disorder predisposes to development of certain types of psychiatric and social pathology in adolescence and in later life. Moreover, although a variety of therapeutic modalities have been advocated and there is strong evidence for the short-term efficacy of some of these such as stimulant medication, there is no hard evidence that over the long haul any type of therapeutic intervention has been shown to successfully alter long-term outcome. Although on the other hand it must be said the proper study of his nature has not yet been carried out. Early intervention with these children is likely to be more effective in preventing some of these secondary problems than waiting for the secondary problems to develop and then treating them. A variety of therapeutic modalities have been discussed in this chapter. Each of them has its place. Their need should be determined by individual analysis of each child and his family.

References

Arnold, L. (1973) The art of medicating hyperkinetic children: A number of practical suggestions. *Clin. Pediat.* 12:35–41.

Baker, H.J., and B. Leland. (1967) *Detroit Tests of Learning Aptitude.* Indianapolis: Bobbs-Merrill.

Bakwin, H. (1949) Cerebral damage and behavior disorders in children. *Pediatrics* 6:271–382.

Barkley, R.A. (1977) A review of stimulant drug research with hyperactive children. *J. Child Psychol. Psychiat.* 18:137–165.

Barkley, R.A., and C.E. Cunningham. (1978) The effects of Ritalin on the mother-child interactions of hyperactive children. *J. Pediat.*, in press.

Bell, R.Q. (1968) A reinterpretation of the direction of effects in studies socialization. *Psychol. Rev.* 75:81–95.

Bender, L. (1938) *A Visual Gestalt Test and Its Clinical Use.* New York: American Psychiatric Association.

Borland, B.L., and H.K. Heckman. (1976) Hyperactive boys and their brothers: A 25-year follow-up study. *Arch. Gen. Psychiat.* 33:669–675.

Campbell, S.B. (1975) Mother-child interaction: A comparison of hyperactive, learning disabled, and normal boys. *Am. J. Orthopsychiat.* 45:51–57.

Cantwell, D.P. (1972) Psychiatric illness in families of hyperactive children. *Arch. Gen. Psychiat.* 27:414–417.

Cantwell, D.P., ed. (1975a) *The Hyperactive Child: Diagnosis, Management, and Current Research.* New York: Spectrum Publications.

Cantwell, D.P. (1975b) Epidemiology, clinical picture, and classification of the hyperactive child syndrome. In D.P. Cantwell, ed., *The Hyperactive Child: Diagnosis, Management and Current Research.* New York: Spectrum Publications.

Cantwell, D.P. (1975c) Familial-genetic research with hyperactive children. In D.P. Cantwell, ed., *The Hyperactive Child: Diagnosis, Management and Current Research.* New York: Spectrum Publications.

Cantwell, D.P. (1976) Genetic factors in the hyperkinetic syndrome. *J. Am. Acad. Child Psychiat.* 15:214–223.

Cantwell, D.P. CNS activating drugs in the treatment of hyperactive children. In J. Brady and H. Brodie, eds., *Controversy in Psychiatry.* Philadelphia: W.B. Saunders, in press.

Cantwell, D.P., and G.A. Carlson. Stimulants. In J.S. Werry, ed., *Pediatric Psychopharmacology—The Use of Behavior Modifying Drugs in Children.* New York: Brunner/Mazel, in press.

Cantwell, D.P., and J.H. Sattersfield. The prevalence of educational retardation in hyperactive children. *Arch. Gen. Psychiat.*, in press.

Clements, S. (1966) *Minimal Brain Dysfunction in Children.* Washington, D.C.: U.S. Public Health Service.

Coleman, M. (1971) Serotonin concentrations in whole blood of hyperactive children. *J. Pediat.*

Conners, C.K. (1973) Rating scales of use in drug studies with children. Special issue, *Psychopharmacol. Bull.*: Pharmacotherapy of Children. Washington, D.C.: U.S. Government Printing Office, pp. 24–84.

Conners, C., E. Taylor, G. Meo, M. Kurtz, and M. Fournier. (1972) Magnesium pemoline and dextroamphetamine: A controlled study in children with minimal brain dysfunction. *Psychopharmacologica* 26:321–336.

Conrad, W., and J. Insel. (1967) Anticipating the response to amphetamine therapy in the treatment of hyperkinetic children. *Pediatrics* 40:96–99.

De Hirsch, K. (1973) Early language development and minimal brain dysfunction. *Ann. N.Y. Acad. Sci.* 205:158–163.

Department of Health, Education and Welfare. (1973) Special issue, *Psychopharmacol. Bull.*: Pharmacotherapy of Children. Washington, D.C.: U.S. Government Printing Office.

Douglas, V. (1972) Stop, look and listen: The problem of sustained attention and impulse control in hyperactive and normal children. *Can. J. Behav. Sci.* 4:249–282.

Douglas, V.I. (1974) Differences between normal and hyperkinetic children. In C. Conners, ed., *Clinical Use of Stimulant Drugs in Children.* Amsterdam: Excerpta Medica, pp. 12–23.

Douglas, V.I. (1975) Are drugs enough to train or to treat the hyperactive child? *Int. J. Ment. Health* 5:199–212.

Douglas, V.I. (1976) Perceptual and cognitive factors as determinants of learning disabilities: A review paper with special emphasis on attentional factors. In R.M. Knights and D.J. Bakker, eds., *Neuropsychology of Learning Disorders: Theoretical Approaches.* Baltimore: University Park Press.

Douglas, V.I., P. Parry, P. Marton, and C. Garson. (1976) Assessment of a cognitive training program for hyperactive children. *J. Abnorm. Child. Psychol.* 4:389–410.

Durell, D.D. (1955) *Durell Analysis of Reading Difficulty.* New York: Harcourt, Brace & World.

Eeg-Olofsson, O. (1970) The development of the electroencephalogram in normal children and adolescents from the age of 1 through 21 years. *Acta Paediat. Scand.* (Suppl.) 208.

Egeland, B. (1974) Training impulsive children in the use of more efficient scanning techniques. *Child Develop.* 45:165–171.

Eisenberg, L. (1968) Psychopharmacology in childhood: A critique. In E. Miller, ed., *Foundations of Child Psychiatry*. New York: Pergamon, pp. 625–641.

Feingold, B. (1973) Food additives and child development. *Hosp. Prac.* 8:11–12, 17–19.

Fish, B. (1975) Drug treatment of the hyperactive child. In D. Cantwell, ed., *The Hyperactive Child: Diagnosis, Management and Current Research*. New York: Spectrum Publications, pp. 109–127.

Gardner, R.A. (1973) Psychotherapy of the psychogenic problems secondary to minimal brain dysfunction. *Int. J. Psychother.* 2:224–256.

Gittelman-Klein, R., D.F. Klein, H. Abikoff, S. Katz, A. Gloisten, and W. Kates. (1976) Relative efficacy of methylphenidate and behavior modification in hyperkinetic children: An interim report. *J. Abnorm. Child Psychol.* 4:361–379.

Gofman, H. (1973) Interval and final rating sheets on side effects. Special issue, *Psychopharmacol. Bull.*: Pharmacotherapy of Children. Washington, D.C.: U.S. Government Printing Office, pp. 182–187.

Goodwin, F., and W. Bunney. (1973) A psychobiological approach to affective illness. *Psychiat. Ann.* 3:19–56.

Humphries, T., M. Kinsbourne, and J. Swanson. (1978) Stimulant effects on cooperation and social interaction between hyperactive children and their mothers. *J. Child Psychol. Psychiat.* 19:13–22.

Jastak, J. (1946) *Wide Range Achievement Test*. Wilmington: C.L. Story Company.

Kehne, C. (1974) Social control of the hyperactive child via medication: At what cost to personality development. Some psychological implications and clinical interventions. Paper read before the annual meeting, Orthopsychiatric Association.

Kellam, S.G., M.E. Ensminger, and R.J. Turner. (1977) Family structure and the mental health of children. *Arch. Gen. Psychiat.* 34:1012–1022.

Kennard, M. (1960) Value of equivocal signs in neurologic diagnosis. *Neurol.* 10:753–764.

Keogh, B. (1971) Hyperactivity and learning disorders: Review and speculation. *Except. Child* 38:101–109.

Knobel, M. (1962) Psychopharmacology for hyperkinetic child—dynamic considerations. *Arch. Gen. Psychiat.* 6:198–202.

Kraft, I. (1968) The use of psychoactive drugs in the outpatient treatment of psychiatric disorders of children. *Am. J. Psychiat.* 124:1401–1407.

Laufer, M.W., and E. Denhoff. (1957) Hyperkinetic behavior syndrome in children. *J. Pediat.* 50:463–474.

Loney, J. Childhood hyperactivity. In R.W. Woody, ed., *Encyclopedia of Clinical Assessment*. San Francisco: Jossey-Bass.

Meichenbaum, D., and J. Goodman. (1969) Reflection, impulsivity and verbal control of motor behavior. *Child Develop.* 40:785–797.

Meichenbaum, D., and J. Goodman. (1971) Training impulsive children to talk to themselves: A means of developing self-control. *J. Abnorm. Psychol.* 77:115–126.

Mendelson, W., N. Johnson, and M.A. Stewart. (1971) Hyperactive children as teenagers: A follow-up study. *J. Nerv. Ment. Dis.* 153:263–270.

Menkes, M., J. Rowe, and J. Menkes. (1967) A twenty-five-year follow-up study on the hyperactive child with minimal brain dysfunction. *Pediatrics* 39:393–399.

Millichap, J. (1973) Drugs in management of minimal brain dysfunction. *Ann. N.Y. Acad. Sci.* 205:321–334.

Minde, K., D. Lewin, G. Weiss, H. Lavingueur, V. Douglas, and E. Sykes. (1971) The hyperactive child in elementary school: A 5 year, controlled follow-up. *Except. Child* 38:215–221.

Minde, K., G. Weiss, and M. Mendelson. (1972) A five-year follow-up study of 91 hyperactive school children. *J. Am. Child Psychiat.* 11:595–610.

Palkes, H., M. Stewart, and B. Kahana. (1968) Porteus maze performance of hyperactive boys after training in self-directed verbal commands. *Child Develop.* 45:165–171.

Parry, P. The effect of reward on the performance of hyperactive children. Ph.D. dissertation, McGill University, Montreal, 1973.

Patternite, C.E., J. Loney, and J.E. Langhorne, Jr. (1976) Relationships between symbolic and SES related factors in hyperkinetic/MBD boys. *Am. J. Orthopsychiat.* 46:291–301.

Patterson, G.R. (1971) *Families*. Champaign, Ill.: Research Press.

Patterson, G.R., and M.E. Guillon. (1968) *Living With Children*. Champaign, Ill: Research Press.

Petersen, I., O. Eeg-Olofsson, and U. Sellden. (1968) Paroxysmal activity in EEG of normal children. In P. Kellaway and I. Petersen, eds., *Clinical Electroencephalography of Children*. New York: Grune & Stratton.

Porteus, S.D. (1969) *Porteus Maze Tests: Fifty Years' Application*. Palo Alto: Pacific Books.

Quinn, P., and J. Rapoport. (1974) Minor physical anomalies and neurologic status in hyperactive boys. *Pediatrics* 53:742–747.

Rapoport, J., and J. Mikkelsen. Antidepressants. In J. Werry, ed., *Pediatrics Psychopharmacology: Behavior Modifying Drugs in Children*. New York: Brunner/Mazel.

Rapoport, J., I. Lott, D. Alexander, and A. Abramson. (1970) Urinary noradrenaline and playroom behavior in hyperactive boys. *Lancet* 2:1141.

Rapoport, J., P. Quinn, G. Bradbard, K. Riddle, and E. Brooks. (1974) Imipramine and methylphenidate treatments of hyperactive boys. *Arch. Gen. Psychiat.* 30:789–793.

Roche, A.F., and T. Jackson. Hyperkinesis, autonomic nervous system acitivty and stimulant drug effects. *J. Child Psychol. Psychiat.*, in press.

Rutter, M. (1966) *Children of Sick Parents: An Environmental and Psychiatric Study*. Maudsley Monograph No. 16. London: Oxford University Press.

Rutter, M., and L. Hersov. (1977) Family influences. In M. Rutter, ed., *Child Psychiatry: Modern Approaches.* London: Blackwell Publications.

Rutter, M., P. Graham, and W. Yule. (1970) *A Neuropsychiatric Study in Childhood.* Philadelphia: Lippincott.

Safer, D.J. (1973) A familial factor in minimal brain dysfunction. *Behav. Genet.* 3:175–187.

Satterfield, J. (1973) EEG issues in children with minimal brain dysfunction. *Semin. Psychiat.* 5:35–46.

Satterfield, J.H., D.P. Cantwell, L.I. Lesser, and R.L. Podosin. (1972) Physiological studies of the hyperkinetic child. *Am. J. Psychiat.* 128:1418–1424.

Satterfield, J., D. Cantwell, and B. Satterfield. (1974) Pathophysiology of the hyperactive child syndrome. *Arch. Gen. Psychiat.* 31:839–844.

Schain, R. (1972) *Neurology of Childhood Learning Disorders.* Baltimore: Williams & Wilkins.

Shaywitz, B.A., D.J. Cohen, and M.B. Bowers, Jr. (1975) CSF amine metabolites in children with minimal brain dysfunction (MBD)—Evidence for alteration of brain dopamine. *Pediat. Res.* 9:385.

Shekim, W.O., H. Dekirmenjian, and J.L. Chapel. (1977) Urinary catecholamine metabolites in hyperkinetic boys treated with dextroamphetamine. *Am. J. Psychiat.* 134:1276–1279.

Shinn, M. (1978) Father absence in children's cognitive development. *Psychol. Bull.* 85(2):295–324.

Silver, L.B. (1975) Acceptable and controversial approaches to treating the child with learning disabilitie? *Pediatrics* 55:406–415.

Snyder, S., K. Taylor, J. Coyle, and J. Meyerhoff. (1970) The role of brain dopamine in behavioral regulation and the actions of psychotropic drugs. *Am. J. Psychiat.* 127:199–207.

Stewart, M., and S. Olds. (1973) *Raising a Hyperactive Child.* New York: Harper & Row.

Stewart, M., F. Pitts, A. Craig, and W. Dieruf. (1966) The hyperactive child syndrome. *Am. J. Orthopsychiat.* 36:861–867.

Waldrop, M., and C. Halverson. (1971) Minor physical anomalies and hyperactive behavior in young children. In J. Hellmuch, ed., *The Exceptional Infant.* New York: Brunner/Mazel.

Weiss, G., J. Werry, K. Minde, V. Douglas, and D. Sykes. (1968) Studies on the hyperactive child V. The effects of dextroamphetamine and chlorpromazine on behavior and intellectual functioning. *J. Child Psychiat.* 9:145–156.

Weiss, G., K. Minde, J.S. Werry, V.I. Douglas, and E. Nemeth. (1971) Studies on the hyperactive child VIII. Five-year follow-up. *Arch. Gen. Psychiat.* 24:409–414.

Welner, Z., A. Welner, M. Stewart, H. Palkes, and E. Wish. (1977) A controlled study of siblings of hyperactive children. *J. Nerv. Ment. Dis.* 165(2):110–117.

Wender, P.H. (1969) Platelet serotonin level in children with 'minimal brain dysfunction.' *Lancet* 1:12.

Wender, P. (1971) *Minimal Brain Dysfunction in Children.* New York: Wiley-Interscience.

Wender, P. (1973) *The Hyperactive Child: A Guide for Parents.* New York: Crown.

Wender, P.M. (1975) Speculations concerning a possible biochemical basis of minimal brain dysfunction. *Int. J. Ment. Health* 4:11–28.

Wender, P., R. Epstein, I. Kopin, and E. Gorden. (1971) Urinary monoamine metabolites in children with minimal brain dysfunction. *Am. J. Psychiat.*

Werry, J.S. (1972) Organic factors in childhood psychopathology. In H. Quay and J. Werry, eds., *Psychopathological Disorders of Childhood.* New York: Wiley, pp. 83–121.

Werry, J.S., G. Weiss, V. Douglas, and J. Martin. (1966) Studies on the hyperactive child III. The effect of chlorpromazine upon behavior and learning ability. *J. Am. Acad. Child Psychiat.* 5:292–312.

Wolraich, M., T. Drummond, M. Salamon, M. O'Brien, and C. Swage. Effects of methylphenidate alone and in combination with behavior modification procedures on the behavior and academic performance of hyperactive children. *J. Abnorm. Child Psychol.*, in press.

Treatment of Emotional Disorders in Children and Adolescents

CHAPTER 28

Learning Disabilities

Jules C. Abrams

Introduction

In view of the obvious importance of the ability to function effectively in school, it is quite unfortunate that year after year, for varied and sundry reasons, so many children experience some type of learning disorder. Probably the single most immediate reason for a youngster's being referred to child psychiatric clinics, child guidance clinics, and child therapists is difficulty in school. Unfortunately, all too often the child is viewed with a kind of tunnel vision, so that extremely important aspects of his unique learning disorder may be ignored. The child is a physical organism functioning in a social environment in a psychological manner. Therefore, it is naive to think of one single cause for learning disabilities. Rather, learning problems are caused by any number of factors, all of which may be highly interrelated.

To someone who has been actively involved for many years in the study of the innumerable factors that influence the learning process, the professional shifts of opinion are alternately significant, amusing, and sometimes dismaying. When psychological causation is most popular, the learning disability field is replete with "functional disorders." Then those involved in learning disabilities are besieged by evidence indicating the tremendous importance of psychogenic factors in determining how well a child will learn and the signficance of these factors in the etiology, diagnosis, and treatment of learning disability. Twenty years ago, if a child had a severe learning disability and was referred to a clinic or a private practitioner, the chances were very strong that following a careful evaluation of his problem, he would be recommended for psychotherapy. Absolutely nothing in the psychological literature could not account for a child's having learning difficulty. Thus we heard such terms as unresolved Oedipal strivings, guilt feelings, conflict over aggression, and familial disharmony as explanations for severe learning difficulties. Unfortunately, all too often after two or three years in therapy the child was discharged with some of his problems resolved but with his learning disorder intact. Psychotherapy may be helpful to some learning disabled youngsters with concomitant emotional problems, but psychotherapy never taught anyone how to read or how to do arithmetic.

Approximately fifteen years ago, the pendulum shifted. Slowly, like a sleeping dragon that had been awakened, this basically amorphous but powerful concept of organicity reared its ugly head. Those professionals dealing with learning disabilities were engulfed by such terms as minimal brain damage, minimal cerebral dysfunction, dyslexia, strephosymbolia, maturational lag, developmental discrepancy, and minimal cerebral desynchronization syndrome. In other words, the clinical situation had been reversed; organic factors overpowered functional factors and emerged as the most common single cause of learning disability in childhood.

Thus we return to the axiom that there is no one cause for learning disabilities. Pearson (1954) has pointed out that anything which interferes with the development of the ego and any of its functions will undoubtedly influence the child's adaptation to life, and one particular aspect of this adaptation—namely, the child's capacity for learning. Belmont (1964) states that a list of the types of learning disorders would double equally well as a list of types of disturbance in total life adjustment, or types of disturbance interfering with various basic ego functions. Still, no one can deny that, all too frequently, there is a tendency for each professional discipline to view the entire problem through its own window of specialization. This often obscures vital factors that may contribute to, or at least exacerbate, the basic difficulty. It is equally invalid to conceive of one mode of treatment, one panacea, applied randomly to all types of learning disorders. Not every learning disabled child requires a special school or psychotherapy or kinesthetic techniques or perceptual-motor training, or for that matter, a regression to crawling along the floor!

What appears to be universal is the fact that when a child experiences difficulty in school, his life is complicated in a number of different ways. Constant failure and frustration may lead to strong feelings of inferiority, which in turn may intensify the initial learning deficiencies. Under the impact of continued failure, the child desperately attempts to defend himself against increasing environmental pressures as well as the growing, gnawing feeling that he is "just plain stupid." Burdened by the fear of further wounding to his own pride, the child may simply withdraw into his own fantasies or may act out aggressively against his teachers or his fellow students. Now he is no longer merely a "learning disability"; he has also become a behavior problem (often at home as well as in school).

Just as sustained learning failure may result in behavioral disturbances, social and emotional conflicts in turn may provide the causative factors in learning disability. A child who is tense, worried, and fearful cannot focus his mind on intellectual pursuits any more than an adult who is consumed with anxiety and worry can. What develops is a continuing series of interactions between the insecurity generated by the lack of success in learning and any emotional instability which may be independent of the learning failure.

Definition

Much of the confusion concerning learning disability has come about because of multiple and varying definitions. Historically, the term "learning disability" was first used by Kirk (1962), who stated that a learning disability refers to a retardation disorder, or delayed development in one or more of the processes of speech, language, hearing, spelling, writing, or arithmetic. Kirk indicated further that the disability resulted from possible cerebral dysfunction and/or emotional or behavioral disturbance. He excluded those disabilities resulting from mental retardation, sensory deprivation, or cultural and instructional factors. Bateman (1965) described children with learning disabilities as those who manifest an educationally significant discrepancy between their estimated intellectual potential and actual level of performance. She related the disability to some basic disorder in the learning processes, which may or may not be accompanied by demonstrable central nervous system dysfunction. She excluded those disabilities secondary to generalized mental retardation, educational or cultural deprivation, severe emotional disturbance or sensory loss.

In 1968, the National Advisory Committee on Handicapped Children stated that learning disabilities may be manifested in disorders of listening, thinking, talking, reading, writing, spelling, or arithmetic. Learning disabilities include conditions that have been referred to as perceptual handicaps, brain injury, minimal brain dysfunction, dyslexia, and developmental asphasia. They do not include learning problems due *primarily* to visual, hearing, or motor handicaps, to mental retardation, emotional disturbance, or to environmental disadvantage. This view of learning disabilities essentially consitututes the definition Congress used in Public Law 94–142: The Education for All Handicapped Children Act of 1975. This is the definition most widely used to identify pupils eligible for specific learning disability services. It is also analogous to the concept of minimal brain dysfunction (see Chapter 25 in this book).

Whatever term is used depends primarily upon the orientation and interests of the individual assessing the problem. When an individual is concerned particularly with a comprehensive diagnosis following a medical model, with the assessment of biological concomitants and antecedents of the condition, and with the role of medical management, "minimal brain dysfunction" is the label of choice. When the individual is concerned primarily with assessment of learning disabilities and techniques of remedial education, "specific learning disability" often becomes the label. The difference and emphasis is reflected in the literature. Authors who write from the medical orientation prefer the term "minimal brain dysfunction" or its equivalent, whereas those who write from an educational point of view tend to use the term "specific learning disabilities" or its equivalent.

It is probably true that when the term "learning disability" is used today, most frequently a condition is described in which there is a specific learning problem that appears to be relatively independent of environmental influences. In other words, the focus of attention is on *specific* learning disability or minimal brain dysfunction. However, if one considers learning disorders in a broader fashion, then there must be included all of the factors influencing the child: psychological, physiological, social and familial (Abrams, In press). In this chapter we will consider learning disorders from the broader perspective. Essentially we define a learning disability as a condition in which there is a significant discrepancy between one's functioning intelligence level and his achievement in one or more of the following areas: listening, speaking, reading, arithmetic, or writing. This definition, although perhaps too broad, has the advantage of not depending primarily upon whether the etiological factors are external or internal.

The definition of learning disabilities as stated in Public Law 94-142 was originally motivated by a desire to highlight a heterogeneous group of children with developmental and academic disabilities and to provide and secure a basis for the systematic provision of financial support for training, research and service delivery. Although some of these goals have been reached, the definition has caused problems of interpretation related to operational implementation. As was stated by the Joint Committee on Learning Disabilities (1976):

1. The definition has led some to assume that learning disabilities represents a homogeneous group of children, when in fact the learning disabled constitute a heterogeneous population.

2. The definition by exclusion of certain handicapping conditions as well as children from different sociocultural and linguistic backgrounds has interfered with a clear understanding of learning disabilities as it is related to these issues.

3. Some state and local educational agencies, by a rigid interpretation of the definition, developed criteria for service delivery that ignored professional preparation and expertise and required delivery consistent with the definition as implied in the law.

4. Identification, assessment, and remediation were keyed to interpretation of the law, with subsequent confusion in all these areas.

The exclusionary factor in particular has caused much confusion and has frequently clouded the issues. For example, it sometimes is very difficult to make the differential diagnosis between an emotionally disturbed child and a youngster with minimal brain dysfunction. At times a child is labeled as dyslexic when in fact the perceptual and conceptual difficulties he manifests are actually representations of inadequate cognitive stimulation in a culturally deprived environment. If we utilize a broader definition as we have done in this chapter, we can successfully avoid these pitfalls. Then specific learning disability or minimal brain dysfunction is looked upon as just one type of disorder in the larger classification of learning disabilities.

Incidence

The confusion regarding the definition of learning disability has resulted in a wide variance in agreement of the incidence of the learning disabled. Figures on the incidence of learning disabilities within public schools range from 3% to 20% depending on the definition and the types of factors taken into account in deriving the figures. When learning disability is defined as in P.L. 94-142, then the incidence is probably close to 3%. Indeed, in counting children, Congress has stated that children with specific learning disabilities may not constitute more than one-sixth of the children counted as handicapped. Another limitation on the count is that a state may not count more than 12% of the number of children aged five through seventeen as handicapped. This means at most only 2 percent of the children in a state may be counted as having specific learning disabilities for allocation purposes.

When the prime definition of learning disabilities involves specific skill deficiencies that cause the child to be educationally retarded in terms of his intellectual potential (the definition used in this chapter), 15% to 20% of the school population may well be categorized as having learning problems. Within inner-city schools, when that definition has been used, incidence figures as high as 40% have been reported.

It is apparent that determining the incidence of learning disability in the school population is a difficult task. All of the problems discussed above regarding definition affect the validity of attempts to count the number of learning disabled children. In addition, etiological classifications are frequently confused with specific symptomatology. At times, distinctions between degrees of defect or severity of a learning disabling condition are inadequate. Finally, the professional orientation of the researcher may influence the estimate, his background and viewpoint perhaps tending to influence choice of sample, etiologic and symptomatic terminology, definition of the condition studied, and/or conclusion.

Etiological Considerations

It is clear that we do not fully understand the relationship between neurological impairment and learning disability (or between neurological impairment and behavioral disorder). There are certain physical and psychological conditions that may predispose a youngster to meet with learning difficulty, but we certainly do not know why. Environmental conditions may have a profound effect upon even constitutional factors, but the quality and quantity of that influence remains obscure. An approach to the disabled learner that takes into consideration the unique interaction of functional and organic factors is most desirable.

An ego orientation with its emphasis on the developmental-interaction approach to learning disabilities has been proposed by Rappaport (1961), Belmont (1964), Abrams (1970), and Adamson (1978). In this way the *interaction* of both neurological and psychological factors can be studied extensively; the factors are not regarded as isolated units. It is true that in other approaches, ego functions—such as perception, concept formation, and language development—have been utilized in diagnosis and remediation. But with an ego orientation, with the constant emphasis on developmental interaction, we are provided the opportunity for treating the child more effectively as a whole person.

Disorders of the Central Nervous System

When a child suffers an insult to the central nervous system prenatally, perinatally, or postnatally, this may constitute a severe threat to the integrity of the organism and may effect deficiencies in the primary ego apparatuses, which in turn interfere with the child's ability to interact with his environment in an adaptive manner. In some cases the defect in the ego apparatuses may result solely from a situation where the child is completely deprived of intellectual and/or emotional stimulation. In order for the ego to develop properly, there are two basic requirements: (1) the primary apparatus—that is, the neurological substrata of the ego, the central nervous system—must be intact; and (2) there must be a proper degree of stimulation in the environment.

Rappaport (1964) has pointed to three major areas of difficulty in children who have suffered an insult to the central nervous system. Under the broad heading of inadequate integrative functions, he discusses problems in perception and concept formation. Here we refer to children who are able to take in stimuli, but who have trouble fitting them appropriately into things they already know. They may have difficulty in categorizing because they have trouble differentiating between essential and nonessential details. These children frequently are able to acquire many facts and even parrot them back. However, they experience a great deal of difficulty when they attempt to apply this background of information to functional situations. They are unable to draw inferences or relate one area of knowledge to another. The major problem is in concept formation; the child can deal with that which is specific and concrete, but he cannot engage in the kind of active mental manipulation that is such an essential aspect of abstract conceptualization or generalization. We refer here also to the child who might be very accurate in handling numbers when these numbers are related to some aspect of himself, but who is unable to make the simplest computations when the numbers do not deal with him directly. This child persistently and consistently makes letter and word reversals long past what might be considered a part of a developmental stage. This child, too, may have a distorted idea of his own self, his own body—how big he is, how he is shaped, and how one body part relates to another. Problems in laterality and directionality are quite common.

A second area of disruptive ego functioning is that of inadequate impulse control or the control of ideas and feelings. These youngsters tend to be hyperactive, hyperdistractible, disinhibited, perseverative, and to show lability of affect and poor motor control. Although these characteristics have been well described in the literature on minimal brain dysfunction and specific learning disability, our focus here is psychodynamic. We view these symptoms as related to deficiencies in normal ego development and not as characteristics related solely to defective neural transmission or specific brain cell malfunction. For example, some "hyperactive" children may show excessive activity as a defense against overwhelming sadness and depression. Sometimes a child can feel so low, so defeated, so helpless that his only recourse is to act out aggressively in what appears to be driven behavior. Another "hyperdistractible" youngster may show severe interferences to attention and to concentration because of anxiety and/or overvalent feelings of inadequacy. Abrams and Smolen (1973), for example, discuss the effects of stress upon the functions of attention and concentration, describing how the organism responds to the impact of sustained learning failure.

Rappaport's third area of ego disturbance in the brain-injured child relates to the defensive maneuvering on the part of the ego in coping with the anxiety brought on by the intense feelings of inadequacy and defectiveness. The child who has experienced early insult to the central nervous system is under tremendous pressure. He feels helpless in the face of his own intense handicap. When he feels this way, he becomes frightened and anxious. As a result, he tends either to be more aggressive, more hostile, or withdrawn. He finds it extremely difficult to understand that he cannot control the world around him. He sees himself as the center of the universe. He is also angry that other people in his environment are not experiencing the same problems that he must strive to overcome. Frequently, there is a retreat into a kind of omnipotence as a defense against the terribly disturbing feelings of damage and defectiveness. To maintain this omnipotence, the child must avoid any challenging situation at whatever cost to himself. He must retreat from learning because any possibility of failure represents a severe threat of further wounding to his pride and self-esteem. Other manifestations of the defective self-concept and narcissistic hypersensitivity are low frustration tolerance, overcompensation, control and manipulation of others, and negativism or power struggles.

The emphasis on the child's ego functioning must also take into consideration the pivotal role of the family, both in terms of its influence in contributing to the learning disorder and the effect of the learning disability on the family constellation. Abrams and Kaslow (1976) point out that there is a mutual interaction; the child's ego development is affected by the environment in which the development takes place; and the learning disability, whatever its etiology, exercises a profound effect on the total family gestalt.

The normal child's acquisition and mastery of basic ego skills during infancy and early childhood evokes a maternal responsive joy and pride. The child is frequently perceived quite literally by the mother as her "product" and represents a personal accomplishment. But when the child is "defective" or lags behind in developing normal functions, he may elicit a different response from the mother. It is as if she asks herself: "How could I have produced this defective, unappealing child?" If, as part of her own personality, she is experiencing a great deal of guilt, she may view the child as punishment for real or imagined transgressions. She may experience hostility, a feeling that is intolerable because she basically loves the child. As a result, she may tend to become overly protective or overly indulgent in order to compensate for the underlying hostility to the child. This may deprive the child of opportunities for growth and development of adaptive secondary ego functions. Instead, the child becomes adept at using his handicap as a way of controlling his parents. In a very real sense he becomes the dependent despot. This manipulative overdependency plays a large role in the power struggles set up between parent and child. The same kind of behavior is ultimately displaced onto the school and becomes a problem between teacher and child (Abrams and Kaslow, 1977).

In summary, the child who has suffered an early injury to the central nervous system may not develop certain fundamental ego skills at the time that he should develop them. This lag in development may bring about an altered maternal response from the environment in that the mother may respond to this offspring not as a wished-for extension of herself but rather as a threat to her own narcissism. This further interferes with the development of secondary ego functions. The disturbance both in ego development and subsequently in the child's ability to learn efficaciously can be alleviated by the proper type of psychoeducational programming along with other adjunctive modes of intervention.

Dyslexia

Dyslexia is a specific type of learning disability characterized by severe problems in the recognition of the printed symbol. Hinshelwood (1917) referred to the condition as word blindness, and he attributed it to a congenital defect in the cerebral cortex. Rabinovitch (1962) prefers the term "primary reading retardation," which he defines as follows:

The capacity to learn to read is impaired without definite brain damage being suggested in the case history or upon neurological examination. The defect is in the ability to deal with letters and words as symbols, with resultant diminished ability to integrate the meaningfulness of written material. The problem appears to reflect a basic disturbed pattern of neurological organization. (p. 74)

The ego functioning of the dyslexic child is, in many cases, almost antithetical to the ego functioning of the brain-damaged child. The dyslexic (or primary retarded reader) does not usually evidence problems of impulse control, nor is he hyperactive and hyperdistractible. Although he does suffer with intense feelings of inadequacy, these feelings are usually evident only in response to the reading situation. In the early years of the reading failure, the child often reacts quite favorably and confidently as long as he need not deal with verbal symbols. It is only when he is made daily to climb over that ten-foot wall of continued frustration for a number of years that his impotence begins to generalize even to those situations that do not require reading ability.

Dyslexia has been termed an idiopathic condition—that is, one whose cause is unknown. There is some evidence today to suggest that developmental dyslexia is a genetically determined constitutional disorder. Nevertheless, this concept would postulate only that there is a genetic predisposition. It does not imply that just because a biological disposition exists in a child that the child will necessarily develop dyslexia. The constitutional disorder may be the sine qua non, the causal condition that is necessary; not every child with this condition will become dyslexic. If in the initial stages of teaching the child to read, one could be made aware of this predisposition, one could probably modify the program in such a way that the difficulties could be circumvented.

The dyslexic child's major problem is symbolization or association. He experiences basic difficulty in the association of common experiences and the symbols (words) representing them. Since reading, in the last analysis, is a process of association, difficulty in this area means that the child will frequently encounter many problems in acquiring a sight vocabulary (a storehouse of immediately recognizable words). The dyslexic child tends to have less difficulty in association when both the visual and auditory sensory pathways are involved, as compared to the making of strictly visual associations.

Perhaps the most pervasive quality of the primary retarded reader is his incapacity for adequate means of expression and for sustained abstract attention. If this child is initiated into reading at a time when his ego deficiencies do not allow him to profit from the normal methods of teaching reading, he almost inevitably experiences failure. It is no wonder that a secondary emotional problem may then ensue, with great discouragement on the part of the child and a negative attitude toward reading. The negative attitude may account for many of those symptoms associated with the dyslexic child. It is no mere coincidence that this child has difficulty with concentration in dealing with only word-like or school-like material. The memory span of these children, when dealing with visual objects rather than letters, is quite superior. Their ability to make visual-visual associations is more than adequate when the stimuli are geometric rather than word-like. It is true that they most characteristically show better achievement in the nonverbal area of an intelligence test rather than in the verbal area. Nevertheless, an analysis of their responses indicates that poor performance in the verbal area is attributable directly to inability to concentrate on abstract stimuli. Concentration on concrete stimuli is superior even to that of achieving readers.

Over the years, much has been written concerning the relationship of visual perceptual problems, spatial orientation, and dominance factors in dyslexia. We have not been impressed with the importance of these factors in the remediation of dyslexia. This is a crucial issue because the parents of these children are exceedingly vulnerable to a host of questionable and expensive cult-oriented treatment approaches. The efficacy of these training methods in facilitating the acquisition of basic academic skills has yet to be established. There are still children today who are asked to walk on balance beams in the belief that this will magically help them learn to read. (Indeed, it might prove helpful if children were required to read books as they engaged in some of these perceptual-motor activities!)

In summary, dyslexia or primary reading retardation is a specific type of learning disability characterized by an associative learning problem, or more specifically, an inability to deal with letters and words as symbols. As a result, the child has tremendous difficulty in developing an adequate sight vocabulary that will permit him to master more advanced word analysis skills and to read with comprehension. The incidence of developmental dyslexia is rare (all too frequently it has been overused and has become a wastebasket term).

Nevertheless, it is a severe problem and is unquestionably exacerbated by the secondary emotional factors that inevitably arise. Gever (1970) points out that excessive failure creates the conditions for more and more failure. The failure experience becomes the etiological and sustaining agent of learning disorders. It is no wonder that the dyslexic child, having developed an aversive attitude toward reading and similar tasks, does so poorly on any task requiring selective attention to abstract or word-like stimuli.

Educational Issues

If we consider learning disabilities in the broad sense, as we have in this chapter, then we must recognize that the vast majority of the children who develop learning disorders do so not because of neurological or psychological shortcomings but because of pedagogical failings. Stauffer (1978) indicates that almost all qualified educators admit that children who are likely to experience extreme difficulty in learning to read can be identified in first grade, if not earlier in the preschool years. Yet most schools continue to devote most of their funds to trying to cure or correct disabilities rather than to prevent them.

Probably the greatest cause for the milder learning problems is to be found in the group of conditions that might be classified as educational. Many reading problems, for example, are brought about by ineffective teaching or some other deficiency in the educational situation. Once the child has begun to have some problem in school, his deficiences are exacerbated because he does not have the skills to acquire new learning. In turn, as pointed out above, he feels inadequate and frustrated, which interferes with his ability to attend and to concentrate and increases the probability that he will not learn.

Probably the major educational issue related to learning deficiency is the all-too-frequent circumstance in which a child is not taught at his true instructional level. Many clinicians and teachers are not trained to evaluate the child's instructional needs and to appraise his proper level of functioning. If, for example, the clinician relies solely upon a standardized test of reading achievement to determine the instructional level in reading, many children will be placed one to three levels above their true instructional level. Frustrated by material that is much too difficult for them, the children, not surprisingly, lose their interest in reading and often withdraw from the reading process.

Many learning problems appear to develop because of an inappropriate match between the capabilities of children and the instructional demands placed on them. An appreciable number of children who arrive at the first grade are not ready to read in the typical program. Many of these children require an extensive period of readiness before they have sufficient skills to cope with the requirements involved in learning to read. If a child is introduced to reading activities before he is ready physically, intellectually, socially, and emotionally, he is not likely to experience success in classroom reading activities.

The importance of effective teaching cannot be overestimated in the etiology of the milder learning disorders. Many factors can contribute to an unsatisfactory teaching experience. The fact that children differ from one another, most times distinctly so but sometimes quite subtly, can be both the boon and the bond of instruction. The range of differences when recognized and utilized is what make teaching and learning exciting and invigorating. If instruction is to truly be differentiated, then the teacher must be properly trained and cannot simply give lip service to the factor of individual differences. Surprising as it may seem, there are still many classes in which children are all taught at the same reading level. Sometimes there is an undue emphasis upon the mechanics of reading to the neglect of the major purpose of reading—that is, reading for meaning. In other situations, administrative policies may either prevent adjustment of instruction to individual differences or not give the teacher sufficient time to provide proper readiness for learning.

Social and Emotional Factors

Psychologists and psychiatrists alike have long recognized that emotional and personality maladjustments occur in conjunction with learning difficulty. Much of the controversy in this area has raged around the chicken or the egg proposition over which is cause and which effect. Most children with severe learning disabilities do have concomitant emotional problems that have resulted from constant failure. Nevertheless, this is not to imply that the converse is not also true. That is, there are social and emotional factors that may result in learning problems.

Pearson (1954) discusses disorders of the learning

process in terms of two major classifications: (1) when the learning process is not involved with the neurotic conflict, and (2) when the learning process is involved with the neurotic conflict. In the first case, he refers to the problem of deflection of attention. Children's conflicts, whether they are perceived consciously as worries, guilt, or shame and embarrassment, or whether they occur in the unconscious portions of the ego, attract the children's attention to themselves and deflect it to a greater or lesser extent from all external considerations. To put it in a slightly different way, the children simply do not have sufficient mental energy available for learning.

When the learning process is involved in the neurotic conflict, the situation is more complicated. It may be that the child has a positive motivation not to learn. It may be that the nature of the child's emotional conflicts is such that it becomes dangerous for him to learn. For example, learning to read may become equated in the unconscious with growing up. If children feel for any reason that to grow up is undesirable and perhaps even dangerous, they may unconsciously resist developing the skills that represent becoming independent. Some children may resist learning because it puts them into a situation in which they must be competitive. If they fear their aggressive impulses, and indeed are unable to differentiate between destructive hostility and acceptable self-assertiveness, they may assume a radically passive posture, almost precluding any possibility of their being sufficiently aggressive to learn.

Some children unconsciously use learning, or rather not learning, as a weapon to express resentment toward the parental figures. This is an effective weapon and one over which the child maintains complete control. Nobody can make him learn if he does not want to. The older child who is angry at his parents may use nonlearning as a two-edged sword—he punishes his parents and also himself. He feels so guilty because of his resentment toward the parents that he must appease his guilt through self-punishment.

An overly harsh superego can lead to a restriction of the ego and abandoning of one activity after another. In one child, for example, there was a tremendous amount of hostility stemming from her feelings of emotional deprivation. She could not aim the hostility outward as she felt it, but instead had to masochistically turn the hostility on herself. One aspect of her hostility was her wish to flout authoritarian dictates. The only way she could achieve that without risking further rejection or emotional deprivation was by being inadequate. That is, when an authority figure told her to succeed, and instead she was inadequate, she was flouting that authority. This is akin to the intrapunitive theme mentioned earlier.

Abrams (1971) formulates an approach to psychogenic learning problems in which the emphasis is upon the pervasive quality of resistance to the reading or learning process. Symbolically the ability to read and success in learning represent an accomplishment that the child at all costs must avoid. Three types of resistances are described: the fear of exploration or "I must resist looking" syndrome; the fear of aggression or "I must resist success" syndrome; and fear of independence or "I must resist growing up" syndrome. Abrams cautions clinicians that only in some cases of severe reading disability is the problem a manifestation of underlying unconscious conflicts that create an actual resistance to the learning process. He emphasizes again the importance of recognizing the multiplicity of factors that can cause learning disabilities.

Belmont (1964) is aware of this and speaks of organic disturbance and maturational disturbances, as well as environmental and neurotic disorders, affecting the learning process. Among the environmental factors he discusses are the child's home and school milieu, the family stability, acts of fate, seduction, the opportunity for identification, and the personality of the teacher herself.

The attitudes of the parental figures toward the child play an extremely influential role in determining his receptivity to the learning process. If the parents have infantilized or overprotected the child, he will not be ready for school. Conversely, some families place undue stress upon the necessity for school achievement. The child learns quickly that it is imperative for him to achieve in order to maintain an adequate affectional relationship with the mother figure. When the child begins to despair of ever completely gaining his parents' approval, he may withdraw from the struggle. It is as if he realizes that his parents are too hard for him to please and that no matter what he does, he will only meet with criticism; he is unable to satisfy them, so why try?

Some children experience difficulty in learning because of inadequate cognitive stimulation during the early years. The culturally deprived child does not experience the same impetus to ego development as is experienced by the child from a more stimulating environment. On the whole, this child has had limited contact with the outside world. He has experienced less opportunity to listen to the kind of complex speech that will enhance his own vocabulary development. His conceptual repertoire is quite limited. In many cases, he develops a language extraordinarily different from the language that he is exposed to in the average school. As a result, he performs less well on the verbal measures that are characteristically used in a typical school situation.

Summary

In the area of *etiological considerations*, we recognize that determining the cause of learning disabilities is no easy task. In many cases, a combination of factors contribute to a child's difficulty in learning. In practically every case, the child's failure itself and his reactions to failure become another sustaining agent in the perpetuation of the learning disability. A viable approach to a comprehensive understanding of the causes of learning disabilities is to focus on the ego functioning of the child—essentially a dynamic-developmental-interaction orientation. Utilizing this viewpoint, we have discussed disorders in the neurological substratum of the ego—the central nervous system; a specific type of learning disability, dyslexia; all important educational factors; and social and emotional considerations as well. When one recognizes the multiplicity of the factors that can effect a learning disability, it is clear that tunnel vision must be avoided at all costs in dealing with the child who is experiencing a learning problem. Only then can we be reasonably assured that our diagnostic, habilitative, and remedial procedures can prove effective.

Diagnostic Considerations

It has been emphasized repeatedly that a unitary approach to the diagnosis of learning disabilities is highly fallible. Learning problems are caused and sustained by any number of factors. In any comprehensive evaluation, one must view the youngster experiencing learning difficulty as a physical organisim functioning in a social environment in a psychological manner. The corrollary to this is that in every child there exists a unique interaction of both functional and organic factors.

The basic hypothesis stated above leads inevitably to the conclusion that a multidisciplinary approach to the diagnosis of severe learning disability constitutes the optimal way of understanding and treating this complicated problem. The major purposes of any diagnostic evaluation are to determine the existence and severity of the learning disability, the specific strengths and weaknesses, and the therapeutic steps needed to ameliorate the condition. In order for diagnosis to be effective, it must also result in accurate communication to the remedial clinician, the therapist, the school and the parent, of sufficient information about the problem so that a profitable program of rehabilitation will result.

In order to comprehend fully all the factors that may be contributing to the child's learning difficulty, information must be obtained in five major areas. First, a detailed history is required to provide the contextual basis for understanding and interpreting all the clinical and test data to be obtained. Second, there should be careful analysis of the child's current physical-social and emotional status. Third, an individually obtained assessment of the child's intelligence is required. Fourth, there must be measures of specific capacity, including perceptual motor skills, associative learning ability, and memory span. Finally, the presenting picture with respect to achievement in each of the academic and communication areas involved must be detailed sufficiently to clarify the specific nature of the child's difficulties and the resources that he has available to him in meeting any learning demands which are made upon him.

History

As already noted, the child's adjustment mechanisms employed at any particular time are a product of the accumulated dynamics of his interaction with his environment since conception. It is important, therefore, to gain as much insight as possible into the sequence of this behavioral development. A detailed history of his growth and development should be obtained as a first step in the diagnostic process. Through interviews with the parents and the child himself, a skillful interviewer can elicit most of the significant information desired. In many instances, especially in getting accurate data in the medical or educational history, it will be necessary to contact the physician, the hospital, or the school to verify information given or to supplement it with additional items of significance. In an occasional case, other family members and/or other professional workers who have had clinical contact with the client may need to be consulted for further data.

Five highly related areas of significance bear careful objective study in obtaining the history of the development of a problem. The first of these pertains to the family constellation itself and the child's positioning within the family group. For each member of the family and others who may be living in the home, information about their age, educational experience and achievement, occupation, general health factors, interests, hobbies, normal daily schedule of activities, and general reading habits should be obtained. A general description of the home itself and the community within which it is located, recreational spaces available, library facilities, reading matter within the home, and work areas suitable for private study are recorded. One should also obtain a brief medical and social history of the mother's and the father's families and nature of the extended family support in the past and present.

Second, all facts pertinent to the prenatal, perinatal, and postnatal development must be obtained. Major importance rightly is attributed to the record if, for example, the child was a small premature infant, or had neonatal bilirubin encephalopathy or meningitis in early infancy. There are traumas that accompany the birth process that will be of interest to the diagnostician. One might almost wish to have a detailed obstetrical history in making an initial assessment of possible brain lesions in the full-term newborn. There is also conflicting evidence concerning the effect of prolonged labor, precipitous delivery, and intracranial pressure at the time of birth, caused by forceps delivery or a narrow pelvic arch in the mother.

Pasamanick and Knobloch (1961) have coined the term "reproductive casualty" to account for the sequelae of harmful events during pregnancy and the birth process; most of the resulting damage to fetuses and newborn infants is in the central nervous system. Because fetal and neonatal deaths are largely associated with complications of pregnancy and/or prematurity, these potentially brain-damaging events might result in children who do not succumb, but go on to develop a series of neuropsychiatric disorders. Depending upon the specific nature and extent of the insult to the brain, the disorders might range from gross neurologic impairment to the more subtle specific and nonspecific disabilities labeled as minimal brain dysfunction and dyslexia. It may well be that the greater vulnerability of the male fetus and neonate may account for the higher incidence of learning problems among boys. (This is in no way meant to minimize the importance of social, emotional, and cultural factors in effecting more learning problems among boys.)

Throughout the country, intensive studies of neonates are being made, many of these dealing with those infants who fail to grow to normal size before birth. The survival of infants seems to be profoundly affected by the birth weight; the lower the weight of newborn, the greater the danger he or she faces. Wessel (1979) presents data to support the construct of a continuum of reproductive casualty in that certain types of delivery clearly increase the likelihood of later impaired or delayed performance. In addition, the findings of his investigation provide evidence that argues strongly for a developmental-interaction approach to the diagnosis of learning disability. An analysis of his results supports the view that both constitutional and environmental factors are responsible for the impact of the birth process and obstetrical medication on the developmental status of the child.

The third area of importance in the history involves the medical and psychological record. Accidents, illnesses, immunizations, and behavioral characteristics noted preceding and following each of these instances should be included. It is often necessary for the clinician to follow up on a recorded medical episode or previous psychological evaluation by contacting the physician or psychologist involved in the treatment for additional data. Once again, of particular significance will be those episodes that appear to have bearing upon subsequent neurological and/or communication functioning.

Fourth, it is important to acquire as much information as possible about the social and emotional development of the child. Knowledge of the phases and stages of personality development is important in any assessment process of the child with learning disability. Genetically, the child's social and emotional adjustment is explored with questions related to his feeding habits, sleeping habits, nervous symptoms, early interpersonal relationships, and first experiences in school.

Finally the entire school record is examined carefully. The child's social and emotional adjustment to his fellow students and to his teacher is reviewed with as much care as his academic performance in each grade. The child's initial reaction to school, regularity of attendance, early symptoms of difficulty, attempts at that point to identify the problem and provide assistance, referrals for diagnosis, tutoring, and remedial treatment—all may have bearing on his current difficulties and should be carefully recorded.

Assessment of Physical Factors

A thorough diagnosis of learning disability should include visual screenings designed to evaluate the coordinate functioning of the eyes. Specifically, the screening should be directed to detect problems of visual efficiency—that is, accommodation, convergence, and the relationship established between accommodation and convergence. The diagnosis and treatment of a visual problem rightly belongs in the realm of the vision specialist who is trained to handle such problems. But the diagnostician of the learning disability should be equipped to screen out visual difficulty that may affect the child's ability to learn. Exclusive reliance on the Snellen Chart is inadequate for detecting problems that might contribute to learning difficulty. Such procedures as the Keystone Visual Screening Test, the Ortho-Rater, or the Massachusetts Vision Test offer more comprehensive methods to detect visual anomalies.

Hearing problems may play a role in the etiology of learning disabilities. Since reading is taught in most schools as a process whereby the child associates printed symbols with speech sounds, the student having a hearing loss is readily confused. Some children do not experience any difficulty in auditory acuity, but are unable to discriminate between similar sounds (auditory discrimination). There is fairly wide agreement that an audiometer should be used to screen hearing. Further assessment of auditory acuity for children includes tests of speech-sound discrimination and informal observations.

It is difficult to interpret the minor signs that are found in a significant number of presumably normal children and yet which are often considered to be "soft signs" suggesting minimal brain damage. Some representative signs are abnormal eye movements, clumsiness, visual-perceptual problems, and articulation defects. The Bender Visual-Motor Gestalt Test (1938) has been increasingly utilized (particularly by school psychologists) to detect the presence of brain damage in children. There needs to be much caution here. Although it is probably true that relatively few brain-damaged children do well on the Bender-Gestalt, it is equally true that not all children who do poorly suffer from neurologic impairment.

Assessment of Social and Emotional Status

A clinical evaluation of the child can be of inestimable aid in understanding the child's strengths and weaknesses relevant to his emotional status. Specifically, the diagnostician in this area is concerned with the child's ability to see things as other people see them, his capacity to relate to other persons, and his effectiveness in dealing with his ideas and feelings in an adaptive manner. The clinician attempts to learn how the child copes with disturbing emotions. He attempts to discern the maneuvers the child employs to bring about desired reactions from others; he also studies the particular defense mechanisms that the child utilizes which may facilitate or impede educational progress. Abrams (1968) states that the ego defense mechanisms are the most important emotional factors affecting learning. He feels that the emphasis in the assessment of the emotional factors related to learning disabilities should move away from the conflicts themselves to the ego defenses erected to cope with these conflicts.

The diagnostician should also give much of his attention to the child's perception of important people in his environment. He is concerned with the child's attitude toward his parents, toward other authority figures including teachers, and toward his own peers. The perception of the child may not necessarily coincide with reality. The child can see the teacher as frightening because of displacement of anxiety. In essence, the diagnostician, through the clinical evaluation of the child, attempts to acquire a clear-cut picture of important factors that would either be etiological or sustaining to the learning disability.

In addition to the clinical observations of the child, psychological testing may make an important contribution to understanding the nature of the emotional factors in the learning disability. For example, the psychologist must determine if there is any significant discrepancy between the child's functioning intelligence level and his potential capacity. Through a careful quantitative and qualitative analysis of inter- and intratest variability, as well as the verbalizations of the child, the psychologist searches for any significant interference to the thinking processes. Individual variations reflecting on the personality of the child are manifested on every subtest of an individual intelligence scale. Let us examine, for example, three different responses to the question: "What is the thing to do if you cut your finger?" (Each of the following responses earn the maximum number of points for a correct answer.) (1) "I would put a band-aid on it." (2) "I would wash it off; I would then put on mercurochrome or iodine; I would get a band-aid and then a bandage; and maybe I would go to the doctor." (3) "How big a cut is it? (Said with intense affect) Was my finger cut off? I guess I would get a bandage or a band-aid, but is it really bad?" These responses reveal unquestionably important personality factors of each child. The first child answers the question immediately, exercising good judgment and experiencing no difficulty in making a decision. The second child, less decisive, must consider many different possibilities; there is almost an obsessive-compulsive quality to the response. The third child shows perhaps an excessive fear of bodily injury (some question of bodily integrity?).

In addition to the formal evaluation of the thinking processes, the psychological assessment will usually include projective testing. The child, in responding to relatively unstructured materials, will project his own ideas and feelings, his conflicts and anxieties, on these stimuli and thereby furnish a kind of x-ray of the personality. By carefully interpreting the results of projective tests, the psychologist may gain very important clues as to the child's general effectiveness in a learning situation.

More specifically, the psychological evaluation will be aimed at assessing the child's ability to organize and synthesize life experience into meaningful goal-directed patterns. It will explore the child's ability to differentiate between what is constructively aggressive and what is destructively aggressive. If this ability is lacking, for example, then the child will not be able to be assertive in the learning situation and will not be able to compete.

The psychological evaluation will also be directed to evaluate the child's attitudes toward dependency, his feelings about anger and rage, his need to inflict punishment upon himself, his level of aspiration, his motivation and his self-concept. In essence, the psychological evaluation should help to determine whether there is truly a psychogenic etiology to the learning disability or if symptoms of emotional maladjustment result from continued frustration and failure in school.

Assessment of Intellectual Factors

Since we have defined learning disability as representing some discrepancy between achievement and intelligence level, the diagnosis must include an individual measure of intelligence. Although a number of such instruments are available, those devised by David Wechsler are most commonly used. In cases of reading disability, they are particularly appropriate, since they combine measures of verbal and nonverbal intellectual abilities and provide a scattering of subtests measuring specific abilities that appear to be highly related to difficulties in reading. In addition to the overall intelligence score and the comparison between verbal and performance tests as a whole, those subtests related to concept formation, perceptual abilities, memory span, and visual-motor associational skills are often particularly helpful to the clinician.

A good clinician uses the results of an intelligence test in much the same way as a detective uses clues to solve a mystery. Nothing is left to chance or just considered an anomaly. The basic principle is determinism; the working assumption is that little if anything occurs by chance. Every subtest score, every single response, and every part of every response must be viewed as significant and as representative of the subject. When a response deviates greatly from what is conventional, this means something much more than the fact that an error has been made. If, for example, one child says: "Columbus discovered America," while another child of the same age responds: "I know you expect me to say Columbus, but actually it was Leif Ericson and his Vikings, while more recently there has been considerable evidence suggesting the Japanese came even earlier," both responses would be scored as correct. Nevertheless, it is clear that we are dealing with two different kinds of personalities.

It is foolhardy to analyze the data obtained from an individual intelligence test strictly on the basis of characteristic test patterns. True, there are clusters of test patterns associated with different types of learning disorders, but this kind of analysis is effective only when it is carried out in a perceptive, nonbiased manner with much attention focused on the dynamic quality of the verbalizations. With this caution in mind, one can more profitably use an intelligence test to detect certain perceptual and conceptual deficiencies that are frequently manifested in various learning disability syndromes. Decker (1964) has discussed the kinds of errors made by the typically brain-damaged child; Abrams (1975), the intellectual patterning expected in two types of dyslexics; and Pikulski (1978), the implications of intelligence-test findings in a variety of cases of reading disability.

Although some diagnostic aspects regarding intelligence testing have been discussed, we have only touched the tip of the iceberg. Intelligence ultimately is nothing more than the social application of ego functions. All that has been written concerning ego development must certainly apply to the development of intelligence as well. For too many years educators have been subjected to outdated mechanistic intelligence models. It is no wonder that so many complain about psychological evaluations and state that this kind of testing is of little value in helping the child. The search for pathological signs has increased but is essentially fruitless (a cookbook approach); the validities of isolated scores and indicators have proved low, fluctuating, and of no practical usefulness. The understanding of what has led to specific thinking processes requires an investment in comprehending all aspects of the child in an integrated fashion.

Assessment of Specific Capacities

Perceptual-motor abilities, while measured to some extent in certain subtests of the Wechsler scales, bear further evaluation. The Bender Visual-Motor Gestalt Test (1938) is the most frequently used measure of perceptual-motor functioning. Several variations of the original procedure for administration and scoring this instrument have been developed. The results are often used to recommend a program of perceptual training. On the other hand, poor performance on the Bender Gestalt test may be ascribed to a number of different factors: perceptual deficit alone, motor dysfunction, inefficient coordination of visual and motor processes, anxiety interference, or simply negativism on the part of the child.

The Frostig Developmental Test of Visual Perception (1963) assesses five areas that may be related to academic skills: figure-ground relationships, eye-hand coordination, form constancy, position in space, and spatial relationships. Motor skills are necessary for adequate performance in each subtest. The DTVP yields a "perceptual quotient" with norms for children from ages four to seven. However, there is little evidence to suggest that the Frostig actually has the diagnostic ability to measure five separate visual perception skills. Some have also questioned whether the skills measured by the Frostig are significantly related to achievement in school.

Several assumptions have been made about the interrelationship between visual perception and motor ability. Some have indicated that visual perception is dependent upon learning gross motor skills. This implies that disorders in gross motor skills should be corrected before training in visual perception is undertaken. If, for example, during his early years a child was handicapped in the development of motility because of inadequate ego apparatuses, he would not be likely to develop a sense of mastery that would also contribute to a sense of identity. In any event, some kind of evaluation should be made of the child's motor development.

We have previously discussed the importance of associative learning ability in the reading process. In order to evaluate associative learning ability, the tests probably most frequently employed are the Gates Associative Learning Test (1928) and the Van Wagenen Reading Readiness Test–Word Learning Cards (1938). Distinct patterns of functioning on these batteries have been used clinically to designate children who are likely to experience extreme difficulty in learning to recognize words when the teaching modalities employed are only a visual or a combination of visual-auditory.

We have also referred to difficulties with attention and concentration as they relate to learning disability. Although some memory abilities are involved in responding to most individual test items in any area, a specific memory-span battery is helpful in identifying the nature of the child's ability to attend to and retain stimuli experienced in different modalities. The Wechsler Memory Scale (1942) or specific memory subtests selected from the Detroit Tests of Learning Aptitude (1941) are often employed. Tests used to measure attention and concentration should be composed of both discrete and related items as well as stimuli presented in various modalities (visual, auditory, or a combination of these).

From a psychodynamic point of view, we may interpret our test findings on attention and concentration in a different way. Rapaport (1946) points out that attention suffers first under the impact of stress, anxiety, and/or overvalent feelings of inadequacy. As long as individuals have at their disposal a reserve of mental energies not specifically tied up with these affects and anxieties, they are able to call upon this reservoir, as it were, and to concentrate. Even at this time the process requires great effort, and individuals may evidence a high degree of stress by the reduction in their spontaneity and creativity. In actuality, their energies are bound up in their defenses and therefore not available for free, passive attending. Nevertheless, they are able to concentrate and still function in a somewhat impaired fashion.

If the stress situation continues beyond a certain

point, people are inevitably forced to exhaust their reserves; they use up the energies that were not intimately associated with conflict and anxiety. It is at this point that concentration, too, becomes impaired. No longer can individuals force themselves to function. It is as if now they are exceedingly vulnerable to the stresses of the environment and the concomitant anxiety.

Kirk and Kirk (1971) suggest that the Illinois Test of Psycholinguistic Abilities (Kirk, McCarthy, and Kirk, 1968) is an effective instrument to assess specific capacities and their connections with language. Possible problems in each of the following areas may be studied: (1) basic processes (input, integration, output); (2) different channels (visual-motor and auditory-vocal); and (3) levels (representational and automatic).

Assessment of Educational Skills

The educational evaluation of the child is of utmost importance in determining the nature of the habilitative and remedial steps to be pursued. Thus it is almost unbelievable that frequently a child with learning disability is evaluated without the benefit of an educational diagnosis.

It is the responsibility of the clinician to determine where the child is functioning in all aspects of language development, such as listening, speaking, reading, and writing. More specifically, he must appraise (a) how well the child's current achievement compares with his intelligence level; (b) how his performance matches up with the performance of other children of his age; (c) what level of material he can be expected to read on his own and where he will most profit from instruction (not to mention where he will be frustrated by the complexity of the material); and (d) how well he can evaluate his own performance and be aware of his own deficiencies.

For many years now it has become generally accepted that the answers to most of the questions stated above can best be elicited by the intelligent use of informal inventories. Although the group reading inventory provides a valuable instrument for determining levels of performance, a much more thorough and diagnostic method is to appraise the performance of each pupil individually. In essence this procedure consists of having the child read orally at sight and then silently from a series of reading selections that increase in order of difficulty. Comprehension is checked by means of factual, inferential, and vocabulary type questions. Information regarding achievement levels and specific deficiencies in language and reading can be gleaned from the proper administration of an informal reading inventory.

In addition to informal evaluation techniques, there are two other major approaches to evaluating reading: criterion referenced measures and standardized reading procedures. The categories are not mutually exclusive. In most cases, criterion referenced evaluation offers more valuable information for instructional planning than does norm referenced evaluation. Two popular standardized tests, the Peabody Individual Achievement Test (PIAT) (1970) and the Wide Range Achievement Test (WRAT) (1965), have serious limitations. For example, the WRAT reading subtest seriously overestimates a child's reading ability and tends to place the child at his frustration level rather than the instructional level.

A number of formal standardized tests are available to assess a child's specific skill strengths and weaknesses in arithmetic. One important aspect that should be considered in selecting such a test is the number of arithmetic subskills evaluated. Those tests that provide a profile of skills will be helpful in planning a program of remediation. The Key Math Diagnostic Arithmetic Test (1971) is one of the most frequently used instruments. The test is individually administered and designed to evaluate math ability from preschool through grade six, with no upper limits for remedial use.

Summary

In the area of *diagnostic considerations* we have stressed the importance of a multidisciplinary approach to the learning disabled child. Competent assessment procedures require that the child be viewed with a sound conceptual framework. There are many possible pitfalls in the evaluation of any youngster with a learning problem. It is certainly important that the observations and testing be perceptive and accurate; the interpretation of both clinical and test findings depends to a great extent upon the competence of the diagnostician. We have reviewed the five major areas that need to be evaluated in understanding the nature of the learning disability and what should be the habilitative and remedial steps to ameliorate the problem. These consist of the history; the physical, social, and emotional status; intelligence; specific capacities; and the educational status. The findings in these areas must not be used mechanically. The experienced clinician recognizes that he is dealing with interactions of factors that operate upon the child in a dynamic fashion. Feeling cannot be separated from cognition, emotion from perception, nor affect from concept formation.

Treatment Considerations

As has been repeatedly emphasized, the approach to learning disabilities used here is rooted in the tenents of psychoanalytic ego psychology, or what we have called the dynamic-developmental-interaction approach. This viewpoint considers varied influences in a child's development as they relate to other aspects of life, rather than assessing each one of them in isolation. It is valuable in exploring the theoretical background of learning disorders and in determining adequate diagnosis and appropriate habilitation or remediation.

In a number of different papers Abrams and Kaslow (1976, 1977) have identified a number of possible intervention approaches, each of which might constitute the "treatment of choice" depending upon a variety of factors. In the ensuing discussion these will be considered and expanded upon.

Special School Placement

When a child experiences a severe learning disability, it may become necessary to consider a special school placement. There are undoubtedly many reasons why a child with severe learning problems may require the setting of a special school. Some of the advantages he encounters in such a setting include smaller classes and more realistic instructional levels. There is usually more teacher personnel with increased sophistication and tolerance for disruptive behavior. The class is generally grouped in such a way that the child with difficulties does not stand out in such great relief as he formerly had in his regular school.

In setting up such a program, the necessity for structure must be kept in mind. The brain-damaged child, in particular, may be disturbed by changes in routine and by unexpected situations. Proper structuring of the child's environment will go far in reducing the child's anxiety level and alleviating the basic tendency to be hyperactive, hyperdistractible, and disinhibited. By a structured environment, we are not talking about a situation characterized by extreme rigidity. Warmth and concern for the child can exist in a setting of structure where the youngster is not overly stimulated. The teacher must be comfortable with structure, be able to establish limitations, and be able to maintain limitations. The manner in which firm limits are applied is extremely important.

Learning Therapy

The thrust of this type of intervention is based on the premise that the experienced teacher can utilize many psychotherapeutic techniques to supplement his teaching skills. Teachers of children with severe learning disabilities must be selected with great care. Waldman (1970) has pointed out that the predominant goal is to help the teacher become a learning therapist. Often an understanding of the child's psychodynamics can help the teacher to respond in an appropriate fashion. Frequently there is a lack of constructive attention to the intrapsychic and interpersonal factors that interfere with the acquisition and utilization of academic skills. These interferences are often similar to conflicts which the child has experienced at home. For example, the same frustration and anger that have been experienced by the parent in his relationship with the child may also be felt by the teacher and, as with the parent, may serve to bring about an inflexible approach to the child that will lessen the teacher's effectiveness. The teacher who expresses anger overtly and punitively, or who tries very hard to teach while feeling great unexpressed frustration, or who feels ashamed and guilty about his anger, cannot be expected to consistently maintain the role of a helping person. While the teacher who is continually in a position of having to face a child who arouses much anger in him may with great strain and effort brush aside or teach through these feelings, he cannot be the steadying influence or auxiliary ego the child needs.

We have found that empathic, intuitive, and experienced teachers can be trained to be more attentive to stratagems that can help the learning disabled child accommodate more readily to the classroom. Following the lead of Waldman (1971), teachers have been trained to use a hierarchy of techniques within four major areas: preventive techniques, which are used in an effort to insure that the child's classroom milieu does not contribute to his ego disruptions; defusion techniques, which are brought to bear when prevention has failed; integrative techniques, which enlist the child's ego in critically examining his behavior so that he can see the pattern which has constantly been tripping him up; and techniques for maintaining contact, which are everyone's province but are especially relevant to the teacher who daily works with the child. Through these techniques, the learning therapist shows the child that he is important to him.

The learning therapist does *not* replace the individual psychotherapist. Rather, the former has a predominant goal to teach the child skills within the context of a good understanding of him and his needs.

Remedial Techniques

When the nature of the child's specific learning disabilities has been adequately diagnosed, the necessary remedial procedures may then be instituted. Multisensory approaches to reading instruction usually attempt to develop reading skills through auditory, visual, kinesthetic, and tactile stimulation. Many children with severe reading disabilities are greatly assisted when the visual-auditory-kinesthetic techniques (VAK) and the visual-auditory-kinesthetic-tactile technique (VAKT) are employed. These are techniques that provide additional sensory reinforcement. Writing or even tracing the word is useful not only because of possible kinesthetic-tactile facilitation of memory but because the child's attention is called to the word. The very nature of the kinesthetic-tactile approach is one that forces concentration and attention. If we postulate that one of the factors interfering with concentration and attention is the child's own anxiety and narcissism, then any technique that will force concentration will be helpful.

By having the child write and read or dictate and read stories that represent his present interests and his past experiences, we are making certain that he is always dealing with concepts with which he is already familiar. Any words he learns in these stories, he should always encounter again in new and different contexts, so that there is a great deal of reinforcement. As the child finds that he can learn and retain words through the use of VAK and VAKT, and as he sees that he is successful in the reading tasks prepared especially for him, greater satisfaction comes from trying than from evading.

The improved attention and concentration usually occur not only within the word learning situations but in other areas as well. Even in listening activities, concentration becomes more important, more worthy of expenditure of energy, because the child is actually concerned about the ideas he can get through concentrating on materials read to him. In reading, the material commands attention because he can get meaning from it, something that may not have been true in the past. Stauffer (1978) has probably described the Fernald technique more effectively than any other author.

The Gillingham approach is also based upon a multisensory technique for learning specific reading skills. In contrast to the Fernald technique, the Gillingham approach emphasizes individual letters.

Additional Therapeutic Modalities

When the child's problems are largely internalized and personality restructuring appears to be advisable, intensive child therapy stands out as the treatment of choice. If the child is ego disturbed, some modifications in traditional clinical practice are warranted. The nature of the child with ego disturbance does not allow him to adapt to the usual approaches employed in psychotherapy as it is traditionally practiced. Rappaport (1961) has excellently described the nature of the therapy employed with a brain-injured child.

A thorough assessment of the child's ego skills may prove fruitless if one does not consider the family constellation in which the child must function. When a child and parents are amenable to help but each needs the treatment and therapist to himself, they should be seen by different therapists who collaborate closely. In other instances conjoint family therapy of child, siblings, and parents is indicated. The reader is referred to Abrams and Kaslow (1976) for more information in this area.

Conclusion

We have emphasized in this discussion that learning disabilities have multiple determinants. The concept of a circumscribed area of learning disability is highly questionable. In actuality, there are many kinds of learning disorders, and each may require different types of intervention. We must recognize further that many children who have experienced severe learning disabilities have packed a lifetime of pain into a few years. Much of this pain has been associated with the struggle to maintain their dignity in spite of an organism that refuses to be efficient. In this struggle, and unfortunately contributing to it, have been relationships with people—parents, siblings, other relatives, peers, well-meaning acquaintances, and teachers. These relationships have often added immeasurable distortions and complications to an already intolerable situation. Consequently, the interpersonal nature of their lives takes on a quality of warpage that drains their energy devastatingly. Without taking these crucial parts of the total picture into consideration when planning a reeducational program, there is little of real meaning to the techniques utilized. The best-thought-out strategies and programs established by the most learned people can have little lifelong value or durable impact if the interpersonal relationship patterns are impersonal, insincere or patronizing. It is the manner in which the contact with the child is maintained that determines the success or failure more than anything else. A psychodynamic, affective approach to children must replace the more traditional orientation, which has separated the cognitive from the emotional realm, a dichotomy that is superficial, to say the least.

References

Abrams, J.C. (1968) The role of personality defenses in reading. In G. Natchez, ed., *Children with Reading Problems.* New York: Basic Books.

Abrams, J.C. (1970) Learning disabilities—A complex phenomenon. *Reading Teacher* 23(4):299–303.

Abrams, J.C. (1971) Emotional resistances to reading. *J. Reading Specialist* 10(4):191–196.

Abrams, J.C. (1975) Minimal brain dysfunction and dyslexia. *Reading World* 14:219–227.

Abrams, J.C. (in press) A psychodynamic understanding of the emotional spects of learning disorders. In B. Keogh, ed., *Advances in Special Education.* Greenwich, Conn.: Jai Press.

Abrams, J.C., and F. Kaslow. (1976) Learning disability and family dynamics: A mutual interaction. *J. Clin. Child Psychol.* 5:35–40.

Abrams, J.C., and F. Kaslow. (1977) Family systems and the learning disabled child: Intervention and treatment. *J. Learning Disabilities* 10(2):27–31.

Abrams, J.C., and W. Smolen. (1973) On stress, failure, and reading disability. *J. Reading* 16:462–466.

Adamson, W. (1978) Questions, definitions, and perspectives. In W. Adamson and K. Adamson, eds., *A Handbook for Specific Learning Disabilities.* New York: Gardner Press.

Bateman, B. (1965) An educator's view of a diagnostic approach to learning disorders. In J. Hellmuth, ed., *Learning Disorders*, Vol. 1 Seattle: Special Child Publications.

Belmont, H.S. (1964) Psychological influences in learning. In *Sociological and Psychological Factors in Reading.* Philadelphia: Temple University Press.

Bender Visual-Motor-Gestalt Test. (1938) New York: Psychological Corporation.

Decker, R.J. (1964) Manifestations of the brain damage syndrome in historical and psychological data. In S.R. Rappaport, ed., *Childhood Aphasia and Brain Damage: A Definition.* Narberth, Pa.: Livingston.

Detroit Tests of Learning Aptitude. (1941) Indianapolis, Ind.: Test Division of Bobbs-Merrill.

Frostig, M. (1963) *Frostig Developmental Test of Visual Perception.* Consulting Psychologists Press.

Gates Associative Learning Tests. (1928) Philadelphia: Reading Clinic, Temple University.

Gever, B. (1970) Failure and learning disability. *Reading Teacher* 23(4):311–317.

Hinshelwood, J. (1917) *Congenital Word Blindness.* London: H.K. Lewis.

Key Math Diagnostic Arithmetic Test. (1971) Circle Pines, Minn.: American Guidance Service.

Kirk, S.A. (1962) *Educating Exceptional Children.* Boston: Houghton Mifflin.

Kirk, S.A., and W.D. Kirk. (1971) *Psycholinguistic Learning Disabilities: Diagnosis and Remediation.* Urbana, Ill.: University of Illinois Press.

Kirk, S.A., J.J. McCarthy, and W.D. Kirk. (1968) *Illinois Test of Psycholinguistic Abilities*, rev. ed. Urbana, Ill.: University of Illinois Press.

National Advisory Committee on Handicapped Children. (1968) *Special Education for Handicapped Children*, First Annual Report. Washington, D.C.: U.S. Department of Health, Education and Welfare, January 31, 1968.

Pasamanick, B., and H. Knobloch. (1961) Epidemiologic studies on the complications of pregnancy and the birth process. In G. Caplan, ed., *Prevention of Mental Disorders in Childhood.* New York: Basic Books.

Peabody Individual Achievement Test. (1970) Circle Pines, Minn.: American Guidance Service.

Pearson, G.H.J. (1954) *Psychoanalysis and the Education of the Child.* New York: Norton.

Pikulski, J. (1978) Factors related to reading problems. In R. Stauffer, J.C. Abrams, and J. Pikulski, eds., *Diagnosis, Corrections, and Prevention of Reading Disabilities.* New York: Harper & Row.

Rabinovitch, R. (1962) Dyslexia: Psychiatric considerations. In J. Money, ed., *Reading Disability: Progress and Research Needs in Dyslexia.* Baltimore: Johns Hopkins University Press.

Rapaport, D. (1946) *Diagnostic Psychological Testing.* Chicago: Yearbook Publishers.

Rappaport, S.R. (1961) Behavior disorder and ego development in a brain-injured child. *Psychoanal. Study Child* 16:423–450.

Rappaport, S.R., ed. (1964) *Childhood Aphasia and Brain*

Damage: A Definition. Narberth, Pa.: Livingston.

Recommendations of the Joint Committee on Learning Disabilities. (1976) Unpublished.

Stauffer, R., J.C. Abrams, and J. Pikulski. (1978) *Diagnosis, Corrections and Prevention of Reading Disabilities*. New York: Harper & Row.

Van Wagenen Reading Readiness Test. (1938) Minneapolis: Van Wagenen Psycho-Educational Research Laboratories, University of Minnesota.

Waldman, M. (1970) Psychodynamics and educational orientation in the special school. *Reading Teacher* 23(4):325–330.

Waldman, M. (1971) Adjunctive programming for special education teacher. Unpublished.

Wechsler Memory Scale. (1942) New York: Psychological Corporation.

Wessel, K. (1979) A prospective study of the relationship between the type of delivery and the use of medication and learning disabilities and ego disturbances in children. Unpublished doctoral dissertation.

Wide Range Achievement Test, rev. ed. (1965) Wilmington, Del.: Guidance Associates.

Treatment of Emotional Disorders in Children and Adolescents

CHAPTER 29

School Interventions: Case Management and School Mental Health Consultation

Irving H. Berkovitz

Introduction

Schools are children's natural habitat between the ages of 4 and 18, with the potential therein for growth or disability. Just as intervention with families is often crucial to help children, so may be the case with intervention in schools. Intervention in schools already does occur from many agencies and individuals of the community. Here I will describe those most possible and useful by child psychiatrists (or other mental health professionals) in private practice or in child oriented clinics and agencies.

While my discussion here may seem to highlight mainly the psychopathology in some children in schools, let me stress as well the positive growth enhancement that occurs during most children's school experiences. The majority of children entering schools find the presence of variably empathic, skilled personnel who assist them to tolerate the stress of separation from familial contexts. While it does not always occur to an ideal degree, many children learn to form satisfying and ego-enhancing relations with nurturant adults, who are not parents or otherwise related.

Children learn to relate to a new and larger group of peers, expanding and strengthening skills of interpersonal relating such as trusting, sharing, reciprocating, accepting disappointment, making new friends, etc. Most schools deemphasize or ignore the affective part of child development and school experience. Understandably, and appropriately, school personnel place a major emphasis on encouragement of cognitive capacities, acquisition of basic information, and development of learning skills and work habits. Developmentally, an important part of building or repairing self-esteem after the early childhood familial influences is the pride in mastery, accomplishment, and self-discipline that can be encouraged by skilled, conscientious educators. The value of learning as a mental health benefit has been emphasized from the days of Witmer and Dewey (Krugman, 1958; Ratner, 1937).

Unfortunately these benefits do not accrue to all children in schools. Various authors (Wickman, 1928; Rogers, 1942; Kellam et al., 1975) cite percentages varying from 7–14% of children in schools as showing "severe maladjustment" and as also needing mental health assistance. These authors mention also an additional 20% of pupils who are at risk but not yet disturbed. School experience, unhappily, at times, can perpetuate or increase these percentages. Most interventions in schools are made with the hope of reducing these percentages. Children are helped by other agencies as well, such as Head Start, probation, welfare, etc. Some of the remarks pertaining to intervention in schools may be relevant to these agencies as well.

Before a clinician enters *any* school setting, the following differences in orientation need to be carefully understood and observed:

Within the school milieu the psychiatrist is no longer on his old familiar "turf," the psychiatric office or hospital, but rather on the "home grounds" of a different but equally important professional in the child's life, the educator. Working with professionals in the field of education—principals, counselors, classroom teachers, etc., requires different skills than one needs in the treatment of patients in the office. These professionals are specialized in areas in which the psychiatrists have little knowledge or experience. Managing a classroom of thirty or more very different individuals, motivating them to learn, judging the limits of their capacity for attention, maintaining a sense of humor in the face of classroom disruptions, etc., and doing this for several hours every day, is a task which requires the highly developed interpersonal skills of most school teachers. (Berkovitz and Newman, 1980a)

Intervention in schools may occur with a variety of structures and purposes:

A. Case Management*:

1. To obtain data for better evaluation and/or treatment of individual child patients.

2. To intervene in school programs for the improvement of adjustment and growth, or to reduce damaging conditions, for individual children in therapy. This intervention may occur on the initiative of the therapist, or at the request of parents or at times of school personnel.

B. Mental Health Consultation:

1. To improve the school psychological milieu for as large a number of children as possible by consulting with the various categories of school personnel, in a case consultation or system-oriented format.

2. To assist school personnel in a staff development or in-service education context and to enhance skills in providing psychological services to students and at times to staff.

C. Child Psychiatric Training

1. To observe normal behavior for a better appreciation of the wide range of children's activities, to expand perspective as a child psychiatrist, and to develop better understanding of children in school.

D. Occasional Volunteer

1. As a citizen and/or parent in school support organizations such as the PTA and parent advisory councils or as volunteer faculty participating in health classes or other classes at the request of school personnel, one's own child, or a colleague providing a school program—for example, sex or drug education, career guidance, group counseling, desegregation assistance, etc.

Case Management

In the case of most children seen by the child therapist for evaluation or treatment of neurotic disorders, little school involvement is usually necessary beyond obtaining the minimum data available in school records. This can be done by letter or phone. In the cases of children with school problems, organic deficit, psychotic disorder, and certainly hyperkinesis, the need for greater school involvement may be more essential. In the case of small, private remedial or even nonremedial schools, this involvement may be fairly simple and easily achieved. In the case of public or parochial schools, it may not in all cases be as simple or as expeditious.

Unavoidably, mental health professionals and school personnel often have different concepts and criteria for designating behavioral pathology and emergencies.

Furthermore, the traditional referral model must be abandoned. In the traditional model the school refers individual children who present behavior difficulties in the classroom to clinics for diagnosis and treatment. Although many children demonstrating behavior disorders in a school are referred for a psychiatric evaluation, a large portion of those that are told to go to psychiatric clinics do not keep the appointments ... communication takes place primarily through written reports following a bureaucratic model that is fragmented, slow and inefficient. The school sends a request for evaluation along with information as to academic status and a translation of the teacher's complaints into psychopathological terms such as "anxious," or "aggressive." Often, unfortunately, these reports fail to give the clinic a real picture of the child's

* This term is often used to indicate case consultation. Here I use it to indicate school-related interventions by the therapist and/or evaluator in behalf of a patient.

life during the school day. The clinic then evaluates the child in its own setting. While the basic psychiatric diagnosis may be accurately defined, the differences in the demands and the general atmosphere of the two settings make it unlikely that the psychiatrist will observe those behaviors that were the school's reason for referral.

The report of the clinic is often couched in psychiatric jargon and it is extremely difficult for the teacher to understand its implications for the educational setting. In addition, the same term may have a different meaning for clinic and school when applied to a specific child. For example, the clinic's recommendation for "individualized attention" may mean an approach to the child that takes into account any special problems and vulnerabilities. The school, however, may have referred this child to begin with because he was demanding "excessive" individualized attention from the teacher. (Chess and Hassibi, 1978)

Outpatient clinics, especially those affiliated with residency training programs, often include an educational consultant on the staff to help child Fellows more expeditiously visit and learn about the school behavior of their child patients. Less well equipped clinics or most private practitioners may have to limit themselves to requesting the usual school data, hoping to avoid some of the communication difficulties described by Chess and Hassibi.

Occasionally parents will request and finance a session or a visit by the therapist with significant school personnel. Some practitioners comfortable in the school milieu will include, as a part of their total evaluation and therapy, one or more school visits to confer with involved school personnel, especially in the elementary grades. In the secondary grades this may be more difficult, since there are usually five to six different teachers and one or two counselors who may be involved with each student. Moreover, these personnel often know the student only sketchily, unless there has been a more complicated school problem. Case conferences in a community setting about children in difficulty often involve several agencies, including schools, and occasionally the child psychiatrist or clinic representative. In some cases, unfortunately, knowledge of a child's involvement with mental health treatment/evaluation needs to be kept from school personnel awareness if there is the suspected presence of anti-mental health attitudes and a likelihood of stigmatizing or scapegoating.

In the first part of this chapter I will deal with the case management approach, which at times is incorrectly labeled "school consultation." Most school consultants feel that the term "school mental health consultation" should be reserved for a specific set of procedures. I will describe these procedures in greater detail in the second part of the chapter. While both approaches have elements of child advocacy, this is more direct and appropriate in the case manangement role.

Despite the most conscientious intentions, a child therapist entering schools for the first time may find the encounter frustrating for some of the reasons indicated above. In order to be able to adapt comfortably from the clinical environment to the school life space environment, experience in consulting with school personnel would help toward both more effective communication and knowing the parameters of the school setting. Opportunities for gaining this experience are becoming more available in many child psychiatry and psychology training programs, or in courses available at postgraduate training centers—e.g., in California (Center for Training in Community Psychiatry, Los Angeles and Berkeley), Massachusetts (McLean Hospital, Belmont), and other places. If a course is not available, a cautious, nonintrusive, respectful approach supported by reading is often constructive and effective.

Let me briefly further distinguish case management from mental health consultation. Mental health consultation is a process of interaction with school personnel which is intended to bring benefit to as many children in the schools as possible. Case management is intended to help the individual child who may be evaluated or treated by the therapist doing the case management intervention. In the course of intervening for an individual child, no doubt some benefits for other children will be facilitated, but this is really not of prime intent.

Historically, therapists working with children have intervened in schools for individual children or to share and extend new mental health knowledge. In the 1930's, as child guidance clinics developed, the work of Gesell, Healy, Kanner, and others kindled an awareness of children's needs which were appreciated by school personnel as well. Educational services incorporating this new knowledge underwent gradual reorganization. In the 1950's, Caplan, Berlin, and others refined the concepts and described various procedures for helping educators and mental health personnel to improve dialogue and mutual understanding. No doubt earlier descriptions exist in the literature, but in 1960 Ekstein and Motto gave three case illustrations of borderline children and intervention in their school programs. They make also a convincing plea for the benefit of public school experience to the borderline, disturbed child.

We have given three case illustrations in which the public school system was utilized in spite of a degree of disturbance in the child which a few years ago would have been thought to prohibit the use of public schools. It may well be true that even today the majority of public schools, and perhaps also private schools, could not undertake the responsibility for such children. As schools learn to make use of professional people in the clinical field, however, and start some training of teachers for this type of work, we find more and more situations where this is possible. Frequently, we find that children with severe borderline conditions or psychotic conditions make excellent recoveries, and may then even make outstanding contributions when they have not been deprived of their chance in school. Rather than thinking of such children as nuisances, as disturbers of normal educational processes, we may wish to think of them as hidden assets. But regardless of whether they are hidden assets they may benefit from treatment, as well as from participation in social activities as much as is possible for them. When the children's true capacity is restored, they will not have lost opportunities for choices because of lack of education. Education and psychotherapy for such children are two aspects, neither of which can replace the other. Either one can be successful only if the other is not disregarded. (Ekstein and Motto, 1960)

The type of intervention described in the three cases is of interest, but cannot be cited here. Recent educational organization, called "mainstreaming," involves reintegrating such children into regular classrooms. Often some were segregated in special education classes, thus losing the benefit of participation with "normal" children.

I would like to refer to two other examples of intervention. The first, described by Rutter (1975), is the case of a 9-year-old girl, Brigitta, who was referred because she had never talked at school, after the first two months there. She had been teased about her foreign accent and slight difficulties in pronunciation. She was diagnosed "elective mutism associated with a high level of specific anxiety in a classroom situation." Two years of individual psychotherapy had brought little change. Rutter concluded that

Nothing was to be gained by searching around for the initial causes. It appeared preferable to focus specifically on the factors in the current situation, which was serving to perpetuate the mutism. Accordingly it was decided to use a behavioral approach in which things should be organized to give maximum encouragement for speaking at school in parallel with a withdrawal of the advantages which had occurred from the mutism . . . there were a series of meetings with the child, with the parents and with the schoolteacher, to work out how to do this. (Rutter, 1975)

Rutter described a very useful program which was developed in the classroom to help reinforce Brigitta's willingness, pleasure, and freedom to talk. He summarized:

The main onus in treatment fell on Brigitta's class teacher who proved very adept at judging how hard to press Brigitta and when to let her be. This is a good example of how when a problem occurs in one situation, away from the clinic, it is important to take the treatment to the situation. Schools are not involved in cooperation with clinic often enough and teachers have a lot to give children with emotional and behavioral problems, if they can be guided as to how to help. (Rutter, 1975)

Yet another and different example of such collaboration was described recently by personnel from the Philadelphia Child Guidance Clinic. (Aponte, 1976). Aponte described "a family-school interview" that included the child with his family and the personnel of the school. This was used especially when the school had referred the child to the clinic and the family saw no problem with the child at home.

An important part of this procedure was the initial interview being held at school. They found that

When we compromise and have the first interview with the child and family in the Clinic, we are apt to meet greater resistance to a school interview. It makes sense to include school personnel when the complaint comes from the school. And, as with the family, we include the key figures in the child's life at school: the counselor, the teacher, and the school principal. In a large institution, the vice-principal occasionally substitutes for the principal. We hold the interview in the school, since it is impractical to expect numerous school staff to come to the Clinic, and because by doing so the school maintains a primary sense of responsibility with the family to find a solution to the problem.

The interview is used principally as a way to find

solutions, rather than to dig for causes of trouble. The therapists attempt to make the interview a practical experience in which the family and school staff will recognize the relevance of their roles as agents of positive change. Although an effective diagnostic tool, the interview is built not on a exploratory, as much as a therapeutic, model.

Just as the mother and father must maintain their parental posture in relation to their child, the teachers have their position to uphold in the face of the therapists' assuming direction of the session. This is a difficult spot for the therapists, particularly when the interview is conducted on school grounds, often in the principal's office. (Aponte, 1976)

Aponte describes a fascinating case example which needs to be read in detail. I shall quote selectively.

The mother of ten-year-old Jerry called the Clinic to ask for an appointment. She said Jerry was fighting in school and not doing his school work.

We called the counselor who had urged Jerry's mother to contact us. She thought the participation of the principal, Jerry's three teachers, and the counselor herself was an unusual request. But she was very concerned about Jerry and would try anything. Her main question, however, was whether our purpose was to try to change the school or to help the boy. She said the staff of another mental health center had gone to the school with attempts to treat the school every time it tried to refer a child for treatment.

This last sentence is an important caution to be kept in mind by anyone dealing with school personnel. Educators in this context *are not patients*, but co-equal professionals, not to be worked *on*, but worked *with*.

Aponte summarizes the goals of the particular family-school interview as follows:

Jerry's ecological context is his personality, his family, the school, and the community with its sociopolitical character. To briefly summarize his predicament: Jerry is an insecure youngster with a tough exterior. He was in a powerless, somewhat isolated position at home, where his father, whom he respected, was not involved in his care, and his mother, who had little control over him, was responsible for him. His brothers, who are older, out-fought him in the competition for each to have things his own way at home. In the larger class at school, Jerry fought his classmates for similar reasons, which only put him in trouble with his teacher and, like his mother, this teacher did not have the strength to handle the challenge Jerry presented. The principal sided with the teacher; Jerry's good work with his other teachers was less conspicuous and was not enough to offset the troublemaking reputation he had already earned. In her effort to help Jerry, the counselor overprotected him and prevented the school and his family from working on Jerry's problems.

The target for the therapists included all of these systems. It was therapeutically economical to have the significant representatives of each of the systems meet face-to-face. With everyone active in the interview, the therapists had the opportunity to learn how they interacted, and the family and the school staff could see for themselves how their relations with one another affected Jerry. Because the Clinic convened the interview, the therapists had the leverage to assume leadership of the session, a strategically necessary but difficult endeavor when one considers that the family and school staff were confronting each other on the school's turf. That the meeting was conducted under the aegis of the Clinic helped neutralize the area of discussion and made possible the most direct and complete communications these people had experienced to date. The therapists were able actively to affect the flow of communications and the patterns of the transactions in this very real encounter of the people involved in Jerry's problems. (Aponte, 1976)

The clinic personnel returned every two weeks. The outcome of the process was described as follows:

The thin hypotheses about his being a ready victim formed a starting point for the development of other hypotheses as the interview progressed. These hypotheses served as the bases for a series of treatment goals: reinvolving the father with Jerry; helping the father to support his wife with the other boys; removing Jerry as the common target of his brothers' aggressiveness; finding a more experienced and forceful home-room teacher for Jerry with whom he would not have a history of conflict; engaging the counselor as a communication link between home and school; and, eventually, changing Jerry's negative image of himself. The work with Jerry, his family, and school lasted several months, and all major objectives were achieved. (Aponte, 1976)

This example is one that not many practitioners at this point in history may be able to duplicate in or out of clinics. There are practical difficulties, including the need for time and travel by the therapists, and initial reluctance of several school personnel taking a large amount of time for one child's problem.

This experience, however, does suggest the special benefit in working so comprehensively with the child's school environment. Also, Rutter's experience may have been easier than Aponte's because English schools have a longer tradition of collaboration with child mental health personnel.

In most cases where a therapist is able to communicate with school personnel, there is a nonspecific value in the alerting of the school person that a child is troubled or in therapy. This will often increase and/or improve the amount of attention and concern from the school person, usually the teacher. This can be helpful at times to the child and may stimulate some benefit. However, occasionally the teacher, or other school person, can be overzealous in an attempt to please the psychiatric authority. They may unwittingly reduce healthy demands on the child, thus reducing the necessary challenge for learning and mastery. At times, stigmatizing of the child may occur. It is best to gauge the judgment and understanding of the school person face to face, rather than over the telephone, before including them extensively as an ally in the therapeutic role. Also, often a teacher or school psychologist will ask for specific recommendations. To provide this by phone or letter may be risking faulty communication.

Many more examples of varying types and degrees of intervention, resulting in a gamut of consequences, could be described. Some are available in the bibliographic references. Some knowledge of the varieties and dynamics of such intervention need to be a part of the fully trained and skilled child therapist's armamentarium.

School Mental Health Consultation

Consultation techniques are skills that can be of help to a successful case-management approach. However, consultation has different goals, entry dynamics, and outcome. It may be considered a subspecialty of child or community psychiatry rather than a part of evaluation and/or therapy. At times, it may evolve from a case-management intervention. For example, the educator may be pleased and impressed with the value derived for better managing the educational as well as psychological aspects of the particular child's needs. The obvious relevance for other children in the school may lead the educator to ask the intervening therapist or another mental health professional to make time for further case consultation, frequently involving additional school personnel also.

Therapeutic Availabilities in Schools

> The ideal mental health climate in a school would be that which provided a success experience for every student wherein he enjoyed learning, gained pride in competency and self-esteem, and built the feeling that people in the world could be truly loving and helpful. Unfortunately, this ideal is often difficult to realize because of factors present in the pupil, the educator, or because of social and financial limitations. In the case of the educator, some of these factors are not difficult to trace. Adequate knowledge of child development is not always provided in the teachers' or administrators' preparatory programs. Many mental health concepts are confusing or contradictory when learned from popular media or even in one's own reading. Subtle attitudes of relating or communicating with children and peers are often not readily perceived without outside assistance. Of paramount importance is the fact that some children are emotionally disturbed and seriously tax the teacher in a class of 25 to 35. Sometimes minimal new knowledge from professionals or peers can strengthen the educator and bring the ideal experience closer for more children. (Berkovitz and Thomson, 1973, p.1)

Usually school personnel do not provide traditional psychotherapy. Some school districts do have mental health clinics to which children are referred for brief therapy, and/or evaluation. The clinics are staffed by personnel who often have also had educational experience. Other than the school orientation, there may be little difference from other child treatment clinics in the community. However, the term "counseling" is more often used in the educational context than the word "therapy."

Before any attempt at referral, counselors or school psychologists may see children in brief (or extended) contacts, which may involve confrontation, reassurance, and occasionally promotion of insight, depending on the dedication and training of the particular counselor or psychologist. Increasingly, schools are providing therapeutic opportunities in group counseling in both elementary and secondary schools. This may be provided with or without support and assistance from outside mental health consultants (Berkovitz, 1975).

These individual or group counseling opportunities, if appropriate and skillfully performed, can be of great aid to young people and families, often avoiding the need for referral and the assumption of the patient role. When the problem is chronic or pervasive in nature, traditional therapy modalities are needed. Most young people's problems, however, are of an adjustment reaction nature, and with timely brief assistance in schools there may be significant improvement in well being, social adjustment, learning, and even family problems (Kaplan, 1975).

The mental health consultant in these cases can provide a service to the psychological support staff of the school system. This service may include a modified type of supervision, didactic lectures, and demonstrations. Some prefer to exclude these types of assistance from the rubric of "mental health consultation." Indeed, there is a distinction, but the value of these types of assistance for the children in schools and the educators, especially support staff, is often immeasurable. A danger is present, however, of encouraging role confusion in some educators, especially teachers, of derogating the values inherent in educational techniques versus those in psychotherapeutic techniques. Ideally, good educational practices can be therapeutic.

Guidance committees or case conference meetings, especially in elementary but also in secondary schools, constitute a valuable quasi-clinical format for consideration of and assistance to disturbed and disturbing children. Typically, the principal, or assistant principal, nurse, school physician (if one is available), counselor, psychologist, teacher, and other relevant personnel are present. Available data on the individual child or children will be presented and recommendations made.

The consultant can be a resource "expert" as well as a facilitator for the discussion to bring out the diagnostic and management skills of the personnel, hopefully avoiding excessive dependency on the consultant "expert." Typically this type of conference will meet for one hour weekly or biweekly, with brief records kept to enable follow-up. In such weekly meetings 40 or more children and/or families can be assisted during a school year; school staff skills are often enhanced as well. Occasionally, but not usually, family members or children may be present. These case-oriented procedures are immensely useful to help hard-pressed educators pay more effective attention to the needs of disturbed students. Assistance to the special education parts of schools will be described later.

In selected instances, convincing administrators and other educators of the need for the above (or other) types of brief counseling facilities and helping to establish these may be an important and appropriate task of the mental health consultant. Rap rooms (Smith, O'Rear, and Cashion, 1975), stand-by rooms (in Denver, Colorado), and so forth have been other in-school forms of assistance found useful in several parts of the country. The drug epidemic of the late sixties and early seventies, the increase of violence and aggression on campus, and other crises have prompted school personnel increasingly to seek the assistance of mental health personnel. In the usual parlance of preventive health, these consultative procedures may be considered secondary and tertiary prevention goals and results, contrasted to the frequently hoped for ideal of primary prevention—i.e. changes affecting children not yet labeled as disturbed. Consultation to school personnel provides the opportunity for all three types of prevention and assistance.

Primary prevention is a goal appropriate to consultation with teachers of "normal" classes. Secondary (or tertiary) prevention may be considered more appropriate to consultation with support staffs who are dealing with children already labeled disturbed or failing in the school context, though they are not yet involved with the clinical mental health system.

Consultation Technique

Entry for consultation may take place in a variety of ways. Occasionally an interested professional can get to know his child's teacher and educators and build a relationship with them, which then expands to more formal mental health consultation (Vanderpol, personal communication). More usually the child mental health specialist is part of a community organization, clinic, or community mental health center that approaches or is approached by school personnel to explore the applicability and scope of mental health consultation. Such mutual exploration can occur deliberately or occasionally accidentally, for example, if the involved personnel were to meet at community meetings or social occasions. Entry rarely involves, initially at least, a specific agenda, goal, or consultee group. This is usually defined in the early meetings and may change as meetings continue. Initial contact may be with the group who will become the consultees. Or a part of the system may arrange for service to yet another group of personnel. For example, the assistant superintendent may make contact to provide a consultant for a group of principals or psychologists. A principal or a school psychologist, on the other hand, may make contact in order to obtain a consultant for a group of teachers concerned with disturbed student behavior, concepts of child psychology, and so forth (Berkovitz, 1970b).

Several practical details deserve attention in this early negotiating phase of the consultation entry. Forman and Hetznecker (1972) bring attention to several:

In our experience, clinics have offered their services free, out of a sense of interest and public service without imposing enough responsibility on the schools for providing or finding funds. In our economic society, services that are paid for are more valued than services that are not paid for. Fees impose the obligation on the service-giver and the service-receiver of evaluating the worth of those services.

The issue of funding may be a difficult one, since most schools have low funds. Another issue may be the full involvement of the administrator, especially the principal.

Frequently it becomes clear that the principal is requesting a program which will not involve him. It is probably obvious to all of us now that any program which does not actively involve the school principal stands a good chance of being doomed to failure, just as individual work with children divorced from the family contact may be fruitless. Furthermore, the principal and consultant may each adopt the "father knows best" attitude, and the very people (teachers, counselors, parents, home and school coordinators, and even pupils) with whom most of the collaborative work will be done may be excluded from these early meetings. A contract is worked out between the bosses and the program is presented to the workers. Chances for sabotage using such an approach are limitless.

Other nitty-gritty points basic to the program may be overlooked: What room will the consultant use? Will it always be available or will he wander, gypsylike, from week to week? Does the consultant get a parking space in the school parking lot? Will teachers always be available at a specified time, and are there plans for adequate classroom coverage? Will the school be open at night if parents' meetings are part of the program? Is there money to pay teachers if the program is conducted after school hours? What is the procedure for resolving the above difficulties? (Forman and Hetznecker, 1972)

Consultation with educators requires the continuing awareness that within the school the primary responsibility for the well-being of the children is with the school professional—administrators and other educators. The goal of the psychiatric consultant is to enhance the ability of administrators, teachers, and support staff to deal with the specific areas of emotional or behavioral disturbance they encounter in the classroom or counseling office and then to expand on these specific cases so that the educators may be able to apply the knowledge generally. The goal is not to convert educators (even support staff) into mental health professionals. The primary task of their profession is education. Ideally the community-oriented child psychiatrist, working within the school on an egalitarian basis especially with teachers and administrators, will increase the awareness of these professionals in the role that the school plays in the social and psychological development of children both toward optimum mental health as well as disturbance (Berkovitz and Newman, 1980a).

A consultant to schools (or any agency) needs to keep in mind that he is a "guest" in the particular agency or system. The "guest" role usually implies courtesy and respect for current operating procedures and personnel, *even if* the consultant has strong disagreement or disapproval. If strong uncontrollable negative attitudes are present, just as in psychotherapy, the consultant may need to request a change of assignment. Since many of us or our children have occasionally had painful experiences in public schools, some consultants may enter schools with an agenda of revenge or rapid reform. Patient, skillful consultation at times does achieve significant reform and/or program change. More rapid changes in school practices can be attempted along political or public media avenues. From the consultee side, envy and/or overexpectation can occur and need attention (Vanderpol and Waxman, 1974).

Early identification of severe psychopathology and appropriate referral is one outcome of consultation that can have an important role in the primary prevention of mental illness. School consultation programs have devised a myriad of approaches to the development of special programs within schools toward the goal of primary prevention. Similarly the goal of tertiary prevention or rehabilitation of psychiatrically troubled youngsters returning to schools is enhanced by an awareness of the special problems these children face. (Berkovitz and Newman, 1980a). The following example may serve to illustrate this process:

> A 14-year-old girl with anorexia nervosa refused to go to school for a period of four months because she was "too fat." This despite a decrease in body weight from her normal weight of 100 pounds to 65 pounds, which at that point necessitated hospitalization. With recovery of her weight to 85 pounds and discharge from the hospital, the patient continued in outpatient psychotherapy but was extremely reluctant to return to her school the following semester because of fear of the questions her classmates would ask. She particularly feared that they would consider her "crazy" because she had been in a hospital, and she worried also about certain teachers whom she feared "had it in for her." (Berkovitz and Newman, 1980a)

A psychiatric consultant working in the school, questioned about the syndrome of anorexia nervosa, was able to explain it to teachers and the principal in a way that avoided the stigma of "craziness" from being attached to the former patient. Discussion focused on specific difficulties this patient would have in getting back to the primary task of learning her subjects because of continued preoccupation with food. Special approaches were devised by the teachers themselves, stimulated by the consultation. As a result, the reentry of the child into the school was accomplished smoothly, and the attitude of school personnel helped with the recovery from the problem of anorexia.

In contrast, another patient with anorexia, who had fully recovered in the sense that her world had returned to normal and she was no longer obsessed with her appearance or eating, returned to a school that had received no psychiatric consultation. Within three weeks she reported to her psychiatrist that she felt that the teachers in her school "don't understand me and I think they hate me." She refused to return to the school and had to be transferred twice more to two additional schools before her education could resume (Berkovitz and Newman, 1980a).

Berlin (1974) has described a five-stage process for school mental health consultation. Descriptions of these stages are only briefly excerpted here. The fuller description provides better clarification.

> The first step centers around developing a good working relationship so that the consultee does not feel suspicious or fearful that the worker will try to uncover unconscious motivations or pry into personal problems.
>
> The second step is an effort to reduce the consultee's anxieties and self-blame, his feelings of failure, frustration, anger, and hopelessness.
>
> The third step is designed to keep the collaboration task-oriented and to prevent the helpless dependency that may follow relief of anxiety. The consideration of etiological factors in the client's troubles and the consultant's diagnostic appraisal of the consultee's ego strengths are used to focus on the first step to be taken by the consultee to help the client. Thus, the teacher is engaged in consideration of how he can engage the student in the learning process. This needs to be a mutual consideration and agreement to work with the child in a particular way that the teacher considers consonant with his own capabilities. In this phase, the consultant needs to be wary of making unilateral recommendations or being seduced into prescriptions about the educative process in which the educator is the expert.
>
> The fourth step, a vital one, consists of follow-up meetings to evaluate, reconsider, modify, and try new approaches in the light of the teacher's experiences and the changes in the child. This enables the consultee to recognize that he can build on every tiny increment of learning, that each minute step is important and meaningful to the child's interpersonal experience and beginning sense of mastery.
>
> The fifth step is the consolidation and disengagement from consultation. As the consultee works more effectively and feels more secure in his capacity to work and help a wider variety of disturbed children, he needs the consultant less. His increasing competence as a teacher, counselor, or administrator leaves him free to call the consultant when and if he needs help. (Berlin, 1974)

Berlin (1974) stresses other awareness useful for prospective consultants.

> Since this is not a casework, patient or client relationship, certain gratifications and rewards inherent in direct work may be missing and may initially make consultation less satisfying. Consultees who are helped to work more effectively usually do not express gratitude. Because they are engaged as collaborators, they often may not recognize that they have been helped. Frequently, the most successful consultation is indicated only by the evidence that the consultee does not require further consultation. As in all interpersonal processes, it is a slow one.
>
> Consultation may be very anxiety provoking if the consultee feels overwhelmed. He may demand from the consultant answers that are not available.

In these circumstances it may be very difficult to recognize that the consultee may be identifying with the attitudes and methods of the consultant as he helps evaluate the situation and begins to look for "bite-sized" approaches. (Berlin, 1974)

Caplan (1970) has written extensively on mental health consultation and has delineated categories of consultation. His writings are comprehensive and cannot be adequately summarized here. He describes consultation as

A process of interaction between two professional persons—the consultant who is a specialist and the consultee who invokes the consultant's help in regard to a current work problem with which he is having some difficulty and which, he has decided, is within the other's area of specialized competence. The work problem involves the management or treatment of one or more clients of the consultee, or the planning or implementation of a program to cater to such clients.

Caplan (1970) further differentiates consultation from other specialized methods such as "supervision, education, psychotherapy, casework, counseling, administrative inspection, negotiation, liaison, collaboration, coordination and mediation." He has delineated four major types of consultation, depending on content and process. Again, these cannot be discussed in adequate full detail, but will be briefly summarized here. Berlin's five stages are relevant especially to categories 1 and 2.

1. *Client-centered case consultation.* The primary goal of the consultation is for the consultant to communicate to the consultee how this client can be helped.

2. *Consultee-centered case consultation.* Here too the consultee's work problem relates to the management of a particular client and he invokes the consultant's help in order to improve his handling of the case. In this type of consultation the consultant focuses his main attention on trying to understand the nature of the consultee's difficulty with the case and in trying to help remedy this.

The aim of this type of consultation is frankly to educate the consultee, using his problems with the current client as a lever and a learning opportunity; and the expertness of the consultant is focused on this task, rather than a client-centered case consultation, on the diagnosis of the client and the developing of a specialist prescription for his treatment.

3. *Program-centered administrative consultation.* The work problem is in the area of planning and administration—how to develop a new program or to improve an existing one. The consultant helps by using his knowledge of administration and social systems as well as his expert knowledge and experience of mental health theory and practice, and of program development in other institutions, in order to collect and analyze data about the points at issue. On the basis of this he suggests short term and long term solutions for the administrative questions of the consultee organization.

4. *Consultee-centered administrative consultation.* Here the primary concern of the consultant is not the collection and analysis of administrative data, relating to the mission of the institution, but the elucidation and remedying among the consultees of difficulties and shortcomings that interfere with their grappling with their tasks of program development and organization.

In addition to lack of knowledge, skills, self-confidence and objectivity in individuals, the problem of the consultees may be the result of group difficulties—poor leadership, authority problems, lack of role complementarity, communication blocks and the like.

Caplan was a pioneer in describing the interpersonal currents of the relationship between consultant-consultee-client, especially in his concept of "theme interference reduction" (Caplan, 1970). Caplan evolved this technique from the conviction that

minor transference reactions of a special type occasionally complicate professional functioning in most people, whatever their state of mental health.

It is not uncommon for unsolved present or past personal problems to be displaced onto task situations and for this to produce temporary ineffectuality and loss of emotional stability in dealing with a segment of the work field. (Caplan, 1970)

This technique is especially relevant in one-to-one consultation where the consultant has the opportunity to observe and ameliorate the biases of the consultee, while discussing the consultee's interactions with clients.

LaVietes and Chess (1969) provide an especially cogent example of the differentiation of the activities of consultation and therapy in consultee-centered consultation. This example came from their training of child psychiatrists in "school psychiatry" at the New York Medical College Child Psychiatry Training Program.

A resident in a supervisory session expressed concern about the teacher's "countertransference."

There is a very greedy child in the group whose incessant efforts to grab everything—food, supplies, adult attention—arouses a withholding attitude on the teacher's part. Her own impulses in these directions seem to have been handled by reaction formation, which makes her vulnerable to the child's extreme behavior. To maintain her own defenses, she is unreasonably depriving toward the child. The supervisor acknowledged the probable validity of the resident's assessment, but wondered how a change could be effected since it was inappropriate and ineffective to deal with the teacher's psychological problems directly, as might be done with a psychiatric supervisee, or to treat the teacher as if she were a patient. In the ensuing discussion, the resident decided he would try to use the teacher's underlying identification with the child to promote more tolerance for him. The supervisor also helped him to see that most persons have similar defenses in one area or another. In an ensuing meeting with the teacher, the resident was able to point out how "starved" and anxious the child was, how difficult it was to deal with him since all of us, including himself, had a distaste for such behavior and wondered speculatively whether it was possible ever to gratify such a child. Such discussion served to promote the teacher's empathy with the child, intellectual interest in the problem, and identification with the consultant's greater willingness to try to satisfy the youngster.

In recent years, consultation is performed in groups more than in a one to one format. Usually the groups include three to fifteen school personnel, meeting weekly, bi-weekly, or monthly at the school site. Sessions last usually 1½ hours, occasionally longer. In this setting, the consultant may better facilitate the consultees' helping one another. Group process skills are useful for the consultant to know, but the consultation ought not be conducted as a group therapy session (Altrocchi, Spielberger, and Eisendorfer, 1965). Usually the attendance of participants is structured as voluntary, but consistency of attendance is stressed when feasible. Many groups in schools meet often for a minimum of 8 to 10 sessions during one semester and occasionally continue from one school year to the next. As Berlin (1974) described, a goal for the consultant may be to withdraw as soon as the consultees gain skills. This may require from six months to two years. In large school districts (over twenty schools), as new parts of the district learn of the consultant's presence, additional requests and new program tasks may develop, thus prolonging the consultant's service.

Depending on finances, a consultant and/or team may function productively in such an assignment for several years, effecting significant learning at all levels of personnel, including teacher aides, counselors, psychologists, nurses, teachers, principals, assistant superintendents, and at times, superintendents and school board members. The interrelating functions of this array of school personnel may at first be confusing to the clinician and may require time and patience to learn. Some helpful descriptions are available (Berkovitz, 1970b; Berkowitz, 1975).

The approaches above presume a group discussion format that is *relatively* free and unstructured. Anecdotal reporting of children's behavior may prevail. Educators are often bothered by a completely unstructured approach, feeling more comfortable with lecture—even if brief—or other educational types of presentation. When mental health personnel satisfy this wish, there can be the risk of a passive experience for the consultee group, and the optimum values of an interactive consultative experience are lessened. A brief introductory set of remarks can at times facilitate a subsequent freer discussion. Perhaps some wary school personnel prefer initially to witness the feared "shrink" on display and at a distance. In oral terms, "tasting" may need to precede "breaking bread" together.

Behaviorally Oriented Consultation

Behaviorally oriented consultants often do provide a more structured set of procedures, at times avoiding the anxiety of less structure. Those behaviorists who have consultation expertise, as well, may beneficially blend the two approaches. Canter and Paulson (1974) described a version of this blending in the context of a college credit course. They felt that

Consultation attendance is typically on a voluntary basis, thus the impact is dependent not only on the consultant's expertise, but the teacher's workload and desire for assistance at that moment. If the teachers feel they need to see the consultant, will they find time to do so? The meaningful continuity that is helpful in educating and training teachers is often lacking due to a limited and often changing audience.

Unit credit from an accredited college for participation in a consultation was hypothesized to be a significant additional motivating factor. The college units would be applicable toward higher educational degrees as well as increased salary from their school district.

The consultation seminar was conducted in twenty 1½ hour sessions held at the elementary school in the spring semester of 1972. Sessions took the form of a modified case-conference consultation. The initial part of each session was conducted along the lines of a traditional consultation model. Teachers brought up current problems they were having in their classes with groups of students or, as most frequently occurred, with an individual child. The teachers were encouraged to ventilate their frustrations in order to deal more objectively with the situation. They received support and encouragement for their efforts from the consultants and each other.

The specific problems that were raised at the beginning of the session—for example, the hyperactive child or the slow learner—served as the focal point for the didactic part of the session that followed. A lecture-discussion approach was used to present specific theories and techniques useful in correcting the problem behavior in question. This style, which precluded the use of a structured lecture format, was used in order to make the didactic material as relevant as possible. To provide immediate feedback to the teachers and to facilitate learning, teachers were observed in their classrooms; the amount of actual observation time varied from ½ hour to a total of 1½ hours during the semester, depending on the desires and needs of the teachers involved.

In order to ensure the functional application of the principles presented, outside requirements were assigned. Teachers were asked to decide on a child in their class who was demonstrating problem behavior. These students were most often those discussed by the teacher during the weekly sessions. The teacher was to conduct a functional intervention with the child in question.

Each intervention consisted of eight steps, which cannot be detailed here.

The teacher was required to go through each of the steps with the child selected and present a written record of the results. The consultants discussed the progress periodically with the teacher and gave feedback and assistance as needed.

The teachers were also assigned required reading in Buckley and Walker (1972) "Modifying Classroom Behavior," Glasser (1969) "Schools Without Failure," and Ginott (1972) "Teacher and Child." A final examination was required that was designed to evaluate and facilitate the practical application of the principles taught during the semester. (Canter and Paulson, 1974)

This is a more structured procedure than most "consultation"—indeed, bordering on didactic learning. The inclusion of "ventilation of frustrations," observation of classes, and the specific agenda of each meeting emerging from the discussion differentiated this from a more formal academic course. The inclusion of required written records, assigned reading, and final exam certainly marked it as more academic. Many teachers liked this part and did pay more attention to the message being put forth. Some teachers rejected it.

The case study quoted by Canter and Paulson (1974) illustrates the type of learning being encouraged. The subject was Larry, a 10-year-old fourth-grade boy.

The teacher reported that the child exhibited inadequate social interaction with his peers, often engaging in physical fights with his classmates. The behavior to be modified consisted of decreasing physical fighting while increasing the appropriate expression of feeling.

Prior to the implementation of the contracted intervention, the teacher appeared to be maintaining the physical confrontations by the contingent attention and verbal dialogue that characteristically followed such episodes. No appropriate avenues were provided to the child for the constructive presentation of his feelings. The frequency of the child's fighting behavior was recorded on a daily basis through baseline and intervention stages. A behavioral frequency record of appropriate feeling talk (expression of displeasure or approval regarding peer interaction) was also kept. The intervention strategy implemented consisted of:

1. A mutually agreed upon contract stipulating the receipt of drawing supplies previously not available to the student for use in the final 15 minutes of the school day contingent on a day without a fight.
2. Every time the child engaged in a fight he was sent from the room to sit in the hall for 5 minutes (timeout) with minimal verbalization on the part of the teacher (on the playground he was sent to sit on a bench for the remainder of the period when he engaged in fighting).

3. The contingent verbal approval by the teacher of all appropriate "feeling talk" during the class meeting.
4. The intermittent use of teacher approval and proximity for cooperative peer play.

The frequency of physical fighting reduced to zero and the frequency of "feeling talk" during the classroom meetings increased.

The lack of fighting and increased verbalization of feelings continued, and 5 weeks after the intervention had begun, the teacher began to phase out the free arts period. Initially the contract was changed to one free period for every 2 days without a fight, then 4 days without a fight, then the free period was completely eliminated. Larry was still encouraged to verbalize his anger supported by the contingent presentation of teacher approval. (Canter and Paulson, 1974)

Jones and Eimers (1975) use behavioral principles to focus on the class as a whole, rather than on individual pupil behavior. They described role-playing to train elementary school teachers to

use a broad range of social skills in dealing with group behavioral management in the classroom. This training reduced disruptive student behavior during both seat work and group discussions . . . (Jones and Eimers, 1975)

Improvement in children's arithmetic learning was demonstrated, as well as greater teacher satisfaction and comfort. This type of satisfaction has been reported with a variety of consultation procedures and styles, but the behavioral approach seems to have a special relevance to the classroom when carefully and humanistically applied. These consultation procedures could be considered teaching new skills and techniques.

A group of teachers who met weekly for anecdotal type of case consultation was described as follows:

The supportive, non-critical attitude of the group seemed to make it possible for the teachers to present their difficulties in a non-defensive manner. Typically, one would come because she was concerned about a child or the disruptive effect one in particular was having on the class. Support always seemed to be available from other teachers in the group who had been confronted with similar problems. It was remarkable to see how the group was sensitive to individual personalities and styles. They seemed to know what would work for one teacher and what would not work for another. The kinds of suggestions offered varied from practical "gimmicks" to observations like "You're letting those kids walk all over you! Let 'em know who's boss!" (Berkovitz and Thompson, 1973, p. 2.)

Certainly some behavioral types of learning occurred in this type of consultation as well, but without a systematic behavioral focus.

Program Consultation and Program Change

While the case consultations described above are useful and essential, there will never be enough available to reach all needy children in any school system. One would hope that program changes would also be developed to improve the system's ability to provide greater health enhancing opportunities for more children.

Most expeditious is when personnel in a district, especially administrators or school board members, realize the need for program changes and take steps to institute these. They may engage a consultant or consultant group for this purpose, as described in Caplan's categories 3 and 4. Some examples of these will be given later in this chapter. One example occurred in one school after a student suicide. This tragic event set into motion the calling in of a consultant to evaluate and redesign the school's mental health practices. Ethnic transition events and pressures have prompted program changes in many schools in the sixties and seventies. Occasionally mental health consultants have been of assistance (Sugar, 1974).

At times program change can develop from case consultation. For example, a consultant met one to two times per month with personnel of a special program for students expelled from regular classes for various types of antisocial behavior. This program in a large urban school district consisted of thirteen separate classes, each meeting in widely scattered off-school sites. Each class consisted of about ten students, usually a majority male. In discussing the individual problems presented by one or two of the more troubled female students, it became apparent that there was insufficient pride in self as a woman and insufficient knowledge of skills associated with cultural female roles—e.g., choice of clothing, makeup, speech, etc. It was an easy step for the consultant to suggest a gathering of the twenty of so female students from the thirteen scattered sites to meet periodically to discuss, consolidate, and amplify the feeling and knowledge of being female. In a sense, this was a "female consciousness raising" group. Adding this type of group to the program brought surprisingly effective benefits and pleasure to students and staff (Berkovitz, unpublished).

Types of Consultation in Secondary Schools

The variety of different ways that educators and mental health consultants have developed to exchange knowledge and skills for better care of children at times boggles and delights the mind. The previously described case consultation experiences are especially relevant to the smaller, more child-oriented elementary schools (200 to 700 pupils, grades kindergarten to sixth). In the larger, more subject-oriented secondary schools (1,200 to 3,000 pupils, grades 7-12), appropriate consideration of the special mental health needs of adolescents are often impeded by organizational as well as size difficulties. Each generation has had its own difficulties peacefully incorporating the new generations of young people. Unfortunately, the educational system does not always optimally assist the process (Miller, 1970; Berkovitz, 1980). Mental health consultation can offer some assistance to this process. Many of the formats and techniques described above are relevant, but additional procedures have been developed in secondary schools.

Also on the following pages, I shall describe briefly and perhaps sketchily, a small sample of the varieties of useful interactions that have come into being between consultants of various mental health disciplines and educators of various categories.

In one junior high school the consultant helped staff to formulate the following programs (Berkovitz and Thomson, 1973, p. 7):

> (a) Group counseling conducted by teachers was arranged for some of the students identified as having problems.
>
> (b) Consultation was provided to the opportunity-room teachers whose students usually presented particularly difficult behavior problems.
>
> (c) A series of meetings was arranged at which designated students could present their problems. The purpose was to help teachers and counselors resolve their problems in working with these children.
>
> (d) Exploratory conferences were to be held with groups of homeroom teachers to discuss philosophies of homeroom guidance.
>
> (e) Plan a mental health curriculum for the school.

In high schools, a similar but somewhat different program was developed by two consultants (Berkovitz and Thomson, 1973, p. 9):

> Both consultants meet every other week with a group composed of the principal, vice principals, guidance counselor, the nurse, registrar, welfare and attendance officer, and the administrators for counselors. These meetings have been discussion periods where staff members were invited to present problems which have perplexed them. From these have grown more general and broad areas of discussion, particularly regarding specific student examples. Several discussions have been held concerning the difficulty that black girls from other districts have been having in becoming integrated into the school population, both academically and socially. The girls' vice principal was encouraged to take advantage of the grouping of these girls to establish "rap" groups for them. She did get one started during the past year. Considerable support was given to the various staff members to help them tolerate anxiety in working with disturbed youngsters. It was also possible to suggest referral resources to them when appropriate.
>
> Another area of discussion was the recognition of the struggle for a sense of identity by the high school students, especially those who were causing noticeable problems. Over a period of time, a number of the staff came to be able to recognize the different sets of values regarding grades and school courses this generation of students holds in contrast to those of the generation of the staff and the consultants. A serious effort was subsequently made to try to establish policy changes to deal with the more diverse problems in curriculum and education for these students, a group different from many that the staff had previously encountered.

In another high school, the consultant provided an extended case consultation (Berkovitz and Thomson, 1973, p. 10):

> There was a four-session consultation centered around helping the teachers handle a severely disturbed girl in the classroom. I met with the teachers, the special education advisor, and the student's counselor who was the main contact person. The content of the meetings included techniques of behavior modification, ventilation of teacher's anxiety, and an exchange of ideas. The outcome was that the student still was not able to be managed in school, but because of her progress, the family was willing to seek long-term treatment. The school was exposed to the consultation process, and the

participants were provided with techniques they could use also with other behavior problems.

Occasionally consultants become involved in the classroom—for example (Berkovitz and Thomson, 1973, P. 12):

a. Discussion with a guidance class of problems relating to drugs and personal development.

b. Meetings with a student curriculum committee regarding more effective means for achieving curriculum changes.

c. Discussion with a student-led "mini-class."

d. Classroom visits and discussions with the remedial reading teacher and aide. The visits included student interviews and suggestions to teacher regarding behavior modification approaches to problem students.

e. Visits to a physical education class and interviews with the teacher and a problem student.

f. Meeting and classroom observation of a teacher in training. This involved sitting in with student "kitchen teams" in a home economics class where teamwork had been impaired by several problem students.

g. Continuing participation in the classroom aide program. This involved visits to elementary school classrooms where high school students served as student aides, and later, discussion with the entire high school class and the teacher who directed the aide training program.

h. Student interviews at the counselors' request and discussion of problem cases with counselors.

i. "Rap" room visits.

Assistance to Group Counseling Programs

One of the school programs with which consultants frequently became involved in secondary schools was the group counseling program. Most schools are currently increasing the use of group counseling as a way of assisting students. Secondary schools are the most active in this direction, and many of the secondary counselors both need and are seeking in-service education opportunities that can help them learn how to conduct counseling groups. Of equal importance is the need for subsequent continuing supervision to maintain quality and satisfaction in their work. Since group techniques have been a part of mental health practice for many years, it is natural that mental health professionals should be of assistance in adapting their use in the school setting.

The use of group techniques in schools is appropriate for assistance to students with unique problems, drug abuse, unwed pregnancy, etc. Such groups are also important to the too-often-forgotten average child who needs to talk about the normal adolescent problems of growing up. In addition, groups can serve as a setting in which to work on problems involving more broad school issues.

In one group program (Berkovitz and Thomson, 1973, p. 13):

It was arranged that four groups would meet for ten weekly sessions with a school counselor and consultant as co-leaders in each group. After eight sessions the consultants felt that the counselors were doing well and should be able to continue without them. The focus in the groups had gradually changed from "What's wrong with the student?" to "What's wrong with the high school climate?"

In another high school (Berkovitz and Thomson, 1973, p. 13):

The consultant and the eleventh-grade boys' counselor conducted a weekly group for girls who were drug abusers. No goals were outlined, since rapping seemed sufficient. Attendance was uneven, but crises usually precipitated a member's return to the group. The members showed their resistance in the group by reading, eating, walking out, having side conversations, insulting group leaders, and calling the group a "class" and a "waste of time." Once, they gave a party. They were always threatening to end the group, but they never did. By the end of the semester, the group had settled down, and members evidenced that they felt close and supportive of one another. They wanted to continue.

In another high school (Berkovitz and Thomson, 1973, p. 14):

Consultants were asked to provide services to a group of high school girls who were having difficulty staying in school. Following a conference with school personnel, a series of weekly meetings was arranged for a group of twelve girls to discuss some of the problems facing them at home and at school. The school nurse and counselor formed a team with us to work with this group. Our goal as consultants was to provide an adequate model from which the school nurse and counselor would be able to learn to conduct groups on their own by the end of the semester. Help was also given them in being able to deal more effectively with some of the student problems they encountered in their duties, such as suicide attempts, pregnancy and drug abuse.

Consultative and some direct services have been given to the Teen Mothers' Program. There has been a program of body awareness and also discussion sessions around the emotional crises of those pregnant teenagers, some of whom are married and some of whom are not. Other services, such as development and referrals for community services, have also been provided. In addition, a few home calls were made with the teacher at her request when interviewing problems associated with their pregnancy. Continuing plans for the groups include: (1) collage therapy; (2) continuing with the body awareness program; and (3) some psycho-drama around everyday situations.

In one high school unit for a group of pregnant adolescents, the consultant provided group counseling weekly.

In these sessions it came out that some of the students felt unconsciously that having a child with a boyfriend guaranteed security and permanence of the relationship. Others of the pregnant teenager group felt that physical abuse from the boyfriend was part of the women's role and showed the man's love. Group counseling helped to change some of these stereotypes. Some of the girls were able to point out to each other the life consequences and future liabilities of some of these beliefs and consequent actions. (McManmon, personal communication)

The previous experiences involved the consultants in collaborative group leadership with the educators. The following is an example of consultants training teacher-counselor teams in a more didactic-supervisory format (Flacy, Goda, and Schwartz, 1975).

The first meeting of 35 teachers who had volunteered to participate in the program was held in October, and from this meeting three training groups were formed.

A part of the consultants' task involved retaining the enthusiasm of the participants while alleviating the need for "pat" answers. The need to "do something" was approached by redirecting the focus toward acceptance of the probability that no student was going to give up drugs solely because of the teacher's efforts. Also, that the teacher should not impose this responsibility on himself. Rather than expecting to solve the psychological problems of the students, each could offer himself as a listener, a sounding board and perhaps a model, creating a climate for new experience to take place within individuals so that alternative behavior could become possible.

At first the teachers worried about role confusion, fearing the students would be hostile toward them as authorities. Encouraged to examine closely their own values and attitudes about drugs, unlawful behavior, authority, and obscene language, they recognized with some humor and relief that much of their anxiety related to their own ambivalence. As a result, they reported feeling more comfortable in handling provocations from group members.

As the student groups got underway, the teachers brought specific situations to the consultation for discussion. Some of these had to do with hostility: group members toward leaders, toward fellow group members, and leaders toward members (this last possibility was introduced by the consultants); resentment stemming from mandatory attendance; long silences; the manipulative group member; confrontation; a curiosity about the leader; how to avoid endless rapping about drugs; reacting to four-letter words; talking about uncomfortable things, and dealing with the student who come to the group "high."

It was noted that with experience the teachers began to recognize when their own emotional involvement was interfering with group process. They were increasingly able to handle situations within their group, or among themselves, relying less on referral and consultation. They often expressed amazement, as these students revealed themselves, at the staggering amount of family chaos and the kinds of home situations in which these young people had to exist. Most leaders showed that they were becoming more sensitive and empathetic toward the students. They were also less preoccupied with the drug-taking than in helping the student deal with his realities, to enlarge his view of possibilities, to encourage him to stand on his own feet, and to use the support of the social network around him.

In summary, this consultation began as in-service training and education. The consultants made no attempt to impart a systematic body of knowledge about techniques, nor to offer specific methods which they felt might only be imitated. The effort was made to promote the self-awareness of the teacher and counselor group leaders without infringing on their privacy; to let them know that it is normal for new leaders to feel inadequate, and that this does not mean they are inadequate; and that common sense and past experience can often serve them well when they feel a lack in skill, knowledge, or self-confidence. (Flacy, Goda, and Schwartz, 1975)

Consultation to Teachers of Children with Special Needs

Teachers in programs for the educationally handicapped (EH), in programs of special education, in child care centers, and in other programs providing education to children with special needs face a large number of challenges in the classroom. These challenges include the special behavior and other needs of children with physical or neurological impediments.

It is of value for teachers in such classes to receive as much knowledge as possible of the physical nature of the problems of the children and as much understanding as possible of the emotional transactions between themselves as teachers and the pupils. It is important also to have help in comprehending the relationships between the parents and their children and between the pupils themselves.

Those responsible for many such programs have requested the services of mental health consultants. Unfortunately, many others are neither aware of the availability of such assistance nor of how to make the best use of it.

In one EH class the consultant combined consultation with leading a demonstration counseling group (Berkovitz and Thomson, 1973, p. 29):

The program this year began as a consultation to six EH teachers from various schools in the district. From this there developed a request to hold counseling groups with fourth, fifth, and sixth graders. Two groups were selected, one with eight boys, and the other with six boys and two girls. These groups met every other week with four adults; the guidance director, the two teachers who taught the children who were in the groups, and the consultant. Each group session lasted one hour and was followed by a half-hour discussion with the teachers. This consultation has been well received by the staff, and in addition, it has allowed for some direct service to selected children. It has given the teachers a chance to see positive therapeutic changes in students in the group, to participate in a group as co-leaders, and to gain confidence in this role. It has also given them a chance to observe useful interventions with the children in the group and given them the opportunity to ask questions about these later.

In a child care center, the consultant was able to help teachers accept the aggression of the young pupils (Berkovitz and Thomson, 1973, p. 29):

This fall began with a staff consisting of an acting head, one teacher formerly with the Center, one part-time older retired teacher, and two new younger teachers who came from experiences with nursery schools for middle-class children. The new teachers were feeling that they had never known such aggressive, hostile children. They described them as destructive with each other and with things, angry and defiant in their response to teachers, and generally out of control. In the early consultation sessions, the teachers were encouraged to express what they were feeling about the youngsters and about themselves professionally, but focus was kept on understanding this "new breed" of child and on meeting the special needs of this group. As histories were reviewed of the present life situations in the families from which the children came, the staff came to comprehend some of the sources of the children's hostility. They realized the need for structure in the program as contrasted to the permissive approach which they had felt to be best in their previous setting. They gradually overcame their guilt feelings about firmness and consistency. The children responded quickly, apparently relieved that their teachers could be unconflicted about controls. Teachers began to take pride in their roles again, and things improved considerably.

In another day care program, the consultant reported (Berkovitz and Thomson, 1973, p. 30):

These teachers have become more understanding in working with parents. They have worked toward being able to conduct interviews with parents by discussing principles of interviewing and reviewing their own interviews to perfect their skills in this area.

Consultation to Special Education Programs

Consultants have been of value in programs for the blind, deaf, aphasic, autistic, crippled, etc. In one school for the deaf (k–12), the child psychiatrist consultant was able to facilitate an especially unique change in the program of teaching. With the assistance of teachers in the early childhood program the consultant determined that the deaf children do not have any or only inadequate words or signs for the important bodily parts, functions, and other human emotions. Important learning and psychological development in every child is tied in with fantasies around fear, anger, separation, sex, and parts of one's body, as well as with the acquisition of reality facts for which word symbols are needed. Therefore, the consultant, with the assistance of teachers, developed a handbook of terms and procedures useful to teachers in understanding the problems and needs of deaf children. The consultant filled a genuine need for a special approach to deaf children that was outside the scope of normal school services usually furnished to deaf children. Another consultant who had himself overcome deafness worked in groups with some of the more disturbed deaf boys and girls. In this secondary school program, as a result of the close group contact there was a remarkable change in attitude relative to authority and in attendance, more concern for others, and reduction of classroom antisocial incidents (Freeman, personal communication).

Consultation Especially With Pupil Personnel Services Workers

Pupil personnel services workers (or support staff), including counselors, nurses, psychologists, and psychometrists represent the prime mental health resource within a school. Many of the types of consultation and assistance with school staff described above are being or have been provided within school districts by these personnel. Fortunately, in many districts, PPS workers also participate in many of the mental health consultation sessions held with other staff members. Such experience helped add to the knowledge of situations faced by the staff and students and has helped to increase the working connections with others. Since the mental health consultant rarely works directly with children within the district, there is no problem of duplication of services.

Group Discussion to Improve Communication between Staff Members

While most communication among teachers is adequate for everyday functioning, there are times when improvement in communication could increase the occupational and personal satisfactions of the staff as well as result in better performance toward children in the classroom. Mental health consultation cannot solve all communication problems, but as is current in many industrial organizations, group discussion of interpersonal factors affords some improvement. Of course this procedure requires a group of teachers and administrators who are willing to engage in this kind of discussion. The discussion is most often job oriented and is not intended to be personal psychotherapy. Individual pupils are discussed to some extent, but the discussion usually involves a greater degree of personal focus than the case discussion models presented in the previous examples.

A consultant working with a group of teachers in this type of process reported as follows (Berkovitz and Thomson, 1973, p. 19):

Two groups of teachers, nine to ten members each, met on alternate weeks, after school, for sessions of two to two and one-half hours during the school year. The purpose of both groups was to promote individual growth in dealing with interpersonal relationships. Each member was to choose his own focus; i.e., relationships with other persons in the school or relationships outside the school which had impact on their ability to function within the school. Discussion was structured occasionally by devices such as role-playing, questionnaires, and check-lists to help refocus the group's thinking. These devices became less needed as the year progressed. The two groups were quite different. One, composed entirely of teachers, working in a team-teacher situation, dealt almost exclusively with interpersonal problems which arose within the team. The second group, consisting of eight teachers, one speech therapist, and one director of preschool education, focused 90% of its time on the problems of relationships outside the group. There was a theme common to both groups of how women can handle the conflicting demands of home and profession. The groups have requested that we continue next year.

Similar types of meetings with administrators can have benefit to children in classrooms, as well as to the administrators themselves. In one small school district, a two-year experience involved about 120 hours of consultant time distributed in over twenty meetings, lasting usually three hours but occasionally as many as ten hours. The group consisted of ten administrators: the superintendent, assistant superintendent, and eight principals. After the experience, some of the participants reported the following (Berkovitz, 1977):

"I was a new principal at a school. When I first arrived there were some days when as many as 18 or 19 students were lined up outside my door awaiting disciplinary action. Now there are none. I have taught my teachers to become better listeners." .. "Reading scores in my school have increased from 26% to 62%, partly as a result of better teacher and principal interaction." ... "I am better at handling emotionally distraught children, and allow them catharsis and expression rather than try to still their feelings." ... "As a result of my leveling with teachers and comparing philosophies of child management, we've become better able to work together. One of my teachers has changed to become fairer in her treatment of problem students. She seeks discussion and explanation before reacting punitively. She has become a more reasonable person." ... "I feel free to take a tough, hard line with my teachers, but even so I am getting few requests for transfers." ... "I can take criticism more easily. As a result, I developed rap sessions with my staff, and I found that my staff perceived me differently from how I perceived myself. Partly as a result of this, I have involved my staff in decisions affecting the school, for example the selection of teacher aides. I like to think I would have done this anyway, but it is possible that it was facilitated through consultation." ...

Evaluation

Evaluation of the results of mental health consultation has always been difficult to quantify. In one paper reviewing 35 consultation outcome studies (17 of which were in schools) between 1958 and 1972, "69% of the studies reviewed showed positive change on the consultee, client, or system or some combination of these" (Mannino and Shore, 1975). Attempts at evaluation should be a part of every consultation program. Two-thirds of the consultees of one school district (ten schools) reported the following changes. These were ascertained in a questionnaire filled out after three years of consultation:

A. Greater sensitivity to feelings of others;

B. Improved ability to listen;

C. Awareness of the behavior norms which are frequent in groups;

D. Greater acceptance of different attitudes and values;

E. Increased willingness to discuss staff problems and personal feelings in an open manner;

F. Changed attitudes towards children with problems. (Berkovitz, 1970a)

Summary

This large variety of experiences between educators and mental health professionals is an example of essential outreach activities by child treatment facilities and/or practitioners. The bulk of disturbed children rarely arrive at clinical services but are available to primary, secondary, and tertiary prevention activities in the schools. In order for a mental health professional to assist in this, it is necessary to overcome the mutual barrier of territorial sensitivities and language problems. While clinical skills are very useful, equally important is the need to develop consultative skills—i.e. dealing in a co-equal relationship with personnel of a different profession.

Certainly many educators are sensitive to the needs to reorganize many aspects of current school structure to help better growth and maturation of young people. The mental health consultant can often join with the energy and momentum of these educators to effect changes, as well as to bring new needs to awareness. Many child psychiatry training programs encourage child psychiatrists to gain expertise in the interventions described above. Some programs encourage skills in consulting with legislators to help improve and draft legislation for children (Berlin, 1976). Current legislation—e.g. P.L. 94-142—offers still unrealized opportunities (and difficulties) for collaboration between educators and child oriented mental health professionals.

Hopefully, child psychiatrists of the future will feel that their skills are as useful in the schools as in their offices, for the benefits of child patients, as well as the general child population.

Acknowledgment

With appreciation to several helpful persons including Jacquie Friedman for unstinting secretarial services and the several unnamed school consultants who supplied me with descriptions of their work.

References

Altrocchi, J., C. Spielberger, and C. Eisendorfer. (1965) Mental health consultation with groups. *Comm. Ment. Health J.* 1:127–134.

Aponte, H.J. (1976) The family school interview: An ecostructural approach. *Fam. Process* 15:303–312.

Berkovitz, I.H. (1970a) Varieties of mental health consultations for school personnel. *J. Second Ed.* 45(3):

Berkovitz, I.H. (1970b) Mental health consultation to school personnel: Administrator considerations and consultant priorities. *J. School Health* 40:348–354.

Berkovitz, I.H., ed. (1975) *When Schools Care: Creative Use of Groups in Secondary Schools* New York: Brunner/Mazel.

Berkovitz, I.H. (1977) Mental health consultation for school administrators. In S.C. Plog and P.I. Ahmed, eds., *The Principles and Techniques of Mental Health Consultation.* New York: Plenum.

Berkovitz, I.H. (1980) Improving the relevance of secondary education for adolescent developmental tasks. In M. Sugar, ed., *Responding to Adolescent Needs*, New York: Spectrum Publications.

Berkovitz, I.H., and L.E. Newman. (1980a) Mental health intervention in the school-world. In D. Cantwell and P. Tanguay, eds., *Clinical Child Psychiatry*, New York: Spectrum Publications.

Berkovitz, I.H., and M. Thomson. (1973) *Mental Health Consultation and Assistance to School Personnel of Los Angeles County.* Los Angeles: Office of the Los Angeles County Superintendent of Schools.

Berkowitz, M.I. (1975) *A Primer on School Mental Health Consultation.* Springfield, Ill., Charles C. Thomas.

Berlin, I.N. (1974) Mental health programs in the schools. In S. Arieti, ed., *American Handbook of Psychiatry*, 2nd ed. New York: Basic Books, pp. 735–744.

Berlin, I.N. (1976) Presidential address to the American Academy of Child Psychiatry annual meeting, Toronto.

Canter, L., and T. Paulson. (1974) A college credit model of inschool consultation: A functional behavioral training program. *Comm. Ment. Health J.* 10:268–275.

Caplan, G. (1970) *The Theory and Practice of Mental Health Consultation.* New York: Basic Books.

Chess, S., and M. Hassibi. (1978) *Principles and Practices of Child Psychiatry.* New York and London: Plenum.

Ekstein, R., and R.L. Motto. (1960) The borderline child in the school situation. In M.G. Guttsegen and G.B. Gottsegen, eds., *Professional School Psychology.* New York and London: Grune & Stratton.

Flacy, D., A. Goda, and R. Schwartz. (1975) Assisting teachers in group counseling with drug abusing students. In I.H. Berkovitz, ed., *When Schools Care.* New York: Brunner/Mazel.

Forman, A., and W. Hetznecker. (1972) Varieties and vagaries of school consultation. *J. Am. Acad. Child Psychiat.* 11(4):699–704.

Kaplan, C., (1975) Advantages and problems of interdisciplinary collaboration in school group counseling. In I.H. Berkovitz, ed., *When Schools Care.* New York: Brunner/Mazel.

Kellam, S.G., J.D. Branch, K.D. Agrawal, and M.E. Ensminger. (1975) *Mental Health and Going to School.* Chicago: University of Chicago Press.

Krugman, M., ed. (1958) *Orthopsychiatry and the School.* American Orthopsychiatric Association.

LaVietes, R.L., and S. Chess (1969) A training program in school psychiatry. *J. Am. Acad. Child Psychiat.* 8:84–96.

Mannino, F.V., and M.D. Shore. (1975) The effects of consultation. *Am. J. Comm. Psychol.* 3:1–21.

Miller, D. (1970) Adolescents and the high school system. *Comm. Ment. Health J.* 6:483–491.

Ratner, J., ed. (1937) *Intelligence in the Modern World: John Dewey's Philosophy.* New York: Random House.

Rogers, C.A. (1942) Mental health findings in three elementary schools. *Educational Res. Bull.* (Ohio State University) 21(3).

Rutter, M. (1975) *Helping Troubled Children.* New York and London: Plenum.

Smith, P.A., W. O'Rear, and A. Cashion. (1975) A survey of rap rooms in five high schools and some student attitudes. In I.H. Berkovitz, ed., *When Schools Care.* New York: Brunner/Mazel, pp. 154–169.

Vanderpol, M., and H.S. Waxman. (1974) Beyond pathology: Some basic ideas for effective school consultation. *Psychiat. Opin.* 11:19–25

Wickman, E.K. (1928) *Children's Behavior and Teachers' Attitudes.* New York: Commonwealth Fund.

CHAPTER 30

Therapeutic and Preventive Interventions in Mental Retardation

John Y. Donaldson
Frank J. Menolascino

Introduction

"Mental retardation refers to subnormal general intellectual functioning which originates during the developmental period and is associated with impairment of either learning in social adjustment or maturation or both" (DSM II, 1968). The diagnosis of mental retardation depends partly on impaired intellectual ability but it should also involve a clinical judgment of the patient's adaptive behavioral capacity, motor skills, and social and emotional maturity.

The primary focus of this chapter will be on the diagnosis, prevention, and treatment of various emotional problems that may be acquired by a retarded child or that may accompany retardation. We will not attempt to summarize all of the sixty or more various diagnostic categories for retardation that were possible in DSM II. Our discussion will cover broad categories of retardation, and we would refer you to the current APA approved *Diagnostic and Statistical Manual* for specific diagnostic considerations.

History

At the close of the eighteenth century and throughout much of the nineteenth century, the care of the retarded was closely linked to psychiatry in that all mental abnormalities tended to be grouped together. The works of Itard, Seguin, and Howe were especially good examples of the type of concern for the retarded that was shown by physicians of that era. As the nineteenth century drew to a close, a number of events came together that tended to separate the retarded patient from the psychiatric patient, from the psychiatrist, and from society itself. These factors included the identification of organic brain defects in many retarded patients, the eugenics movement, the overcrowding of various state facilities, and even the fact that the IQ test made it possible to diagnose mental retardation without a medical evaluation.

This trend was not reversed until the middle of the twentieth century, when four new developments tended to make it possible and increasingly desirable to maintain the great majority of retarded persons in their home communities. These developments included an improved understanding of the process of human development—especially that of attachment, improved methods of medical management of certain psychiatric conditions, the community psychiatry movement, and a variety of social factors, including the efforts of parent groups such as the National Association of Retarded Citizens (Donaldson and Menolascino, 1977).

Many authors have noted that retarded patients

can suffer from virtually the entire range of psychiatric illness seen in the general population (Webster, 1970; Phillips and Williams, 1975). It is important to note that patients having different levels of retardation are more at risk to develop certain emotional problems that are more or less characteristic of their group. We will be discussing these characteristic problems later in the chapter.

The authors consider the following concept to be especially important. In the past, the majority of retarded patients were institutionalized because of acute emotional or behavioral problems (Menolascino, 1967). This was not only unfortunate but inappropriate. The institutions for the retarded were typically without the services of a psychiatrist, and all too often the institution became the final destination for the retarded child. Fortunately, in the great majority of cases, short-term intensive psychiatric intervention can make it possible for the acutely disturbed retarded patient to resume functioning in the community. The recent "right to treatment" court decisions and legislation place an even greater emphasis on this approach (APA Position Statement, 1977).

Theoretical Considerations

Emotional Problems Most Commonly Associated with Different Levels of Retardation

The severely and profoundly retarded. This group of patients is characterized by multiple physical signs and symptoms, a high frequency of multiple handicaps (especially involving gross central nervous system impairment). These severe problems significantly impair the child's ability to assess and effectively partake in ongoing interpersonal-social transactions. By definition, their IQs are below 35. Clinically, these patients manifest primitive behaviors and gross delays in their developmental repertoires. Such primitive behaviors include very rudimentary utilization of special sensory modalities with particular reference to touch, position sense, oral explorative activity, and minimal externally directed verbalizations. In diagnostic evaluation of these patients, one will often note a considerable amount of mouthing and licking of toys and excessive tactile stimulation (e.g., "autistic" hand movements which are executed near the eyes, as well as skin picking and body rocking).

From a diagnostic viewpoint, the very primitiveness of the severely retarded child's overall behavior in conjunction with much stereotyping and negativism may be misleading. For example, when minimally stressed in an interpersonal setting, this group of patients frequently exhibit negativism and out-of-contact behavior initially suggesting a psychotic disorder of childhood. However, these children do make eye contact and will interact with the examiner quite readily despite their very minimal behavioral repertoire. Similarly, one might form the initial impression that both the level of observed primitive behavior and its persistence is secondary to extrinsic deprivation factors (a functional behavior). To some extent this is true in that the retarded child's efforts to adapt to his various sensory and cognitive impairments may hinder further his social functioning.

One group of authors (Chess, Korn, and Fernandez, 1971) has clearly documented the high vulnerability of severely retarded children with the rubella syndrome to psychiatric disorders. It has been noted that without active and persistent interpersonal, special sensory, and educational stimulation (including active support of the parents), these youngsters often fail to develop any meaningful contact with reality, and they may display a kind of "organic autism."

The authors have been impressed by the extent of personality development which the severely retarded can attain if early and energetic behavioral, educational, and family counseling interventions are initiated and maintained. True, they remain severely handicapped in their cognitive and social-adaptive dimensions; however, there is a world of difference between the severely retarded child who graduates from a standing table to a wheelchair with a wide number of self-help skills and those who are aloof and totally lacking in such skills.

Even in well-managed severely retarded individuals, one notes that their problem with language development remains a very significant factor in blocking growth toward more complex personality development. This places them at relatively small risk for neurotic solutions to life problems. Fortunately, these youngsters are nearly always accepted by their parental support systems and peer groups (if adequate evaluations and anticipatory counseling are accomplished), perhaps reflecting empathy for the obvious handicaps which these youngsters display.

The moderately retarded. Children with this level of retardation have many of the wide variety of obvious handicaps noted in the previous group, and they are also easily identified as retarded even by the unskilled observer. Their IQs range from 36 to 52. Their slow rate of development and their specific problems with language elaboration and concrete approaches to problem-solving situations present both unique and marked vulnerabilities for adequate personality development.

In an outstanding study, Webster (1970) viewed these personality vulnerabilities as stemming from the characteristic postures that moderately retarded individuals tend to use in their interpersonal transactions, more autism (selective isolation), inflexibility and repetitiousness, passivity, and a simplicity of the emotional life. This simplicity of emotional life, a cardinal characteristic of the moderately retarded, reflects their undifferentiated ego structures and poses a clinical challenge in attempting to modulate their tendency toward direct expression of basic feelings and wants, as noted in their obstinacy, difficulties in parallel play situations, and so on.

Like the more severely retarded, the high frequency of special sensory and integrative disorders in this group hampers seriously their approach to problem-solving and makes them more likely to develop atypical or abnormal behaviors in a variety of educational or social settings. The limited repertoire of personality defenses, coupled with their concrete approaches, tends to be fertile ground for overeaction to minimal stresses in the external world. Proneness to hyperactivity and impulsivity, rapid mood swings, and temporary regression to primitive self-stimulatory activities are characteristic of their fragile personality structures. Limitations in language development hamper further their ability to fully communicate their interpersonal or intrapsychic distress.

This group of youngsters is more likely than the severely retarded to be rejected by their parents and peers. Their significant attempts to involve themselves in family and neighborhood activities, coupled with the above noted behavioral traits, tend to alienate them from the interpersonal contacts which they so desperately need.

The mildly retarded. Mildly retarded children have a unique set of stresses. Their often nearly normal appearance tends to preclude their easy identification by others even though their IQs are by definition between 52 and 68. This can lead to unrealistic expectations and a series of failures. At the same time, these children are capable of developing some insight into their limitations.

Emotional disturbances in the mildly retarded reflect the well-known residuals of an individual who is labeled as deviant and then becomes caught in the dynamic interplay of disturbed family transactions. The frequent delay in establishing that these youngsters have a distinct learning disability (usually not confirmed until six to nine years of age) is a common source of anxiety for the mildly retarded individual. This is compounded by his inability to integrate the normal developmental sequences at the appropriate time in his life. Usually during the latency period of psychosexual personality integration, the mildly retarded person will have considerable difficulty in understanding the symbolic abstractions of schoolwork and the complexities of social-adaptive expectations from both his family and peer group. It is at this stage they gain some understanding of their lmitations. Unfortunately by early adolescence, they have all too often established an identity that incorporates both retardation and deviance. The vulnerabilities of the mildly retarded are not as likely to be buffered or redirected by loved ones into new interpersonal coping styles that can help correct earlier misconceptions about the self. Without some source of community support and direction, the mildly retarded are at high risk to fail in society.

Emotional and Developmental Problems Associated with Different Models of Care

An alternative way in which to conceptualize the more general problems of the retarded, in addition to the levels of retardation, is to consider the problems that appear to be related to different models of care.

Providing optimal care for the retarded at home, in the community, or in an institutional setting is extremely difficult because there is no "average" retarded child. In a general way, they can be grouped by overall abilities, but one of the most striking things about the retarded is the great variation of abilities often seen within each of these persons. This variability plus the great difficulty the caregivers are likely to have in fully understanding the individual retarded person's abilities and disabilities appears to be the basis for a number of the psychiatric problems seem in the retarded. The most common type of error we have seen in the care of the retarded involves the caregiver having either overly limited or excessive expectations for the retarded person. Errors in either direction appear to contribute significantly to a great many of the psychiatric problems seen in the retarded.

Overly limited expectations. Too few expectations combined with too little effort on the part of the care provider was a care pattern commonly seen in the vast number of institutionalized retarded of previous decades. These children tended to show a pattern of underachievement and a detachment syndrome that is typical of persons raised in barren institutional environments. One common problem characteristic to these children was a profound and often indiscriminately expressed affect hunger. Because these children, particularly the moderately or mildly retarded, often had no experience with significant or meaningful object relations and were accustomed to living their lives amidst large numbers of minimally involved people, their indiscriminate approach to strangers was a serious problem. This lack of "social sense" was often cited as not only part of the syndrome of retardation, but also a reason for continued institutionalization (Donaldson and Menolascino, 1977). Another variant of this detachment syndrome was more often seen in the severely retarded. Instead of indiscriminate approach behavior, this group often withdrew into themselves to develop a pattern of primitive, self-stimulating behaviors that were easily confused with the stereotypic behaviors seen in infantile autism.

Another variant is the situation wherein the caretaker actually did too much instead of too little—an overprotective model. Prior to the availability of community-based programs, parents who were faced with the singularly unhappy choice of sending their child to an institution sometimes felt that the only acceptable solution was to keep the child at home. All too often this was in an isolated part of the home away from the bulk of family or external social contacts. Here the devoted mother tended to the child's every need and in doing so increased his dependency and almost totally eliminated any capability for developing effective social-adaptive functions. This caused even more serious problems when the child's physical maturation or the parents' advancing years made home care no longer possible.

Where the detached mildly or moderately retarded person is "at risk" to become the counterpart of a character disorder in a person of normal intelligence, the overprotected retarded person is likely to show symptoms of inflexibility, autistic thinking, and separation anxiety. This second group may also tend to show stereotypic behavior as a pattern of self-stimulation. As might be expected, the detached previously institutionalized child is "at risk" to show active but indiscriminate behavior in community placement efforts, while the older child with a history of overprotective isolation is at more risk to respond with anxiety and anger to the social and self-help demands of the community or institutional placement that must eventually come.

Excessive expectations. At the other end of the spectrum, we see also retarded children and young adults who show evidence of caretakers having had unrealistically high expectations. One of the most common problems in very young moderately retarded children who do not have physical stigmata is a failure by the parents to recognize their intellectual limitations prior to the normal time for language acquisition. It would appear that one common cause of autistic-like psychoses is the placement of a sensitive, intelligent-appearing, but nevertheless retarded child in a situation where his conscientious parents are doing all the "right" things during the second year of life to facilitate language skills. Verbal demands to learn to name objects often cause the moderately retarded child with a language disability to react with increasing anxiety and a variety of avoidance behaviors that reflect the lack of pleasure they find in verbal interactions. We have seen a number of these children who when detected early (by age 2 or 3) were able to give up their autistic-like behavior as ways were found to relate to them that did not depend on verbal productions. Similar examples of excessive expectations are occasionally seen in innovative institutional or community programs where children who are more severely retarded may be involved with overly intense efforts to maximize their capabilities. In some cases this has resulted in more frequent seizures, and in others we have noted a pattern of autistic withdrawal quite similar to that noted above. One of the most distressing problems with older children in this group are outbursts of violent behavior when excessive expectations have been maintained for too long. All too often such children are placed on high doses of medication in an effort to control aggression that is actually reactive in nature and not a symptom of psychosis.

A related pattern is that of denial of all or part of a child's retardation. This type of parent may attempt to enroll a retarded child in a regular class when it is obviously inappropriate or may discount gross behavioral abnormalities that are often easily managed in a more appropriate environment.

Applicability

We have noted earlier that mentally retarded persons can fall prey to essentially the same types of emotional illnesses that befall persons of normal intellectual ability. Therefore, one can expect to see in the retarded the full range of psychoses, neuroses, personality disorders, behavioral disorders, psychophysiologic disorders, and transient situational disturbances that are noted in the "normal" population (Webster, 1970). In community-based psychiatric programs that provide services for the retarded, it is not unusual to note combined diagnoses such as childhood schizophrenia and moderate mental retardation associated with unknown prenatal influence, or unsocialized aggressive reaction of adolescence and mild mental retardation associated with prematurity.

Practically speaking, certain diagnostic categories such as the neuroses tend to be underrepresented in the retarded, while others are seen with relative frequency (e.g., schizophrenia, the various behavioral reactions, and transient situational disturbances). Those diagnostic entities that are seen most frequently, or that present special problems of diagnosis, will be described in this section.

Childhood Psychoses and Mental Retardation

Psychotic reactions of childhood have presented a major challenge to the clinician since their distinct recognition by De Sanctis (1906). Delineation of types and etiologies was delayed in part by the fact that the psychotic child frequently functions at a mentally retarded level. Early observers believed that all psychotic children "deteriorated." In 1943, "early infantile autism" was described and received much interest, including speculation as to whether it represented the earliest form of childhood schizophrenia (Kanner, 1943). The term "autism" frequently is employed in the differential diagnosis of the severe emotional disturbances in infancy and early childhood. Yet to label a child as "autistic" presents some formidable problems in regard to definition of the term, its specific etiological-diagnostic implications, and the treatment considerations for the child so designated (Ornitz and Ritvo, 1976). All too often the word is used as if it were a diagnosis, a synonym of childhood schizophrenia, or an abbreviation for early infantile autism. Such usage obviously is imprecise and contributes further to the diagnostic confusion which has abounded in the literature concerning childhood psychosis. Autistic behavior, like hyperactivity, should call to mind a differential diagnosis but should not be a diagnosis in itself.

Today there is not the amount of discussion or disagreement concerning diagnosis, treatment, and differential outcome of the functional childhood psychoses or their interrelationships to mental retardation that there was ten to fifteen years ago. A number of follow-up studies (Menolascino and Eaton, 1967) coupled with the literal rediscovery of the wide variety of primitive behavioral repertoires in the retarded and a lack of relative differences in treatment modalities and corresponding patient responses all have tended to mute this earlier clinical fervor. For example, an excellent review of the past relationships between emotional disturbance and mental retardation by Garfield and Shakespeare (1964) addressed almost a third of its content to the relationships between emotional disturbance and mental retardaton. As Creak (1963) and Penrose (1966) have noted, the most common concern in this relationship is not whether the patient is retarded or psychotic, but to determine how much of the condition is attributable to retardation and how much to psychosis. In the seventies, the issue has been clarified, and it is becoming quite apparent that the number of functional etiologies of infantile autism and childhood schizophrenia is quite limited in scope. The reported findings of central nervous system pathology in the psychoses of childhood is the most frequent trend noted in the past fifteen years (Bialer, 1970; Robinson and Robinson, 1965; Rimland, 1964; Rutter, 1965; Rutter, Graham, and Yule, 1970; Menolascino, 1965; Menolascino and Eaton, 1967; Orintz and Ritvo, 1976).

In summary, the clinical reports of the last decade have rather clearly shown several important points: (1) The psychoses of childhood, and particularly that of autism, are strongly associated with dysfunction of the central nervous system. (2) The appearance of psychotic behavior (and/or autistic behavior) and mental retardation in young nonverbal children bespeaks both common etiology and a diminished capacity to tolerate stress. (3) Retarded patients may show stereotyped self-stimulating behavior that resembles autism. (4) Improvement of the psychotic condition in an "autistic" child far more commonly results in a retarded child who is able to interact with others than in a child of normal intelligence.

Personality Disorders and Behavior Disorders

This group of emotional disorders is characterized by chronically maladaptive patterns of behavior (e.g., antisocial personality, passive-aggressive personality, etc.) that are qualitatively different from psychotic or neurotic disorders (DSM II, 1968). Studies reported in the earlier history of retardation tended indiscriminately to see antisocial behavior as an expected behavioral accompaniment to mental retardation. For example, the much-discussed earlier reports on the relationship between retardation and personality disorders (especially the antisocial personality) were at one time couched as a moralistic-legal construct, rather than on definitive descriptive criteria (Barr, 1904). The antisocial personality designation is a diagnosis that is frequently overrepresented in borderline and mildly retarded adults. The comparable diagnosis in children is the unsocialized aggressive reaction of childhood or adolescence. It would appear that behavioral problems of an antisocial nature are more frequently seen in this group for a variety of reasons. The same poverty of interpersonal relationships during childhood that leads to retardation associated with psychosocial deprivation can also lead to impaired object relations and poorly internalized controls. Also, the diminished coping skills of this group often necessitate their performing deviant acts simply to exist. Finally, this group is most likely to be released from institutional settings in young adulthood, thereby graphically illustrating the effects of institutional detachment on personality structure.

It is interesting to note that other personality disorders (e.g., schizoid personality) have been reported only rarely in the retarded. The only other personality disorder in the retarded that has received much attention is the "inadequate personality," even though the application of exact diagnosis criteria would exclude this disorder as a primary diagnosis in mental retardation. The current definition of this personality disorder as a primary diagnosis states: "This behavior pattern is characterized by ineffectual responses to emotional, social, intellectual, and physical demands. While the patient seems neither physically *nor mentally deficient*, he does manifest inadaptability, ineptness, poor judgment, social instability, and lack of physical and emotional stamina" (DSM II, 1968). Unfortunately, this diagnostic category is still frequently overutilized in the retarded.

In summary, while personality disorders do occur in the mentally retarded, they are primarily based on extrinsic factors, have no distinct etiological relationships to mental retardation, and despite persistent folklore, are not increased overall as to their frequency in the noninstitutionalized retarded population.

Psychoneurotic Disorders

There is very little in the older literature (pre-1950) on the frequency and types of psychoneurotic reactions in the mentally retarded. Previous reviews of this facet of emotional disturbances in the retarded suggested that the frequency of psychoneurosis in the retarded is quite low (Deier, 1964; Garfield and Shakespeare, 1964; Robinson and Robinson, 1965; Menolascino, 1967), and the types of psychoneurosis reported are few in number (e.g., anxiety reactions, Menolascino, 1965; phobic reactions, Webster, 1970; and depressive reactions, Gardner, 1971).

Recent studies (Webster, 1970; Chess, 1970; Woodward, Jaffe and Brown, 1970) dispute the concept of neurosis being incompatible with retardation. It appears that much of what was previously considered "expected behavior" in the retarded on closer study has been noted to be quite similar to emotional disturbance in the nonretarded. Each of these studies is quite explicit as to diagnostic criteria and attributes the neurotic phenomena to factors associated with atypical developmental patterns in conjunction with disturbed family functioning. For example, the above noted recent reports of psychoneurotic disorders in retarded children clearly delineated parameters such as the internal defensive tactics of retarded children (e.g., anxiety, fear of failure, insecurity, etc.) against externally derived phenomena such as chronic frustration, unrealistic family expectations, deprivations, etc. Interestingly, each of these reports suggest that psychoneurotic disorders are more common in children of the high-moderate and mild ranges of mental retardation. This trend has prompted speculation that the relative complexity of psychoneurotic transactions is beyond the adaptive limits of the severely retarded patient (Webster, 1970).

Transient Situational Disturbances

Although this rather large category of minor emotional disturbances is perhaps overutilized in the assessment of the nonretarded, it is employed only rarely during clinical assessment of emotional disturbances in the retarded population. The authors feel that such underutilization is one of the major drawbacks of descriptive approaches to the retarded.

DSM II defines transient situational disturbances as being a "category reserved for more or less transient disorders of any severity (including those of psychotic proportions) that occur in individuals without any apparent underlying mental disorders and that represent an acute reaction to overwhelming environmental stress. If the patient has good adaptive capacity, his symptoms usually recede as the stress diminishes . . ."

The reader will note that the transient nature of these disorders is their paramount feature. The sentence "If the patient has good adaptive capacity, his symptoms usually recede as the stress diminishes" poses a recurrent dilemma when one works with a retarded population.

In our experience a great number of emotional and behavioral problems in the retarded are transient in that they are frequently caused by inappropriate expectations or rapid changes in life patterns and do often respond rapidly to environmental adjustments. Even though it may not be possible to use the transient situational diagnosis if one follows the letter of the guidelines for DSM II, it is recommended that the reader will still conceptualize cases in this manner when it is appropriate.

Hyperactivity

Although hyperkinetic reactions are defined as behavioral reactions in DSM II, there is increasing evidence that hyperactivity is a symptom that may have multiple etiologies (Donaldson, 1975).

Hyperactivity in children of normal intelligence may be due to difficulty concentrating on external events in the psychotic child, to lack of cortical inhibition in the child with classical hyperkinesis associated with minimal brain dysfunction and abnormally low anxiety levels, to tension release in the overly anxious child, to increased irritability in the allergic or food-additive-sensitive child, or to alienation from authority in the unsocialized child. The retarded child may suffer from any of the above conditions or they may be seen in combination because of his frequent central nervous system immaturity, difficulty mastering complex situations, and often limited ego strengths. Satisfactory treatment of the "hyperactivity" is dependent on proper identification of the underlying cause. The presence of retardation should not cause the clinician to discount the other possible etiologies noted previously.

Methods

Two major approaches to the treatment of retarded children are described in this section. They include a discussion of a variety of psychiatric management techniques and recommendations regarding the appropriate use of medications.

Systematic Approach to Management.

Careful Diagnosis

The diagnosis of children who are both mentally retarded and emotionally disturbed underscores the necessity of an open-minded approach. This is the first basic principle for the clinician who plans treatment for these youngsters, and it is important to reassess the patient throughout treatment. Often problems are related to multiple etiologies and will require a variety of interventions. Periodic reevaluation often reveals developmental surprises that underscore the need for a flexible diagnostic-prognostic attitude. Social, psychological, and biologic factors contributing to the child's dysfunction must be clearly identified so that the most effective means of intervention can be determined.

Active Family Involvement and Education

The second principle in treatment planning for children with both mental retardation and emotional disturbance is to engage the family through active participation as early as possible. The family is the key to any effective treatment program. The clinician's attitudes and level of interest frequently are the key to success in this endeavor; thus future cooperation (or lack of it) may reflect his unspoken as well as spoken attitudes at the time of initial contact. The therapist needs to convey to the family his willingness to share with its members the facts he learns, not as an end point but as part of the first step in treatment. Treatment plans become a cooperative process that the parents and clinician work out over the course of time. It is valuable to indicate in an early contact that treatment planning rarely results in a single recommendation—it is something that may shift in focus and alter its course as the child grows and develops. Early implementation of diagnostic and treatment flexibility helps develop the clinician's ability to view the total child and encourages referrals to other special sources of help as indicated. This helps to forestall the "doctor shopping" that often occurs if the parents seek a series of opinions concerning some special allied problem.

Much has been written about the grief reactions

of families with handicapped children. Such a reaction frequently occurs in parents of mentally retarded children. Alertness to this grief reaction must be retained by clinicians evaluating these children, and it must not be forgotten at the time of interpretation to parents or in subsequent interviews. Often a failure to grieve is an additional cause of the doctor shopping. Denial can also be seen as a major symptom of a failure to grieve.

Assessment of family interaction and strengths is a necessary part of the total evaluation, since these assets are essential to planning a comprehensive treatment program. Conversely, some of the family psychopathology encountered serves to reactivate their difficulties with the child in question. Several interviews may be necessary to determine the nature of family transactions with their handicapped child.

Principles of Primary and Secondary Prevention

A third consideration in a comprehensive systems approach to treatment is early diagnosis and treatment. In the more severely retarded, this process is likely to occur in conjunction with a medical evaluation during infancy or in the preschool years. In relatively mild cases in disadvantaged families, screening programs within the school or prior to school entry become relatively more important. Much can be done to prevent the alienation of borderline and mildly retarded children if their limitations are identified early. This has the advantage of preventing their suffering the effects of unrealistic expectations and also allows the school to develop appropriate special programs for the child. In all areas, early diagnosis facilitates identification of problems, which in turn is essential if one is to formulate realistic therapeutic goals and overall expectations for the child. If this is done, frustration is reduced and fewer secondary psychiatric problems are encountered. In this sense, prevention becomes a cohesive part of the ongoing work for the child and his family. This total approach requires continued follow-up of the patient. Periodic reevaluation must be done so that appropriate shifts in treatment and overall levels of expectation may be carried out.

Principles of Tertiary Prevention

The fourth principle involves focusing on the maximation of developmental potential. It involves a different type of goal setting from the usual treatment expectation, since the focus must often be on what the child can do rather than anticipation of a *cure*. The goal then becomes one of maximally and at the same time realistically habilitating the patient. If done well, each retarded person will have avoided the problem of inappropriate expectations.

Normalization

The principle of normalization (Nirge, 1969) has literally revolutionized the field of mental retardation. It means the provision of services within the mainstream of our communities. It stands in contrast to the non-normalizing settings of the institutions of the past. The overwhelming majority of retarded are able to enjoy and profit from the rich variety of human experiences that are found in our communities. These include the opportunity to enjoy life experiences in a family setting or a small group home, to have a work or school experience in a location separate from their dwelling, and to have developmentally appropriate activities within the context of a larger community. This trend became federal policy via the deinstitutionalization policy of 1971. It is becoming clear that the great majority of retarded children will remain with their families or in community-based care programs. As a result, a tremendous number of supportive services, including psychiatry, are necessary. In some communities, it may be necessary for the psychiatrist to take the lead in creating such services as group homes for the retarded, day-care programs, family crisis or respite care programs, citizen advocacy programs, or appropriate educational and work opportunities.

A relatively small percentage of retarded patients will require short or long-term inpatient placement for life-threatening behaviors of physical or emotional etiology or for behavior control. For example, profoundly and severely retarded children who have multiple medical handicaps may need placement out of their primary homes for extended training and management. Retarded patients functioning at higher levels may require long-term care when they present with intractable psychotic conditions. Parenthetically, these psychotic retarded youngsters should be treated in mental health facilities in contrast to the nontreatment which they have often received in the large public institutions for the retarded. The special needs of these more handicapped patients typically exceeds the capabilities and expertise of most community-based programs. However, short-term crisis and long-term care inpatient facilities should only be utilized as back-up supportive services to the rapidly evolving community-based programs.

Coordination of Multiple Services

The sixth principle is to coordinate the many services needed for the child. This requires awareness of the various services available in a given community and an attitude which permits collaboration. It necessitates sharing of the overall treatment plan with the child (when appropriate), the family, and with community resources, with special emphasis on the child's teacher. Close attention to the clarity and continuity of communication is essential. Recent federal legislation (PL 94-142 and the 504 Regulation of HEW) mandates the need for an individualized treatment prescription for every retarded child. The psychiatrist may be called on to assist schools and group homes in developing these individualized plans.

Services which emotionally disturbed mentally retarded children may need will range from office psychotherapy in selected instances through many types of specialized medical care, special education placement, and community services. The Section VI on comparisons will amplify the need for a community psychiatry or systems approach which is required to manage these multiple interventions.

Psychopharmacologic Adjuncts to Treatment

The medications used in psychiatry have one common route of therapeutic intervention in that they all affect neurotransmitter activity in some way. The tranquilizers tend to block or diminish neurotransmitter activity while the stimulants and antidepressants tend to enhance the activity of certain neurotransmitters. As a result of the experience with these various drugs over the past twenty to forty years plus more recent studies regarding the metabolism of neurotransmitters in various comparative psychiatric conditions (Murphy and Wyatt, 1972; Wing and Stein, 1973; Rosenblatt, Leighton, and Chanley, 1973), psychiatry has developed an increasing consensus regarding the probable neurotransmitter abnormality in certain psychiatric conditions (Snyder et al., 1974; Cohen and Young, 1977). Thus if the clinician is able to correlate the probable neurotransmitter abnormality in a given psychiatric condition with the pharmacologic action of various psychoactive medications, he will have a high probability of selecting an appropriate medication.

It appears that children without physiologic signs of anxiety who present with impulsive hyperactivity tend to be catacholamine deficient and are likely to respond positively to stimulant or antidepressant medication (Donaldson, 1975). Similarly, physiologically anxious, hyperalert children tend to have high norepinephrine levels and generally respond well to the more sedative phenothiazines, while children with stereotyped ritualistic behavior appear to have high dopamine levels and tend to respond best to the more potent antipsychotic medications. See Table 1 for a more detailed presentation of this medication and symptom correlation. The dosages used in that table are most appropriate for prepubertal retarded patients. After puberty, dosages may be adjusted upward toward more typical adult ranges.

Although many clinicians might argue that medication is not the ultimate answer to the problems of the retarded or that their disadvantages may outweigh their advantages, it is our opinion that the proper use of medication can lead to a dramatic reduction of patient symptomatology in some cases. This is an especially important consideration when unacceptable behavior has caused the family or school to demand immediate movement toward more restrictive placement alternatives.

Comparisons

The treatment of retarded children by psychiatrists places a much greater emphasis on a systems approach or a community psychiatry model than it does on traditional insight-oriented psychotherapy for the identified patient. While many neurotic children or acutely troubled adolescents may require a considerable amount of individual therapy or family therapy oriented toward clarifying communications problems, these patients typically require a somewhat more directive approach. In this respect, the care of the retarded is quite similar to the care of many other dependent populations and can be compared to the community aspects of child psychiatry or geriatric psychiatry.

Many of the emotional problems of the retarded will require that the psychiatrist be relatively active, more direct and concrete in the interview or treatment setting, and also require that he become accustomed to the delayed language development

Table 1
Psychotropic Medications for Retarded Children

Drug	*Dose*	*Indication*	*Apparent Action*	*Potential Problems*
1. Dextroamphetamine (Dexedrine)	5-20 mgm/day	Classical or "stimulus bound" hyperactivity with minimal brain dysfunction (MBD)	Mimic or release norepinephrine	↓ Appetite ↓ Growth ↑ Anxiety ↑ Aggression when given to anxious children
2. Methylphenidate (Ritalin)	10-40 mgm/day	Classical or "stimulus bound" hyperactivity with MBD	Mimic or release norepinephrine	↓ Appetite ↓ Growth ↑ Anxiety ↑ Aggression when given to anxious children
3. Imipramine (Tofranil)	10-25 mgm/day	Classical hyperactivity with MBD, some types of detachment enuresis	↑ brain norepinephrine,† block acetylcholine*	Anticholinergic side effects, ↑ anxiety, ↑ aggression, may unmask latent schizophrenia
4. Chlorpromazine (Thorazine)	10-300 mgm/day	↑ anxiety associated with aggression and/or psychosis	Block norepinephrine,† and dopamine*	Photosensitivity leukopenia—occasional extrapyramidal side effects, tissue deposition with prolonged usage, tardive dyskinesia
5. Thioridazine (Mellaril)	10-300 mgm/day	↑ anxiety associated with aggression and/or psychosis	Block norepinephrine,† dopamine* and acetylcholine*	Headache, depression, weight gain, nasal stuffiness, retrograde ejaculation, tissue deposition, tardive dyskinesia
6. Trifluoperazine (Stelazine)	1-10 mgm/day	↑ anxiety with withdrawal and compulsive features and/or psychosis	Block norepinephrine* and dopamine†	Extrapyramidal side effects, leukopenia, ↑ aggressiveness or hyperactivity in some patients with MBD, tardive dyskinesia
7. Fluphenazine (Prolixin)	1-10 mgm/day	↑ anxiety with withdrawal and compulsive features and/or psychosis	Block norepinephrine* and dopamine†	Extrapyramidal side effects, leukopenia, ↑ aggressiveness or hyperactivity in some patients with MBD, tardive dyskinesia
8. Haloperidol (Haldol)	0.5-10 mgm/day	Organicity with psychosis and ritualistic or stereotyped behavior	Block dopamine,** block norepinephrine*	Severe extrapyramidal side effects, ↑ hyperactivity in some patients, tardive dyskinesia
9. Hydroxazine (Atarax, Vistaril)	30-75 mgm/day	Anxiety, psychophysiologic disorders, allergy	Antihistamine,* sedative†	Some ↓ effectiveness over time, inadequate for more severe conditions
10. Diphenhydramine (Benedryl)	25-300 mgm/day	Hyperactivity 2°, anxiety, allergies	Antihistamine,† sedative*	Drowsiness, some anticholinergic effects, may worsen classical hyperkinesis
11. Diazepam (Valium)	4-15 mgm/day	Situational anxiety	Hypothesized to increase competitive inhibitors of norepinephrine and dopamine—i.e., GABA, glycine	Possible loss of recent memory, ↑ aggression in some children, some potential for dependence
12. Chlordiazepoxide (Librium)	10-40 mgm/day	Situational anxiety	Same as above	Same as Valium except less problem with recent memory loss
13. Phenobarbital	30-240 mgm/day	For grand mal and petit mal epilepsy, situational anxiety	Sedative, anticonvulsant	↑ aggressive behavior in some children—especially with MBD, recent memory loss, potential for dependence

* Pharmacologic activity slight but significant
† Pharmacologic activity moderate
** Pharmacologic activity marked

Table 1 *(continued)*

Drug	*Dose*	*Indication*	*Apparent Action*	*Potential Problems*
14. Diphenylhydantoin Sodium (Dilantin)	5 mg/kg/day up to 300 mgm/day	Grand mal seizures	Anticonvulsant	Leukopenia, gingival hypertrophy, skin rash
15. Primidone (Mysoline)	250-750 mgm/day	Grand mal and psychomotor seizures	Anticonvulsant	Metabolized to phenobarbital, ataxia, drowsiness, worsened hyperactivity or aggressiveness
16. Ethosuximide (Zarontin)	250-750 mgm	Petit mal seizures	Anticonvulsant	Blood dyscrasias, allergic reactions, drowsiness

so often seen in the retarded (Menolascino and Bernstein, 1970; Szymanski, 1977). Some parents of the retarded will need traditional psychotherapeutic approaches as they work through grief or unrelated emotional problems that might interfere with their ability to care for their child. Nearly all parents will require specific information and recommendations regarding the many problems they will face. Here, we would stress the need for long-term support and guidance to help them to most effectively manage a "problem" that has been literally thrust upon them.

In addition to the importance of the psychiatrists being aware of the many community services, he must also be aware of the specific needs of different types of retarded patients. Often conventional programs are not adequate. While the staffing ratio and the degree of supervision required in group home care of mildly retarded adolescents may not differ significantly from that required in group homes for emotionally disturbed or delinquent adolescents, group homes for modeerately or severely retarded patients or those with special medical problems will require much higher staffing ratios, more strict building codes, and greater medical and nursing supervision of the staff.

With regard to younger retarded children who are treated in day-care programs, it is important to provide a diversity of activities that will allow for the varying developmental levels of children. Not only is there likely to be a considerable variation of abilities from child to child, it is not unusual to see significant variability from skill to skill within one child. Again, these special day-care programs for the retarded will require a more intense staffing pattern and a higher degree of staff expertise than conventional day-care programs. A crucial difference in consultation here is the more frequent need to focus on the amelioration of a specific client's adjustment difficulties while simultaneously providing support and curriculum guidance to the program personnel.

In the past, psychiatrists and teachers focused unduly on resolving the retarded child's roadblocks to learning (i.e., the concomitant emotional disturbance) without giving equal attention to the ongoing developmental needs. Parental counseling and individualized therapy with the child can often be interwoven into a developmentally oriented curriculum that focuses on language stimulation and the acquisition of self-help skills. Without this, the child's emotional status may improve while he or she is passing critical developmental periods for skill acquisition. In these challenges, we would strongly recommend mixed modality approaches such as an individual psychotherapy focus on the child and his family, a behavioral modification approach to certain learning tasks; and the utilization of specific medications when indicated.

Most child psychiatrists are already aware of the federal legislation (PL 94–142) mandating that local school systems provide appropriate educational opportunities for all handicapped children. As a result of this legislation, many special programs are already functioning in most communities. Unfortunately, the quality of these services and the specific educational programs developed may vary widely from community to community. It therefore must be the responsibility of each psychiatrist to familiarize himself with the services provided by local programs. The child psychiatrist may be rather surprised to note both the variety and complexity of the excellent community-based programs for the retarded that have come into being during the last ten years. The very newness of these programs demands that the child psychiatrist keep abreast of developments in early childhood education. This aspect of care has not been stressed previously in child psychiatry training programs. Similarly, consultation to the special education programs in the schools demands an awareness of current trends whether one is making specific recommendations regarding the special needs of one child or making recommendations regarding entire school programs.

Families who have elected to keep a retarded child or adolescent at home often can function quite well with the help of the various community support systems that have been described. Nevertheless, these families may find that common life crisis such as death, divorce, unemployment, parental illness, or even a vacation may present almost overwhelming challenges. For this group of patients, a system of respite care can often prevent a temporary crisis from forcing a decision to permanently institutionalize a retarded family member. Because of the special skills required to care for such patients even on a temporary basis, it is not possible simply to ask well-meaning volunteers to take many of these patients into their own home. Often respite care means temporary entry into an existing program for the retarded such as a hostel or properly equipped short-term psychiatric facility. For this reason, it is advisable that such programs maintain a staffing cushion or operate slightly short of capacity so short-term crisis care of this type can be accomplished without undue delay.

It is most common for families to contact a psychiatrist at a time of crisis. When such crisis occurs regarding a retarded patient, the psychiatrist is relatively more likely to become involved in a long-term collaborative relationship with the family. Significant personal satisfaction can come from this type of relationship. The psychiatrist is more likely to have an opportunity to work with an intact family with less parental pathology and a greater capacity to carry out his recommendations than is the case with "pure" psychiatric cases. In addition, added satisfaction can be gained as the psychiatrist is able to note the impact of his efforts to improve the quality of life of both the patient and his family.

This frequently observed quality of family strength provides another important difference in the manner in which a child psychiatrist interfaces with retarded patients and their families. These parents, through their establishment of a national movement of concern over 28 years ago, have become a well-organized force for seeking changes in treatment approaches for their children. Indeed, the majority of the major national changes have come from this parental movement—the National Association for Retarded Citizens. Through this organization the child psychiatrist can help parents in their advocacy for new services, while simultaneously fulfilling his own professional role as a positive change agent on behalf of these children and adults.

Summary and Conclusions

Retarded persons are subject to the same basic types of psychiatric illnesses as the general population. Because of their tendency toward CNS impairment and diminished overall coping ability, they present somewhat greater than average risks for psychosis, long-term behavioral disturbances, and transient situational reactions.

Many retarded persons are unnecessarily institutionalized because of acute emotional problems. In nearly all cases the retarded can be maintained in the community with the help of psychiatrists who are willing to provide short-term and supportive psychiatric care for them and their families.

As with other groups of dependent psychiatric patients—i.e., child or geriatric—the clinician's efforts must frequently be directed as much toward assessing and treating the strengths and weaknesses of the family and community support systems as they are toward the more traditional direct care of the individual patient.

References

American Psychiatric Association. (1968) *Diagnostic and Statistical Manual of Mental Disorders II*. Washington, D.C.: American Psychiatric Association.

American Psychiatric Association. (1977) Position statement on the right to adequate care and treatment for the mentally ill and mentally retarded. Task Force on the Right to Treatment, *Am. J. Psychiat.* 134:354–355.

Barr, M.W. (1904) *Mental Defectives, Their History, Treatment and Training*. Philadelphia: Blakiston.

Bialer, I. (1970) Emotional disturbance and mental retardation: Etiologic and conceptual relationships. In F.J. Menolascino, ed., *Psychiatric Approaches to Mental Retardation*, New York: Basic Books.

Chess, S. (1970) Emotional problems in mentally retarded children. In: F.J. Menolascino, ed., *Psychiatric Approaches to Mental Retardation*. New York: Basic Books.

Chess, S., S. Korn, and P.B. Fernandez. (1971) *Psychiatric Disorders of Children with Congenital Rubella*. New York: Brunner/Mazel.

Cohen, D.J., and J.G. Young. (1977) Neurochemistry and child psychiatry. *J. Am. Acad. Child Psychiat.* 16:353–411.

Creak, E.M. (1963) Childhood psychosis: A review of 100 cases. *Brit. J. Psychiat.* 109:84–89.

De Sanctis, S. (1906) Supra alcune varieta della demenza precoce. *Riv. Sper. Freniat.* 32:141–165.

Deier, D.C. (1964) Behavioral disturbances in the mentally retarded. In H.A. Stevens and R. Heber, eds., *Mental Retardation: A Review of Research.* Chicago: University of Chicago Press.

Donaldson, J.Y. (1975) Some considerations in the treatment of hyperactive children. *Neb. Med. J.* 60:194–196.

Donaldson, J.Y. (1975) and F.J. Menolascino. (1977) Past, current, and future roles of child psychiatry in mental retardation. *J. Am. Acad. Child Psychiat.* 16:38–52.

Garfield, A., and R. Shakespeare. (1964) A psychological and developmental study of mentally retarded children with cerebral palsy. *Develop. Med. Child Neurol.* 6:485–489.

Gardner, W.I. (1971) *Behavior Modification in Mental Retardation.* Chicago: Aldine-Atherton.

Kanner, L. (1943) Autistic disturbances of affective contact. *J. Nerv. Child* 2:217–250.

Menolascino, F.J. (1965) Psychiatric aspects of mental retardation in children under eight. *Am. J. Ortohpsychiat.* 35:852–861.

Menolascino, F.J. (1967) Psychiatric findings in a sample of institutionalized mongoloids. *Brit. J. Ment. Subnorm.* 13:67–74.

Menolascino, F.J., and N.R. Bernstein. (1970) Psychiatric assessment of the mentally retarded child. In *Diminished People.* Boston: Little, Brown, pp. 201–222.

Menolascino, F.J., and L. Eaton. (1967) Psychoses of childhood: A five-year follow-up study of experiences in a mental retardation clinic. *Am. J. Ment. Defic.* 72:370–380.

Murphy, D.L., and R.J. Wyatt. (1972) Reduced monoamine oxidase activity in blood platelets of schizophrenic patients. *Nature* 238:225–226.

Nirge, B. (1969) The normalization principle and its human management implications. In R. Kugel and W. Wolfensberger, eds., *Changing Patterns in Residential Services for the Mentally Retarded.* Washington: Government Printing Office.

Ornitz, E.M., and E.R. Ritvo. (1976) The syndrome of autism: A critical review. *Am. J. Psychiat.* 133:609–621.

Penrose, L.S. (1966) The contribution of mental deficiency research to psychiatry. *Brit. J. Psychiat.* 112:747–755.

Phillips, I., and N. Williams. (1975) Psychopathology: A study of 100 children. *Am. J. Psychiat.* 132:1265–1273.

Rimland, B. (1964) *Infanile Autism.* New York: Appleton-Century-Crofts.

Robinson, H.B., and N.M. Robinson. (1965) *The Mentally Retarded Child: A Psychological Approach.* New York: McGraw-Hill.

Rosenblatt, S., W.P. Leighton, and J.D. Chanley. (1973) Dopamine-B-Hydroxlase: Evidence for increased activity in sympathetic neurons during psychotic states. *Science* 182:923–924.

Rutter, M. (1965) The influence of organic and emotional factors on the origins, natures, and outcomes of childhood psychosis. *Develop. Med. Child Neurol.* 7:518–592.

Rutter, M., P. Graham, and W. Yule. (1970) *A Neuropsychiatric Study in Childhood.* Philadelphia: Lippincott.

Synder, S.H., S.P. Banerjee, H.I. Yamamura, and D. Greenberg. (1974) Drugs, neurotransmitters and schizophrenia. *Science* 184:1243–1253.

Szymanski, L.S. (1977) Psychiatric diagnostic evaluation of mentally retarded individuals. *J. Am. Acad. Child Psychiat.* 16:67–87.

Webster, T.G. (1970) Unique aspects of emotional development in mentally retarded children. In F.J. Menolascino, ed., *Psychiatric Approaches to Mental Retardation.* New York: Basic Books.

Wing, C.D., and L. Stein. (1973) Dopamine-B-hydroxylase deficits in the brains of schizophrenic patients. *Science* 181:344–347.

Woodward, K.F., N. Jaffe, and D. Brown. (1970) Early psychiatric intervention for young mentally retarded children. In F.J. Menolascino, ed., *Psychiatric Approaches to Mental Retardation.* New York: Basic Books.

Treatment of Emotional Disorders in Children and Adolescents

CHAPTER 31

Therapeutic and Preventive Interventions in Juvenile Delinquency

David Zinn

An interest in juvenile delinquency and the difficulties of individual delinquents is a significant aspect of the heritage of child mental health. From its inception the juvenile court has had as its manifest goal treatment and rehabilitation of the youthful offender, and as such has involved workers from all disciplines concerned with the welfare of children: psychiatry, psychology, social work, education. Pioneers such as William Healey, August Aichorn, and Fritz Redl have made fundamental contributions not only to work with the juvenile delinquent but to child treatment in general.

Psychiatric involvement with delinquents, in particular, has centered primarily on consultation with the court, helping to define intervention strategies both in the main and for the individual court client, and on provision of direct service to young people remanded by the court for treatment. What distinguishes this work is not so much the nature of the effort as the context in which it is done. As such, the issue is less distinctive psychopathology or specific treatment techniques than understanding the social and institutional background of delinquency. Currently, however, changes in social policy are occurring which likely will alter considerably the juvenile justice system and mental health activities within it. Further, research is clarifying the significance of delinquent behavior for development and psychopathology. While the precise character of future work is unclear, certain issues and trends are apparent. This chapter addresses three topics: perspectives on delinquency, issues in intervention, and clinical work with the delinquent.

Perspectives on Juvenile Delinquency

General Issues

Delinquency per se is not a psychiatric symptom but a socially ascribed label. A young person engages in some type of proscribed behavior, is arrested (or "taken into custody"), may or may not be "detained," and is adjudicated "delinquent" in the juvenile court. The process is legitimatized in the juvenile codes of the fifty states and rests on social expectations for the behavior of young people and society's view of what is "deviant" for this age group. How, then, can this social process governing behavior of youth be understood from the perspective of child mental health? To what degree are "delinquency" and "antisocial attitudes and behavior" related? Three topics deserve consideration: the historical background of juvenile justice, research on "hidden delinquency" and what it suggests about contemporary youth, and the issue of the chronic offender.

Malmquest (1967) has reviewed the historical background and current structure of juvenile jurisprudence in the United States. This country is unique among industrial societies both in the wide range of juvenile behavior governed by statute and in extending juvenile jurisdiction until age 17 or 18. Indeed, a "juvenile court" and the practice of treating youth differently from adults for certain types of crime—for example, murder—is largely limited to the United States. The juvenile court has evolved out of a nineteenth-century concern for homeless or poorly supervised young people and a belief that their delinquencies, such as they were, could be aborted by a legal institution that supported personal growth. Young people should not be "punished" for their misdeeds but "helped" to develop along more socially constructive lines. Procedural informality was felt necessary to expedite the "helping" or "rehabilitative" process. Associated with this emphasis away from punishment was the incorporation within the juvenile codes of a much broader interpretation of deviant behavior, reflecting, in effect, a legal mandate as to how the young person should "behave" while growing up. Thus juvenile codes typically contain statutes regarding sexual conduct, school attendance, behavior in the home, and the like, as well as those regarding adult criminal offenses such as burglary and assault. Offenses of the former type are generally referred to as "status offenses"; and some states—for example, New York—have revised their juvenile codes to distinguish status offenders, "persons in need of supervision" (PINS), from "delinquents," young people who have committed offenses that would be a crime for an adult. While this is an important clarification, there exists, nevertheless, a bias that to be in juvenile court is to be "delinquent" or antisocial. In fact, a large portion of the work of the typical juvenile court is not with antisocial offenses at all, but with "anti-development" problems such as promiscuity or home truancy.

Self-report questionnaires administered to large groups of young people have demonstrated that within the adolescent age group there is considerable "hidden delinquency"—vandalism, burglary, shoplifting, for example—never coming to the attention of the police (Gold, 1966, 1970; Schwartz, 1977). One longitudinal study of normal adolescents found that almost all these young males at one time or another committed a delinquent act (Offer and Offer, 1975). There is sound empirical bases for assuming that some degree of delinquency, here defined as more typically antisocial acts such as property crimes, are very much a part of the fabric of normal adolescence. Beyond this empirical evidence, however, a review of adolescence in historical perspective suggests that there is a basis for assuming disquiet among contemporary youth. While all societies recognize a period around puberty as a distinctive phase in the life cycle, "adolescence," as commonly understood, is very much a creation of twentieth-century industrial society. The juvenile court act, child labor laws, and mandatory school attendance laws in effect legislated a developmental phase in the midteens, so-called psychosocial adolescence, a time when the young person is considered to be beyond childhood but not yet ready to assume the prerogatives of an adult (Bakan, 1971). This operates through what Elkind (1967) has referred to as the "contract" between parent and child. The child is expected to obey the norms of society, and in return the parents (and society) will support the extended period of development necessary for success in the modern industrial world. Adult authority must be viewed as just for the contract to be binding. Elder (1975) has described contemporary adolescence as a "bridge to adult roles through appropriate socialization and role allocation" involving experiences that guide the young person toward the social maturity required for the contemporary adult. What, though, is current reality? Responding to a loose social fabric, parents (and society) at times can be capricious, sadistic, childishly egocentric, while at the same time demanding behavioral conformity. Institutions providing socialization experiences for adolescents erode in quality and relevance, and adult authority looses its moral imperative (Halleck, 1973). Young people are acutely aware of the pace of social change and the lack of a clear transition to adult roles (Moriarty and Toussieng, 1976). Feelings of oppression are the anticipated consequence of being caught in a web of expectations that are not perceived as personally beneficial (Halleck, 1973). This sense of oppression, in turn, at times will lead to an attack on the perceived aggressor.

To say that feelings of oppression and consequent antisocial attitudes are widespread among the young is not to say, however, that *sustained* delinquency is widespread. Indeed, the converse would appear the case. The self-report surveys noted above find that delinquency among young people is limited both in quality and quantity. Many, if not most, young people commit delinquent acts, including property crimes such as shoplifting and burglary, but this tends to happen only infrequently and not involve violence against persons. On the other hand, there is a group of youth whose delinquency is more sustained as well as directed toward persons. Wolfgang (1970, 1976) followed 9,946 boys born in 1945 and residing in Philadelphia from age 10 to 18. Thirty-five percent had at least one contact with the police, but only 627 boys, 6.3%, committed five or more offenses during their juvenile court ages. This group accounted for 52% of all the delinquencies committed by the entire birth cohort and 53% of the crimes against persons. It appears that a small percentage of youth account for both the majority of delinquent acts and those acts that are truly antisocial.

In summary, the broad scope of juvenile justice legislation within the United States includes what for the mental health professional are three separate groups. There are a large number of young people who commit isolated and relatively trivial delinquent acts, only a small number of which would be expected to come to the attention of the court. A smaller group of young people are defined "delinquent" by society because of home and school truancy, sexual promiscuity, etc. Their problems are more likely to reflect developmental difficulties than entrenched antisocial attitudes or behavior. Finally, there is a much smaller group of youth whose difficulties focus on chronic antisocial conduct.

While it would be helpful to have some quantitative measure of delinquency and juvenile court practice, such statistics as are available have significant limitations. Arrest data, for instance, is based on voluntary collection by the FBI; participation is greater in cities than in rural areas. Further, arrest statistics quantify arrests, not individuals. A small number of highly delinquent youth can bias a larger population. This caveat having been noted, each year over 1,800,000 arrests are made of persons under 18. More than 1,125,000 young people ultimately appear in juvenile court, representing 2.9% of all children aged 10 through 17. The probability of a youth appearing in juvenile court before his eighteeth birthday is 1 in 9, 1 in 6 for males. Juveniles accounted for 26.4% of all arrests in 1973, a significantly greater percent for certain crimes, for example, auto theft (57.1%), burglary and breaking and entering (54.2%), arson (61.5%). The proportions are higher in the cities, less in the suburbs, lowest in rural areas. Excepting prostitution and runaways, boys exceed girls in all categories, though the overall ratio has dropped over the past ten years from 4:1 to 3:1. Proportionately more blacks are arrested than whites (Cavan and Ferdinand, 1975).

Between 1957 and 1971 delinquency cases increased 156%, particularly crimes of violence, homicide, rape, assault, while the population aged 10 to 17 years of age increased only 49%. Further, these rates have continued high despite a drop in the population (Cavan and Ferdinand, 1975). These figures, along with the sense of increasing unrest among the young noted above, suggest that youth are becoming more delinquent. Such a conclusion must be drawn with caution, however. First, the statistics reflect juvenile court practice, not delinquency in the community. Juvenile court referrals tend to be higher in the cities and suburbs, and with the increasing mobility and urbanization of American society, one would expect increasing use of the juvenile courts to deal with behavior heretofore handled informally. Further, much of the increase reflects crimes of violence, hardly related to "unrest" per se. Violence has largely been limited to the ghetto, and the statistical increase in violent crime may reflect increasing movement of youth out of poorly policed areas to ones of greater public visibility and concern. In considering relative rates of delinquency, it is important to note that the FBI statistics date only from 1930, and that the records of cities—for example, Boston and Buffalo—describe periods of violent crime during the nineteenth century. Wolfgang (1978) concludes that the largest amount of variance in rates of violent or "street" crime for the society as a whole can be explained by demographic factors: the higher the proportion within the total population of young people, the group most predisposed to this type of deviance, the larger the rate of violent crime. In this context, historical variations within the youth population are probably less significant.

Conceptual Approaches

Two themes predominate in the literature on delinquency. One, the sociological, begins with the observation that delinquency, particularly violent crime, is most prevalent within the lower-class population. The attempt to explain this association comprises one body of theory about delinquency. The second theme is more diffuse but focuses on the individual delinquent, his psychological functioning, his development, his adaptive failures.

Indeed, Johnson (1959) distinguished between "sociologic delinquency" and "individual delinquency," a distinction still prevalent. The former is thought to arise primarily out of conditions within a particular social milieu—for example, the presence of gangs and delinquent identificatory models—while the latter is a function of the vicissitudes of individual development. At present it appears that this distinction obfuscates more than it clarifies, at least from a clinical perspective, but the two trends first must be reviewed.

Social Parameters

Thio (1978) and Cavan and Ferdinand (1975) have reviewed the sociological literature, and the interested reader is referred to them for a more detailed presentation of this area. In outline, Merton (1957), Cohen (1955), and Cloward and Ohlin (1960) proposed that delinquency could be understood as a consequence of social class membership. Merton argued that the conflict between aspirations for success and the availability of means to succeed within the lower class gave rise to delinquent behavior. Focusing more specifically on juvenile delinquency, Cohen described this conflict in lower-class youth exposed to middle-class values through the schools. He saw the "delinquency subculture" as a defensive attempt to cope with status frustration. Cloward and Ohlin argued that the lower-class youth not only is more likely to be frustrated in legitimate aspirations but is more likely to have access to illegitimate opportunity. The difficulty with this line of thinking is that there is no reliable data to suggest that lower-class youth hold the same level of success aspirations as do middle- or upper-class young people and that they experience the status frustration the theory suggests (Thio, 1978). Further, the self-report studies (Gold, 1966, 1970; Schwartz, 1977) suggest that class relationship is with type of offense and degree of delinquency, not with deviance per se. While entrenched patterns of antisocial conduct appear associated with lower-class membership, impulses toward deviant behavior probably are not. The latter are more relevant from a psychiatric perspective than the former. In this context, Robins' (1966) finding that parental sociopathy is a more potent predictor of antisocial development than class membership is of note. Sutherland and Cressey (1974) drop the issue of lower-class membership and argue instead that delinquency is "learned" in a "delinquent subculture" through a process of "differential association." Young people with delinquent tendencies gravitate together and reinforce and elaborate delinquent behavior. This is less a theory than a truism. The question, rather, is one of relevance. While the group may (and certainly does) reinforce delinquent tendencies, the major clinical issue in understanding delinquency is the deviant impulse, not its propagation.

The theorists noted above approach delinquency in the framework of social forces toward delinquency. Another tradition is to understand delinquency as a breakdown in social control. Hirschi (1969), for example, has approached delinquency from the perspective of a breakdown in "bonding" between individual and society—for example, defects in attachments to others, commitment to conformity, a belief in the moral validity of social rules. This is a view quite compatible with much that will be noted below. There appears to be a trend within the sociologic tradition away from broad structural variables to individual-focused social-psychological constructs.

Individual Parameters: Etiology

Individual-centered research in delinquency can be divided according to conceptual focus into the genetic/physiological, psychodynamic, and developmental psychological approaches, though in actual practice there is much overlap. Biological research has focused largely on two areas; the search for a constitutional or hereditary predisposition toward delinquency and for biological or neuropsychological mechanisms that might predispose toward a delinquent adaptation. While the constitutional approach might be said to have its roots in Lombroso's conception of the criminal as an "atavistic throwback," contemporary issues are the work of Sheldon, the controversy over the XYY chromosome, and modern genetic studies. Sheldon's (1949) work is noteworthy in the observed correlation between mesomorphism and delinquency, confirmed by Glueck and Glueck (1970), but this association can be explained as much through environmental adaptation as a constitutional tendency. Throughout the 1960's there was a spate of articles reporting the association of an XYY chromosome, tallness, and aggressive behavior. More systematic investigation, controlling for earlier methodological errors (Kessler and Moos, 1970), has qualified these observations: XYY males are more likely to be institutionalized, but for crimes against property, not against persons. Their intelligence is lower when compared to XY males as a group, but XY males with lower intelligence are themselves more likely to be institutionalized. The relevant variable, then, would appear to be intelligence, not chromosome complement (Mednick and Christiansen, 1977). While it is generally assumed that hereditary factors are not important in criminality, Mednick presents recent data from Denmark which "lend credence to a hypothesis involving genetic factors in the etiology of psychopathy and criminality." It should be noted, however, that in part this data was developed in a research design involving a rigorous definition of psychopathy applied to an adult sample. "Character neurosis," borderline states, and psychosis were excluded. Thus this intriguing finding would appear to apply to a narrow group within the total delinquent population. Further, as Mednick cautions, Denmark's relatively homogeneous social structure would minimize crime-related environmental dimensions compared to other countries. Mednick postulates that the intervening variable between genetic loading and delinquent behavior is a deficit in response inhibition, itself consequent to low autonomic responsiveness, presumably impairing social learning. Mednick is investigating this hypothesis in a longitudinal study of children whose autonomic responsiveness has been measured. Mednick's hypothesis is consistent with Hare's (1968) report that adult sociopaths have higher thresholds for the perception of pain than nonsociopaths.

A number of correlations are described in the literature: temporal lobe disorders and violence (Pincus and Tucker, 1974); psychomotor epileptic symptoms, paranoid ideation, and delinquent behavior (Lewis and Balla, 1976); neuropsychological deficits and delinquency (Berman and Siegel, 1976); hyperactivity and delinquency (Cantwell, 1978; Satterfield and Cantwell, 1975); trauma to the central nervous system, parental psychopathology, social deprivation and delinquency (Lewis, 1978). There are major methodological problems in definitively establishing such correlations, however. On the basis of a systematic review of the literature, Murray (1976), for instance, argues that the commonly accepted correlation between learning disorders and delinquency is not proven. Further, even when such correlations exist, one must ask whether this reflects an underlying biological predisposition directly producing delinquency or whether the independent variable merely loads toward adaptive failure, in turn leading to delinquency. In the latter case one is left with the conclusion that the inherently limited are inclined toward socially deviant behavior.

The *psychodynamic* tradition in thinking about delinquency has its roots in the work of August Aichorn (1925), who used psychoanalytic insights in a treatment program for delinquent youth in Vienna in the 1920's. While Aichorn was very much a part of the Viennese psychoanalytic professional milieu, it is important to note that his concern with the inner life of the delinquent was very much counter to the rather strict notions of child rearing then prevalent in Austrian society. It was this concern with psychological functioning, conceptualized in the language of psychoanalysis, which is Aichorn's unique contribution and the impetus to subsequent work with delinquents in the United States. Aichorn thought of the delinquent act as a symptom of inner conflict in the context of impoverished identifications and sense of self. Thus Aichorn, and subsequent writers in the psychoanalytic tradition, Alexander (1930), Lampl de Groot (1949), Friedlander (1945) conceptualized their observations in terms of the structural viewpoint in psychoanalytic metapsychology. Generally, the delinquent act was seen as a defensive maneuver by the ego, though in the context of defective identifications.

Simultaneously William Healey (1936) was involved in delinquency research, first in Chicago, then Boston, and focused on the family milieu of the delinquent. He found inadequate models of identification and an environment where potentially delinquent children are scapegoated. Healey's work was extended by Adelaide Johnson (1949, 1959), who described "superego lacunae" in delinquents, deficits in superego functioning consequent to unconscious stimulation by the parents. Johnson's work stimulated considerable investigation by clinicians of a variety of aspects of family functioning and its effects on symptoms in children. Contemporary writers (e.g., Masterson, 1972; Zinner and Shapiro, 1975) have moved beyond focal unconscious processes in families to describe major developmental interferences, projective identifications, double binding, and the like, which leave the young person with an impoverished sense of self. Rather than engender specific deficits in psychological functioning, such interferences lead to general emotional impoverishment. The general trend in psychodynamic thinking has been away from delinquency as a neurotic symptom in the context of psychoanalytic structural metapsychology to delinquency as a character style in the context of object relations theory. It is interesting that the movement of social theorists from the outside in has been mirrored in the psychodynamic tradition by a movement from inside out. There is general recognition that delinquency must be understood in social psychological terms, interpersonal events, rather than strictly in terms of internal psychological structures.

Interrelating both social observation and psychodynamic insight, *developmental psychologists* have investigated a variety of aspects of delinquency. Bowlby (1951) observed the association of severe maternal deprivation, subsequent character impoverishment, and predisposition toward delinquency. He used the term "affectless character" to describe the emotional emptiness, interpersonal alienation, and lack of purpose in victims of maternal deprivation. Subsequent research in early child rearing has not confirmed the necessary correlation between early deprivation and subsequent delinquency, but early rejection is a theme which runs through developmentally oriented delinquency research. Bandura (1958), for instance, uses the term "dependence anxiety" to describe the tension many delinquent young people feel in intimate relationships, believed consequent to early maternal rejection. These young people are internally conflicted over impulses to place themselves in a dependent position, but at the same time fear rejection should such impulses be acted upon. Experience of violence in the home leading to identification with a violent person is believed to be behind a predisposition toward interpersonal violence. Loose discipline in the context of non-nurturing parents is believed to predispose toward delinquency (Glueck and Glueck, 1970; McCord and McCord, 1956, 1959), while rejecting or ambivalent parental relationships associated with overcontrol are believed correlated with autoplastic symptoms. School failure, lowered self-esteem, and a tendency to defend against the pain of this decreased self-esteem are postulated as another parameter (Gold and Mann, 1972). Baumrind (1975) has developed a typology of socialization styles, the delinquent category of which involves harsh, exploitative, arbitrary treatment by the parents, this in the context of their lacking adherence to a principled moral code.

Individual Parameters: Descriptive

One of the difficulties with much of the literature on delinquency is the lack of recognition of what for the clinician is obvious: the heterogeneity in delinquent populations. Two approaches attempt to deal with this problem. One is to study populations of delinquents from the perspective of psychiatric nosology; the other is to use factor analytic techniques to generate type clusters from a variety of observations of members of a population. In the former vein, Kaufman and colleagues (1963) in the 1960's made a distinction between the delinquent who was "impulse ridden" as a character style and the delinquent who was schizophrenic. Lewis and colleagues (Lewis, 1978; Lewis and Shanak, 1978; Lewis and Balla, 1976) found a number of young people in a court sample suffering from schizophrenia or "schizophrenic spectrum disorders," and they argue that clinicians should be more attuned to the possibility of treatable psychosis in delinquent young people. Cocozza (1978) and Chwast (1974) both have described the high incidence of depression in delinquent populations, though there is no evidence that this depression is primary or syndrome-based. Rather, the depression is believed to reflect character impoverishment. Attempting to link delinquents with syndrome-based categories is potentially productive in tying interventions with general psychiatric practice, but there is no evidence that the vast majority of delinquents fall easily into diagnostic categories as currently understood in psychiatry.

Using factor analytic techniques, Jenkins (Jenkins and Glickman, 1947; Jenkins and Boyer, 1967) in the 1940's described three types of delinquents in a group of 500 children: socialized delinquent, unsocialized aggressive, and overinhibited. Socialized delinquents, in contrast to the unsocialized, were more involved in a peer group, and their delinquency appeared to evolve out of this group process. The distinction between socialized and unsocialized was believed to reflect the relative weight of social milieu and early maternal deprivation in determining delinquent behavior. The overinhibited group was seen as more fundamentally neurotic. Jenkins' work was influential in the categories used in DSM-II. A series of studies by Peterson, Quay, and Tiffany (1975) identified four factors significant in a delinquent population: socialized, unsocialized, overinhibited-neurotic, and inadequacy-immaturity. Offer and colleagues (1979) also used factor analytic techniques with a delinquent population to describe four clinical pictures: delinquents who were predominantly narcissistic, impulsive, depressed, or "empty borderlines." Unlike the previous studies, their sample was a group of hospitalized delinquents, permitting more detailed observations, though psychotic, mentally retarded, and brain-damaged young people were excluded.

In summary, there is no one conceptual approach sufficient to "explain" delinquency. In a general way, delinquency can be thought of as a *variety* of behavioral adaptations of individuals, reflecting various biological, developmental, psychological, and social variables sharing one thing in common: the adaptations are socially deviant. From a clinical perspective, the direction of further research would appear to be an increasing refinement of diagnostic typologies accompanied by longitudinal investigation of both their natural course and the degree to which they can be modified by intervention.

Intervention: General Aspects

The Juvenile Court and Corrections

Over the past ten years the juvenile court and corrections programs for youth have been subject to increasing criticism. Large numbers of young people are kept in often deplorable detention facilities while awaiting disposition (Sarri, 1974). Juvenile court dockets are crowded, resulting in perfunctory hearings and lack of attention to individual issues. There are inadequate dispositional alternatives, particularly the availability of psychiatric treatment (Committee of Mental Health Services, 1972; Policy Committee, O.C.S., 1973). These problems in turn have focused attention on the lack of due process protection afforded youth in the juvenile court system (Burt, 1973). What Stone (1975) has called "a failure in the social work emphasis" has lead to a reevaluaton of the legal foundation of the juvenile codes. The juvenile court function is predicated on the waiver of adult procedural protection for the anticipated benefit of "rehabilitative" treatment rather than punishment. If rehabilitation is not offered—indeed, if the juvenile is subject to arbitrary and often harmful treatment by the juvenile justice system—should not he at least be allowed a fairer day in court? Certainly the trend in legal opinion since the Supreme Court's decision in the Gault case is in the direction of more due process protection in the juvenile court. This places a greater burden on the police and juvenile court investigative staff to establish "facts," rather than generate "opinion." The climate witin the court becomes more adversarial. Marginal cases are dropped. Underlying this shift is a reworking of the basic dilemma described by Malmquest (1967). The court is expected both to protect society and to rehabilitate the young person. In theory these goals should have a common juncture in promoting the emotional health of society's youth. The reality, however, is something different: whether from lack of resources or from a more fundamental failure of theory and technique, the system has major limitations. At the same time there is extraordinary social concern with juvenile crime, particularly violent crime. The inevitable trend is for juvenile justice to move more in the direction of a social protective function, for the juvenile courts to be brought more in line with adult criminal standards. Indeed, a model juvenile code developed by the Juvenile Justice Standards Project, a joint effort of the America Bar Association and the Institute of Judicial Administration (Flicker, 1977), proposes eliminating all status offenses from juvenile court jurisdiction, establishing strict due process procedures for the juvenile court, and linking sanctions for juvenile offenses to the adult criminal code.

Paralleling this trend in thinking about the juvenile court has been criticism of traditional corrections programs for delinquents and a movement away from large institutions to smaller community-based facilities. In 1972, for instance, Massachusetts closed all its training schools and opted instead for seventeen group homes scattered throughout the state. These homes are small, involving twenty or so young people, and are staffed largely by nonprofessionals. Given the inevitable confusion surrounding so radical a change, it is too early to gauge accurately the success of the program. Such shifts are propelled by the commonly accepted view that traditional corrections not only are ineffective in preventing crime, but indeed promote a criminal life style in its clients, and are harmful to young people as well. Supporting this contention is the high rate of recidivism commonly reported for corrections programs, generally in the range of 60–70% (Cavan and Ferdinand, 1975). Murray, Thomson, and Israel (1978), however, comment that "to a surprising degree" such a view rests on "undocumented assertions." Most particularly, reports of recidivism commonly ignore preintervention levels of criminal activity, which in mental health terms would mean degree of personal difficulty and tenacity of maladaptation. Murray, Thomson, and Israel (1978) present data based on a study of chronic delinquents in Illinois which support the view that an energetic corrections approach, whether through traditional corrections facilities or a diversion program involving intensive monitoring of the young person's behavior, exercises a "suppressor effect" on subsequent delinquency.

Reviewing these issues of social policy, one is impressed with how much of the argument rests on perception and attitude, rather than systematic study of young people and their problems. Overall, however, it would appear that the juvenile court and corrections increasingly will become less involved with the problems of young people and instead more focused on protecting society from the relatively small percentage of severely delinquent youth.

Alternatives

If legal institutions are to play less of a role, what is to take their place? The problem of delinquency must be seen as but one aspect of the broader social issue of promoting healthy development in young people, and intervention in delinquency should become but one target in a range of mental health services for children and adolescents. The fundamental message of studies documenting widespread delinquent attitudes and behavior among contemporary youth is the failure of social institutions to engage young people and to provide for their needs (Schwartz, 1977). Beyond this generalization, what is specifically relevant for delinquency? Three types of service must be considered: preventive efforts with the preadolescent age group, acute intervention with adolescents, and the issue of the chronic offender.

The central issue in prevention is anticipating which young people are likely to become delinquent and developing appropriate interventions for them. This in turn presumes some knowledge of what "causes" delinquency. Here, of course, one encounters the difficulty noted above: as an interpersonal adaptation, delinquency does not have *a* cause but many contributing factors. Which are the most relevant? There has always been a sense that delinquency is related to poverty and that reducing poverty will reduce delinquency. Beyond the fact that this is an ambitious goal, difficult to realize in practice, it must be recalled that the social class correlation is with street crime, not deviance per se (Schwartz, 1977; Wolfgang, 1978; Thio, 1978); and even here a stronger correlation exists with parental psychopathology (Robins, 1966). Individual and family variables, then, are more likely to precisely predict future delinquency than the necessarily more general social ones. In Britain, West and Farrington (1973), for example, argue that the behavioral problems of future delinquents are evident by ages 8–10 in their "disobedience, quarrelsomeness, and inattention in school." Notable background variables include: being a member of a large family with limited income; below-average intelligence; a parent with a criminal record; negligent parental love and attention. Based on a prospective study of boys identified according to these criteria, West and Farrington found that these factors exert a cumulative effect: the more that are present, the more likely is the young person to be delinquent. Boys having three of the five factors were six times more likely to be delinquent than the general population. In this country the most ambitious efforts at developing predictive indicators have been by Sheldon and Eleanor Glueck (1970). They studied 500 chronic delinquents and 500 nondelinquent boys from the same neighborhood matched for age, IQ, and ethnicity. Delinquency was associated with mesomorphic body build; lower verbal than performance IQ; parental emotional disturbance: family disorganization; poor supervision and negligent love by parents. Based on these observations they constructed a prediction table with high loading for delinquency indicated by: erratic discipline by father; unsuitable supervision by mother; hostility toward boy by mother and father; and lack of integration in family. While the Gluecks argue for the predictive power of their scale, other studies suggest that for a given population, predictive power is no more accurate than the base rate for the population—i.e., the scale is no more potent an indicator than knowledge of the neighborhood (Achenbach, 1974). In a different vein Berman and Siegal (1976) argue on the basis of their observation of the relatively high frequency of neuropsychological deficits in a delinquent as opposed to a nondelinquent population that screening for such deficits in elementary age populations would indicate the young predisposed to adaptive failure and future delinquency. This approach, in contrast to the first two, is based not on actuarial study but on a theory of etiology, delinquency consequent to developmental failure in academic mastery, similar to that proposed by Gold (Gold and Mann, 1972). No prospective study of the utility of this approach has been done, and Murray (1976), moreover, questions the entire concept. Overall, one is left with the impression that prediction of future delinquency is not at a point allowing wide application. Further, virtually all studies have been of delinquent males; very little attenton has been paid to the antecedents of delinquency in females, particularly significant in light of the declining sex difference in delinquency rates.

Assuming that at-risk populations could be accurately identified, what interventions might be attempted? Certainly learning problems in the primary grades could be approached through special education. More interesting, however, is the question of whether a fundamentally aggressive interpersonal stance, the "disobedience" noted by West and Farrington, can be modified in latency. Some of the boys at the Wiltwyck school to be discussed below, were in this age range and did appear to benefit from *intensive residential* care. The evidence of success from other efforts is less compelling.

Critical to acute intervention in adolescence is the development of a broader range of services for this age group. The police and courts are neither equipped nor predisposed to deal with typical adolescent behavior problems. Schonfeld (1971) has described the role that psychiatry and mental health facilities could play in such an effort. Critical to this is more expertise within the mental health professions about adolescent development and psychopathology and a stronger commitment to dealing with this often frustrating age group. Lewis and Balla (1976) rightly criticize overuse of the term "sociopath" by diagnosticians, reflecting essentially a reaction to the behavior rather than an understanding of the individual's difficulties. Indeed, one survey of 110 psychiatric inpatients according to the Research Diagnostic Criteria identified only 7 with "antisocial personality disorder," though many had significant behavior problems (Hudgens, 1974).* Morse (1975) argues for the potential usefulness of the school in supporting adolescent development and as a framework for intervention in adolescent difficulties. Here too, however, the problem is one of a shift in emphasis and commitment. The ideology of secondary school education centers on the teaching of specific skills, with "personality development" a secondary consideration. A new entrant on the adolescent scene is the "youth service agency," offering the advantage of no traditional goal or focus. The concept arises from the deinstitutionalization and deprofessionalization emphasis of the past ten years and has received financial backing from the Juvenile Justice and Delinquency Prevention Act of 1974. It is intended to be a community-based facility that functions to prevent delinquency, particularly status offenses, through direct service to the adolescent population. What this rather general concept means in concrete terms varies enormously from area to area (Little et al., 1977). Agencies may offer individual counseling, group experiences, activity programs of various sorts, including therapeutic camping. The success and viability of this concept has yet to be measured. Overall, the issue in acute intervention, whether through mental health, educational, or youth service agency approaches, is reducing intergenerational distance, providing an interpersonal bridge between childhood and adulthood, while at the same time promoting competence in the individual young person. Central to this task is an appreciation of the special vulnerabilities which individuals of this age group may manifest.

What of the chronic offender? Certainly for the protection of society some form of containment is in order. From a psychiatric perspective there is nothing to suggest that anything less than residential treatment will be effective. And yet, it is precisely this combination of containment and treatment that has fallen on hard times. In part this reflects economic considerations, the enormous expense of maintaining intensive residential programs. Contributing as well is the reluctance of the mental health professions to deal with angry, characterologically alienated youth. A major factor, however, is the belief that such youth are "untreatable." Such a belief operates in the face of a literature suggesting precisely the opposite. Redl and Wineman (1954), Aichorn (1962), and Miller (1964), among others, have described residential programs that dealt successfully with highly delinquent young people. McCord and McCord's (1956) report from the Wiltwyck school is an important example. This school was established to help "psychopathic" or hyperaggressive boys essentially through providing a limit-setting but warm and understanding milieu. On projective measures the Wiltwyck boys demonstrated progressive diminution of aggressive imagery throughout their stay when compared to a matched reformatory group. No long-term follow-up was done, but McCord and McCord did demonstrate emotional responsiveness in a highly delinquent population. Can such responsiveness be the basis for a fundamental shift in character style? No study has yet dealt with this question in a satisfactory manner. One would hope, however, that society's need to incarcerate

*In Warren's (1969) studies of a population of 400 delinquents in California, 46% would be classified as neurotic, while less than 6% could be called antisocial character disorders.

severely delinquent young people would be associated with a moral commitment to make such incarceration as personally beneficial as possible. Berlin (1975) draws a distinction between "authoritarian" and "authoritative" detention. The former focuses on control of the young person and in essence perpetuates an aggressive stance. The latter involves a commitment to values of individual growth and productivity which at least offers the young person an option.

The problem with discussing treatment in this context is the lack of measures of delinquency that can be related to personality variables and hence offer some gauge of treatment outcome. Several efforts in this direction should be noted. Satten and colleagues (1970) have reported an attempt to use "level of ego functioning and organization" as means of differentiating among delinquent boys and hence a guide to intervention. The Quay typology (1975) is the basis for prescription of treatment in a behaviorally oriented program at the federal youth center, and Warren (1969) has developed a classification system of "stages of interpersonal maturity" that is used for differential assignment of treatment within the California corrections system. Such work is an important foundation for more precise intervention with delinquent youth.

Intervention: Clinical Issues

Assessment

Courts often ask the psychiatrist consultant to make a statement about the delinquent's "dangerousness," particularly the potential for violence; and it is important for the clinician to recognize that predictive statements in this area are outside his area of expertise (Stone, 1975; Cocozza and Steadman, 1978; APA Task Force, 1974). From a clinical perspective, evaluation is directed toward assessing treatability of emotional and developmental difficulties and recommending a plan for intervention. Initial questions usually involve the appropriateness of psychological interventions, as opposed to more behaviorally focused modalities, and the question of locus of treatment: family and community based, residential, a psychiatric hospital, a corrections facility. In general, prospects are best to the degree that affect is potentially available in a therapeutic relationship, that the young person experiences an internal push toward developmental growth, in contrast to a passive or defensive stance with regard to age-appropriate tasks, and that he sees others as potentially helpful to him. Few young people with delinquent behavior, certainly those with entrenched patterns of delinquency, will appear to meet these criteria during initial interviews. Most will appear highly defended and quite unengaged with appropriate developmental issues. Two considerations are important, however: the context and process of the evaluation and the particular character of adolescent cooperation. With regard to the former, only in the most obvious situations such as florid psychosis can one make an accurate assessment in a single interview in a detention facility. Quite aside from the problems with this approach in any setting, it should be noted that delinquents have sound reasons for distrusting psychiatrists. Many have experienced multiple evaluations without productive outcome and have come to see the psychiatrist as an agent of the court, an attitude only exaggerating defensiveness. Assessment must be tied to the prospect of some benefit for the young person if the evaluation is to be even reasonably accurate. Several interviews are most always in order, with a clear statement to the young person of the evaluation's purpose and potential benefit to him. The need to maintain at least the illusion of autonomy can be powerful in many basically dependent adolescents; assessment of "cooperativeness' must put verbal statements in the context of behavior. Many adolescents will verbally protest but behaviorally comply. Attention must be paid not only to the individual young person but to the family and community milieu. Intelligence testing and academic achievement measures, including evaluation of possible learning problems, are of help; projective testing, however, usually contributes little beyond what can be obtained from well done clinical interviews.

One approach that has been useful in integrating evaluative information is to attempt to place the young person in one of three broad and sometimes overlapping categories: neurosis, character disorder, or schizophrenic spectrum disorder, each of which can be linked to general treatment concepts. (Consideration of the occasional normal young person who presents for evaluation will be omitted.)

The delinquency of the *neurotic* young person is usually but one aspect of broader difficulties derivative from internalized, structural conflict. Symptoms of the latter, particularly anxiety and guilt, are thinly defended against and take precedence over the feeling of oppression and massive sense of unworth characteristic of the character disorders. Their problems often have situational determinants and their interpersonal behavior may suggest "socialization" defects or pregenital character conflicts, but their ego maturity suggests the capacity to bring troubling affect under internal control.

The difficulties of the *character disordered*, by contrast, focuses on disavowal of personal responsibility, externalizaton of internal feeling states within the interpersonal milieu, and an action orientation to problem-solving, rather than a reflective or verbal one. The young person tends to see himself as a victim, helpless, powerless. Feeling thus, it is internally consistent to see problems determined externally. This reflects early developmental experience. These young people tend to behave toward others as they themselves were treated, frustrating others just as they experienced frustration. Affects are not organized within the self-construct but are experienced in this interpersonal transaction. The manifest rage is in the behavior, not in the internal world. Since these difficulties are a consequence of early problems in nuturing relationships, such relationships in the present symbolically trigger these symptomatic manuevers. Reflecting early withdrawal from relationships and hence growth-inducing experience, autonomous ego functioning, particularly internal use of concepts to modulate affect, is poorly developed. Problems are worked through in action rather than reflection or verbal discussion.

One of the most difficult assessments to make is differentiating so-called reactive and process character disorders. The former is not a true character disorder but an environmental adaptation during adolescence to internal, neurotic decompensation. Family members themselves may experience a regressive pull during a young person's adolescence and may respond to the adolescent's difficulties with defensive behavior of their own. An early adolescent girl, for instance, may defend against incestual longings during puberty by assuming an angry stance toward her father. He in turn may counterreact. Mutually provocative behavior may escalate, become established, and give a character-disordered cast to what is essentially a neurotic problem.

Typologies of delinquents typically have made a distinction between "socialized" and "unsocialized" delinquency, both in contrast to a neurotic type. An internal variable that might account for the former is adaptive fit and vulnerability to disorganization under stress. The developmental background of some character-disordered adolescents has been basically stable and consistent, though traumatizing. As such, their character problems might be expected to have developed adaptive constancy. A more unpredictable and inconsistent developmental experience, by contrast, would impair formation of stable character defenses. The former would appear more "narcissistic," the latter more "impulsive." The "socialized"—i.e., narcissistic—delinquent is one whose development has promoted stable, if interpersonally limited, identity formation, while the "unsocialized"—i.e., impulsive—delinquent is one whose development has not allowed such a consolidation. Both, however, are points on the same continuum.

Character-disordered adolescents generally feel terrible about themselves, see themselves as victims, and are predisposed to rage attacks. As such they are potentially homicidal or suicidal. Some young people, however, have been the subject of particularly brutal treatment early in life and, whether through a total failure to develop human bonds or through identification with a violent parent (or both), are inclined specifically toward aggressive attacks on people. Thus the casual indifference toward others characteristic of narcissistic youth should be distinguished from the capacity to dehumanize, to see people solely as physical objects, characteristic of the potentially homicidal young person. A clue to this differentiation is the uncomfortable feeling aroused in the evaluation by youth in the latter category, a sense of their denial of humanness, often provoking intense discomfort and anxiety (Miller and Looney, 1975). Narcissistic young people, by contrast, more often stimulate rage and a compulsion "to be in control," reminiscent of infantile struggles.

The *schizophrenic spectrum disordered delinquent* is one who experiences internal disorganization, fragmentation of self, and disordered thinking when under stress. Such young people range from the borderline youth who experiences only transient or episodic fragmentation to the process schizophrenic.

Several areas of clinical exploration are helpful in distinguishing these three categories of young people. Regarding interpersonal relatedness, one should inquire directly about the young person's sense of morality. Is some external authority perceived as rational? While criticism of social institutions is hardly evidence for psychopathology, one looks for some concept of an extrapersonal moral order, usually present in neurotics and lacking or limited in the character disordered. The concreteness and tangentiality of schizophrenics and borderlines often prevent them from conceptualizing morality in the abstract or with any depth. Familiarity with Warren's stages of interpersonal maturity (1969) or Kohlberg's moral development scheme (1976) is helpful in conceptualizing this dimension. Many character-disordered young people distort the intentions of others with a tenacity suggesting delusion, but examination of thought process reveals no evidence for a disorder of thinking. The distortions are not so much defects in reality testing as attitudinal styles outside the realm of cognitive processing. The schizophrenic and borderline young person usually will demonstrate, by contrast, inattention and distortion in a variety of situations around different types of tasks. Associative processes are less predictable, more idiosyncratic. Anxiety and guilt are the predominant affects in neurotics, while externally directed rage alternating with depression characterizes the character disordered. Emptiness and absence of affect are more indicative of a schizophrenic process.

Treatment

In general, the neurotic group benefits most from psychotherapy, with group and family work provided on a concurrent basis as needed to provide environmental stability. In particularly disruptive family or community situations short- to intermediate-stay hospitalization may be indicated, particularly with the reactive character disordered group. Also, hospitalization may serve to stabilize the therapeutic alliance. True character disorders can rarely be treated with anything less than a milieu-oriented approach. Psychotherapy in the initial stages involves mainly confrontation of distortions and maladaptive behavior, shading into more internally focused work as the young person responds. Youth with schizophrenic spectrum disorders usually need long-term support, day programs, or 24-hour care depending on level of symptoms, medication, and the opportunity to form relationships around life space tasks. Psychotherapy is less helpful.

Whether through an individual psychotherapeutic relationship or through environmental intervention, delinquent behavior must be interrupted for treatment to occur. The clinician must recognize the enormous gratification accompanying regressive modes of behavior. Rexford (1966) and Miller (1975) offer an important conceptual clarification in this context. "Acting out" should be reserved for use in its historical sense: a defense against remembering—i.e., a specific ego operation. Much adolescent behavior is "acting up"—i.e., discharging internal tension through behavior rather than being organized and inhibited in fantasy. In the presence of such tension discharge, motivation for change will be minimal.

Psychotherapy has been found most consistently useful with neurotic delinquents, but has found application with the character-disordered group as well. Noshpitz (1957) has described the early stages of treatment with such young people. The patient must invest in the therapist, must see the therapist as potentially helpful in restoring a sense of personal effectiveness. In order for this to occur, the patient needs to recognize that the therapist has succeeded where the patient has failed: he has mastered his own impulse life. The basis of the therapeutic alliance is the patient's envy of the therapist's capacity to control internal tension. The therapist must avoid either pity or condemnation, which only colludes with the patient's defensive stance. Once an alliance is established, the treatment process focuses on an exploration of the patient's sense of ineffectiveness and the various ways he behaves so as to maintain this negative view of self. Family and group work with delinquents is no different from the general adolescent patient population. Easson (1967), Rinsley (1971), and Zinn (1979) have described residential and hospital programs.

The tendency to equate adolescent problems with behavior leads to much confusion in the use of the term "behavior therapy." It is generally accepted that a well-defined and consistent social structure is necessary in any milieu for adolescents. Further, a number of modeling techniques (e.g., Sarason and Ganger, 1973) have been described for working with adolescents which have been found relatively more useful than verbal ones with delinquents. Rossman and Knesper (1976) have described the use of behavioral techniques in the early stages of treatment in a psychodynamically oriented milieu. "Behavior therapy," however, should be reserved for those situations where behavioral manipulation is the major modality of intervention, and as such, would be useful for only the most tenacious character problems. Maloney, Fixsen, and Maloney (1978) have described such a program. It should be noted that neurotic and moderately impaired character-disordered young people often fare poorly in behaviorally oriented treatment programs. Strict adherence to a behavior protocol does not allow for fluctuations in the capacities that are a part of growth in these young people.

The use of medications with delinquents, particularly in corrections settings, is the subject of controversy, raising in the minds of some a parallel with Russian treatment of dissidents. Based on considerable expert consultation, Kalogerakis (1978) has drafted guidelines for the use of medications with the institutionalized adolescent; these guidelines do not differ from generally accepted psychiatric practice.

References

Achenbach, T.M. (1974) *Developmental Psychopathology.* New York: Ronald Press.

Aichorn, A. (1925) *Wayward Youth.* New York: Viking, 1965.

Alexander, F. (1930) The neurotic character. *Int. J. Psychoanal.* 11:292–311.

American Psychiatric Association Task Force. (1974) *Clinical Aspects of the Violent Individual.* Washington, D.C.: American Psychiatric Association.

Bakan, D. (1971) Adolescence in America: From idea to social fact. *Daedalus* 100:979–995.

Bandura, A., R.H. Walters. (1958) Dependency conflicts in aggressive delinquents. *J. Soc. Issues* 14:52–65.

Baumrind, D. (1975) Early socialization and adolescent competence. In S.E. Dragastin and G.H. Elder, Jr. *Adolescence in the Life Cycle.* New York: Wiley.

Berlin, I.N. (1975) It can be done: Aspects of delinquency treatment and prevention. In I.N. Berlin, ed. *Advocacy for Child Mental Health.* New York: Brunner/Mazel.

Berman, A., and A. Siegel. (1976) A neuropsychological approach to etiology, prevention and treatment of juvenile delinquency. In A. Davids, ed. *Child Personality and Psychopathology: Current Topics.* New York: Wiley.

Bowlby, J. (1951) *Maternal Care and Mental Health.* Geneva: World Health Organization.

Burt, R.A. (1973) The therapeutic use and abuse of state power over adolescents. In J.C. Schoolar, ed., *Current Issues in Adolescent Psychiatry.* New York: Brunner/Mazel.

Cantwell, D.P. (1978) Hyperactivity and antisocial behavior. *J. Am. Acad. Child Psychiat.* 17:252–262.

Cavan, R.S., and T.N. Ferdinand. (1975) *Juvenile Delinquency,* 3rd ed. Philadelphia: Lippincott.

Chwast, J. (1974) Delinquency and criminal behavior as depressive equivalents in adolescents. In S. Lesse, ed., *Masked Depression.* New York: Jason Aronson.

Cloward, R.A., and L.E. Ohlin. (1960) *Delinquency and Opportunity: A Theory of Delinquent Gangs.* Glencoe, Ill.: Free Press.

Cocozza, J.J., and E. Hartstone. (1978) *Treatment Effectiveness: The Level of Improvement Experienced by Youths While on the Bronx Court Related Unit.* Albany: New York State Council on Children and Families.

Cocozza, J.J., and H.J. Steadman. (1978) *Prediction in Psychiatry: An Example of Misplaced Confidence in Experts.* Albany: Special Projects Research Unit, New York State Department of Mental Hygiene.

Cohen, A.K. (1955) *Delinquent Boys: The Culture of the Gang.* Glencoe, Ill.: Free Press.

Committee of Mental Health Services Inside and Outside the Family Court in the City of New York. (1972) *Juvenile Justice Confounded: Pretensions and Realities of Treatment Services.* Paramus, N.J.: National Council on Crime and Delinquency.

Easson, W. (1967) *Residential Treatment of the Severely Disturbed Adolescent.* New York: International Universities Press.

Elder, G.H., Jr. (1975) Adolescence in the life cycle: An introduction. In S.E. Dragastin and G.H. Elder, Jr., *Adolescence in the Life Cycle.* New York: Wiley.

Elkind, D. (1967) Middle-class delinquency. *Mental Health* 5:80–84.

Flicker, B.D. (1977) *Standards for Juvenile Justice: A Summary and Analysis.* Cambridge, Mass.: Ballinger.

Friedlander, K. (1945) Formation of the anti-social character. *Psychoanal. Study Child* 1:189–204.

Glueck, S., and E. Glueck. (1970) *Toward a Typology of Juvenile Offenders.* New York: Grune & Stratton.

Gold, M. (1966) Undetected delinquent behavior. *J. Res. Crime Delin.* 13:27–46.

Gold, M. (1970) *Delinquent Behavior in an American City.* Belmont, Calif.: Brooks/Cole.

Gold, M., and D. Mann. (1972) Delinquency as defense. *Am. J. Orthopsychiat.* 42:463–479.

Halleck, S.L. (1973) Alienation of affluent youth, revisited. *World Biennial Psychiat. Psychother.* 2:3–21.

Hare, R.D. (1968) Detection threshold for electric shock in psychopaths. *J. Abnorm. Psychol.* 73:268–272.

Healey, W., and A.R. Bronner.. (1936) *New Light on Delinquency and Its Treatment.* New Haven: Yale University Press.

Hirschi, T. (1969) *Causes of Delinquency.* Berkeley: University of California Press.

Hudgens, R.W. (1974) *Psychiatric Disorders in Adolescence.* Baltimore: Williams & Wilkins.

Jenkins, R.L., and A. Boyer. (1967) Types of delinquent behavior and background factors. *Int. J. Soc. Psychol.* 14:65–76.

Jenkins, R.L., and S. Glickman. (1947) Patterns of personality organization among delinquents. *Nerv. Child* 6:329–339.

Johnson, A.M. (1949) Sanctions for superego lacunae of adolescents. In K.R. Eissler, ed., *Searchlights on Delinquency.* New York: International Universities Press.

Johnson, A.M. (1959) Juvenile delinquency. In S. Arieti, ed., *American Handbook of Psychiatry.* New York: Basic Books.

Kalogerakis, M. (1978) *Pharmacotherapy for Institutionalized Adolescents.* Albany: Office of Children and Youth, New York State Office of Mental Health.

Kaufman, I., et al. (1963) Delineation of two diagnostic groups among juvenile delinquents: The schizophrenic and the impulse-ridden character disorder. *J. Am. Acad. Child Psychiat.* 2:292–318.

Kessler, S., and R.H. Moos. (1970) The XYY karyotype and criminality: A review. *J. Psychiat. Res.* 7:153–170.

Kohlberg, L., et al. (1976) *Moral Stage Scoring Manual.* Cambridge, Mass.: Center for Moral Education, Harvard Graduate School of Education.

Lampl de Grott, J. (1949) Neurotics, delinquents and ideal formation. In K.R. Eissler, ed., *Searchlights on Delinquency.* New York: International Universities Press.

Lewis, D.O. (1978) Paper presented at the Annual Meeting of the American Society for Adolescent Psychiatry, Atlanta, May 1978.

Lewis, D.O., and D.A. Balla. (1976) *Delinquency and Psychopathology.* New York: Grune & Stratton.

Lewis, D.O., and S.S. Shanok. (1978) Delinquency and the schizophrenic spectrum of disorders. *J. Am. Acad. Child Psychiat.* 17:263–276.

Little, A.D., Inc. (1977) *Cost and Services Impacts of Deinstitutionalization of Status Offenders in Ten States.* Washington, D.C.: Arthur D. Little, Inc.

Maloney, D.M., D.L. Flixsen, and K.B. Maloney. (1978) Antisocial behavior: Behavior modification. In W.B. Wolman, ed., *Handbook of Treatment.* Englewood Cliffs, N.J.: Prentice-Hall.

Malmquest, C.P. (1967) Dilemmas of the juvenile court. *J. Am. Acad. Child Psychiat.* 6:723–748.

Masterson, J.F. (1972) *Treatment of the Borderline Adolescent: A Developmental Approach.* New York: Wiley-Interscience.

McCord, W., and J. McCord. (1956) *Psychopathy and Delinquency.* New York: Grune & Stratton.

McCord, W., J. McCord, and I.K. Zola. (1959) *Origins of Crime.* New York: Columbia University Press.

Mednick, S.A., and K.O. Christiansen, eds. (1977) *Biosocial Bases of Criminal Behavior.* New York: Halstead Press.

Merton, R.K. (1957) *Social Theory and Social Structure.* Glencoe, Ill.: Free Press.

Miller, D. (1964) *Growth to Freedom.* Bloomington: Indiana University Press.

Miller, D. (1975) *Adolescence.* New York: Jason Aronson.

Miller, D.H., and J.G. Looney. (1975) Determinants of homicide in adolescents. *Adoles. Psychiat.* 4:231–254.

Moriarty, A.E., and P.W. Toussieng. (1976) *Adolescent Coping.* New York: Grune & Stratton.

Morse, W.C. (1975) The schools and the mental health of children and adolescents. In I.N. Berlin, ed., *Advocacy for Child Mental Health.* New York: Brunner/Mazel.

Murray, C.A. (1976) *The Link Between Learning Disabilities and Juvenile Delinquency: Current Theory and Knowledge.* Washington, D.C.: Law Enforcement Assistance Administration.

Murray, C.A., D. Thomson, and C.B. Israel. (1978) *UDIS: Deinstitutionalizing the Chronic Juvenile Offender.* Washington, D.C.: American Institute for Research.

Noshpitz, J.D. (1957) Opening phase in the psychotherapy of adolescents with character disorders. *Bull. Menninger Clin.* 21:153–164.

Offer, D., and J.D. Offer. (1975) *From Teenage to Young Manhood: A Psychological Study.* New York: Basic Books.

Offer, D., R.C. Marohn, and E. Ostrov. (1979) *The Psychological World of the Delinquent.* New York: Basic Books.

Pincus, J.H., and G. Tucker. (1974) *Behavioral Neurology.* New York: Oxford University Press.

Policy Committee, Office of Children's Services. (1973) *Desperate Situation—Desperate Service.* New York: Office of Children's Services, Judicial Conference of the State of New York.

Quay, H.C. (1975) Classification in the treatment of delinquency and antisocial behavior. In N. Hobbs, ed., *Issues on the Classification of Children.* San Francisco: Jossey-Bass.

Redl, F., and D. Wineman. (1954) *Controls from Within: Techniques for the Treatment of the Aggressive Child.* New York: Free Press.

Rexford, E.N. (1966) A survey of the literature. In E.N. Rexford, ed., *A Development Approach to Problems of Acting Out.* New York: International Universities Press.

Rinsley, D.B. (1971) Theory and practice of intensive residential treatment of adolescents. *Adoles. Psychiat.* 1:479–509.

Robins, L.N. (1966) *Deviant Children Grow Up.* Baltimore: Williams & Wilkins.

Rossman, P.G., and D.L. Knesper. (1976) The early phase of hospital treatment for disruptive adolescents. *J. Am. Acad. Child Psychiat.* 15:693–708.

Sarason, I.G., and V.J. Ganger. (1973) Modeling and group discussion in the rehabilitation of juvenile delinquents. *J. Counsel. Psychol.* 20:442–449.

Sarri, R. (1974) *Under Lock and Key: Juveniles in Jails and Detention.* Ann Arbor: National Assessment of Juvenile Corrections.

Satten, J., E.S. Novatny, S.L. Ginsparg, and S. Averill. (1970) Ego disorganization and recidivism in delinquent boys. *Bull. Menninger Clin.* 34:270–283.

Satterfield, J.H., and D.P. Cantwell. (1975) Psychopharmacology in the prevention of antisocial and delinquent behavior. In R. Gittelman-Klein, ed., *Recent Advances in Child Psychopharmacology.* New York: Human Sciences Press.

Schonfeld, W.A. (1971) Comprehensive community programs for the investigation and treatment of adolescents. In J.G. Howells, ed., *Modern Perspectives in Adolescent Psychiatry.* New York: Brunner/Mazel.

Schwartz, G. (1977) *Summary and Policy Implications of the Youth and Society in Illinois Reports.* Chicago: Institute for Juvenile Research.

Sheldon, W.H. (1949) *Varieties of Delinquent Youth.* New York: Harper.

Stone, A.A. (1975) *Mental Health and Law: A System in Transition.* Rockville: National Institute of Mental Health.

Sutherland, E.H., and D.R. Cressey. (1974) *Criminology,* 9th ed. Philadelphia: Lippincott.

Thio, A. (1978) *Deviant Behavior*. Boston: Houghton Mifflin.

Warren, M.Q. (1969) The case for differential treatment of delinquents. *Ann. Am. Acad. Polit. Soc. Sci.* 381:47–59.

West, D.J., and D.P. Farrington. (1973) *Who Becomes Delinquent?* London: Heinemann.

Wolfgang, M.E. (1970) *Youth and Violence*. Washington, D.C.: U.S. Government Printing Office.

Wolfgang, M.E. (1976) Child and youth violence. Paper presented at the Symposium on the Violent Child, Center of Forensic Psychiatry, New York University School of Medicine.

Wolfgang, M.E. (1978) Real and perceived changes of crime and punishment. *Daedalus* 107:143–157.

Zinn, D. (1979) Hospital treatment of the adolescent. In J. Noshpitz, ed. *Basic Handbook of Child Psychiatry*. New York: Basic Books.

Zinner, J., and E.R. Shapiro. (1975) Splitting in families of borderline adolescents. In J.E. Mack, ed., *Borderline States in Psychiatry*. New York: Grune & Stratton.

CHAPTER 32

Treatment of Emergencies in Children and Adolescents

Gilbert C. Morrison

The interdisciplinary team planning emergency psychiatric intervention with children, adolescents, and their families, can reach reliable conclusions about the essential characteristics of the parent-child relationship that enable them to intervene actively in the reorganization of the pathological family interaction. Basically, one cannot conceive of a dynamic short-term psychotherapy that differs from the methods used for intensive prolonged psychotherapy (Kaffman, 1963, p. 205).

Today it is possible to distinguish three types of psychiatric services for severely emotionally disturbed children. Children's psychiatric treatment centers provide intensive, long-term hospitalization with both individual psychotherapy and a well-defined treatment milieu. Brief psychiatric hospitalization provides an opportunity for the remission of the patient's symptoms, the protection of the patient and his family during periods of crisis and exacerbation, and provides a period of rest for the child and the family when they have reached a point of mutual frustration and exhaustion. Following an acute stress or trauma, child psychiatric emergency teams meet with the members of these families, their usual counselors, and their representatives from other community organizations in order to plan a treatment program that will provide protection, support, and skilled psychiatric treatment without the use of hospitalization or separation of the child from his family. This process offers an opportunity for both the child and his parents to gain confidence in their capacity to understand the nature of the emotional disturbance, to define the causes of the problem, to participate in the understanding of and the planning for the resolution, and to experience the important discovery that the family, rather than just the child, is the patient.

Understanding those events in a child's or an adolescent's life that constitute a psychiatric emergency is as important as recognizing emergencies in general medical and psychiatric practice. In many ways this understanding is more difficult because the child or adolescent disguises his problems by behavior rather than by talking about them. The ability to decode the crisis demands looking broader and deeper than the immediate behavioral problem that led to the referral of the child. Most children seen because of psychiatric emergencies are referred for specific behavioral problems despite long-standing manifestations of emotional and developmental problems (Smith and Morrison, 1975). Most children and youths referred for psychiatric emergencies show urgent behavioral symptoms, often in response to well-defined crises in their lives, yet most are poorly prepared for the stresses of normal development (Morrison and Collier, 1969).

In planning for the establishment of an emergency psychiatric service, Morrison studied child psychiatric consultations in the emergency room of a large general hospital as well as "urgent" applications for treatment at an outpatient psychiatric clinic to determine the types of problems presented, the kinds of families, their situation, and their environment. That review revealed that the peak months for application were January through March, and again in August (Morrison and Collier, 1969). Referrals included children with acute anxiety states, school phobia, truancy and school refusal, acute behavioral disorders, adolescent turmoil, hysterical conversion, depression, suicidal attempts or threats, and acute emotional problems associated with drug abuse and physical or mental handicaps. More than 80% of the patients were between the ages of 13 and 17, and twice as many girls as boys were referred. Several hundred consecutive families were studied to determine what types of presenting difficulties brought these families to emergency child psychiatric attention. Suicide attempts and threats, and school refusal (school phobia, truancy, etc.) predominated as the primary causes for referral to the services and constituted approximately half of the applicants. The families seen wished for an easy and rapid solution to long-standing and difficult problems. The parents asked for medication to solve the problem, for hospitalization, and often for placement of the child outside of the home.

The treatment approach to these families is best formulated from an understanding of the history of psychiatric and medical experiences with these crisis-oriented families. The studies found that they often expected immediate treatment. They preferred that something be done to or for them, not by or with them. They insisted on results from a single visit or a few visits to an emergency room or to a doctor's office. Previously, they had often sought and obtained assistance for medical and psychiatric problems in one or a few visits. They usually had been referred for further diagnostic studies or treatment, but had rejected the recommendation or had failed to follow recommended treatment after diagnostic evaluation. To be effective, treatment for psychiatric emergenices must be specific to the symptoms presented and to the limited time that the families will make available. It is sometimes possible to establish a relationship on which a longer-term treatment can be based.

It is becoming increasingly clear to those therapists who are responsible for the planning and development of community mental health services that several levels of psychiatric response are necessary. The first is along the line of the medical emergency room and the social work intake service that provide the first response and function in a triage role. The second is an emergency or crisis service that provides an urgent in-depth child psychiatric evaluation in a brief therapy, family therapy format. The third is a long-term psychiatric treatment facility using individual collaborative psychotherapy with brief or long-term child psychiatric hospitalization. A highly skilled and experienced staff, with each member of of the treatment team able to demonstrate a solid grounding in their discipline, and with additional experience in collaborative psychotherapy and family and group therapy methods, is essential to any approach using emergency psychotherapy.

Rudolf Ekstein, in a significant paper entitled "Brief Therapy Versus Intensive Therapy or: Patient-Oriented Treatment Programs," has summed up these problems by observing, "An intensive-care treatment center tries to deny neither emergency nor long-term needs. . . . Treatment techniques must be modified according to the specific needs of the patient. It is necessary to continue to reduce the ideological and political basis of our clinical activities and to strengthen the scientific by thorough diagnosis, careful training of staff, and appropriate application of the whole range of treatment possibilities" (Ekstein, 1972, pp. 11–12).

History

During the first quarter of the century, psychiatrists, social workers, and other professionals in the juvenile courts and mental hygiene clinics often were confronted by children brought to their services in acute emotional distress. At that time, and in the psychiatric outpatient and inpatient services that developed in the second quarter of the century, the usual response was to use any staff member who was available along with the involvement of all family members who would cooperate. Subsequently, child guidance clinics attempted to provide for urgent emotional problems through the use of the social worker assigned that day to the intake service. The social worker, while providing telephone consultation, also met walk-in families and provided emergency interviews with consultative back-up from the clinic psychiatrist. Such services often were effective, but limited by the skill and experience of the social worker assigned, and the success in catching a psychiatric consultant with time to provide consultation. In the last 25 years, although communities have shown wide variations in the development and effectiveness of their treatment settings, there has been an obvious trend toward the development of separate and enlightened psychiatric services for children. Children's psychiatric inpatient services often have had the same problems as psychiatric hospitals for adults; the progressive separation of the patient from the community and the tendency toward custodial care rather than a planned treatment program.

Emergency psychiatric treatment methods combine the following concepts: the diagnostic and treatment skills of child psychiatrists, combined with the most recent developments in the practice of community psychiatry; the clinical understanding of those families under stress and the development of family therapy; the study of the process of normal grief and mourning, as well as the study of the symptomatology associated with interrupted grief; and the development of crisis intervention methods. Freud, in *Mourning and Melancholia* (1917), identified the normal regression associated with loss, grief, and mourning, and called attention to the susceptibility of individuals to experience pathological mourning and depression. Lindemann (1944) provided further theoretical and clinical underpinnings for crisis intervention and crisis therapy following his careful study and research into the emotional responses of the survivors of the Coconut Grove fire in Boston. His delineation of the stages of normal grief and mourning, and his demonstration of the need for early evaluation and the development of responsive services, continue as the most significant contributions to the development of clinical crisis intervention.

Several authors have considered and have attempted to apply the public health concept of prevention and early intervention to mental health and mental illness (Caplan, 1961; Coolidge et al., 1962; Parad, 1965; Rapoport, 1962). They have defined primary preventive activities which are directed toward the promotion and maintenance of good health; secondary prevention which uses early intervention, diagnosis, and prompt treatment; and tertiary prevention which is directed toward rehabilitation and limitation of disability. In clinical practice, emergency services usually provide early intervention directed toward secondary and tertiary prevention, often serving in a triage role in attempting to determine the most effective level of response, and in attempting to distinguish the optimum potential for prevention of further decompensation. Family therapy, with its roots in child psychiatry through collaborative individual psychotherapy with the child and parents, through various research and clinical group therapy methods, and through research into child development, family behavior and family interactions, has provided another essential support for the development of crisis intervention treatment methods. This history of emergency service for children, youths and their families finds its roots in the earliest services provided for emotionally disturbed and delinquent children and adolescents.

Theoretical Considerations

Theoretical studies by Caplan (1961, 1964), Erikson (1963), and Hill (1949) have laid a foundation for the clinical study and testing (Mattsson, Hawkins, and Seese, 1967) of the concepts of crisis intervention with children and their families, but much of the practical application of this work has yet to be performed and evaluated. Comprehensive studies of individual symptoms, such as school refusal and phobia (Coolidge et al., 1962; Eisenberg, 1958; Malmquist, 1965), suicide attempt and threat (Levi et al., 1966; Mintz, 1966; Morrison and Collier, 1969; Shaw and Schelkun, 1965; Shneidman and Farberow, 1961; Tuckman and Connon, 1962), hysterical conversion (Proctor, 1958), assaultive behavior (Burks and Harrison, 1962), runaway (Robey et al., 1964; Stierlin, 1973), and delinquency (Kaufman and Heims, 1958) have been derived from typical clinical settings. Morrison and Smith (1975a, 1975b) have focused their attention on the emotional dependence of the child in defining an emergency in child psychiatry. They believe that the emotional disturbance in the family as well as in individual members of the family incites crises and leads to distortions or blocks in the emotional growth of the child. They (Morrison and Smith, 1975a) have defined an emergency in child psychiatry as *"that situation in which the significant adults around the child can no longer help him master his anxiety and can no longer provide temporary ego support and control"* (Morrison, 1975, p. 17). Parental absence, anxiety, or helplessness in the face of environmental and developmental problems provoke a situation that is experienced by the child as desertion and isolation. The child's coping maneuvers include withdrawal (suicide attempt, school refusal and drug abuse), projection (assaultive and delinquent behavior), or decompensation (panic and psychosis).

Child therapists are particularly concerned with the role of adults in ego lending and ego support during periods of developmental crisis for the child. Recognizing the natural emotional dependence of children upon adults, we can anticipate the effect of an anxious, disorganized adult upon an anxious, dependent child who may be looking to him for support, security and modes of conflict resolution. We may then hypothesize that those situations in which a significant adult is unable to foster ego growth, to provide ego controls, or to indicate avenues of tension reduction potentially constitute a serious impairment to the ego development of the child. Caplan (1961, 1964) and Lindemann (1944) and others have indicated that successful crisis resolution provides a small but significant emotional development for the individual, potentially enhancing his capacity for meeting later stresses without necessarily affecting recognizable characterologic change.

One finds it essential to return to the concepts of crisis intervention and coping methods in defining a crisis or an emergency in child psychiatry. Caplan (Rapoport, 1962, p. 24) defined a crisis as "An upset in a steady state," emphasizing that an individual strives to maintain an equilibrium through a constant series of adaptive maneuvers. Murphy (1961), in discussing coping styles, noted "individual differences in coping resources and resilience within the child, as well as differences in support from the environment, help to determine which children can weather these stresses sufficiently to permit continued growth, and can develop increasing capacity to reach workable relationships with the environment." Erikson (1963) stressed that the zones of development most seriously blocked or distorted by disintegrative reactions to extreme stress or crisis are apt to be those whose maturation is still incomplete or those dynamically related to the most recently acquired function. During periods of relatively rapid ego development, unresolved crises distort this development and lead to regression, withdrawal, or the utilization of maladaptive defense mechanisms.

Applicability

Burks and Hoekstra (1964) reviewed emergency child psychiatric referrals at the University of Michigan Medical Center in 1961. They found that children who had attempted suicide, those developing a psychosis, and those with an acute school phobia presented *bona-fide emergency situations that required prompt clinic intervention.* They found that referrals often resulted from family crises rather than from an intrapsychic crisis in the child. The approach of crisis theory and the development of treatment methods to involve the entire family as a unit have stimulated a new look at these familiar problems.

Morrison (1969) reported that suicide attempt and threat and school refusal (school phobia, truancy, etc.) predominated as the primary causes for referral, constituting approximately half of the applicants to the emergency psychiatric service for children and adolescents. Other presenting symptoms, listed here in the order of their frequency, included conversion reaction with paralysis, sexual promiscuity (frequently associated with pregnancy), runaway, toxic psychosis from several types of drugs and inhalants, fire setting, manifestations of acute anxiety, incest, killing of pets, and symptoms associated with acute psychosis.

Mattson, Hawkins, and Seese (1967) reported on the results of a retrospective and follow-up study of 170 child psychiatric emergencies seen at the child psychiatric service at the University Hospitals in Cleveland. The student is referred to this study because of the careful demographic and statistical work performed by Mattsson and his co-workers. He reported that there was a concentration of emergencies in the adolescent age range (12–18 years, 83%) and that girls were more commonly seen than boys on an emergency basis (60% versus 40%). He found that the preponderance of girls among the emergencies was due to the marked increase in girl emergencies from age 14 onward, reaching a peak at ages 16 to 18. Boys were referred almost three times as often as girls in the preadolescent group. The acute symptoms responsible for emergency referrals, with each emergency represented only in one category, revealed that suicidal behavior accounted for almost half of the sample, followed by assaultive and destructive behavior, marked anxiety with fears and physical complaints, bizarre and confused behavior, school refusal, truancy and runaway.

Mattsson also reported that more than half of the emergencies were referred because of changes in mood and behavior, such as depression often with suicidal behavior, somatic complaints and fears that indicated emotional conflicts within the child, who, for the most part, had maintained satisfactory control of impulsive behavior toward the environment. The remaining group presented with behavioral manifestations that were more outwardly directed in an impulsive, often unmanageable fashion indicating emotional conflicts acted out; such as, assaultive, delinquent and truanting behavior.

Morrison and Smith (1975a) in an extensive study of child psychiatric emergencies comparing socio-economic groups in public and private practice settings discovered that the immediate crisis in the family often was precipitated by threatened separation, actual object loss, or the anniversary of such a loss. They found that more than half of the children seen in emergency consultation had lost a parent or near relative through illness, hospitalization, marital separation or death within 3 weeks of the onset of their symptoms. Additionally, impending high school graduation or return to school, a family move to a new neighborhood or city, interruption of a close relationship, or hospitalization of a parent also represented significant threats of separation. Threatened and actual separations, the death of a parent, and the loss of members of the extended family should always be considered, and questions about such losses or potential losses should always be explored in the diagnostic evaluation and treatment planning for emergency intervention with children and their families.

Methods

Emergency intervention with children and adolescents involves immediate diagnostic evaluation and therapeutic planning for the child, the parents and their environment. The treatment format utilizes a combination of brief psychotherapy and family therapy methods. An emergency psychiatric program for children and their families can be viewed as focusing attention toward early amelioration of emotional disorders. Mattsson (Mattsson, Hawkins, and Seese, 1967) considers the following criteria necessary for an effective child psychiatric emergency service program: (1) prompt diagnostic evaluation of the child and his family in crisis; (2) clarification for the family of the significant factors that provoked the emergency situation and determined its nature; (3) active involvement of the parents in the treatment plan, with specific and practical direction for immediate alleviation of the child's distress—i.e. giving him adequate protection, ego support, and external control; (4) access to a psychiatric inpatient unit for the small number of children needing admission; (5) clinic facilities for continued study and short-term therapy of the child and his family; (6) optimal collaboration with community agencies, clinics, and schools throughout the emergency treatment period (this implies determining which agency has the main responsibility for the long-term care of the family); (7) flexibility of schedules for psychiatric trainees, social workers, and supervisors in order to meet these needs of the program; and (8) recognition of emergency service experience as a necessary integral part of the training for child psychiatrists and social workers.

The recommended initial diagnostic-therapeutic procedure is a group interview with the child or the adolescent and all significant family members together with a child psychiatric clinical team. The initial family interview focuses on a discussion of the presenting problem and on the formulation of a definition or statement of the nature of the child's or the family's problem. The initial goal is to reach some understanding of the problem that is accepted by the family members and the clinical team. In the initial interview, methods that might be tried to cope with the crisis are considered, and the family is helped to arrive at a working plan or direction for the immediate handling of the acute situation. In order to reevaluate the family situation and to clarify, if possible, the underlying problems in the family relationship that contributed to the crisis, most of these families are seen again as a group from two to five days later, depending upon their need and the nature of the problem. The treatment team works with the families as long as necessary to alleviate the crisis. For some families further therepautic management includes referral for additional psychiatric treatment, such as outpatient collaborative individual psychotherapy for parent and child, inpatient treatment, physical diagnosis and medical management.

Comprehensive studies of children with psychiatric emergencies have involved the diagnostic evaluation of individual symptoms and have been derived from typical clinical settings. During the past decade, specific therapeutic approaches have been developed for familes with children who have symptoms of suicide attempt and threat, school refusal and phobia, hysterical conversion, runaway, assaultive behavior and delinquency, drug abuse and toxicity, or precocious sexuality. Primary preventive treatment approaches also have been attempted with children who are survivors of parental suicide, children who live with acutely psychotic or chronically emotionally ill parents, families who are confronted by a premature birth, children who have manifestions of autism, children who have manifestations of childhood depression, young adolescents who are pregnant, children who have a chronic debilitating disease such as juvenile diabetes or who have a physical or physiological handicap—i.e., those children who we have come to recognize as "children at risk."

There was agreement several decades ago that acute psychotic decompensation, suicidal behavior, and school phobia represented emergencies in child psychiatry. Both psychotic decompensation and suicidal expression, because of potential aggressive action either to the self or to others, fell within the scope of all conditions defined as medical emergencies—i.e., those conditions constituting a threat to biological integrity or life. The recognition of acute school phobia as an emergency situation precipitated consideration for a different definition of an emergency in child psychiatry. Traditionally, child psychiatry had studied the growth and development of the child, and had integrated the understanding of both physical and emotional factors in the child's development and maturation. That recognition and the willingness to attend to factors that interfered with emotional maturation by centering concern upon ego development in all its manifestations, provided the opportunity for the development of the clinical services to meet the needs of "children at risk." The treatment technique of choice used for children at risk is brief family psychotherapy. Several books have been written on the development and application of this therapeutic modality, and all of the findings and recommendations will not be reviewed here. Rather, the treatment technique as modified for the family in crisis will be discussed. For further understanding of the use of brief family therapy in the wide variety of situations in which children are at risk, the following books are recommended: *The Treatment of Families in Crisis* by Langsley and Kaplan; *Crisis Intervention: Selected Readings* by Parad; *Children and Their Families in Brief Treatment* by Barten and Barten; and *Emergencies in Child Psychiatry: Emotional Crises in Children, Youth and Their Families* by Morrison.

The treatment method for these familes with a defined psychiatric problem of a child at risk, usually involves the team approach with a child psychiatrist and a psychiatric social worker. The treatment team is often expanded, depending upon the clinical problem, by the addition of a clinical psychologist, a visiting teacher, a welfare or an agency case worker, a public health nurse, and occasionally by the family's physician, attorney, minister, or priest. In summary, as many representatives of the child 's and the family's environment are invited to attend and participate in the meetings as have been involved in or can contribute to the resolution of the crisis and help further the child's development and maturation.

The treatment approach is based on the clinical observation and understanding that the crisis involves not only the patient with the acute symptoms, but also the family and sometimes the community (represented by appropriately selected participants) as well. The goal of the first interview is to identify the internal stress or the external situation that has provoked or contributed to the crisis, and to clarify the child's clinical symptoms and the family's susceptibility to emotional problems. An assessment is made of the style that each family member uses in meeting his tensions and fears. Within this setting it can be demonstrated how the behavior of each family member distorts or interferes with the communication required for minimal support of the symptomatic child or adolescent. Distortions, incomplete presentations and missing details of a situation related by one member of the family are corrected or modified by other family members or participants present. Long-held secrets have served as an overvalued stimulus to the family tensions. It is difficult to overestimate the importance of poor family communication, individual and family secrets, and private family collusion in the stimulation of symptomatic behavior and family crises. The family's problems and secrets often involve threatened and actual separations and losses. These secrets are experienced as restrictions and qualifications of attention, tenderness, and love by the children and also between the marital partners.

Although the immediate focus is on the current crisis which has brought the family to the treatment situation, the emphasis rapidly broadens to include many other symptoms in the "labeled" patient as well as symptoms in other family members. By the end of the first interview, the diagnostic-treatment team should formulate with the family a definition of the child's and the family's problem acceptable to the members of the family, the representatives of the community, and the clinical team. The immediate goal in family crisis is to reduce the level of tension and the emotional disturbance present in the family. The treatment team activity is directed toward limitation of further regression and attention to beginning stabilization (Langsley and Kaplan, 1968). The initial interview and subsequent treatment interviews are not limited to the usual "therapy hour," but may vary in length from less than a half-hour to many hours in duration. In the first session it is important that the members of the family come to know that the behavioral problems or emotional symptoms leading to the crisis situation are representations of underlying family problems rather than the cause of the family problems.

The treatment team and the community representatives should feel free to make concrete suggestions to the parents as to how they can protect their child in a responsible and realistic fashion. Family tasks can be proposed as a step toward the resolution of the specific crisis, and the family should be assigned activities directed toward the resolution of the current crisis. Specific assignments of "homework" should be made to the parents and to the child or adolescent to work together toward their own solutions of the family's problems. Examples of such assignments include the determination as to which parent will assist the school phobic child in preparing for school attendance, transporting and then remaining temporarily at the school with the child. The child does not have the prerogative of remaining home, but can make requests and negotiate for tension-reducing assistance. The suicidal child can participate in the planning for his own observation and for the appropriate disposal of the tempting drugs in the family's medicine cabinet. The runaway child can participate in planning for temporary living arrangements or modifications in the home stresses. The obvious goal is to include the child in all planning so that there is neither the adults managing a recalcitrant child nor the child manipulating the adults through his symptomatic behavior, the familiar "tail wagging the dog". With adolescents who are moving toward independence of living, school activity and sexual behavior, the entire family should have the home assignment of arriving at age-appropiate rules for dating, driving and work plans consistent with community peer privileges and activities. Family conferences should attend to a reasonable distribution of household tasks and family responsibilities. The family should be expected to attend to tasks rather than symptoms.

The treatment team must be alert to unspoken family alliances and nonverbal communications during the group meetings. Such nonverbal communications and alliances are often the most valuable clues to the disruptive family secrets. It is essential that the family members come to see for themselves that the behavioral problems or physical symptoms leading to the crisis represent underlying family problems rather than being the cause of the family problems. Alternative means of communication, rather than symptomatic expression, are considered with both the children and their parents. Again at some variance with usual clinic and practice approaches, subsequent family meetings are determined by the capability of family members to grasp their problems, and by the confidence of the treatment team that there is an increasing understanding of the family tensions. Subsequent meetings are sometimes scheduled the same day, and occasionally several interviews may occur within a week. The frequency is determined by the confidence or doubts expressed by members of the family or by members of the treatment team. Specific treatment goals or behavioral changes are defined as subsequent meetings are scheduled, and future meetings may be determined by the achievement of treatment goals, or by the presence of new problems that come from family conferences in the home.

Emergency intervention with family crises is not limited to group meetings at the clinic or private office. Home and school visits, meetings at the offices of involved community agencies, and extensive use of phone calls actively contribute to the education of the family in the handling of their emotional crisis. A benefit that must not be underestimated results from the willingness of the crisis team to meet with agencies and schools in their own settings. Such meetings not only demonstrate the willingness of the child psychiatric crisis team to interact with communicty agencies on their own territory, but also serve as inservice training that many agencies would be unable to obtain otherwise, because of large service loads, waiting lists, and long-term commitments. The brief treatment approach demonstrates to the family and to the community representatives that there are effective ways of solving individual and family emotional problems other than by developing physiological symptoms, symptomatic behavioral problems, or the exclusion of a family member by runaway or hospitalization. The family participates in active psychological treatment and education toward adaptive management of future crises.

It has been the experience of crisis services that the clearly stated expectation of participation of all family members, members of the extended family and representatives of involved agencies is sufficient to ensure their participation (Langsley and Kaplan, 1968; Morrison, 1975; Parad, 1961). In addition to the active participation and involvement of parents and other adults important to the child experiencing a psychiatric emergency, effective therapeutic intervention needs other simultaneous activities to support the crisis treatment approach. A few examples will demonstrate the associated activities and will serve to highlight the need for interrelated services for children and their families experiencing emotional difficulties. Suicidal adolescents often have several symptoms representing their various attempts at a solution to their depression and low self-esteem. In addition to overt suicide attempt, there may be associated symptoms, such as school refusal, runaway, sexual promiscuity (with possible pregnancy or venereal disease), drug abuse and toxicity, and physical complications resulting from the method of suicidal expression. There is need for emergency medical facilities, along with the availability of an adolescent inpatient treatment unit or foster home care, a detoxification unit, contraceptive counseling, abortion services if requested, maternity and prenatal health care, and the opportunity for continuing educational or vocational training. Emergency medical facilities are essential not only as back-up medical resources for patients with suicidal expression, but also for those patients with conversion and dissociative reactions, acute psychophysiological symptoms and drug intoxication. Child and adolescent emergency services must maintain an active liaison with juvenile courts, probation departments, and law enforcement agencies for children involved in truancy, runaway, assaultive and destructive behavior, and for children who are the victims of incest or sexual assault. Follow-up and continuing care for children and families who have received emergency psychiatric treatment should be developed to be consistent with our psychological, medical and demographic understanding of those families that are most likely to use or to be referred for emergency services.

These families tend to follow predictable patterns in seeking medical services. Understanding those patterns is essential to the development of such services and the planning of follow-up programs. Crises are often used as a means of communication within the family and as a method of receiving assistance from the family. Morrison and Smith reported on the many similarities found in families that tend to relate through their emotional crises. They observed many similarities among these families regardless of their socio-economic, ethnic or cultural background. Although some differences were noted in the degree of family intactness in terms of the cohesiveness of the family and the presence of parental figures, and some differences were seen in the use of medical services as compared with juvenile court facilities; the similarities were far more prominent. The families expected an immediate resolution of their problems, prompt reduction in their anxiety, and a solution through the use of medication or hospitalization.

A frequent problem in planning follow-up care for these families is the increasing tendency to carefully define psychiatric services by the use of geographic boundaries and catchment areas which delimit services. Crisis-prone families move across city, county, and state lines to follow employment opportunities, to maintain family ties, and to avoid legal and financial entanglements. The development of catchment areas has further complicated the maintenance of lines of communication with these families. Psychiatric and medical services are often geographically delimited by sources of funding support and political divisions. Children's psychiatric emergency services can mitigate the limitation caused by these "boundaries" by providng direct or indirect (consultation) services to several catchment areas.

Comparisons

Psychiatric emergencies of children, adolescents and their families have always been seen by child psychiatric clinics or social work intake services, but the realities of treatment waiting lists and heavy individual staff case loads have made the approach to these families other than optimal. Trained professional personnel with flexibility in their schedules and the immediate availability of the 24-hour emergency room with inpatient facilities are resources found associated with very few child psychiatric clinics. Even where such services can be offered, many families needing urgent help seem unable to tolerate even a few day's delay after their initial contact with a children's psychiatric service or psychiatric emergency unit. Immediate response and continuity of care are essential to emergency intervention with children and adolescents.

Several difficult challenges are apparent to most professionals involved in the use of emergency intervention method. The need for trained and experienced staff with flexible schedules and the demand by the crisis families for immediate solutions to difficult problems are the most obvious challenges. Such names as "the band-aid approach" and "the mental health workers' panacea" reflect the frequency of the family's or the less skilled therapist's wish for a quick solution to difficult human problems. Even a superficial review of the works of Caplan (1961, 1964), Lindemann (1944), Berlin (1970), Parad (1965), Langsley and Kaplan (1968), and Morrison (1975) demonstrates the complexities of the problems and the enormous skill and experience needed to effectively apply emergency psychotherapeutic measures to family crises.

When one considers alternatives to brief family psychotherapy for children and adolescents with acute emotional problems, one must ask, "What symptoms are receiving therapeutic attention?" "How emotionally stable is the child and his family?" and "What are the therapeutic alternatives?" Emotional crises, because of the noise created, have always received a response by one or another of the medical or judicial resources provided in an organized society. Socially disruptive behaviors (runaway, fire-setting, sexual promiscuity) have come to the attention of the juvenile and family courts. Assaultive and homicidal behaviors (including drug abuse at the present time [The Medical Letter, 1977]) have come to the attention of the criminal court system. Educational problems (school phobia, truancy, school disruption) have been the responsibility of our educational institutions and their counseling services. Urgent medical problems (suicide attempt and threat, conversion reactions, psychophysiological symptoms, bizarre or psychotic behavior, and the victims of sexual assault) have been evaluated and treated in hospital emergency rooms and other acute medical facilities. Some behaviors viewed as indicative of serious individual and family disturbance (sexual incest, killing of pets, survivors of parental suicide, and children experiencing acute grief) rarely have come to psychiatric attention, but subsequent emotional and economic costs have been very high. Crisis services have demonstrated an immediate usefulness with their success in preventing or reducing the number of fires set by a child, in preventing suicide and the associated tragedy or suicide attempts resulting in hospitalization, and in reducing drug abuse by appropriate and timely attention to the causes.

A brief review of the history of school phobia can help clarify the kind of clinical and theoretical work that has influenced the receommendation that all members of the family participate in attempting to resolve a psychiatric emergency. Almost five decades ago school phobia was first recognized and described as a specific clinical entity with debilitating consequences. Society had recognized the need for education for all children and had mandated school attendance to a certain age. Initially school phobia was considered only in the context of treatment for the child's anxiety about school attendance. During the following two decades there was an increasing recognition of the phobic child's attachment to his mother and an increasing awareness of the mother's subtle or active participation and contribution to the child's anxiety when absent from the home, so individual psychotherapy of the mother was added. A shift in attention came with the recognition of the mother's fear and anxiety, and emphasis was given to the mother-child dyad in contributing to the school phobia. With increasing attention to the mother, there was the discovery of marriage problems. This in turn focused attention to the husband-wife dyad, and the recognition that the child's father also played a part in the child's phobic symptoms and school anxiety. While some clinicians attended to the pragmatic issues of returning the child to school as quickly as possible, others focused on the treatment of the child's and the family's problems in psychiatric services in or near the school setting, and still others recommended individual intensive depth psychotherapy for each member of the family. School phobia as an aspect of family neurosis came to prominence in the late 1950's, culminating in an elegant paper written by Malmquist (1965). The present understanding of the child's emotional tensions and symptomatic behavior associated with required school attendance need not be rediscovered with each child and family referred for emergency intervention. A similar history of clinical discoveries and understanding can be traced for each of the clinical symptoms seen as child psychiatric emergencies.

The treatment of school phobia, to be effective, needs enlightened school personnel who are able to cooperate and actively participate with the psychiatric emergency team. The flexibility of school personnel is severely tested by the high anxiety exhibited by the child and the parents during the first days of renewed school attendance. For several weeks, each weekend break and intervening holiday reactivates the child's wish to avoid the separation from the home, and stirs similar anxiety in the parents. In marked contrast, truancy needs a different kind of educational or vocational training setting that can catch and hold the adolescent's limited interest.

In evaluating indications for the brief family-oriented therapy method, one can draw an analogy to the usually short treatment for a complicated and extended grief reaction as compared to the treatment for an individual with chronic depression. We can define the stages of a normal grief reaction (Lindemann (1944), pp. 10–12) and can recognize resolving grief as distinguished from an unresolved grief or reactive depression. Symptomatically, one can observe the tears of acute grief and can recognize the description of tightness in the throat, shortness of breath, a need for sighing, an empty feeling in the abdomen, muscular weakness and numbness. One can distinguish acute grief from the symptoms of chronic reactive depression; such as, sleep and appetite changes, early morning awakening, preoccupation with guilt, and feelings of failure.

Experienced clinicians are aware of the importance of recognizing a history of object loss or separation that has contributed to the family's helplessness and the emotional crisis. These crises are responsive to the brief-treatment approach with early intervention and resolution. Conversely, such an approach when used with the chronically disordered family bogs down in endless misunderstandings about descriptions, causes, details and denials. Frustration and suffering are apparent, the quantity of problems can be defined and measured, but the quality of the response and the evidence of progress is lacking. Individual and family psychotherapy is useful for families with chronic and pervasive problems, but brief-therapy is inappropriate for such deep and long-standing problems. Crisis therapy, in response to such chronic difficulties, serves only to delay appropriate treatment for these families and inappropriately utilizes the limited time of the crisis team with endless pursuit of issues that have long since been incorporated into the family's mode of functioning.

Summary and Conclusions

Kaffman (1963, pp. 205–206) has summarized the goals and purposes of brief family therapy by commenting that, "It is not within the scope of a short service of family therapy to bring about basic and extensive alterations in character structure of family members. . . . The therapist's help to all the members of the family, in obtaining focused insight into the nature of conscious and preconscious conflicts, is likely to lead to a readjusted and healthier family interrelationship, to goal modification, and to full use of potential possibilities." He believes that no measures that could contribute to a healthy family adjustment should be avoided by the therapist. He considers therapeutic counseling to be acceptable if the patient or the family is ready to follow advice. Additionally, he stresses the importance of assisting the family to an emotional equilibrium through attention to and relief of clinical symptoms.

Most experienced psychotherapists have had the opportunity to observe many changes in a patient as well as in members of his family when an area of emotional tension and conflict has been explored and relieved through psychotherapeutic means. The crisis therapist has many advantages for achieving such relief: the patient and his family are highly motivated for symptom relief; the therapist is usually viewed as a source of relief and as one who has demonstrated interest in the family's problem by prompt involvement; the individual and family anxiety, although high, can be directed toward the immediate problems and related family conflicts from the past; and the usual characterologic defenses of the members of the family have been modified and realigned by the immediacy of the crisis. All of the foregoing provides an opportunity for powerful leverage toward modification of previously rigid and destructive family interactions. Kaffman has referred to this as the "snowball phenomenon" which can lead to favorable modifications in the child-parent relationship.

Therapeutic results have been reported by Morrison (1975a), Langsley and Kaplan (1968), Parad (1961), and Barten and Barten (1973). These authors have used similar types of modified individual and family psychotherapeutic modalities in treating crisis-prone families. All have emphasized the need for careful planning of follow-up services, as a concomitant part of the treatment and support of families in emotional crisis. Their reports show that the psychiatric treatment programs described are considered very helpful by the majority of the families treated. That result has been reported by Kaffman (1963) as measurable symptom relief. Langsley and Kaplan (1968) have presented information comparing the financial cost of such services, and have tabulated the results of their specific program in terms of the number of hospital days needed and prevented through the use of family crisis therapy. Their report of the emotional and financial costs to families in crisis that have an acutely psychotic adult is similar to estimates of the costs to families that have an acutely disturbed child. The resolution of the family crisis, the avoidance of hospitalization, the resolution of psychiatric symptoms, and the return to school are all important to the emotional development of the child. The short-term family therapeutic approach to children and families in crisis is a useful and constructive means for early alleviation of emotionally crippling symptoms and behaviors, and should be available to all families in need of acute psychiatric care for their children.

In defining emergencies in child psychiatry one not only should focus on the degree or kind of disturbance in the child, but also should scrutinize the kind of anxiety and the degree of helplessness, and disorganization in those adults who are most closely involved with the child in his imnediate life situation. Ackerman (1958) discussed the capacity of one or more family members to contain significant family psychopathology. The concept of the extended family is essential to the recognition of the role of significant extended family members as well as the nuclear family members in the total functioning of the child, his parents and siblings. The treatment method proposed, immediate psychotherapeutic intervention with the child, his family, and important adults in his environment, is based on the developmental model defined. Immediate diagnostic evaluation and treatment utilizes techniques of conjoint collaborative interviewing, brief psychotherapy, and family therapy. Psychiatric attention is directed toward prevention and early alleviation of emotional disorders. The important aspects of such an approach include the immediate appraisal of the child, his family, and his milieu concurrently; the reestablishment or development of communication within the family and the environment by the emergency treatment chosen; the establishment and maintenance of good working relationships with various community agencies, schools, and clinics; and the provision of sufficient flexibility within the treatment program to afford the frequency and intensity of contact to achieve these results.

References

Ackerman, N.W. (1958) Toward an integrative therapy of the family. *Am. J. Psychiat.* 114:727–733.

Barten, H.H. and S.S. Barten. (1973) *Children and Their Parents in Brief Therapy.* New York: Behavioral Publications.

Berlin, I.N. (1970) Crisis intervention and short term therapy: An approach in a child psychiatric clinic. *J. Am. Acad. Child Psychiat.* 9:595–606.

Burks, H.L., and S.I. Harrison. (1962) Aggressive behavior as a means of avoiding depression. *Am. J. Orthopsychiat.* 32:418–422.

Burks, H.L., and M. Hoekstra. (1964) Psychiatric emergencies in children. *Am. J. Orthopsychiat.* 34:134–137.

Caplan, G. (1961) *Prevention of Mental Disorders in Children.* New York: Basic Books.

Caplan, G. (1964) *Principles of Preventive Psychiatry.* New York: Basic Books, pp. 28–30.

Coolidge, J., E. Tessman, J. Waldfogel, and M. Witter. (1962) Patterns of aggression in school phobia. *Psychoanal. Study Child* 17:319–333.

Eisenberg, L. (1958) School phobia: diagnosis, genesis, and clinical management. *Ped. Clin. N. Amer.* 5:645–666.

Ekstein, R. (1972) Brief therapy versus intensive therapy or: Patient-oriented treatment programs. In G.C. Morrison, ed., *Emergencies in Child Psychiatry,* Springfield, Ill.: Charles C Thomas, 1975, pp. 5–12.

Erikson, E.H. (1963) *Childhood and Society.* 2nd ed. New York: Norton.

Freud, S. (1917) *Mourning and Melancholia.* In *Standard Edition,* Vol. 14. London: Hogarth Press, 1957, pp. 237–260.

Hill, R. (1949) *Families Under Stress.* New York: Harper and Brothers.

Hollingshead, A.B., and F.C. Redlich. (1958) *Social Class and Mental Illness.* New York: Wiley.

Kaffman, M. (1963) Short-term family therapy. In H.J. Parad, ed., *Crisis Intervention: Selected Readings.* New York: Family Service Association, 1965, pp. 202–219.

Kaufman, I., and L. Heims. (1958) The body image of the juvenile delinquent. *Am. J. Orthopsychiat.* 28:146–159.

Langsley, D.G., and D.N. Kaplan. (1968) *The Treatment of Families in Crisis.* New York: Grune & Stratton.

Levi, L.D., C.M. Fales, M. Stein, and V.H. Sharp. (1966) Separation and attempted suicide. *Arch. Gen. Psychiat.* 15:148–164.

Lindemann, E. (1944) Symptomatology and management of acute grief. In H.J. Parad, ed., *Crisis Intervention: Selected Readings.* New York: Family Service Association, 1965, pp. 7–21.

Malmquist, C.P. (1965) School phobia: A problem in family neurosis. *J. Am. Acad. Child Psychiat.* 4:293–319.

Mattsson, A., J.W. Hawkins, and L. Seese. (1967) Child psychiatric emergencies. *Arch. Gen. Psychiat.* 17:584–592.

The Medical Letter (1977) Diagnosis and Management of Reactions to Drug Abuse, Vol. 19, No. 3 (Issue 472), February 11, 1977, pp. 13–16.

Mintz, R.S. (1966) Some practical procedures in the management of suicidal persons. *Am. J. Orthopsychiat.* 36:896–903.

Morrison, G.C. (1969) Therapeutic intervention in a child psychiatry emergency service. *J. Am. Acad. Child Psychiat.* 8:542–558.

Morrison, G.C. and J.G. Collier. (1969) Family treatment approaches to suicidal children and adolescents. *J. Am. Acad. Child Psychiat.* 8:140–153.

Morrison, G.C. (1975) *Emergencies in Child Psychiatry: Emotional Crises of Children, Youth and Their Families.* Springfield, Ill.: Charles C Thomas.

Morrison, G.C., and W.R. Smith. (1975a) Child psychiatric emergencies: A comparison of two clinic settings and socio-economic groups. In G.C. Morrison, ed., *Emergencies in Child Psychiatry.* Springfield, Ill.: Charles C Thomas, pp. 107–114.

Morrison, G.C., and W.R. Smith. (1975b) Emergencies in child psychiatry: A definition. In G.C. Morrison, ed., Morrison, *Emergencies in Child Psychiatry.* Springfield, Ill.: Charles C Thomas, pp. 13–20.

Murphy, L.B. (1961) Preventive implications of development in the preschool years. In G. Caplan, ed., *Prevention of Mental Disorders in Children.* New York: Basic Books, pp. 218–243.

Parad, H.J. (1965) *Crisis Intervention: Selected Readings.* New York: Family Service Association.

Parad, H.J. (1961) Preventive casework: Problems and implications. In H.J. Parad, ed., *Crisis Intervention: Selected Readings.* New York: Family Service Association, 1965.

Proctor, J.T. (1958) Hysteria in childhood. *Am. J. Orthopsychiat.* 28:394–407.

Rapoport, L. (1962) The state of crisis: Some theoretical considerations. In H.J. Parad, ed., *Crisis Intervention: Selected Readings.* New York: Family Service Association, 1965, pp. 22–31.

Robey, A., R.J. Rosenwald, J.E. Snell, and R. Lees. (1964) The runaway girl: A reaction to family stress. *Am. J. Orthopsychiat.* 34:762–767.

Shaw, C.R., and R.F. Schelkun. (1965) Suicidal behavior in children. *Psychiatry* 28:157–168.

Shneidman, E.S., and N.L. Farberow. (1961) Statistical comparisons between attempted and committed suicides. In N.L. Farberow and E.S. Shneidman, eds., *The Cry for Help.* New York: McGraw-Hill, pp. 19–47.

Smith, W.R., and G.C. Morrison. (1975) Family tolerance for chronic, severe, neurotic, or deviant behavior in children referred for child psychiatry emergency consultation. In G.C. Morrison, ed., *Emergencies in Child Psychiatry.* New York: Charles C Thomas, pp. 115–128.

Stierlin, H. (1973) A family perspective on adolescent runaways. *Arch. Gen. Psychiat.* 29:56–62.

Tuckman, J., and H.E. Connon. (1962) Attempted suicide in adolescents. *Am. J. Psychiat.* 119:228–232.

Treatment of Emotional Disorders in Children and Adolescents

CHAPTER 33

Treatment of School Phobia*

John M. Berecz

Definitional Considerations

Basic to any meaningful discussion of a psychological disorder is some kind of definitive statement. With phobias, this proves to be a formidable task; various definitions have been influenced by the intellectual climates existing at the times of their proposals. Recently, two general ideas have received attention in definitions: the idea that the fear is perceived by the person as foreign to his personality, and the idea that the fear is out of proportion to the external stimulus.

Kanner (1957) writes: "Phobia shares with other obsessions the feeling of strangeness and the strong desire to be rid of the unwanted, not understood, and utterly disturbing sensation." Friedman (1959) defined a phobia as a fear "which becomes attached to objects or situations which objectively are not a source of danger—or, more precisely, are known by the individual not to be a source of danger." Berkowitz and Rothman (1960) emphasized the fact that "the individual who develops a phobia recognizes the fear as illogical and unreasonable, but does not generally understand why he has the fear and feels helpless in overcoming it." Zax and Stricker (1963) suggest that a phobia involves "an overwhelming and disproportionate fear of some relatively harmless object, situation, or idea." Kutash (1965) says that "there is a persistent, morbid, unreasonable fear exaggerated out of proportion to the danger of the dreaded object or situation."

At this somewhat global level of definition, there is adequate consensus; however, when phobias are examined in detail, the picture becomes very confused.

One major source of confusion is the fact that many writers include in their definitions concepts which are heavily influenced by their own theoretical biases. Wechsler (1929), for example, said: ". . . all phobias represent an unconscious sense of guilt attached to an early memory." Freud (1934) wrote: "Phobias do not occur when the vita sexualis is normal." Cohn (1959) states: "All real phobias carry strong hate toward the parents who have unconsciously deserted the child." Finch (1960) says: "Transient phobias are result of the child's attempts to deal with his Oedipal struggles, during which he projects into the outer world some of his unconscious worries." Kutash (1965) maintains that "The phobia is a symbolic representation of unacceptable libidinal and aggressive impulses."

Confusion also results because the word "phobia" is used to describe such a variety of conditions that it loses much of its definitive value. The fact that all conditions subsumed under the term "phobia" are not similar is implied by Crider's (1949) discussion of the dynamic and behavioristic explanations of phobia. He states: "Confusion to the beginner comes in using the word phobia in both

---

*Portions of this chapter originally appeared in an article entitled "Phobias of Childhood: Etiology and Treatment" published in *Psychological Bulletin*, Volume 70, 1968, pp. 694–720, and appear in the present chapter with permission of the author and the American Psychological Association.

theories, confusion would be lessened if we remember that one type of phobia arises from a conditioned fear whereas the other arises from conditioned anxiety." Even a brief survey of the literature reveals that the term phobia is used in describing many very diverse kinds of situations. It is difficult to assess, for example, what "shooting phobia" in a hunting dog (Haack,1954) and the "phobia of communism" (Perrotti,1949) have in common, save the nonheuristic fact that both designations employ the word "phobia." Studies are found of the phobia of impregnation (Robie, 1935), acarophobia (Wilson and Miller, 1946) nosophobia (Ryle, 1948), nyctophobia (Devereux, 1949), germophobia (Buessmilch, 1950), ailurophobia, ornithophobia (London, 1952), the phobia avoidance of corners of buildings (Brody, 1953), and Mackie (1967) even reported the case of a patient who, as a 14-year old, has developed the inability to tolerate anyone sitting on the left side of her (leftophobia?). In addition to the numerous case studies, it is possible to construct an almost infinite list of phobias by merely appending the suffix "phobia" to various words. Masserman (1946) gives a lengthy, but not exhaustive, list in which he includes, for example, ergasiophobia (activity), pnigophobia (choking), ballistophobia (projectiles), graphophobia (writing), etc. In 1949, Terhune reported that the literature listed 107 specific phobias. Among the phobias included by Kanner (1957) are pyrophobia (causing fire), aichmophobia (pointed objects), paraliphobia (fear of precipitating disaster by having omitted or forgotten something), taphephobia (fear of being buried alive), and even phobophobia (fear of phobias) and pantophobia (multiple obsessive fears of practically everything). In 1964, White said that the medical literature mentioned "literally hundreds" of phobias. Redlich and Freedman (1966) report that Hinsie and Campbell's dictionary lists 200 phobic reactions.

Finally, another confusing factor is that the term "phobia" has carried different meanings in different periods of history, making it necessary to take into account not only the writers' theoretical biases, but also the period in which they were writing. Koegler and Brill (1967) point out that the contemporary term "anxiety reaction" and "phobic reaction" do not correspond completely with the older terms "anxiety neurosis" and "anxiety hysteria."

When dealing with children and adolescents, the issues are further complicated by the tendency to regard psychopathology in children as merely a "miniature replica" of what is found in adults. Various writers have emphasized the qualitative differences between children and adults (Howells, 1965; Warren, 1960).

In summary, the definition of childhood and adolescent phobias is wrought with many difficulties. Definitions typically included elements that reflect theoretical biases, the word "phobia" is used so broadly that its meaning becomes obscured, and disparate historical usages further cloud the issue. These problems are accentuated by the tendency of many to regard implicitly children and adolescents as "little adults." Parochialism, then, would seem a hindrance to progress in the area of childhood phobias. Kanner's (1959) statement that "Child psychiatry, in brief, is a fusion of what used to be a collection of more or less loosely scattered parts" ought to sensitize investigators to the fact that the study of children and adolescents is hampered by fragmentary knowledge in many vital areas and that the phrase "loosely scattered parts" is still an apt description of the field.

When dealing with children and adolescents, there is little good normative data against which to measure whether a fear is symptomatic of neurosis or whether it is a transitory normal fear. Thus, although Finch (1960) contends that "The child with a typical psychoneurotic phobic reaction is one whose phobias are more prolonged or more exaggerated than normal. To be a phobia, a fear must have an exaggerated character which far exceeds realistic expectations." It is not always easy to decide what constitutes a "normal" fear and at what point a fear may be thought of as excessively "exaggerated." At a very practical level, it is probably the child or parent's level of discomfort that brings them into treatment rather than any theoretical considerations.

The clinician, however, needs to have some internal norms for deciding whether a given fear is phobic in quality, and these ought to be based on some knowledge of fears in normal children and adolescents.

Fears of Normal Children and Adolescents

Jersild and Holmes (1935) reported that a large number of children's fears are "outgrown" in the normal course of growth and experience. English and Pearson (1945) described phobias as the "normal neurosis of childhood," reflecting the fact that transient phobias are not pathological. Kessler (1966) states that "Childhood phobias are so common that mild, transient phobic reactions are regarded as a normal part of early development."

These views emphasize the tenuous nature of speculations about children's fears. To the extent that information is available, workers in this area should have a firm grounding in the "normal" fears of children upon which to base their speculations and conclusions regarding phobias.

Well-designed studies of fears in normal children are not prevalent, but a few studies give some tentative ideas. Hagman (1932) interviewed the mothers of 70 children, ranging in age from 23 months to 6 years, and reported the following conclusions: (a) The average number of fears was 2.7; (b) rank order of things feared was dogs, doctors, storms, deep water, and darkness; (c) there was a real tendency for the child to have fears corresponding to those of his mother; (d) there was a correlation of .667 between the gross number of children's fears and the gross number of their mothers' fears. The last two conclusions are difficult to interpret, since there is no way of ascertaining the influence of the mothers' own fears upon the ratings done by her upon her child.

A more recent and better-designed study by Lapouse and Monk (1959) found no significant correlation between mothers' and childrens' fears.

In their extensive studies, Jersild, Markey, and Jersild (1960) interviewed 398 children aged 5 to 12 years and found the rank order of fears as follows: supernatural agents (ghosts, witches, corpses, mysterious events), 19.2%; being alone, in the dark, in a strange place, being lost, and the dangers associated with these situations, 14.6%; attack or danger of attack by animals, 13.7%; bodily injury, falling, illness, traffic accidents, operations, hurts and pains, etc. 12.8%. Cummings (1944) studied 291 British children aged 2 to 7 years and found that 22.2% showed specific fears. Pratt (1945) studied 570 rural children and found the average number of fears to be 7.5% per child, with girls showing a greater number of fears than boys. As the author himself points out, several factors make this study difficult to interpret. Furthermore, it is not possible to compare it with the findings of Jersild et al. (1960), since the fears were scored differently in both studies.

It is difficult from these studies to draw meaningful conclusions, and the dearth of knowledge in this area is one of the real handicaps in the study of phobias of children and adolescents.

The study by MacFarlane, Allen, and Honzik (1954) is one of the most comprehensive and best designed. Their finding that 90% of the children in their study reported fears, emphasized the need for more information about fears of normal children and adolescents as a basis for generalizing about phobias.

Relationship of Fears to Age

Dunlop (1952) concluded that age was unimportant insofar as number, intensity, and distance of causation of fears was concerned. Angelino and Shedd (1953) concluded very broadly, and with reservation, that children of ages 11 to 12 showed a preponderance of animal fears, 13-year-olds showed more school-connected content, while 15- to 18-year-olds showed more concern with political and economic factors. They found that in the upper socioeconomic classes, although there was an overall decrease of fears with increases in age, both girls and boys showed a marked increase in the number of fears at ages 11 to 12. MacFarlane et al. (1954) found that for specific fears, "the frequencies showed definite down trends with age for both boys and girls except for an increase for both at age 11." If their sample is upper class (and it seems that it is) according to the criteria followed by Angelino and Shedd (1953), these two large-scale studies seem to confirm each other.

The general decrease of fears with age is hardly surprising, but needs considerably more clarification in order to be of value. Why there should be an increase in fears at about age 11 is not clear, but it seems interesting that these two studies corroborate each other on that point.

Relationship of Socioeconomic Class to Fears

Angelino, Dollins, and Mech (1956) grouped their 1,100 subjects into upper and lower classes and concluded that there was a positive relationship between socioeconomic background and the number and kinds of fears present. As an example, in the area of safety: lower-class boys feared switchblades, whippings, robbers, killers, guns, and matters of violence, whereas upper-class boys feared car accidents, getting killed, juvenile delinquents, disaster, and other more nebulous events. Lower-class girls feared animals, strangers, and acts of violence, whereas upper-class girls feared kidnappers, heights and a variety of things not mentioned by lower-class girls, such as train and ship wrecks.

Socioeconomic class seems to be an important consideration that has been given short shrift by psychologists studying fears in children. The systematic investigation of this variable is quite incomplete, and the study by Angelino et al. points out a direction for futher research.

Relationship of Fears to Other Behaviors Commonly Thought To be Pathological

MacFarlane et al. (1954) found that the correlates of fears at age 5 in girls indicate that the basis for their specific fears is a generalized anxiety seen in such behaviors as irritability (r=.43), somberness (r=.41), overdependence (r=.35), mood swings (r=.31), insufficient appetite (r=.31), tempers (r=.29), and timidity (r=.29).At age 5, only negativism (r=.32) correlated significantly with fears in boys. At age 3, boys showed the following significant correlations: physical timidity (r=.63) and freedom from illness (r=.42). At 21 months, girls showed the following significant correlates: physical timidity (r=.64), temper tantrums (r=.44), and a negative correlation with overactivity (r=.65). Lapouse and Monk (1959) studied 482 children whose names had been selected from a pool of 1,600 that had been systematically taken from the Buffalo city directory. They were unable to find a statistically significant correlation between the considerable number of fears and worries reported by mothers as occurring in their children and other behaviors (e.g., bedwetting, nightmares, stuttering, tics, etc.) commonly thought of as pathological.

These findings indicate the need for considerable caution in attempting to relate fears and specific behaviors. Most of the correlations in the MacFarlane et al. (1954) study were quite low, and it is well to remember that a correlation of .32 accounts for less than 10% of the variance. Lapouse and Monk (1959) were unable to find any significant correlations.

On a whole, the results of studies of fears in normal children and adolescents are not very gratifying. Although there are hints that fears are related to age, social class, and "pathological" behaviors, the relationships are extremely unclear and much more research is needed in this area. Various criteria are used for determining which fears are recorded, and few longitudinal studies are available. Almost no information about the intensity of fears at various ages, etc. is available. Quite simply, very little is known about the qualitative and quantitative characteristics of fears of normal children and adolescents relative to age and other important variables.

Definitional Considerations Unique to School Phobia

Broadwin (1932) was one of the first to describe the school-phobia syndrome. He characterized it as occurring in a child who was suffering from "deep-seated neuroses of the obsessional type . . . while at school the child thought 'something terrible is happening to mother.' . . . The child felt he must run home to see his mother." Johnson, Falstein, Szurek, and Svendsen (1941) were the first to coin the term "school phobia." Since that time, there has been controversy about all aspects of school phobia, including questions about the usefulness of the term itself. Vaughan (1957) contends that school phobia is basically not a fear of school, but rather a fear of leaving home, primarily a problem of separation from mother. Estes, Haylett, and Johnson (1956) write: "The term school phobia emphasizes a common symptom rather than the underlying nature of the true disorder." Johnson (1957) says: "School phobia is a misnomer, actually it is separation anxiety which occurs not only in early childhood, but also in later years." Davidson (1960) writes: "School phobia is a symptom, not a diagnosis." She suggests that these children are "mother-philes" rather than "school-phobes." Reger (1962) says: "The term school phobia is of questionable utility, because unwarranted emphasis tends to be placed on understanding the label rather than the child with the problem." Radin (1967) implies that the label is misleading when he says: "School phobia involves more complex mechanisms than are ordinarily encountered in phobias."

Since school phobia refers to a reluctance to go to school, some writers use the term interchangeably with school refusal. There is a fairly good consensus, however, on the difference between truancy and school phobia. In Broadwin's (1932) study, he emphasized the fact that the school-phobic child stays with the mother or near home. Vaughan (1957) said that the school-phobic child differs from the truant in being terrified of school: "He may flee school in a panic, but unlike the truant, he dashes straight home to mother." Eisenberg (1958b), points out that the truant cuts classes and spends time away from home. Shaw (1966) writes: "Truancy is an absence from school on rational (if not socially acceptable) grounds, e.g., an encounter with the school bully, sadistic teachers, etc. A phobia is irrational, and changing teachers, etc., only temporarily helps." Waldfogel (1959) gives an excellent definition of school phobia:

School phobia refers to a reluctance to go to school because of acute fear associated with it. Usually this dread is accompanied by somatic symptoms with the gastrointestinal tract being most commonly affected. . . . The somatic complaints come to be used as an auxiliary device to justify staying at home, and often disappear when the child is reassured he will not have to attend school. The characteristic picture is of a child nauseated or complaining of abdominal pain at breakfast and desperately resisting all attempts at reassurance, reasoning, or coercion to get him to school. In its milder forms, school phobia may be only a transient symptom; but when it becomes established, it can be one of the most disabling disorders of childhood, lasting even for years (pp. 35–36).

Shapiro and Jegede (1973) have recently reviewed the historical trend in definitions tracing the early broad conception of school avoidance toward a narrow conception of school phobia and back toward a systems analysis. They suggest that a definition ought to consider the syndrome in relationship to developmental factors, transactional involvements with mother, family, and community; intrapsychic dynamics; and the personal view of the child toward his symptoms. They suggest that consideration of these areas will permit an individualistic tailored therapeutic intervention rather than a uniform approach to a complex symptom.

Frequency

Wakabayashi, Ito, and Ito (1965) found that among Japanese schoolchildren, urban children showed a higher incidence 80/150,967 (.06%) of school refusal than did rural children 11/30,934 (.03%). Ono (1972) also studied school phobia among Japanese schoolchildren and found that among 130,000, 95 children were identified as school phobic and an additional 49 were in the questionable category. Kennedy (1965) gives the rate as 17/1,000 school-age children per year. Kahn and Nursten (1962) said that 2–8% of the referrals in some child-guidance clinics are school-phobic children. They say that in Boston (population 800,000), there are 25 severe cases of school phobia each year. Kessler (1966) observes that while in general boys outnumber girls in child-guidance clinics, most authors (Coolidge, Willer, Tessman, and Waldfogel, 1960; Suttenfield, 1954; Talbot, 1957; Van Houten, 1948) report that school phobias are more common in girls.

The frequency of school phobia is extremely difficult to evaluate, since the figures obtained depend upon so many different kinds of factors (e.g., the kind of community, clinic, referral system, etc.). Obviously, children refused to go to school before 1941 (when the term "school phobia" was coined), but they were probably thought of as truants, delinquents, or just "problem children."

An interesting finding is that school phobia, like other phobias of childhood and adolescence, seems to peak around the onset of adolescence. Morgan (1959) reports the peak age for school phobias to be 11–13. Chazen (1962) reports the peak to be around 11 years.

Theories of Etiology and Treatment

The distinction between etiology and treatment is often quite vague in the literature and frequently not even made. Since most etiological notions have implications for the kinds of treatments to be employed, it is often implicitly assumed that the success or failure of a treatment directly follows from the correctness or incorrectness of the etiological notions upon which it is based. It needs to be emphasized, however, that the successes or failures of treatment procedures are empirical facts quite apart from, and in some cases unrelated to, the etiological theories from which they may have been derived. As such, they carry no vindicative value for these theories; that is, psychoanalysis or behavior therapy may "work" or fail to "work" because of what the therapist does rather than why he does it.

The following discussion will treat the various major theoretical views separately. This is done not in the belief that various "schools" are substantively independent, but rather to facilitate implementation of treatment from a given perspective.

Psychoanalysis: The "Little Hans" Paradigm

In 1909, Freud's account of his treatment of a phobia in a 5-year-old boy (Hans) was published. Although Freud actually saw the boy only once, he presented an analysis based on conversations with the boy's father. Freud pointed out that without the special knowledge by means of which the father was able to interpret the remarks made by the boy, it would have been impossible to conduct psychoanalysis upon so young a child. In this case study, Freud presented the view that the basis for phobic disturbances could be found in the

Oedipus complex. Most analysts have more or less followed his lead. Rachman and Costello (1961) present the rudiments of the theory in the following steps: (a) the child is fixated at the Oedipal or pre-Oedipal level, and the phobic object serves as a substitute for the father, a substitute onto which the fear of the father is projected; (b) the child has sexual desire for the mother; (c) the child has castration fears; (d) the child fears the father; (e) the fears of the father are projected onto the neutral object; (f) the onset of the phobia is generally preceded by a period of privation or sexual excitement; (g) the onset of the phobia is generally preceded by an anxiety attack associated with the phobic object; (h) phobias develop only in people with disturbed sexual adjustment.

Psychoanalytic evidence is generally quite indirect, often involving a number of interpretive steps in the effort to relate empirical observations and theoretical deductions. Although many cases are offered which seemingly support the model, their value in validating the theory is difficult to assess, since the operationalization of the language of theory in terms of observable data is typically not done.

This is not to say that psychoanalytic formulations are not heuristically or programmatically useful, but rather that many of the formulations are presently untestable because they have not been operationalized. The following excerpts from case studies illustrate statements that are untestable because the terms are couched in unoperationalized, theoretical terms. When reading such case studies, it is necessary to distinguish between empirical facts and interpretive or speculative statements.

Bornstein (1935), in discussing the phobia of a 2½-year-old child, stated that a "latent instinctual conflict" was responsible for the phobia. Discussing erythrophobia, Yamamura (1936) stated that "blushing was the manifest protest against a phallic libido." Dosuzkov (1949), writing on the same subject, concluded: The symptom of blushing is a manifestation of regression from the phallic stage, with the use of the displacement mechanism from below upwards. The erotic regression to the component instincts is accompanied by manifestations of exhibitionism and masochism. Object love is tinged with unconscious homosexuality (p. 194). Fenichel (1945) wrote that the content of phobias was not due primarily to displacement, but rather resulted because anxiety was felt in a situation where an uninhibited person would have experienced sexual excitement or rage. He stated: "The fear of falling from a high place connotes danger of being killed . . . the sensation of falling, itself simultaneously representing the sensation of sexual excitement. . . . The simultaneity of punishment and temptation is, as a rule, also the basis for the frequent fear of "going crazy." . . . Experience may have established the equation penis = head, therefore insanity = castration. A child may, depending upon various experiences, connect various ideas with insanity" (p. 197). Feldman (1949) quotes Fador as saying: Women who grow hysterical at the sight of a mouse and jump on a chair disclose the phallic acceptance of the mouse. They are really frightened of a sexual attack: of the mouse running up under the skirt into the genitalia (p. 227). Pinchon and Arminda (1950) discussed a balloon phobia in an 11-month-old girl and concluded that since it had developed while the mother was in her second pregnancy, "the initial phobia indicated the child's destructive impulses toward the contents of the mother's belly." Rangell (1952) analyzed a man with a doll phobia that had begun when he was 3 years old. Rangell concluded that the phobia had resulted from the father playfully bringing the child's hands toward a bas-relief hanging on the wall and then snapping it back and saying "cootchi-coo, musn't touch": The path for displacement was thus laid down . . . "don't touch" was projected outward, displaced from the body to the external world. Instead of not touching the penis, he would not touch the china, the bas-relief, eventually the doll. The return of the repressed is seen in the choice of the object. The doll, though inanimate, is again the human body. The doll is his penis, not to be touched (p. 45). Brody (1953) discussed the case of a man who throughout most of his life experienced a phobic avoidance of corners of buildings. Brody concluded that "The corner represents, unconsciously, the point of contact with the mother's body. Gratification of forbidden incestuous desires is to be found around the corner which is both the promise of, and the barrier against the incestuous wish." Gero (1955) said: "Phobic displacement represents the end product of an initial repression of drives and phantasies." Finch (1960) states that "pyschoanalytic work has shown clearly that the phobic object or animal really represents a projection of an inner emotional problem of which the child is totally unconscious. . . . A boy becomes phobic about Frankenstein's monster or of gorillas. These are projected fears about his conflict with his father and the latter's strength and retaliatory powers" (p. 101).

Although analysts offer accounts rich with clinical detail, the value of these accounts is somewhat diminished for the nonanalytically oriented worker. For example Kraupe's (1948) description of one of his phobic male patients, "He showed marked anal-erotic, sado-masochistic, and bisexual trends, with repressed passive homoerotic impulses," is not very informative in terms of actually observable phenomena which could be used by nonanalytically oriented clinicians or experimenters.

In the anecdotal accounts of these writers, it is difficult to distinguish clearly between etiology and treatment. Their emphasis is on the etiology with the implicit premise that when this is thoroughly understood by the patient the neurosis will recede. The major techniques seem to be the use of interpretation, explanation, and suggestion. This approach is illustrated by Maeder's (1944) treatment of his 7-year-old nephew. Following an attack of measles, the boy developed an extreme fear of dogs. "Knowing that the dog is a sexual symbol," the author suspected that the basis of the fear was a sexual guilt. When questioned, the boy admitted that he had begun to masturbate during his illness. Asked why he was afraid of the dog, he explained that he was afraid the dog would bite his finger. Maeder interpreted this to him as a disguised reference to his penis. He convinced the boy that if he gave up masturbation the danger and consequent fear would disappear. He reported that the next day the phobia disappeared, and that there was no relapse during the next 15 years.

One of Sperling's (1952) comments regarding her treatment of a 2-year-old child with animal phobia illustrates some of the difficulties encountered in assessing the validity of formulations presented in theoretically interpreted terms: "By the mechanism of condensation, all these impulses, wishes, and fears primarily directed toward her mother and brother were condensed in her phobias in accordance with the unconscious identification of nipple-stool-penis-finger." Admittedly, this statement has been lifted from the context of the case, but a close study of the case still leaves one with questions as to how a judgment regarding the validity of this statement would be made. It is an open question whether processes such as condensation and unconscious identification are, as this statement seems to imply, proven phenomena which can be offered as sufficient explanation.

Leonard (1959) discusses her treatment of 2½-year-old Nancy in the following way: "On the fifth visit, I brought a second baby doll. . . . To this I had added a small piece of clay to represent a penis. When Nancy discovered this, she immediately took it off and put the doll back. . . . I repeated to her the story I had told her previously, adding that the reason the little girl did not like the baby was because the baby was a boy and had a penis. . . . This she denied vigorously. 'Boys don't have penis. Girls have penis and Mommy has penis.' I told her in simple language that this was not true. . . . As I talked, I took the doll out of the bag again and replaced the 'penis.' Once more she tore it off and put the doll away. I did not pursue the subject" (pp. 33–34).

Analytic and Neoanalytic Perspectives in the Etiology and Treatment of School Phobia

Probably the most influential view about the etiology of school phobia has been the "separation-anxiety" model. Although this concept is of psychoanalytic origin, writers of various persuasions have recognized the etiological importance of the mother-child relationship for the school-phobic child.

Broadwin (1932) characterized the school-phobic child as thinking while in school:"Something terrible is happening to mother." In their original paper, Johnson et al. (1941) took the anxiety-about-separation approach. They noted three factors that were common in the eight cases they studied:

1. Acute anxiety in the child was manifested in a variety of ways and was precipitated by the arrival of a new sibling, promotion in school, etc.
2. There was an increase of anxiety in the mother due to some simultaneously operating threat to her satisfactions (e.g., economic deprivation, marital unhappiness, illness, etc.).
3. There was always a strikingly poorly resolved overdependent relationship between these children and their mothers.

Klein (1945) saw the main reasons for refusing to go to school as "castration anxiety, masturbation guilt, and aggressive impulses toward the parent upon whom the child is greatly dependent." Jacobsen (1948) studied 30 cases from the files of the Bureau of Child Guidance in New York City and concluded that "symptoms tended to involve mother-centered fears." Pappenheim and Sweeney (1952) discussed the case of a 4-year-old child who refused to go to nursery school in terms of the inability of the mother to allow the child to be autonomous. They discussed how the child exploited the relationship while at the same time he tried to extricate himself from it. Vaughan (1957) said, "School phobia . . . is primarily a problem of separation from mother." Gardner (1956), commenting on a case, said, "Here is a case that to my mind presents in clearest form the major problems of the latency period . . . one of which is fear of the loss—or causing the loss—of the mother." Estes et al. (1956) outlined certain events which they felt were crucial in the development of school phobia: (a) early, poorly resolved dependent relationship between the mother and child; (b) inadequate fulfillment of the mother's emotional needs, usually because of a poor marriage; (c) temporary threat to the child's security; (d) exploitation of this situation by the mother; (e) similar relationship between mothers and their own mothers; (f) expressions of hostility toward the child; (g) development of strong hostility toward the mother; (k) displacement to the teacher so that the teacher becomes the phobic object. Johnson (1957) says: "School phobia is related to some significant precipitating event; when the mother derives less than her share of gratification, she regresses, thus remobilizing an early, unresolved, mutually ambivalent dependency." Kanner (1957) sees school phobia as a variety of separation anxiety. Waldfogel, Coolidge, and Hahn (1957) say that, like the case of "Little Hans" (Freud, 1959a), "school phobia represents anxiety shifted from the basic source to the school. It invariably originates in the child's fear of being separated from mother." Eisenberg (1958b) says that the school-phobic child is usually unwilling to leave home. He discusses a case where he observed a child and mother at the nursery. The mother would watch the child, and when the child would become interested in playing the mother would move closer, wipe the child's nose, check the child's toilet needs, etc. In Eisenberg's apt words: "The umbilical cord evidently pulled at both ends!" Friedman (1959) emphasizes that phobias are "par excellence the neurosis of childhood" and that separation anxiety seems to be responsible for a variety of phobic reactions which in recent years have been called school phobias. Waldfogel (1959) says: Like all phobias, the symptom in school phobia represents a displacement of anxiety. When the anxiety is traced to its source, it is invariably found to originate in the child's fear of being separate from his mother. The child's anxiety about separation is an outgrowth of the mother's own anxiety on this score (p. 37). Berryman (1959) maintained that "in every serious case, the mother can't separate. This is partly because the mother's over-identification with the child brings back her own dislike of school." Davidson (1960) observes: "It first appears that the mother is trying to persuade the child to attend and that the child is refusing to go, but later we see that the mother unconsciouly prevents the child from returning." Coolidge, Tessman, Waldfogel, and Willer (1961) see the problem as derived from the mother's own unresolved dependency on her mother. Lippman (1962) writes: "Our studies indicate that the phobic child is unable to give up dependency ties to mother because of her clinging to him. Neither the mother nor the child knows what is taking place, but both unconsciously behave as though they were unconsciously aware of each other's deeper needs" (p. 131). Weiss and Cain (1964) describe the behavior of mothers and children on the day of admission of these children (school phobics) to a residential treatment center: "Amidst tearful outbursts, screaming, or protests and pleas 'for just another change,' the child clutched his mother who mirrored his anxiety by her own tears, pallor, and frenzied clinging." Berlin (1965) writes: "In such cases, the mother usually feels great anxiety about separation from her child, who has provided her most of her emotional satisfactions—satisfactions she cannot get with her husband." Olsen and Coleman (1967) discussed the case of a 6-year-old child who refused to attend the first grade. They reasoned that he had come to the first grade "without having mastered the 'separation challenge' of kindergarten."

Thus, while there are many variations, most writers regard the mother-child relationship as the most important etiological consideration with respect to school phobia.

Behavioral Theory: The "Little Albert" Paradigm

Although the psychoanalytic literature is quite diverse and rich in anecdotal material with regards to etiology and treatment, behavior theory, on the contrary, has not dealt in such great detail with etiology. Eysenck (1960) states: "A neurotic symptom is a learned pattern of behavior which for some reason or another is unadaptive." With this rather direct approach to observable behavior, it is hardly surprising that detailed anecdotal accounts of etiology are omitted from their discussions. The behaviorists have their counterpart of "Little Hans" in the form of Watson and Rayner's (1920) famous "Little Albert." Wolpe and Rachman (1960) discuss the "Little Albert" case and state: ". . . any neutral stimulus, simple or complex, that happens to make an impact on an individual at or about the time that a fear reaction is evoked acquires the ability to evoke fear subsequently." They describe the etiology of phobias in the following steps: (a) phobias are learned responses; (b) phobic stimuli, simple or complex, develop when they are associated temporally and spatially with fear-producing states of affairs; (c) neutral stimuli which are of relevance in the fear-producing situation are more likely to develop phobic causalities than weak or irrelevant stimuli; (d) repetition of the association between fear situations and the new phobic stimuli will strengthen the phobia; (e) associations between high-intensity fear situations and neutral stimuli are more likely to produce phobic reactions; (f) generalization from the original phobic stimulus to stimuli of a similar nature occurs.

Another widely quoted case which appeared in the early literature is Jones' (1924) study in which she discussed the treatment of a number of children. She reported success using a deconditioning technique with a 3-year-old boy (Peter) who was afraid of white rabbits. Most writers fail to mention the fact that she had success using other techniques as well. Most behaviorists accept the conditioning paradigm as the appropriate one for discussing the etiology and treatment of phobias. They tend to regard phobias of all kinds as conditioned anxiety reactions.

Early Behavioral Treatment

In 1920 Watson and Rayner reported the case study of "Little Albert." In 1924, Jones reported several cases involving the elimination of fear in children. The most widely quoted case is the one involving Peter (age 3), in which an eating response was used to eliminate fear. Jones reports, "This method obviously requires delicate handling. . . . A careless manipulator could readily produce the reverse result, attaching a fear reaction to the sight of food." Jones (1924) used 70 children in all and employed a variety of methods. She found that verbal appeal, elimination through disuse, negative adaptation (repeated presentations of the feared stimulus), and distraction were sometimes effective. With direct conditioning (used with Peter) and social imitation she found success in all cases. Rachman and Costello (1961) discuss these early studies and attempt to integrate them with more recent work.

It is interesting to note that although behavior therapists quote Jones' conditioning success with Peter, they fail to mention that social imitation was also successful. Further, as Rachman and Costello (1961) observe, many of the suggestions and techniques growing out of this early work are being used today. Apparently the Zeitgeist (Boring, 1950) in the 1920s was not prepared for behavior therapy as it is practiced today.

Current Techniques of Behavior Therapy

Much of the work in behavior therapy has been done recently, and a brief survey will be presented of the general area before discussing the treatment of children and adolescents. Eysenck's (1952) paper marks the crystallization of a growing dissatisfaction with psychoanalysis as the treatment for psychological disorders. Wolpe's (1958) book provided further impetus for behavioral techniques. In the writings of behavior-oriented therapists, phobias have received much emphasis. Rachman (1959) reported treating a phobic patient using desensitization. Wolpe (1961) treated phobias in 39 patients. He reports that after a mean of 11.2 sessions 91% recovered. A 6-month to 4-year follow-up of 20 of the 35 patients revealed no relapses. In 1963, Wolpe attempted to determine quantitative relationships between the kinds of phobias he treated. Wolpe presented recovery curves relating the kind of phobia to the number of sessions to recovery. Lang and Lazovik (1963) treated 24 subjects who had snake phobias and reported success. Cooke (1966) later replicated their results. Ashem (1963) reported treating a disaster phobia by systematic desensitization. Kraft and Al-Issa (1965) treated a traffic phobia using learning-theory principles. Wolpin and Pearsall (1965) reported their treatment of a woman with snake phobia. Their procedure represented a departure from the usual desensitization method, since they presented the entire hierarchy in one session. They also used "naive" therapists who had been trained using the manual presented by Lazovik and Lang (1960).

Recently there have been several attempts to look at the "successes" of behavior therapy in a more rigorous way and to evaluate what changes result from various treatment techniques. In an extensive retrospective study of behavior therapy with phobic patients, Marks and Gelder (1965) point out that the considerable claims made for behavior therapy are not without problems. Specifically, they observe: (a) behavior therapy describes widely differing techniques which at the same time have features in common with other forms of therapy; (b) since behavior-therapy techniques have been applied to a wide variety of neurotic disorders, any general statement about the value of these techniques is of limited value; (c) the well-known tendency of neurotic disorders to respond to energetic, enthusiastic treatments with nonspecific methods makes it difficult to assess the results of treatment in the absence of matched control groups. Lang, Lazovik, and Reynolds (1965) used control groups and attempted to assess the contribution of suggestibility to desensitization. They concluded that the results implied desensitization was relatively independent of suggestibility and that the desensitization of specific fears generalized to other fears. Lomont (1965) contended that only one experiment clearly indicated any feature of reciprocal inhibition which could not be attributed to extinction. He concluded that it was still an open question whether the concept of reciprocal inhibition was better than extinction. Rachman (1965) investigated the separate effects of desensitization and relaxation. He concluded that the combined effects of desensitization and relaxation were greater than the separate effects. Davison (1966) compared desensitization, relaxation, exposure without relaxation, and no treatment. He found that only subjects in the desensitization group showed significant reduction in their snake-avoidance behavior. Hain, Butcher, and Stevenson (1966) treated 27 patients with Wolpian desensitization. They reported that 70% showed marked improvement after a mean of 19 sessions. Interestingly, they agreed with the need for controlled studies, but presented their own study without adequate controls. Gelder and Marks (1966) used 27 patients with severe agoraphobias and found that when they used a control group, 7 out of 10 patients improved symptomatically in both the experimental and control groups. They concluded that behavior therapy could produce only limited changes in severe agoraphobia. Gelder, Marks, Wolff, and Clark (1967) discussed the relative merits of desensitization and psychotherapy in the treatment of phobic states. They concluded: "Desensitization and psychotherapy can contribute in different ways to the treatment of phobic patients; neither can be relied on for all patients, and some patients may need both." This concurs with Lazarus' (1966) proposition for "broad-spectrum" therapy in the treatment of agoraphobia.

There seems to be a growing awareness on the part of behavior therapists that simple conditioning models are not sufficient to explain changes in psychotherapy with phobias. Myer and Gelder (1963) suggested that "the application of learning principles is less clear-cut than the theory suggests, since treatment must be carried out by a therapist and the therapist introduces an interpersonal relationship which may itself influence the course of treatment" (p. 27). Lazarus (1966) presents a model which accounts for the interaction of learning-theory with social-interpersonal variables. He points out that agoraphobia depends as much on interpersonal as intrapersonal variables. Thus there seems to be, on the part of behavior therapists, an increasing interest in interpersonal variables relative to the formulation and treatment of phobic cases.

Variations in Behavioral Techniques

Lazarus (1961) adapted Wolpe's systematic desensitization technique to the group treatment of phobic patients. Rachman (1966) attempted "flooding" techniques; that is, he presented stimuli to imagine which evoked an intense response. He found that this did not reduce fear. Wolpin and Raines (1966) treated six women who had snake phobias. Two of the women used the hierarchy but did not relax, two used the hierarchy and tensed their muscles, and two had four sessions near the top of the hierarchy. All six subjects were able to handle the originally feared snakes. Wolpin says that the necessity of either relaxation or hierarchies needs to be reexamined. Strahley (1966) found that forcing subjects to confront fear-evoking stimuli without the benefit of successive approximations was effective. Friedman (1966a) questioned the validity of the assumption that profound muscle relaxation is accompanied by changes in autonomic activity. He therefore used ultra-short-acting intravenous barbiturates (methohexitone sodium) to achieve a predictable degree of relaxation. After an average of 12 sessions, he reported that patients were symptom free. Friedman (1966b) also reported that he used methohexitone in the treatment of a case of dog phobia in a deaf-mute. Since the patient could not communicate except by sign language, Friedman used pictures of dogs, in order of increasing ferocity, and after six sessions the patient was able to look calmly at a color photograph of an Alsatian dog jumping on a small boy. Kirchner and Hogan (1966) report that after listening to taped therapy sessions, significantly more of the subjects in the experimental group lost their fears. Migler and Wolpe (1967) reported using what they called "automated self-desensitization." They taped instructions and had the patient take the tape recorder home with him and use it there.

The experimentation with new methods is an encouraging trend in any endeavor, and although it is difficult to assess the value of these new ideas, due to the small number of subjects used in most cases and the lack of adequate experimental design, it is encouraging to see new techniques being tried.

Modifications of Behavior Techniques for Use with Phobic Children and Adolescents

Over thirty years ago, Weber (1936) reported treating a 19-month-old girl who had a phobia of her own shadow by using a graded desensitization technique. This phobia first appeared when the child had observed her shadow cast by a street lamp. In treating her, Weber used a doll and showed how it cast a shadow while the child sat on her father's lap. The therapist used other objects such as a ball, etc., and the father gradually lowered the child to the floor. She overcame the fear in one session. Bentler (1962) treated an 11½-month-old infant using reciprocal inhibition therapy. In discussing the case she pointed out that many of the behavior-therapy techniques are not feasible with very young children. Getting small children to relax, etc., presents some difficult problems. She suggests the use of drug-induced relaxation, real objects instead of imagined situations, and feeding responses. Based on Harlow and Zimmerman's (1959) work, she suggests the use of body contact with a warm mother as another technique for inhibiting phobic reactions in infants. She also suggests the use of attractive toys paired with the phobic objects in a kind of graded proximity procedure. She treated an infant who had slipped in the bathtub and had become very frightened of water. Toys were placed in the bathtub, and the child was given free access to the bathroom. The kitchen sink was filled with water and toys. There were also toys on the kitchen table, and gradually the table was moved toward the sink. Bentler suggests that the addition of attractive food might have been a useful technique. She reported success with this infant. Lazarus and Abramovitz (1962) suggested the use of "emotive imagery" in the treatment of children's phobias. They defined emotive images as classes of images which are assumed to arouse feelings of self-assertion, pride, affection, mirth, and similar anxiety-inhibiting responses. As in the usual desensitization procedure, the range, intensity, and circumstances of the patient's fears are ascertained and a hierarchy is drawn up. The child is asked to close his eyes and imagine a sequence of events close to real life, but with a story woven around his hero. Lazarus and Abramovitz report that the therapist "can skillfully arouse the child's affective reactions to the necessary pitch." When the child is maximally aroused, the clinician introduces as a natural part of the narrative the lowest item in the hierarchy and proceeds in the usual systematic desensitization. This technique was used with nine patients ages 7 to 14, and seven of them were reported to have recovered after an average of 3.3 sessions.

The studies considered in this section have illustrated the importance of adapting therapeutic techniques for use with children and adolescents. Although many of the ideas seem promising, the present author concurs with Costello's (1967) statement: "Much research and discussion are needed in order to develop rules of behavior modification in children."

Behavioral Techniques Utilized in the Treatment of School Phobia

A number of clinicians have applied behavioral techniques specifically to the treatment of school phobia. Lazarus, Davison, and Polefka (1965) and Patterson (1965) formulated treatment of school phobia in learning theory terms. Blackhan and Eden (1973) presented a case study describing the successful treatment of a young adolescent male suffering from school phobia and gave a brief account of each step of the behavior modification technique utilized. Edlund (1971) described a reinforcement approach to the elimination of a child's school phobia. Hersen (1970) described a three-part behavioral modification program that was successfully utilized with a 12-year-old school-phobic male. Rines (1973) describes the successful treatment of a disturbed 12-year-old girl's school phobia by behavior modification techniques. In this particular case it was felt that the behavioral techniques obviated the seemingly increasing necessity for the child to be hospitalized. Instead, the girl was able to return to school after two months.

One of the most widely utilized techniques in the treatment of phobias in general and also utilized specifically for school phobias is systematic desensitization. Chapel (1967) describes the treatment of a case of school phobia in which the kind of systematic desensitization technique was used in vivo. The child was gradually exposed to the classroom situation and the duration of exposure was gradually increased. Miller (1972) presents a case study in which a 10-year-old child suffering from numerous phobias including school phobia was successfully counterconditioned using systematic desensitization both in vivo and using imagery. Lowenstein studied 12 children whose school phobias were expressed in various bodily ailments and anxieties related to school attendance. He used two matched groups of six children each aged 9 to 14 years and subjected them to either systematic desensitization or discussion sessions. After five weeks of treatment both groups underwent a five-week period of verbal extinction procedure known as negative practice. While both groups improved, a greater reduction in personal distress was experienced by children in a desensitization group. Improvement also was reported in academic work and a six-month follow-up indicated that improvement was maintained. This study would thus seem to indicate that systematic desensitization is a useful technique for the treatment of school phobia. A number of clinical case studies also support this, but Lowenstein's (1973) is one of the few systematic investigations of the effectiveness of desensitization in the treatment of school phobia. Smith (1973–74) describes the characteristics of school phobia and evaluates the effectiveness of various behavioral therapies. She compares operant, classical, and a combination of these conditioning paradigms in terms of the child's return to school, his performance in school after his return, and evidence of symptom substitution. It is concluded that school phobia can be successfully treated by any one of these three procedures. However, further research is needed in the areas of follow-up investigations. Although it is beyond the scope of this chapter to discuss each of these studies referred to, it is probably fair to summarize them by referring to Shaw and Jarvis's (1975) study discussing techniques for eliminating school phobias. Beginning with the thesis that school phobia may be reinforced by the secondary gains of attention, free time, etc., two objectives are recommended. First, it is suggested that the clinician determine how the school phobia is being rewarded and enlisting the aid of parents and school personnel in lessening the attraction of staying home and increasing the attraction of going to school. Second, it is suggested that help be given the client in overcoming fears and deficient interpersonal behavior through desensitization. Most behaviorally oriented clinicians attempt to either decrease the fear of school, decrease the rewards of staying home, or simultaneously work at both. There is less emphasis on the child-parent relationship than is the case with analytically oriented clinicians. The behaviorists tend to focus more on school as the feared object and mother as a reinforcement dispenser. Thus, the emphasis becomes much more environmental and less family focused.

Ayllon, Smith, and Rogers (1970), for example, define school phobia in an 8-year-old black girl as zero or low probability of school attendance. The techniques utilized involved getting the child's mother to withdraw the rewards of staying at home. Then a home-based motivational system was used to reinforce school attendance, and refusal to attend school resulted in punishment. It is reported that school attendance was generated quickly and maintained even after the procedures were withdrawn a month later. No symptom substitution was noticed either by parents or school officials within the nine months of follow-up. This illustrates a typical behavioral approach to the treatment of school phobia, where the clinician focuses on the various reinforcements or punishments in the child's environment and attempts to rearrange the contingencies in such a way that school attendance will be rewarded and staying at home will be punished. Additionally, systematic desensitization or other forms of gradual exposure are used in order to reduce the aversiveness of the school situation. Although there is some focus on the parents, it is basically in order to enlist them in the treatment program as dispensers of reinforcements or punishments rather than delving into the personal family dynamics involving dependence or over dependence in the child and the various subtle nuances of the child-parent relationship. In concluding this discussion comparing the analytic, neo-analytic, and behavior techniques in the treatment of phobias, it is relevant to refer to a case discussed by Leonard (1959). This involved the treatment of a 2½-year-old girl with a phobia of walking. Although Leonard referred to the fact that the child slipped from her perch on the kitchen sink and broke her leg when she was 2 years and four months old, Leonard does not see this accident as sufficient explanation of the phobia. She writes: ". . . an accident, however, is experienced as 'something is being done to me': a castrative punishment. . . . she had also reached the stage when children become aware of the differences between the sexes. . . . with the magical thinking common to children at that age, Nancy must have believed her 'bad' impulses were perceived by her parents and that they let the accident happen in order to punish her.

It is quite likely, too, that Nancy interpreted her penisless state as punishment for some previous 'badness.' The accident had now added insult to injury in symbolisms so well understood by children: retaliation for her impulse to injure her brother—a leg for a penis" (pages 36-37).

This case study amply illustrates where the analysts and behaviorists would part company. The behaviorists would obviously feel that the phobia of walking was due to the accident and that this was sufficient explanation for it. They would probably utilize some successive approximation techniques in which the child would be gradually helped to walk in a progressive series of small steps. As illustrated by the dynamic discussion quoted above, the analysts would see a deeper meaning in the phobia and would tend to treat the underlying dynamics rather than directly work on the behavior itself.

It is the present author's view that analytic, behavioral, and other perspectives are complementary rather than diametrically incompatible. It seems very possible to view phobias as being determined by intrapsychic, interpersonal, and situational factors. In the following paragraphs a number of additional perspectives will be explored with the hope that this will sensitize a clinician to the many possible variations of technique. The issue then becomes not which technique is *the* correct one but rather which technique or combination of techniques will prove to be most useful in a given instance. The search is not for ultimate truth but for appropriateness, usefulness, and effectiveness.

"Action" Therapy

This is not a term used by writers quoted below, but it does characterize an active approach to dealing with phobias. Over forty years ago, for example, Jersild and Holmes (1935) suggested that of all the techniques they studied, the "most effective techniques in overcoming fears are those that help the child to become more competent and skillful and that encourage him to undertake active dealing with the thing he fears." It is of interest to note that even some of Freud's (1959) observations hinted in the direction of these trends. In 1910 he wrote that patients could not resolve their phobias as long as they felt "protected by retaining their phobic condition" (p. 289). Alvarez (1951) suggests that "innumerable persons whose lives are disturbed by phobias could have cured themselves if at the start, they forced themselves to do repeatedly what they feared. . . . In many cases phobias are never conquered because of the inability of the patient to fight hard enough" (pp. 556-557). Ellis (1962) writes: "Espousal of learning theory helped my therapeutic efforts in at least one significant respect. I began to see that insight alone was not likely to lead an individual to overcome his deep-seated fears and hostilities; he also needed . . . action."

Most behaviorally oriented clinicians view phobias as avoidance behavior, and from laboratory findings it is well known that avoidance behavior does not undergo extinction very rapidly because of the very fact that the animal avoids the feared object. This prevents the animal from having contact with the object in a nonfearful situation and prevents affective counterconditioning or extinction to occur. This apparently is what the action oriented clinicians are saying when they suggest that the phobic patient must encounter the feared object in order to overcome the fear.

The action orientation has become especially prominent in the treatment of school phobias because our society demands that children attend school. Consequently, the primary objective in treating the school phobic child is to get him back into the school. There was rather good consensus on this point, although there is some disagreement as to how soon this should be attempted and who ought to be the primary focus of treatment. In the following discussion we will briefly address the issue of how soon the child ought to be gotten back into the school situation, and we will later discuss the issue of who ought to be involved in the treatment process.

Most writers advocate returning the child to school as quickly as possible. Lassers, Nordan, and Bladholm (1973) suggest that parents are often ambivalent about sending or keeping a child at school, but the rapidity with which they could do so is often beneficial to the therapy of both the parent and the child. Klein (1945) suggests that "early attention to getting the child back in school seems important." Jacobsen (1948) suggests that "it is important to get the pupil back in school as soon as possible so the phobia won't become fixed." Lippman (1962) advocates urging the child to return. Spock (1957) writes: "If the child is freely allowed to stay home, his dread of returning to school usually gets stronger . . . so it usually works best for the parents to be very firm about getting him back to school promptly" (p. 409). Weiss and Cain (1964) observe that while the former trend was to let the child stay home from school indefinitely, the trend now is to get the child back in school immediately. Kennedy (1965) advocates early return of the child to school. Eisenberg (1958b) says that the "key to success" is early return. Reger (1962) favors returning the child to school immediately whenever possible. Leventhal et al. (1967) opt for rapid return.

Some workers, although seeing the importance of early return, see certain dangers in this approach and recommend a kind of compromise. Berryman (1959), for example, recommends a gradual returning of the child to school. She suggests taking the child to the building the first day, up the steps the next day, etc.

A few therapists recommend keeping the child out of school for a period of time. Talbot (1957) says: "The first step is to relieve pressure for attendance; then when the tug-of-war is over, treatment can begin." Greenbaum (1964) writes: "In most cases there are advantages in not having children return too early, in the direction of more favorable outcome for continued and successful treatment." Jarvis (1964) implies that a delayed return is best: "When we encounter school phobia, one of our tasks is to evaluate the animosity, often great, among personnel of the school. . . . Work in schools—or indeed any work with children—may attract adults who enjoy sado-masochistic relationships. For such gratifications the child with school phobia is unconsciously singled out, and because of his thinly concealed rage, he is placed in the feared situation long before he can tolerate it without damage" (pp. 411, 418–419). Radin (1967) feels that, in some cases, "premature pressure to return to school may precipitate an underlying psychosis."

Although most therapists seem to favor early return to school, there is not a clear consensus. Those opting for early return seem to imply that any delay would serve to crystallize and strengthen the phobia, while those advocating later return seem to think that pressure on the child might be successful in returning him to school, but that this would be only a temporary kind of solution. As we have seen, there is some disagreement as to how rapidly the child ought to be returned to school, but generally even analysts show a fairly active orientation in attempting to return the child to school. Similarly there is disagreement as to which method is best for returning the child to school, but again there seems to be consensus that the child ought be moved back into the school situation with some degree of rapidity. Waldfogel et al. (1957) was able to work out a situation where the child was tutored at school, although this was done after regular school hours. This might be thought of as a kind of gradual desensitization procedure. Lippman (1962) views school phobia as primarily a family problem, but he advocates the use of ancillary measures such as special school placement; Eisenberg (1958b) favors rapid return and advocates even calling the police if necessary in order to return the child to school. Similarly Rodriguez, Rodriguez, and Eisenberg (1959) did not hesitate in using legal means to return the child to school if the family did not cooperate.

In summary, then, looking at the treatment of phobias of children and adolescents in general, we find some movement in the direction of active intervention. This trend becomes even more pronounced in the treatment of school phobia. It is even likely that historically speaking the emphasis on school phobia and the treatment of it has catalyzed a more active interventional approach to phobias in general. As previously mentioned, the law requires a child to be in school, and this probably catalyzes within the clinician a more active and sometimes even urgent effort to return the child to school.

Family Orientation in the Treatment of Phobias

Although much work, especially in the analytic perspective, has focused upon the child, the recent emphasis on school phobia seems to have brought with it an increasing emphasis on family relationships. Szurek, Johnson, and Falstein (1942) wrote that there was "an increasing awareness on the part of the clinicians dealing with children that the behavior of the child is to be understood only in the context of intrafamilial relations." Koegler and Brill (1967) wrote: "The treatment of school phobia illustrates a basic principle for treatment of all phobias. The family of the patient is usually quite intimately involved and should be involved."

Berryman (1960) described grandiosity as one of the characteristics of the adolescent school phobics she was treating. Levensen (1961) described ten school-phobic middle-class Jewish boys whose personalities were similar to the kind described by Berryman. And Radin (1967) describes the etiology of school phobia in the following way: "The impact of the primary objects upon the child created a shared illusion of primordial omnipotence which flourishes at home. . . . the special kind of nurturance received at home is not available in school, where reward and punishment are based upon realistic performance; hence the illusion is sooner or later dispelled by real or imagined social or academic failure" (p. 127). Radin points out that to consider intrapsychic phenomena primarily in isolation is to acknowledge only a segment of what appears to be a complex. He lists the following steps as part of the etiological cycle: (a) the fostering of infantile omnipotence; (b) evaluation of realistic performance in school exposes the vulnerable child and threatens the omnipotent self-image; (c) child avoids school, where he feels threatened, and hastens home to reestablish his strong and magical position with parental collusion. Leventhal (1964) and Leventhal, Weinberger, Stander, and Stearns (1967) emphasize the role of the child's overvalued and unrealistic self-image.

The consideration of an omnipotent self-image is a somewhat novel and interesting idea whose merits have not been thoroughly investigated. This is included in the present context, however, to illustrate the trend by many clinicians of viewing the patient's dynamics within the family context. This seems to receive clear focus in the treatment of school phobia, where, with the exception of some behavior therapists, most clinicians view school phobia as being related to the family constellation and usually advocate some kind of treatment involving members of the family and sometimes school personnel.

Waldfogel et al. (1957) said: "The main technical problem is the treatment of the mother's unresolved dependency conflicts." Berg and McGuire (1974) used preference scores on a self-administered dependency questionnaire to see whether the mothers of school-phobic adolescents were overprotective. They found that there were raised scores in the 39 school-phobic cases but not in the 58 other psychiatric cases. They interpreted these findings to be consistent with the view that mothers of school phobics prefer their children to be excessively dependent.

An interesting dependency relationship that has been articulated by the analytically oriented clinicians is presented by Silverman, Frank, and Dachinger (1974). They believe that systematic desensitization (primarily a behavioral technique) is only effective to the extent that it activates unconscious merging tendencies. They subjected ten women with insect phobias to a variant of systematic desensitization in which a procedure aimed at stimulating the fantasy of "merging with mother" was substituted for muscle relaxation. The procedure consisted of subliminal exposure of the verbal stimulus MOMMIE AND I ARE ONE during the visualization part of desensitization, whenever the suject's anxiety rose above a specified level. They used a control group of ten other women with insect phobias who underwent the same procedure except that the subliminal message was the neutral one PEOPLE WALKING. They found that on both phobic behavior and anxiety measures, the experimental group manifested significantly more improvement than the controls, and they interpreted this finding as supporting the proposition that the effectiveness of systematic desensitization resides in activating unconscious merging fantasies. This psychoanalytic reinterpretation of systematic desensitization is an interesting illustration of how it is possible to combine various perspectives. In the present context it illustrates the almost symbiotic dependency relationship that is assumed to exist between the phobic child and mother.

In a more traditional behavioral way, Cooper (1973) presents a case study of a 6-year-old school-phobic child where the primary therapeutic agent was the child's mother. In this case, the focus was not on resolving the overdependent relationship that is assumed to exist between mother and child but rather on utilizing the mother as an agent of therapeutic change. A number of writers—for example, Johnson et al. (1941)—have advocated treating the mother and the child simultaneously. These writers believe that in most cases a vicious circle of guilt was operating between the mother and the child, and that the most efficacious type of treatment was a "collaborative dynamic approach to the mother and the child." Waldfogel (1959) wrote: "It is of paramount importance to include the mother in treatment of school phobia. . . . The problem of separation is as great for her as for the child." Davidson (1960) writes: "Mothers all feel like failures and need much help before they can believe in their capacity to be good mothers."

Johnson et al. (1941) suggested that in some cases the fathers as well as the mothers ought to be seen in therapy. Estes et al. (1956) brought both parents into therapy, and Lippman (1962) advocated seeing both parents in treatment with the child. Berryman (1959) said: "It is important to see both parents for the first interview." Kennedy (1965) included a structured interview with the parents. Johnson (1957) emphasized the importance of helping the parents to adjust to their own problems and points out that if the parents do not resolve their problem, another child may be selected as the "neurotic victim." She recommends that as the school-phobic child improves, a close watch be kept on the other children in the family.

Shaw (1966) advised the therapist to "involve himself in the family's complex of psychopathology." In a recent discussion, Skynner (1974) noted that the previous literature on school phobia has tended to emphasize defects in the mother-child relationship to the neglect of the crucial failure of father to help loosen the original exclusive maternal attachment. An approach is described that makes use of a conjoint family technique to achieve this aim.

Takagi (1973) discusses the increasing numbers of school phobics in Japan and relates this to the changing family in an increasingly industrialized society. It is suggested that parents have lost their former roles as organizers and integrators, that the nuclear family is ever smaller, and that ties of kinship to patriarchal authority are disappearing as education is being assumed by school and society. Takagi assumes that this results in emotional and dependent mothers and confused fathers. Yamazaki (1973) interviewed the fathers of 12-to-20-year-old chronic school phobics to determine how the father's personality characteristics affect family relationships. He characterized the fathers as being passive, lacking authority and not being involved in family problems. Although these observations are difficult to evaluate because of their subjectivity and even more difficult to translate from the Japanese culture to North America, there does seem to be consensus that school-phobic children come from families where interpersonal dynamics and authority structures are not clearly operative.

One of the most important persons in the child's environment, the teacher, has received little attention in the treatment of school-phobic children. Most writers present long discussions about the child, the family, etc., but very few devote much attention to the teacher. Waldfogel (1959) is an exception and points out that a child with school phobia poses a threat to the teacher. The irrational character of his fear, which is unresponsive to ordinary kindness and reassurance, gives her a sense of helplessness. Since the child projects the fear to her, she may often see herself as a source of the problem, so the teacher may vacillate between firmness and leniency, thus unwittingly duplicating the mother's ambivalence. Thus helping the teacher to understand herself and the nature of the problem is part of the entire therapeutic effort.

Additionally, many clinicians of a behavioral orientation involve the school personnel in implementing a program of gradual approach to the school or of special rooms where the child can study after school hours, etc. Miller (1972) suggests that underlying family dynamics can aid in diagnosing school phobia and that the physician, school principal, school nurse, and teacher, working as a team, can effectively intervene.

In summary, recommended treatment procedures have varied in terms of how many of the child's relatives they have involved. There has even been an extension of the family concept to include school personnel. There seems to be consensus on the idea that school phobias ought to be handled as interpersonal problems, and this contrasts to some extent with some of the earlier work which emphasized intrapsychic elements and focused exclusively on the child or adolescent.

Follow Up Studies of School Phobia

The follow up studies of school phobic children have yielded conflicting results. Rodriguez et al. (1959) studied 41 cases and concluded that their hypotheses (poor prognosis for older children and the importance of prompt intervention) were confirmed. Coolidge et al. (1964) followed up 66 school phobic children, and of the 47 they were able to locate, they rated 13 as having no limitations, 20 as moderately limited, and 14 as severely limited. They reported that caution seemed to be the theme throughout, with more than half of the subjects leading "colorless, restrictive, unimaginative lives, with delayed or absent heterosexual development, excessive dependency, blunted affect, and a lack of mood swings." Nursten (1963) compared the scores of adult females who had been school phobics as children with presumably normal student nurses and found no significant differences between the groups. Weiss and Burke (1967) followed up hospitalized school phobic children and adolescents and found that although most had graduated from high school, half had significant problems in the following areas: hesitancy about heterosexual ties, circumscription of peer anxiety in the younger subjects, school phobia in older subjects, and depression or withdrawal in adolescents.

It is probably well for the clinician to make a distinction between early-onset school phobia and late-onset school phobia, with the latter representing a much less favorable prognostic picture.

In summary, then, early acute onset accompanying the child's first experiences with school generally suggests favorable prognosis. This kind of syndrome is probably best articulated by the separation anxiety model, where the child's first major experience of separating from his mother—or more generally, the family—is traumatic and results in a phobic reaction to the school situation. With late onset, however, differential diagnosis becomes extremely important, since the clinician must distinguish whether this is simply the reemergence of an earlier school phobia or a pre-psychotic withdrawal or another serious kind of emotional problem being triggered by the emergence of adolescence.

Neurotic versus Characterologic

In their 1962 review, Kahn and Nursten said that Goldberg (1953), Nursten (1958), Bonnard (1959), and Hersov (1960) considered school phobia as a phenomenon manifested by different psychopathological types. Although some of the distinctions are not clear, there has been an interest among some workers in differentiating between two distinct kinds of school-phobic children. Coolidge et al. (1957) distinguished between what they called a "neurotic" disorder, where the anxiety reaction, clinging behavior, etc. is similar to that found in other phobias. They said that this kind of child had a fairly "sound personality." The "characterological type" they pictured as being more seriously disturbed. This kind of school phobia was characterized as having a less acute onset and being the result of character disturbances. The "neurotic" type is seen mostly in young girls, ages 5 to 8, while the "characterological" type is seen in older boys, ages 9 to 12. Others have maintained a similar distinction. Eisenberg (1958a) writes: "When school phobia occurs in adolescence it represents a much more serious intrinsic disturbance of general adjustment." Coolidge et al. (1960) maintain this distinction saying that in the neurotic type there is generally a very favorable prognosis with good management, while in the older group the opposite picture is found. In the latter group, there is invariably an early history of school phobia that subsides and then reappears in adolescence. Weiss and Cain (1964) reported their residential treatment of adolescent school phobics, and they distinguished two groups. In one group, school phobia was "part of a chronic complex of psychopathology." In this group, there were depressive trends, somatic reactions, other phobias, etc. which existed prior to and concomitantly with the school phobia. The other group resembled the typical picture. Kennedy (1965) distinguished between the "neurotic-crisis" type, which was characterized by acute onset in the lower grades, etc., and the "way-of-life" type, which was characterized by incipient onset, family history of neurotic and character disorders, etc. He listed ten criteria for differentiating these groups. The neurotic-crisis type he lists as being determined by: (1) the present illness is the first episode; (2) Monday onset, following an illness the previous Thursday or Friday; (3) an acute onset; (4) lower grades most prevalent; (5) expressed concern about death; (6) mother's physical health in question: actually ill or child thinks so; (7) good communication between parents; (8) mother and father well adjusted in most areas; (9) father competitive with mother in household management; (10) parents achieve understanding of dynamics easily.

The way-of-life school phobia is characterized by the differing ten criteria: (1) second, third, or fourth episode; (2) Monday onset following minor illness, not a prevalent antecedent; (3) incipient onset; (4) upper grades most prevalent; (5) death theme not present; (6) health of mother not an issue; (7) poor communication between parents; (8) mother shows neurotic behavior; father, a character disorder; (9) father shows little interest in household or children; (10) parents very difficult to work with.

Although Kennedy's criteria may not be universally applicable, they do point up the need for distinguishing clearly between a kind of primary early-onset school phobia and later manifestations where school phobia may be part of a larger complex of symptoms including characterological disorders or even be simply an indication of a prepsychotic withdrawal.

Sexual Identity

Some clinicians have stressed the role of sexual identity in school phobia. Levenson (1961) described the treatment of ten Jewish boys with school phobia and said that one of their personality characteristics was inadequate male identification. Lippman (1962) writes: "Girls with school phobia tend to be subtly aggressive and boys passive and withdrawn. In one group at the Wilder Child Guidance Clinic, 3 of the 4 boys enjoyed playing with dolls and one became frankly homosexual in later life." Adams, McDonald, and Huey (1966) report on 21 cases of school phobia, and they observe that scanty attention has been paid to bisexual conflict in the etiology of school phobia. They quote Coolidge, Hahn, and Peck (1957), Burns (1959), Greenbaum (1964), and Malmquist (1965) as having pointed to cases of school phobia where coexistent bisexual conflict occurred. In a follow-up study, Weiss and Burke (1967) reported that in the cases studied there was hesitancy about heterosexual ties.

Although it is difficult to understand clearly how sexual identity relates to school phobia, it seems consistent with the picture of the school phobic coming from a family where basic relationships have been disturbed. Whether this disturbance manifests itself symptomatically as a mutually overdependent relationship between mother and child, or whether, as in the transition occuring in the Japanese culture, it results from confusion of well-established roles, is unclear; but in any case, there is probably a relationship between the inappropriate or confused sexual identity of the child or adolescent and the inappropriate or confused relationships within the family system.

Depression

Shapiro, Neufeld, and Post (1962) discussed a case in which multiple phobias and a severe depression occurred, but they made no attempt to relate these. Roberts (1964) followed up some phobic patients and concluded that there are two distinct etiologies: (a) the psychoneurotic type, which has a poor prognosis; and (b) a superficially similar kind, but one in which the illness is primarily depressive and has a good prognosis. Gehl (1964) was impressed with how frequently depression and claustrophobia occurred together. He concluded that "in states of claustrophobia and depression the subjective experiences of the patients have much in common. In both situations, a closed system configuration exists, and the patient finds it is this closed system that provokes the disturbance" (p.316).

In these studies it is extremely difficult to ascertain the role depression plays relative to phobias. Whether Gehl's (1964) observation is merely appealing at the level of analogy or whether there are substantive similarities remains an open question.

Agras (1959) presented the hypothesis that the basis of school phobia is depressive anxiety. He says that "there is a typical, recognizable family constellation in the disorder which is common to many of the depressive disorders of childhood.... This syndrome is part of the natural history of depressive disorders." Davidson (1960) also stresses the role of depression. She notes a high incidence of deaths or threatened deaths (severe illnesses) preceding onset.

It is of some diagnostic interest here to note that again a number of workers seem to be observing two distinct kinds of phobias. One a more crisis-related phobia, the other a neurotic or characterologic kind that carries a much poorer prognosis. Again, the issue seems to be not so much whether depression is present but rather whether the depression is of a crisis kind or of a more endogenous variety.

If, for example, the child or adolescent has recently experienced severe illness, death of a family member, etc., it would probably still remain prognositcally promising. However, if the depression along with the school phobia seem to be of a much more incipient endogenous variety, the prognostic picture would be much less hopeful.

As all experienced clinicians are aware, depression can also occur concomitantly with anxiety. The issue of whether the depression is primary and the anxiety secondary or whether the anxiety is primary and the depression secondary or whether both are related to the phobia in some complex manner is a difficult differential diagnostic issue. These considerations lead quite naturally to the next section, which is a brief discussion of pharmacological treatment. Obviously, whether or not to use drugs, whether to treat the patient residentially or on an outpatient basis, or whether to rely on behavior modification techniques or more traditional psychotherapeutic techniques depends upon the conclusions obtaining from a careful differential diagnosis.

This concept is nicely illustrated by looking briefly at two studies. Vaal (1973) describes a case in which a 13-year-old male junior high school student who had been absent 94% of the school days voluntarily returned to school as a result of a behavioral contingency contracting procedure. Following this, he had a perfect record of attendance for the remaining three months of school and attendance records for the next year indicated the subject had missed only 1½ days out of 85. Contrasting with this, van Krevelen (1971) feels that the cure of school phobia requires admission to a children's psychiatric inpatient department. These differences in treatment approaches and prognostic opinions are probably a result of working primarily with different target populations. Marine (1973) reports that simple separation anxiety responds to guidance and crisis intervention. However, childhood psychoses with school refusal symptoms requires residential treatment or classes for the emotionally disturbed. In conclusion, then, it seems clear that how one treats a child or adolescent and what the follow-up results are depends very much upon careful differential diagnostic decisions.

Pharmacological Treatments

Imipramine

Gittelman-Klein and Klein conducted a double-blind, placebo-controlled study of the effects of imipramine among 35 6-to-14-year-old school-phobic children. Children and their families were given a multidisciplinary treatment program concurrently with imipramine or placebo treatment. Imipramine (100-200 mg. per day) over a six-week period was found to be significantly superior to placebo in inducing school return and in global therapeutic efficacy. It was found that the imipramine effects could not be detected after three weeks but were clearly present after six. Of ten items rated by psychiatrists at baseline and after six weeks of treatment, four items which reflect severity of the child's phobic behavior were significantly improved by imipramine treatment. However, among the ten items rated by mothers, only one item reflecting depressive mood showed a significant drug effect. On the whole, side effects were not significant.

Saraf, Klein, Gittelman-Klein and Groff compared the incidence, range, and severity of side effects in 65 6-to-14-year-old school-phobic and hyperkinetic children receiving imipramine treatment with those occurring in 37 others receiving placebo. Minor side effects occurred in 83% of the impiramine group and in 70% of the placebo group. Just under 5% of the subjects in the imipramine group had significant side effects, but none were serious enough to necessitate drug withdrawal. The majority of side effects in both groups occurred during the first treatment. The writers pointed out however, that there may be serious idiosyncracies to high dosages of imipramine, suggested by the sudden death of a 6-year-old child receiving imipramine treatment.

Sulpiride

Abe (1975) reported the successful use of sulpiride in treating 16 9-to-17-year-old depressive school-phobic children. Daily doses of 100 mg. for the 10-to-17-year-olds and smaller adjusted doses for the 9-year-olds were found to be effective in that 10 of the 16 children returned to school within a few days and the anxious, depressive, and autonomic symptoms disappeared within one week.

Sodium-Pentothal

Nice (1968) reported the use of sodium pentothal in the treatment of a 10½-year-old school phobic female. The writer reports that sodium pentothal must be used under strict medical control and is recommended only in extreme cases after other forms of therapy have failed.

This very brief glance at pharmacological interventions illustrates the variety of drugs which may be used in helping children and adolescents overcome phobic problems. Whether one uses an anti-anxiety agent or an antidepressive agent or some combination of both again depends upon differential diagnoses and even upon one's basic theoretical perspective regarding the etiology of phobic conditions.

Summary and Conclusions

As must be amply clear from the foregoing discussion, there does not exist a single coherent theory of phobias of children and adolescents. Although many writers define phobias as fears that are unrealistically severe with respect to the precipitating stimuli, it is difficult to define what constitutes "unrealistically severe." At a very practical level, phobias are usually defined with respect to the seeking of treatment. If the fears are incapacitating enough or uncomfortable enough, the parents of the child or adolescent actively seek clinical intervention. Thus not only is there difficulty in defining a phobia with respect to an individual who is labeled the "patient," but whether or not fears are perceived as phobic will depend upon the tolerance of the family or relatives with whom the child lives. In this respect it is somewhat analogous to defining hyperactivity. Whether a child is defined as hyperactive often depends upon the tolerance of the parents for high levels of activity. A child who is "normally hyperactive" but who is living with a depressed mother may find himself in treatment much earlier than a child with the same activity level who lives with highly active parents.

Many definitions are couched in theoretical terms reflecting the biases of their proponents and make communication among clinicians of various persuasions somewhat difficult. Even in such rather extensively studied areas as school phobia the term itself has different meanings depending upon the orientation of the clinicians employing it. Thus the analytically oriented clinician who talks about school phobia is actually describing a different etiological and treatment problem than the behavior therapist who uses the same term in discussing fear of school.

Probably one of the greatest deficits in knowledge is the lack of good normative data relating to changes in the quantity and quality of fears relative to age. In most studies and case reports, there is a confounding of the variable of age with a kind of phobia. An understanding of the normal fears would seem to be important in understanding phobias.

The distinction between etiology and treatment is difficult to maintain because with most case studies the treatment is directly related to the theories of etiology. And when success occurs it is attributed to the correctness of the etiological and therapeutic approach. This of course represents a confounding of two somewhat independent aspects of the problem and fosters the incorrect implication that a certain treatment "works" or fails to "work" because of the correctness or incorrectness of the etiological and theoretical assumptions upon which it is based. Interestingly, if one looks at what clinicians actually *do*, there is a surprising convergence among some very diverse viewpoints such as psychoanalysis and behavior therapy. This is most clearly illustrated in the school phobia work, where psychoanalyst, behavior therapist, and most clinicians in general advocate returning the child to school.

Considering the tremendous gaps in our knowledge and the diversity of theoretical and therapeutic approaches, it seems unwise to adopt a doctrinaire or parochial approach to the treatment of children and adolescents who are suffering from phobias. In treating the school-phobic child or adolescent, for example, there seems to be no theoretical reason for not looking both at the environmental contingencies (punishments and reinforcements) and at the family-child interactions. Whether one focuses most of the clinical efforts upon the mother-child relationship or whether one utilizes the school personnel in reinforcing desired behavior would seem to be more an empirical issue depending upon which variables in the particular situation seem most responsive to change. In other words, analytic and behavioral approaches can be thought of as complementary rather than incompatible or antagonistic. This kind of theoretical flexibility seems specially appropriate in an area where "hard data" is so difficult to come by and where our admitted lack of knowledge is so great.

In my own outpatient private practice, I attempt to utilize as many treatment modalities as possible simultaneously. If, for example, a school-phobic child is brought to me, I attempt to assess the family dynamics, the school and peer relationships, and the biological condition of the patient. In some instances, I will refer the patient for medication, do psychotherapy focused upon family dynamics, and consult with the school in order to facilitate situational changes that may enhance the child's return. In addition to attempting to maintain the therapeutic flexibility, I have become increasingly impressed with the importance of accurate differential diagnosis. In this respect I am encouraged by the more fine-grained analyses that are appearing in the literature with respect to school phobia, for example. At the very least, it seems necessary to realize that the child who is afraid to enter school at the first level is probably struggling with psychological issues quite different from the adolescent who becomes afraid to continue in school at the junior high or high school level. Furthermore, maintaining a distinction between early-onset and late-onset phobias sensitizes the clinician to the possibility of pre-psychotic conditions emerging at adolescence, which may be masked by the presenting symptom of school phobia. By contrast, with the very young child, conditions such as child schizophrenia, autism, major affective disorders, or other severe pathological conditions are less likely to be confused with neurotic phobias. Thus, the danger of inappropriate treatments or delay of appropriate treatments may be less in the young child than in the adolescent. Finally, a somewhat innovative approach that I used in my own practice has been that of finding alternative learning experiences for adolescent school phobics which provide for them meaningful learning experiences without the severe pressures of the classroom situation. One is of course limited by the legal implications of such procedures, but generally speaking, it is possible to work with the authorities and at times circumvent the school classroom by providing a meaningful alternative. There seems to be no compelling reason to insist that all adolescents must attend large classrooms and participate in a typical high school situation. Therefore, if, for example, one can arrange a work oriented program such as secretarial training, key-punch operating, beautician's training, etc., it is possible to help adolescents maintain a sense of worth and usefulness while at the same time providing a respite from the kinds of worries and pressures the peer group may exert upon them. After a year or two in an alternate program an adolescent may then choose either to work, return to high school, or even take the high school equivalency test and continue with college. Although this option is only available with the older child or adolescent, at least one ought to consider whether the most reasonable and therapeutic role is to return the child to school. And in some situations, it may be that an alternative experience is better.

In summary, then, how can we best help children and adolescents overcome phobic problems? Probably by cultivating in ourselves clinical attitudes of openness to a variety of techniques, sensitivity to the tremendous differences between individual patients that we see, and a willingness to be creative and innovative in applying various combinations of techniques. Above all, an awareness of the ignorance-to-knowledge ratio ought to quite naturally result in attitudes of humility and a healthy respect for our limitations. This would foster good relationships with colleagues within and across disciplines, thus setting up the possibilities for consultation with other professionals where difficult cases present themselves. This would be especially true in the outpatient private practice setting, where the team approach is not as likely to occur.

References

Abe, K. (1975) Sulpiride in depressive school phobic children. *Psychopharmacologia* 43(1):101.

Adams, P., N. McDonald, and W. Huey. (1966) School phobia and bisexual conflict: A report of 21 cases. *Am. J. Psychiat.* 123:541–547.

Agras, S. (1959) The relationship of school phobia to childhood depression. *Am. J. Psychiat.* 116:533–539.

Alvarez, W.C. (1951) *The Neuroses.* Philadelphia: Saunders.

Angelino, H., J. Dollins, and E. Mech. (1956) Trends in the fears and worries of school children as related to socio-economic status and age. *J. Genet. Psychol.* 89:263–276.

Angelino, H., and C. Shedd. (1953) Shifts in the content of fears and worries relative to chronological age. *Proc. Okla. Acad. Sci.* 34:180–186.

Ashem, B. (1963) The treatment of a disaster phobia by systematic desensitization. *Behav. Res. Ther.* 1:81–84.

Ayllon, T., D. Smith, and M. Rogers. (1970) Behavioral management of school phobia. *J. Behav. Ther. Exper. Psychiat.* 1(2):125–138.

Bentler, P.M. (1962) An infant's phobia treated with reciprocal inhibition therapy. *J. Child Psychol. Psychiat.* 3:185–189.

Berg, I., and R. McGuire. (1974) Are mothers of school-phobic adolescents overprotective? *Brit. J. Psychiat.* 124:10–13.

Berkowitz, P.H., and E.P. Rothman. (1960) *The Disturbed Child: Recognition and Psychoeducational Therapy in the Classroom.* New York: New York University Press.

Berlin, I.N. (1965) Children. In I.N. Berlin and S.A. Szurek, eds., *Learning and Its Disorders.* Palo Alto, Calif.: Science and Behavior Books.

Berryman, E. (1959) School phobia: Management problems in private practice. *Psychol. Rep.* 5:19–25.

Berryman, E. (1960) The treatment of adolescents—effecting the transference. *Am. J. Psychother.* 14:388.

Blackhan, G.J., and B.F. Eden. (1973) Effective re-entry in a longstanding case of school phobia. *Devereux Schools For.* 8(1):42–48.

Bonnard, A. (1959) School phobia. An address before the Association of Child Psychology and Psychiatry. (In *Am. J. Orthopsychiat.* 32:707–718)

Boring, E.G. (1950) *A History of Experimental Psychology.* New York: Appleton-Century-Crofts.

Bornstein, B. (1935) Phobia in a two-a-half-year-old child. *Psychoanal. Quart.* 4:93–119.

Broadwin, I.A. (1932) A contribution to the study of truancy. *Am. J. Orthopsychiat.* 2:253.

Brody, M.W. (1953) The unconscious significance of the corner of a building. *Psychoanal. Quart.* 22:86–87.

Buessmilch, F.L. (1950) Germophobia in an adolescent boy. *Clin. Psychol.* 1:42–47.

Burns, C.L. (1959) Truancy or school phobia. In *Proceedings of the Fifteenth Interclinic Conference of the National Association for Mental Health.* London: Association for Mental Health.

Chapel, J.L. (1967) Treatment of a case of school phobia by reciprocal inhibition. *Can. Psychiat. Assn. J.* 121:25–28.

Chazen, M. (1962) School phobia. *Brit. J. Ed. Psychol.* 32:209–217.

Cohn, H.N. (1959) Phobias in children. *Psychoanal. Rev.* 46:65–84.

Cooke, G. (1966) The efficacy of two desensitization procedures: An analogue study. *Behav. Res. Ther.* 4:17–24.

Coolidge, J.C., R.D. Brodie, and B. Feeney. (1964) A 10-year follow-up study of 66 school phobic children. *Am. J. Orthopsychiat.* 34:675–695.

Coolidge, J.C., P.B. Hahn, and A. Peck. (1957) School phobia: Neurotic crises or way of life. *Am. J. Orthopsychiat.* 27:296–306.

Coolidge, J.C., E. Tessman, S. Waldfogel, and M.L. Willer. (1961) Patterns of aggression in school phobia. *Psychoanal. Study Child* 17:319–333.

Coolidge, J.C., M.L. Willer, E. Tessman, and S. Waldfogel. (1960) School phobia in adolescence: A manifestation of severe character disturbance. *Am. J. Orthopsychiat.* 30:599–608.

Cooper, J.A. (1973) Application of the consultant role to

parent-teacher management of school avoidance behavior. *Psychol. Schools* 10(2):259–262.

Costello, G. (1967) Behavior modification procedures with children. *Can. Psychologist* 8:73–75.

Crider, B. (1949) Phobias: Their nature and treatment. *J. Psychol.* 27:217–229.

Cummings, J. (1944) The incidence of emotional symptoms in school children. *Brit. J. Educ. Psychol.* 14:151–161.

Davidson, S. (1960) School phobia as a manifestation of family disturbance: Its structure and treatment. *J. Child Psychol. Psychiat.* 1:270–287.

Davison, G.C. (1966) The influence of systematic desensitization, relaxation, and graded exposure to imaginal aversive stimuli on the modification of phobic behavior. *Diss. Abst.* 26:6165.

Devereux, G. (1949) A note on nyctophobia and peripheral vision. *Bull. Menninger Clin.* 13:83–93.

Dosvszkov, T. (1949) A survey of erythrophobia. *Int. J. Psychoanal.* 30:194–195.

Dunlop, G.M. (1952) Certain aspects of children's fears. *Diss. Abst.* 12:34.

Edlund, C.V. (1971) A reinforcement approach to the elimination of a child's school phobia. *Ment. Hyg.* 55:433–436.

Eisenberg, L. (1958a) School phobia: Diagnosis, genesis, and clinical management. *Ped. Clin. N. Amer.* 5:654–666.

Eisenberg, L. (1958b) School phobia: A study in the communication of anxiety. *Am. J. Psychiat.* 114:712–718.

Ellis, A. (1950) An introduction to the principles of scientific psychoanalysis. *Genet. Psychol. Mon.* 41:147–212.

Ellis, A. (1962) *Reason and Emotion in Psychotherapy.* New York: Lyle Stuart.

English, O.S., and G.H.J. Pearson. (1945) *Emotional Problems of Living.* New York: Norton.

Errera, P. (1962) Some historical aspects of the concept, phobia. *Psychiat. Quart.* 36:325–336.

Estes, H.R., C.H. Haylett, and A. Johnson. (1956) Separation anxiety. *Am. J. Psychiat.* 10:682–695.

Eysenck, H.H. (1952) The effects of psychotherapy: An evaluation. *J. Consult. Psychol.* 16:319–324.

Eysenck, H.J. (1960) *Behavior Therapy and the Neuroses.* New York: Macmillan.

Feldman, S.S. (1949) Fear of mice. *Psychoanal. Quart.* 18:227–230.

Fenichel, O. (1945) *Theory of Neuroses.* New York: Norton.

Finch, S.M. (1960) *Fundamentals of Child Psychiatry.* New York: Norton.

Freud, S. (1934) *Collected Papers.* London: Hogarth.

Freud, S. (1909) Analysis of a phobia in a five-year-old. In *Collected Papers,* Vol. 3. New York: Basic Books, 1959.

Friedman, D.E. (1966a) A new technique for systematic desensitization of phobic symptoms. *Behav. Res. Ther.* 4:139–140.

Friedman, D.E. (1966b) Treatment of a case of dog phobia in a deaf mute by behavior therapy. *Behav. Res. Ther.* 4:141.

Friedman, P. (1959) The phobias. In S. Arieti, ed., *American Handbook of Psychiatry.* New York: Basic Books.

Gardner, G.E. (1956) Discussion of O. Krug and S. Lentz, "Collaborative treatment of a mother and boy with fecal retention, soiling, and school phobia." In G.E. Gardner, ed., *Case Studies in Childhood Emotional Disabilities.* New York: American Orthopsychiatric Association.

Gehl, R.H. (1964) Depression and claustrophobia. *Int. J. Psychoanal.* 45:312–323.

Gelder, M.G., and I.M. Marks. (1966) A controlled prospective trial of behavior therapy. *Brit. J. Psychiat.* 112:309–319.

Gelder, M.G., I.M. Marks, H.H. Wolff, and M. Clarke. (1967) Desensitization and psychotherapy in the treatment of phobic states: A controlled inquiry. *Brit. J. Psychiat.* 113:53–73.

Gero, G. (1955) Defenses in symptom formation. *Yearbook Psychoanal.* 10:113–127. (Psychol. Abst. 29:8819)

Gittelman-Klein, R., and D.F. Klein. (1973) School phobia: Diagnostic considerations in the light of imipramine effects. *J. Nerv. Ment. Dis.* 156(3):199–215.

Goldberg, T.B. (1953) Factors in the development of school phobia. *Smith College Stu. Social Work* 23:227.

Greenbaum, R.S. (1964) Treatment of school phobia. *Am. J. Psychother.* 18:616–632.

Haack, T. (1954) Cure of a hunting dog with shooting phobia. *Praxis der Kinderpsychologie and Kinderpsychiatrie* 3:211–213. (*Psychol. Abst.* 30:1385)

Hagman, E. (1932) A study of fears of children of preschool age. *J. Exper. Ed.* 1:110–130.

Hain, J.D., R.H.G. Butcher, and I. Stevenson. (1966) Systematic desensitization therapy: An analysis of results in 27 patients. *Brit. J. Psychiat.* 112:295–307.

Harlow, H.F., and R.R. Zimmerman. (1959) Affectional responses in the infant monkey. *Science* 130:421–434.

Hersen, M. (1970) Behavior modification approach to a S-phobia case. *J. Clin. Psychol.* 26:128–132.

Hersov, L.A. (1960) Persistent nonattendance at school. *J. Child Psychol. Psychiat.* 130:137.

Howells, J.G. (1965) *Modern Perspectives in Child Psychiatry.* Springfield, Ill.: Charles C Thomas.

Jacobsen, V. (1948) Influential factors in the outcome of treatment of school phobia. *Smith College Stud. Social Work* 18:181–202.

Jarvis, V. (1964) Countertransference in the management of school phobia. *Psychoanal. Quart.* 33:411–419.

Jersild, A.T., and F.B. Holmes. (1935) Methods of overcoming children's fears. *J. Psychol.* 1:75–104.

Jersild, A.T., F.V. Markey, and C.L. Jersild. (1933) Children's fears, dreams, wishes, daydreams, likes, dislikes, pleasant and unpleasant memories. In A.T. Jersild, ed., *Child Psychology.* Englewood Cliffs, N.J.: Prentice-Hall, 1960.

Johnson, A. (1957) School phobia: Discussion. *Am. J. Orthopsychiat.* 27:307–309.

Johnson, A.M., E.I. Falstein, S.A. Szurek, and M. Svendsen. (1941) School phobia. *Am. J. Orthopsychiat.* 11:702–707.

Jones, M.C. (1924) The elimination of children's fears. *J. Exper. Psychol.* 7:382–390.

Kahn, J.H., and J.P. Mursten. (1962) School refusal: A comprehensive view of school phobia and other failures of school attendance. *Am. J. Orthopsychiat.* 32:707–718.

Kanner, L. (1957) *Child Psychiatry.* Springfield, Ill.: Charles C Thomas.

Kanner, L. (1959) The 33rd Maudsley lecture—Trends in child psychiatry. *J. Ment. Sci.* 105:581.

Kennedy, W.A. (1965) School phobia: Rapid treatment of 50 cases. *J. Abnorm. Psychol.* 70:285–289.

Kessler, J.W. (1966) *Psychopathology of Childhood.* Englewood Cliffs, N.J.: Prentice-Hall.

Kirchner, J., and R. Hogan. (1966) The therapist variable in the implosion of phobias. *Psychotherapy* 3:102–104.

Klein, E. (1945) The reluctance to go to school. *Psychoanal. Study Child* 1:263–279.

Koegler, R.R., and N.Q. Brill. (1967) *Treatment of Psychiatric Outpatients.* New York: Appleton-Century-Crofts.

Kraft, T., and I. Al-Issa. (1965) The application of learning theory to the treatment of traffic phobia. *Brit. J. Psychiat.* 111:277–279.

Kraupe, F. (1948) Some observations on the analytic group treatment of a phobic patient. *J. Ment. Sci.* 94:77–87.

Kutash, S.B. (1965) Psychoneuroses. In B.B. Wolman, ed., *Handbook of Clinical Psychology.* New York: McGraw-Hill.

Lang, P.J., and A.D. Lazovik. (1963) Experimental desensitization of a phobia. *J. Abnorm. Soc. Psychol.* 66:519-525.

Lang, P.J., A.D. Lazovik, and P.J. Reynolds. (1964) Desensitization, suggestibility, and pseudotherapy. *J. Abnorm. Psychol.* 70:395–402.

Lapouse, R., and N. Monk. (1959) Fears and worries in a representative sample of children. *Am. J. Orthopsychiat.* 29:803–818.

Lassers, E., R. Nordan, and S. Bladholm. (1973) Steps in the return to school of children with school phobia. *Am. J. Psychiat.* 130(3):265–268.

Lazarus, A.A. (1961) Group therapy of phobic disorders by systematic desensitization. *J. Abnorm. Soc. Psychol.* 63:504–510.

Lazarus, A.A. (1966) Broad-spectrum behavior therapy and the treatment of agoraphobia. *Behav. Res. Ther.* 4:95–97.

Lazarus, A.A. and A. Abramovitz. (1962) The use of "emotive imagery" in the treatment of children's phobias. *J. Ment. Sci.* 108:191–195.

Lazarus, A.A., G.C. Davison, and D.A. Polefka. (1965) Classical and operant factors in the treatment of school phobia. *J. Abnorm. Psychol.* 70:225–229.

Lazovik, A.D., and P.J. Lang. (1960) A laboratory demonstration of systematic desensitization therapy. *J. Psychol. Studies* 11:230–242.

Leonard, M.R. (1959) Fear of walking in a 2½-year-old girl. *Psychoanal. Quart.* 28:29–30.

Levenson, E.A. (1961) The treatment of school phobia in young adults. *Am. J. Psychother.* 15:539–552.

Leventhal, T., G. Weinberger, R.J. Stander, and R.P. Stearns. (1967) Therapeutic strategies with school phobics. *Am. J. Orthopsychiat.* 37:64–70.

Leventhal, T., and M. Sills. (1964) Self-image in school phobia. *Am. J. Orthopsychiat.* 34:685–695.

Lippman, H.S. (1962) *Treatment of the Child in Emotional Conflict.* New York: McGraw-Hill.

Lomont, J.F. (1965) Reciprocal inhibition or extinction? *Behav. Res. Ther.* 3:209–219.

London, L.S. (1952) Ailurophobia and ornithophobia. *Psychiat. Quart.* 26:365–371.

Lowenstein, L.F. (1973) The treatment of moderate school phobia by negative practice and desensitization procedures. *Assn. Ed. Psychol. J. Newsletter* 3(3):46–49.

MacFarlane, J.W., L. Allen, and M. Honzik. (1954) *A Developmental Study of the Behavior Problems of Normal Children.* Berkeley: University of California Press.

Mackie, R. E. (1967) The importance of the "left." *Am. J. Psychother.* 21:112–115.

Maeder, A. (1943) Cure of a fear of dogs in a boy of 7 years old. *Zeitschrift fur Kinderpsychiatric* 10:36–39. (*Psychol. Abst.* 18:632)

Malmquist, C.P. (1965) School phobia: A problem in family neuroses. *J. Am. Acad. Child Psychiat.* 4:293.

Marine, E. (1973) School refusal: Who should intervene and how? *Psychiat. Comm.* 14(1):43–51.

Marks, I.M., and M.G. Gelder. (1965) A controlled retrospective study of behavior therapy in phobic patients. *Brit. J. Psychiat.* 111:561–573.

Masserman, J. (1946) *Principles of Dynamic Psychiatry.* Philadelphia: Saunders.

Migler, B., and J. Wolpe. (1967) Automated self-desensitization: A case report. *Behav. Res. Ther.* 5:133–135.

Miller, D.L. (1972) School phobia: Diagnosis, emotional genesis, and management. *N.Y. State J. Med.* 72(10):1160–1165.

Miller, P.M. (1972) The use of visual imagery and muscle relaxation in the counter-conditioning of a phobic child: A case study. *J. Nerv. Ment. Dis.* 154(6):457–460.

Morgan, G.A.V. (1959) Children who refuse to go to school. *Med. Off.* 102:221–224.

Myer, V., and M.G. Gelder. (1963) Behavior therapy and phobic disorders. *Brit. J. Psychiat.* 109:19–28.

Nice, R.W. (1968) The use of sodium pentothal in the treatment of a S phobic. *J. Learn Disab.* 1:249–255.

Nursten, J. (1963) Projection in the later adjustment of school phobic children. *Smith College Stud. Social Work* 32:210–224.

Nursten, J.P. (1958) The background of children with school phobia. *Med. Off.* 100:340.

Olsen, I.A., and H.S. Coleman. (1967) Treatment of school phobia as a case of separation anxiety. *Psychol. Schools* 4:151–154.

Ono, O. (1972) An investigation in a local area. *Jap. J. Child Psychiat.* 13(4):250–260.

Pappenheim, E., and M. Sweeney. (1952) Separation anxiety in mother and child. *Psychoanal. Study Child* 7:95–115.

Patterson, G.R. (1965) A learning theory approach to the problem of the school phobic child. In L.P. Ullmann and L. Krasner, eds., *Case Studies in Behavior Modification*. New York: Holt, Rinehart and Winston.

Perrotti, N. (1947) La phobie du communisme. *Psyche* 2:1374–1379. (*Psychol. Abst.* 23:4309)

Pinchon, R., and A. Arminda. (1950) Fobia a los globos en una niña de 11 meses. (A balloon phobia in an 11-month-old girl.) *Revista de Psychoanalisis* 7:541–554.

Pratt, J.C. (1945) The study of the fears of rural children. *J. Genet. Psychol.* 67:179–194.

Rachman, S. (1959) The treatment of anxiety and phobic reactions by systematic desensitization and psychotherapy. *J. Abnorm. Soc. Psychol.* 58:259–263.

Rachman, S. (1965) Studies in desensitization: I. The separate effects of relaxation and desensitization. *Behav. Res. Ther.* 3:245–251.

Rachman, S. (1966) Studies in desensitization: II. Flooding. *Behav. Res. Ther.* 4:1–6.

Rachman, S., and C.G. Costello. (1967) The aetiology and treatment of children's phobias—A review. *Am. J. Psychiat.* 118:97–105.

Radin, S.S. (1967) Psychodynamic aspects of school phobia. *Comp. Psychiat.* 8:119–128.

Rangell, L. (1952) The analysis of a doll phobia. *Int. J. Psychoanal.* 33:43–53.

Redlich, F.C., and D.X. Freedman. (1966) *The Theory and Practice of Psychiatry*. New York: Basic Books.

Reger, R. (1962) School phobia in an obese girl. *J. Clin. Psychol.* 18:356–357.

Rines, W.B. (1973) Behavior therapy before institutionalization. *Psychother. Theory Res. Prac.* 10(3):281–283.

Roberts, A.H. (1964) Housebound wives—A follow-up study of phobic anxiety states. *Brit. J. Psychiat.* 100:191–197.

Robie, T.R. (1935) The phobia of impregnation and its relation to the psychoneuroses. *Am. J. Orthopsychiat.* 5:318–324.

Rodriguez, A., M. Rodriguez, and L. Eisenberg. (1959) The outcome of school phobia: A follow-up based on 41 cases. *Am. J. Psychiat.* 116:540–544.

Ryle, J.A. (1948) Nosophobia: The twenty-first Maudsley lecture. *J. Ment. Sci.* 94:1–17.

Saraf, K.R., D.F. Klein, R. Gittelman-Klein, and S. Groff. (1974) Imipramine side effects in children. *Psychopharmacologia* 37(3):265–274.

Shapiro, M.B., L. Neufeld, and F. Post. (1962) Experimental study of depressive illness. *Psychol. Rep.* 10:590.

Shapiro, T. and R. Jegede. (1973) School phobia: A Babel of tongues. *J. Autism Child. Schizo.* 3(2):168–186.

Shaw, R.S. (1966) Psychiatric Disorders of Childhood. New York: Appleton-Century-Crofts.

Shaw, W.J., and C.G. Jarvis. (1975) The behavioral counselor's approach to school phobia. *School Applications of Learning Theory* 7(2):9–21.

Silverman, L.H., Frank, S.G., and P. Dachinger. (1974) A psychoanalytic reinterpretation of the effectiveness of systematic desensitization: Experimental data bearing on the role of merging fantasies. *J. Abnorm. Psychol.* 83(3):313–318.

Skynner, A.C. (1974) School phobia: A reappraisal. *Brit. J. Med. Psychol.* 47(1):1–16.

Smith, M. D. (1973-74) The use of behavior therapies in the treatment of school phobia. *Univ. Maryland Counsel. Personnel Serv. J.* 4(1):48–62.

Smith, S.L. (1970) School refusal with anxiety: A review of sixty-three cases. *Can. Psychiat. Assn. J.* 15(3):257–264.

Sperling, M. (1952) Animal phobia in a 2-year-old child. *Psychoanal. Study Child* 7:115–125.

Spock, B. (1957) *Baby and Child Care*. New York: Pocket Books.

Strahley, D.F. (1966) Systematic desensitization and counterphobic treatment of an irrational fear of snakes. *Diss. Abst.* 27(3-B):973.

Suttenfield, V. (1954) School phobia: A study of 5 cases. *Am. J. Orthopsychiat.* 24:368–380.

Szurek, S., A. Johnson, and E. Falstein. (1942) Collaborative psychiatric therapy of parent-child problems. *Am. J. Orthopsychiat.* 12:511–516.

Takagi, R. (1973) The family structure of school phobics. *Acta Paedopsychiat.* 39(6):131–146.

Talbot, M. (1957) Panic in school phobia. *Am. J. Orthopsychiat.* 27:286–295.

Terhune, W.B. (1949) The phobic syndrome: A study of 86 patients with phobic reactions. *Arch. Neurol. Psychiat.* 62:162–172.

Vaal, J.J. (1973) Applying contingency contracting to a school phobic: A case study. *J. Behav. Ther. Exper. Psychiat.* 4(4):371–373.

Van Houten, J. (1948) Mother and child relationships in 12 cases of school phobia. *Smith College Stud. Social Work* 18:161–180.

van Krevelen, D. (1971) Kinder, die nicht zum Schulbesuch zu bewegen sind. (Children who cannot be persuaded to go to school.) *Acta Paedopsychiat.* 38(5-6):161–172.

Vaughan, F. (1954) School phobias. Cited by M. Talbot (1957) Panic in school phobia. *Am. J. Orthopsychiat.* 27:286–295.

Wakabayashi, S., H. Ito, and S. Ito. (1965) The investigation of the actual condition of school phobia or refusal to attend school. *Jap. J. Child Psychol.* 6:77–89.

Waldfogel, S. (1959) Emotional crisis in a child. In A. Burton, ed., *Case Studies in Counseling and Psychotherapy*. Englewood Cliffs, N.J.: Prentice-Hall.

Waldfogel, S., J.C. Coolidge, and P. Hahn. (1957) Development and management of school phobia. *Am. J. Orthopsychiat.* 27:754–780.

Warren, W. (1960) Some relationships between psychiatry of children and adults. *J. Ment. Sci.* 106:815–826.

Watson, J.B., and R. Rayner. (1920) Conditioned emotional reactions. *J. Exper. Psychol.* 3:1–14.

Weber, H. (1936) An approach to the problem of fear in children. *J. Ment. Sci.* 82:136–147.

Wechsler, E. (1929) *The Neuroses*. Philadelphia: Saunders.

Weiss, M., and A.G. Burke. (1967) A 5 to 10 year follow-up of hospitalized school phobic children and adolescents. *Am. J. Orthopsychiat.* 37:294–295.

Weiss, M., and B. Cain. (1964) The residential treatment of children and adolescents with school phobia. *Am. J. Orthopsychiat.* 34:103–112.

White, R. W. (1964) *The Abnormal Personality*, 3rd ed. New York: Ronald Press.

Wilson, J.W., and H.E. Miller. (1946) Delusion of parasitosis (acarophobia). *Arch. Dermatol. Syphil.* 54:39–56. (*Psychol. Abst.* 21:163)

Wolpe, J. (1958) *Psychotherapy by Reciprocal Inhibition*. Stanford: Stanford University Press.

Wolpe, J. (1961) The systematic desensitization treatment of neuroses. *J. Nerv. Ment. Dis.* 132:189–203.

Wolpe, J. (1963) Systematic desensitization of phobias. *Am. J. Psychiat.* 119:1062–1068.

Wolpe, J., and S. Rachman. (1960) Psychoanalytic "evidence," a critique based on Freud's case of Little Hans. *J. Nerv. Ment. Dis.* 131:135–147.

Wolpin, M., and L. Pearsall. (1965) Rapid deconditioning of a fear of snakes. *Behav. Res. Ther.* 3:107–111.

Wolpin, M., and J. Raines. (1966) Visual imagery, expected roles, and extinction as possible factors in reducing fear and avoidance behavior. *Behav. Res. Ther.* 4:25–37.

Yamamura, M. (1936) Psychoanalytic studies of erythrophobia: Part II. *Arbeiten aus dem Psychiatrischen Institut der Kaiserlich-Japanischen Universitat zu Sendai, Tohoku University* 5:13–14. (*Psychol. Abst.* 10:2516)

Yamazaki, M. (1973) A study of school phobia: II. Family dynamics that obstruct socialization of chronic cases with main reference to the personalities of the fathers. *J. Ment. Health* 21:29–48.

Zax, M., and G. Stricker. (1963) *Patterns of Psychopathology*. New York: Macmillan.

Treatment of Emotional Disorders in Children and Adolescents

CHAPTER 34

Depression and Suicidal Behavior

James M. Toolan

Introduction

For many years relatively few papers were written on the subject of depression, even though it has always been the diagnosis of a sizable percentage of patients seen in both inpatient and outpatient services. The situation has changed significantly over the past fifteen years. Numerous clinical studies of depression have been published, inspired by the increased knowledge of the biochemistry of depression, and the beneficial action of lithium and various antidepressant medications. With few exceptions, however, little has been written about depression in children. The first edition of *The American Handbook of Psychiatry* (1959) did not include a single reference to childhood depression, nor did Beck's (1967) monograph or Klerman's (1971) extensive review on depression. The APA's *Diagnostic Statistical Manual II* (1968) does not include childhood depression in its nosology.

Even today the debate continues as to whether children can be diagnosed as being truly depressed—not just moody or unhappy. The situation is further complicated by the fact that the term "depression" is used to refer to a symptom, a syndrome, or a nosological entity. Many clinicians seem unclear as to whether they view depression as a single illness with different signs and symptoms or whether they are referring to several different diseases. In the problem of childhood depression further difficulties ensue; some authors (Rochlin, 1959) have maintained that clinical depression, being a superego phenomenon, cannot occur in children; others have claimed that developmentally, children cannot become depressed—at least prior to the end of the latency years, and stress the fact that the usual clinical signs or symptoms associated with depression in adults do not usually occur in children before mid-adolescence (Rie, 1967). Many observers, while they agree that children are in fact often sad and moody, still question whether children's moods are at all consistent.

Several years ago the writer (Toolan, 1962a) suggested that the basic mood of children is as consistent as that of adults—that infants, children, and adolescents can be diganosed as depressed provided that we employ criteria different from those used for adults. I suggested, for example, that we have learned schizophrenia can be seen at all age levels but that this entity is manifested by markedly differently signs and symptoms in children from those observed in adults, and that this same fact is true of depressive reactions. Just as we have been able to follow many schizophrenic children into adulthood and observe their functioning at different developmental stages, so too have we now observed the developmental stages of depressives. In recent years, a number of authors have described children who remained depressed during the childhood period and who then presented different clinical pictures with age changes (Poznanski and Zrull, 1970; Toolan, 1962a). It would appear from the increasing number of articles on the topic of childhood depression over the past ten years that the theory of developmental changes is becoming accepted more generally. This paper, then, is based on the thesis that children and adolescents become depressed as adults do, but they exhibit different clinical pictures at different ages and stages of their developmental growth (Malmquist, 1971; Toolan, 1962a, 1962b, 1974). It is further based on the premise that many children and adolescents continue to be depressed as adults, and that depression occurring at these early developmental stages is not an entity to be dismissed lightly with "Don't worry, he will grow out of it," which is so often the attitude of well-meaning physicians, teachers, school guidance personnel, and even parents (Poznanski, Krahenbuhl, and Zrull, 1976; Toolan, 1962a, 1962b, 1974).

Therapeutic approaches must naturally be based upon the age of the individual patient, his level of ego development, his intelligence, the defenses used to handle depressive feelings, the attitude of the parents, and the facilities available in the community.

Historical Background

In 1946, Spitz and Wolf described institutionalized infants with symptoms of withdrawal, loss of weight, insomnia, weeping, and marked developmental retardation. Some of these infants continued their decline into stupor and death. Spitz and Wolf coined the term "anaclitic depression" to describe the symptoms they had noted. Goldfarb, writing in the same year, also described social and intellectual retardation in institutionalized children and ascribed the symptoms to emotional deprivation; he did not use the term "depression." Spitz and Wolf theorized that the depression occurring in the institutionalized infants they had observed resulted from a maternal separation of at least three months' duration, occurring when the infant was between six and eight months of age. Engel and Reichsman (1956) in their classic study of a youngster with a gastric fistula, showed that a depressive reaction could be induced experimentally. The infant described improved rapidly when cared for by a single mother substitute. When confronted with a stranger, the child would react with a depressive-withdrawal syndrome, but would recover when once again her needs were met by a familiar person. Bowlby (1960) studied the effect of separation from the mother upon the infant and noted three predictable stages: protest, despair, and detachment. Bowlby used the term "mourning" rather than depression to describe the child's reactions. Despert (1952) was one of the earliest clinicians to describe depression in children and to indicate that the syndrome was more common than usually believed, while Keeler (1954) was among the first to note that children often mask their feelings of depression. Other authors have described occasional youngsters who manifested at an early age the signs and symptoms of depression ordinarily seen in adults. Agras (1959) postulated a relationship between school phobia and childhood depression. Campbell (1955) also related school phobias to childhood depression, which he believed to be a variety of manic-depressive disorder. Sperling (1959) introduced the term "equivalents of depression" in children. Toolan (1962a) described a developmental theory of childhood depression, noting in detail the signs and symptoms of this disorder from infancy through late adolescence. He believed that each age level tended to present depressive feelings in certain characteristic ways. Kaufman and Heims (1958) had earlier related juvenile delinquent acting-out to an unresolved depression.

Cytryn and McKnew (ISA) have divided childhood depressions into three categories: masked depression, acute depression, and chronic depression. They emphasized that masked depression can be evidenced by hyperactivity, aggressive behavior, psychosomatic illness, hypochondriasis, and delinquency, with periodic displays of overt depression. More recently, Poznanski (1970) has discussed the clinical characteristics of overtly depressed children. Malmquist (1971), who wrote an extensive review of the literature through 1971, describes depressive signs and symptoms during the latency years, in older children, and in adolescence. Easson (1977) has recently given an extensive clinical presentation of depression in adolescents. Since much of the early literature addressed itself to the question of whether or not depression occurred in children, it is understandable that there has been very little written on the subject of therapy for depressed children. Anthony (1970) differentiated between two types of adolescent depressives and their treatment. Masterson (1967, 1972) has frequently referred to the need to recognize and treat the abandonment depression in severe character disorders and borderline states in adolescents. Toolan (1962a) attempted to relate therapeutic approaches and techniques to the developmental aspects of childhood and adolescent depression. Malmquist (1977) has recently described therapeutic approaches to depressed children and adolescents.

Therapy

Theoretical Considerations

The therapeutic approaches to be described in this article are essentially based upon a psychoanalytic understanding of personality development, bearing in mind that differences in ego and superego development at various ages will produce diverse clinical pictures, which in turn will necessitate disparate technical approaches. Abraham (1927) and Freud (1917) theorized in their early papers that a harsh, punitive superego turned aggression and hostility against the self, leading to depression. The depressed person was assumed to have identified with the ambivalently loved, lost object. Most psychoanalysts since Freud, undoubtedly influenced by Fairbairn (1954), have theorized that depression follows the loss of a significant love-object, whether the loss be reality or fantasy. Bibring (1953) modified this theory in stating that loss leads to diminished self-esteem, which he believed to be the underlying cause of depression. "Depression can be defined as the emotional expression of a state of helplessness and powerlessness of the ego, irrespective of what may have caused the breakdown of the mechanism which established his self-esteem." He went on to add that the basic mechanism is "the ego's shocking awareness of its helplessness in regard to its aspirations." Sandler and Joffe (1965) have in turn modified Bibring's theory of the significance of self-esteem in depression. They "stress rather the basic biological nature of the depressive reaction, related to pain (and its opposite, 'well-being'), rather than the psychologically more elaborate concept of self-esteem." They also revised the theory of the loss of the desired love-object: "While what is lost may be an object, it may equally well be the loss of a previous state of the self. . . . When a love-object is lost, what is really lost, we believe, is the state of well-being implicit, both psychologically and biologically, in the relationship with the object." They state that as the child grows older, the object-loss becomes of greater significance than the loss of the state of well-being embodied in the relationship with the object. They defined depression "as a state of helpless resignation in the face of pain, together with an inhibition both of drive discharge and ego function."

Several authors (Cytryn and McKnew, 1972; Toolan, 1962a, 1962b, 1974) have referred to the frequent incidence of parental loss, caused by separation, divorce, or death, in the family history of depressed adolescents. Quite often depressed youngsters have been rejected and depreciated by their parents, who have lost interest in their children. Many of these parents have been themselves clinically depressed. Malmquist (1971, 1977) has described the parents of depressed children as demanding conformity and dedication to duty as the price of parental approval. Poznanski and Zrull have also mentioned the increased incidence of parental depression noted in the history of depressed children and adolescents, and have mentioned that such families have trouble handling aggression and hostility. These families often oscillate between aggression and depression, which makes it very difficult for their children to handle these emotions appropriately.

My understanding of the developmental aspect of depression is based on the thesis that depression is a reaction to loss, either of an object or a state of well-being, with feelings of diminished self-esteem and helplessness; such a theory enables us to understand the various manifestations of depressive reactions at different ages. The result of any object loss will depend on the individual's ability to tolerate pain and discomfort, be it physical or mental, and the developmental stage when such loss occurs. The younger the child, the more serious the consequences. The infant may become fixated in his ego development or even regress. At times, the impairment of ego development will hinder intellectual growth. The ability to form adequate object relationships may be significantly impaired. This will interfere with the ability of the individual to identify with significant figures in his life. Such disturbances in the process of identification will adversely affect the development of the superego, ego ideal, and the whole personality structure.

When the loss takes place during latency and early adolescence, the youngster will often exhibit hostility and anger toward the person whom he feels has betrayed and deserted him. This often leads to serious acting-out and delinquency, which may temporarily help ward off painful feelings of helplessness and impotence. These defensive operations unfortunately seldom if ever prove successful and only lead to further conflict with the parents, who become increasingly antagonistic toward the child, who desperately needs their love and support. Some children will inhibit the expression of anger toward their parents and turn it against themselves. Such a child will consider himself to be evil, and such a self-image will also lead to the acting-out so commonly seen in depressed children. Such behavior will reinforce the child's poor self-image, further lower his self-esteem, and increase his feelings of helplessness and depression.

All humans must learn how to cope with loss. This is best achieved by learning how to mourn the loss of a significant person in an appropriate manner and at the appropriate time. Most religions have built-in rituals to help this process. Contemporary society, especially in this country, finds it very difficult to face death and loss, and mistakenly attempts to shield children from the necessary mourning process. If adults are confused about loss and mourning, it is not strange that children are even more so. A child who is not helped to deal with loss will deny his grief and thereby become more liable to depression.

Numerous defensive operations are used by children and adolescents to guard against the painful feelings of depression. Those most frequently encountered are regression, repression, denial, and projection. We often note displacement onto somatic symptoms during adolescence. A reversal of affect is seen in some youngsters. Toward mid-adolescence, significant maturational changes occur in ego functioning, especially in the area of reality testing. The youngster will use denial to a lesser extent; he will see his parents' role in his object loss. This will not only increase his anger toward his parents but will also increase his guilt for having such feelings. The hostile feelings toward the parents become, in mid-adolescence, directed toward their introjects within the youngster, since the superego does not fully develop until mid-adolescence (Toolan, 1960). These changes, plus the knowledge that reality will not change and that he will not regain his lost love-object, reinforce the adolescent's feelings of lowered self-esteem and helplessness and produce the clinical picture of overt depression.

Another factor that contributes to the formation of depression in adolescence is the resolution of the Oedipus complex, with its sense of parent loss. This sense of loss is increased when the child leaves home for the first time for boarding school or college. Many youngsters at that period still need parent substitutes with whom they can relate in order to diminish their feeling of parent deprivation. Others meet this need by relating closely to their own peer group, as is clearly illustrated in the so-called family communes. Those who fail to obtain some close relationship at this period frequently succumb to serious depressive reactions.

In addition to the psychoanalytic theory of depression, we must also consider the biochemical theory of depression and how it relates to treatment with antidepressant drugs and lithium. The current theory is that alteration of catecholamine and serotonin formation may lead to depression. It appears that tricyclic antidepressants may inhibit catecholamine uptake. This has led to the supposition that the subnormal catecholamine function is associated with depression. Such subnormal catecholamine-functioning can be improved by prolonging catecholamine synaptic action with tricyclics, which prevent catecholamine reuptake, or by monomine oxidase inhibitors of catecholamine breakdown. Both groups of medications affect serotonin in a similar fashion. Electroconvulsive therapy also affects the amount of catecholamine in the nervous system, but this therapy is seldom used any longer for depressed children and adolescents. Lithium, it would appear, reduces the quantities of catecholamine and serotonin at the cell receptor level.

Applicability

There are two essentially different approaches (or a combination of the two) for the treatment of depressed children and adolescents. The most significant one is psychotherapeutic. Medication is of value in certain cases (primarily in those older children and adolescents who exhibit oert depressive symptomotology.) Most authorities believe that even when medication is of help, it should be used in conjunction with psychotherapy and not as the only therapy.

The youngest population—those described as anaclitic infants—require neither psychotherapy nor medication but rather a reunion with the mother or a mother surrogate as rapidly as possible. In treating children, the younger the child, the more important it is to have the parents actively involved in the therapeutic process, since often the pathology is essentially their inability to relate properly to their children. This is one of the significant limitations of working with children of any clinical syndrome; unless the parents are actively involved, very little is likely to be accomplished.

It is my theory that children and adolescents who are depressed should be regarded as seriously in need of therapy. Such reactions are seldom transitory and if not adequately treated will continue into adulthood (Poznanski, Krahenbuhl, and Zrull, 1976). I believe further that many depressed children require intensive psychotherapy—not short-term, crisis-oriented help as is so popular these days—and that only competently trained therapists are capable of offering such therapy. As a general rule, the average physician, teacher, guidance counselor, or mental health worker is not capable of providing such highly skilled technical assistance. It requires an individual well trained in child development as well as child psychiatry, who in addition has a sound understanding of psychopharmacology. Unfortunately, such individuals are all too rare, so that in practice many depressed youngsters are frequently given inadequate treatment by poorly trained practitioners. The shortage of competent therapists is one of the reasons why many clinics depend largely upon medication (as is so often the case also in the treatment of schizophrenics); medication is obviously easier, less expensive, and requires less skilled personnel.

Acting-out individuals, especially those already engaged in serious delinquency, may require some type of residential placement where their acting-out can be limited. Unfortunately, very few institutions offer any therapeutic help to such youngsters; many are little better than prisons. As such they are not only of little benefit but may even cause the youngster to become more disturbed and to enter into a lifelong pattern of acting-out.

Methods of Treatment

As already stated, I believe that only highly experienced and adequately trained therapists should work with depressed children and adolescents. The skills required are first of all a sound foundation in normal child development plus a knowledge of the effect that divorce and other losses have on children and adolescents. A special prerequisite in the therapist is the clinical experience to distinguish between a temporary mourning reaction and/or brief periods of unhappiness versus clinical depression. Most adults are inclined to assume that children are generally happy, that few things bother them, and that they will outgrow any problems. Working with depressed youngsters not only requires that the therapist be familiar with the symptomatology of depression as seen in adults, but also to recognize how youngsters handle depression at different developmental stages. The therapist must be able to relate not only to the child but especially to the parents, who are often eager to regard the child's problems as being of a minor nature and due to growing pains, minimal brain damage, or bad companions.

In general, outpatient therapy will suffice; hospitalization is only required when the youngster is suicidal or in a life-threatening situation—e.g., severe cases of anorexia nervosa. Occasionally hospitalization is helpful in order to observe and evaluate youngsters with somatic symptoms masking their depression, such as headache, abdominal distress, and the like. As previously indicated, severe acting-out youngsters may require residential treatment.

The therapist working with depressed youngsters must be keenly aware of his own feelings toward such patients. He may be overly frightened by their suicidal propensities and unnecessarily hospitalize some patients. On the other hand, he may believe that he can omnipotently handle any problem and thus not protect the youngster adequately. Many therapists find it difficult to work with both youngsters and their parents together. In such cases it would be advisable for another therapist to work with the parents and to collaborate closely with the child's therapist. I have come to believe, however, that whenever possible it is preferable for the same therapist to work with the youngster and his parents. This allows for a much deeper understanding of the dynamics operating between child and parents, and diminishes the opportunity for child and parents to play one therapist against another.

Therapists working with depressed children and adolescents can anticipate that certain countertransference feelings will arise. Many therapists may find themselves bored by the apathy and indifference displayed by some depressed youngsters. Others may become frightened when they sense the depth of the patient's despair and helplessness. In turn, the therapist himself may feel helpless or defeated, and resent the patient. If handled therapeutically, these feelings may often be turned to constructive ends; if not, therapy may be destroyed. In many respects, such feelings are similar to the countertransference feelings that borderline and schizophrenic patients often arouse in their therapists. If the youngster is to confront his depressive feelings fully and then work them through, he must face the painful emotions that he has been strongly attempting to deny. Many therapists themselves find this process painful and are only too eager to agree with the patient and his parents that he is feeling better and that there is no need for further therapy. Quite often this happens just before the youngster would be facing his most painful emotions, which he is understandably reluctant to do. In my opinion, if he does not do so, they will continue to handicap the youngster.

I will now attempt to spell out in detail the techniques which are helpful in working with depressed children and adolescents of different ages who exhibit various clinical pictures.

1. *Anaclitic infant.* As already mentioned, Spitz and Wolf (1946) described this syndrome arising in infants separated from their mothers for prolonged periods during the first year of life. Such infants may not only become depressed but also fail to thrive and even die. It is important to be certain that there is no physiological cause for such a syndrome. It is especially important that corrective action not be delayed lest the situation become irreversible. An infant suffering from this syndrome requires reunion with the mother if at all possible; if not, a mother surrogate should be provided to care for him.

2. *Infants with a depressed parent.* Many infants come to the attention of pediatricians because of eating and sleeping difficulties, persistent crying, and colic. A thorough family history will often reveal that one of the parents, more often the mother, is profoundly depressed. In such cases efforts should be directed toward resolving the mother's depression, not only for her own sake but for that of the child, who will exhibit his depression by various other symptoms as he grows older.

3. *Children of divorced parents.* Divorce is an ever-increasing problem in our society, with the rate now in excess of 30% of all marriages. The rate is especially high among couples in their twenties and thirties, many of whom have children who will be affected by the loss of a parent. Almost invariably the child of divorced parents is distressed by the disruption of his home. Unfortunately, few studies have been made of the effect of divorce on children, but those few have indicated that the effect depends greatly upon the age of the youngster (Wallerstein and Kelly, 1975). Many children will regress to much earlier modes of behavior, while others may present symptoms of withdrawal and apathy. Not all of these reactions are permanent, but a recent study showed that one year after a divorce many of the children seen in consultation were still depressed—some even more so than when first examined (Wallerstein and Kelly, 1975). It is obviously important to evaluate such youngsters; fortunately, not all will need therapy, as there would not be enough therapists to satisfy the demand. On the other hand, it is very important not to assume that the adverse reactions following divorce represent a child's normal grief, which will soon pass. Efforts should be directed toward helping the parents anticipate such reactions and to assist the child in coping with his troubled feelings. Unfortunately, the mother of these children is often having a difficult time herself and may have little time to give to the child when he most needs support. Another issue that frequently arises in divorce cases is a bitter custodial battle between the parents, with the child being used as a pawn. Such families need professional help. Here the courts could take the lead, for I believe that children whose custody is in dispute should have counsel appointed to represent *their* rights, which may well be in conflict with those of the parents. Many of these children experience much guilt over the breakup of the parents' marriage, feeling somehow responsible for the situation. Occasionally, brief cathartic therapy may enable the child to rid himself of such feelings and to see the situation more realistically; at other times the child's guilt may become internalized in a true neurotic process, and intensive therapy will be then required.

Clinical Examples

As previously stated, depression manifests itself differently depending upon the age of the child or adolescent affected. In the following clinical examples, I hope to illustrate some of the main syndromes encountered, and my therapeutic approach to them.

1. Many depressed youngsters present a clinical picture similar to that of John, a 12-year-old boy who was obese, encopretic, and enuretic. He had difficulty relating to his siblings and to other youngsters. He was unpopular, and his nickname, "Stinky," summed up the regard in which he was held by his peers. John disliked coming for therapy, trying hard to maintain a pose that all was well and that he could lose weight and stop wetting and soiling himself whenever he wished to do so. He frequently maintained that he was fairly popular, and then would reverse this position and state that he could not understand why he was not better-liked. For a long time John practiced denial and evasion to an extraordinary degree. Slowly he began to admit that he was often unhappy when his friends teased him and when his father humiliated him (a frequent occurrence). John slowly began to trust the therapist, not an easy task for such a youngster. Finally, he was able to disclose a recurrent fantasy that he was lying dead in a coffin as everyone filed by, crying, and lamenting that they were sorry to have treated him so badly. At this point I was able to say that it is understandable to feel sorry for oneself if one has been mistreated, but that this was the first time he had ever mentioned such an idea. He then spoke meaningfully of his parents, of how much he loved his mother and how good she was to him, and then of his father who constantly berated, beat, and bribed him, all to no avail. I indicated that he must have strong feelings about his father's behavior. Suddenly his anger toward his father burst out—he hated him, and would like to kill him, but was terrified of him. We were then able to examine these feelings—how he could not challenge his father directly but could only give vent to his anger by passive-aggressive behavior, which further infuriated the father. John was next able to realize that such behavior hurt him more than the father, and had alienated everyone around him except his long-suffering mother. After a fierce struggle (he did not want to relinquish his angry passive-aggressive behavior toward his father as that would leave the latter victorious,) he began to change. He ceased soiling and wetting, and lost 25 pounds. For the first time he was able to keep up with the other boys in sports, and slowly he became accepted by them. Finally, his sullen, negative behavior diminished. I believe that the turning point in working with John was when he was able to express his miserable feelings and then face the cause of them. I also believe that without therapy, in all likelihood John would have remained an obese individual with a passive-aggressive personality disorder.

It should be noted that one of John's symptoms was enuresis, a most common symptom among pre-adolescent boys. Many clinicians prescribe Imipramine Hcl. at bedtime for this condition, often with good results. The usual explanation of this is that the drug has an anticholinergic effect upon the bladder sphincter. This may be true, but we should bear in mind that many enuretic children may be depressed and therefore respond to the antidepressant action of this medication. A similar situation is presented by some hyperactive children, who are diagnosed as having minimal brain damage (often with little workup) and then placed on this same medication, with occasional good response. Is the favorable result due to stimulation of certain systems of the central nervous system, as claimed by the drug's adherents, or are some of these children also depressed and, not uncommonly, using hyperactive defenses?

2. Charles was referred for therapy by both the headmaster of his school and his father. At 15 years of age, his behavior was very immature. He was arrogant, supercilious, and sarcastic. A bright boy, he was performing well below his academic potential. The main concern of the father was Charles' abuse of drugs. I first saw him just after a holiday, when Charles had been using LSD daily and had had at least two bad reactions. He was the younger of two boys, and had been doing well until his mother's death three years earlier. Following that event (which Charles noted with amazement was not upsetting, even though he had been very close to his mother), Charles lived with his father who, as a hard-working businessman, was frequently away from home. They had a series of housekeepers, none of whom were at all close to Charles. Previously a good student, he began to lose interest in school; while he occasionally attempted to do his academic work, he was unable to sustain his interest. He then became involved with drugs: marijuana, amphetamines, and finally LSD. His father cared for him, but overwhelmed by his own grief and his business concerns, could give Charles little but money to show his affection. When first seen, Charles wished to speak of nothing but drugs and his reactions to them. He was fascinated by my knowledge of drugs and their effects upon himself and others. He appeared jaunty, almost manic at times. His tension was very evident; he was especially troubled by a facial tic. After several sessions, I wondered aloud why he had to be so frantically active—constantly running to see his friends, trying to find a girl, watching television, playing music, popping pills. He seemed surprised at this description of himself and initially somewhat defensive. Then he began to talk about how lonely he felt (an emotion he found very hard to tolerate), especially when his father was away on business and he was alone at home. Girls were magic—if he could be successful with them, all would be well. Although a handsome young man, he was somehow never able to sustain an emotional relationship with a girl. In speaking of them, he began to associate to his mother—how close they had been before her death and how he missed her; for the first time he could grieve over her death. He had a series of dreams concerning her death and burial. Suddenly Charles decided to give up drugs as well as cigarettes; he was going to be the boy his mother knew and cared for.

He did succeed in this, but only to become profoundly depressed as his ability to deny and avoid his depressive feelings collapsed. On two or three occasions he relapsed and turned to drugs, which had the effect of making him feel momentarily better. Only when he realized this fact could he admit to himself that drugs were an escape from depression. He was able to reach out to his father and reveal his need for him, and the father was better able to respond once drugs were no longer an issue of conflict.

The significant therapeutic effort in this case was to help Charles realize the role drugs played in warding off depressive feelings. When he himself was finally convinced of that fact we could then turn to the expression of the feelings that arose following the death of his mother.

3. Sally, a 15-year-old girl, came for therapy upon referral from school, but actually she had arranged the matter herself by telling one of the teachers that she had recently attempted suicide. A tall, slender, attractive girl, she began the first session by reading me a ten-page handwritten letter in which she described her suicidal feelings, her sexual acting-out, her guilt over the latter, her feeling that her parents hated her, and her excessive use of alcohol. She was well aware that she was drinking to narcotize her feelings, and had just made the decision to stop drinking entirely. At the end of the initial session I recall thinking how well Sally had outlined her problems and how, unlike many teenagers, she could realize the main issues rather than slowly working through the defenses being used to avoid facing them. I should have known better. At the next session she began by stating that she had decided she wanted a female therapist, but clearly showed that was not the issue by saying that her parents would insist upon her seeing me. I next saw her parents (at her request). She decided not to attend the session. When next seen, Sally was angry—I had told her parents that she was ill and needed therapy. Actually, I had simply gone over the issues raised by her in her first session. Shortly after this she threatened to discontinue therapy because she was angry at the headmaster, who had recommended me, and who had given her an unfavorable school report.

I realized that Sally was saying two things: (1) although she had consciously sought therapy and was only too well aware of her need for it, she was also frightened; (2) that she was very angry with all adults and especially her parents. When I pointed out the latter fact, she readily agreed, giving many reasons why her parents angered her, all rather superficial rationalizations. I added that I believed I knew a more important reason for her anger. In their session with me the mother had admitted that she had never been able to feel close to Sally. Even during her early years they had battled over every conceivable issue—eating, toilet-training, discipline, and so forth. Sally said that she was amazed that her mother had been so frank with me. I responded that it must have been difficult for her mother, but that she had clearly stated her feeling that this pattern may have influenced her daughter and desperately wanted to undo the damage if at all possible. This was very meaningful to Sally. She began to realize that though she had been emotionally neglected by her mother, she had been loved at the same time. She could face her angry feelings and her guilt more readily, realizing that her mother had acknowledged her own role and wanted to help remedy the situation.

This case illustrates the importance of having contact with the parents. I might in time have come to surmise such a pattern, but here it was, presented openly early in therapy. It further showed the advantage of having the same therapist for parents and child, even though at times he may become a scapegoat—e.g., Sally's anger at me for conveying her needs and feelings to her parents, although it had been at her own request.

The last two cases also illustrate the importance of alcohol and drug abuse and their escape and denial function in the lives of depressed youngsters. The recent trend to regard alcohol and drug abuse as entities in themselves (witness the efforts in many states, as well as in the national institutes, to separate mental health facilities from those dealing with alcohol and drug abuse) raises serious concern. The goal of programs for alcohol and drug abuse is clearly stated: to free individuals from their dependence on these substances. Admittedly, this is a laudatory aim, but we should not be deluded into believing that abstinence solves all problems. In my opinion such abstinence is but the beginning of an individual's changing, not its end.

4. Martin, an 18-year-old college sophomore, was referred for therapy by the college physician after making a very serious, near-fatal suicide attempt by an overdose of medication. Martin was clearly depressed—showing a sad facies, slowed psychomotor activity, difficulty in concentration, and a continuous depressive affect over the past two years. His history is of interest as it evidences so many features seen in depressed young people. Early in life he exhibited significant parental separation anxiety, had difficulty on entering kindergarten and first grade, and refused to stay at summer camp after he had been there only three days. During his latency years he was frequently convinced that he was gravely ill with serious physical diseases, although in reality he was a healthy child. Despite being a strong and well-coordinated young man, he did not enjoy sports of any type. He gradually came to feel more comfortable in the presence of girls rather than boys, but always in a nonsexual fashion. He was an excellent student, but obtained little satisfaction from his success. Toward the end of his high school years his father died after a long, lingering illness. The father's illness was complicated by the fact that the proper diagnosis was not made until months after he began to feel ill, despite his being examined in leading medical centers. As a result, the mother had accused the father of being lazy, and indifferent to the needs of his family. Martin found himself caught in the struggle between them. After his father's death, Martin felt very guilty about his feelings and behavior toward his father during the latter's illness, and gradually became more overtly depressed. He entered college in his hometown, as he was reluctant to go away, and finished the first year with a B average. (His school was one of the best Ivy League colleges, with high academic standards.) He was, however, dissatisfied with his academic performance. At the beginning of his sophomore year he became even more isolated than previously from his fellow students; he felt terrified of the future, and could not even determine the choice of a major field of study, much less make a long-term career decision.

When initially seen, Martin was profoundly depressed and still vaguely suicidal. He had no plans for the future, and his reason for seeking therapy was that everyone said he should do so. He spent the first several weeks of therapy staying at home and seldom venturing out. He was in fact the picture of a classic anhedonic depressive. Even his fantasies and dreams were full of depressive symbolism.

Therapy with such youngsters is difficult, to say the least. Many therapists would have urged hospitalization. I offered it as a definite possibility, but he was terrified of the prospect. He was given an antidepressant medication for two reasons: first, he was so depressed as to make meaningful therapy very difficult; and second, the strong suicidal potential still persisted. Within a month he was clinically less depressed, working at a menial job and beginning to become involved in his therapy. He was still very pessimistic about the future and very isolated from his peer group. Strong encouragement was given him to become more active socially. Since I did not believe that he was truly a schizoid individual, I was not afraid that such a move might backfire. Martin was surprised to find that people (still only females) enjoyed his company, and was especially amazed when one girl became annoyed at his lack of sexual interest in her. He himself wondered whether he was a homosexual; actually he was functioning as an asexual with all libidinal impulses repressed. After a period of approximately six months he began to discuss the painful issue of his father's illness and death. He greatly admired his father's success in his profession and his dedicated hard work, but had sided with his mother in feeling neglected by his father, long before his father's illness brought the issue to the forefront. His parents had had frequent arguments, almost always initiated by the mother who felt neglected, and had threatened to leave and to obtain a divorce. Martin slowly began to understand his ambivalent identification with his father; he loved and admired and respected him, but encouraged by his mother, had also felt neglected and wondered if his father cared at all for him. To make matters worse, communication of personal thoughts and feelings was almost nonexistent within the family. One of the important early components of therapy was his discovery that it was not only acceptable but actually healthy to have feelings, and furthermore, whenever possible they should be communicated to other people. He was able to reexperience his early fears of leaving home—what was happening in his absence? Was mother going to leave father? He then was able to understand that his parents' overprotection of him only allowed these feelings to increase to the point where he was markedly different from and felt inferior to other youngsters.

This case illustrates the fact that severely depressed and suicidal patients can be treated in an outpatient setting. The use of antidepressant medication was probably an important facilitating agent in the therapeutic process. I believe that this is the ideal use of such medication—not as the sole or main therapeutic tool. The technical problems involved in Martin's therapy were: (1) the need to get him involved in therapy, as initially he was too depressed to care; (2) to help Martin realize that emotions and feelings were healthy, as were their expression; (3) to support him when he began to face his mixed feelings about his father and his father's death. (It probably would not surprise too many therapists to learn that Martin's mother tended to discourage his questions about his father and his parents' relationship. Her response to such questions was, "It is best to leave such matters alone—talking about them can do no good.")

5. Jane, a 16-year-old, was first seen while a junior in high school on referral from her physician. She had been complaining of excessive fatigue and apathy for several months and he could find no physical cause for these symptoms. Jane was the fourth and youngest child of elderly parents. Her father had had a serious drinking problem and died when she was nine years of age; she had been very close to him. They lived in an isolated area, and the two of them would spend hours talking and walking together. After his death she became even more isolated from her peers, and spent a great deal of time in fantasy, picturing herself as a great writer or artist. She was unhappy in the regional high school and transferred as a day pupil to a private school; here she was even less successful socially, and began to exhibit hysterical and histrionic behavior.

Jane was extremely reluctant to enter therapy. She would reiterate: (1) she had no problems; (2) if she did have problems, they were all physical in nature; (3) she could not understand why the other youngsters rejected her. Toward the end of the school year she became very depressed and withdrawn. Frequently she either did not go to school or would call her mother to take her home after attending only a few hours. When the school insisted that she either attend or withdraw, she panicked, wanting to be hospitalized and insisting that she had an undiagnosed brain tumor.

Antidepressant medication was tried without success; small amounts of minor tranquilizers helped to keep her anxiety under control. Therapy was aided by the cooperation of both the mother and the school. Although the former was frightened and did not fully understand what was happening to her daughter, she realized the need to help and finally to be firm and not respond to the girl's frantic demands to be taken home from school. During her senior year Jane did improve and became more involved in therapy, but still found it difficult to understand her own role in the company of her peers. She would say, "I'm too mature for the other students here; things will be better when I go away to college."

By the end of high school Jane was off all medication. She had some apprehension about leaving for college, but after a brief period she began to adjust to and enjoy college life. I had tried, but to no avail, to get her to continue with therapy while at college. She refused, insisting that she had no further problems. She was seen over the Christmas holiday and complained of trouble with her roommate, but otherwise she was doing well. In the middle of the spring term she had a definite manic episode which was not drug-induced. Fortunately, she responded to a brief period of hospitalization.

This particular case illustrates the difficulty of working with an adolescent who, though depressed, avoided acknowledging it by somatization and projection. Antidepressant medication was of no assistance. In retrospect, it appears that Jane was a manic-depressive (bipolar type). The only hint of this was the hysterical behavior and the mood swings. Even careful psychologic testing failed to suggest such a diagnosis.

This brings us to the interesting question as to just how common are manic-depressive reactions in children and adolescents. For many years Campbell (1955) believed that this illness was fairly common in young people, but he had little support for his thesis. After a thorough review of the literature on the subject, Anthony and Scott (1960) concluded that it is extremely rare to find a clear-cut manic-depressive illness in adolescents.

The recent interest in manic-depression in adults has renewed interest in the possibility of its occurrence in adolescents. Several authors (Frommer, 1968; Gallemore and Wilson, 1972; Horowitz, 1977) have recently concluded that this illness is much more frequently encountered in adolescents than has been previously recognized. The tendency of American psychiatrists to overdiagnose schizophrenia and schizoaffective disorders has contributed to this problem. Jane, in retrospect, has to be considered a manic-depressive, and I would urge therapists to be alert to the fact that this syndrome may not be so rare in young people as we recently believed. As a footnote to Jane's case, many therapists would have suggested prophylactic lithium therapy; this was recommended, but rejected by the patient, who persisted in believing that the manic episode was a valuable experience related to her use of transcendental meditation.

Although the syndrome of anorexia nervosa is covered elsewhere in this volume, a brief note of it should none the less be made in this chapter. In my opinion, many youngsters with anorexia nervosa are not only struggling to control their fear of obesity by starvation, frequently utilizing obsessive-compulsive defenses, but are actually fundamentally depressed. Until that core of depression can be uncovered, the mere gain in weight so understandably the goal in therapy is only a first step.

6. Agnes was a 17-year-old girl seen for the first time at the beginning of her junior year in high school. Her parents' marriage had begun to deteriorate when she was 9 years old, and a most bitter and acrimonious four years passed before they were finally divorced. During that time Agnes had very mixed feelings toward her parents. She strongly identified with her father, who was a very successful man, and both hated and wanted to protect her mother in spite of believing her lazy and not a good mother. In fact, it appeared that her mother had been going through a serious depression. Agnes was perhaps a few pounds overweight, but not significantly so; however, she decided to diet, and as is typical of anorexics, lost all perspective. She lost 30 pounds, her menses ceased, and she was hyperactive and obsessed with the subject of food. She ritualistically reiterated certain numbers, had to walk through doors in a certain fashion, and used other obsessive-compulsive defenses. Unlike many with this syndrome, Agnes knew she was depressed. Just a week before her first session, while out boating she began to swim away from the boat, but was noticed and rescued. This was clearly a suicidal attempt. A very intelligent girl, Agnes had difficulty concentrating on her school work. She constantly tested her peers; she wished to be close to them but could not believe that anyone might care for her. She was terrified of sexual activity.

Agnes had been seen briefly by another therapist, given a trial of phenothiazine without benefit, and refused to consider antidepressant medication.

Therapy revealed that this girl had introjected both good and bad images of both parents. She felt compelled to achieve (father identification), as if she were her father's slave; hated her mother and yet yearned to protect her and to help her seek therapy. As is typical of many youngsters with this reaction, Agnes had a hypertrophied superego—accusing herself of being a horrible person for minor peccadilloes. Her real "crime" was the anger she felt toward both parents, now introjected in her unconscious. Work with Agnes was a grim experience; she took therapy very seriously—"the most important aspect of my life"—but she refused to realize that her eating habits were health-threatening and even life-threatening. She was often profoundly depressed and gave vent to feelings of helplessness and hopelessness, saying, "What is the use of living? What is there to live for, even if I get better? I will still be empty—nothing."

I briefly refer to this case only to underline the key role that depression plays in many anorexia nervosa cases. I might add that there is more disagreement over how to treat this syndrome than almost any other in the whole field of child psychiatry. Approaches vary from analysis, to drug-oriented therapy (phenothiazine and antidepressants), family therapy (Rosman et al., 1977), and lately behavior modification (Agras et al., 1974) has been strongly emphasized as the treatment of choice. There is little doubt that behavior modification in a hospital setting can quickly reverse the weight loss. However, Bruch (1977) has recently cautioned against the use of this approach, citing cases she has seen after successful weight gain where the patients have been severely depressed and suicidal. This reaction is not surprising, as (1) the underlying depression has not been treated, and (2) the youngster, as Bruch notes, who was so fearful of losing control, has had all initiative taken away from him by the people caring for him.

The approach used in treating depressed children and adolescents thus far described is essentially that of analytically oriented psychotherapy. Emphasis has been placed upon involving the parents in therapy—a necessity if the youngster is residing at home, and desirable and often helpful even if the patient is away at school. Other approaches are widely used. Most community mental health centers and college counseling services offer what can best be described as short-term, crisis-oriented therapy. There has been a remarkable interest lately in short-term therapy, based on analytic concepts (Sifneos, 1972). Most of this work has been confined to adults, or older adolescents in a college setting. It is therefore difficult to state how effective such a technique would be in treating depressed youngsters. However, few depressed children would seem to satisfy the criteria listed by Sifneos (1972) to describe those patients whom he considered suitable for such an approach. The crisis-oriented approach does not attempt to alter basic personality patterns or resolve neurotic depressive operations. It is possible that such a technique may allow a youngster to function better and that as a result he may grow emotionally. All too often, however, such therapy at best may offer temporary assistance, and may at times discourage more intensive therapy.

During the past decade family therapy (Minuchin, 1970) has played an increasingly important role in the entire field of child therapy. In fact at times it almost appears that family therapy may devour the entire field of child psychiatry. Certainly the techniques used conform to many of the principles outlined above. Family therapists include the parents and siblings, and their approach is often very useful in clarifying and altering family dynamics. As such, this therapy should be of assistance in the therapy of depressed youngsters. The tendency to minimize intrapsychic conflicts in this approach raises serious questions as to whether it can fundamentally influence the core of depressive feelings harbored by these children. As already mentioned, there are relatively few articles on the therapy of depression in youngsters, regardless of the approach used. The literature on family therapy has few references to this specific syndrome. There have been several very encouraging reports on the use of family therapy in treating anorexia nervosa, but the depressive aspects of this syndrome have not been mentioned at all. One can only await the test of time to properly evaluate the results of family therapy in the treatment of depressed children and adolescents.

Behavioral modification is another technique that has found widespread acceptance during the past decade. Little in this technique, however, bears on the treatment of depressed youngsters except for the subject of anorexia nervosa (Agras, 1974), where the adherents of this school have claimed very significant results. Bruch, as previously mentioned, has cautioned that this approach may be dangerous. It is difficult for me to perceive how behavior modification can be of value in the therapy of depressed youngsters.

The use of medication has been briefly mentioned. There are relatively few references to the use of medication for depressed children and adolescents in the literature on this subject, and there is little agreement as to its effectiveness. It does appear to be helpful in those youngsters who are overtly depressed and who exhibit the usual clinical symptomatology of depression as seen in adults (Freud, 1917; Frommer, 1968). Almost all references concern the use of one of the tricyclic antidepressants, rather than a monomine exidase inhibitor. The latter, if used, should follow an adequate trial of tricyclics, and then the same food restrictions indicated for adults would have to be followed. This would necessitate the youngster's being a responsible person. Attention should be given to the use of medication for enuretic children (antidepressants) and for hyperkinetic children with presumed minimal brain damage (stimulants and antidepressants). As noted above, some children with these symptoms are undoubtedly depressed. When medication is helpful we are pleased—but we should be careful not to overlook the child in our zeal to improve the symptoms.

There has been recent interest in the use of lithium for depressed youngsters who have a bipolar illness (Horowitz, 1977). As already mentioned, there is considerable debate about the occurrence of manic-depression in children and adolescents. There would appear to be no reason to hesitate to use lithium for this age group if one encounters a true manic-depressive reaction. There have been many reports recently on the use of lithium in treating some unipolar illness, but few in the age group under consideration in this book.

If medication is used, I believe it should be part of the therapeutic process and not the only proceudre employed. This approach to medication is consistent with good clinical practice—that of seeing the patient as a whole, not as just a collection of symptoms. It is also consistent with the therapeutic goal of achieving, if at all possible, alterations in the patient's fundamental defensive operations, rather than aiming at symptom removal or suppression.

Electroconvulsive therapy is used with much less frequency today than before the era of antidepressant medication. This form of therapy should be used (if ever) only as a last resort for depressed children and adolescents when psychotherapy and medication have failed and overwhelming depressive symptomatology remains, especially if there are suicidal tendencies.

Mention should be made of the role of residential placement (including hospitalization) in the therapeutic approach to depression in children and adolescents. Hospitalization, as noted earlier, can be useful for observation and evaluation of youngsters when somatic symptoms are present or when the suicidal risk is high. Most authors who mention therapy of depressed children do not recommend hospitalization. Masterson (1972), in his work with borderline patients and those with severe character disorders (many of whom he considered to be suffering from abandonment depression), initially recommended hospitalization as the treatment of choice. He has of late begun to work with similar patients on an outpatient basis. Certainly the cost, plus the shortage of hospitals capable of providing such care, make hospital confinement of limited value except in extreme circumstances. Residential placement for acting-out youngsters is often indicated; when any youngster is beyond the control of his parents, placement has to be considered. Continued acting-out only exacerbates the underlying problem and makes the likelihood of successful resolution that much less probable. Institutionalization offers the opportunity of limiting the patient's acting-out, giving him an opportunity to confront his problems. Unfortunately, very few institutions provide adequate therapy; all too many are necessarily custodial institutions which use a form of behavior-modification therapy, rewarding good and punishing bad behavior. For many delinquent youngsters, placement only enables them to meet other older and more delinquent youngster, who may help them become more adept and "successful" delinquents.

It is notoriously difficult to evaluate the effect of any one form of therapy for emotional and mental problems, especially concerning psychotherapy.

Because of the changes that different ages produce in youngsters, evaluating the effects of therapy for children and adolescents is even more unreliable. To complicate the matter further, there have been almost no long-term follow-up studies done on depressed children and adolescents. This is not strange, since even now the existence of this syndrome is still being debated.

On a personal note, I have been interested in and worked with depressed youngsters for the past fifteen years. Reviewing my records, children and adolescents with a diagnosis of depression make up almost half of the patients I see in that age category. This figure is comparable to an estimate of 40% given by Masterson (1972), while Frommer (1968) estimates 25% of his youthful patients suffer from depression. Although my personal cases represent too small a number for any significant statistical analysis, I will say that the proportion of depressed children and adolescents is definitely larger than that of youngsters with other neurotic reactions and character disorders.

Summary and Conclusion

It is my thesis that there is a definite clinical entity of depression in children and adolescents, but that the signs and symptoms are not only different from those seen in adults but vary with different age levels. I believe further that this syndrome exists in significant numbers, probably to an extent similar to that presented by depressive reactions in adults. It is important that this syndrome be recognized as early as possible, for depression is not only a most painful emotion with which to contend but one which may cause an afflicted youngster serious difficulty in his adademic life by reason of his inability to concentrate. Depression can affect his relations with his peers to a significant degree, and if acting-out behavior ensues, as it so often does, it can lead to serious delinquent behavior, sexual promiscuity, and illegitimate pregnancies, as well as alcohol and drug abuse. Last, but far from least, it can lead to suicide.

Numerous therapeutic approaches are used in the field of child psychotherapy, including the therapy of depression. It is this author's firm belief that when a child or adolescent is truly depressed, the treatment of choice is individual, psychoanalytically oriented therapy, provided that the parents are also involved in a similar therapeutic program, if possible with the same therapist. Even if the child is living away from home, some contact with the parents on the part of the therapist is important. Medication at times may be a useful adjunct to such therapy. The role of family therapy for depressed youngsters is still untested. I believe that good residential facilities (those with a therapeutic program in fact and not just in theory) can play a very important role in the therapy of depressed, acting-out youngsters.

It is also my thesis that when the depression of children and adolescents is not properly treated, it continues to take its toll, leading to life-long depression, delinquency, and substance abuse. However, when depressed youngsters receive proper therapy the results are truly rewarding. As one patient stated, "When I wake up in the morning these days the sun is shining—before, it was always dark and gloomy."

One last word: as important as therapy is, prevention of depression in young people is even more so. If my thesis is correct—that depression results from the diminished self-esteem caused by loss of significant love-objects in a child's life—then we should be alert to the effect that the present high divorce rate is likely to produce upon youngsters from disrupted families. It is unlikely that anything is going to lower the divorce rate; all evidence seems to indicate that it will become even higher. We can, however, help parents, courts, teachers, and others involved with young people to become more aware of the possible lasting effects divorce can produce and thereby minimize the damage to children from marital breakdown.

Suicidal Behavior

Introduction

Suicide and suicidal attempts (Toolan, 1962a, 1962b, 1974) are not rare in childhood and adolescence, and of late have been increasing at a frightening rate. This fact has only begun to be appreciated even by professionals in the field due to the mistaken belief that children and adolescents to not experience true depression and hence are unlikely to commit suicide. Freud early exploded the myth of sexual innocence in children; the myth of childhood happiness has lasted much longer and has been even more difficult to shatter. A glance at suicidal rates in the United States clearly shows that the number of suicides among adolescents has seen the greatest rise of any age group. The suicidal rate for persons aged 15 to 19 in 1950 was 2.7 per 100,000; by 1973 that rate had reached 7 per 100,000. Suicides among the 20-to-24-year age group in 1950 numbered 8.1 per 100,000; in 1973 this rate had risen to 14.8 of every 100,000 persons, and at present exceeds the rate of suicides in the population as a whole, which is 12 out of every 100,000 people.

Formerly, the rate for suicide was highest among the elderly and lowest among the young; it now appears that the rates are being reversed. Similar figures for suicide among the young are found in many other countries. In the United States, suicide at present rates as the fourth leading cause of death in the 15-to19-year age group, being surpassed only by accidents, malignant neoplasms, and homicide. It must also be borne in mind that all reported rates for suicide are underestimated—more so for children and adolescents than for adults. Many well-meaning individuals, including physicians and medical examiners, are loath to label the death of a youngster a suicide unless they can visualize "the smoking gun." Numerous obvious cases of suicide are labeled accidents. The Suicide Prevention Center of Los Angeles has estimated that up to 50% of all suicides are disguised as accidents. Since we have become increasingly aware that many accidents are attempts at self-destruction, and also know that accidents currently lead all the causes of death in childhood and adolescence by a large margin, the inference to be drawn is obvious. Certain accidents are especially suspect as being suicidal in nature, such as one-car accidents. In the few incidences where psychological autopsies have been performed following an accident, this conclusion has been dramatically supported. At times the intention of the victim may be ambivalent, but it is none the less present in a significant number of cases. Males consistently outnumber females in *death* by suicide in all age groups throughout the world. To some extent this may reflect the fact that men use more violent methods of suicide such as hanging or shooting themselves. Females tend to use wrist-slashing and overdosing with medication as preferred suicidal methods, where a larger margin for error exists and a subsequent higher rescue rate occurs.

If statistics for suicide itself are unreliable, the figures on suicidal attempts are almost entirely worthless. Most communities do not require the keeping of such statistics, and even hospital records are notoriously inadequate in recording definite suicide attempts as contrasted to overdoses of medication taken by confused patients. One thing is certain—many more people attempt suicide than succeed. Another fact which holds true throughout the world is that females consistently outnumber males in *attempted* suicide.

Historical Background

There have been surprisingly few studies on suicidal attempts by children and adolescents. In 1937, Bender and Schilder, working at Bellevue Hospital in New York, described 18 youngsters under 18 years of age who had either threatened or attempted suicide. The authors felt that these children were trying to cope with intolerable living situations, which caused them to become very angry and in turn to experience feelings of guilt about their anger. In 1959 Balser and Masterson, working in a private psychiatric hospital, reported that of a group of 500 adolescent patients, 37 had attempted suicide. In 1960, while at Bellevue Hospital, I (1962a) reviewed the statistics on children and adolescents who had either seriously threatened or actually attempted suicide. 102 out of 900 admissions fell into that category—a much higher rate than that reported by Bender and Schilder twenty-three years earlier in the very same setting. A breakdown by age groups showed that 18 youngsters were under 12 years of age, and 84 were between 12 and 17 years. The youngest child in this series was only 5 years of age. Further analysis of the youngsters in this group showed that the majority came from disorganized and chaotic homes. Less than one-third had both parents present in the home; fathers were conspicuous by their absence. It was of interest that first children were represented to a disproportionate degree. When I examined the diagnostic categories, the vast majority were suffering from behavioral and character disorders. As a group, they were immature, impulsive youngsters reacting violently and often excessively to various stresses; by far the majority consisted of angry youngsters—the anger usually directed toward parents or parent surrogates, for what was often genuine neglect. This anger had become introjected as guilt and depression and diminished self-esteem. Many of the females used suicidal behavior as an attempt to manipulate or to punish another person. There were a few individuals who used suicide as a dramatic effect, to call attention to their needs—a "signal of distress."

In 1964 Schrut studied 19 adolescent suicidal patients. He described them as a very hostile, self-destructive group, and postulated a mechanism similar to that offered by this author—namely, that the child felt neglected and therefore was angry at the parents, and his resultant behavior in turn usually aroused the parents' anger.

Another type of suicidal patient is represented by the frustrated perfectionist. Studies of suicidal college students by Blaine (1975) and Nicoli (1967) reveal that these young people are often first-rate students who nevertheless are dissatisfied with their academic performance. Since they cannot tolerate being less than perfect, their unrealistic drives are often unattained, with the result that they turn to self-destruction.

Theoretical Concepts

When one works with parents of children who have attempted suicide it is not uncommon to encounter the reaction: "He really didn't mean to kill himself—he doesn't even know what death means." It is of interest that the children, when questioned, are usually very definite about their intentions until they encounter such a reaction from the parents. This is just another instance of adult unwillingness to be realistic about children. A child's idea of death may be somewhat different from that of an adult, but most children from the age of five or six have a fairly realistic idea of death. One might add that adults have equally vague ideas as to what constitutes death—concepts ranging from living forever with God in heaven, to transmigration of souls, to the belief that death is total annihilation of the person. Many children and adolescents who attempt suicide have often mentioned the idea of doing so previously, and many have even made earlier attempts. Also, suicidal youngsters have often run away from home, with the fantasy, "You'll be sorry for what you have done to me." A good number have been seen by physicians and mental health workers prior to the suicidal episode. It is still amazing at this late date to hear the statement "People who talk about suicide never attempt it." No notion could be further from the truth. Another fact which emerges in studying suicidal children is that they are often not asked, even when in therapy, whether they are suicidal. Unless asked, many will be reluctant to volunteer the information. Occasionally one still hears the old rubric "If you ask a child about suicide you may suggest it to him." This is patently absurd; children are no more suggestible than adults. If they were, we would not need so many mental health workers and correctional institutions.

The first step in working with suicidal youngsters (as with suicidal patients of any age) is to evaluate as best one can the suicidal risk. This is a challenging task with any patient but even more so with children and adolescents. The parents and occasionally other involved persons often complicate the issue further by insisting it was all a mistake and that the child did not know what he was doing. It is also not unusual to find the parents very angry at the child—"How could he have done this to me?" For these reasons it is often desirable to place such a youngster in a hospital setting for a period of evaluation and observation. This disrupts the interaction between the child and parents and allows more objective personnel, such as nurses, to observe the child's behavior. A general hospital is preferable and usually available in every community for it allows the child to be near home, rather than a psychiatric hospital which is often some distance away.

When suicidal children and adolescents are seen shortly after a suicidal attempt, they often appear to be angry rather than depressed as are most adults in such a situation. This should not mislead the examiner, as most youngsters under 14 to 15 years of age do not overtly evidence the signs and symptoms of depression and often use anger as a cover for depressive feelings. Psychological testing is often of assistance in these cases, but here again one will find an angry protocol rather than a depressed one.

This period of evaluation should not only include the children but the parents as well, especially if there is the possibility that the child can return home. It is also helpful whenever possible to interview friends, teachers, or clergy who may be involved with such a youngster. Parents are often the last people to know how a child feels. I always inquire whether a diary has been kept and ask for permission to read it; girls especially tend to pour out their most important feelings in such writing. Information thus obtained is often useful in convincing parents that their child has been seriously contemplating suicide for some time. It is very important to get a good, detailed history of the events leading up to the suicidal attempt. If a youngster carefully plans to take an overdose of medication when alone in the house, not expecting anyone to return for several hours, it is obviously a more serious attempt than one who cuts his wrists in front of his parents.

If a period of hospitalization is used for evaluative purposes, it should last for at least a week. It is a well-known phenomenon that immediately after a suicidal attempt many patients have purged themselves temporarily of their depressive feelings and may appear almost euphoric. When dealing with students at a prep school or college, the school infirmary is the ideal location for such a period of evaluation. An advantage of using this facility is that the student can continue to attend classes and thereby one can determine his ability to continue in an academic institution.

At the end of this observation period a therapeutic plan should be determined. Some youngsters are either so disturbed or their homes so chaotic that placement in a hospital or residential institution is desirable. The majority, however, can return home or remain in school if therapy is provided. I firmly believe that everyone who attempts suicide requires therapy. Some will scoff at this statement and reply, "What? Even those who use this behavior to punish or manipulate another person?" The answer is an emphatic yes. Anyone who resorts to such drastic behavior to convince another person is either severely dependent, insecure, or frightened by an overwhelming feeling of loneliness. Any of these entities, in my opinion, require help. It is my personal experience that difficulties encountered by the physician in treatment lie not so much with the young suicidal patient (most of the time they are only too willing to accept help) but with the parents, who wish to pretend that everything is fine, or with the school authorities who are frightened of allowing such youngsters to remain with them lest they make another suicidal attempt. I believe that if the youngster is capable of functioning academically and a therapy plan can be arranged, he should continue in school. If, however, the youngster cannot concentrate, or school itself is the overwhelming problem, a medical leave of absence is indicated.

No one treatment plan will be suitable for all youngsters who attempt suicide. In general, I base treatment on the premise that depression is always present, and advocate the use of the same methods as have been discussed in the section on therapy for depressed children and adolescents. Once again, it is imperative that parents be involved, even when the youngster is away from home. All too often the parents may be frightened initially, and want help for the child, but when things have improved somewhat they may urge them to discontinue therapy. For example, a 16-year-old girl who was both depressed and had suicidal ideation requested therapy. Her father, a professional man, was totally in favor of the plan; in fact, even though he was aware that my schedule was very full, he emphasized his daughter's need and asked me to see her at least twice a week. Within a month, he was pointing out to his daughter the expense of therapy. Fortunately, I was able to meet with him and his daughter together to resolve the issue, which really did not exist since he was well provided with insurance coverage. He then admitted that he felt uncomfortable with the thought that his daughter "was so sick as to require intensive treatment."

As was also mentioned in the section on therapy of depression, medication may be of great assistance in treating those youngsters who are overtly depressed (cf. Martin, in section on therapy of depression). Such medication may, if efficacious, facilitate the patient's ability to engage in the therapeutic process and also help reduce the suicidal risk. We must bear in mind that antidepressant medication, even when effective, takes two to three weeks to produce its full therapeutic effect. Those suicidal youngsters who are essentially clinically angry do not seem to respond well to antidepressant medication.

In any discussion of medication for suicidal patients, mention must be made of the use of sedation. Many suicidal and/or depressed persons have difficulty sleeping. Unfortunately, barbiturates are usually prescribed; not only are they a danger to life if used by suicidal patients, but there are better ways to improve the altered sleep pattern. Tricyclics are very useful, and if a sedative is needed, flurazepam hydrochloride appears to be the safest to use at present.

The question of duration of therapy and type of therapy can be determined only after a thorough evaluation and diagnostic workup. Both individual and family therapy are used (cf. section on therapy of depression). If medication is prescribed it should be as an adjunct to therapy, rather than the sole method. As a general rule, the same principles of therapy previously discussed *re* depressed children and adolescents would apply to suicidal youngsters. By and large, the same qualities and training needed in a therapist for depressed children and adolescents would be required for the treatment of young suicidal patients. One should not overlook the fact that the therapy of suicidal patients takes a toll of the therapist. He may find himself frightened of the burden of suicidal risk, and find himself ruminating about such patients. He may fear that his reputation will suffer if one of his patients should commit suicide, especially if the youngster comes from a well-known family. Possibly some therapists would do better not to work with suicidal patients. As a general rule, it is wise for most therapists not to have more than one or two acutely suicidal patients in therapy at the same time, lest the therapist become emotionally depleted. In my opinion, the same criteria hold true in selecting a therapist for young suicidal patients as for depressed youngsters: the situation requires an individual with sound training in child psychiatry and child development as well as a good knowledge of depressive and suicidal ideation in young people and a knowledge of psychopharmacology. Unfortunately, relative few such therapists exist.

There is no way that one can evaluate the results of therapy with suicidal youngsters, or for that matter, of suicidal patients of any age. Follow-up studies in psychiatry are uncommon, and when we look for follow-up statistics on suicidal patients they are even more rare. There have been a few such studies of suicidal adults who have had psychiatric hospitalization, but the vast number of suicidal patients never see a psychiatric hospital. Follow-up studies of suicidal children and adolescents are almost nonexistent. We do not even have a baseline of suicidal youngsters who have had therapy, as opposed to those who have not had therapy of any kind.

Under such circumstances I can only give an impressionistic report based on my own clinical experience. Certainly the majority of youngsters who attempt suicide never get adequate treatment. Most of them survive. How many untreated patients continue to lead depressed lives, to abuse alcohol and drugs, to exhibit acting-out and delinquent behavior? In my opinion, a sizable percentage develop as emotionally handicapped persons. As a general rule, those suicidal youngsters whom I have personally had in therapy have done very well. Once in therapy they tend to become quite involved, pleased that someone has taken their situation seriously. Their prognoses (not only for survival but for successful resolution of underlying problems) on the whole has been quite good.

Summary

Suicide and suicidal attempts have been widely ignored in children and adolescents. The sober fact is that the rate of suicide in the 15-to-19 and 19-to-24-year age group is increasing more rapidly than that at any other age. Many attempts at suicide are made by college students, often those who are considered outstanding academically. It is imperative that we abandon the myth that children do not become depressed, ergo do not commit suicide. Every suicidal attempt, no matter how manipulative, should be taken seriously. Suicidal youngsters, as well as suicidal adults, should have a period of evaluation, either in a school infirmary or a general hospital. It is of the utmost importance to include the parents in the evaluative workup, and to include them in any subsequent therapeutic plan. There is a definite tendency on the part of adults, especially parents, to underestimate the significance of suicidal behavior on the part of youngsters.

The author has defined his concept of suicidal behavior as a manifestation of depression, and has outlined a procedure to be followed in the evaluation and therapy of suicidal children and adolescents.

References

Abraham, K. (1927) Notes on the psychoanalytic investigation and treatment of manic-depressive insanity and allied conditions. In *Selected Papers*. London: Hogarth.

Agras, S. (1959) The relationship of school phobia to childhood depression. *Am. J. Psychiat.* 116:533–536.

Agras, S., D.H. Barlow, G.G. Abel, and H. Leitenberg. (1974) Behavior modification of anorexia nervosa. *Arch. Gen. Psychiat.* 30:279–286.

American Psychiatric Assocation. (1968) *Diagnostic and Statistical Manual of Mental Disorders*, 2nd ed. Washington, D.C.: American Psychiatric Association.

Anthony, J. (1970) Two contrasting types of adolescent depression and their treatment. *J. Am. Psychiat. Assn.* 18:841–859.

Anthony, J., and P. Scott. (1960) Manic-depressive psychosis in childhood. *J. Child Psychol. Psychiat.* 1:53–72.

Arieti, S., ed. (1959) *American Handbook of Psychiatry*, Vo. 2. New York: Basic Books.

Balser, B., and J.F. Masterson. (1959) Suicide in adolescents. *Am. J. Psychiat.* 115:400–405.

Beck, A.T. (1967) *Depression*. New York: Hoeber.

Bender, L., and P. Schilder. (1937) Suicidal occupations and attempts in children. *Am J. Orthopsychiat.* 7:225–234.

Bibring, E. (1953) The mechanism of depression. In P. Greenacre, ed., *Affective Disorders*. New York: International Universities Press.

Blaine, G.B. (1975) Presentation at Workshop on Psychotherapy with Suicidal Adolescents, Society for Adolescent Psychiatry, Los Angeles, California.

Bowlby, J. (1960) Childhood mourning and its implications for psychiatry. *Am. J. Psychiat.* 118:481–498.

Bruch, H. (1977) Anorexia nervosa. In S.C. Feinstein and P. Giovacchini, eds., *Adolescent Psychiatry*, Vol. 5. New York: Jason Aronson.

Campbell, J.D. (1955) Manic-depressive disease in children. *J.A.M.A.* 158:154–157.

Cytryn, L., and D.H. McKnew. (1972) Proposed classification of childhood depression. *Am. J. Psychiat.* 129:149.

Despert, J.L. (1952) Suicide and depression in children. *Nerv. Child* 9:378–389.

Easson, W.M. (1977) Depression in adolescence. In S.C.

Feinstein and P. Giovacchini, eds., *Adolescent Psychiatry*, Vol. 5. New York: Jason Aronson.

Engel, G.L., and F. Reichsman. (1956) Spontaneous and experimentally induced depressions in an infant with a gastric fistula. *J. Am. Psychoanal. Assn.* 4:428–453.

Fairbairn, W.R.D. (1954) *An Object-Relation Theory of the Personality.* New York: Basic Books.

Freud, S. (1917) *Mourning and Melancholia.* Standard Edition, Vol. 14. London: Hogarth Press, 1949.

Frommer, E.A. (1967) Treatment of childhood depression with antidepressant drugs. *Brit. Med. J.* 1:729–732.

Frommer, E.A. (1968) Depressive illness in childhood in recent developments in affective disorders. A symposium. A. Cappen and A. Walk, eds. *Brit. J. Psychiat.* special publication #2, pp. 117–136.

Gallemore, J.L., and W.P. Wilson. (1972) Adolescent maladjustment, or affective disorder? *Am. J. Psychiat.* 129:608–612.

Goldfarb, W. (1946) Effects of psychological deprivation in infancy and subsequent stimulation. *Am. J. Psychiat.* 102:18–33.

Horowitz, H.A. (1977) Lithium and the treatment of adolescent manic-depressive illness. *Dis. Nerv. Syst.* 38:480–483.

Kanner, L. (1960) *Child Psychiatry.* Springfield, Ill.: Charles C. Thomas.

Kaufman, I., and L. Heims. (1958) The body image of the juvenile delinquent. *Am. J. Orthopsychiat.* 28:146–159.

Keeler, W.R. (1954) Children's reaction to the death of a parent. In P. Hoch and J. Zubin, eds., *Depression.* New York: Grune & Stratton.

Klerman, G.L. (1971) CLinical research in depression. *Arch. Gen. Psychiat.* 24:305–319.

Ling, W., G. Oftedal, and W. Weinberg. (1970) Depressive illness in childhood presenting as a severe headache. *Am. J. Disab. Child.* 120:122–124.

Malmquist, C.P. (1971) Depression in childhood and adolescence. *New Eng. J. Med.* 284:887–893; 955–961.

Malmquist, C.P. (1977) Psychodynamic treatment of childhood depression. In E. Usdin, ed., *Depression.* New York: Brunner/Mazel.

Masterson, J.F. (1967) *The Psychiatric Dilemma of Adolescence.* Boston: Little, Brown.

Masterson, J.F. (1972) *Treatment of the Borderline Adolescent—A Developmental Approach.* New York: Wiley-Interscience.

Minuchin, S. (1970) The use of an ecological framework in the treatment of a child. In E. Anthony and C. Koupernick, eds., *The Child in His Family.* New York: Wiley.

Nicoli, A.M. (1967) Harvard dropouts: Some psychiatric findings. *Am. J. Psychiat.* 124:105–112.

Poznanski, E.O., and J.P. Zrull. (1970) Childhood depression. *Arch. Gen. Psychiat.* 23:8–15.

Poznanski, E.O., V. Krahenbuhl, and J.P. Zrull. (1976) Childhood depression—A longitudinal perspective. *J. Am. Acad. Child Psychiat.* 15:491–501.

Rie, H.E. (1967) Depression in childhood: A survey of some pertinent contributions. *J. Am. Acad. Child Psychiat.* 5:653–685.

Rochlin, G. (1959) The loss complex. *J. Am. Psychoanal. Assn.* 7:299–316.

Rosman, B.L., S. Minuchin, R. Liebam, and L. Baker. (1977) Imput and outcome of family therapy in anorexia nervosa. In S.C. Feinstein and P. Giovacchini, eds., *Adolescent Psychiatry,* Vol. 5. New York: Jason Aronson.

Sandler, J., and W.G. Joffe. (1965) Notes on childhood depression. *Int. J. Psychoanal.* 46:88–96.

Schrut, A. (1964) Sucidal adolescents and children. *J.A.M.A.* 188:1103–1107.

Sifneos, P.E. (1972) *Short-Term Psychotherapy and Emotional Crisis.* Cambridge: Harvard University Press.

Sperling, M. (1959) Equivalents of depression in children. *J. Hillside Hosp.* 8:138–148.

Spitz, R., and K.M. Wolf. (1946) Anaclitic depression: An inquiry into the genesis of psychiatric conditions in early childhood. *Psychoanal. Study Child* 2:313–341.

Toolan, J.M. (1960) Changes in personality structure during adolescence. In J.H. Masserman, ed., *Science and Psychoanalysis.* New York: Grune & Stratton.

Toolan, J.M. (1962a) Depression in children and adolescents. *Am. J. Orthopsychiat.* 32:404–415.

Toolan, J.M. (1962b) Suicide and suicidal attempts in chldren and adolescents. *Am. J. Psychiat.* 118:719–724.

Toolan, J.M. (1974) Depression and suicide. In S. Arieti, ed., *American Handbook of Psychiatry*, 2nd ed. New York: Basic Books.

Wallerstein, J.S., and J.B. Kelly. (1975) The effects of parental divorce—Experiences of the preschool child. *J. Am. Acad. Child Psychiat.* 14:600–616.

Treatment of Emotional Disorders in Children and Adolescents

CHAPTER 35

Running Away and the Treatment of the Runaway Reaction

Richard L. Jenkins

Introduction

Running away is a time-honored method that adolescents have used to escape from parental control, sometimes with good reason, more often simply in pursuit of adventure and/or independence. In the last century "running away to sea" was a traditional method for boys to escape parental dominance. However, in recent decades running away from home on the part of the adolescents has assumed epidemic proportions, noticed particularly in suburbs and middle-class neighborhoods (Shellow et al., 1967; Ambrosino, 1971; Chapman, 1976). It resulted in regions such as Haight-Asbury in San Francisco becoming inundated with young runaways, who were then exposed to the "hippie" culture. The runaway adolescent is often the willing or even the eager victim of the commerce in illegal drugs. This results in drug-related crime, chiefly crime to get money to buy drugs. It results in some incidence of addiction, although the addicting drugs, such as heroin, are not as widely used by runaways as are some other drugs. It results in the spread of infectious hepatitis. The epidemic proportions of running away and the resultant casual living have contribuged to the rapidly rising rate of venereal disease among the very young, and of course to the unwanted pregnancies. The runaway adolescent is typically an easy victim, particularly when attracted to drugs, as was witnessed by the discovery of the bodies of some thirty adolescent boys in Texas—the victims of sexual murders. On the other hand, the rootless and runaway adolescent or young adult may be drawn into crime, particularly by a self-righteous and charismatic leader such as Charles Manson.

The epidemic of runaways from middle-class homes would develop only in an affluent society. It has been pointed out that the ability of Charles Manson's girls to make "delicious meals" from what they could retrieve from garbage cans could occur only in a land of plenty.

The following are reasons adolescents may give for running away from home:

- The desire for adventure.
- The desire for independence or for "freedom" as the adolescent sees it. This concerns particularly the freedom to associate with companions of his or her choice, who are often disapproved by parents.
- The desire for sexual freedom.
- The desire to drink beer or other alcoholic beverages.
- The desire to smoke pot (marijuana) or to use drugs.
- The desire to escape from a brutal, overcritical, or alcoholic parent person.
- The desire to be relieved of pressure toward school achievement or conforming behavior.

An important distinction in relation to running away is whether the individual is *running to* or *running from*. The power in influence of the peer group is central for most of those who are *running to*. It is the freedom, the girlfriends or boyfriends, the parties, the group use of alcohol or other drugs that is likely to be the magnet here. Conflicts between these children and their parents is most likely to be over the parents' objection to such activities.

It might be pointed out that all peoples have made some use of drugs that change the way the person feels if indeed they have knowledge of such drugs. Our own culture has long made use of caffeine in coffee, tea, and cola, of nicotine in tobacco, and of alcohol for such purposes. The younger generation has added cannabis and a wide variety of chemicals with varying effects. The new chemical always arouses suspicion from the older generation, and often justly so. Cigarettes have added enormously to our health problems. Alcohol is our major drug problem at present, with very deleterious effects upon family members as well as on the individual himself. Alcohol has been the drug of the older generation, not of the younger. Perhaps this is changing, in that alcohol is increasingly popular with the younger generation. Alcohol is widely related to violent and irresponsible actions. Cannabis seems to stimulate such actions in very few people.

Besides those adolescents who are *running to*, there are those adolescents who are *running from*. Such running is usually from a parent, a severe father or stepfather, a critical mother or stepmother.

Running away from home is usually a benign event. Most juvenile runaways soon return home. Because of their numbers, the hardships they encounter, and their need for shelter and food, runaway houses or shelters have been established in many cities. Such houses may require communication, usually by phone, with the parents of runaways, and sometimes their permission for him or her to stay. Usually there is a time limit, often a week, on how long the youngster can stay in the runaway houses or shelter. Most runaway children return home. Some repeat their running away. A few are able to support themselves by legitimate work in the community. Others support themselves by begging, stealing, selling drugs, or prostitution.

The running away of a child or adolescent is usually invariably an indication of a problem or need within the family, relating to the other members of the family as well as to the runaway child. Help through counseling for *both* child and parents is always indicated. In most cases the problems can be ameliorated, if not resolved, through family therapy.

Runaway reaction is a diagnostic term that is limited to a particular group with a somewhat internalized or ingrained tendency to solve problems by running away.

History

The term *runaway reaction of childhood (or adolescence)* first appears as a diagnostic category in DSM-II, the revised *Diagnostic and Statistical Manual of Mental Disorders* of the American Psychiatric Association (1968). Here it is one of the behavior disorders of childhood and adolescence. The characterization of the behavior disorders is as follows: "This major category is reserved for disorders occurring in childhood and adolescence that are more stable, internalized and resistent to treatment than transient situational disturbances, but less so than psychoses, neuroses and personality disorders. This intermediate stability is attributed to the greater fluidity of all behavior at this age."

Under the behavior disorders in DSM-II are listed the *hyperkinetic reaction of childhood (or adolescence)*, the *withdrawing reaction of childhood (or adolescence)*, the *overanxious reaction of childhood (or adolescence)*, the *runaway reaction of childhood (or adolescence)* (Jenkins, 1971, 1973), the *unsocialized aggressive reaction of childhood (or adolescence)* and the *group delinquent reaction of childhood (or adolescence)*. Of these six *behavior disorders*, only the last three commonly lead to involvement with the police and the courts.

The characterization of the *runaway reaction* in DSM-II is as follows: "Individuals with this disorder characteristically escape from threatening situations by running away from home for a day or more without permission. Typically they are immature and timid, and they feel rejected at home, inadequate, and friendless. They often steal furtively." It is necessary for the diagnosis that the individual *characteristically* escape from threatening situations by running away from home.

It is worth while to consider the relation of the *runaway reaction* to the two other behavior disorders that bring adolescents and children into conflict with the law.

The group delinquent has a basic socialization, acquired in early childhood, usually through his contact with a nurturant and caring mother. He typically has lacked the guidance of an effective and interested father, has lived in a delinquency area, is a product of a large family, has gravitated to the street, and there become a part of a street gang, which then tends to become a delinquent gang by a natural process of growth.

By contrast with the *group delinquent reaction*, those children and adolescents showing the *unsocialized aggressive reaction*, and in particular the *runaway reaction*, have commonly experienced a lack of early nurturing and have failed to develop an adequate capacity for a reciprocal, friendly, interpersonal feeling and relationship with others. They are, as a consequence, egocentric and lacking in compassion, unhappy, fearful, or hostile, and often bitter in their relation to other human beings. The Minnesota Multiphasic Personality Inventory (MMPI) and the Parent-Child Relations Questionnaire (PCR) tend to differentiate these groups (Shinohara and Jenkins, 1967; Tsubouchi and Jenkins, 1969), at least from the *group delinquent reaction*.

If a rejected child has good musculature and is somewhat protected against the outside world from the consequences of his own actions by his family, he is likely to become an *unsocialized aggressive* individual. If his rejection has been more profound, if he has no special compensating abilities, then his courage is likely to be more completely broken and the end product may well be the chronic runaway that we know as the *runaway reaction*.

While DSM-II is the first use of *runaway reaction* as a diagnosis, a similar group was recognized by Herbert Quay (Quay, 1966; Quay, Morse, and Cutter, 1964, 1966) in his factor analytic studies of delinquent boys. His *behavior category 1*, (*BC-1*), *inadequate*, *immature*, conforms to the pattern of the *runaway reaction*, except that not all of his boys have run away—as yet.

The basic problem of these children is one of lack of confidence and security in parent persons, with resultant lack of ties, lack of confidence, fearfulness, and fear of staying at home for reason of actual or anticipated parental severity. In general, running away from home is often a more or less normal exploration of the outer world and may be a venturesome activity. What distinguishes the *runaway reaction* is not venturesomeness, but rather timidity; not exploration, but rather flight.

A statistical clustering study of 300 boys in the New York State Training School for Boys (Jenkins and Boyer, 1967) disclosed three significantly different groups. There was one group of socialized delinquents, called in DSM-II *group delinquent reaction*, characterized by gang activity, cooperative stealing, and undesirable companions. There was one group of unsocialized aggressive delinquents, characterized by assaultive tendencies, defiance, bullying, active homosexuality, and destructiveness. There was one group of runaway delinquents characterized by stealing in the home, repeatedly running away from home overnight, and staying out late at night. When three groups were selected on the basis o the presence of these traits, it was found that the runaway delinquents were significantly characterized by emotional immaturity, apathy, and seclusiveness. The study contained seven indicators of the degree of stability in the home or the degree of pathology there. One of these, *child with both parents*, was interpreted as showing stability, six of them as showing less in the way of stability. These were *only child*, *parental rejection*, *illegitimate child*, *child presently in other family*, *unwanted child* (at birth), and *foster child* (past or present). In every one of these indices, the *group delinquent reaction* showed the most favorable home background and the *runaway reaction*, the most unfavorable. One item, *overprotection by the parents*, was highest in the unsocialized aggressive and lowest in the unsocialized runaway group.

Theoretical Considerations

A basic characteristic which seems common to children showing the *runaway reaction* is a high degree of fearful egocentricity, a gross lack of trust, and a lack of empathy or the capacity to feel for others. Trust grows out of being taken care of and having one's emotional needs met. Sympathy for others grows out of having one's own emotional needs met and learning through cuddling, affectional exchange and play activities and tasks in common with others, to feel *with* others, to be empathetic and compassionate.

As was revealed by the study just cited, the children showing the *runaway reaction* have been the most lacking of the three groups in normal parenting. They are conspicuously lacking in trust and in empathy. Such a lack cannot fully be compensated for later. Loyalty is lacking, as well as trust. It is particularly important that those dealing with adolescents showing the *runaway reaction* be open, fair, consistent, and predictable. When loyalty cannot be used, the *self-interest of the adolescent* must be utilized by some type of behavior modification approach.

Since the basic problem is a gross lack of early socialization, those public measures that reduce the risk of unwanted, unwelcome children are probably the most important preventive public health measure. When infants are born to immature teenage girls who do not want motherhood, then a decision must be made as to whether to seek to give support to the mother and help her to accept the maternal role or whether it would be preferable to encourage severance of the maternal tie by adoption or otherwise. Probably the most important indicator here is the desire of the mother herself to keep the child, when indeed such desire is present, but it should be dealt with in a fashion in which she understands and, so far as possible, accepts the responsibilities of motherhood if she undertakes them.

Actual running away from home does not usually develop before the teenage period, although the character structure lending itself to this course develops decidedly earlier, and we have reported a notable example of an 11-year-old boy who was a wanderer for 22 years (Jenkins and Stahle, 1972).

As with any problem with children, in treatment one seeks to understand causes and to influence the behavior of the child. Some children run away because they are beaten or otherwise severely treated with great frequency at home. Some parents with rather limited resourcefulness seem able to develop no means of control other than severe punishment. Some parents are frankly rejecting of their children. Often, one parent is accepting and the other is severe, and the child has great difficulty in understanding or adjusting to a confusing situation of this sort.

If it is an unbroken home, and there are repeated runaways by the child or adolescent, then with the possible exception of a few brain-damaged children, it is rather safe to assume that there is severe pathology in the home relationships. If it is a broken home and a child wishes to be with the other parent, repeated running away to seek to accomplish this purpose is not at all difficult to understand.

One of our most repetitive runaways sought always to join the home of his grandmother, where he had spent his earliest years. After this period, he was not able to reconcile himself to the parental home, and not without some good reasons.

Relatively speaking, compared with other forms of actions classified as delinquent, running away is less uncommon and probably less pathological in teenage girls than in teenage boys. The fantasy of rescue by some prince charming leads unhappy teenage girls into many unwise actions in which they are or may be victimized.

Applicability

An ancient recipe for rabbit stew begins: "First you must catch the rabbit." One can hardly treat the adolescent showing a *runaway reaction* in his absence. In this regard there is a very ominous prospect as a result of the present children's rights movement. In general, its advocates insist that status offenses are not delinquency, and often they would deprive the juvenile court of any power over the status offender, including the unmanageable child and the chronic runaway adolescent. This would deprive the community of any means of dealing with this problem. The runaway boy may be supporting himself by burglary, the runaway girl by prostitution or by selling drugs. It is usually an easy matter for the police to apprehend a runaway as a runaway. If it is necessary to catch the runaway adolescent committing a burglary, committing prostitution, or selling drugs before they can be apprehended, then we will find ourselves sheltering a school for young criminals in every city.

Treatment in the Child's Own Home

The form treatment takes will depend to some extend on the location of the adolescent. Prevention or early treatment is always preferable to late treatment. If possible the child should be treated in his own home. This inevitably will demand the cooperation of his parents. If the adolescent is too much troubled by anxiety and if the therapist has effective influence with the parents, sometimes the adolescent can be persuaded to seek out the therapist or the therapeutic setting in a clinic rather than running away. If the family problem is severe, the objective is to prevent the adolescent from running away further, then the boy or girl *must* have someone to turn to for help or even refuge in place of running away.

Naturally, such problems cannot be resolved without work with parents as well as with adolescent.

Louise A. Homer (1973) reported work with twenty runaway girls. Seven out of the twenty were classified as running *from* and thirteen as running *to*. Among the seven running from an unfavorable family situation, six were successfully treated through the use of family therapy, plus insight-oriented individual treatment. Only one of these six had any occasion to return to the juvenile court, and this was on another charge that was dismissed after she remained out of further difficulty with the law. In the one case remaining, this treatment seemed helpful but proved insufficient. She continued to run away from home and was committed.

These seven girls who were running *from* seemed to fit into the picture of the *runaway reaction of adolescence*, although no diagnoses were offered.

The thirteen girls who were running *to* probably should not be classified as instances of the *runaway reaction*, but rather of the *group delinquent reaction*. "These girls were running to places and people who provide a variety of experiences that they are forbidden at home: sex, drugs, liquor, truancy, and a peer group that was usually involved in other more serious crimes. These girls expressed minor grievances with their parents, but seemed to feel in general that the home situation was not much different from anyone else's." The members of this group probably do not belong in the *runaway reaction of adolescence*.*

In some cases the home conflict cannot be sufficiently amerliorated with the adolescent in his or her own home. If adequate treatment resources are available in the community, placement in a group home or halfway house or shelter house may be acceptable to parents and to the adolescents while the process of treatment is undertaken. A foster home is less likely to be accepted by the parents or to work out with the adolescent, for foster-home placement usually implies to parents that their own home is inadequate or unfit—an admission they may be unwilling to make. On the side of the adolescent, placement in a foster home asks the adolescent to put down personal roots in a home with new parent persons at a time of life when reduction of ties of family dependence and family control is the logical step. This is swimming upstream.

For the foregoing reasons, the more impersonal controls of the group home or halfway house are likely to be better accepted by the adolescent than the more personal controls of the foster home. The group home or halfway house also does not imply (as does the foster home) that the problem is solely in the parental home.

Methods

The treatment of the *runaway reaction*, like treatment in general, begins with a careful history and diagnostic study. A rather frequent contributing factor is some slight and usually nonlocalizing damage to the central nervous system related frequently to a history of anoxia at birth or to maternal toxemia during pregnancy and sometimes reflected in grand mal seizures in infancy or childhood or other more gross or clear signs of central nervous system abnormality.

Some runaways, even though repeated, related to a recent unhappy situation in the home such as the mother's marriage to an alcoholic and perhaps brutal stepfather and the child's consequent repeated runaways. Of course, the prospect in such an acute reaction is much more favorable than in a chronic one, if corrective measures can be taken and are taken. Parental quarreling may lead to repeated runaways and sometimes can be resolved by marriage counseling or family therapy.

Removal of the adolescent from the home may give family problems an opportunity to quiet down, and for parents and adolescents alike to assess the positive factors in the parent-child and child-parent relationship without the heat of immediate conflict over the negative ones. Some combination of family group therapy with individual therapy where needed may make the family relationships again workable. Parents often need to learn to be less overbearing. The adolescent may need to learn to

---

* For the reader's interest, Louise Homer states that nine of these thirteen girls were not successfully treated in the community and had to be committed for institutional treatment. Four were successfully adjusted without commitment. "Of these four, one did not return to court on a runaway charge or any other charge; two returned one time each on a runaway charge; and one returned twice on a runaway charge. These girls were also running to the pleasures of the runaway's world. They were, however, sufficiently anxious about the consequences (possible commitment) of their behavior to curtail their running to the extent that they returned few, if any, times to court. These four girls also had difficulty with setting limits, but were able to respond to the externally placed limits established by the therapist. They were less impulsive than the other nine and were able to forgo the pleasures experienced while being on the run for the real pleasures and real freedom that came from not being committed to the department of youth services. In a real sense, two goals were mutually established by the therapist with each of these girls; 1) not to be committed, and 2) to wait until the age of 17 to leave home, to forgo the immediate pleasures of independence until it was legally acceptable to leave school, to set up one's own apartment and get a job."

express dissatisfaction with specific matters in a reasonable way, before dissatisfactions build up to the point of emotional explosions or runaways.

One element which is quite general among the chronic runaway adolescent is a very poor self-image. If one can cultivate any areas of skill, of achievement as a basis for some self-pride and self-belief, the prospects for successful treatment are very much improved—particularly if one can persuade parents to give some real positive recognition and encouragement to these achievements by the adolescent. Some positive appreciation by the peer group—which has usually been lacking for these youngsters—is also of great value in self-belief, and self-respect must be very gently cultivated.

Residential Treatment

A distinction can be made between those adolescents who, although they cannot be maintained in their own homes, are willing to remain in a group home or shelter care during a period of treatment. In these cases the treatment of both child and family is viewed as a separate task and the removal of the child from the home serves merely to reduce the tension between adolescent and family to make treatment possible. On the other hand, when the pattern of running away has become so much internalized as a part of the adolescent that it continued even in this setting, then residential treatment center or a training school for delinquents is indicated. Residential treatment centers are likely to stress treatment, and training schools are likely to stress training. Both are needed. In either case, a necessary ingredient is a program with a degree of supervision to reduce the individual's temptation to run away, to make the attempt to run away unlikely to be successful. Even adolescents who do manage to run away can be treated successfully if they are returned without too much delay.

As a group, children and adolescents showing the *runaway reaction* are self-centered, fearful, and mistrustful of others. While there is very much a place for lending a sympathetic ear to the unhappy feelings and unhappy stories of these children, yet in those in whom the family ties are absent or are too ambivalent, slow progress must be made toward the individual assuming responsibility for himself or herself at least in the sense of assuming responsibility for his or her own behavior. This can be a frightening matter for an already frightened, timid adolescent. A steady and steadying framework of control, even though resented, is constructive. The control must be benign, but it must be consistent and effective. The key word is dependability.

Within this framework, the individual must be encouraged, step by step, to assume responsibility for himself and his own behavior and must receive some recognition and reward for it. Inevitably, with his limited capacity for postponing gratification or for working toward a goal, he will feel that the rewards do not come soon enough, or are insufficient, or both. Control must be maintained patiently and must remain benign in the face of the individual's resentment of this control. A great deal of individual attention is needed, and often a verbal statement of the adult's interest is very needful. It should be honest, and should not be given unless the adult can feel it at the time. It is better to try to build more slowly than to try to build on false assurance.

It is important to seek to cultivate and expand any constructive area of aptitude or skill the individual may show—and to give him recognition for it. These individuals particularly have a profound need for developing some belief in themselves.

Ultimately the effort must be directed toward helping these adolescents recognize their own best interests in a stable social structure and seek to work toward them. The individual who has little to give others must learn to look after himself without expecting others to give them a type of relationship that he cannot return because he lacks that degree of feeling for others. With such persons we can afford to consider ourselves successful if we can help them learn to keep out of trouble with the law.

Comparisons

The treatment of the *runaway reaction* is substantially more difficult than the treatment of the *group delinquent reaction* and somewhat more difficult than the treatment of the *unsocialized aggressive reaction*.

The adolescent showing the *group delinquent reaction* is likely to have much hostility toward adult authority, but he has some sense of give and take, some capacity for loyalty. His loyalty can be won by fair, reliable treatment and help in meeting his problems, and that loyalty can be nurtured and used in modifying his behavior.

The adolescent showing the *unsocialized aggressive reaction* typically lacks loyalty or the capacity for very much empathy. Usually he has at least a belief in himself and his own toughness. He is not easily defeated or discouraged and he will and can learn at least to serve his own interests by adapting to a structured situation. Then he can learn skills and tools other than aggressive attack for use in interpersonal relations.

The adolescent showing the *runaway reaction* typically trusts no one and *does not believe in himself*. Much effort must be expended to give him a better self-image if treatment is to be successful.

Summary and Conclusions

Running away from home is a common occurrence among adolescents today. It usually reflects a desire for adventure or an unwillingness to live within parental rules. It does expose adolescents to risks of being victimized or being enlisted for delinquent acts. Although a runaway is most often a benign occurrence, revisions of the juvenile justice laws which would strip juvenile courts of the power to deal with status offenses are ominous for the future.

The *runaway reaction* is a diagnosis justified for only a small fraction of runaway adolescents who *characteristically* escape from threatening situations by running away from home for a day or more without permission. If the adolescent is to return to his home, work will always need to be done with the parents as well as with the adolescent. Placement out of the home in a group home or treatment institution is often necessary to temporarily reduce conflict with the parents and to make treatment possible. We must further recognize that there are a number of cases in which the adolescent will never be able to make an adjustment in his or her own home and in which we must work toward some arrangement for independent living as they approach adult life.

Addendum

Present plans are that the diagnosis of the *runaway reaction* in DSM-II will be replaced by the diagnosis of *conduct disorder, undersocialized nonaggressive type* in DSM-III. This will correspond rather closely with the BC-I (inadequate immature) group of Quay, and may be diagnosed in children who have never run away, as well as in the chronic runaway child.

References

Ambrosino, L. (1971) *Runaways*. Boston: Beacon Press.

American Psychiatric Association. (1968) *Diagnostic and Statistical Manual of Mental Disorders*, 2nd ed. (DSM II) Washington, D.C.: American Psychiatric Association.

Chapman, C. (1976) *America's Runaways*. New York: Morrow.

Homer, L.E. (1973) Community-based resource for runaway girls. *Social Casework* 54:473–479.

Jenkins, R.L. (1971) The runaway reaction. *Am. J. Psychiat.* 128:168–173.

Jenkins, R.L. (1973) *Behavior Disorders of Childhood and Adolescence*. Springfield, Ill.: Charles C. Thomas.

Jenkins, R.L. and A. Boyer. (1967) Types of delinquent behavior and background factors. *Int. J. Soc. Psychiat.* 14:65–76.

Jenkins. R.L., and G. Stahle. (1972) The runaway reaction: A case study. *J. Am. Acad. Child Psychiat.* 11: 294–313.

Quay, H.C. (1966) Personality patterns in preadolescent delinquent boys. *Ed. Psychol. Measure.* 26:99–110.

Quay, H.C., W.C. Morse, and R. L. Cutter. (1964) Personality dimensions in delinquent males as inferred from the factor analysis of behavior ratings. *J. Res. Crime Delin.* 1:33–37.

Quay, H.C., W.C. Morse, and R.L. Cutter. (1966) Personality patterns of pupils in special classes for the emotionally disturbed. *Except. Child.* 32:297–301.

Shellow, R., J.R. Schamp, E. Liebow, and E. Unger. (1967) Suburban runaways of the 1960's. *Mon. Soc. Res. Child Develop.* 32(3):1–51.

Shinohara, M., and R.L. Jenkins. (1967) MMPI study of three types of delinquents. *J. Clin. Psychol.* 23:156–163.

Tsubouchi, K., and R.L. Jenkins. (1969) Three types of delinquents: Their performance on MMPI and PCR. *J. Clin. Psychol.* 25:353–358.

Treatment of Emotional Disorders in Children and Adolescents

CHAPTER 36

Treatment of Drug Abuse

Merritt H. Egan

Introduction

Every society of which we have record has had herbs, drugs, medicines, and so forth it has used to allay pain, suffering, misery, or on the other hand, to seek a new high of pleasure. Drugs often become part of the ritual by which people gain relaxation from the stresses of life. Throughout history, also, they have been involved in certain religious rituals. The recent drug abuse epidemic is not new but another phase in man's use and abuse of drugs.

Drug misuse/abuse in children and young adolescents rarely fits the psychiatric stereotypes seen in the adult addict population (e.g., hard-core drug addict who cares only for immediate narcissistic gratification). Rather, it is an "adaptive and defensive choice made by a young person for a combination of intrapsychic, familial and social reasons." For instance, children and adolescents commonly take drugs for curiosity, because they are depressed, have major ego deficits, or have been subjected to deprivation, inconsistency, and/or rejection (Proskauer and Rolland, 1973).

Others have defined drug abuse as an excessive or persistent use of a drug beyond medical needs which is usually characterized by an overpowering desire to increase the dose for psychologic and/or physiologic reasons. The partial cross-tolerance and cross-dependence of some drugs permits substitution of one drug for another and complicates the diagnosis and the treatment problems.

There has been such confusion about the term "drug abuse" that the National Commission on Marihuana and Drug Abuse recommended that the term be discarded and that increased emphasis be placed on drug use—learning how to use drugs appropriately rather than destructively (Farnsworth, 1974). Addiction in the old sense of the term concerned itself with psychic or behavioral dependence (habituation), physical dependence (associated with withdrawal), tolerance, and behavioral toxicity. The term "addiction" is not acceptable because it has a variety of meanings. More exact terms now in common usage are physical dependence and psychic or psychological dependence—a spelling out of the various properties of any particular drug. Physical dependence is associated with a withdrawal syndrome and psychic dependence has to do with how much the individual craves and seeks the drug. More recently, we have become increasingly concerned with behavioral toxicity—the risk to the drug abuser and the public when someone partakes of a drug. This relates to the capacity a person has under the influence of a drug to perceive reality, make decisions, solve problems, etc. For example, glue sniffing has zero physical dependence and withdrawal symptoms but 4+ behavioral toxicity. In contrast, heroin has 4+ physical dependence and withdrawal symptoms but very little behavioral toxicity. LSD and methamphetamine has essentially zero physical dependence and withdrawal symptoms but has 3–4+ behavioral toxicity, including paranoid psychotic type behavior. The various aspects of addiction as they relate to each classification of commonly abused drugs are summarized in Table 1.

The word "drug" now refers to a highly active substance taken for pleasure (rather than therapeutic purposes) and usually carries with it the implication of illicitness and danger. On the other hand, substances taken for therapeutic purposes are more properly called "medicines" (Naftulin, 1971).

People may be classified into the following categories:

1. Those who have no drug experience (nonusers).

2. Those who regularly use mild stimulants such as caffeine, nicotine, etc. These usually have little toxicity but may injure organ systems. This category includes the majority of the world's population. The use of these substances is continued mainly because of primary psychological dependence and to avoid negative symptoms. There is a drug reward connected with the use, at least initially.

3. Those who use, on a voluntary or pseudotherapeutic basis, potent psychoactive drugs. These may be subdivided into occasional, regular, or

Table 1
Basic Characteristics of Commonly Abused Drugs

Substance	Source(s)	Physical Dependence	Withdrawal Reaction	Psychic Dependence	Behavioral Toxicity*	Halluci-nations	Other Effects†
Stimulants							Insomnia
Amphetamines and related sympathomimetic amines	Synthetic (diet pills, etc.)	0	0	+++	+	+	Hypertension Arrhythmias
Methamphetamines (speed)	Synthetic	0	0	+++	+++	+ to ++	Acute psychosis
Cocaine	Synthetic	0	0	+++	+++	+	
Hallucinogens							Prolonged psychosis
Lysergic acid diethylamide (LSD)	Synthetic	0	0	+ to ++	++++	++++	Brain damage Chromosomal breaks Suicide & accident
2, 5-dimethoxy, 4-methyl-amphetamine (STP) (DOM)	Synthetic	0	0	+ to ++	++++	+++	"Bad", long "trip" Suicide, Accidents
Mescaline (Peyote)	Cactus	0	0	+ to +++	++	+++	
Psylocybin	Mushrooms	0	0	+ to +++	++	+++	
Myristicin	Nutmeg	0	0	+ to +++	++	++	Liver and kidney damage
Marihuana (THC, pot, grass, bang, hashish)	Synthetic, Hemp plant (cannabis sativa)	0	0	+ to +++	+ to +++	++	Insidious personality effects
Sedative-Hypnotics							Liver cirrhosis
(alcohol, barbiturates, meprobamate, glutethimide)	Synthetic Medicines	+ to ++++	+++ to ++++	+++	+ to ++	Alcohol++	Neurological disorders Accidents
Narcotic Analgesics							
Heroin—Morphine	Oriental Poppy	++++	+++	++++	+	+	Respiratory and circulatory depression, endocarditis, thrombophlebitis
Demerol	Synthetic	+++	++	+++	+ to ++	+	
Methadone	Synthetic	++	++	++	+?	0?	
Organic Solvents							
Glue sniffing, etc.	Plastic cements Lacquer thinner Lighter or cleaning fluid, nail polish or remover, gasoline, etc.	0	0	+ to +++	++ to ++++	++	Varies with solvent. Visceral and bone marrow damage Sudden death.

* Effects are dose related and ratings refer to situations commonly seen with heavy usage.

† Frequent, chronic use of any of these drugs may be associated with persistent mood changes & personality deterioration. See Text.

heavy users. Drugs that are commonly abused by the drug abusing segment of the population are stimulant drugs (such as cocaine, amphetamine, methamphetamine, phenmetrazine); hallucinogens (such as LSD, marihuana, mescaline, STP, DMT, PCP, etc.); depressant drugs (such as alcohol, other hydrocarbons, barbiturates, and other sedative-hypnotic-like drugs, morphine and morphine-like analgesics); inhalants (such as model-airplane glue, paint thinner, gasoline, industrial solvents, amyl nitrite, ether, aerosol sprays, etc.); and anticholinergics (such as atropine, scopolamine, antihistamines, etc.).

4. Those who use medicines for therapeutic reasons. Here there is no abuse, minimum harm, and perhaps maximum reward from a medicinal point of view. These have minimal social consequences.

In a recent study of 100 young psychiatric inpatients, ages 8–25 years, it was found that 49% of these patients were tabulated as heavy users (Westermeyer and Walzer, 1975). Heavy users were defined as including at least one of the following use patterns during the year prior to admission: (1) alcohol intoxication on three or more days of the average week; (2) daily cannabis use; (3) recreational use of any other illicit drug—i.e. LSD, heroin, mescaline, STP, etc.—on more than three occasions during the past year; (4) nonprescription use of any prescription drug—for example, barbiturate, amphetamine, morphine,—on more than three occasions during the previous year. Heavy users in comparison to other patients were found to have more unemployment, divorce, separation, problematic social events, and fewer neurotic diagnoses and social resources at the time of admission.

Drug abuse in the past has had other definitions than those we have given above and undoubtedly they will be different in the future. This has led Einstein and Quinones to define drug abuse as "the use of particular drugs in particular ways for particular reasons which are contrary to agreed upon rituals in a given community at a given point in time" (Einstein and Quinones, 1971). The importance of this definition is highlighted by the present legalization of tobacco and alcohol (which have major known harmful effects and are our greatest drug problems) contrasted with society's controversy about marihuana and our obsessive-compulsive attention to certifying new medicines for professional use or chemicals to be used in the preparation of food, etc.

As the drug epidemic progressed, it was necessary to define and describe poly-drug-users (Halikas and Rimmer, 1974). In a study of 100 regular marihuana users, it was found that 48% of subjects used two or less other drugs and 52% were found to have used more than two other drugs (mean 7.5). Two important patterns of drug use were found to be significantly associated with multiple drug abusers: (1) lower age of first illicit drug experience; (2) higher likelihood that the first illicit drug they ever tried was not marihuana. Other factors that have been found to be antecedents of multiple drug use are early sexual activity, substantive adolescent-parental conflicts, adolescent antisocial behavior, police contact, homosexual experiences, self-defeating behavior in adolescence, poor adolescent adjustment, higher incidence of truancy and drop-out problems, and more school socialization problems.

History

The pattern of drug abuse over the centuries was greatly changed in recent decades by chemical technological breakthroughs leading to the formulation of many new compounds. It was hoped that these new compounds had magical properties and could prevent or cure many illnesses. Troubled people with limited abilities to solve their problems who were looking for rescue fantasies turned to drugs for the alleviation of misery or for the attainment of exhilarating experiences.

In the seventies it was observed that a relatively high proportion of children and adolescents who use illicit or psychoactive drugs have mothers who take similar chemicals (Archibald, 1970). A child's chances of abusing drugs rise substantially when his mother is a drug user. In one study, 33% of young marihuana users had mothers who used barbiturates, 12% had mothers who used stimulants, and 36% had mothers who were taking tranquilizers. In another study, it was found that 46% of mothers of speed users take tranquilizers, 32% used stimulants, and 43% used barbiturates. It appears that if parents routinely use drugs or certain medications such as tranquilizers that it will sharply increase the likelihood that their children will be drug abusers. However, such studies should be compared to controls.

In 1970 the Federal Controlled Substances Act (Public Law 91–513) was passed which required persons to register if they were to manufacture, import, export, or dispense controlled substances which were classified under five schedules.

Stimulants

In the sixties reports began to show that excessive consumption of amphetamines can produce serious psychiatric complications. These may vary from severe personality disorders to chronic psychosis (Griffeths, 1966). From Japan came reports after World War II of 2,000,000 amphetamine addicts (Lemere, 1963). In some of these, they demonstrated that amphetamine can produce permanent organic brain damage (Tatetsu, 1963). The amphetamine psychosis of chronic users has been described repeatedly and consists usually of paranoid ideation, hallucinations, and compulsive behavior. One must consider amphetamine psychosis in patients who manifest psychotic symptoms and are on amphetamines.

Hallucinogens

In the sixties with the availability of d-lysergic acid diethylamide (LSD) there were a flood of articles on the use of this psychotomimetic drug. It was reported in 1968 that one of every five students on the Yale and Wesleyan campuses had used hallucinogenic drugs at least once in his/her life time, and a majority of all nonusers reported knowing somebody who had used hallucinogens. A sizable minority reported having seriously considered trying them (Imperi, Kleber, and Davie, 1968). It had taken approximately 38 years from the time that LSD was synthesized in 1938 by Stoll and Hofmann until it had become widely used and a common household word. Even though we had initially thought that LSD induced a "mild psychosis" resembling schizophrenia, we learned that it had little relationship to schizophrenia except that many of the symptoms were similar (AMA Council on Mental Health, 1967).

In the sixties reports began to come in that LSD caused chromosomal damage in human leukocytes. In 1967 (Cohen, Marinello, and Back) it was reported that LSD quickly produces chromosomal damage in vitro in the first or second division of cultured leukocytes. Studies of patients on LSD dosages ranging from 80 to 200 micrograms showed a chromosomal breakage rate of 12% compared to the normal of 3.7%. Other reports showed an increase in chromosomal abnormalities in leukocytes of LSD users compared to drug-free controls and also an elevated breakage rate in children exposed to the drug in utero (Egozcue, Irwin, and Maruffo, 1968).

In 1971, a followup survey of 247 persons who had received LSD revealed that it becomes less effective with continued use and in the long term its use is almost always self-limiting (McGlothlin and Arnold, 1971). This is undoubtedly one of the principal reasons why drug abusers have gone to other chemicals. When this is combined with the possibility of organic and chromosomal damage, the payoff is usually not great enough for its continued use.

A significant development was the Drug Control Act of 1970 (PL 91–513) which authorized the appointment of a National Commission on Marihuana and Drug Abuse. In summary, the commission reported that marihuana is a national problem and society does not know what to do about it. The life style of heavy users is often unconventional and they may develop organ injury (for example, diminution of pulmonary function). The commission also found that marihuana inhibits expression of aggressive impulses and does not lead to physical dependence.

The Commission's report did not contribute greatly to our knowledge of or control of marihuana use. On the one hand, it recommended liberalization of federal and state laws applying to the use of marihuana but then spoke of some of the dangers of its continued use. We have learned that drug use can not be controlled by laws.

A study of 38 individuals (ages 13 to 24) who had smoked marihuana 2–3 times a week all showed adverse psychological effects and some manifested neurologic signs and symptoms (Kolansky and Moore, 1971). Eight of the 38 demonstrated psychoses, 4 attempted suicide, 13 of the 18 female patients became sexually promiscuous while using marihuana, and 7 of these became pregnant. Researchers found no evidence of predisposition to mental illness in these patients. It was their impression that moderate to heavy use of marihuana in adolescence even without predisposition to mental illness may lead to decompensations ranging from mild ego disturbances to psychosis.

The above findings should alert us to problems of the future in view of the fact that the Marihuana Commission found that 24 million Americans had used marihuana even in 1972.

In a 10% sample of the UCLA undergraduate student body, it was found that drug use is extensive and the use of all other drugs is associated with use of marihuana (Hochman and Brill, 1973). The use of all drugs (other than marihuana) tends to be transitory in college students usually. It was felt that marihuana does not cause the use of other drugs but almost everyone who uses other drugs also uses marihuana. As individuals are frequently more willing to experience marihuana intoxication, they also are more willing to try other drugs. Marihuana users began sexual experience at an earlier age, saw themselves as more experienced, had more sexual experiences, suffered more venereal disease, and had a more liberal attitude towards sex than the nonusers.

It appears from many studies that as the age polarization in our society increases, the peer group becomes stronger and increasingly tends to neutralize the parental influence. This is especially true if the family of origin is pathological. This is a fact that must be kept in mind as we think about prevention and treatment.

Mild tolerance and physical dependence may develop when the more potent preparations of cannabis are used to excess; however, tolerance and physical dependence are virtually nonexistent for occasional or moderate regular users (McGlothlin, 1964). There are apparently no serious deleterious physical effects that we have been able to measure from moderate use of marihuana. However, excessive indulgence in Eastern countries contributes to a variety of ailments, including the precipitation of transient psychoses. Unstable individuals may experience a psychotic episode from even a small amount of marihuana; although they typically recover within a few days, some psychoses triggered by marihuana may last for months. In Eastern countries where marihuana is taken in large amounts, many observers feel that it is directly or indirectly responsible for many psychiatric hospital admissions.

On January 31, 1971, the Secretary of Health, Education and Welfare submitted a summary report to Congress concerning marihuana and health. This report emphasized that there was increasing evidence that frequent, heavy use of marihuana is correlated with a loss of interest in conventional goals and with the development of lethargy.

In 1972 a significant study was made of 720 hashish smokers identified among 36,000 people in the U.S. Army (Tennant and Groesbeck, 1972). The researchers found that the casual smoking of less than 10 to 12 grams of hashish monthly resulted in no ostensible adverse effects other than minor respiratory ailments. They found few panic reactions, toxic psychoses, and schizophrenic reactions unless hashish was consumed with alcohol or other psychoactive drugs. However, if over 50 grams per month of hashish were used, these patients often had a chronic intoxicated state characterized by apathy, dullness, and lethargy with mild to severe impairment of judgment, concentration, and memory.

It appears that there is a continuum of effects paralleling the dosage and frequency of marihuana use. Cannabis studies that do not identify the type of material, the amount of the chemical constituents, and the assay standards used ought to be ignored.

Narcotic-Analgesics

A significant new method in treatment of heroin addiction was described in 1965 (Dole and Nyswander). In a study of 22 people who had been addicted for periods of 1–15 months, it was found that when they were given maintenance doses of methadone, they lost their hunger for heroin. If they did take heroin, they got no thrill out of it. The problem was that methadone, a synthetic narcotic drug, is in itself addictive. It is inexpensive and can be taken orally. Other advantages were that it had few side effects and it is relatively long acting. Therefore, patients could be stabilized on a single daily dose under medical control. Further, they found that many patients could function more normally in the community and at work.

Theoretical Considerations—General Principles and Assumptions

Understanding the drug-abusing teenage psyche is necessary if one successfully is to treat the drug abuser. A study of 100 adolescents who were actively misusing drugs (who requested consultation from a voluntary mental health service) revealed similar characteristics as follows (Geist, 1974): (1) an unrealistic sense of trust in and demand for human love among people. (2) a tendency to deny the reality of time. For instance, adolescents have prolonged reversal of night and day, complain that history is irrelevant, and periodically refuse to anticipate future needs. (3) a flight from inner reality. (4) a tendency towards severe depression. The teen often has a hopeless feeling about himself that is manifested by his lack of care of his own body. (5) a tendency to isolate the process of physical sexuality from psychological mutuality. (6) a tendency toward behavioral passivity. This manifests itself in the life style and in the complaints of parents that their child sleeps all the time, sits and stares, eats meals in his room, etc.

The drug-using teenager frequently expresses the desire to get away, to turn life off, step outside the world, etc. His philosophy often is one of nonexistence. He seems to want to get away through drugs, running away, or leaving his family, etc., and hibernate with the hope that at a later time he can be resurrected without the problems that now attend him. It is probably these feelings that led to the development of crash pads and other holding environments that are sympathetic to the adolescent's philosophy and have the promise of health, a better future, and isolation from and perhaps antagonism toward the establishment.

Family Dynamics

The dynamics of family life in drug addicts/abusers has been studied by several workers. The following are frequently reported findings:

A. Regarding the family of origin

1. Frequently there has been parental deprivation in the form of parent-child separation or death of a parent. In a study of 76 amphetamine abusers, 17 to 36 years of age, nearly 50% had suffered bereavement or separation from a parent before 16 years of age.

2. Mother's dealing with the child is often overindulgent and permissive. This may be interpreted by some as a loving relationship but on another level may be seen as a form of rejection. This is confirmed by other studies demonstrating that the parent-child relationship is often dominated by a lack of love, increased hostility, and the unfortunate "present" of the parent to the child of excessive autonomy. The long-range relationship tends to confirm a basic rejection of child by the parent. This is often denied by superficial defensive actions but confirmed as one looks at the life cycle in toto. The parents and children often end up rejecting each other even though a surface reaction-formation may hide this basic dynamic. The often-described long-term close relationship of the addict to the parents is probably more related to his or her inadequacy and dependency than to a loving relationship.

3. Fathers are often alcoholic, relatively uninvolved with the family, weak, controlled by the mother, and essentially absent. The father's relationship with his daughter is often inept, indulgent, and marked by sexual aggressiveness if not incest.

4. Mother's superficial close relationship to a son addict is often not only a defense against her fundamental difficulty in accepting the child but is also determined in part by her lack of a satisfactory relationship with her husband.

5. If the parents use drugs—for example, alcohol, tranquilizers, amphetamines, barbiturates, etc.—the chance of the child's abusing drugs is greatly increased (even 7 to 10 fold).

6. If a child has friends who use drugs, chances are increased the child will abuse them also. If friends and parents use drugs, the incidence is further increased. However, if the parents are not addicts or abusers and the family relationships are healthy and strong, then a drug-using peer group usually has little influence on the child.

7. Parent-child communication is usually poor and the parents often view the child as weak. They often infantilize him and covertly encourage him to find an escape rather than cope with frustration. This is undoubtedly determined by thier own outlook on life and the two-directional identification between the generations.

8. Drug-using children often serve to maintain a homeostatic condition in the family in many ways. One of these is to divert attention from the mother-father conflict to the addict/abuser child.

9. Drug misuse often originates when a child begins to move away from the family. The child fears being on his own, and drug use in part may be designed by the child to not only alleviate his pain and bring pleasure but to draw the parents closer together.

Hence, the literature on the surface is confusing. Does the mother have increased love for the addict/abuser or less love than is found in normal parent-child relationships? Understanding the dynamics of the relationships helps us clear the confusion. The parents often have difficulty accepting and giving to the child, and this is camouflaged by mother's surface actions—defenses against her basic feelings of ambivalence for the child.

B. Regarding family of marriage and children

1. There is sometimes a "flight" into marriage. Only one-half as many male addicts marry as in the general population; yet those who do marry have an increased rate of multiple marriages. Parents often relate in such a way as to push the child out of the home (and sometimes marriage results), but later parents often on some level encourage the child's divorce and return to the home. This maintains the child's dependency and symbiosis.

2. Addict/abusers in marriage often relate with

their spouse in a manner similar to the way he or she related to the parent of the opposite sex in the family of origin.

3. Those who have children are often incapable of rearing them, and there is a higher percentage of children born out of wedlock and adopted out than in the general population.

Attachment, Separation, and Adjustment

The universal phenomena seen in humans of attachment, separation and adjustment is seen in pathological proportions in the mother-child relationship of heroin addicts. Studies of the degree of symbiosis have shown that between 6 and 16 years of age mothers of heroin addicts have an even higher degree of attachment than mothers of schizophrenics, who have a higher degree of attachment than the mothers of normal children. Possible explanations are: (1) The husband-wife relationship often does not meet the marital partner's needs. This often encourages a closer association with the child. (2) Mother has a need to prove she is an adequate mother as a defense against her ambivalence about the pregnancy originally.

One sees in the adolescent who compulsively and indiscriminately uses drugs the repetitive process that alternates between staying dependent and gaining independence. Again, this phenomenon may explain why some workers observe increased contact between addicts and the family of origin and others see less contact. They may be observing different aspects of a total phenomena which encompasses both forces. The user often is overinvolved with the parent of the opposite sex and is seen as ill, incompetent, unable to be independent and leave home, and in need of money and psychological sustenance. This idea agrees with the fact that there is an increase in drug misuse in single-parent families. It suggests also that as we espouse nonmarriage that this may have an effect on the incidence of drug misuse.

On the other hand, the drug misusers may have left home, run away, be seen as distant and independent. This may be determined by a reaction-formation against dependence—an escape from a desire for close physical contact with the parent of the opposite sex. It also may be part of a rebellion and self-assertion seen in adolescence. This is especially so if the core feeling of inadequacy is present without the self-confidence and assets to be strong in healthy ways. This emphasizes that the core, primary preventive treatment must be to increase the competence of the family and the individual.

Ingested materials are associated with one's mother, and in the deprived adolescent, who is disturbed, drugs may be a substitute for a mother's presence and acceptance. Frequently, the basic pathology that is found in teenage heavy drug abusers is lack of maternal nurturance—and especially the failure of one parent to protect the child from the irrational sexual and aggressive demands of the other parent. Thus the drug user often is looking for something and/or someone to whom he can attach.

The above theoretical formulation may help us understand a commonly seen clinical situation—namely, the relationship of the addictor and the addict. The addictor is a person who gains social and nonsocial rewards from encouraging the drug addiction of another individual. A therapist should determine who the addictor is and what his relationship is with the addict. Then this relationship is explored with the patient. As the therapeutic relationship evolves, the patient is helped to shift his dependency from the addictor to the therapist. When this has been accomplished, one can help the patient see how he has been victimized. Hopefully, also the addictogenic person can be brought into therapy (Little and Pearson, 1966).

Etiology

Freud, in his description of civilization and its discontents, said that life is hard with many disappointments, pains, and unpleasant tasks. We seek palliative remedies. These may be: (1) diversion of interest to sports, animals, hobbies, etc.; (2) substitute gratifications in the form of art, music, sex, nature, accomplishments, etc. When these pleasures of life and others are not enough to neutralize the pain of life, some people use intoxicating substances.

Vital in determining our course of prevention and treatment is some understanding of the etiology of drug abuse. There is no easy explanation, and there are various causes depending on the individual. Among those that seem to be frequently operant are the following:

1. A person seeks pleasure, a wish for a feeling of greater power or ecstasy. He may be seeking sensualism—hoping for an aphrodisiac.

2. Sometimes drug abuse is a symptom of rebel-

lion—an unhealthy attempt to grow up. Also, youth observe that adults pass laws against youth drugs but none against their own—a source of adolescent anger.

3. The fear of failure or failure itself is often a contributing factor. They may feel an intolerable excessive amount of stress from unpleasant inner conflicts, other relationships and/or circumstances and wish to escape from these.

4. Sensationalism seems to contribute to drug taking and increases potential user's curiosity. The mass media communications and the big to-do about drugs in the sixties and seventies undoubtedly increased the use of drugs. We created in effect a multi-million-dollar drug advertising campaign. Youth characteristically have some difficulty learning from others and have a predilection to try everything and avoid any feelings of weakness; hence, there is a good deal of denial and pseudo-omnipotence demonstrated in taking drugs.

5. Some are seriously disturbed, are unable to gather drug data or appropriately evaluate it. Neurotics may use drugs for irrational reasons.

6. Peer pressure is a strong factor in many cases. The desire not to be "chicken" is real in the early teen years particularly.

7. Pressure from pushers and the desire for a relationship are also factors. Drugs may seem to the user to offer not only the payoff of drug effects but individual and group relationships in the drug culture that have often been lost in the community and family and are vital to his functioning. Drugs offer also a simple way of life which often centers around the obtaining and using of drugs—a displacement from complex problems.

All these and more may be in the mind of the potential drug user/abuser. Since his circumstances are usually far from ideal—usually somewhat desperate, since he is willing to take almost any gamble, and since he feels he is incapable of solving complex issues by any means short of a simple solution—because of all of these factors and others, the pill popper may feel drugs are not only worth the chance but the only way for him to go.

Ours—A Chemical Society

There has not been a society that has not had its major problems with regression in one direction or another. There have been no societies that to one degree or another have not taken recourse to drugs, but there has not been a society that has "made it" on drugs. Ours is a more chemical society than any in history, but we are not likely to find the solution to most of life's problems via this avenue.

It will be unwise if we emphasize drugs as a separate problem. They should be considered along with other unproductive and self-defeating behaviors. However, some separate specialized treatment facilities seem to be in order for those who have become addicted. A major part of our overall game plan should be one of prevention, or we will end up on an endless treadmill. We should see the abuse of drugs as a desperate symptom, the prodromals of which we should have heeded long ago and must do so now.

Jargon

It is often helpful to know the elementary drug abuse jargon. Table 2 is a reasonably complete glossary of the same (Evens and Clementi, 1977).

Prevention—Natural Highs

A key to the prevention of adolescent users is to help them find true, natural highs—experiences in living, not in drugs. A diversification of interests and facilitating accomplishments to the end that genuine satisfactions are received are paramount. Then these individuals as a society are less likely to seek magical relief from misfortunes or pleasures from chemicals. These principles are expanded later in this chapter.

The Real Drug Problem

In our deliberations we must remember that alcohol is the major drug abuse problem, with more than 8 million people seriously affected in the United States.

Attitudes Toward Drugs

There are two competing attitudes toward drugs, the roots of which are found in the struggle between the generations: (1) drugs are either a great blessing and are going to make us more powerful and potent and cure our ills; and (2) they are a great curse that is going to injure our physical apparatus and pollute our morals, etc. As a young patient comes for therapy, these two attitudes must be kept in mind if one is going to relate effectively.

Table 2
Compendium of Drug Abuse Jargon

Street Name	Definition
Ab	Abscess which forms at site of injection
Acapulco Gold	Mexican marijuana (extremely potent)
Acid	Lysergic acid diethylamide (LSD) or other hallucinogens
Acid Head	One who takes LSD on a regular basis
Alley Juice	Methyl alcohol
Amidone	Methadone
Angel Dust	Phencyclidine hydrochloride sprinkled on parsley or marijuana
Bag	A small quantity of either heroin or cocaine packaged in cellophane envelopes
Bang	The exhiliration experienced after drug administration
Barbs	Barbiturates
Benn	Amphetamine sulfate
Belongs	On the habit
Bennies	Benzedrine (amphetamine sulfate)
Bernies Flake	Cocaine
Bhang	Marijuana, smoking pipe
Binge	An extended period of continued consumption of alcohol
Bitter	Paregoric
Black Beauties	Amphetamines
Black Hash	Hashish containing opium
Black Russian	Hashish (potent, dark)
Black Stuff	Opium, prepared for smoking
Blackjack	Paregoric which has been prepared to be injected
Blanks	Poor quality merchandise
Blotter Acid	LSD on paper
Blow Charlie or Snow	Sniff cocaine
Blow Horse	Sniff heroin
Blow Weed	To smoke marijuana
Blue Birds	Amobarbital capsules
Blue Devils	Amobarbital capsules
Blue Heaven	Amobarbital capsules
Bogart	Not to pass the "joint" to a neighbor
Bombido	Injectable amphetamine
Bombita	Methamphetamine
Boy	Heroin
Brick	Marijuana compressed, usually for purposes of transport
Brody	A fit or spasm staged by an addict to elicit sympathy
Browns	Amphetamine tablets
Bull Jive	Marijuana heavily cut with tea, catnip, or other impurities
Bummer	A bad trip or experience
Burned	Received fake narcotics
Burned Out	Sclerotic blood vessel from too many injections; relative overdose; addict who tires of abuse "hassle" and tries to stop drug abuse
Bush	Marijuana
Busted	To be caught, usually arrested, by local authorities or to be caught by parents
Businessman's Special	Methamphetamine; dimethyltryptamine (DMT) (hallucinogen)
Butter	Marijuana
Button	Peyote button; tops of marijuana plant flower
C	Cocaine
Caballo	Heroin
Cactus	Peyote
Cadet	New addict
California Sunshine	LSD (hallucinogen)
Can	One ounce of marijuana
Candy	Barbiturates; pills in general
Candyman	Dealer or pusher of addicting drugs
Canary	Pentobarbital
Cashing-A-Script	Getting a forged or bogus prescription order dispensed
Cartwheels	Amphetamine tablets
Catch Up	Withdrawal process
CD	Glutethimide tablet
Cecil	Cocaine
Charlie	Cocaine
Chief	Mescaline
Chippin'; Chipper	Subcutaneous administration of small dose of heroin; "weekend user" who used drugs less than daily
Cleared Up	To have withdrawn from drugs
Coasting	Under drug influence

Compendium of Drug Abuse Jargon (continued)

Street Name	Definition
Cohobe	DMT in powdered seeds (hallucinogen)
Coke	Cocaine
Cokomo (Kokomo)	Cocaine
Cold Turkey	Withdrawal process
Come Down; Crash	Dissipation of drug effects
Connect	Make a purchase
Cook It Up	To prepare a drug for injection
Cooker	The apparatus used to heat and dissolve a drug prior to injection (spoons or bottle top)
Cop	To obtain a small quantity of a drug
Coffin	Tobacco
Co-pilots	Amphetamines
Courage Pills	Barbiturates
Cranks	Methamphetamine
Crap	Heroin of weak potency
Crystal	Methamphetamine
Cube (The)	LSD
Cut	To adulterate with agents such as quinine, milk sugar
Daytop Lodge	Drug abuse treatment center directed by ex-addicts
Dealer	One who sells drugs
Deck	Packet of cigarettes, narcotics, etc.
D (Big)	LSD
DET	Diethyltryptamine (hallucinogen)
Diane	Meperidine hydrochloride
Dexies	Dextroamphetamine sulfate (Dexedrine)
DMZ	Benactyzine (hallucinogen)
DMT	Dimethyltryptamine (Businessman's Special) (hallucinogen)
Doe	Methamphetamine
Dolls; Dollies	Methadone
DOM	4-methyl-2,5-Dimethoxyamphetamine (stimulant—STP)
Doodee	Heroin
Double Trouble	Combination of both amobarbital sodium and secobarbital sodium
Doper	Regular drug abuser
Downers	Sedatives, usually barbiturates
Dreamer	Morphine
Dream Stick	An opium pipe
Dropped	Consumed a drug abuse agent
DT's	Delirium tremens (acute alcohol withdrawal syndrome)
Duds	Bags of heroin containing no narcotic agent
Dust	Heroin; cocaine
Dust of Angels	Phencyclidine base (hallucinogen)
Dynamite	High grade narcotics; heroin, cocaine
Dummy	Drug purchase without purported content
Emma (Miss)	Morphine
Emsel	Morphine
Eyeopeners	Amphetamines
Fag	Tobacco
F-40s	Secobarbital
Fix	To inject drugs; satiate addictive needs
Fizzies	Methadone tablets
Flake	Cocaine
Flake Out	To pass out from drug use
Flash	Rapid, intense, euphoric reaction
Flower	Marijuana
Flying Saucers	PCP, phencyclidine (hallucinogen)
Footballs	Amphetamine tablets
Flashback	Recurrence of some feature of a previous LSD experience
Freak	An addict who enjoys playing with the needle
Freak out	To be intensely affected by something
Ganja	Jamaican marijuana
Garbage	Poor quality merchandise
Garbage Head	Individual who takes any kind of drug
Gear	Drugs in general
Gee Head	Paregoric user
Get It Together	To become mentally organized
Get Off	To initially experience the effects of a drug
Gift of the Sun God	Cocaine
Glad Rag	Cloth or handkerchief that is saturated with a material to be inhaled

Compendium of Drug Abuse Jargon (continued)

Street Name	Definition
	(eg, for use in glue sniffing)
Gold Dust	Cocaine
Goofballs	Amphetamine
Gram	Quantity of hashish
Grass	Marijuana
Grasshopper	A marijuana user
Greezy Addict	Drug abuser who will take any drug, anytime
Griffo	Marijuana
H	Heroin
Habit	Dependence upon drugs
Happy Trails	Cocaine
Hard Stuff	Morphine
Harry; Big Harry; Hairy	Heroin
Hash	Hashish (THC), resin from top of Cannabis sativa
Hash Oil	Concentrate extracting hash
Head	User of drugs
Hearts	Amphetamine
Heavenly Blue	LSD (hallucinogen)
Heavy Grass High	Strong, stuperous reaction to marijuana
Hemp	Marijuana (Cannabis sativa or indica)
High	Stimulant trip
Hikori, Kikuli, Huatari, Wokouri	Peyote
Hit	Make a purchase; take a drag
Hitting Up	Injecting drugs
Hocus	Morphine
Hog	Phencyclidine mixed with vegetable material; veterinary tranquilizer
Holding	Drugs are in user's possession
Hooked	Addicted to drugs
Hop Head	Person who smokes opium; addict
Horror Drug	Belladonna preparations
Horse	Heroin
Hot Shot	Poisons concealed in injectable narcotics for the purpose of homicide
Hype	A needle addict
Ice Cream Habit	Small, irregular drug use
Idiot Pills	Barbiturates
In Action	To seek narcotics
In-Betweens	Barbiturates, in combination with amphetamines
Indian Hay	Marijuana
In Flight	To be very high from drugs, especially methamphetamine hydrochloride (Methadrine)
J	Marijuana cigarette
Jabber	A needle addict
Jammed Up	An overdose
Jive	Marijuana
Joint	Syringe and needle; one stick of marijuana; or an opium smoker's den
Jolly Babies, Beans	Amphetamine
Joy Juice	Chloral hydrate
Joy Popping	Narcotic injections under the skin
Joy Powder	Heroin
Juice	Alcohol
Juice Freak	One who prefers alcohol
Jugs	Injectable amphetamines
Junk	Narcotics
Junkie	Heroin abuser
Kick	Euphoria
Kick Inducers	Cough elixirs (alcohol)
Kicking	Withdrawal process
Kilo	Two pounds of marijuana
Kif	Marijuana
Lay	An opium den
Layout	Equipment for injecting drugs; opium smoker's outfit
Leaf (The)	Cocaine
Lemon	Bad or fake dope
Licorice	Paregoric
Lid	¾ oz of marijuana
Lid Pollers	Amphetamines
Lords	Hydromorphone hydrochloride
Love Drug	MDA (methyldioxyamphetamine)
LSD	Lysergic acid diethylamide (hallucinogen)
Luding Out	Stupor produced from alcohol and methaqualone
Lumber	Marijuana stems which are found in an ounce of marijuana
M	Morphine

Compendium of Drug Abuse Jargon (continued)

Street Name	Definition
MDA	3, 4-methyldioxyamphetamine (hallucinogen)
Mainliner	One who injects directly into the vein
Mary Jane	Marijuana
Mesc	Mescaline (hallucinogen)
Mescal Button; Mescal Beans	Peyote; mescaline
Mescalito	Peyote; mescaline
Meth; Methedrine	Methamphetamine
Mickey Finn	Chloral hydrate and alcohol
Mindblower	A hallucinogenic drug
Monkey; Morf; Morpho	Morphine
Mother	The drug peddler
Moonshine	Ethyl alcohol
Mooters	Marijuana
Mountain Dew	Alcohol
Mud	Stramonium preparation mixed with carbonated beverage
Muggles	Crude marijuana before rolled into cigarette
Mushrooms; Sacred Mushrooms; Magic Mushrooms	Psilocybin (hallucinogen)
Mutah	Marijuana
Mohasky	Marijuana
Mu	Marijuana
Narcs	Federal narcotics agents
Nemmies	Yellow capsules of pentobarbital
Nickel Bag	A five-dollar bag of a drug
Nimbie; Nimbles	Barbiturates
Nose	Cocaine
Odyssey House	Drug abuse treatment center
OD	Overdose; death
On	Using drugs
On the Nod	Drowsiness from narcotics
Ounce	30 grams of marijuana
Outfit	Narcotic injection equipment
PCP; Peace Pill	Phencyclidine (hallucinogen)
Panama Red	Hashish; marijuana
Papers	Papers usually used to roll a marijuana cigarette. Popular brands include: Zig-Zag, Wheatstraw, Papel del Trigo, Bambu, Job, Roach, Tops
Peace	STP
Peaches	Amphetamine tablets
Peanuts	Barbiturates
Pearly Gates	Morning glory seeds
Phoenix House	Drug abuse treatment center
Pep Pills	Amphetamines
Pethidine	Meperedine hydrochloride
Phennies	Barbiturates
PG; PO	Paregoric
Pimp's Drug	Cocaine
Poppies	Flowering plant from which opium is derived
Pot	Marijuana
Quill	Matchbook cover for sniffing cocaine
Rainbow	Amobarbital and secobarbital capsule (red and blue)
Reader	Presciption order
Reader With Tail	Forged prescription order
Reds; Red Devils; Red Birds (capsules)	Barbiturates, secobarbital
Reefer	Marijuana cigarette
Rich Man's Drug	Cocaine
Roach	Butt of marijuana cigarette
Roll	To make a marijuana cigarette
Roses	Amphetamine tablets
Royal Blue	LSD
Run	Period of stimulant abuse
Rush	Rapid, intense, euphoric reaction
Safe	Addict feels protected from problems and challenges of life during trip
Scag; Scat; Smack; Stuff	Heroin
Schoolboy	Codeine
Score	To establish a connection with a dealer
Script	Prescription order
Script Writer	Sympathetic physician; one who forges Rx orders
Seggy; Seccy	Barbiturates
Seni	Peyote
Serenity	STP
Sharps	Needles
Shoot Up	To inject drugs
Shooting Gallery	Place where addicts inject drugs
Sickie	College student using drugs

Compendium of Drug Abuse Jargon (continued)

Street Name	Definition
Skin Pop	Intradermal or subcutaneous injection
Sleepers	Barbiturates
Snappers	Amyl nitrite ampules
Snarf	Nasal inhalation of cocaine
Snort	Inhalation through nose
Snow	Cocaine
Sopors (R)	Methaqualone
Spaced; Spaced Out	Altered consciousness
Splash	Methamphetamine
Speed	Methamphetamine usually, but may be any stimulant
Speed Freak	Amphetamine abuser
Speedball	Heroin and cocaine mixture; also Percodan and methadrine
Spoon	A gram of cocaine
Stardust	Heroin with cocaine
Star Spangled Powder	Cocaine
Spike	Needle for injection
Stash	Collective term for the accumulation of marijuana paraphernalia
Stepped-on	Process of diluting abuse drugs
Stick	Marijuana cigarette
Stoned	Under the influence of narcotics
Straw; Smoke; Splim	Marijuana
Straight	Describes one who avoids the use of drugs
Strung Out	In need of a fix, sedative, trip; hangover
STP	Dimethoxymethylampheta mine (DOM—hallucinogen)
Sugar	LSD; heroin
Syndicate Acid	STP (hallucinogen)
Synthetic Marijuana	Phencyclidine (hallucinogen)
Sweeties	Phenmetrazine hydrochloride (stimulant)
Synanon	Drug abuse treatment center, directed by ex-addicts
Tab	General term to describe drug of solid dosage
Texas Tea	Marijuana
THC	Tetrahydrocannabinol (hallucinogen in marijuana and hashish)
Toke	Inhalation of smoke
Tops	Peyote
Track Drivers	Amphetamines
Tracks; Turkey Trots	Marks and scars from the use of a hypodermic needle
Tranquility	STP, hallucinogen
Travel Agent	LSD seller
Trips; Trippin'	High mediated by LSD
Unkie	Morphine
Uppers	Stimulants
Wake-up	Amphetamines
Wasted	Under influence of drugs
Water Pipe	Device for bubbling smoke through water for cooler inhalation
Wedding Bells	LSD
Weed	Marijuana
White Lady	Heroin
White Lightning	Ethyl alcohol; also name for a specific speed drug (or amphetamine)
Whites	Amphetamine tablets
White Stuff	Morphine; heroin
Windowpane	LSD
Wired	Intoxicated state due to marijuana
Yellows; Yellow Jackets	Pentobarbital capsules
Yen Sleep	Somnolent stage during drug withdrawal

Drug Use and Sociopathy

It has been demonstrated that heavy drug use is strongly correlated with sociopathy (Westermeyer and Walzer, 1975). This is to be expected as we review the deprivation often found in the early life of heavy drug abusers. This helps us understand why many hesitate to get involved with drug abusers. It explains also in part why the treatment of many drug abusers is so difficult.

Treatment Attitudes

One study has shown that patients with drug abuse problems are reluctant to seek medical help, and when they do, they often don't open up (Chappel, 1973). Some physicians, including some psychiatrists, are hesitant to treat drug abusers. Indeed, medical institutions unless they specialize in this area often find an excuse for turning such patients away. The drug culture sees the average medical doctor as a very easy person to con into giving them prescriptions for therapeutic medications that are used illegally and injudiciously as drugs. It has been estimated that 50% of legitimately produced amphetamines or barbiturates in the United States are diverted into illegal drug use. The average medical doctor and pharmacist has limited knowledge of the drug scene. Hence, the drug cultures send their straightest-looking person for prescriptions. They call this "passing script."

New Developments

Three new developments have changed the treatment of drug dependence (Chappel, 1973).

1. Effective chemotherapeutic substitutes have been developed. Legal drugs are substituted under medical supervision for the abused drug. The substitute is cross-dependent with the drug of dependence. Methadone as a substitute for heroin is the most common example of this.

2. There have been many advances in drug detection technology. This includes: (a) urine screening using thin-layer chromatography to detect amphetamines, barbiturates, morphine, codeine, and methadone; (b) positive findings in the urine screen are followed by qualitative or quantitative confirmatory tests using methods such as gas chromatography or ultraviolet spectrophotometry; (c) blood analyzing for barbiturates, glutethimide (Doriden), meprobamate, diazepine (Valium and Librium), salicylates, etc., using ultraviolet spectrophotometry, colorimetry, or gas chromatography. Table 3 summarizes therapeutic and toxic levels of some commonly abused drugs.

3. Training of former drug users as paraprofessional mental health workers to work with addicts has been of help in the treatment of addiction.

Use of these new developments can contribute greatly to the treatment of drug abusers.

Applicability

There are many attempts to classify youthful drug users. A large segment uses drugs because of curiosity. They are experimenting with life as well as drugs and are coming more and more under the influence of peers and are more and more antagonistic toward the establishment. These are usually the children and adolescents who have tried alcohol and tobacco in the past and now are trying other drugs in addition. They usually do not constitute a major problem and can be helped and guided if relationships are healthy.

Another group of drug users is psychoneurotic or depressed. In this subclass the individual is stressed and he often looks for relief by using drugs. This is less likely to happen if he has a healthy family, peer group and religious or other community affiliations that can help him pick up the pieces when his world seems to fall apart. This is a group that can often be helped with psychotherapy.

A major group that offers the greatest challenge is associated with serious mental illness. These usually come from a more deprived background. They have more serious personality problems and are more likely to be psychotic or have a major personality disorder. They seek drugs with the hope of alleviating their stress, but the opposite usually happens (Nichtern, 1973).

The variability in the reported incidence of drug abuse is influenced by the geographical area, age, and section of society that is studied. Some reports indicate that the use of drugs and alcohol is increasing among young people of both sexes. In the last decade there has been a tendency for the drug culture to include younger and younger children, and some studies show that the junior high school age, which is full of stress, contains a large reservoir of drug users. An additional fact that may contribute to this and should be understood in the planning of prevention and treatment programs is that most junior high school students operate on a

Table 3

Drug	*Specimen*	*Approx. Therapeutic Level mg/100 ml*	*Toxic Level mg/100 ml*	
Amitriptyline (Elavil)	Blood Urine	0.01-0.03 0.5-1.5	0.1-0.5	
Nortriptyline	Plasma	0.003-0.016	0.8-2.6 (F)	
Amphetamine	Blood Urine	N.D.	0.05 (F., I.V.) 0.4 (F., I.V.)	
Methamphetamine	Blood Urine	N.D.	0.06 (F., I.V.) 0.01 (F., I.V.)	
Chlordiazepoxide (Librium)	Serum	0.25-0.80	2.0-5.0	
Diazepam (Valium)	Serum	0.1-0.6	1.5-3.0	
Barbiturates	Serum		Barbiturate Alone	Barbiturate Plus Ethyl
(a) Secobarbital (short-acting)		0.01-0.1	1.0-3.0	1-2.4 (F)
(b) Amobarbital (intermediate-acting)		0.03-0.5	3.0-5.0	1-3 (F)
(c) Phenobarbital (long-acting)		0.5-1.5	7.0-10	1-5 (F)
Ethchlorvynol (Placidyl)	Blood Urine	1.0-2.0 2.5-10.0	10.0-20.0 20	
Glutethimide (Doriden)	Blood Urine	0.05-0.7 Trace	2.0-3.0 (3.0 F) 0.5-2.0	
Meperidine (Demerol)	Blood	0.01-0.1	1.0-3.0 (1.0 F)	
Imipramine (Tofranil)	Serum Urine	0.01-0.06 0.05-2.0	0.1-0.5 (0.2 F) 7.5-10	
Meprobamate (Miltown, Equanil)	Blood	0.5-1.5	5.0 (F)	
Methadone	Blood		0.02-0.03 (F)	
Methaqualone (Quaalude)	Plasma	0.2	0.5 (F)	
Methanol	Blood	0.0 (Normal)	75-125	
Lysergic Acid Diethylamide (LSD)	Urine	5.50 ug/liter	5-50 ug/liter	
Morphine	Blood Urine	0.01-0.05 0.05-2.0	0.1-0.5 5.0-20.0	
Phenothiazines (Chlorpromazine, Trifluoperazine, Promazine, Thioridazine)	Serum Serum (overdose cases) Urine	0.01-0.05 0.1-0.5 0.5-2.0 (metabolites)	0.1-0.5 0.5 (F) 5.0-10.0	
Propoxyphene	Plasma	0.02-0.03		
Thioridazine)		(metabolites)	5.0-10.0	
Propoxyphene (Darvon)	Plasma z	0.02-0.03	0.2 (F)	

F=Fatal   I.V.=Intravenous   N.D.=None Detectable

Adapted from: "Laboratory Aids in Toxicological Problems," Norman Weissman, Ph.D., Bio-Science Laboratories, Van Nuys, California 91405.

cognitive level closer to concrete thinking, whereas high school students usually are capable of more introspection and abstraction (Hamburg, Kraemer, and Jahnke, 1975).

There are many studies that show that there is far greater involvement with drugs in young psychiatric patients than in controls. The involvement concerns not only greater use of drugs, use of more drugs, but also chronic dependency upon drugs and a life style that revolves around obtaining and using drugs.

On the other hand, a nationwide study of 1,357 enrollees and 440 staff members in 19 Job Corps centers (which presumably represents disadvantaged young people) shows that in the main they disapprove of drugs and that drug use is not epidemic among them (Nelson, Kraft, and Fielding, 1974). It showed also that this presumably high risk population is poorly informed about drugs. The use of drugs among this segment of mankind is thought to be no higher that that reported in many high schools and colleges. Although the Job Corps enrollees in the main disapproved of drug use, this did not include marihuana.

Clinical experience has shown that the affluent youngster may be just as directionless as the ghetto teen. Often the higher socioeconomic level child has excessive competition with his parents. The goals his parents set for him may be so high that he is discouraged. He may not be able to muster the energy to satisfy his own needs and society's demands. Hence, although the pressures are qualitatively different, he may be stressed quantitatively as much as the deprived child and as a consequence may turn to drugs. Affluence is not sufficient to prevent drug use. It provides limited human satisfactions. One has to have more than money earned by father in order to cope in this world.

Most of the studies about incidence have concerned themselves with psychiatric patients and often psychiatric inpatients. In 1967 (Cohen and Klein, 1970) a study at Hillside Hospital reported a drug abuse incidence of 31% in consecutive admissions under age 25 years. In 1971 another study conducted at the same hospital found a 60% incidence of drug use in the 15-to-25-year age range (Blumberg et al., 1971).

More recent similar studies of psychiatric patients under 30 have shown that approximately half of them had abused drugs. Of those over 30, the incidence is less and tends to be approximately 25%.

Various studies have compared drug users and non-drug users. This knowledge is useful in preventive programs. For instance, those who use drugs tend to date earlier, run their own informal social parties, tend to be more gregarious; are not involved in organized activities, sports, or homework; do not agree with parents, teachers, or other social institutions as much; are more interested in the social aspects of school than the intellectual; are not active in religious activities; and perhaps most important of all, are very critical of and apparently are not influenced by drug education programs (Hamburg, Kraemer, and Jahnke, 1975). Another study demonstrates that using any drug before the age of 15 years predicts with great accuracy future serious drug involvement such as the use of barbiturates and narcotics (Shearn and Fitzgibbons, 1972).

Experience has shown also that if a person has been a poly-drug-user, has used narcotics, hallucinogens, or a volatile substance, then he is more likely to be an extensive abuser and probably is using drugs at the present time. The high incidence of drug abuse among those who are psychiatrically disturbed and the high use of psychostimulants and barbiturate-tranquilizer type drugs (which are available on prescription) suggest that physicians need to use great discretion in prescribing and following up on the use of drugs in their patients (Fischer et al., 1975).

Treatment Methods

Stimulant Drugs (Cocaine, Amphetamine, Methamphetamine, Phenmetrazine, etc.)

Amphetamine abuse illustrates the one thing that is constant about the drug abuse scene—it is constantly changing. In the early seventies the amphetamines were one of our biggest drug abuse problems, and now in many areas they seem to be out of style and occupy a much less important position in the total drug abuse picture in many areas.

Stimulant medications, particularly "speed," have considerable behavioral toxicity. Persons under their influence may be dangerous and many commit acts against humanity and property. This is in contradistinction to the crimes committed under narcotics, which are mainly against property to support the habit. There is also a high homicide and suicide rate. Patients who have taken large doses of amphetamines must be supplied adequate protection for themselves and others.

Amphetamines may be ingested, snorted, or injected. The latter provides a faster, more intense "Flash" than oral intake. Another favorite technique is "balling," where the drug is instilled into the vagina before intercourse. Some individuals feel too intense from amphetamine intake alone and prefer to use "purple hearts" which is dexamyl (dextro-amphetamine sulphate and amobarbital). Some have mixed methamphetamine and heroin and injected them together. Others after they have had a "speed run" come "down" on heroin, which often leads to a new addiction.

Amphetamines may produce symptoms such as hyperalertness, euphoria, etc., or panic reactions, or psychotic symptoms, or the side effects of chronic high dosage, or death from overdose. Under the influence of amphetamines, a person has racing thoughts, dry mouth, hyper-reflexes, anxiety, tachycardia, sweating, and often a sensation that bugs ("crank bugs") are crawling under the skin. His blood pressure is often elevated. He usually has a mild tremor, and may run some fever.

If the dosage of speed is raised too rapidly, a person may develop a syndrome that has been called "over-amped." The individual is conscious but is unable to move or speak. His pulse, temperature, and blood pressure are elevated, and occasionally there is chest distress.

A "speed run" has varying effects upon orgasms and ejaculations. In some people these are delayed or impossible to achieve and may result in a marathon of sexual activity in an effort to achieve an orgasm. Others report an absence of sexual interest on amphetamines. Sometimes use of amphetamines causes a panic reaction. The patient literally wants to climb the wall.

Patients on amphetamines may not only be agitated, but many manifest an agitated psychotic state with paranoid delusions and hallucinations which can be both auditory and visual. Usually they continue to be oriented and have fair memory and intellectual functioning. An amphetamine chemical psychosis clears spontaneously with time—usually within two to three weeks. If this does not happen, then the diagnosis may be in question. There may be an underlying functional psychosis.

If a person has been "speed tripping" for days, he may manifest the side effects of chronic high dosage. He may appear emaciated and exhausted because of the anorexia, sympathominetic activity, and the constant alertness and hyperactivity that the amphetamine-like drugs produce.

Other side effects that have been reported in chronic high doses of amphetamine are cerebral hemorrhages, cardiac arrhythmias, necrotizing angitis, parenchymal liver damage, and brain cell injury. One may encounter severe abdominal pain mimicking acute surgical abdomens which may be a diagnostic problem. Also to be observed occasionally are dyskinesias (including jaw grinding), and when needles are used, viral hepatitis may occur. The paranoid state comes sooner or later to all high dose users. As one has more "runs," the paranoid state emerges earlier and earlier (Cohen, 1975).

An amphetamine overdose may produce all of the symptoms listed above including restlessness,

Table 4

Agent	*Effects*
Hallucinogens (LSD and mescaline)	Dilated pupils, reflex hyperactivity, anxiety symptoms
Marihuana	Chemosis, dilation of conjunctival blood vessels, rapid pulse, dry throat, normal pupil size, hunger for sweets, difficulty remembering what one is going to say
Anticholinergics	Dilated unreactive pupils, blurred vision, flushed face, reflex hyperactivity, anxiety symptoms, dry mouth, warm, dry skin, tachycardia and fever, foul breath
Central Stimulants	Rapid pulse, increased blood pressure, increased sweating, increased motor activity (variable), paranoid behavior
Opiates	Miosis
Inhalants	Delirium (impaired judgment, orientation, memory and motor skills)

tremor, hyper-reflexes, rapid respirations, confusion, assaultiveness, hallucinations, panic states, arrhythmias, hypertension or hypotension, circulatory collapse, nausea, vomiting, diarrhea, abdominal cramps, as well as convulsions, coma, and death.

After speed is discontinued, there are often overwhelming feelings of fatigue and depression accompanied by insomnia, depressive affect, and gastrointestinal symptoms. Some have reported that the tricyclic medications help under these circumstances. One must recognize that the patient is depressed and should be given a maximum of a week's supply, since an overdose of tricyclics may have serious and possible fatal complications (Cohen, 1975).

The treatment of a person with an amphetamine psychosis includes hospitalization. The symptoms may last for weeks, and there is a high violence tendency (towards self and/or others) due to the hallucinations, paranoid ideas and ideas of reference. Depression often follows a "speed trip." Also, a bad trip is not easily talked down as is usually the case with hallucinogens. Because the amphetamine psychosis is often accompanied by extreme paranoia, it's well to remove such patients from threatening people such as policemen. They should be around those who can give them knowledgeable supervision so as to avoid sensory deprivation and a consequent exacerbation of their symptoms.

Many drugs have been used to help with the panic states and the psychotic-like symptoms. These include the phenothiazines which attenuate the effects of LSD if given after the effects are established. The phenothiazines are not antagonists to LSD. If these are used, it is more difficult to know whether or not the patient with psychotic-like symptoms is a latent psychotic (who has been precipitated into an overt attack with amphetamines) or whether he has a pure chemical psychosis. Chlorpromazine is an aid in helping talk a person down and is a semi-specific antidote for amphetamine psychosis. However, a caution is in order. It's important to observe the patient for atropine-like symptoms, in which event chlorpromazine should be used cautiously, if at all, since it also has an atropine-like effect. An anticholinergic crisis may be reversed by physostigmine. An overdose of physostigmine may cause a cholinergic crisis. One can not be certain that a person has been on amphetamines or that they have not been on several drugs or that the drug was pure. Pushers sometimes sell what they have and label it what the buyer desires. Hence, in case of doubt, phenothiazines should not be used, or in any event, used very cautiously or in small doses with resuscitative equipment and proper medications on hand.

Others have reported that the aggressive, agitated patient is often helped by giving secobarbital (Seconal) by mouth and repeating it as indicated until the patient begins to come off his "high."

A reasonable approach to the amphetamine highs seems to be as follows. One should try to establish verbal contact by offering reassurance and defining reality. If the patient has severe ego disruption and does not respond to the above, then conservative use of phenothiazines should be considered in combination with the verbal interaction. Some have found haloperidol as the drug of choice in lysing an amphetamine psychosis rapidly. Others reason that because of the danger of the anticholinergic effect and because they believe the phenothiazines' beneficial action is through its sedative effect, it is wiser to use paraldehyde, diazepam, or short-acting barbiturates to avoid the possible complications of anticholinergic potentiation (Taylor, Maurer, and Tinklenberg, 1970).

The treatment of an amphetamine overdose is difficult. It concerns itself with the standard overdose procedures of gastric lavage, sedation, perhaps with barbiturates, treating the hyperthermia and hypertension, acidification of the urine, which increases amphetamine excretion, and consideration of hemodialysis and peritoneal dialysis if necessary. The blood pressure usually decreases with sedation. Some have used phentolamine (Regitine) for severe, acute hypertension (Greenblatt and Shader, 1974).

Cocaine produces gregariousness, hyperactive behavior, tachycardia, racing thoughts, twitching, euphoria, and at times a chemical psychosis. There may be a sensation of "crank bugs." Treatment consists of sedation if necessary. Sodium phenobarbital has the advantage of being an anticonvulsant. Often even when a patient reports that he has had only one drug such as cocaine, he is very likely to have had other drugs such as other stimulants, hallucinogens, or heroin (Wikler, personal communication). Therefore, one is well advised to use caution and restraint regarding the co-administration of drugs to patients with drug-induced disease.

Hallucinogenic Drugs (LSD, Marihuana, Mescaline, STP, Dimethyltryptamine ("DMT") and Others)

The hallucinogens may produce symptoms similar to those effected by stimulants. For example, they may produce excitation, anxiety, panic, psychotoxicity, disorders of behavior, loss of control, misperceptions, depersonalization, hallucinations, delusions and depression. Distortion of the senses occurs early on the dose response curve. With cocaine and amphetamines, a much higher dose and usually intravenous administration are necessary to induce psychotic behavior (Chapel, 1973).

The safest method of treating a hallucinogenic "trip" is "talking down." Some administer chloral hydrate or diazepam orally. Others use short-acting barbiturates such as phenobarbital. The patient should be housed in a quiet, well-lighted room under observation. Apparently, deaths from LSD overdose are rare or never seen, but deaths do occur due to psychotoxicity resulting in suicide and/or homicide.

2,5-dimethoxy, 4 methly-amphetamine (STP or DOM) causes many bad trips. In these, the patients are more anxious and panicky because of the stimulant-like effect of this amphetamine congener. The symptoms and signs are high pulse rate, palpitations, and sweating. The patient may feel as if he is having a heart attack. The treatment is the same as described above for hallucinogenic trips. Phenothiazines should be avoided.

Professionals see few "bad trips" because friends have learned effectively how to talk a "high" person down. "Talking down" should include reassurance that the patient is not losing his mind. He should be told repeatedly that he is feeling as he is because of the drug and that when its effects wear off he'll feel better. It helps to give him concrete, simple information again and again such as where he is, what has and is happening, and what will happen. There are fewer "bad trips" now because drug users are more knowledgeable about what to expect and hence don't freak out so often. It is thought now that "bad trips" are usually due to acute anxiety reactions which are more likely when one is neurotic and especially if one is unacquainted with the effects of the drug.

Although there have been many explanations of "flashbacks," it is thought now that they never existed. They were described originally by Dr. David E. Smith in 1968 to 1973 when he was on the San Francisco scene. He saw many "flashbacks" and publicized them and suggested what he thought was the cause with the name. Subsequent studies have shown that "flashbacks" are seen especially in anxiety neurotics. Those who had bad trips on LSD have subsequent anxiety attacks and they remember how very upset they were on the hallucinogen and relive the trip. Dr. Smith feels that it is not a physiological phenomenon but a neurotic one that was initially a misunderstood phenomena that reached massive proportions through advertising.

Marihuana (Tetrahydrocannabinol—THC)

Common symptoms seen with marihuana use are chemosis, hunger for sweets, difficulty completing a sentence (can't remember what he was going to say), increased pulse rate, and dry throat. Users rarely come to emergency rooms or to physician's offices because an overdose is rare. Sometimes a patient develops a panic reaction and becomes agitated. There may be paranoid thinking, hallucinations, delusions, and feelings of depersonalization in the chronic abuser using high doses (similar to an LSD "trip"). In a group, heavy partakers tend to talk at each other and often no one seems to understand the other. There are episodes of laughter periodically but often they can not remember what they are laughing at.

The final information concerning the effects of marihuana is not in yet, even though it has been studied extensively. Probably the different results from marihuana use in the United States compared to those reported in other countries concerns itself with how much THC is used and for how long. For instance, in countries where it has been used for thousands of years in large doses, the natives can pick out the chronic marihuana users because of their indolence and lack of goal direction. Recently there have been reported changes in female sexual functioning and andogenic production with chronic use of marihuana. The chronic smoker tends to develop respiratory difficulties beginning with bronchitis. We are now seeing those who have been chronically intoxicated with marihuana for 15 or 20 years. Those who are stoned all the time usually have a poly-drug syndrome. They often use a good deal of alcohol plus many other drugs and usually have basic emotional and mental problems.

When one is chronically intoxicated (30 days or more) there develops a tolerance to the euphoric effect and in its place comes apathy, irritability, neglect of one's personal habits, and failure to complete tasks. This has become known as the amotivational syndrome. Users sit and smoke pot and meditate. Treatment for this state is hospitalization, withdrawal, and all that rehabilitation encompasses. There should be sparse use, if any, of sedatives or chlorpromazine (Wikler, personal communication). The basic treatment is that of the fundamental emotional problem.

The treatment for a "bad trip" is the same as for other hallucinogens, that is, "talking down" (Chapel, 1973).

Depressant Drugs (Alcohol, other Hydrocarbons, Barbiturates and Non-barbituric Sedative-hypnotics, Some Anti-anxiety Agents, Morphine and Morphine-like analgesics, etc.)

The depressants reduce mental and physical functioning. The psychotoxic condition following their use may result in personal injury or disorders of behavior. Unlike the stimulants, the depressants can cause loss of consciousness and motor function and thereby exert some degree of control over excessive intake of the drug (Seevers, 1968).

When one chronically abuses depressants, he is faced with two phenomena—tolerance and physical dependence. By tolerance we mean that the drug action is modified and it takes a greater and greater dose in order to obtain similar results. As one is exposed to larger amounts of depressant drugs, a state of physical dependence develops. This is a condition of latent hyperexcitability which manifests itself by increased nervous activity when the drug is terminated.

There are two distinct types of abstinence syndromes. The morphine abstinence syndrome is produced by termination of morphine intake (and morphine-like drugs) and is associated with yawning, rhinorrhea, lacrimation, sweating, dilated pupils, and restlessness 12 to 16 hours after the last dose. Later, other symptoms such as muscular aches, twitches, abdominal cramps, vomiting, diarrhea, anorexia, and spontaneous ejaculations in the male and profuse menstrual bleeding in the female may develop.

The morphine abstinence syndrome, although subjectively distressing, is rarely life threatening and withdrawal can be accomplished without much difficulty, usually using codeine (rapid reduction method) or methadone substitution. The second syndrome is that of alcohol-barbiturate abstinence. This differs from the morphine type in several respects. One must have prolonged continuous administration of large doses over months for the syndrome to develop. The syndrome is characterized by delirium, hallucinations, tremor, hyperthermia, and grand mal seizures. It is intense and may be life threatening. Withdrawal must be done gradually over several weeks. It may be induced by alcohol, the barbiturates, minor tranquilizers (but not phenothiazines) and other depressants listed below. The drugs that produce the syndrome may be used interchangeably by substitution to suppress the syndrome induced by the withdrawal (Seevers, 1968).

"Downers"

"Downers" include barbiturates, non-barbituric sedative-hypnotics such as methaqualone (Quaalude), ethchlorvynol (Placidyl), glutethimide (Doriden), etc., and anti-anxiety agents such as diazepam (Valium), chlordiazepoxide (Librium), and meprobamate (Equanil, Miltown, etc.).

Secobarbital, pentobarbital, glutethimide (Doriden), and meprobamate can produce deep coma and death with relatively small doses. Chlordiazepoxide, diazepam, and flurazepam (Dalmane) are less dangerous and produce little respiratory or cardiovascular depression even after relatively large doses. Fatal poisoning with this latter class of drugs is less common (Seevers, 1968).

In the fully conscious patient who has recently ingested a "downer" overdose, syrup of ipecac (not fluid extract of ipecac) is usually effective in inducing vomiting. Apomorphine is more consistently and rapidly effective than ipecac but may produce unwanted central nervous system depression. In the unconscious patient, gastric lavage should be performed with an endotracheal tube with a cuff. Interestingly, in overdoses of glutethimide and meprobamate, a patient may wake up and then subsequently lapse back into deep coma. Hence patients who have ingested significant quantities of these should be hospitalized even if they seem awake because of the possibility of a rebound effect. This pehnomenon has been explained on the basis of delayed absorption or release of the drug from the entero-hepatic circulation or mobilization of the drug from lipid storage sites (Seevers, 1968). In order to avoid the withdrawal syndrome of any of the barbiturates or alcohol, pentobarbital (Nembutal) is often used. It produces sufficient intoxication and avoids an abstinence syndrome if the dose of pentobarbital is decreased gradually each day.

A word of caution is indicated in the treatment of patients who have taken a large dose of downers. It may or may not make him unconscious as expected. The provisional diagnosis may be an "overdose." The usual treatment is given him and he is sent home. The next day he is admitted with convulsions. The real diagnosis was physical and psychic dependence with great tolerance, and he should have been admitted and treated as an addict not just as an overdose.

There is no good antagonist for a "downer" overdose. Treatment consists of general measures such as maintaining respiration, vasopressors, fluids to support the circulation, use of osmotic diuretics (such as furosemide-Lasix), dialysis if necessary, antibiotics, and treatment of possible hyperthermia and cardiac arrythmias (Chapel, 1973).

Alcohol

Alcohol use is very common among teenagers, and there are many 16-year-olds who have been drinking for many years. Hence we are beginning to see more complications of alcohol abuse in older adolescents and young adults. Visual and auditory hallucinations in 16-year-olds after days of drinking are more and more common.

Alcohol hallucinosis is characterized by auditory hallucinations. The patient often has ideas of persecution and reference and is distrustful but oriented. The treatment includes hospitalization, and sometimes phenothiazines are indicated. Some believe it is a schizophrenic reaction released by alcohol.

Acute alcoholic excitement is characterized by an acute psychotic-type reaction with great excitement, combativeness and hallucinations of sight. It is often brief and self-limited, but is a serious condition that may result in coma or death. Treatment consists of paraldehyde until the symptoms subside.

Alcoholic delirium tremens is seen in chronic alcoholics during withdrawal and after a heavy bout of drinking and may be seen from a day to a week after the last drink. It is rarely seen under 30 years of age. Such patients present with disorientation, fears, visual and sometimes auditory hallucinations, tremors, tachycardia, and sweating. It is a dangerous condition and it may last for a week. It can be fatal and the patient is sometimes suicidal. Treatment consists of hospitalization, attention to fluid and electrolyte balance, and judicious administration of paraldehyde (Greenblatt and Shader, 1974). Some physicians prefer chlordiazepoxide or diazepam, and believe the barbiturates are too toxic. Paraldehyde has the disadvantage that it is noxious to patients and medical staff and inappropriate for parental administration due to gluteal irritation. There is some evidence that the phenothiazines should be avoided, since they are associated with increased incidence of seizures and occasionally with hypotension which can be a serious complication. The alcoholic should also be given thiamine intramuscularly, since he may develop an acute encephalopathy due to thiamin deficiency that can become irreversible if not treated. Within 48 hours of cessation of drinking, seizures may occur. Opinions differ as to whether dilantin is useful in preventing or arresting seizures.

Antabuse helps a small number of people who want to control their drinking. It is toxic and can't be used with those with kidney or cardiovascular disease. In a teenager it often doesn't work because he refuses to continue taking it. The teenage boy often has a reaction formation against feeling dependent upon a doctor and his medication, and besides, he wants to continue drinking. He often rationalizes that he can "do it" by himself—dependence upon a medicine threatens his ego.

Opiates

In recent years an acute dose of heroin has been reported as the commonest cause of death in New York City among men 15–35 years of age. An overdose of heroin may be intentional, accidental, or poisons may be concealed in injectable narcotics for the purpose of homicide—a "hot shot." The signs and symptoms of opiate overdose include apnea, decreased respiratory rate, cyanosis, absent reflexes, stupor, coma, myosis, and a urine screen positive for opiates. With severe overdosing, pulmonary edema and respiratory arrest may result. Pulmonary edema should be treated with an orthopnic position and a diuretic such as furosemide (Lasix). Pressor amines may be needed for hypotension. Digitalization is considered by some clinicians. Intubation, tracheostomy, and continuous positive pressure ventilation with an oxygen concentration of at least 40% may be indicated (Chapel, 1973). A specific narcotic antagonist such as naloxone hydrochloride (Narcan) can be useful. This will counteract or prevent excessive respiratory depression from drugs with a morphine-like effect (for example, heroin, morphine, dilaudid, methadone, demerol, etc.). A caution is in order. If the opiates are not the cause of the coma, then antagonists such a nalorphine (Nalline) and levallorphan (Lorfan) may cause respiratory depression with repeated doses. For instance, in barbiturate poisoning this is a danger that must be taken into account. Narcan doesn't produce respiratory depression and hence appears to be the antagonist of choice (Greenblatt and Shader, 1974). Secure physical restraints should be applied before a narcotic antagonist is injected because often the patient becomes combative as he emerges from an opiate-induced coma. The patient must be observed for at least 24 hours, since the respiratory depression may reoccur within several hours because the opiate antagonists are eliminated much more rapidly than heroin. If the patient is physically dependent on the opiate, excessive use of antagonists may precipitate an opiate abstinence syndrome.

The substitution of methadone in the treatment of opiate addiction is a major innovation. One mg. of methadone equals in abstinence suppressing potency 2 to 4 mg. of morphine sulphate or 1 mg. of heroin or 0.5 mg. of hydromorphone (Dilaudid). The patient may be stabilized with methadone over a 2-to-3 day period as the opiate is withdrawn.

Methadone proponents claim that it increases the number of people who are able to go to school and work, facilitates functioning in the family, and decreases the street use of heroin. Methadone blocks the craving for heroin, and one does not get much of an effect even if he takes heroin, etc. Indeed, the result is aversive. He pays for the heroin but doesn't get a "high." But other drugs do not have a cross-tolerance and so the patients may use alcohol, barbiturates, Valium, etc.

Another means of treating the opiate addict is through therapeutic communities. These are treating a few thousand patients whereas methadone programs are treating perhaps a hundred thousand patients in the United States. The therapeutic communities confront the addict with his problems, do not believe in medication substitutes such as methadone, and rely upon the motivation of the addict. It's usually necessary for him to continue in the therapeutic community for one or two years in order to get satisfactory results. The Phoenix House in New York City and Odyssey House in various cities are examples of this type of program.

Darvon is similar in chemical structure to methadone. It can be looked upon as a weak methadone and is sometimes used to detoxify those who are on morphine sulphate or demerol. Naloxone hydrochloride (Narcans), a narcotic antagonist, reverses the effects of an overdose.

There are many medical disorders found in drug addicts. In a study of 200 patients admitted to the Bernstein Institute Medical Inpatient Unit in New York, of which 126 were under 30 years of age, the following incidence of complications were noted: 30.5% had acute hepatitis; 27.5% had infections; 11.5% came in for detoxification; 7.5% had diabetes mellitus; 6.0% had pulmonary disease; 5.0% had taken an overdose; 4.0% had cardiovascular disease; 3.5% had gastro-intestinal disease; and 3.5% had venereal disease (White, 1973). These figures emphasize how important it is to do a thorough medical workup on addicts.

Inhalants (Model-airplane Glue, Paint Thinner, Gasoline, Industrial Solvents, Amyl Nitrite, Ether, Aerosol Sprays, etc.)

The volatile solvents are classified as anesthetics along with ether and alcohol. They may produce temporary periods of stimulation before depression of the central nervous system occurs. The earliest symptoms consist of slurred speech, dizziness, unsteady gait, and drowsiness. The clinical picture may progress on to delirium, mental confusion, emotional lability, and impaired thinking. Respiration may be depressed, pupils dilated, heartbeat accelerated and they may develop a cough. Some manifest what has been called a "glue sniffer's rash" around the nose and mouth. Occasionally, the patient is impulsive, excited, irritable and may develop injuries during this period of overactivity. As the brain is further affected by the drugs, the patient may develop hallucinations and delusions. After a euphoric high, the patient usually falls asleep. The period of intoxication may last from a few minutes to an hour or two (Cohen, 1975). A partial tolerance develops with daily use although no withdrawal syndrome has been described. Psychologic dependence is present.

The usual abuser is likely to be a boy from about 7 to 17 years of age. The course may be a few times at sniffing and then giving the habit up, or it may persist until the late teens, when they usually abandon sniffing. However, many then use other drugs chronically, especially alcohol and barbiturates. There are a number of reports of organ systems damage (brain, liver, kidney, bone marrow). There have been many deaths resulting from "sniffing," most of them being due to aerosol abuse. Death is usually caused by respiratory or cardiac arrest. Aerosols may occlude the airway by freezing the larynx, or some have postulated that the pulmonary alveolar surface is frozen, which prevents the transfer of oxygen. Sometimes inhalants are sprayed into plastic garment bags and these are pulled over the head to achieve a higher concentration of volatile material. Accidental death may result.

One optimistic note is that one model-airplane cement manufacturer has added a small amount of synthetic oil of mustard to its preparation. The amount is insufficient to produce nausea under normal usage, but it is unpleasant when the contents are used for sniffing. Another producer claims to have developed an airplane glue that is nonintoxicating when inhaled. The problem is that the variety and availability of other inhalants in every kitchen, laundry, and bathroom are innumerable (Cohen, 1975).

Treatment is difficult because most of these children come from disorganized homes. The self-image must be changed from that of a loser and loner to a person who is someone and is loved. Many suggestions have been made along these lines elsewhere in this chapter. Treatment is concerned with prevention mainly, but for the patient who is already afflicted, we have no better treatment than rehabilitation, education, control of drugs, adequate supervision at home and at school, appropriate school curriculums, and psychotherapy.

Comparisons

Although the family dynamics discussed above seem to agree with clinical experience, it should be pointed out that the overprotective syndrome—i.e., close mother-child relationship and distant mother-father relationship—is one of the most frequent triangular family arrangements in America and has been described as etiological in many other syndromes. Better controlled studies comparing the family of origin of addicts/abusers with drop-out populations who do not use drugs are needed. Also, we must answer the question: Why do other children reared in overprotective families avoid drug misuse?

Drug-using families often overlook drug use in their offspring, or covertly or overtly encourage it, or interfere with the treatment of it. Interestingly, cures rarely result if the treatment program does not have the family's full support.

Normal, non-drug-abusing families show that parents have an increased capacity to love and do love children more and for healthy reasons. There is also increased husband-wife solidarity, stronger family relationships, many healthy family traditions, friendlier parent-child relationships, with greater priority given to having and caring for children. Parents in these healthier, normal families do not covertly or overtly encourage drug use. Children's needs are met so that there is less need to soothe over disappointment or find pseudo-satisfactions and pleasures in the use of drugs. Children are better prepared for life—have better problem-solving techniques.

Decades ago, drug abuse was a minority, low socioeconomic, ghetto problem, but now it has spread to all peoples. Treatment is concerned mostly with identifying the particular needs of an individual and meeting them, no matter what segment of the population or what individual is affected.

There are three parts of the drug problem—namely, the casual drug user or experimenter, the regular drug user, and the chronic user who usually gets on to narcotics (mainly opiates). These are different problems and require different treatment approaches. Additionally, we must understand the chemistry and pharmacology of stimulants, hallucinogens, depressants, narcotic-analgesics, anticholinergics, etc.

The custom of segregating drug abusers into treatment facilities separate from other diagnostic psychiatric categories has its pros and cons. Drug abusers and addicts are not readily accepted by the professions or society. In theory, drug abuse is a symptom with other underlying problems and should be treated in regular clinics, hospitals, and other institutions by trained personnel. This often is the treatment of choice for the casual and regular user, but the chronic user and the addict have special problems and often need special facilities, personnel, therapy and long term follow-up.

The advent of multiple drug usage has demanded the development of a multitude of treatment facilities. These range from intensive inpatient care for overdose and withdrawal, through regular hospitalization, day hospitalization, therapeutic community, vocational rehabilitation, family therapy, group therapy, to individual therapy, etc.

A mental status examination assists one in diagnosing cerebral intoxication. In the mildly affected patient one may find normal memory, orientation, and perception. The positive findings may include decreased coordination, judgment, attention span, and ability to concentrate. There may be slurred speech, fine tremor, unsteady gait and balance. The person's feelings may be exaggerated in that he is more depressed, irritable or optimistic than is normal. Speed of thought may be increased with stimulants or decreased with depressants but eventually both decrease the ability to think clearly and abstract appropriately. If a patient has more severe cerebral intoxication, he may then suffer a deficit of memory, judgment, and ability to calculate, as well as be excessively labile emotionally.

Casual Drug User

The casual drug user relates to drugs somewhat as a fad. This has been one of the main causes of the drug abuse pandemic in the United States. The Japanese pandemic of methamphetamine undoubtedly included many casual users and was reduced from two million to two thousand users by using three factors: (1) massive education so that the nonusers (who subsequently came in contact with the drug or users) had some data upon which they could make a rational decision; (2) treatment services; (3) intensive law enforcement. The younger the patient, the more the local community must be involved. The casual drug user is usually relatively healthy and gives up unwise drug practices even as he finds himself sexually and in other ways. Healthy relationships and guidance is usually sufficient to avoid further drug involvement.

Regular Drug Abusers

Our first consideration is the prevention of a person becoming a drug abuser as outlined elsewhere in this chapter. Next, we must be concerned with medical emergencies produced by drug ingestion, whether they be overdose suicide attempts or accidental miscalculation of dose. Most medical-psychiatric facilities are capable of handling these circumstances. The even more challenging task is the long-term treatment after the emergency is over.

Psychotherapy with adolescents is frequently not an easy task, but to treat the drug-using/abusing adolescent is even more difficult. He is often unmotivated, breaks appointments, has anti-dependency anger, makes excessive demands, and is frequently seriously disturbed (often sociopathic) and creates a series of crises so that the therapist has greater difficulty getting to the core of the problem.

Of vital concern is the therapeutic relationship (Geist, 1974). A therapist must be available, skilled, and devoted if he is to be important enough to be a patient's transition object between drugs and a healthier life. Before one discusses the drug problem with a teenager, it is usually wise to develop a firm relationship or the patient may terminate therapy or attempt suicide or his core mental illness may become more overt.

The therapist should recognize the healthy, active strivings in the patient's thoughts and actions, even though in the main most of these may be destructive initially. Eventually, therapy gets to the point where the therapist is able to point out that when the teen does the opposite of what someone advises, he is acting just as dependently as if he did everything they said. Subsequently, one can compare the present problems with those of early childhood and suggest that these are preventing the patient from attaining the desired adult life style. As the relationship replaces the drug as a transitional object, there is usually a decrease in the use of drugs. A regression may occur when the therapist is out of town or when an important heterosexual relationship dissolves. Drug-using patients use heterosexual relationships to act out the transference, as additional transitional relationships to help them gain independence, as an attempt to get close to another human sexually and psychologically, and as an attempt to cope with the anxiety associated with loss of one's childhood, parents, therapist, etc. (Geist, 1974).

There is a need with a drug-using adolescent even more than with the average teen patient to be a down-to-earth, friendly, human therapist who can share his own beliefs and feelings—tell the patient something about himself if this seems desired.

The older adolescent, who has sociopathic tendencies and is addicted to drugs, may begin to play adult-type addict games. He has to become a "con" artist in order to maintain his life style. He uses this ploy also in dealing with the therapist. He may try to manipulate with praise, centering the interview on the therapist, playing the therapist's insight game, or with hypochondriacal symptoms. Or he may coax for sympathy when he repeatedly disregards prescribed treatment. The therapist must recognize the various "games" the patient plays, discuss and do something about them—i.e. use consistent limit setting in an inpatient setting when necessary (Levine and Stephens, 1971).

Chronic User (Includes Narcotics Usually)

The confirmed narcotic addict is difficult to manage, and there are several therapeutic schools of thought (Pierce, personal communication).

1. Psychiatric approach. Open communication

and psychotherapy is used with addicts who will stay put and participate in rehabilitation programs because they are motivated. Most addicts can not handle this type of treatment.

2. Institutionalization. Conventional rehabilitation staff, counselors and correction officers are used as co-counselors. Personnel from the ex-addict organizations are used to sensitize the staff as to what is going on.

3. The interdisciplinary approach. All of the disciplines cooperate to withdraw the patient from the addicting drug, help him reestablish family and extra-family relationships, develop a marketable skill, etc.

4. Ex-addicts' program. Ex-addicts treat those who are addicted with apostolic-type zeal. They often feel that their program is the only way to solve the problem. They are totally committed to abstinence and do not believe in drug substitution.

5. Drug maintenance. The most prominent example is the treatment of morphine-like drug addicts with the methadone maintenance program. A street addict is converted into a "square addict" (a methadone addict). This is seen as only an answer and not the answer, and other aspects of the problem must be approached also.

6. Drug antagonists. There are several heroin antagonists available at the present time, such as Naloxone (Narcan) which does not further depress respirations.

7. Ambulatory care. Halfway houses are used together with other approaches to help the addict.

A combination of the above may be used, or at one point a certain approach is indicated and later is replaced by a more appropriate treatment approach.

Prevention

Cope or "Cop-Out"

One of the principal factors that leads to the use of drugs is failure or fear of same. If children do not learn how to cope they are likely to "cop out." In the past we have been preoccupied with health dangers of drugs and the epidemic that was upon us. In addition to these activities, we must get on with the major task of helping people cope with the problems with which they are besieged. We must be concerned with the challenges and sometimes mental anguish that many children and teens face and aid them. Otherwise, life becomes unbearable and they may seek chemical help. We must help them re-evoke or attain initiatives and skills. We must encourage them to attain or regain confidence and self-respect. This will be done mainly from assisting them in attaining accomplishments commensurate with their potentials. They must be seen as individuals with capabilities and talents and hence be given from their earliest years appropriate responsibilities and decisions. This is done first in the family and then in our schools, churches, etc. We must help them see the problems, use their talents to overcome them, take appropriate responsibilities gradually before they are expected to function independently. We must let them gradually gain strength so that they can see the day when they can take over from us. Hopefully, they will have sufficient success that they can anticipate even greater success in the future and see the achievement of their goals. Then they will do more than sit back, criticize, protest, do nothing constructive, and act as if they (without experience, training, education or help from us) have the ability to face this life and handle its problems. Such attitudes often lead to failure, isolation, alienation, and anomie. If we don't make success a possibility, they are likely to expend 90% of their energy opposing their predecessors. They will be strong and independent in unhealthy ways even if their main observable asset is opposing whatever their elders say.

We must help each teen find a place of satisfaction in this world—succeed to the maximum of his abilities. We must help him find himself in positive ways or he is likely to feel he is a nothing, excel in negativism, become great in his own mind only. He may become functionally psychotic or attain rapid chemical psychosis with drugs.

The Family

The neglected, rejected child from an unhealthy family is at high risk for drug abuse. Although problems often appear in the junior high and high school years, the ground work for drug abuse is often laid in the years prior to this. We must create strong families where teens can go for security, peace, protection, and serenity. Families must compensate for the speed of living, competition, disappointment, failure, difficulty in finding one's self, and lack of closeness. Almost every major drug problem in children and teens is associated with a major family problem. Often the teen needs a close human relationship and yet no one is available at home. Inappropriate heterosexual relationships and drugs are often substituted for healthy human relations. The best deterrent to drug use is an individual's value system, getting one's needs met in healthy activities, being reared in a healthy family that helps one develop self control and gain success in life. We can not effectively enforce drug laws nor determine what millions of people put into their mouths. The main legal effort must be to make dangerous drugs unavailable and the family task is to develop healthy personalities.

Parent-Child Relationships

Often a crucial factor in the life of the drug abuser is the inadequate relationship he has with his parents. Whatever can be done to promote more responsible parenthood would be a significant step toward prevention of drug abuse.

If there is a healthy relationship between the parents and the child, they are able to explore attitudes and values in the family and society. They are able to discuss goals and the means of reaching them, so that there is more success and less failure in the day-to-day living and playing together. Healthy families are able to explore effective normal conduct or ineffective, neurotic, beatnik-type conduct, or bizarrely unrealistic, psychotic-like living, and how these increase or decerease one's difficulties in life. Parents are able to use gentle reasoning, personal example, longitudinal case histories of friends, neighbors, and relatives in order to help a child correct prejudices and misconceptions and abandon childhood patterns. They can help a child revise his goals and values and adopt a realistic, productive, rewarding, mature style of life.

Few factors, if any, are more important for the healthy develpoment of a child than that the parents and children stay friends. This is facilitated if the parents have such maturity that their principal pleasure is obtained by assisting, in a wise manner, a child's growth and individuation. If a parent is struggling for his own existence and is competitive with the children, then this is not likely to happen. If a friendly relationship is present, then the teen can identify with the parents and can learn from them. Then the child has a secure personal relationship that is appropriately modified toward healthy independence as the child grows up. Then there is less need to join the "off-beats," the "downbeats," or even the "up-beats" in order to achieve a relationship. If there is not such a parent-child relationship and the teen is unable to join a healthy group, then he is very likely to join an unhealthy one, even if he must do what he knows is wrong and even if it hurts him more than it does his parents. If the relationship with the parents is a healthy one, then the teen can accept the parents' conscience to a large degree and with indirect help can control his acts through this critical period.

Second Lines of Defense

The same principle applies to teacher, leaders, and others in the community who are sometimes more important than the parents themselves. These leaders must stay friends with the teenagers, or they can be of no positive influence and may be detrimental. A principal goal in this relationship is to help the adolescent be successful, find his talents, and learn how to relate appropriately with his family, the same and the opposite sex, authority figures, and society. Staying friends, talking the same language,learning to solve problems are principal objectives of a healthy family. This is a seven-day-a-week job—not a fishing trip once a year. The overall goal is to prepare the offspring to live happily and successfully. Warm human relationships are a much better deterrent to drug abuse than the latest information about heroin from New York City, important as education is.

As a child grows and develops, sometimes the parents are unable to relate to him. Or even in the healthy child, he begins looking to people outside his family for influence. He may have difficulty weaning himself from his parents but can do so more successfully if he has an appropriate substitute. Hence, the key people in the environment become increasingly important at this time. They can help him fight failure or fear of same, help him be successful, and he is much less likely to need to rebel or retreat. If he finds this type of person, then he is much less likely to need an addictogenic friend or a drug group with whom he can find some degree of security and acceptance.

Prominent among the needs of the teenager is a school that has a model curriculum. If a school has a comprehensive curriculum where all students can fit in and be successful, then their needs are met, they have increased self-esteem and are more likely to be successful in school as well as life.

Religious institutions often are of great assistance in this regard also, especially if they present an accepting attitude and a healthy group with whom the adolescent can be accepted and identify.

As a child grows and solves his family status

problems, hopefully he begins working on his social status goals and grows increasingly closer to peers. They have more and more influence with him. If the parents have a healthy relationship with him, then he is likely to identify with a group that has mores similar to those of his parents. Healthy youth groups are vital in helping a teen meet his needs, wean himself from his parents and give him support in facing viscissitudes of life. A teen who is alienated from his parents is often closer to abusing drugs, and he is more likely to align himself with teens who have problems similar to his own. Those who treat drug abusers have recognized this for decades as they have used ex-drug abusers or ex-addicts in the treatment program. Often these teens and adults are at the center of the counter-drug youth efforts. The main difficulty with this approach is that once a person is a drug abuser or is addicted to drugs, professionals can never be certain that he has mastered the problem. Healthy clubs, hobbies, sports and social grops, etc. are a boon to normal adolescent development, and adults should facilitate youth going into any healthy direction they desire in this regard. Such a course prevents or helps with alienations that teenagers often feel. Such an approach is much more profitable than the fear-of-drugs model, which does not work. Education about drugs using the fear model may backfire if the person has a need for self-flagellation, an urge toward self-destruction or a yen for dangerous, irrational adventure.

Life Must Be "Possible" and Hopefully Fun

Difficult as it is, it is usually easier to handle the acute emergencies of drug abuse and overdose than it is to prevent them. The latter is a complicated task and requires a longitudinal effort of great magnitude. As a child grows up, if he finds life miserable, sees little hope for a change in the future, if his pleasures are few and his pain is great, then he becomes desperate and is more likely to seek pleasure however he can find it. His life may begin to revolve around the immediate task of finding an experience and/or drug that will relieve his pain, boredom, or hopelessness and give him pleasure. He has the ability to pursue immediate pleasure but not the strength to adhere to the reality principle. Seeking a pusher, finding a drug, obtaining the money to buy it, is a relatively simple task compared to the talents and energies that are necessary to obtain long-range healthy goals that return delayed pleasure of much greater magnitude.

It frequently comes down to this: Where does one get his needs paid off? Is there some possibility that he can achieve, fit in, and relate with healthy people, or does he search for pleasure elsewhere in the drug world? Parents, educators, community leaders must make life of the healthy variety possible and probable. We must make it a reality for the deprived and disadvantaged as well as the privileged, for the affluent as well as the effluent, for those with less than average talents as well as for the gifted. We must educate for a world of great complexity, but this alone will not assure children against disaster. We must have the example and teachings of a healthy family. If we as teens or parents fail to plan, prepare, learn, and adapt to the exigencies of this world, then we may be planning for some degree of failure, retreat, acting out; or some form of beatnikism may result. It is under such circumstances that the risks of using intoxicating substances to ease the excessive pains of life and gain euphoria are high. Life has plenty of healthy, new experiences that one can try, things to learn, matters to be curious about. There are social, athletic, artistic, and musical events, etc—many ways that one can use to get healthy highs. These are major immunizations against drug abuse if they are used wisely.

Education

In the early years of the epidemic of drug abuse, we frequently fell back upon education as our main approach. Undoubtedly, it does have some effect on some people, but mainly upon the nonuser of drugs. If a person is of a mind to learn, he may gain through education information that gives some degree of immunity when the possibility of drug use arises. Drug abuse is not rational; therefore, education seldom helps the present user. The decision to use drugs is not a thinking one but is usually made because of one's friends or the circumstances in which one finds himself. Doctors have the highest rate of drug abuse, and yet they know the most about it. Education is a tool that we should use at the proper time, in an appropriate way and with the people with whom it is most likely to have influence.

For those who are seeking relief from the pressures of life, sometimes education backfires. It may introduce them to a drug they can use to gain their instant relief, which sometimes amounts to an instant chemical psychosis. Although this sometimes gives immediate pleasure, its long range effect is to make life even more impossible and a vicious cycle may be initiated.

We can approach the education about drugs from two points of view. (1) If we make too much of it, we may reinforce the use of drugs—in effect advertise drug use. It may increase curiosity and experimentation. This we saw at the height of the drug abuse epidemic. The more we did about it, the more we talked about it, the more treatment facilities, the higher was the incidence of drug abuse. At times it seems that when we fight an ill in inappropriate ways it reinforces the effect. The paradoxical, dominant transmission process comes into play. That is, the more we decry a certain practice, the more interest there is in it, the more some people want to try it. (2) On the other hand, if too little information is given about drug abuse, then our population does not know the dangers, and ignorance is not likely to be bliss. There is a fine point in education about drugs which determines whether or not the paradoxical, dominant transmission process comes into effect (which may actually reinforce the use of drugs) or whether the problem is approached in such a manner that we talk about drugs—not drug abuse—to the end that we convert the interest into a healthy understanding of drugs. This might mean less tobacco, less alcohol, and a more sensible pattern of using legal medications and the avoidance of illegal, harmful drugs. At the same time that we are engaging in an educative-preventive program, we must help children develop healthy alternatives to a chemical existence. This will need to be done on a person-to-person approach in addition to school assemblies of 2,500 students being lectured to regarding drug abuse.

Conclusions

Throughout history, drugs/medicines have been used by man. Whether their use is approved or disapproved has been defined often irrationally by what the prevailing society wanted. It is difficult to define healthy drug use, misuse, abuse, and addiction on a quantitative continuum. Similarly, it is difficult to determine when a chemical is being misused and when it is medication to ameliorate disease. Many drug users are in effect attempting to self-medicate themselves for a condition they usually don't understand.

The best test as to whether a person is abusing the use of a drug is to objectively examine its effects upon him. We must answer the questions: Does it increase or decrease his well-being—i.e., physical, mental, social, economic, etc.?

If the drug has lost its psychoactive effect, is being taken to relieve negative symptoms and is difficult to discontinue, then it probably is not having a salutary effect on this individual—i.e., the drug is being abused. It appears that the crucial difference between those who use chemicals for benefits and those who abuse them is found in the strength of the inidividual and his family.

We must differentiate the short-term effects from the long-term ones. Drugs/medications may have a salutary effect initially, but later not only lose this but produce negative effects. For example, paregoric used in the short term may stop diarrhea, but in the long term it may appear to the subject that the opiate must be taken to prevent negative symptoms—the diarrhea produced by withdrawal of paregoric. The long-term excessive use of coffee loses its pharmocologic stimulus and becomes a necessity in order for the person to function in the morning. A dependent relationship has developed. Similarly, coffee may be needed to prevent or terminate gross hand tremors or to stimulate the bowels sufficiently to have a bowel movement after long excessive use—i.e., 20 cups per day or more. When an abuser reaches the point of minimal psychoactive effect from the drug, he often increases the dose, frequency of intake, or potency in an effort to again achieve the previous effect, not realizing that the only way he can reclaim the psychoactive high is to decrease or cease the use of the drug temporarily.

We will always have drug users and abusers. Therefore, we will need medical emergency facilities, physicians trained in this area, hospital wards, and other institutions to aid those who are abusing drugs or have become addicted to them. It will always be necessary that we have laws and enforcement of same in order to control the availability and distribution and use of drugs in ways that are detrimental to our society.

However, there are those who feel that legal prohibition only exacerbates abuse of drugs, that legal efforts interfere with social control of drug use, and that society can not control by law what one will or will not put in his mouth. They feel that social and individual control are the only means available for drug control. It will always be necessary for us to have psychotherapists and other knowledgeable persons help those with problems concerning drugs and life to find healthier alternatives. However, if we rely solely upon these alternatives, it will require a greater proportion of our energies than we can afford. Of necessity, we must understand the causes of drug abuse and addiction and prevent the development of same. In the sixties we saw evidence of a critical mass of drug abusers developing that affected our society in a major way. Behind this army of chronic drug users, abusers, and addicts was a critical mass of failure or fear of failure and other causes of drug abuse. If a person thinks well of himself, gets his needs met in healthy ways, and has healthy interpersonal relationships, he is less likely to retreat from life by abusing drugs. If children get payoffs in healthy ways, there will be less need for payoffs through drugs.

Our future concerns need to concentrate more on healthy interpersonal and family life and less upon specific drugs, since there will always be a series of new compounds with which to contend.

The core problem and solution to the drug problem may well come back to basics such as: How do we help children grow up in a healthy manner and adequately face life?

Summary

The serious drug use problems are usually found in children and adolescents who come from homes in which they have been deprived in some way. A crucial difference between those who use chemicals for benefits and those who abuse them is found in the personality strength of the individual and his family. Emphasis should be placed on how to use medications appropriately rather than destructively. Prohibition only has not been very successful in modifying drug use. Social and individual control must be added to our armamentarium.

Table 1 summarizes the basic characteristics of commonly used drugs—i.e., source, physical dependence, withdrawal reaction, psychic dependence, behavioral toxicity, hallucinations, and other effects.

In the contest between the family and the peer group for influence on the adolescent, the former has lost ground. Age polarization in our society and the need to be strong in a society in which it is increasingly difficult to be strong in healthy ways have also contributed to the increased use of drugs in the young.

Some studies show that those who misuse drugs are more likely to have abnormal, chaotic family relationship—i.e., mother indulgent, father weak and uninvolved, and a weak mother-father marital relationship. The parents and peers are more likely to misuse drugs. The user is less likely to marry, or if he marries, more likely to be divorced and have multiple marriages than controls. The user often duplicates the relationship with the parent of the opposite sex (in the family of origin) in the choice and relationship with the spouse. The user more often than controls is unable to successfully carry out the responsibilities of parenthood.

It is unwise to deal with drugs as if they were a problem separate from other unproductive and self-defeating behaviors.

A glossary of drug jargon is given in Table 2. Drug vocabulary moves on to new terms rapidly.

For many reasons, many physicians have hesitated to become involved in the treatment of drug abusers/addicts. Medical doctors' special knowledge in this area is vital and should be expanded to prevent, treat, educate and solve the quandries we are in regarding drug abuse.

The development of effective chemotherapeutic substitutes, advances in drug detection technology and the use of former abusers of drugs as paraprofessional mental health workers to work with addicts are major advances in the treatment of drug dependency. Table 3 lists therapeutic and toxic levels of commonly used drugs.

Drug use before the age of 15 predicts with considerable accuracy the high possibility of future serious drug involvement with substances such as barbiturates and narcotics. A person who has been a poly-drug-user, used narcotics, hallucinogens, or a volatile substance, has a high probability of being on drugs at the present time and is likely to be an extensive abuser.

The methods of treating patients on stimulants, hallucinogens, depressants, and inhalants is discussed. Stimulant drugs such as speed have considerable behavioral toxicity, and hence patients on large doses of these must be supplied protection for themselves and others less they commit acts against humanity or property. Crimes committed under narcotics are mainly against property to support the habit.

A self-limiting, agitated, psychotic state may be precipitated by high doses of amphetamines, especially if taken intravenously.

"Flashbacks" frequently associated with the use of LSD are now thought to be anxiety attacks in anxiety neurotics.

Depressants produce some psychotoxicity. Because they can cause loss of consciousness and motor functioning, they exert some degree of control over excessive intake assuming the patient has not overdosed in a massive way initially. The two types of abstinence syndromes are discussed. In the treatment of an overdose of glutethimide or meprobamate, a patient may wake up and subsequently lapse back into coma; hence, those who have ingested significant quantities of these should be hospitalized. In the treatment of patients who have taken large doses of "downers," one must be sure that the basic diagnosis is not physical and psychic addiction. If such a patient is misdiagnosed, treated as an "overdose," and sent home, he may subsequently develop convulsions and other withdrawal phenomena.

The decision about the use of a particular drug should be made on the basis of the short- and long-term effects—i.e., does it increase or decrease one's physical, mental, social, and economic well-being? There is a cultural blindness to the effects of our frequent excessive use of common psychoactive drugs such as alcohol, tobacco, and coffee. Abused drugs often have a short-term psychoactive, pleasurable effect. Then with increased dose and frequency they often lose this result and produce negative symptoms. The psychoactive high can only be achieved by discontinuing or decreasing the frequency of the use of the drug. However, the common pathway for almost all drug abusers, once the psychoactive high begins to be lost, is to increase the frequency, dosage, or potency of the drug in an attempt to gain a "high" and to temporarily avoid the negative symptoms. Or they may search for another psychoactive drug.

Many believe that attempts at legal control of drugs interferes with social control and that social and individual control is the only method of ultimate control. Probably, some users can be reached by one method and others by another method of control.

Prevention is the ultimate method of changing the main problems of drug misuse. The etiological factors of drug abuse are discussed and the preventive and treatment programs are built around these. The core of these is to work with families and each individual to develop assets to the point that they are able to face life's vicissitudes successfully and to be able to get natural highs from life's abundant sources—i.e., interpersonal relationships, art, music, sports, hobbies, work, nature, accomplishment, etc. Children must be taught to think well of themselves, and we must work with them to meet their needs. Such pleasures go far beyond the satisfaction offered by chemical substitutes.

References

AMA Council on Mental Health and Committee on Alcoholism and Drug Dependence. (1967) Dependence on LSD and other hallucinogenic drugs. *J.A.M.A.* 202(1):141–144.

Archibald, H.D. (1970) Child's addiction likelier if mother is pill taker. *Pediat. News* 4(12):

Blumberg, A.G., M. Cohen, et al. (1971) Covert drug abuse among voluntary hospitalized psychiatric patients. *J.A.M.A.* 217:1959–1961.

Chapel, J.L. (1973) Emergency room treatment of the drug-abusing patient. *Am. J. Psychiat.* 130(3):257–258.

Chappel, J.N. (1973) Attitudinal barriers to physician involvement with drug abusers. *J.A.M.A.* 224:1011–1014.

Cohen, M., and D. Klein. (1970) Drug abuse in a young psychiatric population. *Am. J. Orthopsychiat.* 40:448–455.

Cohen, M.M., M.J. Marinello, and N. Back. (1967) Chromosomal damage in human leukocytes induced by lysergic acid diethylamide. *Science* 155:1417–1419.

Cohen, S. (1975a) Amphetamine abuse. *J.A.M.A.* 231:414–416.

Cohen, S. (1975b) Glue sniffing. *J.A.M.A.* 231:653–654.

Dole, V.P., and M. Nyswander. (1965) A medical treatment of diacetylmorphin (heroin) addiction: A clinical trial. *J.A.M.A.* 193:646–650.

Egozcue, J., S. Irwin, and C.A. Maruffo. (1968) Chromosomal damage in LSD users. *J.A.M.A.* 204(3):122–126.

Einstein, S., and M.A. Quinones. (1971) Difficulties in treating the drug abuser. *Nat. Acad. Sci.* 2:1450.

Evens, R.P., and W. Clementi. (1977) Compendium of drug abuse jargon. *J. Fam. Prac.* 4:67–72.

Farnsworth, D.L. (1974) The young adult: An overview. *Am. J. Psychiat.* 131(8):845–852.

Fischer, D.E., J.A. Halikas, J.W. Baker, and J.B. Smith. (1975) Frequency and patterns of drug abuse in psychiatric patients. *Dis. Nerv. Syst.* (30):550–553.

Geist, R.A. (1974) Some observations on adolescent drug use: Therapeutic implications. *J.Am. Acad. Child. Psychiat.* 13:54–71.

Greenblatt, D.J., and R.I. Shader. (1974) Drug abuse and the emergency room physician. *Am. J. Psychiat.* 131(5):559–562.

Griffeths, J. (1966) A study of illicit amphetamine drug traffic in Oklahoma. *Am. J. Psychiat.* 123:560–572.

Halikas, J.A., and J.D. Rimmer. (1974) Predictors of multiple drug abuse. *Arch. Gen. Psychiat.* 31:414–418.

Hamburg, B.A., H.C., Kraemer, and W. Jahnke. (1975) A hierarchy of drug use in adolescence: Behavioral and attitudinal correlates of substantial drug use. *Am. J. Psychiat.* 132(11):1155–1164.

Hochman, J.S., and N.Q. Brill. (1973) Chronic marijuana use and psychosocial adaptation. *Am. J. Psychiat.* 130(2):132–140.

Imperi, L.L., H.D., Kleber, and J.S. Davie. (1968) Use

of hallucinogenic drugs on campus. *J.A.M.A.* 204(12):87–90.

Kolansky, H., and W.T. Moore. (1971) Effects of marihuana on adolescents and young adults. *J.A.M.A.* 216(3):486–492.

Lemere, F. (1963) Amphetamine addiction in Japan. *J.A.M.A.* 185:151–153.

Levine, S., and R. Stephens. (1971) Games addicts play. *Psychiat. Quart.* 45:583–592.

Little, R.B., and M.M. Pearson. (1966) The management of pathologic interdependency in drug addiction. *Am. J. Psychiat.* 123(5):554–560.

McGlothlin, W.H. (1964) Hallucinogenic drugs: A perspective with special reference to peyote and cannabis. Personal communication.

McGlothlin, W.H., and D.O. Arnold. (1971) LSD revisited: a 10-year follow-up of medical LSD use. *Arch. Gen. Psychiat.* 24:35–50.

Naftulin, D.H., ed. (1971)*Drugs and Our Youth*, rev. ed. Los Angeles: Department of Psychiatry, Division of Continuing Education, U.S.C. School of Medicine.

Nelson, S.H., D.P. Kraft, and J. Fielding. (1974) A national study of the knowledge, attitudes and patterns of use of drugs by disadvantaged adolescents. *Am. J. Orthopsychiat.* 44(4):532–537.

Nichtern, S. (1973) The children of drug users. *J. Am. Acad. Child Psychiat.* 12:24–31.

Pierce, L., chairman of the New York State Narcotics Division, personal communication.

Proskauer, S., and R.S. Rolland. (1973) Youth who use drugs. *J. Child Psychiat.* 12(32):47.

Secretary of Health, Education and Welfare. (1971) Marijuana and health: A report to the Congress. *Am. J. Psychiat.* 128(2):81–111.

Seevers, M.H. (1968) Psychopharmacological elements of drug dependence. *J.A.M.A.* 206:1263–1266.

Shearn, C.R., and D.J. Fitzgibbons. (1972) Patterns of drug use in a population of youthful psychiatric patients. *Am. J. Psychiat.* 128(11):65–71.

Tatetsu, S. (1963) Methamphetamine psychosis. *Folia Psychiat. Neurol. Jap.* 7 (Suppl.):377–380.

Taylor, R.L., J.I. Maurer, and J.R. Tinklenberg. (1970) Management of "bad trips" in an evolving drug scene. *J.A.M.A.* 213:422–425.

Tennant, F.S., and C.J. Groesbeck. (1972) Psychiatric effects of hashish. *Arch. Gen. Psychiat.* 27:133–136.

Westermeyer, J., and V. Walzer. (1975) Sociopathy and drug use in a young psychiatric population. *Dis. Nerv. Syst.* (36):673–677.

White, A.G. (1973) Medical disorders in drug addicts: 200 consecutive admissions. *J.A.M.A.* 223:1469–1471.

Wikler, A., professor of psychiatry and pharmacology, Department of Psychiatry, University of Kentucky, Lexington, Kentucky, personal communication.

Part VI
Preventative and Psychotherapeutic Interventions in Child Psychiatry

Treatment of Emotional Disorders in Children and Adolescents

CHAPTER 37

Psychoanalytic Perspectives on Vulnerable and High-Risk Young Children

J. Alexis Burland
Theodore B. Cohen

Introduction

Psychoanalysis discovered late in the last century that adult neurotic conflicts were derived from neurotic conflicts in childhood, that as poets had known already, the child is father to the man. But this initial psychoanalytic discovery from work with adults related to neurotic structures, that is to psychosexual drives, particularly from the Oedipal stage of development, the anxiety they engendered, and the symptomatic means selected to cope with that anxiety.

Over the past forty years psychoanalytic research has broadened and deepened its understanding of the psychological life of the child and has revealed that there is much more to it than merely sexuality and neurotic conflict. The child is father to the man in many ways in addition to psychosexually, relating also to the stability and efficiency of his ultimate mental equipment, his self-esteem, and his capacity to relate to other people. It is of interest that children have been developing in our midst for many centuries and yet it is only recently that this unknown domain has begun to be explored directly. Closer than the moon, even closer than the depths of the seas, the minds of children seem to most people not only mysterious but impenetrable. As though they had no meaning, the words and action of children are often ignored or dismissed, even by a society that may shower its children with unprecedented material benefits. It is not surprising that most research in this area has consisted to a large measure of simply *listening* to children, carefully and thoughtfully enough to learn their language as much as possible. Resistances to the information gained from child development research suggest a need to divorce one's self from the events and the language of these years—selectively, of course, as everyone loves a happy, laughing baby. Perhaps it is the pain, unhappiness, and helplessness of childhood people wish to forget; perhaps it is the allure of wishes to return to the illusion of safe and protective lapdom; or perhaps it is the civilized adult mind reluctant to enter the primitive and fantastic world of the child's mentality. Whatever the reason, the vulnerable and at-risk child is the loser, for in his life these immature states tend to predominate.

Psychoanalytic developmental psychology has been pioneered and elaborated by many researchers, including Benedek, Bowlby, Erickson, A. Freud, Glover, Greenacre, Hartmann, Hoffer, Jacobson, Kris, Lampl de Groot, Piaget, Sandler, Spitz, Winnicott, and especially Mahler and her co-workers, to whom we are grateful for formulating the constructs in terminology most used today in understanding early childhood development.

Another important factor has contributed to the growing interest in the early years of life. The "widening scope of psychoanalysis" with its willingness to work with those more developmentally arrested than the so-called normal neurotic patient, has brought a new population into the psychoanalyst's office. There has been an associated increased understanding of the psychogenetics and psychodynamics of such mental states.

These researchers have described the "birth of the mind," the sequence of events that occur particularly in the first three years of life that shape the basic mental equipment with which the child eventually confronts among other things, for instance, the challenge of the Oedipal psychosexual pressures from within when they arise in later childhood.

Development is the product of the interaction between maturation and environmental influence, be it facilitating or not. The cognitive and neuromuscular equipment of the newborn is immature. It matures according to a prearranged timetable and in a prearranged sequence. The psychological structure that will eventually oversee and operate this equipment and that develops as it matures, as well as the state of the equipment itself are receptive to influence by the nature of the parenting, especially at first the mothering, the child receives. An adequately endowed child with "good enough" parenting care develops "normally."

The concepts of "vulnerability" and "at risk" relate to the children who are not so fortunate. As defined by Solnit (1975), *vulnerability* refers to inherent susceptibilities and weakness, active or latent, immediate or delayed. It is the opposite of *invulnerability*, which can be thought of as a strength, a resiliency, a capacity to cope adequately with stress. Being *at risk* refers to a child's precarious situation in the face of undue stress. When the child is seen to be at risk, the likelihood of a disadvantageous outcome to development is increased.

These concepts are relative and interrelated. That is, vulnerability and invulnerability are opposite poles of a continuum; being precariously at risk relates not simply to the nature of the risk but also to the relative quantity of compensatory supports, including the degree of vulnerability or invulnerability available to the child. Further, a child growing up in an at-risk situation often becomes developmentally interrupted or aberrant—becomes, in other words, vulnerable as the result of failure to develop his coping equipment adequately.

A related concept formulated also by Solnit is that a vulnerable child tends to evoke a disproportionate amount of negative responses from his environment, creating, in other words, an at-risk situation in addition to his original vulnerability. For example, a congenitally handicapped newborn is more frequently exposed to rejecting attitudes than a healthy one.

Vulnerability can be the result of congenital malformation, limited or perceptually handicapped cognitive equipment, preordained delays in neurological maturation, blindness or deafness, etc. Also included would be a variety of poorly understood seemingly inherent ego disturbances, such as a poor capacity to neutralize aggression, an inadequate stimulus barrier, or a hyperreactivity to stimuli. At-risk situations would include being born in a war-ravished country or into a broken family; the most common at-risk situation would have to be being born of neglective if not abusive parents, inadequate at the task of parenting, more often than not socioeconomically disadvantaged.

Vulnerability may reveal itself early in life in subtle ways. One or more aspects of motor development may be delayed, even though other aspects are not. Eye contact, initially primarily with the mother, may be fleeting and inconsistent. The "dialogue" (Spitz, 1965) between mother and infant may be slow to establish. The infant may seem to withdraw and appear relatively unresponsive to sights and sounds. There may be excessive headbanging and rocking, self-stimulating activities that go hand in hand with inconsistent connection with the environment. A mother's poorly explained anxiety or feelings of rejection about her infant may reflect, of course, problems of the mother, but may also reflect perceptions she has made of her infant too subtle even for her to be more explicit about. Kron and his associates (Kron, Stein, and Goddard 1963; Kron et al., 1977) have reported success with a device that measures the sucking patterns of newborns. Subtle irregularities or inconsistencies in sucking patterns, perceived when magnified by their equipment, have been regularly associated with eventually more readily confirmed vulnerabilities. Vulnerablity may also reveal itself blatantly, and early, in which case means can be instituted promptly to attempt to compensate. Fraiberg's work with blind children is an example (Fraiberg, 1968, 1971; see also Burlingham, 1975); in her writings on the subject she has made specific recommendations as to how, for example, special forms of physical contact and activity can be used to aid the blind child in his efforts to orient himself spatially in a world he cannot visualize.

At-risk situations can also be at times difficult to identify. Socioeconomically advantaged families are well known for their capacity to appear more adequate at parenting than in fact they might be.

But the at-risk situations with which those in the mental field come in contact most often are readily identifiable and are usually associated with the economically deprived segment of the community.

Although mental health facilities in one way or another have been working with this population since the turn of the century, there is no question but that the community mental health and mental retardation movement has increased the extent of this contact. Part of its initial design was to reach out into the poverty pockets of the community and through what was hoped would be preventive means lessen the impact of poverty on the psychological development of children growing up in such high-risk situations. It is experience with this movement that has both highlighted the importance of the problem and conributed data useful in the elaboration of theory and means of therapeutic intervention.

As might have been expected when dealing with at-risk situations, the social activist becomes as involved as the mental health clinician. This confrontation between politician-sociologist and behavioral scientist is often stormy. At one extreme is the view that the disadvantaged are blobs of clay molded by a destructive environment, and that therefore nothing short of a total restructuring of that environment will be effective. That, in fact, to "entrap" the disadvantaged into a mental health system that is itself a part of the destructive forces that placed the disadvantaged child in the at-risk situation in the first place is to be avoided. Such a view rejects psychological testing, the use of A.P.A. nomenclature, and even keeps to a minimum the use of traditionally trained professionals. Any comments or views relating to the disadvantaged person's active participation in his fate is viewed as a derogatory moral judgment and is vehemently rejected. At the other extreme would be a view that puts emphasis upon the intrapsychic determinants of behavior and relies upon the already accumulated body of knowledge about mental functioning. Such a view would minimize the potential effectiveness of social activism, reject the hapless victim theory of the disadvantaged, and support long-term individual psychotherapeutic work with each patient as the only possible remedy.

The "truth" is probably somewhere in between the two extremes. The conflict between the two points of view is real and frequently intense. Hopefully the conflict will lead to dialogue which will lead to resolution of the conflict.

Among those points of view concerning vulnerability and risk which attempt to take into account both intrapsychic and experiential factors is the psychoanalytic one recounted in this chapter. Much of what appears in it comes from the biannual meetings of the American Psychoanalytic Association's ongoing discussion group on the vulnerable and at-risk child, a function of that association's special committee on social issues. These discussion groups have been meeting for some 11 years now and are attended by psychoanalysts from around the world who are actively involved in work with this population. Clinical observations and innovative or experimental programs have been described and discussed. Nonanalyst researchers and clinicians working in this field have also been invited to participate. It is one of the longest-standing ongoing scientific forums in which this subject has been debated.

Nevertheless, it should be emphasized that at this point there remains much to be learned. The diagnostic, dynamic, and developmental understanding of the vicissitudes of vulnerability or high risk are increasingly more readily conceptualized; or conversely, the psychogenesis of certain clinical pictures, tracing the later behavior patterns to the vulnerabilities and risks experienced in infancy, can be more readily determined. But it is in the area of therapeutic intervention, be it in infancy, childhood, adolescence, or adulthood, individually or within the family, singly or in groups, that the greatest need for further research is felt.

The mental health professional in this field, therefore, needs to play many roles. He must be a perpetual student of what has already been learned about human behavior and a sophisticated theoretician in order to understand adequately that large and complex body of knowledge. He must be a researcher and innovator, searching for new insights to build upon the old. He cannot work alone in his private office, either. He must be a consultant to agencies who need his knowledge, a visitor to hospitals and schools, a teacher of those hoping to follow in his footsteps, even a lobbyist and social activist when his community is legislating unwisely or inadequately. And all of this is in addition to being a clinician, for it is in the office, with the vulnerable and at-risk patient, that the ideas, theories, and even dreams are finally truly tested. Such a multifaceted role is harder for the psychoanalyst than for the psychiatrist and psychologist, and possibly easiest for the social worker. The various mental health professions have much to learn from one another.

In this chapter certain theoretical issues related to the conceptualization of developmental interruption will first be discussed, including the differentiation between Oedipal and earlier-than-Oedipal conflicts, and the assessment of developmental progress by means of an ego function profile, determination of levels of object relationships, and evidences of the persistence of infantile forms of narcissism. Finally a syndrome of developmental arrest will be described.

In the section on application of psychoanalytic developmental theory, the discussion will touch on infant psychiatry, research into the development of communications, psychosomatics, the effects on children of divorce and psychotic parents, deafness, neglect, and abuse, the importance of early diagnosis, use of day care and nursery schools for early diagnosis and intervention, and the problem of teenage pregnancy and parenthood.

Finally, a brief discussion of methods of treatment will touch on traditional child guidance services, psychoanalysis, and the community MH/MR movement.

Theory

The vulnerable and at-risk child is far more prone to suffer developmental interruptions than neurosis. A child entering the Oedipal phase handicapped by developmental problems is not likely to cope adequately with psychological stresses characteristic of that phase, so Oedipal neurotic symptomatology is not infrequent. But it is more of a by-product than the central or core problem, and therapeutic measures directed exclusively at these more superficial neurotic symptoms even if effective leave unmodified the more significant underlying ego structural problems. It is perhaps for this reason that psychoanalytically oriented therapists versed mainly in work with neurotic conflict report frustrations and disappointments when confronted with the population of the developmentally arrested.

Developmental and neurotic conflict can be clinically differentiated from one another despite the overlapping that can occur. The mother of the mother-father-child Oedipal triad is a different mother psychologically speaking from the mother of the mother-infant dyad. For the latter, there is poor or incomplete differentiation between mother and child, and the relationship is characterized by an affective charge that is larger than life and peculiarly intense. The anxiety experienced within the relationship is either annihilation or separation anxiety, both devastating in the image they evoke. Internal objects—especially the mental image of the "good" mother who is adequate in her various roles of caretaking—are not yet stable, and are prone to collapse under the stress of separation or anger. Intimate attachment to the mother is a precondition for narcissistic stability, so that separations or conflicts between mother and child bring with them a profound sense of internal insecurity. The cognitive style of such children is characterized by immature perceptions of reality.

For the child who has adequately met the earlier developmental challenges, the Oedipal phase and its triadic relationships are confronted by a relatively stable ego, one that is aware of and able to cope with the differencces between internal and external reality. Narcissistic support systems are sufficiently independent that conflict with the parents does not threaten mortification. Castration anxiety is prominent, a less devastating form of anxiety than developmentally earlier forms. The father has entered the psychological life of the child as a true other person rather than as a second, but less contaminated mother, father's most frequent role in the years when dyadic attachments predominate.

The ego-adequate Oedipal child has the equipment with which to deal with the phase-specific social, interpersonal, sexual and conflictual challenges. The child who is not ego-adequate tends to regress and can even experience ego fragmentation. He converts castration anxiety into annihilation anxiety, and contaminates Oedipal competitive strivings with infantile forms of destructiveness and sadism.

For the neurotic child, reconstructive work deals primarily with anxieties concerning sexual discoveries and the romantic fantasies involving the triadic cast of characters. For the developmentally arrested child, reconstructive work focuses on the need for and sense of frustration about mothering, and fears of disaster precipitated by separation situations.

Interruptions of psychological development fall into three categories, each long familiar to students of psychoanalytic theory as areas of interest but only in the past three or four decades illuminated to a point of understanding.

First, the development of those mental functions subsumed in the structural theory under the term "ego," those functions that mediate between the internal and the external worlds. In common parlance, these functions add up to "coping mechanisms." As life is a challenge with which one has to cope, one's repertoire of coping skills determines how one meets that challenge. Therapy is also a challenge, and how one copes with it, too, will be determined by the level of ego functioning. Based upon the conceptualizations proposed by Beres (1956), these functions can be listed as follows:

1. The relationship to reality, including the perception of reality, the ability to adapt to reality, and the ability to sense reality and, as it were, feel real.

2. The regulation and control of the instinctual drives. This includes not simply the inhibition of gratification but also its reality-appropriate delay or sublimation, or the elaboration of compromises which take into account more than just internal need alone. Further, not only instinctual drive derivatives pressure the mental apparatus for gratification; there are also narcissistic needs, defensive needs, and object needs.

3. The capacity for object relationships. The development of this capacity has been studied extensively by Mahler (1968, 1975) and will be discussed at greater length below. Object relationships may be defined as predominantly loving affectual interactions with another person who is perceived as an objectively separate and independent individual. This interaction involves giving and receiving, and is sufficiently stable that the affectionate bond survives separations and intervals of conflict.

4. The thought processes. That is, the capacity to understand what is happening in one's life, to be rational, to be aware of differences and similarities and to understand cause and effect relationships, to be able to learn, to make decisions, to understand the past and plan for the future, in the broadest meaning of the term, to think.

5. Defenses against anxiety. Internal needs in the process of their fulfillment threaten one with anxiety, call forth the ego mechanisms of defense, including, for example, repression, reaction formation, isolation, projection, introjection, intellectualization, etc.

6. The "autonomous functions of the ego" first discovered by Hartmann (1939). Certain mental capacities have been thought to develop free from conflict, and to have the capacity to resist contamination by conflict. These would include perception, locomotion, use of the hands, memory, speech, aspects of thinking, etc. Work with the developmentally arrested child is revealing that these functions can be contaminated and made conflictual perhaps more so than was originally believed.

7. The synthetic function of the ego, the capacity to pull together the bits and pieces of an individual's psychological life into a relatively consistent and stable whole. One's sense of identity reflects this funtion, as does the elaboration of character structure, be it symptomatic or not.

These functions are primitive if in existence at all at birth, and develop as a result of the unfolding of inherent maturational sequences, especially of the neuromuscular apparatuses; but their development is also influenced by the quality of nurturing care, even in the earliest months of life. It is not surprising that the commonest at-risk situation is inadequate mothering. Where a lag in ego development is felt to be the primary problem, therapy must be ego growth promoting, involving the evocation of a nurturing interaction. This contrasts with the therapy of a neurosis, where nurturance and growth are not central but more or less objective internal exploration is the rule. Where vulnerability is characterized by genetically determined CNS aberrance or CNS damage due to perinatal injury, the neuromuscular apparatuses themselves can be affected and ego development lag is a secondary phenomenon, though still one that requires attention.

The second major category of developmental interruption is that of object relationships, mentioned above as the third cluster of ego functions. It is itself a complex facility, built up of many parts, and evolved according to its own developmental sequence. The research of Mahler and her associates has illuminated this aspect of childhood development, explicated at its fullest in her book *The Psychological Birth of the Human Infant*, coauthored with Pine and Bergman (see also Burland, 1975).

The human infant is helpless at birth, and depends for survival upon the ministrations of a caregiving person. A dependency-related biological-interpersonal dimension persists throughout life as a result, whether it is revealed in the eventual rewarding capacity for gratifying relationships or in a distortion of or resistance against them. The newborn's helplessness leaves him at the mercy of the quality of care he receives from his caretaker, a truly at-risk situation unless the mother is adequate, or "good enough" in her functioning.

The infant lives at first almost exclusively within

its splanchnic vegetative system. Within a few weeks after birth (within a few days, according to some observers), the perceptual conscious system begins to awaken, and increasingly over ensuing months the infant responds to tactile, visual, and auditory stimuli as well. This shift to the sensory-perceptual system is fostered by the ministrations of the mother. The more adequate, consistent, and in particular affectively responsive the mothering care, the more rapidly and fully this process proceeds. The most profound developmental interruption in the capacity for object relationships is seen in childhood autism, in which this shift either does not occur or does so in a markedly distorted manner. The movement out of the autistic shell and into libidinal investment in the symbiotic dyad peaks at five to six months of age. The term "symbiosis" is here used not in its usual biological sense to refer to an objective interdependence. Instead, it is used to convey what is believed to be the subjective view of the infant, intimately and intensely involved with and responsive to the mothering person, but not yet cognitively mature enough to be aware of the separateness that objectively exists between them.

The symbiotic experience brings about its own dissolution as it fosters ego growth and physical maturation, and thereby ushers in the process of separation-individuation, that is, the growing awareness of objective separateness from mother and the development of a personal individual identity. During the first subphase of this process, during the latter half of the first year, one can observe the infant's efforts at differentiating himself from his mother. He experiments with distance from her, then with reapproaching her. He familiarizes himself with her, scrutinizing her face, for instance, with great intensity. He engages in the exploration of the familiar and the unfamiliar in his immediate world. Yet he remains dependent upon mother, and also aware of her presence. It is hypothesized that certain altered states of consciousness—religious ecstasy, *déjà reconté*, the Isakower phenomenon, etc.—reflect primitive "memory traces" from this phase of development in which perceptions of external reality are first being differentiated from perceptions of internal reality.

Toward the end of the first year of life, there is an increased emotional investment in the musculoskeletal apparatus and the exercise of such relatively new functions as locomotion, perception, and learning. During this second subphase of separation-individuation the toddler practices these new skills with manic affect, throwing himself into activity with abandon. He appears not to be deterred by the bumps and scrapes he suffers from his incessant and impetuous practicing; he may even welcome them insofar as they serve to aid him in his efforts at defining the boundaries of his body. He seems on the surface oblivious to mother's presence and absence; however, the intensity of his activities decreases when mother is not present, and he periodically seeks brief contact with her for what had been called refueling. His affect speaks for his innocent sense of omnipotence, rooted in part in the persistent delusion of shared omnipotence with the symbiotic love object; it is also expressive of the intense narcissistic investment in his physical apparatus. Many clinicians will recognize to what extent this resembles one form childhood depression takes—the almost hypomanic defensive flight into pressured play and constant activity, with denial of all vulnerability or dependency.

This situation is short-lived, however. At the age of fourteen to sixteen months the toddler discovers the fact of his objective separateness from his mother. Maturation of the perceptual conscious system along with progress in cognitive development as a whole makes unavoidable the development of separate mental images of himself and of his mother, these images replacing the sense of the symbiotic dual unity. He discovers the extent to which he is a separate, small, and relatively helpless individual, often apart from mother, and alone. His faith in mother as an omnipotent, omnipresent protective guardian is shattered. His sharing in that omnipotence is therefore also ended. His narcissism suffers a severe blow, an event whose vicissitudes have been studied by Kohut (Kohut, 1968, 1969, 1971, 1977; see also Kernberg, 1975) (see below). At the same time his budding identity as a separate individual and the narcissistic gratifications of independent function push him even further toward autonomy. There is created then an intrapsychic conflict between regressive longings for refusion and the simultaneous thrust toward individuation and self-reliance. This conflict shows itself in the distress and contradictory push-pull behavior that characterizes the mother-child interaction during this, the rapprochement subphase of development, named as such because of the approach behavior the child shows in contrast to his seeming indifference to mother during the preceding practicing subphase. The resolution to this developmental conflict involves the development of a new kind of relationship with mother, one that is loving but predicated on separateness and independence. This relationship is increasingly verbal, in contrast to the nonverbal, archaic language of affects that characterized the previous developmental subphases. Thus starts the road toward object constancy. Resolution of the rapprochement conflict is never complete; the struggle to accept mortality and to resolve closeness-apartness issues continues, of course, throughout life. In fact, complaints in this area may be the most frequent reason for seeking psychiatric help at present.

Vulnerability and/or risk situations can impede this developmental process. It should be added that as in all aspects of psychological development remnants of each phase persist, and the capacity for reactivating more immature modes of functioning exist in almost all people. One can argue that such a capacity can add pleasure to some dimensions of a person's life. Love relationships, for instance, can evoke affects and attitudes reminiscent of the dyadic mother-infant relationship, as can the appreciation of music and nature. In the practice of therapy the capacity to identify with the patient's subjective state—to "tune in," as it is now called—also involves a selective regression to certain modes of interaction in which the lines differentiating self and other are blurred and communications are at least in part nonverbal.

When developmental interruptions interfere with functioning or cause more psychic pain than pleasure, one can view them as psychopathological. But in some instances it can be hard to define the dividing line between significant disturbance and the occasionally painful or pleasurable evocation of infantile psychological states.

The third category of mental phenomena which more commonly reflect problems in development have been alluded to in the discussion of the rapprochement subphase of the separation-individuation process; namely, narcissism and the metamorphosis from its early infantile state into its more mature forms. Kohut (1968, 1969, 1971, 1977) has written extensively on this subject from the vantage point of work with adult patients; his feelings integrate well with Mahler's observations on developing children. Narcissism can be defined as one's emotional investment in one's self, and it can be loving or hostile, primitive or sophisticated, reality-based or fantastic. It can be a predominant preoccupation for an individual or of little conscious importance to him in his conscious day-to-day life. It can be gratifying or a cause of great pain. A certain quantity of adequate self-esteem is considered essential for normal psychological operation. Remnants of infantile forms of narcissism may persist without necessarily causing difficulties in function; in fact, adaptive and functional ambition often contains more than a modicum of infantile omnipotent yearnings.

The newborn's narcissism is dependent upon the mother's loving investment in her child. No where is this more evident that in the six-month-old child, laughing and kicking his legs with glee, as his mother, in eye-to-eye contact, leans over him, stroking or tickling him, lovingly attending to his needs, talking to him of her love and admiration for him. Narcissism at this developmental level can be seen as equivalent to a state of bliss as the infant basks in mother's loving attentiveness to him. When maternal emotional deprivation exists, infantile narcissism fails to develop adequately. Spitz (1945, 1946) has written extensively on this subject. At its extreme, unloved infants die. A lesser form, so-called failure to thrive, is seen commonly in neglected children, with apathy, weight loss, and lack of growth.

This dependent trend in narcissism persists throughout life, but is then joined by a new form of narcissism related to the child's growing self-reliance, independence, and autonomy. As in the practicing subphase of separation-individuation, the toddler becomes enraptured increasingly in what he believes he can do on his own. The rapprochement subphase then confronts him with the impossibility of remaining narcissistically dependent upon mother, a painful but also potentially liberating discovery when accompanied by the development of those physical, social, cognitive, and emotional skills that allow for a sense of independent accomplishment. There is an accompanying change in the tone of the narcissistic investment in one's self as well, from megalomanic and omnipotent to more realistic and socially aware self-regard.

This developmental shift from the more infantile anaclitic sources of narcissistic supplies to the sources dependent upon individuality can be interrupted by a variety of factors. Vulnerabilities that interfere with skill development, such as problems with sight or hearing, or crippling musculoskeletal handicaps tend to keep the child more reliant upon infantile narcissistic supplies, even when his vulnerabilities tend to limit these suplies by evoking rejection rather than acceptance from his caretakers. There is risk when parenting is not sufficiently tolerant, understanding, and supportive during the "terrible twos," the time when the child is struggling with the narcissistic injuries resultant from the discovery of his objective separateness. When this developmental shift fails to occur, these is a tendency to cling to infantile narcissism and to attempt to extract such supplies in later relationships. Kohut has illuminated the clinical picture and problems of the patient who persists in his attempts to recreate dyadic narcissistic attachments in which either his self-worth is mirrored back to him as if by the loving mother, or he is as if fused with an overidealized mother substitute. He seeks to achieve grandiosity at the expense of his realistic identity.

The development of the ego function, the development of the capacity for object relationships, and the developmental shifts of narcissism are aspects of childhood that exist concomitant to the psychosexual developmental processes. Anna Freud's concept of developmental lines is useful in affording one an overview of the depth and breadth of the infantile experience and the significance of events during these germinal years.

A recognizable clinical syndrome has been described (Burland, 1977) which can be used as an example of developmental arrest secondary to vulnerability and/or risk. It is seen most commonly among the lower socioeconomic class deprived and neglected child. Similar clinical pictures are noted among the blind and the deaf, particularly when compensatory supports have not been a part of their rearing. It has also been noted in children from materially comfortable homes, but ones characterized by disorder and unstable relationships. The primary element leading to the disorder is a relative lack of emotional investment in the infant by the mother, regardless of its basis.

The syndrome can be called "mindlessness" because of its clinical picture. Children suffering from it tend not to learn in school; in fact they show little inclination to learn in any situation. Typically they score 80 on the WISC with evidence of average potential. They engage in a wide assortment of antisocial, egocentric, destructive, self-destructive, and sexually perverse activities. They are unresponsive to most forms of discipline other than physical ones, which, if severe enough, usually send them into brief episodes of severe depression. They alternate in mood between inappropriate hypomania and inconsolable despair. They relate promiscuously around immediate need gratification. They are obsessed with a dysmorphic, primitive, sadomasochistic fantasy life. They are eventually rejected by all who know them, including—if not especially—their family; this is even though at first many of them reveal a superficial seductive charm. When younger, the "mindlessness" is most prominent; nonstop, unthoughtout, unstructured, pleasure-focused frenetic rather than joyful unmodulated activity. As they grow older, and their personality crystalizes, the hedonistic perverse and explosive qualities gain greater attention. There is no official diagnostic label for these children. Some psychologists tend to mislabel them as simply instances of minimal brain dysfunction. What might be called the countertransference label is "unsocialized overaggressive reaction of childhood." The most appropriate psychodynamic label would be depressive character disorder with pathological narcissism. Using the current developmental theories outlined above, these children can be understood as follows:

1. From the vantage point of the ego, the relationship to reality is poor, with incomplete self-other differentiation, difficulty in assessing what is realistically appropriate and difficulty evolving adaptive patterns of behavior.

2. The drives are both primitive and poorly controlled. Instant drive gratification, in fact, is a major source of infantile narcissistic gratification, an illusion of persistent fusion with the gratifying (feeding) mother. For this reason when they are frustrated they suffer narcissistic injury. Polymorphous perversity prevails. Interestingly enough, conscious phallic-Oedipal drive derivatives often seem quite unconflicted. Nevertheless, there is usually coexisting sexual repressions, and neurotic symptoms, inhibitions, and anxiety.

3. These children relate to others as part-objects: as candy machines, roller coasters, or monkey bars; as soft, warm dolls or as sexual toys; and they do so promiscuously. With the preponderance of self-other relationships and a failure to acknowledge objective separateness from the omnipotent mother, development of an identity is hindered. Internal relationships are unstable. Because deprivation led to a failure to establish a libidinal attachment to the mother in the first months of life, positive introjects are poorly structured and are promptly dissolved by negative feelings. Hungry as they are, they cannot internalize true object love from others; their meal consists primarily of the re-ingestion of projected images. That is one of the most difficult problems in the treatment of infantile and negative projections. Because of the developmentally determined unrelatedness, these

children have also been said to suffer from an "autistic character disorder," a term that conveys the cause, the major symptom, and the greatest obstacle to cure of the syndrome.

4. The intellect and the autonomous functions are poorly developed or are contaminated; emotionality predominates over thoughtfulness.

5. Defenses against psychic pain are unstable, and there is a preponderance of such primitive defenses as splitting, projection, and introjection.

6. There is a particular prominence of hostility, destructiveness, and sadomasochism in the behavior and fantasy life of these children. The destructiveness one sees is not so much a drive problem per se, but is instead an ego-structural one, related in particular to issues of narcissistic rage and negative introjects. When such a child rages, for example, it is almost always clearly a response to separation anxiety perceived in part as a narcissistic injury. At its worst, some of their destructiveness is an acted-out projection of the intrapsychic fragmentation they fear, not unlike the psychotic. In classical ego psychology terminology, neutralization of aggression (see Hartmann, Kris, and Loewenstein, 1949) is deficient.

7. The narcissistic injuries of rapprochement have not been surmounted. Narcissistic supplies of an infantile sort are what they primarily seek from others. They strive to reestablish infantile omnipotence. Their constant failure to do so leads to a constant undertone of narcissistic injury and depression. In many children one sees what might be called a defensive regression from the depression of rapprochement to the hypomania of the practicing subphase, with its strong but invisible umbilical connection to the symbiotic partner. Infantile omnipotence is delusionally assumed in such cases, contributing to the "mindlessness."

A treatment program is based upon the diagnostic assessment: a detailed assessment of the specifics of the developmental arrests these children suffer pinpoint those areas where developmental supports are needed.

Application

Developmental insights such as those just mentioned that attempt to explain the dynamics of the consequences of vulnerability and risk in young children are currently being utilized to assist in the design of preventive and therapeutic programs. The ones to be described have at least some psychoanalytic input; there are others, of course, that do not.* This work is ongoing; the state of the art has not reached the point where tried and true recipes for intervention can be recounted. Developmental psychology itself is still a young science; in fact, it is from work with the vulnerable and at-risk child that much data can be accumulated to help refine its concepts, a never-ending task. Theory and practice are reciprocally related, each confirming, correcting, and illuminating the other; for this reason those who work in this field most appropriately think of themselves as researchers.

The modes of application of psychoanalytic developmental theory to problems of vulnerability and risk can be recounted under the following headings: research and the further elaboration of basic theory; early diagnosis of vulnerability and the potential for risk; early treatment, and "prevention," although what is hoped will be preventive more often than not turns out to be treatment of already ongoing problem; and treatment of older children, adolescents, and adults when vulnerability and/or risk have already had their effect in the form of significant developmental arrest.

Child observational studies and data accumulated from service programs continue to enrich developmental theory. *Infant psychiatry* as a subspecialty is growing in prominence as techniques are devised for the study of children in this precommunicative stage of development. "Breaking the primal repression barrier" is an expression that has been used in referring to efforts in work with older children and adults by which memories from very early life experiences are reconstructed from the affect-laden but cognitively primitive and fragmentary mental phenomena believed to be derived from them. A similar communications barrier exists in direct observations of very young children. A dictionary of infant communication is not really possible, of course, although repeated exposure to infants does educate the observer so that in time much more of his mental contents can be perceived with fair confidence. The researcher learns, in time and with experience, to utilize more of his own subjective affective responses to the infant in a

* Many of the innovative programs mentioned in this section were described at recent meetings of the Vulnerable Child Discussion Group of the Committee on Social Issues of the American Psychoanalytic Association. They were reported by Elsie Broussard, J. Alexis Burland, Claire Cath, Theodore Cohen, Eleanor Galenson, Yvon Gauthier, Jerome Karasic, Paulina F. Kernberg, Gilbert Kliman, Roy Lilliskov, Dale Meers, Herman A. Meyersburg, Shere Samaraweer, Louise Sandler, Moisy Shopper, Brandt Steele, and Judith Wallerstein.

manner not unlike that which characterizes the mother's part in a good mother: infant "dialogue" in the sense that Spitz meant when he used the term. The practice of the new field of infant psychiatry with its clinical work, its conferences, and its exchanges of ideas will hopefully continue to improve techniques of communication directly with infants and indirectly via reverberation with one's own infantile past.

Theoretical research has attempted to clarify aspects of the *development of communications* from its nonverbal, somato-visceral, affective mode through various behavioral stages to the eventual primarily verbal model that characterizes later functioning. Viewed as such, communication is seen as a much more multifaceted experience than focus exclusively on verbal content would suggest. Earlier modes of communication can persist, both in normal and conflicted situations, so that attention to nonverbal aspects must be paid to perceive all that is being communicated. The infantile coexistent with the adult is more readily recognizable, and the interaction between sender and receiver deepens. Understanding better the psychologically significant events of early childhood aids in identifying communications concerning them.

Studies of certain at-risk situations strive to identify specific aspects of development that are more susceptible. *Asthmatic children* (Gautier et al., 1977), for instance, have long been considered specifically at risk in terms of the development of autonomy and constructive aggression because of the necessary increased dependency and the anxiety associated with the asthmatic attacks. Studies using developmental insights, however, have indicated that it is possible for asthmatic children to avoid problems in these areas, that it is not the asthma itself that places the child at risk as much as it is the reactions of the people involved, in particular the mother, and the interpersonal interactions which result. A more rational preventive and managment program can be devised based upon such insight.

Although it would be impossible to assess accurately the number of children in this country who are living through the dissolution of their parents' relationship, we do know that over a million children a year experience their parents legal *divorce*. The number is increasing. Considering the size of the population, it is surprising there has been little definitive research into the effects divorce has upon the involved children. One notable exception has been the work done since 1971 by Judith Wallerstein and Joan B. Kelly in California based upon the study and treatment of 131 children and adolescents before, during, and after their parents divorce (Wallerstein and Kelly, 1977; Wallerstein, 1977; see also Anthony, 1974).

Their work details the effects divorce may have upon the psychological development of the involved child. It also describes the more common reactive symptom picture such children present, with their short- and long-term reverberations. And they describe the variety of reality challenges the situation of divorce presents to the child. They also make specific recommendations as to modes of therapeutic intervention.

The age of the child is a factor determining the impact of divorce upon him. The younger the child, the greater the damage. In the Wallerstein study, almost half of the preschoolers had worsened psychologically between seven months after the divorce and eighteen months after the divorce. By contrast, a third of the adolescents showed this late response.

The age of the child also determines the nature of the developmental interruption that ensues. Psychoanalytic developmental theory details the specific vulnerabilities related to specific phases of development. The very young child's budding narcissistic stability is readily hurt as it is dependent upon family stability; as a result of the loss of the nuclear family, the child's nuclear self (Kohut) is damaged. At its worst, the result is rage, detachment, guilt, depression, hypochondriasis, shame, and low self-esteem. There may be a disruption in the normal development of the conscience due to the absence of the needed parent, with persistence of infantile superego precursors and associated poor control of destructive impulses.

Symptomatically, children of divorce even under the best of circumstances feel a keen sense of abandonment. There is usually a regressive response, with somatization, confusion, and even disorientation, insomnia, and nightmares. The short- or long-term grieving for the missing parent is associated with rage displayed toward the remaining parent or some other family member. The missing parent is overidealized but simultaneously devalued, this latter being strongly influenced by the attitudes of the remaining parent. The child may run away from home, often to the other parent, or resist going to school. There often results an enduring hopeless yearning for the reunification of the parents, persisting even after remarriage. Mood swings can be extreme, alternating between dark despair and unheralded aggression, reflecting the swings from feelings of helpless vulnerability and defensive grandiosity. In the latter mood the child convinces himself that he is responsible for the divorce, a thought which only then causes such guilt that the child must assuage it through self-inflicted injury or illness. Socially, the child feels shame about being "different" from his peers. He may attempt to cast a peer in the role of the missing parent, often working through his disappointment by seeing to it these relationships also end in rejection.

The parents contribute a great deal to the stresses put upon the child. The conditions under which the divorce occurs can be even more traumatic than the simple fact of the divorce itself. Children too often represent prizes, or are vehicles for what are actually punitive financial demands; this was clearly evident in half of the divorces Wallerstein studied. The child is often used to spy on a former spouse, or the withholding of his visits are used to punish. An angry parent may see or imagine disliked qualities of the missing spouse in the child, and displace onto him anger toward that spouse. The seductive parent may cast the child into the role of the spouse with the false promise of an Oedipal triumph with resultant sexual confusion on the part of the child. The child's own Oedipal longings are stimulated by such a situation, of course, so that he can become an active participant, albeit unconsciously, in such a situation.

The child's dependency upon the remaining parent continues. The degree and quality of the anger, depression, and preoccupation of this caretaking parent influences the nature of the parenting they can deliver. The young child is particularly vulnerable during the initial period of disequilibrium; when this lasts for several years, the cumulative impact upon his psychological development can be great. The remaining parent may lean on the child for emotional sustenance, or require he support the contention that the absent parent is the villain in the piece. The child is then placed in the situation of having to give more than he receives.

A child with preexisting vulnerability has special problems with family rupture. If psychological development has not proceeded well due to chronic parental inadequacy, or if the child suffers a physical handicap or chronic illness, dependency needs and attachment to one or both parents is particularly intense. Fears of abandonment are greater than usual, there is a greater ease of regression, and there is already a tendency towards depression, shame, and guilt.

Adolescents, on the other hand, with but a few exceptions did not feel responsible for their parents' divorce. But they saw the event as personally extraordinarily painful. In keeping with the concerns specific to the adolescent phase of development, they experienced doubts about their own adequacy as future marital and sexual partners. Anxiety about the likelihood that they too would be unable to sustain a marriage led many to believe they would never marry. In some adolescents there was instead an anxiety-motivated premature entry into heterosexual activity. A process akin to mourning the lost parent was seen to be necessary. This process occurred in tandem with the normal adolescent developmental relinquishment of the parental introjects, a process that also entails a kind of mourning. Behavior disorders commonly reflected the failure of completion of such a mourning process.

It should be added that when the parental divorce is expressive of an active attempt at coping and achieving mastery over an intolerable marital situation, at its best divorce can offer the child an opportunity to facilitate development. But supports are still necessary to maximize this potential; the stresses and reactions outlined above can still operate to interfere with such an eventually positive outcome.

Wallerstein has formulated a divorce-specific profile designed to determine the extent of the threat to the child's development. It includes a careful history obtained from the parents, and direct observations of the child both individually in the office and in school.

Modes of intervention were designed to meet the needs of the child as determined by this individual assessment.

Where the child's normal coping mechanism proved insufficient, support was needed to reestablish his ability to function. Siblings, other family members, often teachers were called upon. When this was unavailable or proved to be insufficient, short-term psychoanalytic psychotherapy was utilized, combining the usual therapeutic process with needed support and with an emphasis upon clarification and education to counter the disequilibrium, confusion, and fragmentation. An understanding of the normal developmental needs of the child is essential in understanding the ways these needs are not met due to the divorce. Both parents and children were seen individually. Four-year follow-up studies indicated that this intervention had been helpful.

Goals for work with adolescents also stressed support of preexisting coping mechanisms and clarification. But in keeping with normal adolescent developmental processes, there was also an attempt to increase the psychological distancing from the parental conflicts and to lessen the loyalty conflict. Divorce can interrupt the adolescent's "second individuation" (Blos), as it reentangles him in parental affairs just as he strives to pull away from them.

When there was the threat of kidnapping or physical harm, or homicidal threats, or the danger or actuality of symptomatic sexual behavior, it was felt necessary to remove the child from the situation. Making the situation safe and stable in such extreme situations was a long-term task, involving extensive psychotherapeutic intervention.

Every child of divorce is at risk and needs a caring person with a clear understanding of his situation and his perception of it. Sensitive and sensible support by a relative, friend, or professional may minimize the destructive aftereffects, especially when combined with the assurance of continuing parental support once the acute disruptive effects of the divorce have subsided.

The current practice of discharging increased numbers of psychotic adults has caused new problems for the children of these patients when they return home to them.

E. James Anthony (1974) has been studying *children of psychotic parents* for over ten years. Such children show an increased incidence of problems, including developmental interruption, psychoses in the making, parapsychoses such as folie à deux with the psychotic parent, and symptoms of ego weakness such as massive de-differentiations. There was noted an increased incidence of psychoses starting in adolescence.

In their study, complex profiles were devised to evaluate genetic, constitutional, developmental, physical, environmental, and experiential factors in order to predict the likelihood of disturbance in the hopes of instituting preventive measures as early as possible.

As might be expected from the insights of developmental psychology, vulnerability to later disturbance was correlated with problems of logicality, reality testing, identity formation and disordered fantasy content, all facets of the reality ego disordered in the psychotic parent and dependent upon the relationship with the parent for their normal development in the child.

A young child requires for the development of his nuclear self what Kohut has called an empathic-responsive human milieu, a mother who can react appropriately to her child's needs and a father who can be idealized. In the dialogue between parent and child, the child's expanding exploratory attempts at contact require a positive mirroring response. A psychotic parent, shallow in affect and prone to pseudoemotion disconnected from recognizable reality, cannot offer such a response to his or her child. A feeling of interpersonal failure can result for the child with interruption of the normal developmental consolidation of the self.

Parents who involve their children in their psychoses through aggressive or seductive behavior or who include their children in their delusional systems are contrasted with parents who withdraw into noninvolvement. In the latter instances, the child is more able to turn to the more adequate parent for nurturance and love, and for assistance in developing a more objective view of the psychotic parent. The child who becomes able to be curious about and compassionate for the ill parent—attitudes dependent upon on optimal amount of distancing—has the better prognosis. Daughters have the most difficulty resisting the identificatory pull from their psychotic mothers.

Corrective intervention, to be successful, must be aimed at reducing the child's susceptibility to engulfment by the magical thinking and delusions of the ill parent. The child's ego resources must be strengthened, especially his self-confidence and sense of competence, his realistic body image, and the clarity of self and object differentiation. Such ego supportive therapy was felt by Anthony to be a part of the technique of classical psychoanalytic psychotherapy.

Growth of the reality ego was noted as an indicator of response to therapy. Competence in daily functioning improved first; improvements in realistic thinking and the stability of identity developed later. External behavior, in other words, was modified more readily than internal structure, something to remember when early behavioral improvement leads one to feel therapy might be terminated. The more the improvement in the psychotic parent and the other family members, the more the important in the child.

Grunebaum (1977) describes findings similar to those of Anthony. In control studies, although the psychotic parent (all mothers in his population) did not benefit, the children clearly did profit from long-term ego-supportive reality-oriented therapy provided by a stable contact person. Trustful, supportive relationships were an important element of the therapy, stressing reality and rationality, single-minded and unequivocal communications, and feelings directly correlated with experience. This can be viewed as an attempt to offer compensatory empathic-responsive human milieu. Their findings suggested such intervention would be necessary for the many years spanning the child's development into a sufficiently self-reliant young adult to be protected from the psychotic parent's impact. This fact stresses the role of therapist as substitute for the psychotic parent, something different from the usual role of therapist.

The effects of *deafness* (Shopper, 1976) on the child and his family have also been studied. Parental guilt and problems in communication are central. Conflict among professionals as to the correct educational approach for the deaf frequently catches the deaf child and his family in the center. Socialization is interfered with; peers are poorly related to, and behavior tends to be idiosyncratic and frequently explosive. It is felt that the greatest threat to normal development of the young deaf child is disruption of the mother-child relationship due to the communication problem, the mother's guilt, and the vulnerable child's evocation of negative feelings on the part of the mother. Preventive programs should focus in this area.

Parental neglect and abuse have been studied more extensively than most other at risk situations. It is usually, although not exclusively, accompanied by socio-economic deprivation. Abuse is currently the recipient of a great deal of attention, especially in the popular press. This may help in obtaining funding for programs in this area, but it often encourages oversimplified thinking about this complex problem.

A syndrome of child abuse has been described by Steele (1970, 1977; Steele and Pollock, 1968) and is characterized by inadequate attachment between mother and child, related to deficiences in the parenting the mother received in her early life. In mother's fantasies concerning her child, before or after his birth, negatives predominate, the mother often projecting images of her own supposed deficiencies onto the child. The children are misperceived as being older and more capable of self-restraint and reason than they in fact are, with the resultant unrealistic expectations placed upon them. Abused children reveal eventually low self-esteem, a poor sense of identity, and excessive and unresolved dependency yearnings. There is also a diminished ability to seek and to have pleasure which often evolves eventually into moral masochism.

The effects of socio-economic deprivation as an at-risk situation have also been studied. There is often accompanying racism. Severe problems with passivity and aggression result. It can be difficult determining what is "pathological" rage and what is an appropriate response to a severe at risk situation. Indeed, though to the professional's eye the occurrence of symptoms is pandemic, to those within the community itself there is a striking tolerance for such behaviors and a marked reluctance to identify them as "sick" or calling for psychiatric help. Meers (1970) feels the socioeconomic factors are so great any program of intervention must include their remediation as well.

Theoretical research proceeds as well. Psychoanalytic developmental psychology is young enough that basic concepts are rethought and revised, and clinical work with altered theoretical foundations results in altered clinical perceptions. For instance, changes in the understanding of development result in changes in reconstructive work in the clinical setting, and consequently there are changes in interpretations. The resultant alteration in the course of the therapeutic process in turn leads to further fine tuning of developmental theory. In a related vein, the shift from an instinctual drive orientation to an ego orientation, clinically and theoretically, has altered clinical perceptions and therefore practice and theory. Object relations theory in particular, with its focus on the internal image associated with drive, rather than on the drive alone, has led to changes in the practice of therapy many view as valuable.

Early Diagnosis: Developmental conflicts are best prevented or at least challenged as early as possible. Early diagnosis is therefore a practical aspect of any program with developmental problems as its target.

Programs for early diagnosis have been recently given prominence in federally funded programs, in part thanks to lobbying efforts on the part of child development specialists. The Early and Periodic Screening, Diagnosis and Treatment Program ("EPSDT") is designed to service ultimately the 14 million children eligible to receive Medicaid assistance. But there have been delays in its institution, and it has come under heavy criticism from critics of the current state of the art of mass screening. It has even been criticized by civil libertarians concerned with issues of invasion of privacy. A new program, Comprehensive Health Assessments and Primary Care For Children ("CHAP"), has been proposed by the Carter administration as a revision of EPSDT, and with over twice the funds allotted. It will remain to be seen how much more effective the new proposal will be.

Local school districts in various communities devise innovative programs to identify problem children early. In one such district, mass screening of some 25,000 children revealed 35% of them had developmental immaturity, another 5% of them to a severe degree. Once identified, appropriate educational strategies or treatment programs are suggested related to the specific developmental handicaps each child presents.

In one innovative study dealing with pregnant women, screening procedures seek to measure fantasies mothers have about their soon-to-be-born or newborn children. Based upon what has been learned from future child abusers' fantasies about their children, a group of potential abusers can be identified, and an appropriate program instituted relating to those developmental problems such mothers reveal.

Early treatment is, of course, related to early diagnosis. Most early diagnosis programs include an early treatment service aspect as well.

Many such programs are associated with *day care* and *nursery school* settings. Referrals are by concerned parents, pediatricians, mental health centers, etc., or from within the school system itself. Extensive developmental assessment strives to identify the nature of the interruption or lag for the individualization of the treatment plan. The children and their parents then participate in a special class setting. In some programs, the psychiatric or psychoanalytic consultant works directly with the child, often within the classroom itself, interpreting about and attending to the child's developing ego, building on strengths, viewing ego weakness as something from which the child will grow out of. In other programs, the psychiatrist or psychoanalyst works with the staff, interpreting for them the children's problems and suggesting individualized management approaches. Counseling with the mother is usually an important part of the program. The entire special class staff is viewed often as part of the treatment team, even including maintenance staff who frequently have contact with the children.

Other programs have been instituted for children with more specific vulnerabilities, such as for those with autism, deafness, blindness, etc. One program for autistic children was based upon the concept that the assumed neurochemical deficit which causes the disorder does so by blocking the infant's perception of his mother's nurturing care. Accordingly, the child was exposed to massive quantities of rocking, holding, and nurturing attention, as if to compensate for the deficiency in perception. Early results were promising, but funding was interrupted due to government fiscal problems. This is not an unusual end for such programs.

Prevention fades into early treatment, of course. Genetic counseling and family planning are examples of "true" prevention, although in practice this, too, frequently involves a therapeutic interaction with the parents.

Teenage pregnancy and parenthood are on the rise (Sarrel and Lidz, 1969; Sarrel, 1971). They are also of increasing concern to private and public social welfare and health agencies and organizations, to observers of and commentators on the social scene, and to legislators on the local, state and federal levels. It has been estimated that 20% of live births are to teenage mothers, most of them unwed. In one northeastern United States city with a population of two million, there were 2,046 births to mothers 17 years and under in 1976, 567 of which were to mothers under the age of 15. Such births are of concern for several reasons, prevention of physical, emotional, and developmental problems in the children being paramount. The incidence of prenatal complications, prematurity, and infant mortality are greatest in this population. For instance, in one study, infant mortality occurred in 40 of 1,000 cases, as opposed to 17 in 1,000 cases of births to adult mothers. When teenage pregnancy leads to marriage, the divorce rate can be reportedly as high as 95% in some populations. An increased understanding of childhood psychological development makes clear the factors, though varied, which can lead to teenage pregnancy. They tend to be those factors that contribute to an inadequate capacity for parenthood in the mother and therefore a higher risk of developmental problems for the child. In fact, among lower socioeconomic populations an "unwed mother's syndrome" has been described by Lidz in which inadequate mothering leads to the same depressive, narcissistically injured personality in the child as in the mother; the child then eventually for the same reasons becomes an unwed teenage inadequate mother herself, perpetuating a cycle as it were. Crime, learning problems, mental illness—elements that contribute both to significant social problems for the community and to a very low quality of life for the individual—are endemic in this population (a fact detailed by Meers).

The roots of teenage pregnancy are many and varied. They include social, economic, cultural, educational, and personal factors. Certain populations are better known and understood than others, and health care agencies situated or designed to deal specifically with them have given professionals an opportunity to observe and work with them.

Among the middle-class population, one tends to see adolescent girls in rebellion against parental values, often accompanied by hurt and anger over the discovery of parental fallibility and hypocrisy, a discovery that is so much a part of the adolescent experience. One also sees adolescent girls unconsciously complying with parental unconscious expectations of failure and immorality. One of us (A.B.) has seen several adopted girls, rejecting of their adoptive parents, who become pregnant in unconscious identification with their natural mother, who they assume to have put them up for adoption as they were unwed and an adolescent when they gave birth to them.

Perhaps the group most studied in recent years is the inner-city lower-socioeconomic group, largely but not exclusively black. A syndrome can be described within this population. It is characterized by an apathetic, depressed, lonely mother, yearning for the gratification of never-gratified infantile needs for fusion and nurturance. She is narcissistically depleted as a consequence of her own mother's inability to invest in her, and therefore has little to invest in turn in others. She has low self-esteem, which she expresses directly in a life-long pattern of underachievement and failure. She often becomes pregnant accidentally or out of ignorance of the facts of conception. Frequently, the baby's father is himself struggling to achieve an operational identity, one which gratifies his masculine phallic narcissism in the face of his disappointments and his own record of school and work failure. He demands she bear him a child to thus prove his worth. In many instances sexual activity itself is almost compulsively engaged in, as it itself is a phallic narcissistic confirmation of his existence. Once she "discovers" she is pregnant, she believes she wants the child, and resists all efforts to have it aborted. Her needs, like those of the baby's father, are narcissistic and infantile; she clings to the illusion of the fusion and nurturance she seeks through motherhood, and she experiences her capacity to bear a child as confirmation of her existence and meaning.

As can be seen from the above, prevention by contraception is a far more difficult task in this population than many health and social welfare agencies working with them had initially hoped. The advances in the science of contraception are all too readily nullified by the stubborn resistances to their use. It has been found that contraception and abortion are most successfully employed among educated women who find personal fulfillment through activities other than child-bearing, such as work, school, friends, etc. The unwed adolescent future mother in the ghetto, a very different kind of woman, is too passive as a result of her deep sense of helplessness and worthlessness, and child-bearing is too important for her and for her sexual partner. It is not unusual to see worsening of depressive symptomatology as a reaction to enforced contraception. That effective contraception is available, or that the mechanics of contraception are made known in school and neighborhood, is therefore not always enough. For the inner-city depressed and apathetic teenager, or the defiant middle-class adolescent, or for the adolescent seeking to live out a mother's real or imagined fantasies about her, the forces working against contraception can be very great. Contraceptive counseling, therefore, has to be based on the psychodynamic understanding of their resistances if it is to succeed at all. One proceeds as one does in the psychotherapeutic setting, not as one does in a classroom. Such counseling must be more therapeutic than educational.

The same holds true for mental health programs for the teenage mothers. These programs are increasing in number. Interestingly enough, according to some observers, this contributes to the increased incidence of teenage pregnancy by implying a kind of social sanction of it by offering services for it. These services strive to start working with the mothers, and the fathers when possible, early in the pregnancy. Services are offered around the birth of the child, on occasion accompanying the mother to the delivery room. And the services continue for the mother and her child for varying lengths of time after the birth. Some programs are designed to continue offering services until the child has started school, at which time the mother often continues in care with a younger child.

These programs seek to educate the young parent about pregnancy and childbirth, about infant care, about nutrition, about family planning for the future. They also seek to assist the young mother in coping with her many reality problems: finding housing if necessary, dealing with rejecting or critical relatives, dealing with the frequently stormy relationship with the child's father or with other male friends, planning the resumption of education if it was interrupted, arranging for public assistance or food stamps, etc. But the nature of the problem makes necessary the aspects of these programs which is most critical—namely, its psychotherapeutic function. The "style" of the agency as a whole is one part of the system that delivers this service. The design or profile of any facility dealing with the needy, immature, and vulnerable adolescent mother must be nurturant and supportive. A strictly classroom-lecture educational program is as frustrating and discouraging to these girls as the classrooms they fled in the process of becoming mothers. Offices are made cozy and homelike. A large room is furnished like a family room, with stereo and TV set, with carpets and comfortable chairs, and with a good supply of toys and play-equipment. Staff usually dresses informally. Food and beverage are always available. This is more important than many think. It has been frequently observed that the needy young mother is fiercely competitive for the food her infant receives, even when she is the one doing the feeding. When she feels she has "enough," or that there is more available to her, this competitiveness is moderated.

The interaction between the young mother and her assigned therapist serves as the focal point of the mother's contact with the agency. It reflects and personifies the agency's approach to their clientele. The therapist can individualize the patient in a way the agency as a whole cannot. As pregnancy and motherhood are life events, and as each mother deals with them according to her own repertoire of coping mechanisms, whether successful or not, each mother's own repertoire must be individually uncovered and assessed.

Similarly, being a patient at such an agency, with such a particular set of problems—intrapsychic, interpersonal, realistic, and social—is also a life event. These mothers bring to the therapeutic relationship not only their needs but also the same repertoire of coping mechanisms, many of which are self-defeating and obstructionistic. It is within the therapeutic relationship that these resistances can be identified and confronted. The resistances to help that these mothers can present are both frustrating and discouraging for the staff on the one hand, and on the other hand the arena in which the most effective therapeutic work can take place.

Immaturities in the development of the capacity for object relationships is a frequent problem encountered and a difficult resistance to deal with. The needy ghetto mother relates around need gratification. This can be observed in her relationship with her child: when he is giving more than he is demanding—that is, when he is cute and loving and responsive, or when he is in bed with mother acting like a cuddly doll so that her loneliness is abated—she can invest some feelings in him. But when he is demanding and unrewarding—such as when he is in acute distress, screaming the loudest, and in fact needs her the most—she withdraws her investment in him, rejects him, ignores him, or worse, becomes overly punitive and abusive. In the relationship with her therapist, such a mother "drops out" figuratively or literally as soon as the more or less constant glow of supports she demands is interrupted, or when whe is asked implicitly or explicitly to give of herself more than she thinks she is receiving.

In some instances, the mother who seeks fusion with her sexual partner and her child also seeks fusion with her therapist. Usually for narcissistic gain she needs to overidealize the therapist and then see herself as one with him in a self-object relationship. This, of course, a kind of illusory reestablishment of the mother-infant relationship she seeks the most. As Kohut has written, the therapist has no choice but to accept this role, although without going so far as to encourage or intensify it. He then uses his elevated status to increase the impact of his efforts at encouraging the development of improved individual skills and competencies, and therefore self-assurance, so that the original need for the self-object bond with the therapist will be eventually diminished.

The immature mother reveals a multiplicity of ego developmental deficits as well. The capacity to mobilize stable defenses against anxiety, frustration, or depression is limited, so that she is prone to be overly sensitive and explosive. Cognitive and intellectual functioning is below inherent capacity, so there is a tendency to emotional explosion and action rather than thought in response to stress and challenge. External reality is perceived subjectively more than objectively, and events and people around them are misinterpreted. Drive and need gratification are such an important source of narcissistic gratification that the capacity to delay gratification is underdeveloped.

As in work with ego-developmental arrest generally, the role of the therapist is to permit the mother to reveal her inadequacies and then in the context of a narcissistically supporting positive relationship kindly and diplomatically discuss them objectively, offering alternative and more mature modes of function in word and action with which she can identify.

It has been said of abusive but also generally inadequate mothers that they need what their children need: good mothering. Though oversimplified, the statement has much truth to it. As has been detailed above, the therapeutic approach includes the establishment of a positive narcissistic transference, support for less than adequate coping mechanisms, the establishment of an identificatory relationship, the experience of nurturance, (as opposed simply to the classroom learning of methods of nurturance), and the encouragement of such sources of secondary narcissism as parenting, educational, and social skills. From such a developmental approach, the eventual achievement of improved self-sufficiency leads hopefully not only to an increased capacity for mothering but also to a natural termination of the therapy program. The process, however, is a slow one, taking years, not months, and requires a therapist with great skill and sensitivity as well as theoretical and technical sophisitication. For a para-professional to carry such a case, as is usually what occurs in the social agencies that deliver this service, the professional consultative supports must be strong and steady.

Treatment programs for the long-term consequences of vulnerability and risk are best conceptualized as no different from any adequate psychiatric treatment program. That is to say, treatment is individualized on the basis of a careful and thorough diagnostic assessement; and ideally the full repertoire of treatment modalities should be available so that all varieties of need can be met.

Certain syndromes of vulnerability and risk have achieved much in the way of current attention, including, for instance, child abuse, teenage pregnancy, learning disability and "hyperactivity." Unfortunately, attention in the popular press tends to oversimplify rather than illuminate the issues involved. When dealing with such striking behavioral entities there is an unfortunate tendency to assume that if one piece of a picture is the same—that is, the presenting complaint—all other aspects of the picture will also be the same; all "hyperactive" children or all child abusers are assumed to be alike in all specifics. A single standardized treatment program is then offered them, the treatment program for child abuse, etc. Individual differences are overlooked; and in particular treatability is not assessed, and preparations are not adequately made to identify and deal with the resistances or deficiencies in those personality characteristics that contribute to a good outcome from any therapeutic program.

Finally, such a presenting-complaint focused picture of a patient does violence to the idea of the whole person and raises question as to the adequacy of the theoretical conceptualizations utilized in the creation of such a program. The "compleat mental health professional," be he psychiatrist, psychoanalyst, psychologist, or social worker, is the one best equipped to cope with these as well as with any other patient. It is with this in mind that one can say treatment programs, even for this special population, should follow standard procedures applicable for all problems in mental health.

The classical psychoanalytic therapeutic aim, dating from its early work with the psychoneuroses, focused on making conscious the unconscious conflict, this work being accomplished against resistances expressed particularly within the transference. With an increased appreciation of the role of persistent developmental interruption, even as a precondition in some so-called normal neurotics, but especially with the increasingly frequent use of psychoanalytic therapy with the primarily developmentally arrested, treatment is now also viewed as a developmental process. The patient in such cases uses the analyst more as a dyadic ego auxiliary, at least initially; only later in treatment are neurotic conflicts mobilized to be dealt with in the classical style. Reconstructions focus on developmental issues. Character analysis is utilized more than content analysis. This is still a controversial issue, in part as some classicists prefer to reserve the term "psychoanalysis" only for work with neuroses. But call it what you will, this remains an ongoing area of clinical research. Much of this work is done with those suffering from the after effects of vulnerability and risk.

As the above suggests, the application of developmental insights to problems related to vulnerabiltiy and risk is in a stage of early development itself. As research in early development continues innovative programs evolve which themselves contribute to the research process. Only a small sample of the activity in the field can be suggested in this overview of a new and exciting field.

Methods and Comparisons

The use of more or less *established treatment programs* in dealing with the consequences of vulnerability and risk might seem easier to discuss. Scattered around the country are well-known and long-standing programs dealing with specific problems; such as Fraiberg's and Burlingham's work with blind children (Burlingham, 1975; Fraiberg, 1968, 1971). But the motivation and funding to work with so unrepresented and often unreachable a segment of the community as the vulnerable and at-risk child are largely a product of the relatively recent social concern with those who have been underrepresented in the health care and other social systems. Some clinics and some private practitioners have and still do work with this population. For instance, at a recent conference on child abuse, findings were presented from the *psychoanalysis* of an adult who had been severely abused as a child; at another conference, excerpts were presented from the psychoanalysis of an inner-city child. However, it is the *community mental health and mental retardation centers*, just over a decade old, that assume most of the responsibility for working with them. This is certainly true for the socioeconomically deprived, the largest portion of the vulnerable and at-risk population. The MH/MR centers are a heterogeneous lot. Their funding regulations are such that the services they deliver have greater variability than their program planning, at least on paper, promises. The tasks they are to perform, a cross section of inpatient, outpatient, and education services, are defined more carefully than those factors contributing to quality of service. The heaviest criticism leveled against them is concerning the alleged disparity between their frequent high cost per patient contact and the questionable adequacy of the service they deliver.

The final common pathway in any health delivery system is the individual therapist, the "front line troop" who works face to face with his patient. Therapy is a complex art, based upon the complex science of human behavior. It is also an emotionally and intellectually draining task. One's day is filled with emotion-laden confrontations that call for high quality and knowledgeable improvisation. It also calls for much in the way of tolerance, self-control, and inner strength. The major criticism of many of the MH/MR programs relates to their failure to direct themselves to this issue. Many are designed from their inception to maximize the use of lesser-trained and inexperienced therapists, with often token supervision by those skilled in the field. As unfortunately is true of many bureaucracies, the larger centers often put too much emphasis on paperwork, procedural mechanics, and the needs of the computer; the nature of the funding often dictates this. As a consequence the individual professional identity of the therapist comes second to their expected subservience to the system. Inservice training and continuing education are essential for therapists at all levels of expertise in this young and changing field, but is especially vital when a therapist's formal education has been rudimentary; yet too few hours are set aside for them and a spirit of "studentship" is insufficiently fostered. Although the full repertoire of therapeutic services should be available, the limitations of the staff proscribe this. The establishment and maintenance of *professionalism* among the therapist staff members is rarely given high enough priority. Professionalism can be defined as the state in which a therapist's personal identity and self-esteem are intimately connected to the excellence of his skills and knowledge in his chosen craft. What professionalism one usually sees in a MH/MR center is often the result of an individual therapist's own personal need surviving in spite of center procedures. Where this has been increasingly realized, there is often greater encouragement, for instance, to pursue further undergraduate or postgraduate education; but the funding supports making this possible are not always secure.

The MH/MR center movement is a gigantic and somewhat disorganized experiment. The nature of what they hope to accomplish, with the population they attempt to reach, can be viewed as experimental as well. The MH/MR centers were not created because of the availablity of knowledge and skills required to succeed in their appointed tasks. They arose out of what was felt to be a sociopolitical need, with the expectation that the necessary knowledge and skills would be found, created, or invented. Such is the challenge and responsibility for those who work within them. That excellence of service has not been achieved at least as yet should come as no surprise. One can only hope that those responsible for the future of the MH/MR movement will learn from their mistakes.

As was part of its original plan, the clinical and private practice models remain a part of the MH/MR center's system, although in varying degrees. Some existing clinics and services were simply administratively connected to the new MH/MR centers in their catchment areas. Psychiatrists and psychoanalysts, in private practice for part of their day and with the individual doctor-patient model clearly in mind, consult and even occasionally deliver the same services directly to MH/MR center patients as they do to their private patients.

Reports have been made from one MH/MR center serving a lower-socioeconomic community of a developmentally arrested inner-city child suffering from the "mindlessness syndrome" being seen in psychoanalysis by a psychiatric consultant (Burland, 1977). This is not a unique situation, although undoubtedly an unusual one; similar instances have been reported elsewhere. But it is not as frequent a practice as it should be. The particular kind of in-depth exploratory research that is part of a psychoanalysis is needed to further illuminate the psychodynamics of the consequences of deprivation, neglect, and abuse.

Therapeutic techniques in working with the developmentally arrested also need to be further refined, and this is best done in the intensive therapy situation. The insights from developmental psychology offer new guidelines that are of decided value. For instance, the developmentally arrested child must be met at his level of relationship if rapport is to be established. A fuller understanding of the infantile varieties of pre-object relationships, or of persistent infantile narcissistic attachments, aids in this endeavor. Reconstructive work, whether it serves merely as a guide for the therapist or is a part of the interpretive process, is aided immeasurably by an improved acquaintance with the wide variety of significant experiences that are a part of the earlier years of life. The psychoanalytic treatment of such children is too time-consuming and expensive, and is practiced by too small a number of therapists for it to be used routinely or even frequently. But it has been therapeutically effective when it has been able to put to use clinically the recent developmental insights; it has been less clinically successful when the therapist's repertoire of developmental conceptualizations has been limited to those relevant to neurotic structures. It has also proved valuable as a research tool when practiced by therapists involved in the further elaboration of developmental theory.

Conclusions

This brief overview of psychoanalytic perspectives on the vulnerable and at-risk child has attempted to convey a flavor of the experimental, if not venturesome, nature of work in this field. Though much is known and much that is effective is being done, there is more to learn and many children still not in receipt of the services and attention they require.

To a large measure, the money and human effort expended in this field is in response to what was a sociopolitical perception of an insufficiently attended to need. The demand for service came ahead of the science for performing that service. Among those who have entered this field, some before it was as "popular" as it is today and some after, has been a group of psychoanalysts whose work has been recounted in this chapter. There have been others less skilled and less knowledgeable, who have contributed less; there have been others equally skilled who have contributed as much. Hopefully it has been conveyed that progress in work with the consequences of vulnerability and risk will proceed best where what is known can act as a foundation upon which to build what is being discovered.

References

Anthony, E.J. (1974a) Risk-vulnerability intervention model for children of psychotic parents. In *The Child in His Family: Children at Psychiatric Risk*, Vol. 3. New York: Wiley, pp. 99–131.

Anthony, E.J. (1974b) Children at risk from divorce: A review. In *The Child in His Family: Children at Psychiatric Risk*, Vol. 3. New York: Wiley, pp. 461–477.

Anthony, E.J. (1974c) The syndrome of the psychologically vulnerable child. In *The Child in His Family: Children at Psychiatric Risk*, Vol. 3. New York: Wiley, pp. 529–544.

Beres, D. (1956) Ego deviations and the concept of schizophrenia. *Psychoanal. Study Child* 11:164–235.

Burland, J.A. (1975) Separation-individuation and reconstruction in psychoanalysis. *Int. J. Psychoanal. Psychother.* 4:303–335.

Burland, J.A. (1977) The syndrome of "mindlessness" in deprived children. Paper presented at Vulnerable Child Discussion Group of the American Psychoanalytic Association meeting in Quebec, April 28, 1977.

Burlingham, D. (1975) Special problems of blind infants: Blind baby profile. *Psychoanal. Study Child* 30:3–13.

Fraiberg, S. (1968) Parallel and divergent patterns in blind and sighted infants. *Psychoanal. Study Child* 23:264–300.

Fraiberg, S. (1971) Separation crisis in two blind children. *Psychoanal. Study Child 26:355–371.*

Freud, A. (1965) Normality and Pathology in Childhood. New York: International Universities Press.

Freud, A. (1936) *The Ego and the Mechanisms of Defense.* New York: International Universities Press (rev. ed., 1966).

Furman, E. (1974) *A Child's Parent Die.* New Haven: Yale University Press.

Gautier, Y., et al. (1977) The mother-child relationship and the development of autonomy and self-assertion in young (14–30 months) asthmatic children: Correlating allergic and psychological factors. *J. Am. Acad. Child Psychiat.* 16(1):109–131.

Grunebaum, H. (1977) Children at risk for psychosis and their families. *Psychiatric Spectator*, Sandoz.

Hartmann, H. (1939) *Ego Psychology and the Problem of Adaptation.* New York: International Unversities Press, 1958.

Hartmann, H., E. Kris, and R.M. Loewenstein. (1949)

Notes on the theory of aggression. *Psychoanal. Study Child* 3/4:9–36.

Kernberg, O. (1975) *Borderline Conditions and Pathological Narcissism.* New York: Jason Aronson.

Kohut, H. (1968) The psychoanalytic treatment of narcissistic personality disorders. *Psychoanal. Study Child* 23:86–113.

Kohut, H. (1969) Forms and transformations of narcissism. *J. Am. Psychoanal. Assn.* 14:243–272.

Kohut, H. (1971) *The Analysis of the Self.* New York: International Universities Press.

Kohut, H. (1977) *The Restoration of the Self.* New York: International Universities Press.

Kron, R.E., M. Stein, and K.E. Goddard. (1963) A method of measuring sucking behavior of newborn infants. *Psychosom. Med.* 25:181.

Kron, R.E., S.L. Kaplan, L.P. Finnegin, M. Litt, and M.D. Phoenix. (1977) Behavior of infants born to narcotics addicted mothers: Effects of prenatal and postnatal drugs. In J.D. Rementeria, ed., *Drug Abuse in Pregnancy and the Neonate.* New York: C.V. Mosby, pp. 129–144.

Lidz, R.W. (1976) Woman: Fertility and self-realization. Paper presented at Western New England Psychoanalytic Society.

Mahler, M. (1968) *On Human Symbiosis and the Vicissitudes of Individuation.* New York: International Universities Press.

Mahler, M., F. Pine, and A. Bergman. (1975) *The Psychological Birth of the Human Infant.* New York: Basic Books.

Meers, D. (1970) Contributions of a ghetto culture to symptom formation. *Psychoanal. Study Child* 25:209–230.

Parens, H., and L. Saul. (1971) *Dependence in Man: A Psychoanalytic Study.* New York: International Universities Press.

Sarrel, P.M., and R.W. Lidz. (1969) Contraceptive failure—Psychosocial factors in the unwed. In M. Calderone, ed., *Manual of Contraceptive Practice.* Baltimore: Williams & Wilkins.

Shopper, M. (1976) The effect of a deaf child on family structure. Paper presented at Vulnerable Child Discussion Group of the American Psychoanalytic Association meeting in Baltimore, May 6, 1976.

Sarrel, P. (1971) Siecus Study Guide No. 14: *Teenage Pregnancy: Prevention and Treatment.* Sex Information and Education Council of the U.S.

Solnit, A.J. (1975) Vulnerability and deprivation in early childhood. Paper presented at the Vulnerable Child Discussion Group of the American Psychoanalytic Association meeting in Los Angeles, May 1, 1975.

Spitz, R. (1945) Hospitalism. An inquiry into the genesis of psychiatric conditions in early childhood. *Psychoanal. Study Child* 1:53–74.

Spitz, R. (1946) Hospitalism: A follow-up report. *Psychoanal. Study Child* 2:113–117.

Spitz, R. (1965) *The First Year of Life.* New York: International Universities Press.

Steele, B.F. (1970) Parental abuse of infants and small children. In E.J. Anthony and T. Benedek, eds., *Parenthood.* Boston: Little, Brown.

Steele, B.F. (1977) Psychoanalytic observations on attachment and development of abused children. Paper presented at the Interdisciplinary Seminar—Child at Risk: Child Abuse, American Psychoanalytic Association, Quebec, April 30, 1977.

Steele, B.F., and C.B. Pollock. (1968) A psychiatric study of parents who abuse infants and small children. In R.E. Helfer and C.H. Kempe, eds., *The Battered Child.* Chicago: University of Chicago Press.

Wallerstein, J., and J.B. Kelly. (1977) Divorce counseling: A community service for families in the midst of divorce. *Am. J. Orthopsychiat.* 47(1):4–22.

Wallerstein, J. (1977) Brief interventions with children in divorcing families. *Am. J. Orthopsychiat.* 41(1):23–29.

Winnicott, D. (1953) Transitional objects and transitional phenomena. *Int. J. Psychoanal.* 34:89–97.

Treatment of Emotional Disorders in Children and Adolescents

CHAPTER 38

The Nature of Child Abuse and its Treatment

Linda E. Feinfeld

Definition and History

The term "child abuse" includes a variety of behaviors ranging from simple neglect to physical or sexual assault to willful murder. It is a "new" phenomenon in that until child welfare laws were passed starting in the late nineteenth century, children were considered their parents' chattels and their upbringing was not a matter of public concern. Strict punishment was often the norm, as embodied in the motto "Spare the rod and spoil the child." Child labor was common, and children were often valued for the work they could do. In some cultures children were even sold into slavery, and some even practiced infanticide. Even in more civilized societies if a child was accidentally killed, the offense was rarely recognized and the offender even more rarely brought to trial. Records from nineteenth-century England show hundreds of infanticides by accidental "lying over." This seems to have raised few eyebrows, especially since the majority of the victims were girls.

There were always some voices of protest. In ancient Greece, Socrates espoused a rational and humane mode of education. Jean Jacques Rousseau and Charles Dickens publicized the need for reform in their days, beginning the movement we are still experiencing. In the 1930's and 40's radiologists began publishing cases of "unrecognized trauma" in young children, but it wasn't until 1962, when Kempe and his co-workers described the battered child syndrome, that the phenomenon of child abuse became openly recognized. Recently the mass media have publicized sensational cases so that nearly everyone is aware of the problem.

Over the years medical practitioners have described patterns of nonaccidental trauma inflicted on children. Pediatricians can readily spot cigarette burns and bruises. Radiologists know to look for unexplained subdural hematomas and multiple fractures in different stages of healing, as well as metaphyseal fragmentation and periosteal changes from hemorrhage and calcification with resultant abnormal new bone growth which is the result of forceful pulling and twisting of an infant's limbs, but not all abused children are so easy to recognize as the ones with obvious trauma. Gross neglect, with malnutrition and failure to thrive and chronic, infected diaper rash can be seen, but not subtler forms of neglect. Sexual abuse can occasionally be detected on clinical examination, but it is rarely reported early and in any case usually leaves no telltale evidence. The definition of child abuse is therefore a legal one, including all forms of neglect, nonaccidental trauma, murder, sexual assault, and incest.

Epidemiology

The exact incidence of child abuse is unkown. With increasing awareness of the problem, more and more cases are being reported. In 1962 in New York City less than 1,000 cases were reported, of which about 10% died. In 1973 there were 19,000 reported cases of suspected abuse. More recent estimates are that there are between 150 and 300 cases reported per 1,000,000 population each year. The majority of cases reported are from the lower socioeconomic classes, but whether this reflects the true incidence or a bias against reporting suspected abuse among the middle classes is uncertain. It is known that economic difficulty, poor housing, and crowded living conditions are all stress factors that increase the risk of violent acting out of impulses.

Characteristics of Abusers and Abused

There are many factors contributing to the occurrence of child abuse. Initially all the blame was placed on the parents, but it is now recognized that it often involves a combination of abuse-prone parents, a vulnerable child, and a crisis situation. Generally only one parent is the abuser, while the spouse either tacitly agrees or feels helpless to prevent the attack on the child. Mothers have been implicated somewhat more often than fathers. Sometimes the abuser is a stepparent who projects his hostility toward his new mate onto the child, and similarly, sometimes the abuser is a friend of the parent. Most often the abusing parent was the victim of abuse as a child and never developed a sense of being valued and cared for duing his own early years, with resulting narcissistic injury. Such a development leads to severe ego pathology with a narcissistic-borderline personality organization. This immature and egocentric person looks to her child to fill the void in her life and make her feel loved and wanted. When her baby cries, as all babies do, the mother perceives it as another in a long line of rejections and failures. With poor impulse control this leads to anger against the child and violence.

It was commonly thought that child abusers were mentally ill. Statistically, less than 10% have a diagnosable mental illness such as schizophrenia or depression. By far, the great majority suffer from a character disorder with marked hostility, narcissism, and poor impulse control, but otherwise lead normal lives. The incidence of alcoholism or drug abuse is far less than one might suspect. There is a somewhat greater proportion of the mentally retarded among child abusers than in the general population, since a low IQ allows for fewer coping mechanisms.

Abuse-prone parents have also been described as socially isolated, suspicious individuals who have few supports within the community and shy away from contact with the outside world.

Characteristics of the Child

The child most vulnerable to abuse is often the youngest in the family and is often seen by the parent as somehow different, especially a child with a physical deformity, a birth defect, cerebral palsy, mental retardation, or a chronic or debilitating illness. Children with disabilities often make the parents feel guilty that something they did might have caused the problem. The child's visibility is also a constant reminder to the parents of their narcissistic injury in not having a perfect child. Often an abused child may not be physically different, but is perceived by the parent as different. An irritable, colicky baby can be a problem, as can an active baby whose mother likes quiet babies (or vice versa). Sometimes the child's sex or birth order will remind the parent of a hated and rivalrous sibling or other family members, or the child may be unplanned and unwanted. The child may come too early in a marriage, or at a troubled time for the parents. The parents may feel guilty that they resent the child and this can be an aggravating factor. In addiition, a child who is chronically abused becomes accustomed to it and may learn to behave in such a way as to bring abuse upon itself in order to get what little attention is available from the parent. Similarly, a child may make a scapegoat of himself unconsciously as a way to hold a shaky family together.

An abused child isn't necessarily vulnerable because of certain physical or emotional characteristics. In certain situations even a perfectly normal child might be at risk for abuse. Any situation that puts stress and strain on an abuse-prone parent will increase the risk. Depending on the individuals involved, a stressful time might develop when one is tired or ill, during a visit from parents or in-laws, during a marital crisis, or at a time when the caretaking parent feels unloved and unsupported by the spouse, during times of financial difficulty, or at any other time when a parent is unusually anxious, needy, or angry. A particularly violent parent may require very little to be pushed into an abusing situation, while a more patient person may be provoked by a combination of a vulnerable child and extremely trying circumstances.

Most violent abuse occurs with children under the age of three. If these children survive and grow, they develop with serious personality problems. Being handled with little affection inhibits the development of a sense of basic trust. These children have narcissistic character pathology with serious ego deficits, including the inability to form close relationships, a sense of neediness, poor self-concept, and a pervasive sense of failure. They frequently have academic difficulty in school and are social misfits. They become troublemakers and are labeled "bad kids."

The Nature of Child Abuse

Child abuse is rarely an ongoing, constant event in a household. True, there are some parents who persistently use brutal punishment, but by far the great majority of abuse occurs as sporadic incidents. A frequent story is that of the mother who has reached the limits of her tolerance for her child's crying and lashes out, throwing the child across the room. Remorsefully she takes the child for medical attention, but gives a sketchy or contradictory history that does not account for the nature of the injury seen. She may be amnesic regarding the actual attack or may try to cover up what she has done. Often the parents will doctor-shop or go to several different hospitals in order not to be found out. The parents may seem like responsible, concerned people, but there is always the danger that a new stress will provoke further violence. The events may be isolated, but the pattern is often repeated.

As stated previously, the abused child is generally less than three years old. Young preverbal children express their needs through crying. Unfortunately, a young, needy mother with low self-esteem may want her child to love her, show her gratitude, and take care of her emotional needs. When the infant cries, it is perceived as a rejection, or worse, as a reprimand similar to what she received from her mother. She may identify the child with her mother and take out her hostility on it. She expects the child to anticipate and conform to her needs. Amazingly, many childen perceive this in their mother and will try to comply and comfort her. But a young child has his or her own needs and therefore cries. Enraged parents have been known to beat their children with all manner of instruments, causing bruises, subdural hematomas, and even death. Some parents will pull and twist an infant's limbs in an effort to have it hold still during diapering or feeding. Some parents have inflicted burns and other mutilations.

The patterns of neglect are somewwhat different. Generally the neglectful parent is of low intelligence and low socioeconomic status and doesn't know better. Such a parent may have no idea what to feed a child or how much or how often, especially as nutritional needs change with age. The parent may not know how to diaper and may not care. Neglect tends to be constant rather than episodic. Sometimes the parent may neglect just one child while caring for the rest because of various psychological factors which make that child emotionally significant and vulnerable. More often, all children are neglected equally. In a large family, the older children may be better fed by virtue of their size. They are more adept at grabbing whatever food is available and pushing away the younger children. Frequently the parents feel helpless and unable to cope. They may be isolated socially and unwilling to seek outside help.

Sexual abuse also follows a distinct pattern. It generally involves a girl and other male members of the family. Occasionally a boy may be molested by older males, but almost never by older females.

The intrapsychic taboo against mother-son intercourse is by far the strongest and is rarely violated. The nature of incest correlates with the age of the child. A young child may be hugged and fondled or the adult may have the child manipulate his genitals. Intercourse is rare with a pre-pubertal child. Incest generally occurs when the parents are weak and inadequate in fulfilling their adult roles. The passive, withdrawn mother may have abdicated as her husband's sexual partner while encouraging her daughter in covert ways to be a companion to her father. The girl usually enjoys the special attention she gets by this and will comply in order to obtain affection and ward off threatened punishment if she doesn't. She also may be aware that by filling her mother's role she is keeping the family together and may sacrifice herself to this cause. The father is usually an ineffectual man with character pathology and poor impulse control. Often he will feel guilty about his relationship with his daughter and coerce her into remaining silent about it. The girl is generally loyal to her family and fearful of medical personnel, which makes it difficult for her to seek help.

Diagnosis, Prevention, and Treatment

The first step in treating the abused child and his parents is to make the diagnosis of child abuse. This can be done only if emergency room personnel and physicians in practice maintain a high index of suspicion and look for telltale signs and symptoms. It is a rare parent that readily confesses to beating a child. Many parents felt guilty and will bring the child for medical attention. Often they will have a genuine concern for the child's well-being and remorse for what they have done, but it is not easy to admit to inflicting injury to one's child. The examining physician will notice bruises, lacerations, burns, or fractures, often of different ages and in different stages of healing. Examination will reveal no blood dyscrasia or chronic medical conditon that would predispose to pathological fractures.

Child abuse must be suspected. When the parents are carefully questioned they will give a history that is often vague and contradictory. Their explanation, such as, "Johnny fell down the stairs" or "Pamela touched the stove when my back was turned," does not account for all the physcial findings. They may reveal that they have been to several hospitals or consulted several doctors for the various injuries.

The first and most important step when child abuse is suspected is to admit the child to the hospital. This removes the child from the noxious and potentially lethal home situation. It also allows time for a more careful assessment of the home situation than can be done on an emergency basis.

Second, all fifty states have laws requiring that physicians and often other medical personnel report any suspected cases of child abuse or neglect to their local child welfare agency. Some doctors are reluctant to report such cases for fear that they might inconvenience the parents, or worse yet, incur their hostility and precipitate a lawsuit. However, since the law requires reporting of every suspected case, the physician cannot be sued for obeying the law. The doctor may be liable to civil lawsuit or guilty of criminal neglect if he fails to report the abuse. There have been a few cases where parents sued and won when a medical practitioner failed to report abuse and thereby failed to protect the child from the parents! A common misconception about instituting proceedings in family court is that it is the equivalent of a criminal action. In most states it is not. Except in cases of murder, very little action, if any, is taken against the parents. Generally the courts simply assign protective custody of the child or children. Often the children are kept in the home with supervision of the parents. When they are removed, the hope is usually to return them to the parents as soon as possible.

After a case is reported, the local child welfare agency sends someone to evaluate the family and home situation. The aim is to examine the condition of the home—i.e., clean or in disarray and needing repairs—and the facilities the parents have for taking care of the children. The parents are examined to determine their attitudes toward their children and the nature of any incidents that have occurred. Other children in the family as well as neighbors are interviewed to corroborate evidence of abuse. Workers look to see whether the children are bathed or dirty. In extreme cases they may have lice or chronic infected diaper rash. The investigation may take a few days or a few weeks. Often the workers are impeded by the family's lack of cooperation. Abusive parents have become that way because they themselves had no support system they could turn to when their child became difficult to manage. They tend to be withdrawn, socially isolated and suspicious. They may not show up for appointments, and when the worker schedules a home visit, she may find no one at home. That she has the law on her side often makes it harder for parents to trust her.

In conjunction with the official agency investigation, many hospitals also maintain a child abuse team, usually consisting of a pediatrician, a psychiatrist or a psychologist, and a social worker. Such teams quickly become expert at doing an in-depth evaluation of suspected abuse cases. The child is examined physically and psychologically while the parents' psychological make-up and social network is explored. After they detemine that injury or neglect did occur, their job is to elicit answers to several key questions: under what circumstances did the injury occur, to only one child or to all, and is it likely to recur?

The circumstances of the stress can vary greatly. One parent may become violent only when many stresses build up, such as loss of a job, loss of a spouse, pressure from in-laws, a sick older child, and an unwanted baby with colic who is crying and uncontrollable. Another parent may be retarded or disorganized, and unable to cope even with the ordinary demands of parenthood. Usually all the children of such a parent will be neglected, malnourished, and dirty. But what of the household in which only one child is the victim? Then the investigating team must look for factors that make that child different, either in reality or in the eyes of the abusing parent. This last question is perhaps the hardest to answer. The abusive parent rarely wants to hurt her child. Neglect generally occurs out of ignorance, while violence occurs under circumstances in which the parent feels provoked and anger flares up. Since these people then become somewhat amnesic about the violent episode, it may be almost impossible to reconstruct the precipitating events. Also the parents may sincerely desire never to harm their children again, but will nonetheless lose control and get carried away, in spite of well-intentioned promises.

All these factors require careful consideration and a great deal of time and effort on the part of the abuse team, especially since the parents will rarely cooperate voluntarily. To overcome this, some authors have advocated an approach that demands that the parents come to the professionals' offices rather than vice versa. The parents may face the loss of the child or children if they don't comply.

When the abuse team has compiled its report, the family-court judge decides on a course of action. If the child has been removed from the home, the question is whether the child can be safely returned, and if so, will the parents need supervision. Or should the child be placed in a foster home or custody given to another relative, perhaps a grandparent? The child's physical well-being is usually given primary consideration, with foster care being a frequent choice. Unfortunately, the abused child has a strong need for the parent's affection, even if it is coupled with violence, and experiences separation from the parent as a further rejection.

Treatment

When the full report is compiled, the judge will weigh the various factors and order some placement of the child,. and when available, treatment for the parents and sometimes the child.

There have been many approaches to treatment, with varying degrees of success. The goal of turning an abusive parent into a loving, considerate parent is unrealistic. Most people consider a more reasonable aim is to return the child to the home with reasonable assurance that he or she won't be subject to further injury. One of the most useful approaches to treatment has been to "mother the mother." Since abusive parents were themselves generally abused as children, they tend to have many ego deficits and character pathology that makes them poor mothers or fathers. Partly they do not know how a good parent should act, and partly they lack the inner resources needed to provide adequate emotional nurturance for their children. Nurturing, supportive therapists hope that by making the parent feel appreciated, needed, and worthwhile they can strengthen the parent's ego so that he or she in turn will be able to give more to his or her children. One highly successful program, at least in the short run, actually admitted the abusive mothers with their children to the hospital. The staff focused its energy on the mothers, giving them praise, encouragement, and support. The mothers in turn could extend their more positive feelings about themselves to their children and become better mothers. As the women felt greater self-confidence and the beginnings of pride in themselves, the children benefited. The major drawback of this program was that it was expensive.

Most therapeutic approaches to child abuse use an outpatient setting. Here, compliance may be more variable, since abusive parents tend to be isolated and mistrustful. Often the threat of losing their child to the court's custody will bring them in. The favorite modality is group therapy, in which the members share their personal experiences with one another while the therapist gives encouragement and support. Parents learn that they are not alone in their problems and help one another learn new and different ways of coping with the child, who is trying to express its needs. They can learn from the group leader and from each other that the cry may be a signal that the baby is hungry or tired or in pain, and that there are ways in which they as parents can alleviate the child's discomfort and stop the crying. If all efforts to comfort the baby fail, they can also learn alternatives to acting out their frustrations and hitting the baby.

If the group members do not have ideas, the leader can suggest such things as changing the baby's position or closing the door to the baby's room, or if all else fails just getting out of the house and going for a walk. Often group members are encouraged to exchange phone numbers so that they have someone to call in a crisis. Many medical centers also maintain emergency hot lines that abuse-prone parents can call when their tempers flare or difficult situations develop. In some centers the therapists give the parents their home phone numbers so that they can be contacted at any time. It is often a life-saving measure for potentially violent parents to have one or more people they can rely on and call when they feel enraged or overwhelmed.

Such emergency resources are essential to maintain. Another vital service is the provision of emergency child care. This can take the form of a 24-hour babysitting service where the parents can leave their children at any time when they are afraid they might hurt the child if he or she stayed at home. Where no babysitting service is available, the hospital assumes this role by admitting the child when violence is threatened.

Another approach to treatment of the battered child is family therapy. Here the focus is not on any individual person but the family as a unit and the interactions of the family members. The goals would be to pinpoint how the child or children provoke the parents and how the parents respond. With this knowledge the members of the family can try to develop new ways of relating to each other so that they each feel more wanted and worthwhile, lovable and loving. Individual psychotherapy of the parents has been done. Most ego-deficient people can benefit from supportive therapies. Careful evaluation should be done before attempting any insight-oriented therapy because most abusive parents are not good candidates for an analytic approach.

Few programs have attempted to treat children out of the family context. Those that do work with children age five and older who show faulty ego development as a result of the violent handling the child has received. An abused child with personality pathology would be treated with supportive or reconstructive individual therapy designed to permit ego development with subsequent individuation and independence. These children require patience on the therapist's part because they generally lack a sense of basic trust and are slow to develop rapport. With kindness and caring they may eventually develop a sense of self-worth. Older children may learn insight into their behavior and their parents, which may enable them to avoid situations in which their parents may become provoked and abusive. Ultimately these children should grow to be thoughtful adults who can use rational means to handle their own anger. Hopefully they will deal with their own children in a more peaceful manner, thus breaking the generational cycle of abuse.

With older children it is best to work with the schools as well. The existence of a problem is often picked up by the teachers, who may then bring it to the attention of the school nurse or the psychologist. Once the problem has been diagnosed, it is very useful to encourage the teachers to be more supportive of the child and help him not only to learn how to study but also how to win the acceptance of his peers and of himself.

Neglect

As mentioned previously, patterns of neglect tend to be different from those of violence. Neglectful parents tend to be that way because of ignorance. Generally they are on the lower end of the spectrum of intelligence. Sometimes they are of normal intelligence but are suffering from a mental disorder that impairs judgment. Sane, intelligent people generally seek advice and guidance from friends, relatives, and child health care professionals. Abusive neglect occurs when parents either do not know how to care for children because they do not know where to turn for help and/or cannot comprehend the help they receive or because they cannot consider the needs of their children due to some inner conflict.

Treatment of neglect usually consists of educating the parent(s) whenever possible. Often a visiting nurse, homemaker, or babysitter is sent into the home to supervise and help the mother. If the parents are incapable of learning, custody of the child may be given to a grandparent or other relative, if appropriate, or else the child is placed in foster care. When a parent is psychotic, then appropriate psychiatric treatment is offered. The child is preferably given in custody to another relative either temporarily or permanently. Since separation is felt by the child as punitive, the goal is to return the child to the home whenever possible and as quickly as possible, but the child should be returned to the parent only with supervision of the parents.

Sexual Abuse

Cases of sexual abuse are more complicated. Most adults would be horrified at the thought of their child being sexually molested, and of course there are strong taboos against incest. The most common patterns of sexual abuse are mother's boyfriend–daughter, stepfather–daughter, father–daughter, brother–sister, and neighbor–child. Many of these involve incest and are particularly hard to identify and therefore hard to treat. The parents are often weak and ineffectual in their parental roles. The mother may be tacitly encouraging her husband and daughter, but would openly deny it or may even be unaware of her role. In treating such a family, one must first win the confidence and trust of the various members in order to sort out what role each is playing. The therapist must be especially careful not to place the blame on any one person. He or she must examine how the members interact within the context of the whole family. Often the therapy involves the family as a unit, but psychopathology in each person can be treated individually. Goals of therapy include not only the cessation of the sexual activity, but also helping the parents to become more effective individuals with a better ability to assert themselves and be stronger in their roles as parents, adults, and responsible leaders of the family.

Prevention

There are several aspects to the prevention of child abuse. First, it is necessary to recognize who is an abuse-prone parent. This can sometimes be observed right on the maternity ward by an astute nursing staff. Most new mothers are nervous and uncertain, but most are eager to learn the job of mothering. A rejecting or reluctant mother can easily be recognized.

Staff should also become suspicious of a parent who talks about discipline for his or her newborn or about a "bad" baby. Unfortunately, since violence against children usually occurs when the parent becomes enraged in a situation where they feel overburdened and unsupported, this cannot be seen until the mother is home with her baby and is faced with the demands of caring for it.

A teenage mother is still a child herself and will need plenty of help and guidance in undertaking the responsibility of caring for a baby. Similarly, a retarded mother needs careful, explicit, and repeated instructions, and even then may be unable to handle changing demands. Some retarded parents may be able to learn child care; many will need supervision; some will never be able to manage and should not be given their children.

Once a person is known to be violent or potentially violent with his or her children, then every effort must be made to prevent further violence. If the parents can recognize what stresses them and under what circumstances they feel they can no longer cope, then they can learn how to avoid those situations whenever possible. If they can learn to call for help before going out of control, child abuse hotlines can be lifesaving.

Also it is essential to identify vulnerable children and offer them special protection. In some circumstances it may be necessary to remove them from the home temporarily. In some cases psychotherapy aimed at changing irritating personality traits can help. With a handicapped child, a special program to aid the child may also take some of the burden off the parents. Special situations in which a vulnerable child—or for that matter, any child—is at risk should also be identified and circumvented. Parents and their children should be aware of whatever resources are available: emergency telephone numbers of therapists, friends, and relatives; emergency child care facilities, be they 24-hour drop-in centers or hospital wards or friendly neighbors.

As previously stated, abuse runs in families, with abused children learning harsh methods of child rearing from their parents and using them on their own children. With this in mind, hospital staffs should be especially concerned when previously abused children have children and should offer counseling, love, and guidance. The best prevention would be the successful treatment of abused children and their families so that they could grow up with healthier, more intact egos, feeling self-confident and capable. They in turn would be able to raise their children in a more accepting and nuturing manner, thus breaking the generational cycle.

References

Bell, G. (1973) Parents who abuse their children. *Can. Psychiat. Assn. J.* 3:223–228.

Bennie, E., and A. Sclare. (1969) The battered child syndrome. *Am. J. Psychiat.* 7:975–979.

Brown, J., and R. Daniels. (1968) Some observations on abusive parents. *Child Welfare* 2:89–94.

Caffey, J. (1946) Multiple fractures in the long bones of infants suffering from chronic hematoma. *Am. J. Roentgen.* 56:163.

Chase, N. (1976) *A Child Is Being Beaten.* New York: McGraw-Hill.

Child Abuse and Neglect: Model Legislation for the States. (March 1976) Report #71. Denver: Education Commission of the States.

Fontana, V. (1975) Child maltreatment and battered child syndromes. In Freedman et al., eds., *Comprehensive Textbook of Psychiatry II.* Baltimore: Williams & Wilkins.

Gil, D. (1970) *Violence Against Children.* Cambridge, Mass.: Harvard University Press.

Green, A., R. Gaines, and A. Sandgrund. (1974) Child abuse: Pathological syndrome of family interaction. *Am. J. Psychiat.* 8:882–886.

Green, A. (1978) Psychopathology of abused children. *J. Am. Acad. Child Psychiat.* 17:92–103.

Green, A. (1978) Psychiatric treatment of abused children. *J. Am. Acad. Child Psychiat.* 17:356–371.

Helfer, R., and C.H. Kempe. (1968) *The Battered Child.* Chicago: University of Chicago Press.

Kempe, C.H., F. Silverman, B. Steele, W. Droege-Muller, and H. Silver. (1962) The battered-child syndrome. *J.A.M.A.* 181:17-24.

Kempe, C.H., and R. Helfer, eds. (1972) *Helping the Battered Child and His Family.* Oxford: Lippincott.

A Look at Child Abuse. (1976) National Committee on Child Abuse. Chicago.

Schmitt, B., ed. (1978) *The Child Protection Team Handbook.* New York and London: Garland STPM Press.

Smith, S., R. Hanson, and S. Noble. (1973) Parents of battered babies: A controlled study. *Brit. Med. J.* 4:388–391.

Spinetta, J., and D. Rigler. (1972) The child-abusing parent: A psychological review. *Psychol. Bull.* 77.

Walters, D. (1975) *Physical and Sexual Abuse of Children: Causes and Treatment.* Bloomington: Indiana University Press.

Treatment of Emotional Disorders in Children and Adolescents

CHAPTER 39

Therapeutic and Preventive Interventions with Blind Children

Cecily Legg

In writing of the treatment of young blind children, the intention is not to imply that the visual deficit represents a diagnostic label or that blindness limits the range of pathology encountered. Blindess is recognized as an inescapable and pervasive factor that affects the life and personality of the individual. In this chapter, discussion centers on the young, congenitally blind child who has not achieved adaptive ego functioning, and who, when brought to the psychiatric's office, may have the appearance of autism or mental retardation. If the blind patient is a young child, he almost always presents with severe ego deficits. Whereas when an older blind child is brought for psychiatric evaluation, he may have been able to achieve a limited but somewhat adequate organization of the ego, and may present with a neurosis. An observation or trial period may be needed in order to establish a differential diagnosis in regard to autism, psychosis, retardation, or organicity. Since blind children take much longer than sighted children to show change, such a trial period needs to be longer than just a few weeks. Careful and explicit discussion of this with the parents is needed; as too often a lengthy observation is misunderstood by them and becomes thought of as a treatment process. When careful history taking and observation suggest that a potential exists for further unfolding of ego functions, a psychoanalytically oriented therapy is suggested to be the treatment modality of choice. This therapy will need to be modified with such parameters as are indicated by the degree of severity of the disturbance. It must be recognized that in the initial stage treatment will have to be largely an educative process. It may be many months before treatment can more nearly approximate psychotherapy as that term is generally understood. As the preventive uses of psychiatry become more freely utilized, early intervention in the form of parent counseling may be made available to the parents concurrently with the confirmation of an infant's blindness. The scope of parent counseling need not be limited to working solely with the conflicts and sadness evoked by the child's handicap, important and inescapable as these are. The counseling can serve also an educative purpose, helping parents to recognize and use techniques that will promote the child's adaptive use of important ego functions.

Blindness, fortunately, is a rare occurence in our child population. All too easily, therefore, we speak or write of "blind children" in a somewhat definitive manner, as if to imply the notion that all blind children can be considered in a single category. This is obviously not so. Nevertheless, it can be predicted that lack of vision can inevitably, to a greater or lesser extent, intrude upon the unfolding of a child's expectable developmental sequences, thereby nudging him into some alternative or substitute pathway. The degree of adaptiveness each individual blind child is able to achieve is predicated upon many variables, both inner and outer, as is the case with sighted youngsters. An understanding of the altered developmental pathways to be found in association with congenital or early acquired blindness is a help in therapeutic, educational, or preventive work with blind children.

The term "blindness" may be used to signify varying degrees of visual impairment, anywhere along the continuum from total lack of vision to the limited amount of vision still within the definition of legal blindness. For purposes of the present discussion, blindness will be understood as meaning either complete lack of vision or so little visual perception that the subject will have to learn braille and will be dependent on this method for reading and writing. A child may be born blind or acquire blindness at some later time, in which case vision may have deteriorated slowly due to degenerative or disease process, or have been experienced dramatically as a sequel to a sudden unexpected injury or trauma. Unless stated otherwise, our reference will be to blindness present at birth or soon thereafter, or to early adventitious blindness, by which we mean, blindness that has occurred before the child is into his fifth year. The population principally referred to will be young children without multiple handicaps and without established diagnoses of gross brain damage or ineducable retardation. That is to say, the population most likely, with present knowledge, to be responsive to and helped by interventions of a preventive or psychotherapeutic nature.

Historical Background

Few references relating to blindness in childhood can be culled from the psychiatric literature earlier than the 1950s, the same is not true, of course, of pedagogic literature. Considerable writing by educators had already been published. Most of the contributions appearing in psychiatric journals since 1950 have been written from a dynamic viewpoint, mostly by child psychoanalysts. For reasons to be discussed later, such an approach seems to offer a promising means of furthering the understanding of the developmental issues at risk from blindness, as well as affording an avenue by which to reach and help the child therapeutically. It therefore becomes less a matter for surprise that child psychiatry seems to have been tardy in offering its services to blind children. For in the forties, child psychoanalysis was still in its own infancy. Burlingham (1941) was the first to report on the application of psychoanalytic insights to the observation of blind children. It is possible to identify further contributory influences to the seeming "neglect" of blind children before the forties. The small number of such children in the population at large did not constitute a pressure group demanding attention. Their problems could be avoided all too easily. But more significantly, these children presented a confusing diagnostic picture, since those brought to psychiatrists frequently presented with bizarre behavior patterns and with an appearance of psychosis or severe retardation. They did not seem likely to respond to interventions of a psychotherapeutic nature. Kanner's (1949) contribution to the study of infantile autism led the way to a rethinking of diagnostic categories. After this, the severely disturbed blind child was more likely to be distinguished from the child with bizarre, inappropriate behavior resembling him, but arising from a different etiology.

By the mid and late 1940's, child psychoanalysis was an established and recognized treatment modality ready to meet the dilemma of the blind child. This timely readiness coincided with the increase in the number of young blind children; many of the prematurely born infants able to be kept alive by administration of oxygen were later found to have retrolental fibroplasia. Before the association between the level of oxygen administration and retrolental fibroplasia had been defined, the emphasis was placed on the factor of prematurity. In a Chicago study of 295 preschool blind children, Norris, Spaulding, and Brodie (1957) reported a diagnosis of retrolental fibroplasia and coexisting prematurity for 209 cases—i.e., 71% of their study. For several years the retrolental fibroplasia group were regarded as somewhat distinct from children whose blindness had a different aetiology. However, as Fraiberg (1975) points out, when the literature increased, "a striking uniformity" could be noted between the autistic-like children in her New Orleans group and those described by Parmalee (1959), Norris (1957), and Keeler (1958). It could now be seen, she writes, that "the clinical picture of deviant ego development was not associated with any specific etiology for the blindness." In Canada, Keeler's work pointed to a relation between the gross abnormalities found in some blind children and an insufficient emotional stimulation in the earliest months of life. In England, the careful developmental studies of Burlingham and her co-workers were pointing to similar findings—Burlingham (1961, 1964, 1965), Sandler (1963), Nagera and Colonna (1965), and Wills (1965, 1970).

On this side of the Atlantic, the developmental dilemma of the blind child continued to be scrutinized by Fraiberg (1968, 1971c, 1975), Fraiberg and Adelson (1973), Fraiberg and Friedmann (1964), and Fraiberg, Siegel, and Gibson (1966). It may seem, from the foregoing, that all thoughts of working psychotherapeutically with these children were put on one side while the developmental data was so painstakingly gathered in. This is not so. The picture of the delays, divergences, and adaptations peculiar to the development of blind children that unfolded in therapy sessions were then used to enrich and understand information gleaned from the direct observations in home and nursery school. In writing of the development of young blind children, the authors have drawn extensively from case material in nearly every instance. In fact, one of the first cases to be reported in detail in the literature is that of Omwake and Solnit (1961). Further case studies are those of Fraiberg (1971b, 1976), and Bennett (1973). The Hampstead Clinic took a series of young blind children into treatment, and references to many of these cases are found in the developmental studies already cited, some have been reported more individually—Burlingham and Goldberger (1968), Colonna (1968), and Lopez (1974).

In the process of gathering and scrutinizing developmental information within the conceptual framework of a psychoanalytic approach, possibilities of early intervention to further enhance more adaptive ego development evolved. Fraiberg (1971a) and her co-workers in Ann Arbor began a program of intervention in infancy, helping mothers to find ways of meaningful and pleasurable interaction with their blind children, thus furthering the child's development. In Hampstead, a small nursery school group was started with the usual nursery school equipment and routines adapted and matched to the needs of young blind children. Thus we can say that in the last three decades there have been three main thrusts in work with young blind children. Namely, developmental studies, psychotherapeutic interventions and treatments, and early preventive work.

Theoretical Considerations

It may be asked why so little has been said about other approaches to the problems of the blind child, why such a biased picture is being given? The question is justified and the answer is simple: a computerized library search (skeptically received and augmented by further personal research) yielded very little reference to work with young blind children on other than a dynamically oriented one-to-one basis. Thompson (1974, p. 13) writes, for instance, that "to date there are no publications on the use of T.A. theory and techniques with blind people, and very little literature on group treatment of the blind." Although Thompsom reports beneficial results from group work with young adults, we would not expect this with blind children. The blind child referred for help is most often either not ready for inclusion in nursery or grade school, or only precariously maintaining himself there with considerable support from understanding and supportive adults. His need is for painstaking clarification of his confused external reality followed by interpretation of libidinal conflicts. The literature of behavior therapy has been found to contain only rather brief references to blind children. Martin and Iagulli (1974) report a successful modification of middle-of-the-night tantrums in a 4-year-old severely mentally retarded blind child. Behavior modification would seem a valuable resource for such a child, but less helpful in the case of the potentially well endowed, but confused, child with libidinal ties, who can respond to ego-building techniques.

Another question to be raised is why is there an emphasis on young children? Are older children not treated? What of the latency aged or adolescent youngster? It is a fact that the literature to date does focus on the young child, it should not be over looked that many of these children remained in treatment, however, until chonologically in latency. It is further true that the two most published groups (Ann Arbor and Hampstead) have focused on the young child. Other writers, notably Blank (1957), have documented work with adolescents. It seems that either parents tend to seek professional counseling themselves, on learning of the infant's visual defects, or that help is sought for the blind child as developmental lags and deviances become increasingly difficult for the parent to disguise or to manage. It seems possible that when help is not sought in the early years the situation may, in many cases, deteriorate beyond the state of effective intervention. It can be presumed that when a blind adolescent is responsive to psychotherapy, early development has been sufficiently adaptive to have allowed relative psychic progress to be made.

Because of the wide geographical scattering of blind children and the difficulty of providing special learning situations for these children on an individual basis, a tendency has often been to start quite young children in residential groups. For many children, the stress of separation from libidinal objects is too great an adaptation to the new situation and is made only at considerable cost to further psychic development. Without vision, object constancy is not achieved within the usual limits, the early dependency on adults continues more intensely and for a longer period than with sighted children—thus making the child uniquely vulnerable to separation.

Suitability for Treatment

As in all work with children, it is preferable that the child be referred as soon as the problem is identified. As mentioned above, this may be when the blindness is first known or may not be until the child has demonstrated aberrant behavior. Assessment of blind children is often complicated by questions of organicity, although neurological workups and EEG studies may be negative, deficits in cognitive functioning may still give rise to questions of CNS impairment, not easy to resolve. If gross organicity is present management techniques will probably be recommended. Many blind children have autistic-like features, not infrequently it is also necessary to rule out the possibility of associated deafness. While a marked degree of deafness would probably rule out a trial of psychotherapy, a moderate degree of retardation need not necessarily do so. Burlingham and Goldberger (1968), and Lopez (1974) report on work with retarded children. As always, in work with children, the parents' ability to support the treatment is a vital consideration. These are parents who have already been "cheated" by getting a sightless child, and who are unconsciously, if not consciously, guilty vis-à-vis the child's problems. It is essential for the progress of therapy that the evaluator's findings and predictions are clearly and simply stated to the parents. It is not unusual for a blind child to refuse, for many weeks, to stay with the therapist without the parent. When this seems a likely contingency, it should receive prior discussion with the parent to avoid frustration for the mother, who may envisage already that the sessions will serve as a break from her constant caretaking, perhaps the chance to have a peaceful coffee with a book or to make an uninterrupted phone call.

Briefly then, work with a blind child has to be undertaken with guarded prognosis, often with a trial period and with regular review. Gains may be small and will certainly be slow. The therapist may need to work not only with the parents, but also with the child's teacher and other significant caretakers.

Treatment of Blind Children

The literature describes some of the adaptations and modifications of techniques that have been employed in work with blind children, illustrating the amount of flexibility that can go hand in hand with a correct appreciation of basic tenets and principles. The use of such parameters has not been haphazard, but has been based on an understanding of developmental delays and the distortions in cognitive processes brought about through lack of vision. The extent to which a therapist may need to modify the usual procedure obviously depends on the severity of the child's maladaptiveness and disturbance. Just as with sighted patients, the readiness of the young patient to be left alone with the unfamiliar therapist and the child's freedom to communicate with a new person will be dependent on many factors. Add to these the impossibility of his visually checking the person and surroundings to which he has been brought and the need for facilitating techniques becomes apparent. Before the child can check out the office by moving around it and completely exploring it on his own, a relationship may first have to be built up with the therapist. In the meantime, the child relies on auditory cues and even smells to learn about his enviroment. One 7-year-old child reacted strongly to a lofty, sparsely furnished office. He claimed that something happened to people's voices in there. Another child was upset by the smell of an office, but could not explain that the disturbing smell, a slight mustiness, evoked memories of an occasion of temporary separation from mother. Both of these experiences could happen to a sighted child who might also take some weeks in conveying them to us, but who would, in the meanwhile, have been less overwhelmed by this experience because of the other information gained by visual means.

It is not that elaborate arrangements have to be undertaken in order to make the usual office a suitable place in which to work with a blind child, but rather that the therapist needs to become more aware of the different characteristics of it than he generally is; particularly is it necessary for him not to block out the offstage sounds, those coming from the office next door, from the corridor, and from outside the builidng. Offstage does not exist in the usual sense of the term, for the blind child the distance to which hearing reaches represents the boundaries of the child's present situation, rather than the unseen wall of the room. This extension of the office has to be recognized by the therapist, too.

As the child struggles with forming a conceptual framework in which to better organize his experience and make sense of his wider surroundings, the therapist may occasionally find it appropriate to take the patient outside the office and help him explore the neighborhood. Within the office, rather little is needed in the way of equipment. In selecting the play materials, some objects small enough to be held comfortably in one hand should be chosen. Variation in the textural characteristics and in the sound making possibilities of the items made available should be taken into account. Elaborate toys should be avoided, these only confuse the child.

The foregoing comments lead to a consideration of the therapist—are there particular requirements to be met before one is equipped to treat a blind child? Kessler (1966) has suggested that work with children calls for "some ability to accept ambiguity, to be willing to imagine and guess what is going on in the child's mind." An ability to accept a high degree of ambiguity and uncertainty may be called for if the therapeutic relationship is to be established with a blind child. The therapist will have to be prepared to recognize other, less usual meanings to some pieces of a blind child's behavior. For instance, the quiet, inactive, seemingly withdrawn child may not be depressed, but may be listening intently, piecing together an impression of his surroundings from minimal auditory clues. The unexpected, unrecognized, or painfully associated to sound cannot be checked out visually with an immediate lowering of anxiety. In moments of silence a blind child may fear that the therapist has forgotten about him or has even fallen asleep. One patient, who liked to have the therapist knit as a means of keeping check on her wakefulness, panicked when the therapist sewed instead of knitting. It was found that the sound of the needle going through stiff material had been understood as meaning that a kitten "with scratchy claws" was in the office. Thus, in working with a blind child, the therapist has to become accustomed to listening for unusual possibilities, signals that may provoke either anxiety or pleasure conveyed through commonplace noises. Not only sound effects but speech itself has to be decoded; the blind child's seeming competence in the use of sighted language is soon found to be false. Without vision, words acquire other meanings. A blind child's therapist needs to have some of the qualities of a skillful detective, not least an abundance of patient perseverance.

Developmental Patterns: Significance for Therapy

In working psychotherapeutically with any child, it is necessary for the therapist to be well informed in developmental matters. As already emphasized, blindness can cause alterations in ordinary areas of development, both on the side of the libido and the ego, and not on any one stage or phase of development alone, but on all.

The probability, occasionally even the certainty, of congenital blindness may be known from birth, or not for some while thereafter. The parents' affectual response, whether expressed or denied, brings about an alteration in their cathexis of the child; parenting of a blind child is a serious narcissistic injury. From early days the fact of blindness acts on the infant's human environment as well as directly on the unfolding of the infant's own developmental pathways. The intrusiveness of blindness into the building up of early object relationships has been fully documented in the literature. The arduous task of building object relations when only nonvisual clues can be used has been studied in detail. The interferences are subtler than they at first appear. Problem areas are interwoven in a complex manner manifested by a delay in the process of separation-individuation and in the reaching of object constancy. The inevitably prolonged dependency on the primary libidinal object is reflected in many sectors of the child's development, as, for instance, in loss of self-esteem and cathexis of the self at those times when the object is temporarily less available. Because of the blind child's actual need of the object as protector from external danger, he has to be handed from one caretaker to another. The compliance he shows for this necessary arrangement may sometimes give an appearance of promiscuity in object relationships, but in fact he has a strong libidinal attachment to his primary object. The fact is, circumstances force him to cling to substitutes whenever the real objects are absent from him.

Among those blind children brought for help it is a usual finding that their libidinal development lags considerably behind that of their sighted peers. Nagera (1965) comments on the rootedness of blind children in the early pregenital stages, the move into the phallic-oedipal stage does not at all imply that drive gratification and autoerotic activities pertaining to the oral and anal phase will tend to disappear, or even to recede notably into the background. Nagera suggests that blindness interferes with the child's facility for finding "new means of gratification, both in drive discharge and ego activities." Not only does development proceed more slowly, the old means of gratification are clung to and experienced alongside the new to a greater extent than is usual. The influence of blindness infiltrates into the sphere of ego functioning in both obtrusive and unobtrusive, subtle ways. The blind child's hesitancy to move around freely is understood by Burlingham (1965) as a "control of free movement—an essential mode of self-protection," and as an intentional closing off of "a pathway which, under ordinary circumstances, constantly serves the discharge of the boundless energy which is present in the young." The strenuous efforts a blind child makes in order to recognize inanimate objects and the constant attention he pays to nonvisual clues in order to keep orientated in space are easily disrupted by affectual experiences. When possible, the evaluation of a blind child should include an opportunity to observe him on familiar home territory, as well as in the office.

An area of success most open to a blind child and generally freely encouraged by the parents is that of language. Yet this can so often be a barrier of unique vulnerability for him. In considering the effect of blindness on the ego, Klein (1962) speaks of two kinds of deprivation: "a specific sensory restriction or deficit, and, in addition, an isolation in the environment." This latter, he points out, represents "an assault on the synthetic function of the ego itself." The child copies and uses the language of the sighted world, but with a different frame of reference. The context in which a word is used may be understood, but not the concept; as for example, when a 9-year-old blind girl several times spoke of being embarrassed. The word was appropriately used, but a change of voice to careful imitation of the mother's caused the therapist to ask the meaning of the word. With a sigh came the question "Don't you know either?" When these children are able to use language more personally, we note how often their frame of reference is to their own body or to some feeling or toileting situation. A 6-year-old, telling about a visit to the zoo, described an elephant's leg as seeming like shredded wheat, her favorite breakfast cereal.

The importance of verbalization for early ego development is indisputable, it is therefore necessary to ask in what way lack of vision interferes with language development. Fraiberg (1977), using the Bayley Scales, gives a detailed comparison of language acquisition in sighted and blind (but otherwise intact) children. An interesting finding of her study is that "to name a need or want is not more difficult for a blind than a sighted child." In the Bayley Scale item "Uses words to make wants known," the study group infants are within the ranges of the sighted infants. Fraiberg points to the exogenous nature of stimuli leading to needs and wants. For a sighted child, the experiencing of a need or want may evoke a picture, whereas a blind child will have to make use of some other form of mental representation in which qualities of the wished-for object are derived from nonvisual cues, but this form of representation can also lead to the naming of the need or wish. The blind infant encounters difficulty, however, with an earlier item of "two words," and may lag 6 months behind sighted norms on this level. Fraiberg suggests that this may be explained on the basis that the first words used by sighted infants are largely nominative; some difficulty in naming and labeling is to be expected when recognition can only be achieved through nonvisual perception. The achievement of blind infants also falls below the Bayley median by almost 6 months for the item "sentence of two words"—that is, the putting of two words signifying two concepts together. Fraiberg sees this lag as probably resulting from a difficulty in concept formation: "Without vision, the child must take a long circuitous route to the construction of a world of objects (and naming them), and to the attribution of action and qualities for things and persons (two word sentences)."

Another consequence of blindness—namely, the delay in gaining independent mobility—also has repercussions on language development. The young blind child has to go to his surroundings to learn about them, he cannot take them in visually. As he becomes more mobile it is not uncommon for a coincidental increase in vocabulary skills to be noticed. The blind child uses speech adaptively for purposes the sighted child does not need to (Burlingham, 1961). Whereas the sighted child can keep eye contact with his human environment, the blind child relies heavily on verbal contact. The young blind child distinguishes people by verbally collected data; hence the repetitive and endless questions, "What is your address, your phone number, who do you live with?" It is noted that blind children do not develop a language based primarily on nonvisual experience, but strive to imitate sighted language, this often receives reinforcement from parents who may see such language as adaptive to sighted norms. Only when the environment is facilitating in this respect can use be made of more experiential language. The blind child's difficulty in building up nonvisual conceptualizations of everyday surroundings and events is graphically illustrated by Burlingham when discussing verbalization in a nursery school group of blind children.

It is possibly in relation to aggression that the newcomer to work with blind children may be most easily misled. The blind child's peculiar dependency on his objects influences him to inhibit overt aggression toward them. Yet this may not at first seem to be the case. The child's behavior may be considered quite aggressive. This may seem so on two counts: an older child may still be in the anal sadistic phase of development, and the manifest aggression be phase specific. Nagera (1965) speaks of the need of distinguishing this "from aggressive behavior of a more organized type of response which is phase independent." It is this latter type of aggression that the blind child inhibits. Again, the child's aggressivitiy toward his peers may seem quite marked until it is realized that a chronologically older child may be acting as a toddler, and may not have achieved the ability to experience empathy for the feelings of peers. The foregoing comments leave much unsaid, and are only intended to stress the need for continual ongoing concern with developmental issues whenever evaluation or treatment of blind children is being undertaken.

Treatment Process

When starting treatment with a blind child, the prerequisites are the same as for a sighted case: namely, a diagnosis (however provisional), stated aims, and a treatment plan, with the recognition that these can be revised, modified, or expanded, and are to be subject to periodic review. The therapist can be thought of as the provider of a space in which the patient can become safe enough and free enough to share his problems, with freedom to utilize almost any means he chooses for communication, providing it is not destructive to person or property. The task of the therapist is generally understood as being to further the uncovering process, to assist in the verbalization of feelings, thoughts, and fantasies, so that interpretation of defenses, wishes, and fantasies will allow unconscious instigators of behavior to enter consciousness, and thereby become more amenable to control by the conscious ego. Treatment of a blind child, as of any ego-defective child, calls for modification of the technique followed in the case of children who are reacting to early developmental interferences or presenting with an infantile neurosis. Omwake (1961) gives a vivid picture of the meaning of treatment for a 3½-year-old blind child: it became "an avenue for the child to leave her shut in an infantile world in order to unfold her very considerable capacities that had been hidden under a cover of autistic retardation." With such a child, the therapist's first task has to be a slow, painstaking building up of a relationship in which the child can feel safe enough to tolerate temporary separation from the primary libidinal object; this endeavor may take many weeks, much patience and ingenuity. However, the therapist has to be prepared for a curious turn that events may take as a relationship forms, for as with sighted autistic children, the first sign of a meaningful relationship to the therapist may be in the form of aggressive attacks. Omwake notes that for these children "aggression, whether libidinized or not, is often the first permissible or useful instinctual tie to the object outside of themselves."

As the young patient, in whatever time it takes, begins to accept the invitation to play, even greater demands will be made on the therapist's ingenuity, imagination, and acceptance of personal fallibility. A way has to be found to enter the child's world, to decode the fragmentary, chaotic, and seemingly nonsensical verbalizations that may accompany equally baffling body movements and gestures, as the blind child struggles to translate into action, to dramatize, and to share vignettes of his experience. The blind child's experiences are not framed within a visually informed context, but lack the continuity and organization afforded by vision. These discreet experiences are expressed in the form of attenuated, isolated fragments that have to be recognized for what they are and given meaningful connections by the therapist. Omwake noted further that the chaotic, repetitive, regressed play and verbalizations may represent memory traces which erupt without being organized by the ego. These children often have a good memory, in a limited sense. They store discreet pieces of information for years, but not in a flexible, adaptive way that is of service to the ego in problem-solving. From the foregoing, it can be seen that for some time the focus of the treatment will be centered on ego function.

An ego function of particular importance is that of language. The ability to descriptively associate the coarseness of elephant's hide to a rough-textured breakfast cereal suggests than an experiential language is being built up that can serve for a meaningful communication between sighted and nonsighted. The therapist working with a blind child becomes accustomed to accepting the child's "as is" use of sighted language, to working with the child's distortion of sighted concepts, and however slowly, to helping the child to a more meaningful metaphor. Much tact has to be exercised in challenging the child's use of sighted concepts, for not only are blind children shamed by their imperfect grasp of sighted concepts, they are also at times frustrated by the sighted person's inability to serve as full enlightener. An inescapable poignancy for a sighted therapist is the reality of a no man's land located between the boundaries of two distinct modes of perceiving and experiencing. The therapist of necessity spends more time clarifying and educating than is appropriate generally in working with sighted children. Young blind children may come into treatment talking in garbled, nonsensical seeming sentences or phrases. In decoding these garbled communications, the therapist reocgnizes the unusual uses to which blind children put language. The sighted child's easily evoked visual memories are substituted for by auditory memories which may be verbalized out of context and unassociated to by the child. Moreover, verbalization seems to serve to replace in auditory form the constant visual input of the sighted, to substitute for eye contact with the caretaking adult, and maybe to keep active an inner auditory built mental representation of libidinal objects. This writer recalls one small girl who in treatment hours kept up a constant singsong of "cup saucer, spoon fork, fish dish." Before proceeding to the work of decoding and eventual interpretation, the therapist had to be willing to join in this singsong, which then took the quality of an alternating two-voice litany. Only in very gradual steps could the progress be made via this litany to the kitchen at home, the mother who worked there, and the near panic experienced by the child at times when away from mother, an overwhelming fear of never being able to find mother again. Thus the therapist becomes attuned to the idiosyncratic language of the blind child and in interpretating phrases interpretations in language that makes use of as many nonvisual concepts as possible.

The therapist will need to help the child sort out many confusions about external reality, and this has to be achieved before instinctual matters, fantasies, and conflicts can occupy the stage. In illustration of this, reference can be made to the phobias of blind children; as Nagera (1965) points out, many blind children are afraid of animals at an age when in sighted children we expect to find that the phobic animal represents the oedipal rival. In the blind child, the fear of animals may serve an appropriate, adaptive aspect in terms of self-preservation; for a blind child can hardly tell by the sound of a dog's bark the size of the dog, its behavior, whether playful or aggressive, whether or not it seems likely to advance and bite. Until the ego has learned to cope more adaptively with external reality, psychic energy has to be drained off for purposes of dealing with the immediate environment. Nagera (1965) finds that this need to master the external dangers may so occupy the child that it "outweighs the importance of the internal dangers, represented by the impulses and other drive representatives." As against the threats of the outside world, "the inner world is a source of safety and gratification to the blind child." Nevertheless, the fantasy life of these children lacks the richness of the sighted child. This may reflect the low level of ego development achieved, but furthermore, the blind child cannot afford the luxury of retreat into fantasy, he has to maintain constant vigilance against the unseen but omnipresent discomforts that may be experienced at any moment from his surroundings. Added to this, the need for fantasy may be diminished by the amount of direct drive satisfaction indulged in by these children.

Reaction to the growing awareness of blindness and the painful experience of working through feelings of longing, anger, jealousy, helplessness, and hopelessness are an inescapable poignancy in the treatment of blind children. It may be that this crucial matter is not spontaneously brought by the child, but has to be introduced by the therapist. It is seldom a very open topic in the home, and although much may have been overheard from adult conversations, it remains for the child a closed topic in the same sense that sex, death, and other adult matters may. As one 7-year-old remarked to her therapist, "But I wouldn't want to mention that to parents, it's not the thing to do." Burlingham (1961) draws the parallel between "the effect sexual enlightenment normally has on children in freeing their curiosity and intelligence from inhibitions," and how for blind children, "once they are allowed to talk about their blindness, the way to the exploration of other secrets seems to be opened up for them." Considerable linking will be found in the child's conception of sight and sex; both tend to become recognized as attributes and advantages of the adult world. Blind children commonly think of getting sight when they grow up, the permanence of blindness, its continuing reality has to be grappled with not once but many times. On each new developmental level understanding of blindness is added to, gains new significances and evokes the old feelings of envy, anger, and despair which have to be reworked.

Psychological testing was not discussed earlier because the young child in need of therapy is so often not yet testable; this can be done later when planning for the child's integration into a formal school setting is initiated. Although parents should be actively involved in negotiating the entry into school, in most cases it will be necessary for the therapist to be available for consultation with the teaching staff. It is highly desirable that therapy not be stopped simultaneously with a major change in daily routine, such as entry into school or changes from one school to another.

In discussing the treatment of young blind children, the focus has been on the congenitally blind. In conclusion, a few comments should be added to include the adventitiously blinded. When a useful degree of sight has been experienced, even if only for the first 18 months, the earliest ego organization has been given a valuable start denied the congenitally blind. Despite the trauma, shock, and confusion caused by the loss of vision, the advantages of an early opportunity for ego organization on a visual level remain a significant factor in later development.

An area of future usefulness can be anticipated, namely, postoperative psychotherapeutic intervention with congentially blind children who by means of surgery have sight restoration. Segal and Stone (1961) describe the psychic problems encountered in the case of a 6-year-old girl who had successful surgery for bilateral cataracts. Valvo (1971), writing mainly in reference to adults, points to the need for these patients to "be followed from a dual point of view: psychotherapeutic to cope with the depression they show frequently; and didactic to help them with adequate visual exercises."

Summary

Treatment of blind children has been discussed from the limited standpoint of the young congenitally blind child who has not achieved adaptive ego functioning and may present with the appearance of autism or retardation. It has been suggested that the treatment modality of choice is a psychoanalytically oriented therapy, modified with the introduction of such parameters as are called for in accordance with the severity of the disturbance. In the early months, the process may have to be largely of a reeducative nature, only later progressing more nearly to psychotherapy. By concentrating on the problems of the young blind child, who will almost always present with severe ego deficits, it is not meant to imply that this is the only pathology to be encountered in blind children. Some children who are seen later may have achieved a useful degree of ego organization and may seem to have problems of a more neurotic nature. Even so, the therapist can expect to find the fact of blindess entering into every aspect of the case, and having to be worked with on all levels, in all structures. It has been shown that, although ideally, blind infants and their parents should be worked with preventively. Nevertheless, when needed, considerable help can often be given during late childhood. Evaluation of blind children may raise difficult questions of differential diagnoses in regard to autism, psychosis, retardation, and CNS involvement. It is often necessary to have a trial period of treatment, but this should not be restricted to a few weeks, since these children need time.

The therapist working with blind children has to come to terms with the fact that the space in which therapist and child communicate represents a no man's land, it belongs to neither side: for one side cannot really know the meaning of sight, and the other side has only limited knowledge of blindness.

References

Bennett, M.E. (1973) A study in a case of congenital anophthalmia. *Am. J. Psychother.* 27: 529–538.

Blank, H.R. (1957) Psychoanalysis and blindness. *Psychoanal. Quart.* 26: 1–24.

Burlingham, D.T. (1941) Psychic problems of the blind. *Am. Imago* 2: 43–85.

Burlingham, D.T. (1961) Some notes on the development of the blind. *Psychoanal. Study Child* 16: 123–145.

Burlingham, D.T. (1965) Some problems of ego development in blind children. *Psychoanal. Study Child* 20: 194–208.

Burlingham, D.T., and A. Goldberger. (1968) The reeducation of a retarded blind child. *Psychoanal. Study Child* 23: 369–390.

Fraiberg, S. (1968) Parallel and divergent patterns in blind and sighted infants. *Psychoanal. Study Child* 23: 264–300.

Fraiberg, S. (1971a) Interventions in infancy: a program for blind infants. *Am. Acad. Child Psychiat.* 10: 381–405.

Fraiberg, S. (1971b) Separation crisis in two blind children. *Psychoanal. Study Child* 26: 355–371.

Fraiberg, S. (1971c) Smiling and stranger reaction in blind infants. In J. Hellmuth, ed., *Exceptional Infant*, Vol. 2. New York: Brunner/Mazel, pp. 110–127.

Fraiberg, S. (1975) The development of human attachments in infants blind from birth. *Merrill Palmer Quart.* 21:315–334.

Fraiberg, S., and L. Fraiberg. (1977) *Insights from the Blind.* New York: Basic Books.

Fraiberg, S., and D. Freedman. (1964) Studies in the ego development of the congenitally blind child. *Psychoanal. Study Child* 19: 113–169.

Fraiberg, S., B. Siegel, and R. Gibson. (1966) The role of sound in the search behavior of two blind children. *Psychoanal. Study Child* 21: 327–357.

Keeler, W.R. (1958) Autistic patterns and defective communication in blind children with retrolental fibroplasia. In P. Hock and J. Zubin, eds., *Psychopathology of Communication.* New York: Grune & Stratton, pp. 64–83.

Kessler, J.W. (1966) *Psychopathology of Childhood.* Englewood Cliffs, N.J.: Prentice-Hall.

Klein, G.S. (1962) Blindness and isolation. *Psychoanal. Study Child* 17: 82–93.

Lopez, T. (1974) Psychotherapeutic assistance to a blind boy with limited intelligence. *Psychoanal. Study Child* 29: 277–300.

Martin, J.A., and D.M. Iagulli. Elimination of middle of the night tantrums in a blind retarded child. *Behav. Ther.* 5: 420–422.

Nagera, H., and A.B. Colonna. (1965) Aspects of the contribution of sight to ego and drive development. *Psychoanal. Study Child* 20: 267–287.

Norris, M., P. Spaulding, and F. Brodie. (1957) *Blindness in Children.* Chicago: University of Chicago Press.

Omwake, E.B., and A.J. Solnit. (1961) It isn't fair: the treatment of a blind child. *Psychoanal. Study Child* 16:352–404.

Parmelee, A.H., C. Fiske, and R. Wright. (1959) The development of ten children with blindness as a result of retrolental fibroplasia. *A.M.A. J. Child Dis.* 96:198–200.

Sandler, A.M. (1963) Aspects of passivity and ego development in the blind infant. *Psychoanal. Study Child* 18:343–360.

Segal, A., and F.H. Stone. (1961) The six-year-old who began to see: Emotional sequelae of operation for congenital bi-lateral cataract. *Psychoanal. Study Child* 15:481–509.

Thompson, S.H. (1974) Insight for the sightless: A TA group for the blind. *Transactional Anal.* 4:13–17.

Valvo, A. (1971) Sight restoration after long-term blindness: The problems and behavior patterns of visual rehabilitation. New York: American Foundation for the Blind.

Wills, D.M. (1965) Some observation on the blind nursery school children's understanding of their world. *Psychoanal. Study Child* 20:344–364.

Wills, D.M. (1970) Vulnerable periods in the early development of blind children. *Psychoanal. Study Child* 25: 461–480.

Treatment of Emotional Disorders in Children and Adolescents

CHAPTER 40

Therapeutic and Preventive Interventions with Deaf Children

Moisy Shopper

Since the hearing, speech, and language problems in the deaf pose overwhelming and far-reaching problems for communication and education, the consideration of the emotional problems of the deaf child is often viewed as an expendable luxury. The two readily identifiable deficits, the lack of hearing and the inability to communicate by spoken language, are so basic and crucial to social intercourse and learning that energetic therapeutic efforts directed at correcting these deficits are self-evident. Audiometric testing, the fitting of sophisticated hearing aids for the augmentation of residual hearing, and their utilization for the teaching of oral speech has been a major mode of approach in deaf education. Teaching a profoundly deaf child to communicate via spoken language when the deaf child has never heard spoken language is indeed a huge undertaking both practically and conceptually. There are those (oralists) who believe the deaf child must learn to make his way in a predominantly hearing speaking world. As a result, a vigorous program of training in speech reading (lip reading) and spoken communication is initiated as early as possible. The emotional problems of the deaf, and the emotional factors inherent in the teaching/learning situation, are often given cursory mention if at all in the training of deaf educators. Those problems recognized as emotional are assumed to be the *result* of the sensory and communicative deficiencies (Freeman, Malkin, and Hastings, 1975), a theoretical position that then increases the zealousness of the therapeutic educational efforts.

The neglect of emotional problems by deaf educators is matched by an equally pervasive neglect of the deaf by those with knowledge of emotional difficulties. Since so much of psychiatric investigation and therapy hinges on the ability to communicate through spoken language, the deaf have not been seen as easy subjects for either therapy or research. Oral language of the deaf is not only difficult to listen to because of voice quality but also hard to understand. A psychiatrist's interpretive comments tend to be presented succinctly and must be understood with exactitude. The *gist* of the meaning, for which the average speech reader settles, is too imprecise to have therapeutic effectiveness. Even with hearing patients, misunderstandings and distortions are common. A hearing child will often attempt to shout down a therapist's remarks or will place his hands over his ears. The deaf child's negative response is exceeding effective; he simply closes his eyes or reguses to look at the therapist. Many techniques of therapy used with hearing patients are not directly transposable to the deaf child or deaf adults.* However, the pioneer

* Neto, quoted by Levin (1977), presents the "psychoanalysis of a deaf-mute" which necessitated many changes in what is often considered classical technique, changes which lead Levin to consider it more "psychoanalytically oriented psychotherapy."

work of Rainer and Altschuler (1966), who worked psychiatrically with hospitalized as well as outpatient deaf adults is a striking exception to this neglect. For the psychiatrist to learn a second language (finger spelling and/or manual communication) is very arduous and not undertaken lightly. Facility in manual communication to the degree that one can be effective therapeutically takes several years of dedicated and committed effort (Levin, 1977, personal communication). There is sufficient ethnocentricity and egocentricity in the average psychiatrist for him to make the seemingly reasonable demand of the deaf patient that communication take place in the therapist's primary language rather than in the patient's, although under unusual circumstances (the flight of European analysts in the 1930's to the United States) the psychiatrist adopted the patient's mother tongue. Despite these difficulties there is a growing interest in the developmental and emotional problems of the deaf. Friedman, Cannady, and Robinson (1971) conducted longitudinal studies with congenitally deaf girls on the development of psychic structures; Schlesinger and Meadow (1972) applied psychoanalytic concepts (Erikson's epigenetic table) to the developmental stages of the deaf children; Galenson et al. (1977) have established a therapeutic nursery within the Lexington School for the Deaf in New York.

Synchronous with the emotional problems of the deaf child are the emotional stresses on the parents, siblings, and total family equilibrium. These may be somewhat diminished by placing the child in residence, but for those families with a deaf child at home, the effects are those of cumulative trauma. Unfortunately the recognition of these emotional problems and the therapeutic efforts directed to family members is minimal (Shopper, 1976).

While there is a tendency to consider deaf children as a single homogeneous group, varying only in the profoundness of their deafness, it is important to differentiate at least two groups: the deaf child of deaf parents and the deaf child of hearing parents. Each can be further subdivided by the presence or absence of deaf siblings. The hearing child of deaf parents also has certain problems, reviewed and studied by Arlow (1976) and Bene (1977). The deaf child of hearing parents may be at a somewhat greater disadvantage than the deaf child with deaf parents. In the latter, the diagnosis of deafness may be made much easier, since parental anxiety about the genetic transmission of the deafness is usually high despite the fact that only about 10% of the children of deaf parents are born deaf. Some deaf parents prefer a deaf child, whereas others consider it a major disaster. Nevertheless, the deaf parent compared to the hearing parent is not as shocked nor as unfamiliar with deafness. At the same time, they have a greater facility and acceptance of nonverbal and manual modes of communication. With many hearing parents, the diagnosis of the child's deafness is frequently delayed until there is significant delay of speech, which to many pediatricians is the "objective" evidence needed to justify testing. In other instances it is not the pediatrician but the parents who have significantly delayed the diagnosis. Since despite their many astute observations, they never took the final step to conclude that their child was indeed deaf. For some, deafness is preferred to what they had fantasied or been told (autism, mental retardation), since deafness offers the possibility of remediation and rehabilitation. These possibilities are construed by some parents and even some professionals as implying that the deafness can be "cured." The reliance on speech reading and oral communication as *exclusive* educational techniques which will then enable the deaf child to "function in the hearing/speaking world" often coincides with *unconscious* motives to deny and "undo" the deafness. The promise of early parental and professional intervention, the use of sophisticated hearing aids and oralism, if overly optimistically presented, impede the gradual acceptance and integration of the child's life-long deafness (Vernon, 1973). What is needed is a process, much akin to mourning, of parental working through—a working through supported by a tactful confrontation with the realities of deafness. Seldom told to parents is the fact that on the average 30% of deaf children leaving deaf schools at age 16+ are functionally illiterate, 60% leave having achieved no higher that fifth grade, and only 50% attain tenth-grade level (McClure, 1966).

Once deafness is diagnosed and the child labeled as "defective," it is not uncommon for parents to become significantly saddened and to mourn for the lost idealized (i.e., hearing) child (Solnit and Stark, 1961). The mother's reaction of intense rage, guilt, disappointment, and inadequacy culminate in frequent withdrawal, rejection and anger toward the child. During this period, the mother's capacity to relate effectively and empathically to her child are markedly impaired—a crucial disruption of the mother/child relationship. Fathers often use typical rationalization to distance themselves from the child and/or blatantly deny the deficit.

It is difficult to estimate the degree of impaired

mother/child relationship that exists as a result of the deaf child's sensory deficit. However, it is known that audition is a well-developed sensory modality in infancy that is *only later* surpassed by the visual modalities (Shopper, 1978; Wolff, 1963; Fraiberg, 1969). Nevertheless, there are many occasions when the auditory modality is superior—namely, at times of darkness and at times when distance and room arrangement does not allow for visual contact. Further, the impediments to spoken communication lead readily to a sense of mutual isolation, a situation that can all too easily eventuate in even further rejection of the child. Many authors (Altschuler, 1974; Lesser and Easser, 1972; Rothstein, 1975; Rainer, 1976; Galenson et al., 1977) consider it highly probable that the many educational and emotional handicaps of the deaf adolescent and adult are the result not only of the specific communicative difficulties but also of a disturbed mother/child interaction.

In short, the parents suffer a loss of confidence and ability in their capacity to nurture and rear their child. The assistance of the pediatrician in these instances could be extremely helpful (Solnit and Stark, 1961), were not the parents' prior experiences often unsatisfactory. Many parents bring the pediatrician observations suggestive of the infant's auditory deficit and are told that they are overly anxious (neurotic) about their child or that the infant is too young to be meaningfully tested. When the diagnosis of deafness is finally confirmed, the parents' observations are validated, but the pediatrician as a source of parental support for advice in the rearing of a deaf child is severely undermined.

A third of the parents consulting a physician for suspected deafness of the child were told nothing was wrong. Sixty percent consulted four or more physicians before receiving a definite accurate diagnosis (Meadow, 1968). My own experience in reviewing the experiences of a small group of deaf clients of a social agency is similar. Unfortunately, too few pediatricians are sufficiently knowledgeable concerning the diagnosis of deafness, much less the problems and psychological issues in rearing a deaf child. In fact, the American Academy of Pediatrics position paper, while highlighting the physician's responsibility in management, suggests referring parents for information to organizations representing only one side of oral communication/total communication choice and even fails to mention the existence of a controversy. Even among those physicians whose training and experience enable them to diagnosis deafness, there is often inadequate training in helping and counseling the parents (Fellendorf and Harrow, 1970).

Involvement in an infant/parent program provides many opportunities for support and benefit. The parent meets other parents whose children are also deaf and spontaneously, or with staff encouragement and structure, form an informal support group. Parents are relieved that there is an institution and/or professionals whose expertise will help them and their child. The program, exercises, and training will serve to build a sense of hopefulness and eventual mastery. However, not all intended support by staff is experienced as support by the recipients. For example, when the parent/infant program prescribes particular activities as "homework," the mother's sense of inadequacy is confirmed: her intrinsic "maternal instinct" and intelligence is inadequate to rear this child. Instead of doing what seems natural and what other parents do with their children, she must rely on the expertise of highly trained professionals, and to that degree there is an abrogation of parental function and a diminution of parental confidence. When the child relates better to staff and to the program, the mother may not necessarily be overjoyed but perceive it as a verification of her own inadequacy and ineptness. These feelings may be further exacerbated by the staff's natural motivation to be successful with the child and to demonstrate the superiority of their training and abilities, almost as if they are competitive with the parent.

Many professionals in deaf education often advise that the child be in residence in an institution for deaf education. The rationale is that the child will be taught around the clock by trained staff as well as having the advantages of peer relationships with other deaf and hard-of-hearing children. Some parents are convinced, and readily relinquish custody of their children to the institution. Despite sadness, they feel confident that this is right and beneficial for their child. Institutionalization may also coincide with the parents' wishes to be free of the burden of rearing a "defective" child, as well as tapping any unconscious feelings of rejection and riddance. For families living outside those metropolitan centers with special facilities for deaf education or whose special school districts have a meager or no program for the deaf, institutionalization may represent the only choice. While many families do move to a community where excellent deaf education is available, this option is not available to many other families.

Obvious in the institutionalized child, it is nonetheless equally true of the home-based deaf child, parental confidence, responsibility, and nurturance diminish with the concomitant increase in the educator's input and influence. Although not intended as such, the school* and staff become a parent surrogate, one which rivals and at times supplants the actual parents. It is for this reason that *any consideration of the emotional life of the deaf child must encompass a thorough study of the nature and experiences of the deaf child's educational program*. Programs for the deaf have to be assessed from the vantage point of prevention of emotional problems, and whether specific educational techniques exert a psychologically beneficial or adverse influence. Furthermore, the realization that the deaf education program is in fact a parental surrogate, and as such also a parental model, helps to explain the marked distortions and deviance when the deaf child, now an adult, attempts to parent his/her own children.

In some instances, the decision to institutionalize may mean a concomitant commitment to a particular form of deaf education—i.e., oralism, manualism, total communication. Some institutions are totally committed to the oral approach, while many schools are committed to total communication. If one has to rely on the nearest or least expensive school, the parent, although dissatisfied with the type of education, may have no educational alternatives. When parents contemplate the educational choices available to them, they are confronted more by intense polemics and prejudices than by facts concerning the advantages and disadvantages of the oral method and the manual/total methods. To simplify, the oralists argue that the deaf child has to live in the world of the hearing and frequently add the philosophical concept that it is speech alone which separates man from animal. The manual/total schools argue that a profoundly deaf person cannot rely on speech reading for adequate communication and must have the language of signs and finger spelling as a first language in order to learn spoken and written language and to communicate with deaf peers.

In Missouri, parents contemplating schools are confronted with a well-defined oral school of prestigious proportions, or the publicly supported special school where total communication and manual skills are taught but only after the fifth grade—i.e., to the failures of the oral program. Accordingly, anyone in the total communication program has already been labeled a failure, thus confirming the popularly held stereotype that to use "dumb talk" (signs) is indeed dumb and stupid.

There has always been a push toward mainstreaming deaf children—i.e., the placement of a deaf child in ordinary hearing classrooms. For many deaf youngsters, and parents alike, mainstreaming is thought of as a panacea and/or the criteria for success—"success" defined in terms of the adequacy of oral education or in the ability now to become integrated into the "hearing world." For both the deaf youngster and his parents, mainstreaming may also carry the meaning that the deafness has now been "cured"—i.e., the deaf child is now like everyone else. The "invisibility" of the auditory handicap makes the denial of the deafness a much greater and more frequently used mechanism than, for example, in blindness or an orthopedic handicap. In October 1975, Public Law 94-142, the Education of all Handicapped Children Act, was passed mandating that local school districts prepare individualized educational programs for all of their handicapped children, that the handicapped be educated under the "least restrictive environment," and that they are to be integrated or mainstreamed wherever possible. While the rationale of this act is laudable and serves to correct practices of gross discriminatory isolation and exclusion, there may be serious problems with mainstreaming.

The education of a deaf child is a sufficiently exacting and specialized task as to require a great deal of special training. Nevertheless, it is expected that the ordinary classroom teacher will become knowledgeable enough to act in an appropriate educational manner for the deaf child. Not only is it questionable that a teacher will develop this expertise for the one or two children that may be in her classroom in a particular year, but it is questionable whether the motivation or the flexibility exists to change even obvious aspects of his or her teaching style. For example, speaking while facing the blackboard or the occurrence of classroom discussions with participants either to the side of our behind the deaf student only bewilder and further isolate the deaf student. The willing and ready acceptance of a mainstreamed deaf child may conceal the staff's denial and/or ignorance of the problem and of the adjustments that have to be made for the deaf child.

Few hearing individuals recognize that even under the best of circumstances and with the best of lip readers, the deaf student can catch only 15% to 20% of that which is spoken. Two-thirds of the 42

* With prolonged contact, transference to an institution (as opposed to an individual) is a common occurrence (Reider, 1953).

sounds in the English language are either invisible or look like other sounds on the lips. Vowels, the most important sounds, are the most difficult to "read." The visible sounds must be grasped in the fleeting instant of their production (Hardy, 1970). Is 15–20% sufficient for learning new material? Does the mainstreamed child need the emotional support of other deaf students, or will he find himself mainstreamed into a position of increased isolation? Speech readers tend to convey the impression that they have understood everything rather than suffer the narcissistic humiliation of acknowledging their deficit and handicap.* If some children are trained in manual forms, are there sufficient numbers of sign language tutors and interpreters, who will be present in the classroom to help deaf youngsters (Greenberg and Dolittle, 1977)?

Whether some of the problems will be overcome by mainstreaming the child from the very beginning of his educational career is yet to be ascertained. For a youngster who has been in a deaf education institution of whatever persuasion, in residence or living at home, the transition to a hearing classroom has to be extremely traumatic. Not only must regular staff and hearing children be prepared, but there must be an ample and available supply of resource people. However, for the mainstreamed child there is not only the usual stress of changed classrooms, changed schools, changed friendships, but the child is also under marked pressure to adapt successfully to a setting that is either a hostile, a ridiculing, or at best an uncaring environment. Several deaf educators interviewed by Greenberg and Dolittle anticipate that only 10% or 15% will be successfully mainstreamed. Again, the parents are faced with a crucial decision in their deaf child's life, a decision for which they do not have the technical expertise, and so must rely on the advice of the experts, if only they would agree (Reichstein, 1976). Thus aspects of parental functioning are surrendered to the experts, but as more professional controversy enters the public domain, the omnipotence of the expert is diminished, the omniscience doubted.

The ordinary guidelines and standards of expected behavior by which parents measure the growth and development of their children are absent for the parents of the deaf child. The Gesell standards, Dr. Spock's advice, as well as other developmental guidelines, are not adequately standardized for the deaf population. This is compounded by the difficulties in relying on the standard batteries of psychological and achievement tests, since adequately trained testers are scarce, especially in mainstreamed schools, and tests are not standardized for the deaf (Levine, 1974). Even when parents compare their deaf child with other deaf children, the problem is not a simple one. The deaf child population is a heterogeneous one, there being different types of deafness, different degrees of residual hearing, and wide differences in the educational approaches. The parent has to endure a high degree of uncertainty as to whether his child is at full potential educationally, socially, or psychologically.

*A beautiful but sad example is Carson McCuller's *The Heart is a Lonely Hunter.*

Oral-Manual Controversy

If one accepts the principle that a therapeutic program should be initiated as soon as the diagnosis of deafness is confirmed, the choice of such a therapeutic program is then of crucial importance. While I do not wish to engage further in the polemics regarding oral-manual education and thus antagonize a significant portion of the special education/deaf community, as a child psychiatrist and psychoanalyst, I feel I must state my viewpoint, prejudice,* and the reasons therefore. Furth (1973) has put the matter succinctly. "This [oral-manual] controversy, which is as old as deaf education, colors all educational considerations; any major decision or change concerning educational practices implies some stand. It is much more than a difference in teaching methods; it touches the very core of deaf people's existence. Indeed, in its extreme form, oralism in nothing less than the denial of deafness" (p. 34). Nevertheless, many schools are committed to the oral approach and frequently begin speech reading (lip reading) even in their preschool program. There is the implicit assumption that speech reading improves with training and that such training should start early; however,

*I should add that I have no personal or familial experience with deafness and that my interest stems from my study of audition in normal early development and from the chance contacts of clinical psychoanalysis (one patient with a deaf parent; another with a deaf child). I do have a prejudice resulting from personal experience with bilingualism (English as a second language), which leaves me somewhat in favor of total communication, although the two issues are only very roughly analogous. However, Charrow and Fletcher (1974) discuss English as a second language of the deaf child.

research does not confirm this assumption. Nevertheless, many parents are advised to take the Tracey Clinic Correspondence Course in speech reading sessions with their preschoolers. Farwell (1976) believed that the intense commitment of deaf educators to speech reading often interferes with research in this area. Apparently, speech reading is a skill where we have yet to understand the factors involved in its success and failure.

Several shortcomings and deficiencies have been noted concerning speech reading. Proficiency at best may mean that only about 30% of what is spoken is understood by the deaf child. Deaf children cannot use speech reading to communicate with one another. There is considerable delay before the child's level of proficiency in speech reading leads to the establishment of meaningful communication with the parents. As a result, the parent-child relationship often has to flounder as best it can for many years without the benefits of intelligible communication.

As early as 1959, Sharoff makes a plea that mothers be allowed to communicate with deaf children by means of signs. He notes the work of Ruesch and Kees (1956), who when speaking about a hearing child state that "an impoverishment of communication and character development can be observed in those children who grow up in surroundings where the verbal was emphasized too early and when messages expressed in nonverbal terms were left unanswered."

This article is too brief to go into the various forms, advantages, and disadvantages of the various methods of manual communication. These may be found in the more specialized literature (Schlesinger and Namir, 1978). Among adults in the deaf community, signing is the preferred mode of communication, and it is the individual trained solely in oralism who once again feels isolated and excluded.

Signing is also the natural language of the peer group. Although many schools attempt to prohibit signing, some even punitively, the children use it surreptitiously and idiosyncratically. If we can extrapolate from ethology and normal child development, peer interactions are a crucial part of socialization and contribute to developing ego structures. Reliance solely on oralism hampers peer communication to a marked extent. To the extent that peer interaction can somewhat mitigate the adverse effects of sensory deprivation and absent mother/infant relationship (Suomi, Collins, and Harlow, 1973), the obstacles to peer interaction and the impairment of peer relationships are of greater significance to the deaf child than to the hearing child. It is bad enough that many deaf children have difficulties in engaging in the play and games of hearing children (so many games depend on the speech and/or audition), but for deaf preschoolers to be only minimally able to communicate with one another is a sizable and significant disadvantage of oral education and one often ignored by its proponents.

Special Problems in Deaf Development

It is difficult to impossible for the average hearing adult to imagine the condition of the infant deaf at birth. Not only is the child experiencing partial sensory deprivation but misses out on the many verbal interactions with the mother that signal, calm, soothe, stimulate, or simply inform the child of the parental presence. Rainer (1976) states that "we can only conjecture . . . how this trait [a shallow and undependable sense of object] relates to the lack of the very early anxiety reducing quality of mother's voice . . . , to the absence of the voice as an external object-defining stimulus in early weeks, or to the frightening inability to hear the mother singing, talking or announcing her presence when out of sight" (p. 122). Rainer is similar to others who can clearly perceive the issues raised but often offer conjecture instead of resolution. Unfortunately, psychiatric and psychoanalytic interest, research, and observation is embryonic. Accordingly, the problems and their treatment should be discussed and regarded as tentative and preliminary to more exacting investigation. While the need for certain therapeutic and/or preventive interventions are in many instances self-evident, I would like to emphasize the need for early, continuous, and intensive monitoring of the deaf child *as well as* the other family members (in my view this includes the deaf school) and the vicissitudes of family dynamics.

Parenting and Empathy

Rothstein (1975) regards the diagnosis of deafness as a pediatric emergency requiring therapeutic intervention as soon as possible. As a result, he has designed a therapeutic nursery for the deaf infant where infant and parent attend two to three 1½ hour nursery sessions/week and are observed by a staff member. Individual and group therapy are available as needed. The mothering abilities of the deaf mothers of the deaf infants were markedly different from those of the hearing mothers (Galenson et al., 1977). The deaf mothers did not or could not engage in reciprocal play, and precociously foster self-bottle feeding (by two or three months of age) with either child or bottle propped in the crib. When held by the deaf mother, the child is positioned so that he faces away from the mother. With solids, self-feeding is discouraged and the child is spoon-fed well into the second year. The mothers tend to be the unempathic, unpredictable, and overly harsh disciplinarians. When the child displays autonomous strivings and initiative, fights with the mother result in which the deaf child is the loser. These findings demonstrate the difficulties of deaf mothers in achieving a mutual, empathic, and nurturing relationship with the child. Further, when they do interact with the child, they seemed to have little regard for their child's bodily integrity, pleasure in self-mastery, and autonomous strivings.

Obvious determinants of this type of maternal behavior are the deaf mother's own experience with her own mother, as well as the distortions in personality development secondary to hearing loss and communication handicaps. In addition, I must add the pervasive influence of the deaf mother's surrogate parenting—namely, the deaf education institution. For reasons mentioned earlier, the educational institution and its multitude of professionals unknowingly but readily appropriate the parenting role and functions. Unfortunately, many schools are characterized by a lack of empathy with the child, endless intrusions into the child's budding autonomous self, and a disciplinary attitude that blurs the distinction between dedication and therapeutic fervor.*

The initiation of locomotion creates a crisis for the deaf child and his parents. In a sense the child has unequal ego development—i.e., motility is excellent, but impulse control, reality testing, cognitive understanding, etc., lag far behind. The usual "terribleness" of the "terrible two" toddler stage usually recedes as proficiency in language and verbalization (Katan, 1961) help establish a mutuality of understanding and a reduction of conflicts. With language, a parent can explain (dangerous, hot, or forbidden) and have a fair chance that the child will understand and gradually accept the parental restriction. With communication absent, the parent has to rely on actual physical interference with the child's activity—i.e., a marked impingement on the child's growing autonomy. The verbal hearing child can internalize parental restrictions, whereas the deaf child proceeds with less internalization and requires greater external controls. As a result, with the deaf child, disagreements over simple matters are the rule, and temper outbursts secondary to frustrations and misunderstandings abound. Obviously, the problem is more intense in the oral parent/child dyad than in the signing parent/child dyad. Harris (1978) measuring response time and number of errors on the Matching Figures Test, the time taken and score of the Draw-a-Person Test as indices of impulse control, found that the deaf children of deaf parents had greater impulse control than the deaf children of hearing parents. He attributed this difference to the early use of manual communication in the deaf parent group. Harris notes that it is the "reflective" child rather than the "impulsive" deaf child who tends to obtain higher achievement scores. It seems sensible to me that the hearing parents, possessing greater ego assets than the young child, should undertake the pain and difficulty of adjusting to the child's deafness, much in the same manner that the sighted parent needs to adjust to the tactile/auditory world of the blind child (Fraiberg and Freedman, 1964; Fraiberg, Siegel, and Gibson, 1966). The child's natural spontaneous gesturing forms the *anlage* for signing in much the same way that babbling is the *anlage* for learned oral speech.

* Schools and parents often do not appreciate fully the degree to which they attempt to control and coerce the child's body as an implicit but integral part of deaf education. The wearing of a hearing aid, the attentiveness to the teacher's lips (entailing gross motor *im*mobility), the positioning of lips, mouth and tongue in the production of specific sounds, plus the endless practice, drilling and repetition demanded by teachers and parent, are experienced by the deaf child as marked interferences in their autonomy. However, unlike the hearing child, the deaf child's negativism and autonomous strivings run counter to the educational task, and if pronounced, lead to educational retardation and failure. The combination of negativism, impaired communication between parent and child, and immature affect control produce unimaginable frustration and hardship for all—child, parent, and educator.

Psychopathology

The psychopathology of the deaf depends on a multiplicity of factors. To isolate one etiological factor—namely, the absence of oral speech and comprehension—and to regard it as the sole handicap is not only to simplify unduly but similarly to simplify and prejudice our educational endeavors and goals. We should not fail to consider: (a) the grief, mourning, and ultimate acceptance of the child's deafness by the parents; (b) the impairment of the mother-child interaction secondary to the absence of the mother as a perceptual auditory modality; (c) the absence of certain aspects of feedback from the child to the parent; (d) the mother's rejection and avoidance of the child for being deaf (Radford, 1973); (e) the mother's patience and tolerance and willingness to expend extra physical and emotional effort on the deaf child (Bloom, 1963); (f) the pervasive impact of early residential education and early education school-home efforts; (g) the nature of staff's attitude toward the child's disability and the emotional impact of the educational techniques used. Unfortunately, the adult deaf have been studied more thoroughly psychiatrically than deaf children and adolescents, the focus in the latter being on the educational tasks. It is as though only after the limits of education are considered reached, that the problems and personality difficulties of the deaf are subsumed under the heading of "emotional"/"psychiatric." Rainer (1976) characterized the deaf as "impulsive, immature, limited capacity for empathy, a tendency to express feelings in motor actions and relatively shallow object relationships, poor insight, especially into the consequences of their behavior." To these we should add their sense of isolation, loneliness, and underlying rage at being deaf (Levin, 1977). Interestingly, these qualities are often to be found in the *hearing* child of deaf adult parents. (Tendler, 1975, quoted by Arlow, 1976). Tendler notes that impulse controls and reality judgment are relatively poor in these hearing children, and that they tend to think in global and concrete ways—i.e., similar to their deaf parents. This is corroborated by Witkin (1965). There is a growing body of research differentiating deaf children into two groups depending on the hearing status of their parents. The deaf child of deaf parents is superior in psychosocial development (Stuckless and Birch, 1966) and more mature, responsible, social, and willing to attempt communication with strangers (Meadow, 1967) than the deaf child of hearing parents.

Affect Control

Temper outbursts, anger, and rage are frequent and troublesome symptoms in deaf children, since they have many more occasions to become angry and fewer ego resources with which to cope with these feelings. The hearing child can obey the parent's sharply stated "no" and "don't" and learn from an explanation of the prohibition and an offer of a future or substitute gratification. The prohibition is gradually internalized. In contrast, the deaf child brings less understanding to the situation, less internalization, a poorer mother-child interaction (Demark, 1966), and the parent must often control the deaf child bodily rather than verbally. To the degree that verbalization (Katan, 1961) augments control of affect, despite the best of oral schooling, the child's verbal abilities in the first 3 to 5 years are meager indeed.

One deaf adult whose siblings and parent I interviewed extensively, terrorized her family with her rage outbursts, a rage that contrasted sharply with her seemingly good nature, obedience, and adaptation at the school for the deaf and later when she was mainstreamed in high school. Whatever resentments were felt in the school situations could be controlled, but only to the extent of delaying (until home) and displacing (family members) rather than modification and integration of the rage.

A young man in late adolescence seen in psychotherapy avoided signing (in which he had been trained), sought out hearing friends only, and was enraged at himself and his parents for his deafness. He had gotten in some bar-room brawls, had physically assaulted his sister when he was living in her household, and used the threat of physical force to manipulate his parents to acceed to his wishes for money, car, etc.

Sibling Relations

The presence of a handicapped child in a family cannot help but upset the dynamic equilibrium in that family. It may markedly influence the planning and spacing of additional children. One family refused to chance another pregnancy fearing another deaf child; another family decided on another child shortly after the diagnosis of deafness was made, as though to "replace" the deaf child with a normal one; while another family devoted themselves selflessly to the tasks of raising a deaf child, only planning another when the deaf child was firmly established in school.

Even though subsequent hearing siblings may be considerably younger than the deaf child, it is not long before the hearing child surpasses the older deaf sibling educationally and psychologically. Accordingly, the younger hearing sibling both takes and is given more responsibility in the household and often has responsibility for the care and supervision of the older deaf sibling. For example, a three-year-younger latency hearing sibling in a peer play setting would explain games, directions and happenings to the older deaf sibling, as well as act as a translator of often unintelligible vocalizations, oral speech or sign language. A younger sister often "ran interference" for an older mainstreamed deaf sibling in high school, only to have her (necessary) interventions disparaged and resented by the older deaf sibling. On other occasions, the older deaf child would babysit for the younger hearing siblings, but one of the latter would remain awake in case the bell or phone rang. Such role reversal was understandably fostered by the parents, ambivalently enjoyed by the younger hearing siblings, and markedly resented by the older deaf sibling. In terms of day-to-day life, the rearing of the deaf sibling entails enormous effort, time, money, and hardship, often eclipsing the needs of other family members. Many of the hearing siblings erect strong reaction formations against their anger at the deaf sibling. In late adolescence, the reaction formation is manifest in frequently choosing a professional role in the education and training of the handicapped. One hearing sibling chose to become an educator of the mentally retarded rather than the deaf, "since even though I know a lot about deafness, I have too many memories of my sister to be able to work objectively."

Sleep Disturbance

Since vision is the only perceptional distance modality for the deaf, bedtime and its accompanying darkness (lights out) often exacerbates separation problems for the young deaf child. While the hearing child is capable of continued auditory contact with the parents despite darkness (Shopper, 1978), the deaf child is in a situation of almost total sensory isolation once put to bed with lights off. Children often overdress or utilize transitional objects (teddy bears, blankets) to afford themselves a "tactile presence" (Shopper, 1978) in their attempt to cope with their separation anxiety. Others attempt to enter the parental bed or if rebuffed often find a comfortable spot on the floor near the parental bed in the middle of the night.

These problems are markedly diminished in an institutional dormitory setting, where other children are close by and lights are dimmed but not out.

Adolescence

Adolescence is a difficult time for the average hearing child; many aspects of deafness accentuate certain problems or create special ones for the adolescent. Even with excellent educational progress, there are many areas where the adolescent requires the presence of a hearing person (often a family member) or an interpreter; the achievement of a sense of independence and competence is thus compromised. The support that adolescents provide for one another in their gradual break with their parents is difficult for the deaf adolescent, who if able to mainstream academically cannot do so socially. Instead, the deaf adolescent must recognize that he is a member of a minority community and one that is often devaluated, ridiculed, and misunderstood. The inability of the deaf adolescent to spend hours on the telephone, while a boon to parents, is a major handicap socially. Members of the deaf adolescent community may be scattered geographically, and are not readily accessible. One's deafness, deemed the significant difference for exclusion from the majority group, becomes hated, denied, and disavowed. The pursuit of social and sexual acceptance by the hearing is replete with frustration, envy, and rage. 85–95% of the deaf who marry, marry deaf; 25–43% never marry (von der Lieth, 1978).

The choice of a vocation presents special difficulties, since certain jobs are almost impossible for the deaf, while others require technical knowledge and/or higher education not easily obtainable for the average deaf adolescent. Not only are there long-range vocational problems, but even the more simple issue of finding a suitable after-school or summer job is especially difficult for the deaf. The absence of earned money, the view of oneself as unemployable, and the necessary but overdone continued involvement of the parents—all serve to impede the successful resolution of dependency/independency conflicts, and the formation of a healthy self-regard.

Sexual Problems

The deaf adolescents' need for sex education transcends instruction in psychological and anatomic processes. Not only do attitudes and values need to be conveyed but also all the social skills so necessary in all preliminary heterosexual encounters. A recent survey of the nation's residential centers for the deaf indicated that one out of three offered no sex education program, while 15% of those which did indicated that sex education was offered "as needed"—a euphemism for a crisis-oriented approach rather than a planned program (Fitz-Gerald and Fitz-Gerald, 1976). Deaf children at residential schools are exposed to various forms of sexual stimulation—autoerotic, pornographic, homosexual, and heterosexual. Many overt sexual activities among residents occur unbeknownst to school personnel. While the sexuality of the deaf is no different from that of the hearing adolescent, the deaf often lack the intellectual understanding of sexual matters, the reading skills for self-education, the social sophistication, and the psychological structures for the channeling and integration of their sexual impulses. For those using sign language, the signs for sexual functions markedly resemble obscene gestures, which makes "talking" about sex that much closer to doing sexual things, while the hearing person using the sign language of sex may experience a modicum of embarrassment. Parents and adminstrators, fearful of adolescent sexual activity, often use prohibition, avoidance, and surveillance rather than more effective measures such as education, sex-role modeling, and social role playing. Rainer, Altschuler, and Kallmann (1963) noted that sexual delinquency is found to a greater degree in the adult deaf population, while their clinical cases showed a 10% incidence of homosexual tendencies. Whether this is a result of residential living, psychosexual immaturity, or lack of heterosexual partners is not stated. The general impression is that the deaf have greater problems of sexual adjustment (Schlesinger and Meadow, 1972), but little specific research has been done in this sensitive and difficult area.

In any event, those factors leading the average parent to neglect the sex education of their normal children operate to an even greater degree in the deaf, while the needs of the deaf for the healthy management of their sexual life are far greater than those of the average hearing adolescent. Yet the courses are few, the topics taught are fragmentary and incomplete, and specially trained teachers are scarce.

Psychosis and Deafness

The issue of childhood psychosis is a complex one, even in the absence of deafness. When we attempt to examine the young deaf child, either clinically or with psychological tests, we would be tempted to consider many of the children psychotic, atypical, or borderline. However, as Youniss (1967) points out, the longer you work with a child to help him understand the requirements of the examination tests, the better the performance. The child appears to think less concretely, nonperservering, capable of logical thought, appropriate affectively, etc. If the examiner and/or child lacks sufficient ability to engage in effective communication (through whatever modality) the only data is the child's behavior and adults' reports. For most psychiatrists, such limited information combined with a major perceptual deficit that distorts the normal course and landmarks of child development would be regarded as insufficient for a confident diagnostic designation. Undoubtedly, many deaf children are operating at a behavioral psychotic level and are not labeled "psychotic." Rather they are regarded as "poorly educated" or as having "emotional problems in learning," the peculiar behavior then being secondary to the communication deficits. This may be best, since many educators would have difficulty with a child labeled as "psychotic" even though they could deal with identical behavior if conceptualized as the result of "language impairment." Of the many standard texts I consulted on deafness in children, only a workshop report (Sonnega, 1967) even mentioned psychosis in the deaf child. Sonnega has been unable to make a diagnosis of schizophrenia in the preschool period and has been unable to find anyone else who could make such a diagnosis. Even in the seemingly straightforward IQ testing, there is considerable debate whether the standard IQ tests even with their nonverbal performance portions are a valid indicator of a deaf child's IQ (Levine, 1974; Gerweck and Ysseldyke, 1975). The issue of psychosis is best summed up by Altschuler (1974): "Unfortunately, there is no psychiatric hospital in the country geared to study the special problems of deaf, disturbed children. As a consequence, comparable reports as to the prevalence and types of illness—let alone their prognoses—do not exist. . . ."

Perhaps the best criteria of a favorable therapeutic course is the capacity of the child to establish sustained and continuous contact with another person over time. In some of the "educational dumping grounds" where seemingly hopeless, angry, wild deaf children abound, no one has had the time, skill, or patience to make contact. Accordingly, an optimistic stance and an avoidance of rigid diagnostic categories should permeate therapeutic efforts lest adverse conjectures and premature diagnostic labels become self-fulfilling prophecies.

Treatment of the Deaf Child

The formulation of treatment plans for the deaf child is exceedingly complex, since we are dealing not only with a perceptual deficit and its concomitant impairment in communication and language, but also with a familial response to deafness, plus the variability in quality and quantity of resources from other disciplines (audiological, linguistic, educational, legal) existent in the local community. Notwithstanding the sharing of many crucial experiences, to overgeneralize and stereotype the deaf child is fraught with error, since there may be considerable variation in the degree of residual hearing, the age at which the deafness is diagnosed, the age of onset of hearing-aid use, the participation in parent/infant programs, choice of educational philosophy, etc. These, together with the uniqueness of the parents' resources and responses to the child and his deafness, interact to produce a wide range of behavioral and psychological differences. Public Law 94-142 will make more services available to the deaf child, but as with all well-meaning laws, the bureaucratic structure may prefer to package one or two treatment regimens and mold the child to fit. While the law clearly allows and encourages an individualized educational plan and one in which the parents provide input and subject to their approval, it is doubtful that time and energies of existent staff will allow such individualization; nevertheless, it is often best and necessary.

Vernon (1969) estimates that 10–12% of deaf children exhibit severe emotional and/or behavior problems, a figure five times the expected; this represents only the most obvious disorders, the visible tip of the iceberg. Psychological/psychiatric services must be included in formulating the total plan.

The treatment of the deaf child can best be viewed developmentally. Verbal and nonverbal communication of the average mother-child are drastically disrupted when the parent suspects deafness and later by the confirmation of the diagnosis. The need to restore such communication quickly has prompted many in deaf education to initiate parent/infant programs, enrollment being encouraged as soon as deafness is diagnosed. Infant/parent programs conceived solely by audiologists and speech pathologists emphasize language-oriented play activities, listening, early home practice with the Tracy Clinic curriculum, the preservation of babbling, and the reinforcement of verbalization attempts. While emphasizing the need for the child's early educational involvement, there has *not* been a concomitant increase in the exposure and training of teachers of the deaf in early childhood education. Northcott (1973) found that only 5 of 119 teachers instructing deaf infants reported an early childhood concentration. It is to be hoped this situation will be corrected.

To focus predominantly on language/communication skills ignores Greenstein's (1975) finding that language acquisition (ages 10 months to 40 months of age) is dependent *not* on methods or types of the mother's presentation of language, but on the *affective* interaction between mother and child. Accordingly, psychotherapeutic efforts should precede and/or be concomitant with a language program and be directed at removing the tension, anger, guilt, rejection, etc., that psychologically separate the mothers from their infants, (Stein, Merrill, and Dahlberg, 1974; Connor, 1976; Rothstein, 1975). This issue is discussed in greater detail by Solnit and Stark (1961). The reported linguistic superiority of deaf children of deaf parents (Vernon and Koh, 1970) may be attributed in part to the greater acceptance and empathy (even at times prenatally) by the deaf parents of their child's deafness, resulting in greater eye contact, object relatedness, and learning.

The customary staff of a parent/infant program has to be supplemented by clinically trained child psychologists and child psychiatrists who not only furnish direct services (diagnostic, evaluative, therapeutic) but also supervise teachers and educators and become part of the total therapeutic/research team (Connors, 1976).

The use of parent groups is helpful in reducing the sense of isolation, uniqueness, and ignorance in the parents as well as helpful in sharing experiences (problems/solutions) in child rearing. It also may provide a platform for the expression of feelings and thoughts that might not be understood or deemed acceptable by any but those in a parent's group led by a trained and noncritical professional.

Fathers are frequently spared or excluded from many areas of parent involvement and assistance. While the father's rejection of the deaf child may be just as strong as that of the mother, and in the long run just as detrimental, it is nevertheless easily concealed by seemingly realistic rationalizations. Some fathers devote their parenting time to the other children and consign the deaf child to the care and supervision of the mother not only for the home academic language exercises but for other areas of interaction as well. The immediate and long-term effect of an affective father loss has been well documented (Lamb, 1976). The absence of an involved and caring male is compounded by the fact that the professionals in deaf education are predominantly female, a situation poor for girl students but horrendous for the boy. When the resources for male gender identity formation and masculine identification are minimal, it becomes difficult for the deaf male child to learn from a female teacher or to submit to her discipline and care. Negativism and hostility often result. As a result, the tendency toward behavior and aggressive problems found even in hearing boys is exacerbated markedly for deaf males. This area can be improved in three ways:

1. Strenuous attempts to involve the father in the parenting of the deaf child, emphasizing the father's affective response to the child and his deafness. If simple education and exhortation are insufficient to secure father involvement, referral for treatment is necessary even though it may be perceived by the father as a trifling matter, one for which the father may have little or no motivation; it is nevertheless a crucial matter, particularly for the boy. Deaf male adolescents (8) seen at a family agency (Rosenthal, 1975) plus several from my own practice *all* showed severe problems in their self-image as males, an impaired sense of masculinity, and a disrupted to absent father/son relationship.

2. The involvement of more males in the field of deaf education, particularly at the preschool and primary grades. Since this hinges on many political factors within the field, not the least of which is money and prestige, this represents a long-term solution. A more immediate and short-term solution is the use of male high school and college students as aides in the classroom. Not only would father surrogate relationships be established, but many males might like the field and choose to obtain additional training.

3. The enrollment of the deaf in a sports program early on. While important for all deaf children, boys often find in sports some of the masculinity not otherwise available in the pure educational setting. Further, there is a tendency for parents to "generalize from the narrow range of tasks that (deaf) children actually cannot do, and assume there is a much larger spectrum of tasks of which he is incapable" (Meadow, 1976), an assumption which then becomes a self-fulfilling prophecy. To the extent that the parents' image of their child is as a defective, and that the child's growing awareness of his deafness will foster the establishment of a defective body image, it would be important to both child and parents to have a strong and realistic sense of bodily competence to compensate for the defect and to offset the child's own tendency to generalize his defect. There are many areas of noncompetitive and nonhearing-dependent sports (tumbling, gymnastics, swimming, diving, track and field, etc.) where the average deaf child can attain on par with the hearing child. An active sports program in a school for the deaf necessitates changes in the attitude and philosophy of the educators, so that they engage in "total education" rather than just language education. If schools are unable or unwilling to mount a physical activity program, the resources of the community should be utilized to their fullest.

Early Communication

As mentioned earlier in this paper, the establishment of effective communication between parents and child, and among the preschool peer group, is sufficiently crucial to be, in my mind, a determining factor in the early use of manual communication. While readily learned by the child, parents need to be counseled as to the importance of early and effective communication in order to secure their motivation for the learning of a "foreign" language (sign) at an advanced age. The learning task is especially difficult if manual communication is viewed as a devaluated language (a view often found among oralists) or as making visible (i.e., sign language) the "invisible defect." The visibility of signing is incompatible with the maintenance of deafness as an "invisible defect" and with the emotional denial of deafness and all that it implies. Fortunately, more public education, greater visibility of the deaf, more captioned TV programs, and the National Theatre of the Deaf are helping undo the stigmatization of the deaf and reducing the need to hide deafness in order to "pass" in the hearing world. The forms of manual languages, their linguistic and theoretical significance, and their use in deaf education are extensively reviewed by Bonvillian, Charrow, and Fletcher (1973) and Schlesinger and Namir (1978).

The psychiatric treatment of the deaf child has to be a multidisciplinary team effort, has to include the total family (Robinson and Weathers, 1974; Shapiro and Harris, 1976), and has to be undertaken by child psychiatrists who have taken the effort to become knowledgeable about deafness, even to the point of acquiring manual communication proficiency. Psychotherapy of the individual child must be combined with the awareness of all the other aspects of the child's milieu even more so than one is accustomed to do in child work. The child psychiatrist must have the skills to work with other disciplines in structuring and coordinating that milieu to therapeutic advantage. Basic communicative skills, taken for granted in the hearing child, have to be evaluated in depth and fully. For those children who use signs, the psychiatrist must also, or else secure a trained interpreter.* In using an interpreter, there is a clear tendency for the transference to be split between therapist and interpreter or to focus entirely on the interpreter, particularly if the interpreter signs at the same time the psychiatrist speaks. The patient no longer has eye contact (relatedness) to the therapist, but is watching the hands and face of the interpreter for the simultaneous translation. My preference is to speak briefly to the patient, then have my remarks signed and spoken by the interpreter, and then continue in short translatable phrases. The patient thus has his speech reading (of the therapist) augmented by sign (translator). The psychiatrist is also provided with an excellent opportunity to learn sign, which, when included in one's comments to the patient, go far toward increasing rapport. Concomitantly, one's difficulty and initial ineptitude in signing give the treating psychiatrist an empathic and experiential understanding of the deaf child's handicaps in communication.

When the patient has marked problems in learning *any* mode of communication, one is inclined to consider the patient a poor candidate for individual treatment. Yet it may be that emotional problems have interfered significantly in the learning of a mode of communication. Thus the focusing on the resolution of these emotional factors, even in the face of rudimentary communication skills, is often the only hope of improving these skills. In effect, psychotherapy is necessary to prepare the patient for psychotherapy, clearly a painstakingly slow process.

Group therapy has been utilized successfully with adult hospitalized deaf adults (Rainer and Altschuler, 1966), but it is doubtful whether this could be an effective treatment modality with latency age or even adolescent deaf. Schlesinger and Meadows (1972) devote an entire chapter to mental health services for the deaf but make no mention of group therapy.

* Many communities have a registry of certified interpreters for the deaf.

References

Altschuler, K.Z. (1974) The social and psychological development of the deaf child: Problems, their treatment and prevention. *Am. Ann. Deaf* 119:365–376.

Arlow, J. (1976) Communication and character: A clinical study of a man raised by deaf-mute parents. *Psychoanal. Study Child* 31:139–163.

Bene, A. (1977) The influence of deaf and dumb parents on a child's development. *Psychoanal. Study Child* 32:175–194.

Bloom, F. (1963) *Our Deaf Children.* London: Heinemann.

Bonvillion, J.D., V.R. Charrow, and K.E. Nelson. (1973) Psycholinguistic and educational implications of deafness. *Human Develop.* 16:321–345.

Charrow, V.R., and J.D. Fletcher. (1974) English as the second language of deaf children. *Develop. Psychol.* 10:463–470.

Connor, L.E. (1976) New directions in infant programs for the deaf. *Volta Review* 78:8–15.

Demark, J. (1966) Mental illness and early profound deafness. *Brit. J. Med. Psychol.* 39:117–124.

Farwell (1976) Speech reading: A research review. *Am. Ann. Deaf* 121:19–30.

Fellendorf, G.W., and I. Harrow. (1970) Parent counseling, 1961–1968. *Volta Review* 72:51–57.

Fitz-Gerald, D., and M. Fitz-Gerald. (1976) Sexual education, survey of residential facilities for the deaf. *Am. Ann. Deaf* 121:480–497.

Fraiberg, S. (1969) Libidinal object constancy and mental representation. *Psychoanal. Study Child* 24:9–47.

Fraiberg, S., and D.A. Freedman. (1964) Studies in the ego development of the congenitally blind child. *Psychoanal. Study Child* 19:113–157.

Fraiberg, S., B.L. Siegel, and R. Gibson. (1966) The role of sound in the search behavior of the blind infant. *Psychoanal. Study Child* 21:327–357.

Freeman, R.D., S. Malkin, and J.O. Hastings. (1975) Psychosocial problems of deaf children and their families: A comparative study. *Am. Ann. Deaf* 120:391–405.

Friedman, D.A., C. Cannady, and J.S. Robinson. (1971) Speech and psychic structures: A reconsideration of their relation. *J. Am. Psychoanal. Assn.* 19:765–779.

Furth, H.G. (1973) *Deafness and Learning: A Psychosocial Approach.* Belmont, Calif.: Wadsworth.

Galenson, E., R. Miller, E. Kaplan, and A. Rothstein. (1977) Assessment of development in the deaf child. Paper presented to the Interdisciplinary Colloquium on Emotional Problems of the Deaf at the American Psychoanalytic Association, December.

Gerweck, S., and J.E. Ysseldyke. (1975) Limitations of current psychological practices for the intellectual assessment of the hearing impaired: A response to the Levine Study. *Volta Review* 77:243–248.

Greenberg, J., and G. Dolittle. (1977) Can schools speak the language of the deaf? *New York Times*, December 11, p. 50.

Greenstein, J.M. (1975) Methods of fostering language in deaf infants. Final report to HEW Grant #OEG 0-72-539.

Hardy, M. (1970) Speech reading. In H. Doris and S.R. Silverman, eds., *Hearing and Deafness*. New York: Holt, Rinehart and Winston.

Harris, R.I. (1978) The relationship of impulse control to parent hearing status, manual communication, and academic achievement in deaf children. *Am. Ann. Deaf* 123:52–67.

Katan, A. (1961) Some thoughts about the role of verbalization in early childhood. *Psychoanal. Study Child* 16:184–188.

Lamb, M.E. (1976) *The Role of the Father in Child Development*. New York: Wiley.

Lesser, S.R., and R.B. Easser. (1972) Personality differences in the perceptually handicapped. *J. Am. Acad. Child Psychiat.* 11:458–466.

Levin, F.M. (1977) Insight-oriented psychotherapy with the deaf. Presented to Interdisciplinary Colloquium on Emotional Problems of the Deaf, at the meeting of the American Psychoanalytic Association, December, New York.

Levine, E. (1974) Psychological tests and practices in the deaf: A survey of the state of the art. *Volta Review* 76:298–319.

McClure, W.J. (1966) Current problems and trends in the education of the deaf. *Deaf American* 18:8–14.

McCullers, C. (1940) *The Heart Is a Lonely Hunter*. New York: Houghton Mifflin.

Meadow, K. (1967) The effect of early manual communication and family climate on the deaf child's development. Unpublished Ph.D. dissertation, University of California at Berkeley.

Meadow, K. (1968) Parental response to the medical ambiguities of deafness. *J. Health Social Behav.* 9:299–309.

Meadow, K. (1976) Personality and social development of deaf persons. *J. Rehab. Deaf* 9:1–12.

Northcott, W. (1973) Competencies needed by teachers of hearing impaired infants, birth to 3 years and their families. *Volta Review* 75:532–544.

Radford, P. (1973) Changing techniques in the analysis of a deaf latency boy. *Psychoanal. Study Child* 28:225–248.

Rainer, J.D. (1976) Some observations on affect induction and ego development in the deaf. *Int. Rev. Psychoanal.* 3:121–128.

Rainer, J.D., and K.Z. Altschuler. (1966) *Comprehensive Mental Health Services for the Deaf.* Department of Medical Genetics, New York State Psychiatric Institute, New York.

Rainer, J.D., K.Z. Altschuler, and F.J. Kallman, eds. (1963) *Family and Mental Health Problems in a Deaf Population.* New York State Psychiatric Institute. New York: Columbia University Press.

Reichstein, J. (1976) Letter to the editor. *Am. Ann. Deaf* 121:1.

Reider, N. (1953) Type of transference to institutions. *Bull. Menninger Clin.* 17:58–63.

Robinson, L.D., and O.D. Weathers. (1974) Family therapy of deaf parents and hearing children: A new dimension in psychotherapeutic intervention. *Am. Ann. Deaf* 119:325–330.

Rosenthal, C. (1975) St. Louis Jewish Fmily and Children's Service, personal communication.

Rothstein, A. (1975) Preventative mental health program at the Lexington School for the Deaf. In D. Lairnan, ed., *Needs of the Emotionally Disturbed Hearing Impaired Child.* N.Y.: Deafness Research and Training Center.

Ruesch, J., and W. Kees. (1956) *Nonverbal Communication.* Berkeley: University of California Press.

Schlesinger, H.S., and K.P. Meadow. (1972) *Sound and Sign: Childhood Deafness and Mental Health.* Berkeley: University of California Press.

Schlesinger, I.M., and L. Namir, eds. (1978) *Sign Language of the Deaf: Psychological, Linguistic and Sociological Perspectives.* New York: Academic Press.

Shapiro, R.J., and R.I. Harris. (1976) Family therapy in treatment of the deaf: A case report. *Fam. Proc.* 15:83–96.

Sharoff, R.L. (1959) Enforced restriction and communication: Its implications for the emotional and intellectual development of the deaf child. *Am. J. Psychiat.* 116:43–45.

Shopper, M. (1976) The effect of the deaf child on the narcissistic equilibrium of the family. Presented to the Workshop on the Vulnerable Child, Annual Meeting of the American Psychoanalytic Association, Baltimore.

Shopper, M. (1978) The role of audition in early psychic development, with special reference to the use of the pull-toy in the separation-individuation phase. *J. Am. Psychoanal. Assn.* 26:283–310.

Solnit, A., and M.H. Stark. (1961) Mourning and the birth of a defective child. *Psychoanal. Study Child* 16:523–537.

Sonnega, J.A. (1967) Diagnostic evaluation of hearing impaired children. In J.D. Rainer and K.Z. Altschuler, eds., *Psychiatry and the Deaf.* Social and Rehabilitation Service, U.S. Department of Health, Education, and Welfare.

Stein, L.K., N.H. Merrill, and P. Dahlberg. (1974) Counseling of parents of hearing impaired children: A psychotherapeutic model. Unpublished paper presented at American Speech and Hearing Association Convention, Las Vegas.

Stuckless, E., and J. Birch. (1966) The influence of early manual communication on the linguistic development of deaf children. *Am. Ann. Deaf* 111:452–460.

Suomi, S.J., M.L. Collins, and H.F. Harlow. (1973) Effects of permanent separation from mother on infant monkeys. *Develop. Psychol.* 9:376–384.

Vernon, M. (1969) Sociological and psychological factors associated with hearing loss. *J. Speech Hearing Res.* 12:541–563.

Vernon, M. (1973) Psychological aspects of the diagnosis of deafness in a child. *Eye, Ear, Nose, Throat Monthly*, February, p. 52.

Vernon, M., and S.D. Koh. (1970) Early manual communication and deaf children's achievement. *Am. Ann. Deaf* 115:527–536.

Von der Lieth, L. (1978) Social-psychological aspects of the use of sign language. In I.M. Schlesinger and L. Namir, eds., *Sign Language of the Deaf.* New York: Academic Press.

Witkin, H. (1965) Psychological differentiation and forms of pathology. *J. Abnorm. Psychol.* 70:317–336.

Wolff, P. (1963) Observations of the early development of smiling. In B.M. Foss, ed., *Determinants of Infant Behavior*, Vol. II. New York: Wiley.

Youniss, J. (1967) Psychological evaluation of the deaf child: Observations of a researcher. *Eye, Ear, Nose, Throat Monthly* 46:458–464.

Index